P9-EAJ-844

Handbook of
Experimental Pharmacology

Volume 107

Editorial Board

G.V.R. Born, London
P. Cuatrecasas, Ann Arbor, MI
H. Herken, Berlin
K. Melmon, Stanford, CA

SCIENCE LIBRARY
UNIVERSITY OF THE PACIFIC
STOCKTON, CA 95211

Physiology and Pharmacology of Bone

Contributors

A.-B. Abou-Samra, D.C. Anderson, H.C. Anderson, R. Baron,
W. Born, F.R. Bringhurst, E. Canalis, M. Centrella,
M. Chakraborty, D. Chatterjee, P.D. Delmas, J.A. Eisman,
E.F. Eriksen, D.M. Findlay, J.A. Fischer, H. Fleisch, J.K. Heath,
W. Horne, H. Jüppner, M. Kassem, H.M. Kronenberg,
L.E. Lanyon, A. Lomri, L. Malaval, T.J. Martin, T.L. McCarthy,
F. Melsen, D.C. Morris, L. Mosekilde, G.R. Mundy, K.W. Ng,
S. Nussbaum, A.M. Parfitt, M. Peacock, J.T. Potts, Jr., L.G. Raisz,
J.-H. Ravesloot, V. Rosen, G. Segre, K.C. Shoukri, A. Vesterby,
J.M. Wozney

Editors

Gregory R. Mundy and T. John Martin

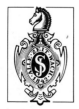

Springer-Verlag
Berlin Heidelberg New York London Paris
Tokyo Hong Kong Barcelona Budapest

Professor GREGORY R. MUNDY, M.D.
Division of Endocrinology and Metabolism
Department of Medicine
The University of Texas Health Science Center
7703 Floyd Curl Drive
San Antonio, TX 78248, USA

Professor T. JOHN MARTIN, M.D.
University of Melbourne
Department of Medicine, and
St. Vincent's Institute of Medical Research
41 Victoria Parade
Melbourne 3065, Australia

With 116 Figures and 27 Tables

ISBN 3-540-56293-1 Springer-Verlag Berlin Heidelberg New York
ISBN 0-387-56293-1 Springer-Verlag New York Berlin Heidelberg

Library of Congress Cataloging-in-Publication Data. Physiology and pharmacology of bone / contributors A.-B. Abou-Samra . . . [et al.]; editors, Gregory R. Mundy and T. John Martin. p. cm.—(Handbook of experimental pharmacology; v. 107) Includes bibliographical references and index. ISBN 3-540-56293-1 (Berlin):—ISBN 0-387-56293-1 (New York) 1. Bones—Physiology. 2. Bones—Pathophysiology. 3. Bones—Effect of drugs on. I. Abou-Samra, A.-B. II. Mundy, Gregory R. III. Martin, T. John. IV. Series. QP88.2.P48 1993 616.7'1071—dc20 92-42565

This work is subject to copyright. All rights are reserved, whether the whole or part of the material is concerned, specifically the rights of translation, reprinting, reuse of illustrations, recitation, broadcasting, reproduction on microfilm or in any other ways, and storage in data banks. Duplication of this publication or parts thereof is permitted only under the provisions of the German Copyright Law of September 9, 1965, in its current version, and permission for use must always be obtained from Springer-Verlag. Violations are liable for prosecution under the German Copyright Law.

© Springer-Verlag Berlin Heidelberg 1993
Printed in Germany

The use of general descriptive names, registered names, trademarks, etc. in this publication does not imply, even in the absence of a specific statement, that such names are exempt from the relevant protective laws and regulations and therefore free for general use.

Product liability: The publisher cannot guarantee the accuracy of any information about dosage and application contained in this book. In every individual case the user must check such information by consulting the relevant literature.

Typesetting: Best-set Typesetter Ltd., Hong Kong

27/3130/SPS-5 4 3 2 1 0 – Printed on acid-free paper

List of Contributors

ABOU-SAMRA, A.-B., Endocrine Unit-Wellman 5, Massachusetts General Hospital, Boston, MA 02114, USA

ANDERSON, D.C., Department of Medicine, Faculty of Medicine, The Chinese University of Hong Kong, Prince of Wales Hospital, Shatin, N.T., Hong Kong

ANDERSON, H.C., Department of Pathology and Oncology, University of Kansas Medical Center, Kansas City, KS 66103, USA

BARON, R., Departments of Orthopaedics and Cell Biology, Yale University School of Medicine, 333 Cedar Street, New Haven, CT 06510, USA

BORN, W., Research Laboratory for Calcium Metabolism, Department of Orthopedic Surgery and Medicine, University of Zürich, CH-8008 Zürich, Switzerland

BRINGHURST, F.R., Endocrine Unit-Wellman 5, Massachusetts General Hospital, Boston, MA 02114, USA

CANALIS, E., Departments of Research and Medicine, Saint Francis Hospital and Medical Center, 114 Woodland Street, Hartford, CT 06105, USA and The University of Connecticut School of Medicine, Framington, CT 06105, USA

CENTRELLA, M., Department of Medicine, University of Connecticut School of Medicine, Farmington, CT 06032, USA

CHAKRABORTY, M., Departments of Orthopaedics and Cell Biology, Yale University School of Medicine, 333 Cedar Street, New Haven, CT 06510, USA

CHATTERJEE, D., Departments of Orthopaedics and Cell Biology, Yale University School of Medicine, 333 Cedar Street, New Haven, CT 06510, USA

DELMAS, P.D., INSERM Unit 234 and Department of Rheumatology and Metabolic Bone Disease, Hôpital E. Herriot, Pavillon F, F-69437 Lyon Cedex 03, France

EISMAN, J.A., Head, Bone and Mineral Research Division, Garvan Institute of Medical Research, St. Vincent's Hospital, Sydney NSW 2010, Australia

ERIKSEN, E.F., University Department of Endocrinology and Metabolism, Aarhus Bone and Mineral Study Group, Aarhus Amtssygehus, DK-8000 Aarhus C, Denmark

FINDLAY, D.M., University of Melbourne, Department of Medicine, and St. Vincent's Institute of Medical Research, 41, Victoria Parade, Melbourne 3065, Australia

FISCHER, J.A., Research Laboratory for Calcium Metabolism, Departments of Orthopaedic Surgery and Medicine, University of Zürich, CH-8008 Zürich, Switzerland

FLEISCH, H., Pathophysiologisches Institut, Universität Bern, Murtenstraße 35, CH-3010 Bern, Switzerland

HEATH, J.K., University of Melbourne, Department of Medicine, and St. Vincent's Institute of Medical Research, 41 Victoria Parade, Melbourne 3065, Australia

HORNE, W., Departments of Orthopaedics and Cell Biology and Molecular Physiology, Yale University School of Medicine, 333 Cedar Street, New Haven, CT 06510, USA

JÜPPNER, H., Endocrine Unit-Wellman 5, Massachusetts General Hospital, Boston, MA 02114, USA

KASSEM, M., Aarhus Bone and Mineral Study Group, University Department of Endocrinology and Internal Medicine, Aarhus Amtssygehus, DK-8000 Aarhus C., Denmark

KRONENBERG, H.M., Endocrine Unit-Wellman 5, Massachusetts General Hospital, Boston, MA 02114, USA

LANYON, L.E., The Royal Veterinary College, University of London, Royal College Street, London NW1 0TU, Great Britain

LOMRI, A., Departments of Orthopaedics and Cell Biology, Yale University School of Medicine, 333 Cedar Street, New Haven, CT 06510, USA

MALAVAL, L., INSERM Unit 234, Hôpital E. Herriot, Pavillon F, F-69437 Lyon Cedex 03, France

MARTIN, T.J., University of Melbourne, Department of Medicine, and St. Vincent's Institute of Medical Research, 41 Victoria Parade, Melbourne 3065, Australia

McCARTHY, T.L., Department of Medicine, University of Connecticut School of Medicine, Farmington, CT 06032, USA

MELSEN, F., Aarhus Bone and Mineral Study Group, University Institute Pathology, Aarhus Amtssygehus, DK-8000 Aarhus C., Denmark

MORRIS, D.C., Department of Pathology and Oncology, University of Kansas Medical Center, Kansas City, KS 66103, USA

MOSEKILDE, L., Aarhus Bone and Mineral Study Group, University Department of Endocrinology and Metabolism, Aarhus Amtssygehus, DK-8000 Aarhus C., Denmark

MUNDY, G.R., Division of Endocrinology and Metabolism, Department of Medicine, The University of Texas, Health Science Center at San Antonio, 7703 Floyd Curl Drive, San Antonio, TX 78248-7877, USA

NG, K.W., University of Melbourne, Department of Medicine, and St. Vincent's Institute of Medical Research, 41 Victoria Parade, Melbourne 3065, Australia

NUSSBAUM, S., Endocrine Unit-Wellman 5, Massachusetts General Hospital, Boston, MA 02114, USA

PARFITT, A.M., Bone and Mineral Research Laboratory, E&R 7, Henry Ford Hospital, 2799 W. Grand Boulevard, Detroit, MI 48202, USA

PEACOCK, M., General Clinical Research Center, Indiana University School of Medicine, University Hospital, 5595, 926 W. Michigan Street, Indianapolis, IN 46202-5250, USA

POTTS, J.T., Jr., Endocrine Unit-Wellman 5, Massachusetts General Hospital, Boston, MA 02114, USA

RAISZ, L.G., Division of Endocrinology and Metabolism MC-1850, The School of Medicine of the University of Connecticut Health Center, 263 Farmington Avenue, Farmington, CT 06030-1850, USA

RAVESLOOT, J.-H., Departments of Orthopaedics and Cell Biology and Molecular Physiology, Yale University School of Medicine, 333 Cedar Street, New Haven, CT 06510, USA

ROSEN, V., Genetics Institute, 87 CambridgePark Drive, Cambridge, MA 02140, USA

SEGRE, G., Endocrine Unit-Wellman 5, Massachusetts General Hospital, Boston, MA 02114, USA

SHOUKRI, K.C., Division of Endocrinology and Metabolism MC-1850, The School of Medicine of the University of Connecticut Health Center, 263 Farmington Avenue, Farmington, CT 06030-1850, USA

VESTERBY, A., Aarhus Bone and Mineral Study Group, University Institute of Pathology, Aarhus Amtssygehus, DK-8000 Aarhus C., Denmark

WOZNEY, J.M., Genetics Institute, Inc., 87 CambridgePark Drive, Cambridge, MA 02140, USA

Preface

Why have another book in the bone-calcium field? When the idea was first raised that this important area of biomedical research should be given more attention in the review literature, we felt that comprehensive texts recently published and in press were directed at more general audiences and did not address in detail some of the important areas of current investigation. As this field has grown and matured, information has accumulated at such a rapid rate that it has become impossible to keep abreast of all areas by reading the original articles in the scientific literature. Accordingly, we believed there was a void which could be filled by a collection of essays on specific topics in which significant progress had recently been made. Thus, this book is meant to be an up-to-date account of specific topics by investigators at the forefront of their areas of research. We have tried to review major areas of basic science in the field which have an impact on our understanding of the diseases of bone and mineral. We hope that you will agree that the authors have done an outstanding job, and will find the volume as stimulating to read as we have.

San Antonio, TX, USA

GREGORY R. MUNDY

Melbourne, Australia

T. JOHN MARTIN

Spring 1993

Contents

CHAPTER 2

Bone Remodeling and Bone Structure
E.F. ERIKSEN, A. VESTERBY, M. KASSEM, F. MELSEN, and

CHAPTER 3

Biology of the Osteoclast
R. Baron, M. Chakraborty, D. Chatterjee, W. Horne, A. Lomri,
and J.-H. Ravesloot. With 7 Figures 111

CHAPTER 4

CHAPTER 5

CHAPTER 9

Pathogenesis of Osteoporosis

L.G. RAISZ and K.C. SHOUKRI. With 1 Figure..................... 299

CHAPTER 10

Vitamin D Metabolism

CHAPTER 11

Bisphosphonates: Mechanisms of Action and Clinical Use
H. FLEISCH.. 377

CHAPTER 12

Paget's Disease
D.C. ANDERSON. With 20 Figures 419

CHAPTER 13

Hyperparathyroid and Hypoparathyroid Bone Disease
M. PEACOCK. With 15 Figures 443

CHAPTER 14

Skeletal Responses to Physical Loading

L.E. LANYON. With 4 Figures 485

CHAPTER 17

Parathyroid Hormone-Related Protein: Molecular Biology, Chemistry, and Actions

CHAPTER 18

Pathophysiology of Skeletal Complications of Cancer
G.R. MUNDY and T.J. MARTIN. With 1 Figure 641

Contents

CHAPTER 20

Bone Morphogenetic Proteins

CHAPTER 1
Calcium Homeostasis

A.M. PARFITT

A. Introduction and Scope

Calcium carries out two types of function in the body. At the gross macroscopic level it is the main constituent of the solid mineral that gives bone its
rigidity and strength, a prerequisite for the evolutionary transition from
invertebrate to vertebrate life. The presence of mineral crystals is the most
distinctive feature of bone as a tissue; despite the present neglect of these
topics by most students of calcium metabolism, the composition, structure,
and physicochemical properties of the mineral have important metabolic as
well as mechanical consequences (GLIMCHER 1984). The amount of calcium
in the body depends mainly on total bone mass, which is partly regulated
in accordance with biomechanical needs by the cells whose function is described
in the next three chapters. At the submicroscopic and molecular levels, ionic
calcium is essential for a wide variety of cellular functions, of which a
detailed account is beyond the scope of this text (NORDIN 1988). Calcium
moves into and out of cells along molecular channels that can be opened or
closed. Abrupt spikes in the very low intracellular concentration of calcium,
spreading rapidly from one region of the cell to another, serve as a versatile
signaling mechanism (LIPSCOMBE et al. 1988). Consequently, intracellular
calcium is not subject to homeostatic control except in the gross sense that a
large excess of calcium may lead to, or at least accompany, cell death.

Calcium in blood, which is the main focus of this chapter, is the link
between the macroscopic and the molecular levels of organization. The
extracellular concentration of calcium must be stabilized in the interests of
its intracellular functions, and this stability is accomplished to a great extent
by the movement of calcium ions between interstitial fluid and bone at
quiescent bone surfaces. The large body of knowledge concerning this
process, accumulated between about 1950 and 1970, has all but disappeared
from current texts, and its reinstatement will be an important component of
this chapter. Extracellular calcium concentration is also influenced by gains
or losses of calcium via the bone remodeling system (Chap. 2), the gut, and
the kidney (Fig. 1). Tubular reabsorption of calcium shares with the bone
surface the regulation of plasma calcium, and net calcium absorption and
net loss of calcium from bone via remodeling are disturbing signals to which
the bone surface and the kidney must respond.

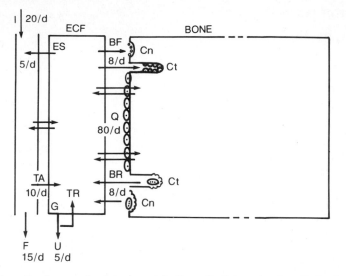

Fig. 1. Overall scheme of calcium metabolism. *I*, dietary intake; *F*, fecal excretion; *G*, glomerular filtration; *TR*, tubular reabsorption; *U*, urinary excretion; *ES*, endogenous secretion; *TA*, total absorption; *BF*, bone formation subdivided into shallow (cancellous, *Cn*) and deep (cortical, *Ct*). *BR*, bone resorption subdivided into shallow (*Cn*) and deep (*Ct*). *Q*, quiescent bone surface. *Single arrows* denote irreversible processes, *paired arrows* denote reversible processes. *Numbers* refer to fluxes in mmol/day

These fluxes are all influenced by hormones whose secretion is partly governed by the plasma calcium level (Fig. 2). For parathyroid hormone (PTH) or parathyrin, and calcitriol, the secretory relationship to calcium is reciprocal, whereas for calcitonin the relationship is direct. The interactions between PTH and calcium will be examined from the physiologic and regulatory perspectives in some detail, but the other calciotropic hormones will be considered quite briefly, since they are of lesser importance for plasma calcium homeostasis and full descriptions are given elsewhere in this book. Calcium is closely linked with phosphate, the other major constituent of bone mineral. Like calcium, the major ionic species of phosphate in body fluids is divalent, and it is affected by each of the calciotropic hormones. Unlike calcium, most phosphate is intracellular and its plasma concentration is not closely regulated, being determined mainly by renal tubular reabsorption (Parfitt and Kleerekoper 1980a). Nevertheless, calcium homeostasis can be affected by movements of phosphate, sometimes in parallel with calcium, sometimes independent of calcium. No known hormone has as its main function the regulation of phosphate, but each of the calciotropic hormones has effects on phosphate as well as calcium (Parfitt and Kleerekoper 1980a).

Understanding the physical chemistry of divalent ions needs consideration of the thermodynamic concept of ion activity. The electrostatic

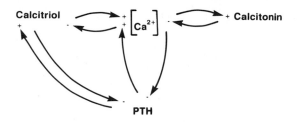

Fig. 2. Relationships between ECF free calcium and calciotropic hormones. *PTH*, parathyroid hormone. *Signs* indicate directional effect on the dependent variable resulting from an increase in the independent variable

field around each ion restricts the mobility of other ions and reduces their potential for chemical reaction, referred to as activity or effective concentration (W.F. NEUMAN and NEUMAN 1958). The ratio of effective to actual concentration, or activity coefficient, varies with pH and temperature, but is mainly a function of total ionic strength. In blood, these factors each have narrow ranges so that ignoring activity coefficient corrections to plasma concentrations does not much affect the interpretation of relative differences. But activity coefficients are both lower and more variable for divalent than for monovalent ions and are important for the physicochemical state of interstitial and intracellular fluids, and for the equilibria between interstitial fluid and bone mineral, and so for both mineralization and calcium homeostasis. Activity coefficients are also relevant to the genesis of both soft-tissue calcification and calcium-containing renal calculi. These and other pathological states are to some extent the costs of maintaining calcium homeostasis (NEER 1989), but will not be considered further in this chapter.

As well as the nonspecific effects of ionic charge, there are also specific effects due to ion pair formation (PAYNE and WALSER 1959). For most strong electrolytes, the constituent ions are either aggregated into crystals, linked by covalent bonds as amorphous solids, or fully dissociated in aqueous solution. Weak electrolytes in solution remain partly undissociated and can also exist in another state, in which specific ions of opposite charge are held together by an electrostatic force but remain in solution. Such ion pairs are conveniently referred to as complexes, although the association is electrostatic rather than covalent. Multivalent ions form ion pairs more readily than monovalent ions. The reversible equilibrium between free ions and ion pairs can be described in terms of the law of mass action and hence by an association constant, as for other chemical equilibria. Ion pair formation has an important effect on the free calcium level in blood and is relevant to both the aggregation and dissolution of bone mineral.

B. Concepts of Homeostasis

Walter Cannon coined the term "homeostasis" 60 years ago to designate the physiological mechanisms responsible for the fixity of the internal environment postulated by Claude Bernard (Yates 1982; Moore-Ede 1986). With the emergence of cybernetics as a unifying scientific discipline (Weiner 1948), homeostasis came to be thought of exclusively in terms of stability achieved by control loops based on negative feedback. A more general mechanism of regulation is reciprocal causality, with two variables linked by two different functional relationships in which dependent and independent status are interchanged (D.S. Riggs 1963; Yates 1982). These functions can be of any mathematical form, provided that they are monotonic and have slopes of opposite sign so that they intersect at only one point, referred to as the equilibrium operating point (Yates 1982). Negative feedback represents the special case where direction can be specified by designating only one of the variables as the subject of control (Yates 1982); in this case the equilibrium operating point becomes the set point for the controlled variable. In man-made systems governed by negative feedback, the set point corresponds to a particular state or setting of a physically real component of the system, such as a thermostat (D.S. Riggs 1970; Yates 1982), but the setting is ultimately the result of human choice, which is external to the system. In biologic systems, there may be no counterpart to the thermostat as a physical entity (D.S. Riggs 1970; Cecchhini et al. 1981); nevertheless such systems display target values that must have contributed to reproductive success and survival, and so are not arbitrary.

In all negative feedback systems, whether factitious or of natural occurrence, the target value and the means whereby it is selected must be distinguished from the mechanisms for correcting deviations from the target value. For example, an automobile cruise control operates in the same manner, no matter what speed is desired. Likewise, one steers a boat in the same manner, whatever compass course one chooses to follow. The same distinction is important in pathophysiology. For example, some patients with chronic wasting diseases have stable asymptomatic hyponatremia, but retain the ability to inhibit antidiuretic hormone secretion and to excrete additional free water (Flear and Singh 1973; DeFronzo et al. 1976). Such patients appear to have undergone a resetting of the "osmostat" (DeFronzo et al. 1976), so that the control system defends a low plasma sodium level as if it were normal, most likely because the maintenance of cell volume in the face of reduced levels of intracellular protein and other constituents requires a lower than normal extracellular sodium concentration (Deane 1966; Flear and Singh 1973). Because PTH is involved both in setting the "calciostat" and in correcting deviations from the prevailing value, the distinction between them has, with few exceptions (Mundy 1989), generally not been recognized, even though it is crucial to the understanding of calcium homeostasis (McCance 1954).

Negative feedback can rest on three basic types of linear control mechanism (D.S. Riggs 1970). With proportional control, the corrective response is directly proportional to the error signal; if only a binary on-off response is possible, as with a household thermostat, the proportionality is manifested by the relative durations of the on and off states. With derivative control, the response is proportional to the rate of change of the error signal and with integral control the response is proportional to the cumulative summation of the error signal. Proportional control permits attainment of a new steady state with acceptable delay, but some persistent error is unavoidable. With derivative control, the response is initiated more rapidly, but the error correction cannot be sustained, and with integral control the response is initiated more slowly but is ultimately more effective, since steady state error can be eliminated. The relative importance of proportional, derivative, and integral control in the parathyroid hormone response to calcium (NEER 1989; GRANT et al. 1990), and the plasma calcium response to parathyroid hormone (BRONNER 1982; NEER 1989), have been studied with inconclusive results that will later be discussed in more detail.

Under the ideal conditions of traditional homeostatic theory, deviations from stability are supposed to be due either to imperfections in the control system or to inaccuracies of measurement. But oscillation, both short-term and long-term, is an essential feature of all physiologic systems (MOORE-EDE et al. 1982; YATES et al. 1987)! Fortunately, it is possible to acknowledge the existence and importance of oscillation without fully grasping the underlying mathematical complexities (GLEICK 1988), such as polytonic functions, bifurcations, and nonlinear differential equations (YATES 1982; YATES et al. 1987). Current control theory gives less importance than in the past to reactive regulation by negative feedback, with recognition of the importance of predictive or anticipatory regulation, in which corrective action is initiated at the same time as, or even before, the perturbation (MOORE-EDE 1986). This is possible if a physiologic process that creates a demand also ensures that the demand is satisfied (PARFITT and KLEEREKOPER 1980a), or if both signal and apparent response are entrained to the same clock (MOORE-EDE et al. 1982). A physiologic clock that oscillates spontaneously is an example of temporal self-organization, a concept that has been applied mainly to biochemical or nonliving systems (NICOLIS and PRIGOGINE 1977; GOLDBETER and DECROLY 1983), but which finds increasing application to physiology in general (YATES 1982; YATES et al. 1987) and to calcium homeostasis in particular (STAUB et al. 1989). With this change in emphasis the concept of homeostasis is gradually being supplemented by the concept of homeokinesis (YATES 1982; YATES et al. 1987).

C. Extracellular Fluid Free Calcium: The Controlled Variable

Plasma, the readily accessible component of extracellular fluid (ECF), is in direct contact only with the cells of the blood and the vascular endothelium. All other cells of the body are immersed in interstitial fluid, which is generally inaccessible. These components of ECF, separated only by the capillary walls, are in osmotic equilibrium and differ mainly in their protein content. Proteins can affect ion concentrations in three ways (PARFITT and KLEEREKOPER 1980a): by occupying space so that concentrations in plasma differ from those in plasma water, by behaving as anions at the normal pH of the blood, and by specific ion-binding affinities. Each organ regulates the composition of its own interstitial fluid for its own special needs, but in many organs the capillary endothelium is more permeable to protein than is generally supposed, and the average interstitial fluid protein concentration is at least 50% of the plasma level ((PARFITT and KLEEREKOPER 1980a; AUKLAND and NICOLAYSEN 1981). Much of the so-called interstitial fluid is not fluid at all, but gelatinous because of the space-filling and water-adsorbing properties of ground substance macromolecules, mainly proteoglycans (PARFITT and KLEEREKOPER 1980a; ENGEL and CATCHPOLE 1989). These are long-chain polymers with many $^-$COOH and $^-$SO$_3$H groups that have high binding affinity for calcium at physiologic pH, so that small changes in their physicochemical state or in pH could significantly modify the amount of calcium that they sequester within their domains.

The plasma concentration of calcium represents not only the plasma itself but the entire pool with which it is in equilibrium (BRONNER 1982; NEER 1989). This includes not only the interstitial fluid but most of the extraskeletal calcium. The calcium content of organs other than bones varies from 1 to 10 mmol/kg tissue (PARFITT and KLEEREKOPER 1980a; NORDIN 1988). Much of the tissue calcium is bound to ground substance macromolecules or to acidic phospholipids in cell membranes, but most of the variation between organs reflects differences in the kind and amount of connective tissue, which determines the susceptibility of the organ to dystrophic calcification with increasing age. The exchangeable or miscible pool for calcium is about 100–150 mmol (PARFITT and KLEEREKOPER 1980a; NEER 1989) and includes all the calcium in ECF, most of the cell membrane and connective tissue calcium, and about 0.3% of the calcium in bone; the latter will be considered in more detail in Sect. G.VI. For most ions the size of the pool determines the extent of change in plasma concentration that results from short-term gains or losses of the ion in question, but the complexity of the exchanges between ECF and bone preclude such a simple relationship.

Of the total calcium in plasma, about half is associated with various anions and about half is free (Table 1; PARFITT and KLEEREKOPER 1980a). The free fraction is usually referred to as ionized, an inappropriate term because all calcium in the body is in ionic form and associates with other ions by means of ionic rather than covalent bonds. Calcium that forms ion pairs with inorganic anions such as bicarbonate or phosphate, or with low-molecular-weight organic anions such as citrate or lactate, is collectively known as complexed calcium; the Ca-HCO$_3^+$ ion pair is the largest component (HUGHES et al. 1984). Both free and complexed calcium will cross biological or synthetic membranes, so together they constitute the diffusible

Table 1. Plasma calcium fractionation

		Ionized (1.2; 50%)	
	Free (1.2; 50%)		Diffusible (1.5; 62%)
Total (2.4; 100%)		Complexed (0.3; 12%)	
	Bound (1.2; 50%)		Nondiffusible (0.9; 38%)
		Protein bound (0.9; 38%)	

Representative values in millimoles per liter in parentheses, together with percentages of total; each column = 2.4 = 100%.

or ultrafiltrable calcium (Table 1). Protein-bound calcium is nondiffusible and nonultrafiltrable; about 85% is bound to albumin and about 15% to various globulins. Normally only about 10%–15% of the binding sites on albumin are occupied. It is generally held that only the free fraction is physiologically active, but activity for some components of complexed calcium has not been firmly excluded (TOFFALETTI and BOWERS 1979); certainly several calcium complexes influence the urinary excretion of calcium. Nevertheless, only the free calcium concentration in plasma influences PTH secretion and so is subject to homeostatic control (TOFFALETTI et al. 1991).

The homeostatic precision with which a plasma constituent is controlled is usually inferred from the variability within the normal range, expressed as the coefficient of variation ($CV = SD/mean*100$). This method is simple and logical, but is unsuitable for comparing the performance of homeostatic systems, since it takes no account of the magnitude of the disturbing signals to which the homeostatic system must respond (D.S. RIGGS 1963, 1970); from this standpoint, carbon dioxide is the most efficiently regulated constituent of the ECF. The term "normal range" is currently unfashionable, but it remains a more appropriate term than "reference range" when the emphasis is on the physiologic rather than the diagnostic significance of a measurement. As usually determined, the normal range CV includes components due to analytic imprecision, between-person differences, and within-person variation. The relative contributions of these components are different for each analyte. For example, total alkaline phosphatase displays substantial biochemical individuality, such that the population-based reference range (CV 21%) is three times larger than the average individual reference range (HARRIS 1981). This reflects not only the large individual differences in bone turnover, but also its short-term stability in each individual, and the absence of any direct homeostatic regulation of alkaline phosphatase.

Much of the nonanalytic variation in total calcium concentration is the result of its dependence on albumin (PEDERSEN 1972; R.B. PAYNE et al.

1979). Adjustment for albumin eliminates most of the population variation in total calcium due to age and gender differences, much of the variation between persons, and almost all the individual variation due to posture and exercise (PEDERSEN 1972; PARFITT and KLEEREKOPER 1980b). Only free calcium, whether measured directly or inferred indirectly from albumin-adjusted total calcium, can be used for the study of calcium homeostasis. By either method, the normal range CV is about 3% (PEDERSEN 1972; R.B. PAYNE et al. 1979). Based on quite limited data, the between-person CV is about 2.5% and the within-person CV about 1.5% (HARRIS and DeMETS 1971; PEDERSEN 1972; LADENSON and BOWERS 1973; R.B. PAYNE et al. 1979; LARSSON and OHMAN 1979). The variability is even less for plasma sodium concentration (HARRIS et al. 1970), and for both ions the narrowness of the ranges justifies their description as normal, since some biological disadvantage must reside in higher or lower values that was avoided by natural selection. The significant differences between individual mean values, or set points, have a partly genetic basis since the differences are smaller between siblings than between members of different families (R.B. PAYNE et al. 1986). Persons differ not only in their set points but in the magnitude of variability about the set point (HARRIS and DeMETS 1971; LADENSON and BOWERS 1973; LARSSON and OHMAN 1979).

The indices of both between-person and within-person precision are based on blood samples taken at the same time of day, usually in the early morning after an overnight fast, which gives no information on changes during the day. Free calcium concentration is highly susceptible to acid-base status, first, because the binding of calcium by albumin is pH dependent and, second, because changes in HCO_3^- concentration cause parallel changes in the $Ca\text{-}HCO_3^+$ ion pair and reciprocal changes in free calcium (HUGHES et al. 1984). During the alkaline tide that accompanies increased gastric acid secretion, free calcium concentration can fall by as much as 5%, but recovers spontaneously after about 1 h (HUGHES et al. 1977). More surprisingly, there is a stable circadian rhythm in free calcium concentration with a peak at about 10:00 a.m. and a nadir at about 7:00 p.m. with an amplitude of about 6% of the mean value (MARKOWITZ et al. 1981, 1988). In other studies, more complex oscillations were found, of greater amplitude in women than in men (CALVO et al. 1991). Plasma sodium concentration also displays a circadian rhythm, but the amplitude is less than 2% (WISSER et al. 1981). The free calcium rhythm is more complex than a simple response to circadian changes in the secretion of calciotropic hormones (MARKOWITZ et al. 1988; CALVO et al. 1991), and its homeostatic significance will be mentioned briefly in Sect. G.VIII.

D. Parathyroid Hormone: The Controlling Variable

In any control system based on negative feedback, a change in the controlled variable must be detected (afferent loop) and transduced into an effector

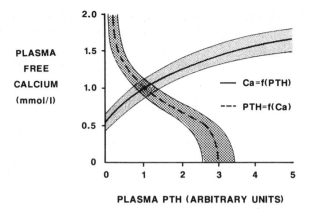

Fig. 3. Reciprocal causality between free calcium and PTH. The intersection between two mathematical functions, one describing free calcium as dependent on PTH, and one describing PTH as dependent on free calcium, determines the equilibrium operating point; this is also the set point for free calcium as the controlled variable. Small changes in the parameters of the equations give rise to bands rather than lines, of which the overlap determines the limits of variation between subjects. The functions depicted were estimated from limited available data and are intended to be illustrative rather than definitive (PARFITT 1982). Note that time is not included in either function, and that each point represents a separate steady-state relationship. (Reprinted from PARFITT 1987 with permission)

response that counteracts the initial change (efferent loop). For the control of ECF free calcium, these operations are provided by the secretion of PTH by the parathyroid gland (Chap. 15), with lesser contributions from calcitriol (Chap. 10) and calcitonin (Chap. 16). The relationships between PTH and free calcium are an example of reciprocal causality as defined in Sect. B. For an adequate description of the steady-state behavior of the system, it is necessary to express as mathematical functions, first, how PTH as the dependent variable is related to calcium as the independent variable and, second, how calcium as the dependent variable is related to PTH as the independent variable (PARFITT 1969d, 1987; MORGAN 1973). Since both variables are subject to circadian variation (MARKOWITZ et al. 1988; CALVO et al. 1991), the functions should preferably be based on average values over a 24-h period, but few such data are available. The intersection of the curves representing these two functions defines the equilibrium operating point, which corresponds to the set point for the controlled variable (Fig. 3). For both curves, each individual point should represent a separate steady-state relationship. The general shape of each curve is known with reasonable confidence (PARFITT 1982), but the most appropriate mathematical representation and the numerical values of particular parameters can only be approximated.

Because they describe steady-state relationships, neither function in Fig. 3 includes any reference to time. Separate mathematical functions, expressing the time courses of the PTH response to calcium and the calcium response to PTH, are needed to describe how quickly and effectively the system responds to a perturbation; a great deal of temporal data are available, but they have not yet been conveniently summarized in mathematical form. Two pairs of equations, one without and one with the inclusion of time as an independent variable, would correspond to the two functions of PTH in determining the set point, and participating in the correction of deviations from the set point (PARFITT 1976b). The effects of all influences on PTH other than calcium, and all influences on calcium other than PTH, could be incorporated into the model by changing the parameters of the equations, if these were known. Neither pair of functions would include any explicit reference to mechanisms, so that the underlying molecular events could be different for equations that define the steady state and equations that describe the transient responses. This distinction is more important for the efferent than for the afferent loop, since the effect of calcium on PTH involves only one organ, but the effect of PTH on calcium is mediated by multiple target organs with responses that cover a wide range of time scales (PARFITT and KLEEREKOPER 1980a; BRONNER 1982; NEER 1989; MUNDY 1989).

I. Afferent Loop: Effects of Calcium on PTH Secretion

The relationship between PTH secretion (dependent) and plasma free calcium concentration (independent) is a sigmoid curve of which the middle steep segment is centered on the normal range (Fig. 4a). In vivo such a relationship, representing the combined secretion from all glands, has been found both in several animal species (BLUM et al. 1974b; Fox 1991) and in human subjects (SEGRE et al. 1981; GARDIN et al. 1988; BOUCHER et al. 1989; BRENT et al. 1988). The results are the same with current assays for intact hormone as with older less specific assays, and the same for either gender (BRENT et al. 1988). A sigmoid relationship has also been found in vitro, representing the aggregate contribution of all cells in a tissue slice or in a dispersed cell preparation (BROWN et al. 1979b, 1987; CANTLEY et al. 1985), and the response of single cells studied by the reverse hemolytic plaque assay (FITZPATRICK and LEONG 1990). In individual patients with primary hyperparathyroidism, very similar responses to calcium were found in vivo and in the dispersed cells from the excised adenoma studied in vitro (BROWN et al. 1979a). The agreement between in vivo and in vitro studies is especially striking since the former are based on serum concentrations of hormone, whereas the latter are based on amounts of hormone released into the medium by a defined number of cells in a defined time period. There is little variation in the metabolic clearance of the intact hormone, and the relationship between secretion rate and plasma concentration is predictable (NEER 1989). When free calcium concentration is changing rapidly, the PTH responses are more complex as will be described later, but when calcium is stable the PTH response is stable (GRANT et al. 1990; SCHWARZ et al. 1990),

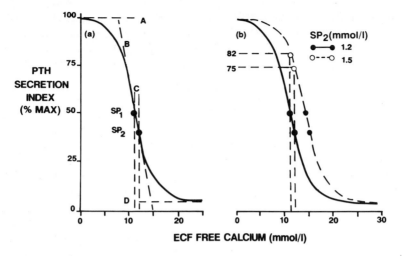

Fig. 4a,b. Parathyroid secretory set point. Sigmoid relationship between index of PTH secretion and ECF free calcium concentration. The form of the relationship is the same whether the index of secretion is the quantity of hormone released into the medium (in vitro studies) or the serum concentration of hormone (in vivo studies). Note that the sigmoid curves represent steady state, not transient, responses, so that each point on the curve denotes a separate steady-state relationship. On the left (a) are indicated the parameters used by BROWN (1983) to define the mathematical form of the curve: *A*, maximum secretion rate; *B*, slope of curve at the steepest segment; *C*, set point; *D*, minimum secretion rate. The set point is conventionally defined as the ECF free calcium corresponding to 50% of maximum hormone secretion (SP_1), but this definition is arbitrary. A more physiologic definition of set point is the value of the controlled variable to which the PTH cell responds as normal (SP_2). In this example, SP_1 = 1.12 mmol/l, SP_2 = 1.20 mmol/l. On the right (b) is shown the effect of an increase in SP_2 from 1.2 to 1.5 mmol/l. The parathyroid response will be the same as the response of parathyroid cells with a normal set point to a free calcium that is reduced to 0.9 mmol/l, so that at a normal value for free calcium PTH secretion will increase to 75% of maximum at the normal physiological set point (1.20) and to 82% maximum at the arbitrary set point corresponding to 50% suppression (1.12)

fulfilling the requirement for defining the steady-state characteristics of the system.

The most widely used mathematical representation of the sigmoid relationship is a logistic curve defined by four parameters, maximum and minimum levels of PTH, the calcium level corresponding to 50% of maximum PTH, referred to as the set point, and the slope of the curve at the set point (Fig. 4a; BROWN et al. 1987; BROWN 1983). Each of these parameters needs separate discussion. The term set point has already been used for the target value of plasma free calcium concentration as the controlled variable, and the relationship between these two usages of the term must be clarified. The choice of 50% suppressibility for the secretory set point is convenient but arbitrary (BROWN et al. 1987). Sigmoid curves with different set points, but with the same values of the other three parameters, differ only in location along the horizontal axis (Fig. 4b), and this location could be specified equally well by any point defined in a consistent manner. From the physiologic standpoint, the secretory set point represents the value of the controlled variable that the individual parathyroid cell "recognizes" as normal and attempts to defend (BROWN et al. 1987; PARFITT et al. 1991b); this defense is facilitated by locating the set point close to the middle of the steepest portion of the curve, so that small changes in free calcium in either direction elicit a large change in PTH secretion (BROWN et al. 1987).

Stated another way, it is the secretory set point of the average parathyroid cell that determines the set point for the controlled variable. Consequently, the between-person differences in free calcium set point and the genetic influence on that set point must reflect between person differences in secretory set point that have a genomic basis. Whatever evolutionary pressures led to the selection of a particular range of values for free calcium in preference to alternative possibilities, they acted on the genomic control of the parathyroid secretory set point, presumably via the various proteins concerned in the maintenance and recognition of concentration differences for calcium between the inside and the outside of the parathyroid cell (PARFITT 1969d; WALLFELT et al. 1988; SEELY et al. 1989a; GYLFE et al. 1990). This is why the values are species specific; for example, the set point in both senses is higher in the rabbit than in other mammalian species (WARREN et al. 1989). The increased secretory set points found in most patients with primary hyperparathyroidism also most likely have a genomic basis (PARFITT et al. 1991b), whether they result from germinal or somatic mutation. There are also at least three nongenomic influences on secretory set point, which is reduced in the nonadenomatous glands from patients with primary hyperparathyroidism, presumably as an adaptive response to chronic hypercalcemia (BROWN et al. 1981), increased in some patients on long-term lithium therapy (SEELY et al. 1989b), and increased in some patients with chronic renal failure as a result of calcitriol deficiency (DUNLAY et al. 1989).

The variability in maximum secretion between subjects is concealed by the usual practice of setting this value to 100%. The justification for this is that normal and abnormal parathyroid cells differ consistently in set point but not in maximum secretion, which was $10-12 \, ng/10^5$ cells per hour for normal glands, but varied from 3.2 to $30 \, ng/10^5$ cells per hour for adenomas (BROWN et al. 1979b). The reason for this wide variation in secretory capacity and its homeostatic significance are unknown (CANTLEY et al. 1985). Obviously, differences expressed in this way are independent of the number of cells, but similar variability of peak secretion in vivo must partly reflect differences in gland size (PARFITT 1969d, 1982; BENSON et al. 1986). The existence of a minimum rate of hormone secretion that is not suppressible by calcium is enigmatic (MAYER et al. 1976). It is not due only to the release of biologically inactive fragments at high calcium concentrations, since it is found also with assays for intact PTH, although its magnitude is much smaller, amounting to about 5% of the maximum value rather than 20% as with the older assays (BRENT et al. 1988). The minimum rate may be related to a cycle of synthesis, packaging, and release of hormone by individual cells (PARFITT and KLEEREKOPER 1980a). This concept was first proposed many years ago (SHANNON and ROTH 1974) on the basis of ultrastructural appearances that have recently been challenged as artifact (MARTI et al. 1987), but intermittency of hormone secretion has been confirmed by the plaque assay (FITZPATRICK and LEONG 1990). A minimum rate of secretion by a cell population would result if the next secretory period by an individual cell could be delayed but not indefinitely postponed.

When plasma free calcium is changing, its effects on PTH secretion are more complex. At any level of calcium, PTH secretion is greater when the calcium level is changing rapidly than when it is changing slowly (ADAMI et al. 1982; GRANT et al. 1990) and, at the same rate of change, PTH secretion is greater when the calcium is falling than when it is rising (ADAMI et al. 1982; CONLIN et al. 1989). Both of these phenomena may be regarded as forms of derivative control. The initial rise in PTH in response to a fall in free calcium is very rapid; occurring within 20 s in the cow (BLUM et al. 1974a) and within a few minutes in other species (FOX and HEATH 1981; ORWOLL et al. 1986; GRANT et al. 1990; TOFFALETTI et al. 1991). This probably reflects release of stored hormone; when stable hypocalcemia is maintained for 1 h ("calcium clamp"), the abrupt initial rise is followed by a slow fall (FOX and HEATH 1981), attaining a stable PTH response after about 1 h (SCHWARZ et al. 1990). PTH secretion probably stops abruptly soon after an increase in plasma calcium, and the fall in blood level of the intact hormone depends on its half-life, which is about 5–10 min (FOX and HEATH 1981; ORWOLL et al. 1986; GRANT et al. 1990). Less rapid changes in either direction involve changes in intracellular hormone degradation (PARFITT and KLEEREKOPER 1980a; HANLEY and AYER 1986; NEER 1989) and in the proportion of cells that are in a secretory phase (PARFITT and KLEEREKOPER 1980a; FITZPATRICK and LEONG 1990). There is a circadian rhythm in PTH secretion with a consistent peak during the night and a less consistent peak earlier in the day (MARKOWITZ et al. 1988; LOGUE et al. 1990; CALVO et al. 1991), possibly reflecting neuroendocrine regulation (KRIPKE et al. 1978; LOGUE et al. 1990). With more frequent sampling, PTH secretion is episodic with 1–6 pulses/h (FOX et al. 1981; HARMS et al. 1989; KITAMURA et al. 1990). Neither short- nor long-term fluctuation in PTH is fully explained by, or fully explains, the circadian rhythm in free calcium mentioned earlier (MARKOWITZ et al. 1988; CALVO et al. 1991).

A final point of homeostatic importance is the relationship between the control of hormone secretion and the control of cell proliferation in the parathyroid gland (PARFITT and KLEEREKOPER 1980b; PARFITT 1982; PARFITT et al. 1991b). An increase in PTH secretion is usually sufficient to reverse a short-term perturbation, but in some disorders the efficacy of PTH in raising ECF free calcium is subject to sustained impairment (PARFITT and KLEEREKOPER 1980b; NEER 1989; MUNDY 1989; LLOYD et al. 1989; Parfitt 1990b), symbolized by a downward shift in the curve representing the efferent loop of the system in Fig. 3. A parathyroid cell that is forced by a chronic hypocalcemic stress to maintain a higher than normal rate of hormone synthesis and secretion has lost the physiologic advantage of operating on the steep portion of the sigmoid curve close to the set point, and is no longer able to defend effectively against any further fall in ECF free calcium (PARFITT 1969d). Such a cell will be better able to achieve its goal of restoring the controlled variable to the secretory set point if it multiplies. This is why the invariable long-term response to hypocalcemia is an increase in parathyroid cell number or hyperplasia (PARFITT and KLEEREKOPER 1980a; PARFITT 1982, 1990b; LLOYD et al. 1989). Eventually, secretion by the whole organ can be maintained at an increased level, even though secretion by individual cells is normal because they are operating close to their set point. As a result, PTH secretion correlates better with the magnitude of the negative calcium load than with the plasma calcium level (NEER 1989). Hyperplasia is the means whereby the parathyroid glands add integral control to the proportional and derivative controls that are usually sufficient for short-term regulation (PARFITT 1969d, 1982; NEER 1989).

II. Efferent Loop: Effects of PTH on Free Calcium

The relationship between plasma calcium (dependent) and PTH secretion (independent) is curvilinear (Fig. 3; PARFITT 1982). It is impossible to bring about sustained changes in PTH secretion except by manipulating plasma calcium, so that the general form of the relationship has to be deduced from measurements in subjects with spontaneous differences in PTH secretion. In patients with surgical or idiopathic hypoparathyroidism and undetectable levels of intact PTH, the albumin-adjusted total calcium is about 1.5 mmol/l (PARFITT 1972; WILSON et al. 1988). In normal subjects, corresponding values are respectively about 40 pg/ml and 2.4 mmol/l, and in patients with mild primary hyperparathyroidism they are respectively about 120 pg/ml and 2.8 mmol/l (BILEZIKIAN et al. 1991 and unpublished data). In the latter group, indices of hormone secretion and the severity of hypercalcemia remain unchanged over many years (PARFITT et al. 1991a). These data indicate that the same increment in steady-state level of PTH produces a successively smaller increment in steady-state plasma calcium (Fig. 3). This exemplifies the general principle in endocrinology that subjects who are deficient in a hormone are more sensitive to its effects than those with normal or increased levels, although for no hormone has this qualitative relationship yet been given adequate quantitative expression. That complete deficiency of PTH reduces plasma calcium only by about a third suggests that PTH amplifies an existing process rather than turning on a completely new process (COPP 1964); the significance of this will be returned to in a later section.

When synthetic human PTH is given in high dose by continuous intravenous infusion over 24 h to human subjects, there is a linear increase in ECF free calcium of about 0.014 mmol/l per hour, the rise being detectable within 4 h (FRIEDLANDER and SEGRE 1988). How long this response would continue is not known, but, as mentioned earlier, chronic hypersecretion of PTH is accompanied by chronic hypercalcemia (PARFITT et al. 1991a). This is associated with increases, direct or indirect, in all the plasma-directed calcium fluxes described in Sects. F and G (PARFITT and KLEEREKOPER 1980a; BRONNER 1982; CHARLES et al. 1986; BROWN et al. 1987; NEER 1989; MUNDY 1989); the underlying biochemical and molecular mechanisms are considered at length in Chap. 15. PTH increases intestinal calcium absorption indirectly by stimulating the production of calcitriol, the active metabolite of vitamin D made in the proximal nephron (Chap. 10), and increases tubular reabsorption of calcium directly by an action on the distal nephron. PTH increases whole body rates of resorption and formation as a result of increased remodeling activation (CHARLES et al. 1986). PTH also enhances the transfer of calcium out of bone by several processes (see Sects. G, H). These effects are supplemented by inhibition of proximal tubular reabsorption of phosphate, which leads to a fall in plasma phosphate, increased dissociation of the Ca^{2+}-$HPO_4^=$ ion pair, and increased effectiveness of PTH on bone (SOMERVILLE and KAYE 1982).

Depending on the magnitude, time course, and kinetics of these responses (NEER 1989), they make different contributions to the two main homeostatic functions of PTH to correct short-term deviations from the set point and to determine the long-term value of the set point for ECF free calcium (McCANCE 1954). The short-term responses are transient and conceptually simple. A quantity of calcium is withdrawn from or added to the ECF pool, a corrective process is initiated, and an equivalent quantity of calcium is replaced or removed with restoration of the status quo (Fig. 5). Almost all work on calcium homeostasis, experimental or theoretical, has been directed to elucidating the components of this short-term corrective process (PARSONS 1976; BRONNER 1982; NEER 1989; MUNDY 1989). But of greater biological and clinical importance is the long-term mechanism for determining the set point (Fig. 5). By precisely what means does a sustained increase or decrease in PTH secretion impose a sustained increase or decrease in set point? Only a few investigators have clearly formulated this crucial question, and recognized that indefinite continuation of the short-term corrective process, whatever its nature, does not provide the answer (HOWARD 1956; MORGAN 1973; NORDIN et al. 1975; PARFITT and KLEEREKOPER 1980a).

The effects of PTH on calcium absorption could begin within 12 h, but are not usually apparent for about 2 days (NEER 1989). The delay includes the time needed for calcitriol production to increase significantly (4–6 h;

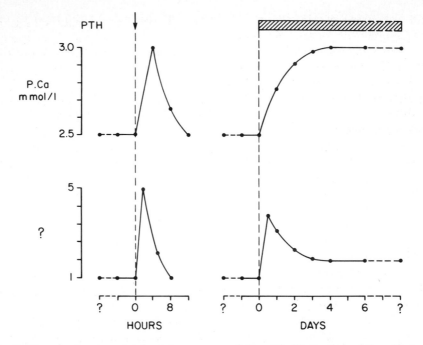

Fig. 5. Transient versus steady state response. Schematic illustration of the effects of a single dose of PTH *on the left*, and of continued administration of PTH *on the right*. *Upper panel* depicts changes in plasma calcium, and *lower panel* depicts changes in some hypothetical experimental variable such as number of osteoclasts or amount of lactate produced. (Reprinted from Parfitt 1979a with permission)

Friedlander and Segre 1988; McElduff et al. 1990), and the time taken for calcitriol to induce new protein synthesis in the intestinal mucosal cell (6–12 h; DeLuca 1983). The magnitude of the effect depends on the availability of calcidiol as a substrate for calcitriol synthesis and the dietary intake of calcium. The effect of PTH on distal tubular reabsorption of calcium is evident within 1 h (Law and Heath 1984), but the expected fall in calcium excretion may initially be masked by increased sodium excretion and consequent decreased proximal tubular reabsorption of calcium (Roelen et al. 1989). The magnitude of this response depends on the prevailing rate of urinary calcium excretion, and a significant effect on plasma calcium is unlikely for several days (Neer 1989). The effect of PTH on tubular reabsorption of phosphate is apparent within 1 h or less, but the earliest detection of a fall in plasma phosphate has varied from 30 min (Roelen et al. 1989) to 24 h (Friedlander and Segre 1988).

The rapid correction of deviations from the calcium set point is accomplished mainly by changes in net calcium release from bone by various mechanisms; the contributions from the gut and the kidney are much slower. The effect of PTH on bone has a fast component of relatively small magnitude apparent within minutes, and several slower components of larger magnitude with onsets in hours or days. The rapid hypercalcemic effect requires the presence of calcitriol, varies inversely with the prevailing level of plasma phosphate, is augmented by prior administration of calcium, and is preceded by a very early fall in plasma calcium, which is probably a reflection of sudden movement of calcium into bone cells (PARFITT 1976b; PARSONS 1976). The earliest effect is probably mediated by the lining cell-osteocyte syncytium described in Sects. G.III and IV, since PTH increases the efflux of calcium from the same bone surface location as receives calcium from plasma (GRUBB et al. 1977), and produces a variety of acute changes in both lining cells and osteocytes (TALMAGE et al. 1970; PARFITT 1976b). Other components of the rapid hypercalcemic effect of PTH are a transient acceleration of bone resorption as a result of stimulating the activity of existing osteoclasts, and a transient deceleration in bone formation as a result of depressing the activity of existing osteoblasts (PARFITT 1976b). These cellular mechanisms, together with contributions from other bone cell types, will be described more fully in Sect. G. The slower hypercalcemic effect depends on increased production of new osteoclasts consequent on increased activation of bone remodeling (Sect. G.I and Chap. 3).

The long-term effect of PTH to change the set point for calcium can only be accomplished by a mechanism that allows a new steady state to be established (HOWARD 1956; MORGAN 1973; NORDIN et al. 1975; PARFITT 1976b, 1979a, 1987). What is required is a pair of opposed calcium fluxes of large magnitude, an inward flux directed toward the ECF that is active, regulated by PTH, and capable of being sustained indefinitely over a wide range of values, and an outward flux directed away from the ECF that is passive but dependent on the calcium concentration. If the inward flux can be defined as a function of PTH (f[PTH]) and the outward flux as a linear function of calcium (k[Ca]), then in a steady state, if all other fluxes are balanced:

$$f[\text{PTH}] = k[\text{Ca}], \quad \text{so that} \quad [\text{Ca}] = f[\text{PTH}]/k \tag{1}$$

If k remains constant, then steady-state ECF free calcium will be dependent on steady-state PTH in accordance with some mathematical function (Fig. 3). As will be more rigorously established in subsequent sections, the necessary pair of fluxes exist only in the kidney and the bone. In the kidney, passive concentration-dependent efflux is provided by glomerular filtration and active PTH dependent influx by tubular reabsorption. In the bone, both concentration-dependent efflux (from ECF) and PTH-dependent influx (to ECF) occur at quiescent bone surfaces. Most previous investigators have assigned a primary role to only one of these, usually the former (MORGAN 1973; NORDIN et al. 1975), less commonly the latter (HOWARD 1956), but both are essential (PARFITT and KLEEREKOPER 1980a; PARFITT 1976b, 1979a, 1987). Consequently, the set point determination by PTH is based on changes in the apparent threshold for tubular reabsorption of calcium, as explained in Sect. F, and in the blood-bone equilibrium, as explained in Sect. G.

III. Short-Term Regulation as a Function of Parathyroid Status

The efficiency of plasma calcium regulation depends on the interaction of the afferent and efferent loops just described. The efficiency in normal subjects was previously characterized as between-person CV (2.5%) and within-person CV (1.5%), but few comparable data are available in patients with abnormal levels of PTH secretion. In both hypoparathyroidism (Parfitt 1972) and hyperparathyroidism (Nussbaum and Potts 1991), between-person differences depend mainly on differences in the severity of PTH deficiency or excess, and provide little information on regulatory efficiency. In dogs, total parathyroidectomy increases the between-individual CV for total plasma calcium by about fourfold (Copp et al. 1961), as predicted from a simpler model of reciprocal causality based on linear rather than curvilinear functions (Morgan 1973). It is common clinical experience that in patients with hypoparathyroidism plasma calcium is more variable than in normal subjects and is more susceptible to the effects of varying dietary intake of calcium or phosphate (Parfitt 1988b). In patients with primary hyperparathyroidism who have had a sufficient number of serial measurements, the average within-person CV is about 3.5% for albumin-adjusted total calcium (Parfitt et al. 1991a) and about 2.5% for free calcium measured directly (Edmondson and Li 1976), but the circadian variation is similar in timing and magnitude to normal subjects (LoCascio et al. 1982). The data indicate that PTH deficiency substantially impairs the precision of set point determination as well as reducing the set point, and that PTH excess modestly impairs precision as well as increasing the set point.

Short-term error correction for plasma calcium has been the subject of extensive experimental investigation (Copp et al. 1961, 1965; Copp 1964; Bronner and Stein 1992) by studying the rate, duration, and completeness of recovery from either positive loads (infusion of calcium) or negative loads (infusion of a chelating agent such as EDTA). In human subjects there has been no systematic study of complete recovery from calcium infusion, although 50%–60% of a rapidly administered load is removed in 2 h (Melick and Baird 1967). But both in dogs (Sanderson et al. 1960; Copp et al. 1961) and in rats (Bronner and Stein 1992), the recovery curves from positive and negative loads are virtually mirror images. In normal human subjects, complete recovery from EDTA-induced hypocalcemia takes about 10 h from the end of a 2-h infusion (Parfitt 1969c). Recovery in adult rats and in cows is of comparable duration, but mature dogs need only about 6 h to restore the pre-infusion values; in all three species recovery is faster in younger animals (Parfitt 1969c). These studies were all carried out before accurate measurement of PTH was possible. The only intact PTH measurements made during

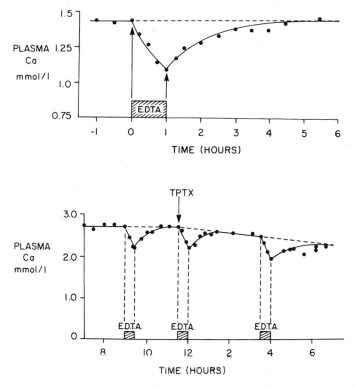

Fig. 6. Changes in plasma unchelated calcium in response to infusion of EDTA in a chronically parathyroidectomized dog (*upper panel*), and immediately before, immediately after, and 4 h after acute parathyroidectomy in a dog (*lower panel*), redrawn from Copp et al. (1961) with permission. Note that recovery occurs to a plasma calcium value appropriate to the contemporary level of PTH, even though no increase in PTH secretion can occur

recovery were not related to time (CONLIN et al. 1989), and there has been no study in any species relating the kinetics of recovery from induced hypo- or hypercalcemia to changes in PTH secretion measured simultaneously.

The role of the parathyroid gland in error correction can be approached indirectly. After parathyroidectomy (PTX), plasma calcium falls at a rate that is species specific and to a lesser extent age dependent. In the dog, if EDTA is infused during the post-PTX fall in plasma calcium, recovery occurs to the value corresponding to the time after PTX, at a rate only slightly slower than in intact dogs (PARFITT 1976b, 1979a; Copp et al. 1961; Copp 1964; Fig. 6). If EDTA is infused after attainment of the new steady-state plasma calcium, recovery of the initial value is usually complete, but slower than in normal dogs. If the plasma calcium is raised by oral or intravenous calcium administration to a value higher than would be expected for the aparathyroid state, recovery from EDTA-induced hypocalcemia is markedly impaired (SANDERSON et al. 1960; PARFITT 1969c), but, if the plasma calcium is raised by the continuous infusion of PTH, recovery is much less impaired (PARFITT 1976b). These data indicate that recovery depends mainly on the presence of PTH in the circulation at a concentration appropriate to the pre-infusion plasma calcium level. Even if PTH secretion cannot increase, complete recovery is possible, albeit at a slower rate than normal, and at the slowest rate if PTH is absent altogether. The presence of parathyroid glands able to increase secretion improves the rapidity of the response, but is not a prerequisite for complete recovery. Although not verified by PTH measurements, this interpretation is consistent with the delayed restoration of normocalcemia after EDTA infusion in asymptomatic patients who have apparently recovered from tetany following thyroid surgery (PARFITT 1969c).

E. Other Calciotropic Hormones

Almost all hormones have some effect on bone or bone mineral metabolism, but by convention calcitriol and calcitonin are grouped with PTH as the calciotropic hormones. PTH-related peptide (Chap. 17) also belongs to this group, but will not be discussed here since it does not appear to be involved in normal post-natal plasma calcium homeostasis. Grouping these hormones together has the disadvantage of suggesting that they are of equal importance; in fact, their functions are complementary but different, and do not challenge the central importance of PTH in plasma calcium regulation. Calcitriol production shows the same reciprocal response to changes in plasma calcium as does PTH secretion, and can be used as a pharmacologic replacement for PTH (PARFITT 1988b). But if this was its physiologic function, calcitriol would vary inversely with a primary change in PTH (via its effect on calcium) as a compensatory response, rather than varying directly, as is observed (Fig. 2). Calcitriol behaves as an agent of PTH, and as a modifier of its effects on target cells, and not as an independent regulator of calcium. In a similar vein, soon after its discovery, calcitonin was temporarily promoted to equal status with PTH on the basis of their reciprocal responses to changes in plasma calcium (COPP 1970), but it is now evident that plasma calcium regulation is not the result of a balance between the opposing effects of PTH and calcitonin.

I. Calcitriol

The rate of calcitriol synthesis depends on the availability of calcidiol as substrate, the activity of the 1α-hydroxylase enzyme in the proximal nephron, and the amount of functioning renal tissue. 1α-Hydroxylation is stimulated by an increase in PTH, by vitamin D depletion, and by hypophosphatemia (PARFITT and KLEEREKOPER 1980a; NEER 1989), and is inhibited by the converse changes in these agents. The increase in calcitriol production that occurs in response to reduction in dietary calcium is mediated both indirectly by increased PTH secretion and directly by hypocalcemia (WEISINGER et al. 1989). Calcitriol levels increase during growth, pregnancy, and lactation, partly because the hormones that accompany the increased demand for calcium (growth hormone, estrogen, and prolactin) have independent effects on 1α-hydroxylation (PARFITT and KLEEREKOPER 1980a); stimulation of PTH secretion is minimal or absent if dietary calcium is adequate. Indirect evidence suggests that calcitriol is also produced locally by intestinal and bone cells in a manner that is less subject to physiologic regulation and more substrate dependent (PARFITT 1990b). Calcitriol has a short half life, but the details of its further metabolism are not fully understood.

Calcitriol acts like a steroid hormone, binding to a nuclear receptor and stimulating the synthesis of a family of calcium-binding proteins (calbindins)(DeLUCA et al. 1990); some of these, like the intestinal calcium-binding protein (calbindin-D_{9k}), are well characterized; others are of uncertain nature and function. In addition, calcitriol promotes the entry of calcium into its target cells by a mechanism that does not depend on new protein synthesis and so is more rapid (NEMERE and NORMAN 1990). Calcitriol deficiency and excess tend to be accompanied by the same directional changes in plasma calcium level, but the effect of calcitriol on calcium differs from the effect of PTH on calcium in several respects. First, the range over which calcitriol status can vary with little or no effect on plasma calcium is relatively wider than for PTH, and the width of the plateau varies considerably between subjects. Second, even at the extremes the effect of calcitriol on plasma calcium is less predictable than the effect of PTH. Third, hypercalcemia due to calcitriol excess is associated with poorer short-term and long-term stability than hypercalcemia due to PTH excess (PARFITT 1979a). These differences reflect the primary role of PTH in determining calcium set point, a process to which the contribution of calcitriol is normally permissive rather than regulatory. Nevertheless, in patients with PTH deficiency, calcitriol (or some other metabolite of vitamin D) can return the calcium set point to normal (PARFITT 1988b), and allow a close to normal defense of the set point in response to EDTA infusion (PARFITT 1976b).

In the intestine, calcitriol increases calcium (and secondarily phosphate) absorption by stimulating active calcium transport out of the mucosal cells at the basal pole; the plasma calcitriol level is the major determinant of calcium absorption in the absence of intestinal disease (DeLUCA et al. 1990). In the kidney, direct effects of calcitriol on calcium and phosphate transport are inconsistent and of uncertain physiologic importance (NEER 1989) except for the likely need for calbindin-D_{28k} to permit active calcium reabsorption (BRONNER 1989). In the bone, calcitriol increases both the activity of existing osteoclasts and the recruitment of new osteoclasts from precursor cells (STERN 1990), but evidence for the coupled increase in bone formation expected from increased remodeling activation is not as clear as with thyroid or parathyroid hormones (see Sect. G and Chap. 2). Indirect evidence suggests that calcitriol facilitates mineralization of matrix by enhancing mineral transport by osteoblasts (PARFITT 1990b). Calcitriol acts synergistically with PTH to enhance non-osteoclast-mediated calcium release from bone (PARFITT and KLEEREKOPER 1980a). Such effects on calcium transport may relate to the presence of calbindin-D_{9k} in bone (BALMAIN 1991). Calcitriol decreases the secretion of PTH, both indirectly by raising the plasma calcium level, and also by a direct action on the parathyroid gland via some mechanism unrelated to a change in plasma calcium (SLATOPOLSKY et al. 1990).

II. Calcitonin

No essential function has yet been found for calcitonin in man, and it may be a vestigial hormone since, unlike PTH and calcitriol, steady state plasma calcium shows little or no change with either complete absence or a large excess of calcitonin, to neither of which has any harmful effect been unequivocally ascribed (BRONNER 1982; AZRIA 1989). Calcitonin secretion is stimulated by an increase and inhibited by a decrease in free calcium, the opposite relationship to PTH. Calcitonin secretion is also increased by several gastrointestinal hormones including glucagon and gastrin, and (at least in the rat) by feeding (TALMAGE et al. 1980, 1983). Calcitonin acts on the bone remodeling system to reduce activation (see Sect. G.II and Chap. 2). This effect seems to be sustainable indefinitely with exogenous calcitonin given for the prevention and treatment of osteoporosis (AZRIA 1989; PARFITT 1990c), but with excessive endogenous calcitonin production the effect may be overcome in the long term by secondary hyperparathyroidism (MELSEN et al. 1989). The best-known effect of calcitonin is to decrease plasma calcium, partly because it transiently reduces the activity of existing osteoclasts, of which it is the most potent known direct inhibitor (CHAMBERS et al. 1986). But this effect is readily detectable only if many osteoclasts are present, which is rarely the case in the adult human skeleton (AZRIA 1989). Calcitonin also reduces the efflux of calcium from bone by a non-osteoclast-mediated mechanism (TALMAGE et al. 1980), probably involving the syncytium of bone-lining cells and osteocytes described in Sects. G. III and IV.

In several species, calcitonin is needed for the earliest homeostatic response to induced hypercalcemia (JAROS et al. 1984); this represents a form of derivative control, but the biologic importance of slightly earlier correction of hypercalcemia is uncertain (BRONNER 1982). In rats with or without renal failure, the presence of calcitonin blunts the calcemic response to PTH (RODRIGUEZ et al. 1991). In treated athyroid patients, the rise in plasma calcium induced by slow calcium infusion is greater and recovery is somewhat delayed (WILLIAMS et al. 1966; ANAST and GUTHRIE 1971), possibly as a result of calcitonin deficiency, but recovery from a rapid infusion is unimpaired (MELICK and BAIRD 1967). The most plausible function of calcitonin is to permit more efficient utilization of absorbed calcium and phosphate (TALMAGE et al. 1980, 1983). Postprandial secretion of calcitonin restricts calcium efflux from bone, thus maintaining both PTH secretion and renal conservation of calcium. Calcitonin also promotes the entry of phosphate into bone, thus accomplishing the temporary storage of calcium and phosphate in the bone fluid. Whatever the physical and chemical nature and location of this labile storage form of calcium, its release at night (when PTH secretion increases) would permit normocalcemia to be maintained without net loss of bone. This mechanism is speculative but makes physiologic sense and is consistent with a large body of evidence. Calcitonin may alsó contribute to the circadian periodicity of ECF free calcium (STAUB et al. 1989; TALMAGE et al. 1983), which is discussed in Sect. G.VIII.

F. External Balance and Turnover of Calcium

The net difference between all routes of gain and loss of substances by the body is the external balance (PARFITT and KLEEREKOPER 1980a). After birth, all body constituents are ultimately derived from the diet, so that gains are determined by net absorption (Fig. 1). Losses occur in the urine and to a much smaller extent from the skin. Consequently, the difference between net absorption and urinary excretion, the two components of external turn-over, determines the external balance, which in turn determines the rate of change of body content; since 99% of body calcium is in bone, this is equivalent to the rate of bone loss or gain. Turnover can take place only via the blood, so that the components of external turnover also influence the plasma and ECF composition; the homeostatic implications of this influence will be considered later (Sect. F.III). The external balance for calcium should be zero in healthy adults, provided it is averaged over an appropriate time. During growth, the external balance is normally continuously positive, but after about age 45 years, because of involutional bone loss, the "normal" balance becomes negative to the extent of about 1.5 mmol calcium daily in women and somewhat less in men.

I. Dietary Intake and Intestinal Absorption

The requirement of a nutrient is the lowest intake that permits maintenance of zero balance, whereas an allowance is the intake that meets the require-ment for at least 95% of the population. Calcium requirement is relatively higher than for other nutrients because of less complete absorption, the existence of a minimum obligatory loss of calcium in the urine, and the need to maintain normocalcemia without sacrificing bone (HEANEY 1986). Mean calcium requirement estimated by the external balance method is higher in women than in men and increases with age in both sexes and after menopause in women, mainly because of decreased absorption efficiency. The actual dietary intake of calcium is normally between 6 and 30 mmol/day, tends to fall with age, and is lower in women than in men.

Net calcium absorption is the difference between dietary and fecal calcium, and also the difference between total calcium absorption and the calcium in gastric, biliary, pancreatic, and intestinal fluids, collectively referred to as endogenously secreted calcium (PARFITT and KLEEREKOPER 1980a). The most commonly used index of the efficiency of absorption of ingested calcium is so-called true absorption, the component of total absorption that is derived from the diet, rather than from endogenous secretion. However, there are many pitfalls in the isotopic determination of true absorption and only net absorption has metabolic and nutritional significance (SHEIKH et al. 1990). At a normal intake, net absorption is about 25% of intake, "true" absorption about 40% of intake, and total absorption (including absorption of endogenously secreted as well as ingested calcium) about 50% of intake. The rate of intestinal calcium absorption is greatest in the duodenum, but the amount absorbed is greatest in the jejunum and ileum (PARFITT and KLEEREKOPER 1980a).

At low and normal intakes absorption is mainly by saturable active transport via the transcellular pathway (PARFITT and KLEEREKOPER 1980a; BRONNER 1990), a process governed by calcitriol. At high calcium intakes, PTH secretion and calcitriol production are suppressed, and absorption is mainly by nonsaturable passive diffusion via the paracellular pathway (PARFITT and KLEEREKOPER 1980a; NELLANS 1990); absolute net absorption increases with intake even though fractional net absorption declines. When intake is reduced, fractional net absorption increases immediately, and there is a further increase for several weeks or months because of increased PTH secretion and calcitriol formation, but absolute net absorption declines and may become negative if intake falls below 2–4 mmol/day. Adaptation to altered intake is always incomplete, so that its effects are blunted but not eliminated (SHEIKH et al. 1990). Adaptive increases in both fractional and absolute calcium absorption, partly due to increased calcitriol synthesis, and partly to other mechanisms that are poorly understood, occur during growth, pregnancy, and lactation, times of greatest physiologic need (PARFITT and KLEEREKOPER 1980a; HEANEY 1986).

II. Renal Excretion

All constituents of the urine are ultimately derived from either the diet or the contents of the body. If external balance is zero and losses from the skin are disregarded, the rate of urinary excretion is equal to net absorption, any difference between them representing a gain or loss by the body. For the preservation of body composition, the function of the kidney is to match urinary excretion to net absorption over a wide range, which for calcium is about 1–10 mmol/day. But for the regulation of plasma concentrations, its function is to supply components of the extracellular fluid by the process of tubular reabsorption, which for calcium amounts to about 250 mmol/day (PARFITT and KLEEREKOPER 1980a; Fig. 1). The fundamental expression of renal physiology is that the excretion of a substance is the difference between the filtered load and tubular reabsorption (counting tubular secretion as negative reabsorption). As applied to calcium, this expression can be written:

$$U_{Ca} = UFP_{Ca} \cdot GFR - TR_{Ca}$$

which can be rearranged:

$$UFP_{Ca} = U_{Ca}/GFR + TR_{Ca}/GFR \tag{2}$$

where U_{Ca} is urinary excretion, UFP_{Ca} is plasma ultrafiltrable concentration, and TR_{Ca} is tubular reabsorption of calcium. The ultrafiltrable or nonprotein-bound calcium includes both free ionic calcium and complexed calcium (Table 1).

For many substances renal tubular reabsorption is limited by the capacity of the transport mechanism, giving rise to a *Tm* (tubular maximum). It is most useful to express *Tm* per unit of glomerular filtration rate (*Tm*/GFR), which is an index of maximum reabsorption per unit of functioning renal tissue or per nephron (PARFITT and KLEEREKOPER 1980a). The concept can be illustrated geometrically by plotting U_x/GFR against P_x (Fig. 7a). The curvilinear lower segment of the line relating these two variables is the splay region, which probably reflects the nonlinear relationship between transport rate and intraluminal concentration (PARFITT and KLEEREKOPER 1980a; BIJVOET 1977). Above the splay region $TR_x/GFR = Tm_x/GFR$, and the linear upper segment has a slope of unity. The renal handling of both phosphate and magnesium conforms closely to this model (PARFITT and KLEEREKOPER 1980a), but for calcium some modification is needed. The titration curves for calcium resemble those for phosphate and magnesium in having a threshold, a curvilinear lower segment, and a linear upper segment, but the slope of this is always less than unity (about 0.5), so that no *Tm* can be demonstrated (Fig. 7b), even though calcium reabsorption is known to be active and saturable (PARFITT and KLEEREKOPER 1980a).

One approach to this paradox (Mioni et al. 1971) is to resolve calcium reabsorption into two components: a fractional (gradient-limited) component related to the slope, which increases progressively with the plasma level, and an absolute (capacity-limited) component related to the intercept, which reaches a *Tm* (Fig. 7c). An alternative approach (D.M. MARSHALL 1976) is a single-component model in which the K_m is so high that the plasma level needed to attain transport saturation is incompatible with life. A third approach, more complex but more flexible, combines features of both the others (BIJVOET and HARINCK 1984). The two-component model makes more obvious physiologic sense, since it corresponds to the distinction between sodium-dependent and non-sodium-dependent components of tubular reabsorption, but the gradient-limited component of reabsorption is

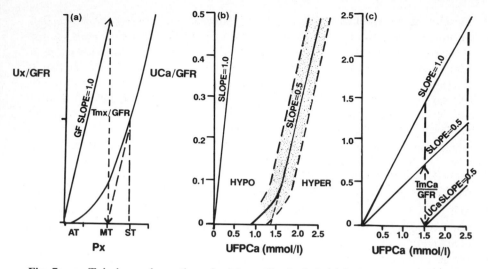

Fig. 7a–c. Tubular reabsorption of calcium. On the left (**a**) is the standard Tm/GFR model of tubular reabsorption of substance X. U_x/GFR, urinary excretion per unit of glomerular filtrate. P_x, plasma concentration. These variables are expressed in the same arbitrary units, but different scales. The diagonal line with a slope of 1.0 represents the glomerular filtered load as a function of plasma concentration. The relationship between the variables is curvilinear below the saturation threshold (ST) and linear with slope of 1.0 above this value. The plasma concentration corresponding to zero excretion is the appearance threshold (AT), and the plasma concentration corresponding to the extrapolation of the linear segment is the mean threshold (MT), numerically equal to Tm/GFR. In the middle (**b**) is shown a representative model for urinary calcium excretion per unit of glomerular filtrate as a function of plasma ultrafiltrable calcium (UFP Ca), both expressed in millimoles per liter. The general form of the relationship resembles panel (**a**) except that the slope does not increase above 0.5. The *shaded section* encloses the range in normal subjects determined by calcium infusion; values to the left of this range occur in hypoparathyroidism, and values to the right in hyperparathyroidism. On the right (**c**) is shown one possible explanation for conformity to a Tm/GFR model without attainment of a slope of 1.0 (after MIONI et al. 1971). It is assumed that 50% of the filtered load is reabsorbed by a gradient-limited mechanism, the amount reabsorbed increasing in proportion to UFP Ca (--). Further reabsorption is by a separate capacity-limited mechanism that includes the component susceptible to control by PTH (---). An alternative explanation is that the saturation threshold for calcium is too high to be experimentally demonstrated. See text for further details

substantially higher than 50% (BIJVOET and HARINCK 1984), so that the observed titration slope cannot reflect only the capacity-limited component (Fig. 7b,c). The single-component model permits a unified concept of tubular reabsorption of many substances (BIJVOET and HARINCK 1984), and enables a "notional" Tm_{Ca}/GFR to be calculated, which is empirically useful in clarifying the pathogenesis of hypercalcemia. Whatever the intrarenal mechanism, an increase in PTH secretion shifts the relationship to the right, and a decrease shifts it to the left without altering the slope (Fig. 7b; PARFITT and KLEEREKOPER 1980a).

The calcium concentration in glomerular filtrate is about 60% of the plasma level. Normally, about 80%–90% of the filtered load is reabsorbed in the proximal tubule and loop of Henle by gradient-limited processes that are linked in various ways to sodium reabsorption (PARFITT and KLEEREKOPER 1980a). An increase in dietary sodium intake leads to expansion of ECF volume and reduction in tubular reabsorption of sodium; a parallel reduction in tubular reabsorption of calcium leads to renal wasting of calcium, increased PTH secretion, and increased calcitriol production (GOULDING et al. 1986). A decrease in dietary sodium intake leads by a converse series of events to fall in calcium excretion; the mechanisms whereby calcium reabsorption is coupled to sodium reabsorption are poorly understood. The duration of these effects on calcium is unknown, but their magnitude diminishes with time, presumably because they are overridden by mechanisms that specifically subserve calcium homeostasis (PARFITT and KLEEREKOPER 1980b). Most physiologically important adjustments of calcium reabsorption take place by capacity-limited processes in the distal tubule and collecting duct, which are unrelated to sodium. At these sites calcium reabsorption, normally amounting to about 10% of the filtered load, is dependent on the presence of calbindin-D_{28k} (BRONNER 1989), and is increased by PTH and by thiazide diuretics and decreased by metabolic acidosis and by phosphate depletion.

In the steady state, urinary excretion of calcium must equal the sum of net intestinal absorption of calcium (NA_{Ca}) and net loss of calcium from bone (NLB_{Ca}). Changes in tubular reabsorption cause short-term transient changes in calcium excretion, but cannot be the direct cause of long-term, steady-state changes, for which there must be a change in the delivery of calcium from one or other of the two sources previously mentioned. In response to a change in the net intestinal absorption of calcium or net bone resorption, the corresponding change in urinary excretion is largely accomplished by altered tubular reabsorption, with only a small change in the plasma calcium level, because of reciprocal changes in PTH secretion. Renal conservation of calcium occurs more promptly than for sodium, but is ultimately less efficient, and the lowest rate of urinary excretion compatible with maintenance of normocalcemia is usually about 1 mmol/day, varying inversely with PTH secretion and directly with dietary protein and sodium intake (PARFITT and KLEEREKOPER 1980a; HEANEY 1986). Calcium loss is much higher during complete starvation because of metabolic acidosis (PARFITT and KLEEREKOPER 1980b). The minimum urinary excretion, together with endogenous fecal calcium excretion and calcium lost in sweat and desquamated skin, comprises the obligatory calcium loss, usually not less than 5 mmol/day.

III. Role of Intestine and Kidney in Calcium Homeostasis

It is evident that the paired fluxes needed to determine the calcium set point in accordance with Eq. 1 are not located in the intestine. Although absorption by the transcellular pathway provides active calcium influx that is controlled indirectly by PTH, the magnitude of the flux is small and is often exceeded by passive absorption along the paracellular pathway, and the total influx via both pathways is much too dependent on dietary calcium to be the primary means of determining the set point. Furthermore, the amount of endogenously secreted calcium depends more on the volumes of gastric, biliary, pancreatic, and intestinal secretions than on the plasma level of calcium, and so cannot function as a concentration-dependent efflux. A transient increase in net absorption may contribute to short-term error correction, and a long-term decrease may contribute to the defense against disequilibrium hypercalcemia resulting from increased bone resorption (PARFITT and KLEEREKOPER 1980b), but the main purpose of calcium absorption is the maintenance of calcium balance and the preservation of bone mass (HEANEY 1986). From the standpoint of plasma calcium homeostasis, calcium absorption functions more as a disturbing signal than as an agent of regulatory control (BRONNER 1982).

As mentioned previously, the kidney, unlike the intestine, is the site of paired fluxes of the requisite magnitude (c. 250 mmol/day) and kinetics. Comparison of Eq. 1 with Eq. 2 indicates that k is represented by GFR and f[PTH] by TR_{Ca}, but with several qualifications. First, a constant proportional relationship between UFP_{Ca} and [Ca] must be assumed, which becomes progressively less accurate as [Ca] deviates further from the normal range (PARFITT and KLEEREKOPER 1980a). Second, an adjustment must be made to Eq. 1 for U_{Ca} as a component of external balance, equal in the steady state to $NA_{Ca} + NLB_{Ca}$ as explained earlier. Third, it is not TR_{Ca} but rather Tm_{Ca}/GFR that is functionally related to PTH, so that f(PTH) is not independent of k as is assumed by Eq. 1. Consequently, as GFR falls with age or with disease, the load component of UFP_{Ca} given by $(NA_{Ca} + NLB_{Ca})$/ GFR becomes progressively more important, and the reabsorptive component $(TR_{Ca}$/GFR) progressively less important. Finally, it is only the capacity-limited component of calcium reabsorption, about 25 mmol/day, that is directly related to PTH, so that the relationship between PTH and whole kidney Tm_{Ca}/GFR is inevitably complex and inconstant.

The role of the kidney in adjusting the calcium set point in accordance with changes in steady-state PTH secretion was deduced from the results of calcium titration curves obtained from subjects with reduced, normal, and increased levels of parathyroid function (PEACOCK et al. 1969). The actual values of the slopes and intercepts of the titration curves must reflect the fall in PTH secretion that would have occurred during the infusions, at least in the normal and hyperparathyroid subjects. Surprisingly, no investigator has compared calcium titration curves with intact PTH levels measured at the same time. Conceivably, the effects of PTH on calcium reabsorption could change more slowly after a fall in PTH than after a rise. But rigorous determination of the functional relationship between PTH and Tm_{Ca}/GFR would require calcium infusions performed during PTH administration at varying doses to parathyroidectomized animals of suitable species, such as the dog. Another reason for inaccuracy in published values for Tm_{Ca}/GFR is that calcium infusion is natriuretic (BIJVOET and HARINCK 1984), and the consequent sodium depletion would increase whole kidney Tm_{Ca}/GFR as explained earlier.

These reservations about the precise mathematical form of the equation Tm_{Ca}/GFR = f[PTH] do not invalidate the concept that this relationship provides one means for PTH to influence calcium set point, but, in addition to the qualifications expressed earlier concerning the relationship between Eq. 1 and Eq. 2, there are many other reasons for doubting that this can be the entire explanation for set point determination. Since sodium balance influences calcium reabsorption, at least in the short term, exclusive reliance on this mechanism would make the calcium set point too vulnerable to the vagaries of sodium metabolism. Thiazide diuretics increase calcium reabsorption and occasionally cause hypercalcemia in patients with abnormal calcium metabolism (PARFITT 1969a), but rarely cause more than slight transient increases in ECF free calcium in normal subjects (STOTE et al. 1972). In pseudohypoparathyroidism, a condition with impaired responsiveness to PTH at multiple target sites (LEVINE and AURBACH 1989), tubular reabsorption of calcium is normal, both basally (PARFITT 1979b) and during calcium infusion (PARFITT 1978), but there is chronic hypocalcemia that cannot be adequately explained by decreased bone resorption or by hyperphosphatemia (PARFITT 1979a,b). The same apparently paradoxical combination of abnormalities is found in some patients with vitamin D depletion and osteomalacia (RAO et al. 1985). Consequently, for a complete explanation of set point determination, the domain of PTH must be extended to the bone, and specifically to the quiescent bone surface (PARFITT 1976b, 1979a, 1987).

G. Bone and Bone Mineral in Relation to Calcium Homeostasis

Bone is a specialized connective tissue with a matrix of collagen fibers embedded in ground substance, rendered hard by the deposition of mineral crystals that contain calcium, phosphate, carbonate, and magnesium ions in an approximate molar ratio of 40:25:5:1 (PARFITT and KLEEREKOPER 1980a). All traffic of mineral ions and water between bone and extracellular fluid takes place at surfaces, of which the internal or endosteal surfaces are the most extensive (PARFITT 1983). Cancellous and endocortical surfaces are in contact with bone marrow, but intracortical surfaces surround the contents of haversian canals which are in continuity with the marrow cavity but do not contain either fatty or hematopoietic marrow. The metabolic activity of bone is largely determined by its surface to volume ratio (FOLDES et al. 1991), by its age and mineral density, and by the composition and vascularity of the adjacent soft tissue. All bone surfaces are in one of three metabolic states (Fig. 1): resorbing, forming, or quiescent. Resorbing surfaces are covered by osteoclasts, cells that simultaneously digest collagen, depolymerize ground substance macromolecules, and dissolve mineral, with an irreversible outward flux of calcium and other minerals of bone. Forming surfaces are covered by osteoblasts, cells that synthesize and deposit the constituents of bone matrix in successive layers, each of which becomes mineralized about 2 weeks later, with an irreversible inward flux of minerals. Resorbing and forming surfaces and their associated cells are the means whereby bone volume is controlled by the remodeling system.

I. Aspects of Bone Remodeling

The process of bone remodeling is fully described in Chap. 2, but some aspects of particular relevance to the theme of this chapter will be summarized briefly. The replacement of small volumes of old bone by new throughout adult life is brought about by the continued repetition of a cyclical process of excavation and repair, each episode extending over about $0.2\,mm^2$ of bone surface and lasting for a period of 4–6 months (PARFITT 1983, 1984, 1990c). At any one time only about 10%–20% of the surface is involved, but, as existing cycles are terminated and new ones begin at other sites, all the surface is involved about once every 2–5 years, which is the average time interval between successive activation events at the same location (PARFITT 1992). The first step in the cycle is the focal activation of a segment of the quiescent surface described later; the lining cells retract to expose the bone, and mononuclear osteoclast precursors are attracted by chemotaxis to congregate and fuse. The team of newly formed osteoclasts erodes a microscopic cavity about $50\,\mu m$ in depth within a few weeks and then disappears. A team of new osteoblasts assembles within the cavity and refills it more or less completely with new bone over the next few months. Some of the osteoblasts die and disappear, some become buried in the new bone as osteocytes, and some undergo terminal transformation to lining cells (PARFITT 1990a); the bone surface is now restored to its previous quiescent state, and (in the young adult) previous location.

Resorption and formation always occur successively in the same location and always in the same order; the coupling between them probably depends in part on the release of a macromolecular constituent of bone matrix that stimulates the proliferation and differentiation of osteoblast precursors. For both resorption and formation, it is important to distinguish between recruitment of new cells and the function of existing cells; the former can have long-term effects on the rates of resorption or formation, whereas the latter can have only short-term effects on these rates. Unlike resorption, bone formation occurs in two successive stages. Matrix synthesis begins first and determines the volume of new bone but not its density; mineralization begins about 10 days later and determines the density of new bone but does not alter its volume, because water is displaced by added mineral (W.F. NEUMAN and NEUMAN 1958). The thickness of the layer of new osteoid progressively increases before the onset of mineralization and progressively decreases thereafter. The last matrix formed by the terminal osteoblasts, before they undergo transformation to lining cells, becomes the endosteal membrane. The rates of matrix and mineral apposition are most rapid at the beginning and progressively decline; although they are systematically out of step, the rates averaged throughout a complete cycle are identical (PARFITT 1990a).

The rate of bone turnover is determined by the rate of remodeling activation and the local surface to volume ratio. For the whole skeleton, the average rate of turnover is about 10%/year; for a total skeletal calcium of 30 000 mmol, this corresponds to about 8 mmol/day. The rate of bone loss is determined by the rate of remodeling activation and the extent of focal imbalance between the depth of erosion and the thickness of new bone, which together determine the net difference between the whole body rates of resorption and formation (PARFITT 1992). This is 0–0.2 mmol/day in adults less than 50 years of age, about 1.5 mmol/day for a few years after menopause, and 0.5–1 mmol/day in older women and in men. Since 99% of total body calcium is in bone, the calcium balance that results from bone remodeling must in the long term be the same as the external calcium balance. The rate of remodeling activation, and hence the rate of turnover, is increased by PTH, thyroid hormone, growth hormone, and probably calcitriol, and decreased by estrogen and calcitonin. The purpose of bone remodeling is unknown, but since the most obvious difference between the bone removed and the bone replaced is in their age, the most plausible function of remodeling is prevention of excessive aging of bone (PARFITT 1990c).

Because of the time between the beginning of resorption and the end of formation in each cycle, remodeling is accompanied by a temporary deficit of bone (PARFITT 1980, 1988a). The aggregate volume of all such deficits at a particular time is the remodeling space. Together with osteoid and incompletely mineralized new bone, the total reversible mineral deficit at a normal rate of turnover is about 300 mmol, or about 1% of total body calcium. The magnitude of the deficit changes in proportion to the whole body rate of remodeling activation. Following a sustained change in activation, it takes about 6 months to establish a new steady state, during which the magnitude of the reversible mineral deficit will change progressively to the value corresponding to the new rate of turnover, with a consequent change in total body calcium in the opposite direction to the change in rate of activation. Long-term changes in the reversible mineral deficit can result from changes in the duration of any of the components of the remodeling cycle. Short-term changes in the reversible mineral deficit can result from changes in the rate of erosion into bone by existing osteoclasts, or in the rate of mineral apposition by existing osteoblasts.

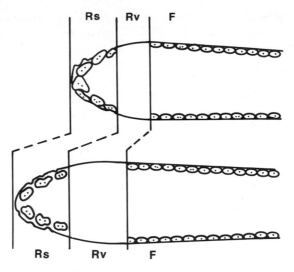

Fig. 8. Possible mechanism for short-term contribution of remodeling system to calcium homeostasis. *Upper panel* shows in diagrammatic form an evolving osteon moving from right to left with a cutting cone of osteoclasts in front (*Rs*, resorption) followed by a transitional zone (*Rv*, reversal), followed by a closing cone of osteoblasts (*F*, formation). *Lower panel* shows the same osteon some time later during which the cutting cone has advanced faster than the closing cone, with a consequent increase in the transitional zone and in the volume of the remodeling space

II. Role of Bone Remodeling in Calcium Homeostasis

The primary purpose of osteoclasts and osteoblasts is to subserve the mechanical rather than the metabolic functions of the skeleton by means of growth, modeling, remodeling, and repair. For this purpose, the most important aspect of their function is the volume of bone resorbed or formed by each cell unit during its active life span, or cell capacity; the rate at which the work proceeds, a reflection of cell vigor, affects the time taken to complete the work but not the quantity of work ultimately performed (Parfitt 1976a, 1984, 1990a, 1992). It is the independence of capacity and vigor that enables osteoclasts and osteoblasts to participate in calcium homeostasis by contributing to short term error correction without compromising their long-term role in controlling bone volume. To clarify this point, consider the organization of a typical cortical remodeling unit or evolving osteon (Fig. 8). On the average the longitudinal rates of erosion and refilling are the same, about 25 μm/day (Parfitt 1983). This is the rate at which the entire unit advances through the bone, maintaining the same spatial relationships between its constituent parts and the same magnitude of the three components of the reversible deficit. In cancellous bone the temporal relationship between resorption and formation is similar, although the spatial relationship is less apparent.

In the short term these relationships are not invariant but elastic. For example, a 60% increase in the rate of advance by existing osteoclasts throughout the skeleton for 4 h to the level normally found in dogs (PARFITT 1983) would release an additional 0.8 mmol calcium (8 mmol/day*0.6*4/24), reflecting a corresponding increase in the reversible deficit (Fig. 8). The same proportional reduction in the rate of advance of osteoblasts for the same time would have the same result. In either case, this extra deficit could be repaired quickly and would have no effect on the outcome of the remodeling transaction when the remodeling unit had completed its evolution. The figures given are purely illustrative, but are consistent with a large body of experimental work (PARFITT 1976b); however, the lining cell-osteocyte complex, described later, probably makes a larger contribution to short-term error correction. The concertina-like relationship between resorption and formation within each remodeling unit, although hypothetical, could produce changes in bone mineral balance of the right magnitude to accomodate the normal circadian changes in external calcium balance, in which a cumulative positive balance of about 1 mmol during a 16-h period of feeding and activity is followed by a negative balance of about 1 mmol during an 8-h period of sleep (PARFITT 1981).

But although the remodeling system can contribute to short-term error correction, it cannot be concerned in the long-term determination of free calcium set point (PARFITT 1976b, 1979a, 1987). To put the same point with different emphasis, long-term steady-state hypercalcemia, as in primary hyperparathyroidism, cannot be explained by the indefinite continuation of the mechanisms responsible for the short-term hypercalcemic response to PTH (PARFITT 1979a). The regulation of bone volume and mass and the regulation of plasma calcium are independent. Low, normal, or high levels for plasma calcium can each coexist with low, normal, or high values for bone resorption, bone turnover, and external calcium balance. For example, the increases in these three variables are much greater in hyperthyroidism than in hyperparathyroidism, although the increase in plasma calcium is much smaller (PARFITT 1979a). In patients with both hypoparathyroidism and Paget's disease, persistent hypocalcemia coexists with a large increase in bone resorption and turnover (PARFITT 1976b, 1979a). In mild primary hyperparathyroidism, inhibition of bone resorption with a bisphosphonate causes a transient decline in plasma calcium, but after a few months the initial values are restored although PTH secretion has increased (ADAMI et al. 1990).

The fundamental reason for the independence of bone resorption and steady state plasma calcium is the temporal and spatial coupling between resorption and formation during the unfolding of individual remodeling units (PARFITT 1984, 1990a, 1992). Although acute calcium release from bone could be characterized as a mathematical function of PTH, the response does not fulfill the requirement of being indefinitely sustainable, since long-term calcium release depends more on the rate of remodeling activation than on the focal imbalance at each remodeling site (PARFITT 1984, 1990a, 1992). The frequency of activation is influenced by so many other factors, hormonal and nonhormonal (PARFITT 1990c), that it cannot satisfy the unique relationship to PTH required for set point determination in accordance with Eq. 1. It was the recognition that calcium set point could not be determined by bone resorption that prompted the assignment of this function to the renal tubular reabsorption of calcium (NORDIN et al. 1975), but, as already explained, this is not the entire explanation.

Even if PTH was the dominant regulator of remodeling activation and long-term calcium release from bone, a concentration-dependent calcium efflux would be needed for the application of Eq. 1. Although the plasma calcium level can influence bone mineralization in young rats (STAUFFER et al. 1973), in the adult human, whole body bone formation is determined mainly by the rate of remodeling activation; it is uninfluenced by plasma calcium and so cannot function as a concentration-dependent efflux. The combination of substantially increased net bone resorption and increased concentration-dependent efflux by the kidney will certainly produce hypercalcemia, but the calcium levels are unstable, highly susceptible to sodium-dependent changes in calcium reabsorption, and subject to rapid progression because of the vicious circles induced by a reduction in GFR (PARFITT 1979a). Clearly, this is not the way in which an increase in PTH secretion produces a corresponding increase in calcium set point, since in most patients with mild primary hyperparathyroidism the degree of hypercalcemia does not change with time (PARFITT et al. 1991a). For a satisfactory explanation of calcium homeostasis, it is necessary to consider how calcium ions can move in and out of bone by mechanisms that are unrelated to bone remodeling.

III. Quiescent Bone Surfaces

In contrast to young growing animals, in which most free bone surfaces are either forming or resorbing, in the adult of large animals, including man, it is usual for at least 80% of the cancellous bone surface and at least 95% of the intracortical bone surface to be inactive with respect to bone remodeling (PARFITT 1983, 1984; Fig. 1). The structure of the quiescent bone surface is complex and resolvable only by electron microscopy (MATTHEWS 1980). At the outer edge of the mineralized bone matrix is the lamina limitans, a thin layer of matrix that is more electron dense than the regular bone matrix adjacent to it (SCHERFT 1972; LUK et al. 1974; VANDERWIEL et al. 1978; MILLER et al. 1980). The difference in density is obscured by mineral, and so is discernible only after decalcification. The lamina limitans consists of organic material of uncertain composition, but probably containing glycosaminoglycans as well as collagen, adsorbed onto the regular bone matrix. The quiescent bone surface is covered by a layer of extremely thin (0.1–1 μm) and flat cells with elongated nuclei (VANDERWIEL et al. 1978; MILLER et al. 1980; MILLER and JEE 1987); these lining cells were first recognized by Edwards Park in the metaphyses of growing children and referred to as the "periosteum of the trabeculae" (Howard 1956). The lining cells are one of the modes of terminal differentiation of osteoblasts, but represent a distinct phenotype (Miller and Jee 1987), and constitute much the largest fraction of the surface cells of bone. The average duration of quiescence between successive episodes of remodeling is about 3 years in the human ilium, so that the average age of a lining cell is about 18 months (Parfitt 1992), but in most other regions of the skeleton where turnover is much lower the average lining cell will be much older.

In two-dimensional sections, the lining cells have profile lengths of $40-60\,\mu m$, corresponding to surface areas of about $2000-5000\,\mu m^2$ and surface densities of about $200-500/mm^2$; the cell area tends to increase and the cell density to decrease with age (Miller et al. 1980). There are few organelles except in the cytoplasm adjacent to the nucleus. The lining cells are often joined by gap junctions and sometimes overlap, but they do not form a completely continuous layer, although the gaps between them are not usually greater than $5-10\,\mu m$ across, and collectively account for no more than 5% of the total quiescent surface. These apparently bare areas are always located some distance from the nearest bone marrow capillary, structures which frequently run in close proximity to he nuclei of the lining cells (Miller and Jee 1980). Because of their osteoblast lineage, lining cells probably retain the same hormonal receptors and responsiveness but, at least in adult remodeling bone, they appear to have lost the ability to synthesize collagen and should not be referred to as osteoblasts, resting or otherwise. Nevertheless they remain able to synthesize proteins other than collagen (Kaye and Henderson 1988). Fine processes from the lining cells extend into the canaliculi and make contact by gap junctions with similar processes extending from the osteocytes, cells which represent another mode of terminal differentiation of osteoblasts.

Between the lining cells and the lamina limitans is a thin $(0.1-0.5\,\mu m)$ layer of unmineralized connective tissue (Matthews 1980; Miller et al. 1980). The collagen fibers of this endosteal membrane are packed in smaller bundles and oriented more randomly than in the bone matrix, and are fewer in number with relatively more amorphous ground substance than in bone. The endosteal membrane, although it never mineralizes, is sometimes erroneously referred to as osteoid (Raina 1972; VanderWiel et al. 1978), a tissue that it may resemble under light microscopy, but which is clearly different at the ultramicroscopic level. The boundary between the endosteal membrane and the lamina limitans is one plausible location for the accumulation of circulating macromolecules that are selectively taken up by bone, such as albumin (Triffitt and Owen 1977) and α_2-HS glycoprotein (Triffitt et al. 1978). On bone surfaces adjacent to fatty (yellow) marrow, the lining cells are separated by a similar connective tissue layer from the thin cytoplasm of the fat cells. On bone surfaces adjacent to hematopoietic (red) marrow, the fat cell cytoplasm is replaced by the squamous cells of the marrow sac

(MENTON et al. 1982). The entire thickness of tissue separating the marrow from the bone (two layers of cells and two layers of connective tissue) is only $1-2\,\mu m$.

IV. Circulation of Bone, Macro and Micro

Bone has an abundant blood supply, with estimates ranging from 10 to $20\,ml/100\,g$ per minute, or from 10% to 25% of the cardiac output (PARFITT and KLEEREKOPER 1980a; CHARKES et al. 1979; BROOKS 1987). Even the lowest figure is far higher than is needed to support the metabolic demands of the tissue. Vasoconstriction magnifies the effect on plasma calcium of both positive and negative loads (COPP and SHIM 1963), which suggests that the accessibility of labile calcium in bone is dependent on blood flow (W.F. NEUMAN et al. 1968). The passage of mineral ions and water from blood to bone can be traced through arterioles to the capillaries adjacent to the bone surface and in haversian canals. Transfer across the capillary wall is by passive diffusion; at low flow rates the extraction of bone-seeking substances is limited by flow, so that the clearance increases in proportion to flow, whereas at high flow rates extraction is limited by diffusion, so that clearance increases proportionately less than flow, and the extraction ratio falls (TOTHILL et al. 1985). The subsequent course is through the ground substance of the connective tissue in the bone marrow or within haversian canals, and then through or between the cells lining the bone surfaces to enter the ECF compartment adjacent to the bone (MATTHEWS and MARTIN 1971; PARFITT and KLEEREKOPER 1980a). The close proximity of the marrow capillaries to lining cell nuclei was mentioned earlier.

The composition of the bone fluid compartment has never been determined in vivo by direct measurements. In vitro equilibration experiments with powdered bovine bone (W.F. NEUMAN 1969) suggested that the concentrations of calcium and magnesium in the bone ECF were about one-third of those in plasma and the concentration of potassium much higher (PARFITT and KLEEREKOPER 1980a), but higher concentrations of divalent ions could be maintained by cellular activity in vivo, as will be discussed in Sect. G.VIII. Some investigators find much more potassium in bone than can be accounted for by the mineral or by the cells (M.W. NEUMAN and NEUMAN 1980), whereas others do not (PINTO and KELLY 1984), probably because of differences in the methods of calculating intra- and extracellular water from the volumes of distribution of putative markers. The former result is supported by estimation of cell number from DNA content; furthermore, a large excess of potassium at the surface of bone has been demonstrated by the scanning ion microprobe in conjunction with secondary ion mass spectrometry (BUSHINSKY et al. 1989). The concentration of albumin in bone fluid is also about one-third that in plasma, so that the proportion of free to protein-bound calcium would be the same in both fluids (OWEN et al. 1973).

The fluid between the lining cells and the bone surface extends via surface pores into the lacunar-canalicular system, where it forms a thin film that separates the osteocytes and their processes from the bone (MATTHEWS and MARTIN 1971). Fluid movement in this thin layer is aided by cilia protruding from the cell surface (FEDERMAN and NICHOLS 1974), but fluid probably also moves along the microfilaments within the intracanalicular processes. In perilacunar and pericanalicular bone, the collagen fibers are more loosely packed and less densely mineralized, and the mineral is more soluble, and more easily removed by acid. Consequently, the bone is more permeable than is found elsewhere and so is more accessible to mineral exchange. These differences are maintained by the osteocyte and do not persist after the cell dies (PARFITT and KLEEREKOPER 1980a). From the canaliculi (diameter, 200 nm) radiate microcanaliculi (diameter, 50 nm) that form channels between adjacent bundles of collagen fibrils (PARFITT 1976a). The surface area for exchange between the hydration shell of the crystals of bone mineral and the bone ECF is more than 30 times greater at the canalicular-lacunar level than at the bone surface, and more than 3000 times greater at the microcanalicular level (PARFITT 1976a).

Little is known of the microcirculation through bone except that it is rapid; in the rat, all osteocyte lacunae can be reached by tetracycline within 30 min (PARFITT 1976a). Even large molecules such as horseradish peroxidase (M_r, 40 000) freely enter the bone ECF (DOTY et al. 1976), and proteins such as albumin (M_r, 68 000) can be found in some osteocyte lacunae within 15 min (OWEN et al. 1973). About 80% of bone water is extracellular, and is completely exchangeable (EDELMAN et al. 1954), but because of its intimate relationship to the crystals and the small size of the microcanaliculi much of the water cannot be penetrated by medium-sized molecules such as polyethylene glycol (M_r, 4000) (M.W. NEUMAN and NEUMAN 1980). In old and fully mineralized bone, the only water that remains is in the hydration shells of the crystals, and the spaces between adjacent crystals are so small that ionic diffusion is too slow to be detectable, and even water itself takes many hours to reach equilibrium (EDELMAN et al. 1954). Water probably percolates from the surface through the microcanaliculi and possibly even smaller channels (ARNOLD et al. 1971; PARFITT 1976a) and is somehow pumped by the osteocytes along the canaliculi, either within or around the cell processes (ARNOLD et al. 1971). The syncytium of osteocytes and lining cells forms a nonvascular transport system that facilitates ionic exchange between ECF and bone.

V. Bone Mineral: Composition and Structure

The solid mineral phase of bone consists of small hexagonal crystals, plate-like in shape and of variable size (MORADIAN-OLDAK et al. 1991), approximately 2–5 nm in thickness, 10–80 nm in width, and 15–150 nm in length (1 nm = 10 Å). The lattice structure of the crystals, which is the three-dimensional arrangement of the constituent ions in space, conforms to that of naturally occurring minerals called apatites, the general formula of which is $3(Ca_3(PO_4)_2)Ca.X_2$ (McLean and Budy 1964; Posner 1988). This is not a molecular formula, but specifies the relative proportions of the smallest number of ions needed for one unit cell, the imaginary parallelopiped that represents the repeating unit of the crystal structure. In bone mineral, the dimensions of the unit cell are $0.94*0.94*0.69$ nm, and the lattice structure is mainly hydroxyapatite ($X_2 = OH_2^-$) with traces of fluorapatite ($X_2 = F_2^-$). The substantial amount of carbonate may be adsorbed to the surface of the crystal or substituted for phosphate in the crystal lattice, or for hydroxyl groups ($X_2 = CO_3^{2-}$) to form carbonate-apatite (McLean and Budy 1964; Posner 1988; Glimcher 1990); the labile CO_2 of bone is probably in the form of bicarbonate (Green and Kleeman 1991).

Large perfect crystals of hydroxyapatite such as may be produced in vitro have a molar Ca/P ratio of 1.67, but in vivo the Ca/P ratio is always lower (McLean and Budy 1964; Glimcher 1990). The crystals are relatively calcium deficient and are so small that at least 25% of the calcium ions are in surface positions, and the crystal surface area is at least $100 \, m^2/g$ (W.F. Neuman and Neuman 1958; McLean and Budy 1964). Because of the small crystal size, bone mineral solubility varies with the crystal surface/volume ratio (Best 1959). The exact composition of bone mineral is indeterminate, because some of its constituent ions can be replaced by other ions of approximately the same radius, and at some lattice points the ions (especially calcium) may be missing altogether, producing minor defects in the shape of the crystals which do not affect the overall structure (W.F. Neuman and Neuman 1958; Posner 1988). Crystals of small size containing lattice defects are referred to as poorly crystalline because they generate weak X-ray diffraction patterns, but, contrary to an earlier view, bone mineral does not contain a quantitatively significant noncrystalline or amorphous component (Glimcher 1990). Nevertheless, small amounts of various types of non-apatitic mineral with a lower Ca/P ratio cannot be ruled out by current methods. Furthermore, in very young bone, a significant proportion of the total phosphorus content is present as HPO_4^{2-}, rather than as PO_4^{3-} (Bonar et al. 1985); it is described as being in a "brushite-like" configuration, but not crystalline brushite ($CaHPO_4.2H_2O$).

Bound to the surface of each crystal is a thin film of water, the hydration shell; because of the small size of the crystals the volume of associated water is relatively large (W.F. Neuman, Neuman 1958; McLean and Budy 1964; Green and Kleeman 1991). In vitro, interactions between bone mineral and aqueous solutions involve four processes: diffusion into the hydration shell, exchange within the layer of ions bound to the crystal surface, exchange with ions occupying surface positions in the crystal lattice, and exchange with ions in the crystal interior. These represent four regions of decreasing accessibility and increasing time to attain equilibrium. The same four processes probably occur in vivo. The composition of the hydration shell reflects

Table 2. Chemical reactions involved in a possible scheme of mineralization[a]. (Reprinted from PARFITT and KLEEREKOPER 1980a, with permission)

	Overall	
$10Ca^{2+} + 6HPO_4^{2+} + 2H_2O$	$\rightleftharpoons$	$Ca_{10}(PO4)_6(OH)_2 + 8H^+$ Hydroxyapatite
	Possible steps	
1. $4Ca^{2+} + 4HPO_4^{2-}$	$\rightleftharpoons$	$4CaHPO_4$ Secondary calcium phosphate
2. $4CaHPO_4 + 2Ca^{2+}$	$\rightleftharpoons$	$2Ca_3(PO_4)_2 + 4H^+$ Tertiary calcium phosphate
3. $2Ca_3(PO_4)_2 + 2Ca^{2+} + 2HPO_4^{2-}$	$\rightleftharpoons$	$Ca_8(PO_4)_4(HPO_4)_2$ Octacalcium phosphate
4. $Ca_8(PO_4)_4(HPO_4)_2 + 2Ca^{2+} + 2H_2O$	$\rightleftharpoons$	$Ca_{10}(PO_4)_6(OH)_2 + 4H^+$ Hydroxyapatite

[a] Note especially the generation of H^+ ions at steps 2 and 4; the reactions will be halted if these are not neutralized or removed.

the composition of the bone ECF, so that any ion in the circulation will be represented, although not necessarily in the same concentration. Penetration into the crystal is possible only for ions within a limited range of sizes and shapes. Potassium and chloride are restricted to the water of the hydration shell, but sodium can enter the crystal surface. Magnesium ions cannot penetrate to the interior of the lattice but their exact location is unknown. For the ions foreign to hydroxyapatite, only strontium, radium, and fluoride can penetrate into the crystal interior (W.F. NEUMAN and NEUMAN 1958).

The initial mineral deposits have a Ca/P ratio of only about 1.3, consistent with the transient occurrence of intermediate forms (Table 2), as have been demonstrated during mineralization in vitro (EANES 1985). Although mineralization represents a phase transformation rather than a chemical reaction (GLIMCHER 1990), it would be easier to attain the structural order of hydroxyapatite in successive steps rather than all at once (W.F. NEUMAN 1980). The scheme in Table 2 involves only the sequential addition of the calcium and phosphate ions present in ECF, and makes obvious the necessity for removal of H^+ ions in order for the process to proceed to completion (PARFITT and KLEEREKOPER 1980a). Based on thermodynamic activity products, ECF is in the region of metastability, and so is undersaturated with respect to brushite, the most plausible candidate for the mineral first formed (W.F. NEUMAN and NEUMAN 1958; W.F. NEUMAN 1980; EIDELMAN et al. 1987). Absent the possibility of spontaneous precipitation, the initial step in mineralization is most likely heterogeneous nucleation by collagen (GLIMCHER 1984). The crystals first formed are located within the hole zones of the collagen fibrils, but these can accommodate only crystals as long as 40 nm and as wide as 3 nm, and longer and wider crystals are located on or between the fibrils, aligned with their long axes parallel to them (WEINER and PRICE 1986; WEINER and TRAUB 1989).

Extracellular fluid is supersaturated with respect to hydroxyapatite (W.F. NEUMAN and NEUMAN 1958; EIDELMAN et al. 1987); consequently once started, primary mineralization proceeds rapidly so that the density of the bone increases to about 70% of the maximum possible within a few days, mainly by multiplication of the number of crystals. The solubility of bone mineral and its relationship to the ionic composition of ECF will be considered further in Sect. G.VIII. During secondary mineralization, bone density continues to increase slowly for many years, mainly by an increase in the size and perfection of existing crystals, but the rate of mineral acquisition declines in parallel with the availability of space. Consequently, as bone ages its density and crystallinity increase and its water content, permeability, and accessibility to systemic ECF decrease (W.F. NEUMAN and NEUMAN 1958; PARFITT 1992). The average lifespan of an individual moiety of bone is determined by its distance from the nearest quiescent surface and the probability that remodeling activation will occur on that surface (PARFITT et al. 1987), and in different locations can vary from a few years to several decades.

VI. Movement of Calcium Ions in and out of Bone

It was mentioned earlier that about 0.3% of the calcium in bone, or about 75–100 mmol, was included with most of the extracellular calcium in the miscible or exchangeable pool. This is defined as the aggregate of calcium atoms within which, after equilibration, the concentration of a radioactively labeled tracer of calcium is the same as in plasma, and changes at the same rate as in plasma, which is the only accessible component of the pool (HEANEY 1976). The definition was framed in terms of atoms rather than ions to gain generality: an ion is a charged atom or group of atoms. The apparent size of the pool is influenced by the frequency of sampling after introduction of the tracer and the accuracy of the radioactivity measurements, but is more dependent on the choice of mathematical model to which the data are fitted (J.H. MARSHALL 1969; MASSIN et al. 1974; HEANEY 1976; JUNG et al. 1978), and most dependent on the time for which the measurements are continued, with estimates varying from 50 mmol at 1 h to 175 mmol at 72 h (PARFITT 1969c, 1976a). The time dependence of the exchangeable pool size is a reflection of the continuous spectrum of residence times of individual calcium atoms in bone, ranging from minutes to decades (PARFITT 1976a). Consequently, any choice is arbitrary, but the chosen value of 75–100 mmol for rapidly exchangeable calcium in bone is quite representative (MILHAUD 1962; HEANEY 1964; J.H. MARSHALL 1969; B.L. RIGGS et al. 1971; MASSIN et al. 1974; JUNG et al. 1978; REEVE 1978; CHARLES et al. 1986).

Before discussing the location, magnitude, mechanisms, and homeostatic significance of the fluxes between blood and bone implied by this phenomenon, the ambiguity of the term "exchange" must be addressed. In the strictest sense "exchange" refers to the "equal and opposite rates of transfer of calcium atoms to and from a single microscopic volume of bone" (ROWLAND 1966). This definition is most applicable to iso-ionic exchange between a mineral crystal and its immediate fluid environment (W.F. NEUMAN and NEUMAN 1958). Each lattice position in a crystal can accommodate only one ion, and exchange occurs when, as an expression of their thermal energy, one ion jumps out of the crystal and another ion of the same species simultaneously jumps into the vacant lattice position. Because exact mass balance is maintained throughout, this process cannot alter the concentration of the exchanging ion in the fluid, and so cannot contribute to homeostatic regulation. But "exchange" can also be used in a less strict sense for the reciprocal translocations that occur in any reversible process that can attain dynamic equilibrium; mass balance is maintained at equilibrium but not during the transition between one equilibrium state and another. In such a system, the net flux in either direction represents the balance between opposing fluxes of larger magnitude, and "exchange" in this sense occurs continuously, not just at equilibrium. Examples include diffusion across membranes, the uptake and release of ligands at binding sites, and the dissolution and growth of crystals (W.F. NEUMAN and NEUMAN 1958). This looser meaning of "exchange" is more relevant to physiology and is used throughout this text, unless otherwise stated.

Examination of bone by radioautography at different times after labeled calcium administration shows that rapid initial uptake occurs over all free bone surfaces including cancellous, endocortical, intracortical, and periosteal (PONLOT 1960; DHEM 1964; ROWLAND 1966; J.H. MARSHALL 1969; B.L. RIGGS et al. 1971; LACROIX 1962, 1972). With time, the intensity of radioactivity gradually declines over most of the bone surface, but rapidly increases at sites of bone formation because labeled calcium ions are trapped beneath the continual deposition of new mineral, and rapidly decreases at sites of bone resorption because labeled calcium ions are promptly removed. Most work was done on cortical bone (Fig. 9; PONLOT 1960), and the sites of focally intense uptake, located around haversian canals, were referred to colloquially as "hot spots," or (more accurate in three dimensions) "hot rods" (J.H. MARSHALL 1969). But the same phenomenon was observed in cancellous bone (Fig. 10; DHEM 1964). The life span of a hot spot depends on the half-life of the isotope used; with radium, hot spots can persist for decades if the bone is not resorbed. The surface radioactivity continues to fade, partly because of return to the circulation as the blood specific activity falls, and partly by slow transfer into deeper regions of bone which gradually acquire an evenly distributed diffuse radioactivity, most likely by radial diffusion from canaliculae and slow penetration into the interior of crystals (J.H. MARSHALL 1969; GROER and MARSHALL 1973). Loss of this activity occurs very slowly by exchange in the strict sense as well as by resorption, which must be allowed for in the interpretation of radiokinetic methods for measuring bone turnover (J.H. MARSHALL 1969; HEANEY 1976).

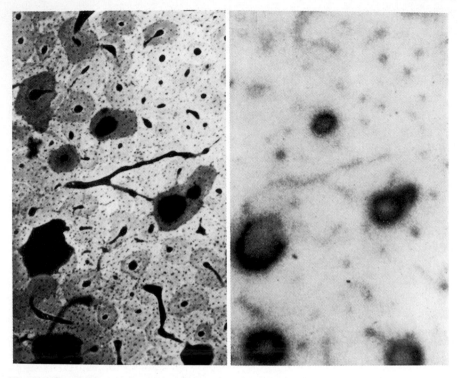

Fig. 9. Comparison of microradiograph *on left* and radioautograph *on right* of a transverse ground section of the tibia of a dog, 7 h after injection of ⁴⁵Ca. Five osteons currently forming show intense uptake (*hot spots*), but all haversian and Volkmann's canals are also labeled, regardless of degree of mineralization or state of remodeling. (Reprinted from Ponlot 1960, with permission)

At one time it was believed that rapidly exchangeable bone calcium was confined to young, recently formed, bone in which secondary mineralization was not yet completed; comparison of radioautographs with microradiographs indicates that hot spots are invariably associated with young low-density bone (Figs. 9, 10). But the early activity extends over the whole surface, regardless of age or degree of mineralization; evidently, rapid exchangeability is a function of proximity to the circulation and not of the physical properties of the bone mineral (Ponlot 1960; Dhem 1964; Rowland 1966; B.L. Riggs et al. 1971; Lacroix 1962, 1972). Consequently, the exchangeable calcium in bone is located at quiescent bone surfaces, at which, except for completion of secondary mineralization at some locations, there is no net calcium flux in either direction (Parfitt 1987). Assuming that rapid exchange is confined to calcium ions in surface positions in the crystal lattice, the exchangeable calcium can be estimated to extend to a depth of approximately 1.5 μm in both the rabbit and the dog (Rowland 1966). With the same assumption,

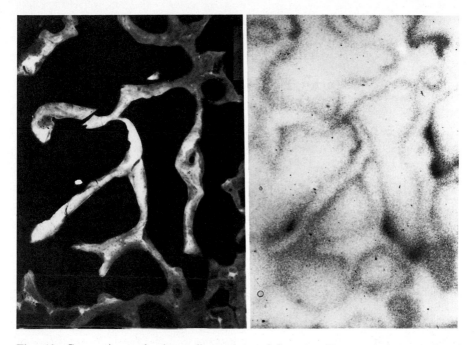

Fig. 10. Comparison of microradiograph *on left* and radioautograph *on right* of cancellous bone from the caudal vertebra of a cat, 7 h after administration of ^{45}Ca. The structures shown differ because the sections are adjacent, not identical. There is intense uptake at sites of bone formation, and less intense but evenly distributed uptake over all other regions of surface, regardless of degree of mineralization or state of remodeling. (From original supplied by A. Dhem, reprinted from PARFITT 1981, with permission)

and using values for the surface to volume ratio in human bone (FOLDES et al. 1991), a depth of 2.0 μm can be calculated, but the assumption under-estimates the variety of components of exchangeable calcium. The fall in specific activity of the blood and the rise in specific activity of the surface become equal at about 2 h in the rabbit, 20 h in the dog, and several days in terminally ill human subjects (B.L. RIGGS et al. 1971), thereafter falling together. Uptake and release can be described by a single rate constant, so that the surface calcium behaves as a single compartment (GROER and MARSHALL 1973).

Since exchangeable bone calcium is located at quiescent surfaces, its composition and behavior must reflect not only the physicochemical complexity of the mineral, but also the structural complexity of the quiescent surface. As well as occupying surface positions in the crystal lattice, labile calcium ions are bound to the crystal surface in hydrated form and dissolved in all the subdivisions of bone water between the crystal and the outer border of the lining cells, including the hydration shell, the bulk water in the immediate vicinity of the crystal, and the bone ECF. Some labile calcium must be bound to macromolecular constituents of the endosteal membrane, and to noncollagenous constituents of the bone matrix such as osteocalcin; preferential calcium binding is a likely function of the lamina limitans. Labile calcium is probably present in particulate or vesicular form within the lining cells (DZIAK and BRAND 1974). The electron-dense granules found in bone ECF are an artifact of specimen processing, but are a reproducible consequence of increased mineral storage (MATTHEWS et al. 1980). As well as exchanges involving all these constituents, movement of calcium ions can occur as a result of crystal growth or dissolution, changes in crystal perfection as a result of hetero-ionic exchange, and shifts in the proportion of minerals of different composition (Table 2). The relative importance of these mechanisms is unknown, but collectively they provide abundant scope for exchange as the basis of a shifting dynamic equilibrium between blood and bone.

The magnitude of rapid calcium exchange at the quiescent surface is not known with certainty because the correspondence between kinetic and anatomic compartments is conjectural. Some early estimates were as low as 40 mmol/day, or as high as 150 mmol/day (PARFITT 1976a). A non-compartmental method of greater precision, based on transit times, gave a mean value of 80 mmol/day in osteoporotic women, and 100 mmol/day in healthy men (REEVE 1978). Even the lower figure is ten times higher than the average daily flux due to remodeling-based bone turnover (8 mmol/day) and three times higher than the component of the fluxes in the kidney that is susceptible to regulation by PTH (25 mmol/day). It would be remarkable indeed if much the largest calcium flux in the body was of no physiologic importance, and yet a recent publication by a learned society, purporting to provide young physicians with, inter alia, a comprehensive description of the pathophysiology of bone and mineral disorders (FAVUS 1990), contains virtually no reference to it. This neglect probably stems from the extreme delay between the discovery of the phenomenon between 25 and 35 years ago, and the general acceptance of its long-term homeostatic significance, which still rests mainly on inferential reasoning rather than on experimental demonstration (MUNDY 1989).

VII. Blood-Bone Equilibrium and Its Homeostatic Function

The previous discussion established the existence of a labile pool of calcium ions at quiescent bone surfaces that is in dynamic equilibrium with the ECF. The pool evidently functions as a short-term buffer, taking up or releasing calcium as needed to correct gains or losses of calcium by the ECF; the buffering ability is a function of the intact organism and cannot be reproduced in an isolated perfused limb (RODAN et al. 1967). The kinetics of recovery of plasma calcium levels from positive or negative calcium loads in a variety of species are broadly consistent with the values for pool size and flux rates deduced from plasma radiocalcium disappearance curves (Copp et al. 1961, 1965; Waron and Rich 1969; Parfitt 1969c, 1976b; D.H. Marshall 1976; Bronner and Stein 1992). Net transfer of calcium into the pool presumably reflects a rise in bone water calcium content, the availability of spare binding sites for calcium, and net growth of existing crystals. Net transfer of calcium out of the pool presumably reflects a fall in bone water calcium content, the release of calcium from binding sites and net diminution of existing crystals; because different calcium ions are now at the crystal surface, the pool does not have a fixed size. The participation of exchangeable bone calcium in short-term regulation of plasma calcium has been recognized for many years (Howard 1956; Talmage et al. 1970; Parfitt and Kleerekoper 1980a; Bronner 1982; Neer 1989), and is not in serious dispute, although much remains to be learned about the physicochemical, hormonal, cellular, and molecular mechanisms involved. But less obvious and less widely recognized is the role of the blood-bone equilibrium in set point determination as well as in error correction.

The existence of a narrow normal range for ECF free calcium concentration and of a complex mechanism for ensuring that each person's free calcium remains within this range could only have come about if it conferred some evolutionary advantage. There must be good biological reasons why ECF free calcium in the human species is close to 1.2 mmol/l, rather than 1.0 or 1.4 mmol/l. Whatever those reasons are, they ensured that the secretory set point for PTH, as the controlling variable, was the same as the biologically desirable set point for ECF free calcium, as the controlled variable. To these two kinds of set point must now be added a third, the set points of the target cells for PTH in kidney and bone, by which the determination of ECF free calcium set point is accomplished. For bone, the set point is the calcium concentration at which the inward and outward fluxes at quiescent bone surfaces are in equilibrium, such that, if plasma calcium falls below the set point, there is net influx from bone, and if it rises above the set point there is net efflux to bone. For kidney, the set point is equivalent to the mean threshold for tubular reabsorption. It cannot be a coincidence that the parathyroid gland normally defends the same set point as do the bone and the kidney, and the only possible explanation is that PTH regulates the set point for blood-bone calcium equilibration as well as the set point for tubular reabsorption of calcium.

Further evidence that this must be the case comes from the consideration of calcium homeostasis in primary hyperparathyroidism. First, in the absence of overt perturbation, the precision of plasma calcium regulation, both short term and long term, is almost as good as in normal subjects (Edmondson and Li 1976; Parfitt et al. 1991a). But if the blood-bone set point was not increased, there would be no equilibration, since calcium would continue to flow into bone until all surfaces had attained the highest possible density, and could no longer contribute to regulation. Second, defense of the increased ECF calcium set point in response to overt perturba-

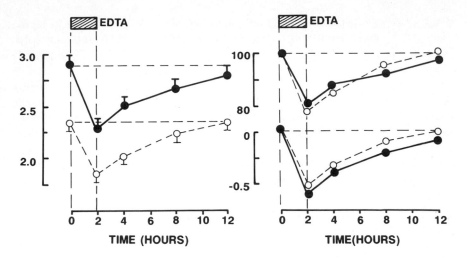

Fig. 11. Recovery from experimental hypocalcemia in primary hyperparathyroidism. Changes in plasma unchelated calcium after infusion of EDTA for 2h (PARFITT 1969c). Left-hand panel, original data (mmol/l); right-hand panel (*upper*), data expressed as percentages of preinfusion value; right-hand panel (*lower*), data expressed as absolute deviations from preinfusion value in mmol/l. Data from five patients with surgically confirmed primary hyperparathyroidism shown as *closed circles* joined by *solid lines*. Data from four healthy subjects with normal parathyroid function shown as *open circles joined by interrupted lines*. Note that the postinfusion value in the patients with hyperparathyroidism is virtually identical with the pre-infusion value in the normal subjects

tion is both qualitatively and quantitatively similar to defense of the normal set point in normal subjects. For example, after EDTA infusion, restoration of the preinfusion plasma calcium is almost as rapid in patients with hyper-parathyroidism as in normal subjects (Fig. 11); if the sequential values are expressed as percentages of the initial value, or as absolute deviations from the initial value, the two curves are remarkably similar. But if the blood-bone set point was not increased, lowering the calcium to a normal value, as in Fig. 11, would elicit no release of labile calcium since, from the stand-point of the bone surface, plasma calcium would need no correction. Although the data are less complete, exactly analogous arguments apply to the responses to calcium infusion.

If blood-bone equilibration occurs at a high plasma calcium level in hyper-parathyroidism and at a normal plasma calcium level in euparathyroidism, then logically it must occur at a low plasma calcium level in hypo-parathyroidism. Indeed, as mentioned earlier, the low basal calcium level in the hypoparathyroid dog is restored, albeit more sluggishly than normal, after EDTA infusion (COPP et al. 1961) and the maximum rate at which calcium can be supplied by bone, when it is continuously removed from the ECF, is only modestly less than normal (TALMAGE et al. 1970). After

Table 3. Explanations for simultaneous biologic equilibrium and chemical disequilibrium at quiescent bone surfaces. (Reprinted from PARFITT 1987 with permission)

A.	Pump-leak	1. Active calcium efflux
		2. Active potassium influx
		3. Active proton influx
B.	Solubility	1. Local proton production
		2. Metastable precursor of hydroxyapatite

calcium infusion, there is a greater rise in plasma calcium and a slower fall in the hypoparathyroid than in the normal state (SANDERSON et al. 1960), but the eventual attainment of the preinfusion level is dependent on uptake by bone as well as by urinary excretion (D.H. MARSHALL 1976). PTH is evidently regulating the operation of some process that proceeds at a low level in the absence of PTH. Patients with hypoparathyroidism who are adequately treated with vitamin D are able to repair EDTA-induced hypocalcemia as rapidly and completely as normal subjects (PARFITT 1969b). It is impossible to account adequately for all these observations unless the level of blood-bone equilibration, or bone set point, varies directly with the prevailing level of PTH, and this effect of PTH can be duplicated by some metabolite of vitamin D, probably calcitriol.

VIII. Blood-Bone Equilibrium: Physicochemical and Cellular Mechanism

To establish the existence of a relationship between PTH and the set point for blood-bone equilibration is a simple exercise in logic based on reductio ad absurdum, but exactly how PTH is able to accomplish this task remains a mystery. An equilibrium between a solid and a liquid phase has to be described and explained in terms of physical chemistry, whereas the effect of PTH, whether direct or indirect, has to be initiated by an action on cells. The question posed by the Neumans on the first page of their classic monograph more than 30 years ago: "How can a vitamin and a hormone influence a solubility equilibrium?" (W.F. NEUMAN and NEUMAN 1958) still lacks an adequate answer. The bulk of the bone mineral is much too insoluble to be in equilibrium with ECF (W.F. NEUMAN and NEUMAN 1958); this is why secondary mineralization continues until ionic diffusion is restricted by the scarcity of water. Before the effect of PTH can be considered, this physicochemical disequilibrium must be reconciled with the biological equilibrium revealed by radiocalcium kinetics and radioautography. Two classes of explanation have been proposed (Table 3; Fig. 12; PARFITT 1987). Pump-leak theories assume that bone ECF is in equilibrium with hydroxyapatite, a concentration gradient for calcium between systemic ECF and bone ECF being maintained by active transport of calcium or some other ion, by lining cells under the influence of PTH. Solubility theories

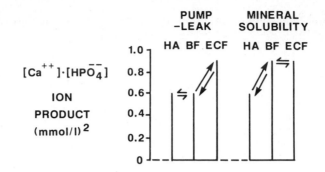

Fig. 12. Comparison between two classes of theory of blood-bone equilibrium. *Each panel* shows three ion activity products of secondary calcium phosphate (brushite), corresponding to the solubility of hydroxyapatite (*HA*), postulated to exist in the bone fluid (*BF*), and experimentally determined in the extracellular fluid (*ECF*). According to pump-leap theories, HA and BF are in equilibrium and the concentration difference between ECF and BF is maintained either by active efflux of calcium or by redistribution of calcium in accordance with the electrochemical gradient generated by active influx of potassium or protons. According to mineral solubility theories, ECF and BF are in equilibrium, and the solubility of surface mineral is increased by local proton production or by the presence of some more soluble precursor of HA in metastable form. A weakness of both types of theory is the need for some additional mechanism to account for differential regulation of calcium rather than phosphate. (Reprinted from PARFITT 1987 with permission)

assume that bone ECF has essentially the same calcium concentration as systemic ECF, but that the solubility of the surface mineral in contact with bone ECF is increased in some way by PTH. The two classes of theory are not mutually exclusive and elements of both may be required.

The greatest attraction of pump-leak theories is the ease with which they provide for regulation in accordance with Eq. 1, since there will be concentration-dependent efflux from systemic ECF into bone ECF, balanced by PTH-dependent influx from quiescent bone surfaces to blood (PARFITT 1976b, 1987). The ability of such opposed fluxes to account for much experimental data on calcium homeostasis has been shown by both simple (D.S. RIGGS 1966) and complex (JAROS et al. 1980) mathematical models. The gaps between lining cells, large enough to permit the rapid passage of macromolecules, would impose a formidable energetic requirement on the postulated pump (BRONNER and STEIN 1992). Nevertheless, the most securely established feature of the bone surface is active inward transport of potassium (SCARPACE and NEUMAN 1976a) and the presence of a remarkably high concentration of potassium in the outermost layer of the mineral, which is dissipated by death of the cells (BUSHINSKY et al. 1989). There is also an electrochemical gradient positive on the bone fluid side that is increased by PTH (PETERSON et al. 1985).

The first pump-leak theory postulated an outwardly directed calcium pump (TALMAGE et al. 1970), but such a pump is inconsistent with the electrochemical gradient. Experimental searches for a calcium pump have been largely unsuccessful (W.F. NEUMAN et al. 1979; M.W. NEUMAN 1982), although the effects of metabolic inhibitors both in vitro (W.F. NEUMAN et al. 1979) and in vivo (McCARTHY and HUGHES 1986) suggest that a modest fraction of calcium efflux from bone is the result of cellular activity. Furthermore, in the rat, calcium efflux is consistently higher on the inner side of the calvarium than the outer (W.F. NEUMAN et al. 1977). The second pump-leak theory attributed calcium flux from bone to active potassium flux into bone, but, if this is inhibited by ouabain, the electrochemical gradient is unaffected (WIRTH et al. 1986) and calcium fluxes are even increased (SCARPACE and NEUMAN 1976b). The third pump-leak theory proposed an active flux of protons toward bone (McGRATH et al. 1986), but the proposal was based on theoretical considerations without experimental confirmation, and PTH decreases rather than increases proton movement into bone (BUSHINSKY 1987).

If the calcium concentration in bone ECF is the same as in systemic ECF, as postulated by the solubility theories, the fluxes in both directions would be passive and Eq. 1 would not apply, but the blood-bone equilibrium can be described in terms of the uptake and release of calcium by binding sites at the bone surface (BRONNER and STEIN 1992). At equilibrium, the free energy of the binding sites will be zero, and ECF free calcium will be equal to the half saturation constant (K_m). Designating the binding sites as B:

$$[Ca^{2+}.B] = K_m[Ca^{2+}]*[B], \quad \text{and} \quad [Ca^{2+}] = K_m[Ca^{2+}.B]/[B] \qquad (3)$$

At half saturation $[Ca^{2+}.B]$ (occupied sites) and $[B]$ (unoccupied sites) will be equal, so that $[Ca^{2+}] = K_m$. Regulation of the bone calcium set point by PTH requires that PTH controls the average value of K_m, either by changing K_m for all sites of a single class, or by changing the relative proportions of different classes of binding site with different affinities for calcium (BRONNER and STEIN 1992). It is likely that most of the binding sites are related to the surface mineral, and the affinity of a particular form of bone mineral for calcium can be regarded as an inverse function (not necessarily linear) of its solubility.

The first solubility theory postulated that surface mineral solubility was increased by local production of protons (M.W. NEUMAN 1982), with a pH gradient between bone fluid and systemic ECF due, not to active transport, but to continuous metabolic production of some organic acid, lactate seeming the most plausible (W.F. NEUMAN et al. 1978). If the bone fluid PTH was as low as 6.8, equilibration with bone mineral could reproduce the observed calcium and phosphate levels in blood in a variety of different conditions (NORDIN 1961; MACGREGOR 1964). PTH increases lactate production, but the amount produced is inconsistently related to the magnitude of any calcium flux (W.F. NEUMAN et al. 1978; RAMP and McNEIL 1978). Furthermore, the pH gradient is unlikely to exceed 0.1 unit (M.W. NEUMAN and NEUMAN 1980), too small a difference to raise the solubility of hydroxyapatite to the level required for equilibration with systemic ECF, or to account for the electrochemical gradient. The most plausible current theory is that the surface mineral in equilibrium with the bone fluid is some more soluble precursor of hydroxyapatite (Table 2; W.F. NEUMAN 1980; M.W. NEUMAN 1982; W.F. NEUMAN and NEUMAN 1985; M.W. NEUMAN et al. 1987). No such precursor mineral has been consistently detected in bone, but even the most sophisticated methods would be unable to exclude the presence of a separate mineral phase constituting only 0.3% of the total, the approximate proportion of the mineral that is exchangeable.

Although plausible arguments based on solubility relationships have been advanced for octacalcium phosphate (MACGREGOR and BROWN 1965; MACGREGOR 1966), a more likely candidate for this regulator phase is brushite, the hydrated form of secondary calcium phosphate that is probably the first mineral formed (W.F. NEUMAN 1980). Brushite is unstable, tending to undergo spontaneous autocatalytic transformation to hydroxyapatite probably via a series of intermediates that include tertiary calcium phosphate and octacalcium phosphate (M.W. NEUMAN 1982; NORDIN 1961; Table 2). These transformations can be inhibited and brushite stabilized by acid production (W.F. NEUMAN and BAREHAM 1975), by several noncollagenous proteins such as osteocalcin and osteonectin that can adsorb to the surface of bone crystals and are known to be produced by bone cells (MENANTEAU et al. 1982; W.F. NEUMAN et al. 1982; Doi et al. 1989), and by a variety of small molecules including magnesium, citrate, phosphocitrate, and pyrophosphate (M.W. NEUMAN et al. 1987). A role for pyrophosphate at quiescent bone surfaces in the regulation of bone remodeling was proposed many years ago (JUNG et al. 1973); a role in maintaining the homeostatic function of the quiescent surface is more in keeping with its evanescent nature (PARFITT and KLEEREKOPER 1980a).

This theory has several interesting and potentially important implications. First, unlike hydroxyapatite, the solubility of brushite is affected by small changes in pH of the magnitude detected in bone fluid, and to an extent that could have physiologic significance (W.F. NEUMAN and BAREHAM 1975; W.F. NEUMAN and NEUMAN 1985). Second, the existence of nonapatite mineral of varying solubility at bone surfaces could be related to the calcitonin-dependent labile storage mineral mentioned earlier (MATTHEWS et al. 1980; TALMAGE et al. 1980, 1983). Third, control of the brushite-hydroxyapatite transformation in both time and space could provide a physicochemical basis for a self-organizing system (STAUB et al. 1988), and intrinsic periodicity of the complex system comprising lining cells, bone fluid, and a variety of ions, crystals, and macromolecules could account for the circadian oscillation in plasma calcium, and enable anticipatory homeostasis in addition to reactive homeostasis (BRONNER 1982; PARFITT 1987, 1989; STAUB et al. 1989). Finally, the theory provides links between the separate functions of set point determination and error correction, and between the cellular and the physicochemical aspects of calcium homeostasis.

None of the theories discussed has yet been shown to account for the control by PTH of the bone calcium set point. PTH has both acute (LEMON et al. 1982) and long-term (REEVE 1978) effects consistent with an increase in K_m in Eq. 3, but the mechanism remains unknown. Changes in the proportion of hypothetical binding sites of different K_m have been attributed to changes in the shape of osteoblasts brought about by PTH (BRONNER and STEIN 1992), but in human bone osteoblasts occupy too small a fraction of the surface for this to be a plausible means of determining the bone set point. PTH does alter the shape of bone surface cells, but in different species and experimental circumstances the outcome can be either a decrease (JONES and BOYDE 1976) or an increase (MATTHEWS and TALMAGE 1981) in the apparent size of the gaps between them; whether chronic hyper- or hyposecretion of PTH is accompanied by persistent changes in lining cell morphology is unknown. It seems more likely that PTH alters the solubility of the surface mineral by regulating bone fluid pH by lactate production (SCHARTUM and NICHOLS 1961; W.F. NEUMAN et al. 1979), or by changing the rate of production or destruction of one or more of the stabilizers previously mentioned, and so controls K_m for the whole surface. This effect of PTH on bone set point could be partly mediated by indirect mechanisms (PARFITT 1976b), which could explain why phenomena observed in the whole animal cannot be duplicated in the isolated perfused limb (RODAN et al. 1967), and why none of the known direct effects of PTH on bone cells provides a completely satisfactory explanation for set point determination.

H. Integration of Skeletal and Mineral Homeostasis

Bone carries out two main types of function: a mechanical function that depends on its rigidity and strength and a regulatory function that depends on its content of mineral, particularly calcium. A major theme of this chapter is that these two functions are carried out by different cell systems. The mechanical function is provided by the remodeling system, comprising osteoclasts and osteoblasts and their precursors, that removes and replaces whole volumes of bone and so determines bone mass. The regulatory function is provided by the homeostatic system, comprising lining cells and osteocytes and their connections, which controls the blood-bone equilibrium. Both of these systems can move calcium ions in and out of bone, but the characteristics of the fluxes produced by the two systems are quite different (Table 4). Obviously these systems are not totally independent. Transient changes in the function of osteoclasts and osteoblasts can subserve a short-term homeostatic function, and sustained changes in remodeling space can meet longer term needs for calcium. Both short- and long-term changes in the remodeling system can also give rise to pertubations to which the homeostatic system must respond. But there are closer and more subtle relationships that need more detailed discussion.

Table 4. Comparison of two mechanisms for movement of calcium ions into and out of bone. (Reprinted from PARFITT 1989 with permission)

Characteristic	Remodeling system	Homeostatic system
Location	Active surfaces	Quiescent surfaces
Mechanism	Wholly cellular	Partly physicochemical
Scale	Microscopic	Ultramicroscopic
Kinetics	Irreversible	Reversible
Duration of cycle	Months	Hours
Timing	Intermittent	Continuous
Magnitude[a]	Small	Large
Capacity[b]	Large	Small

[a] Of daily fluxes.
[b] For meeting sustained long-term demand.

The first link between the two systems arises because bone calcium balance must be equal to external calcium balance, of which the components are related to plasma calcium via Eq. 2 (PRAFITT 1981). Disregarding the usually small changes in soft tissue calcium, in a steady state urinary calcium excretion is equal to the sum of net absorption of calcium and net loss of calcium from bone, so that Eq. 2 can be expanded:

$$UFP_{Ca} = NA_{Ca}/GFR + NLB_{Ca}/GFR + TR_{Ca}/GFR \qquad (4)$$

Consequently, any change in one term of this equation must be accompanied by changes in one or more of the other terms. For example, a decrease in net absorption of calcium must be accompanied by a corresponding increase in net loss from bone or in tubular reabsorption, or both, if plasma calcium is to remain unaltered. Similarly, an increase in net loss from bone must be accompanied by a decrease in net absorption or tubular reabsorption, or both. Changes in PTH secretion are one of the means by which these adaptive adjustments take place, but, in some circumstances, the adjustment is a manifestation of anticipatory rather than of reactive homeostasis (PARFITT and KLEEREKOPER 1980a,b).

Control by PTH of both tubular reabsorption of calcium and the blood-bone calcium set point is important, or else one component of the homeostatic system would be constantly attempting to counteract the other. Consequently, the renal threshold for calcium and the blood-bone set point are normally close together, the difference between them determining the obligatory loss of calcium in the fasting state (PARFITT 1987). If for any reason the threshold is too far below the set point, obligatory calcium loss is increased, and plasma calcium can be maintained only by increasing the net flow of calcium from gut or bone. Since adaptive increases in calcium absorption are usually of small magnitude and the homeostatic system has only limited capacity, in practice this usually means an acceleration of bone loss. From this perspective, the function of the regulated, non-sodium-dependent component of tubular reabsorption of calcium is to allow the homeostatic system to determine the calcium set point without impairing the ability of the remodeling system to conserve bone (PRAFITT 1979a, 1981).

The mobilization of calcium from bone in order to satisfy the requirements of extraskeletal homeostasis and balance Eq. 4 is accomplished by a hierarchy of different mechanisms, each with its own characteristic rate, capacity, and time scale (PARFITT 1981). Moment to moment movement of calcium between blood and bone occurs across or between the cells lining quiescent bone surfaces; equilibration between blood and bone serves to maintain the plasma calcium at a level which is normally the same as the level set by the tubular reabsorption of calcium. Net gains or losses of calcium over a few hours or days, as in the normal circadian changes in balance, are mediated by a short-term storage and release mechanism which does not involve structural changes in bone, such as the concertina effect at existing remodeling sites or the calcitonin-dependent storage mechanism. Satisfying a calcium need of up to 10 mmol/day, which lasts for several weeks or months, as during the adolescent growth spurt, pregnancy, or lactation, is accomplished by an increase in bone turnover and consequent increase in reversible mineral deficit, comprising remodeling space, osteoid tissue, and newly formed low density bone, with no permanent loss of bone volume. Finally, a calcium need which exceeds about 1500 mmol or lasts for longer than about 1 year, as when adaptation to reduced intake or impaired absorption fails, can only be met by an irreversible loss of bone, which results from the difference between the volume of new bone structural units and the volume of the cavities in which they are formed.

The second link between the two systems is that maintenance of the homeostatic capability of bone is one of the principal functions of remodeling (W.F. NEUMAN and NEUMAN 1958; W.F. NEUMAN and BAREHAM 1975), which provides the biological justification for the participation of PTH in both systems. The assumption of no net calcium flux at quiescent surfaces is only an approximation to the truth, since it ignores the process of secondary mineralization. This requires a slow net influx of calcium equivalent to about 10%–15% of the total bone formation rate, or about 1%–1½% of the total calcium exchange. Part of this influx corresponds to the slow irreversible transformation of brushite to hydroxyapatite at the bone surface. The gradual decline in the rate of transformation, and the accompanying depletion of brushite from the surface associated with mineral maturation, reduces the contribution of a particular region of surface to overall calcium regulation as it gets older. But brushite lost by transformation to hydroxyapatite at one location is replaced by the production of brushite as a result of formation of new young bone elsewhere on the surface, so that the circadian cycles that subserve calcium homeostasis are integrated with the much longer cycles that subserve bone remodeling.

References

Adami S, Muirhead N, Manning RM, Gleed JH, Papapoulos SE, Sandler LM, Catto GRD, O'Riordan JLH (1982) Control of secretion of parathyroid hormone in secondary hyperparathyroidism. Clin Endocrinol (Oxf) 16:463–473

Adami S, Mian M, Bertoldo F, Rossini M, Jayawerra P, O'Riordan JLH, Lo Cascio V (1990) Regulation of calcium-parathyroid hormone feedback in primary hyperparathyroidism: effects of bisphosphonate treatment. Clin Endocrinol (Oxf) 33:391–397

Anast CS, Guthrie RA (1971) Decreased calcium tolerance in nongoitrous cretins. Pediatr Res 5:668–672

Arnold JS, Frost HM, Buss RO (1971) The osteocyte as a bone pump. Clin Orthop 78:47–55

Aukland K, Nicolaysen G (1981) Interstitial fluid volume: local regulatory mechanisms. Physiol Rev 61:556–633

Azria M (1989) The calcitonins: physiology and pharmacology. Basel, Karger

Balmain N (1991) Calbindin-D_{9K}: a vitamin-D-dependent, calcium-binding protein in mineralized tissues. Clin Orthop 265–270

Benson L, Rastad J, Wide L, Akerstrom G, Ljunghall S (1986) Stimulation of parathyroid hormone secretion by EDTA infusion – a test for the differential diagnosis of hypercalcaemia. Acta Endocrinol (Copenh) 111:498–506

Best JB (1959) Some theoretical considerations concerning crystals with relevance to the physical properties of bone. Biochim Biophys Acta 32:194–202

Bijvoet OLM (1977) Kidney function in calcium and phosphate metabolism. In: Avioli LV, Krane SM (eds) Metabolic bone disease, vol I. Academic, New York

Bijvoet OLM, Harinck HIJ (1984) The assessment of renal calcium reabsorption. In: Massry SG, Maschio G, Ritz E (eds) Phosphate and mineral metabolism. Plenum, New York, pp 111–126

Bilezikian JP, Silverberg SJ, Shane E, Parisien M, Dempster DW (1991) Characterization and evaluation of asymptomatic primary hyperparathyroidism. J Bone Miner Res 6:S85–S89

Blum JW, Fischer JA, Schwoerer D, Hunziker W, Binswanger U (1974a) Acute parathyroid hormone response: sensitivity, relationship to hypocalcemia and rapidity. Endocrinology 95:753–759

Blum JW, Mayer GP, Potts JT (1974b) Parathyroid hormone responses during spontaneous hypocalcemia and induced hypercalcemia in cows. Endocrinology 95:84–92

Bonar LC, Grynpas MD, Roberts JE, Griffin RG, Glimcher MJ (1985) Physical and chemical characterization of the development and maturation of bone mineral. In: Butler WT (ed) The chemistry and biology of mineralized tissues. Proceedings of the 2nd international conference on the chemistry and biology of mineralized tissues, Ebsco Media, Birmingham, Alabama, pp 226–233

Boucher A, D'Amour P, Hamel L, Fugere P, Gascon-Barre M, Lepage R, Ste-Marie LG (1989) Estrogen replacement decreases the set point of parathyroid hormone stimulation by calcium in normal postmenopausal women. J Clin Endocrinol Metab 68:831–836

Brent GA, LeBoff MS, Seely EW, Conlin PR, Brown EM (1988) Relationship between the concentration and rate of change of calcium and serum intact parathyroid hormone levels in normal humans. J Clin Endocrinol Metab 67: 944–950

Bronner F (1982) Calcium homeostasis. In: Disorders of mineral metabolism, vol II. Academic, San Diego, pp 43–102

Bronner F (1989) Renal calcium transport: mechanisms and regulation – an overview. Am J Physiol 257 (Renal Fluid Electrolyte Physiol 26):F707–F711

Bronner F (1990) Intestinal calcium transport: the cellular pathway. Miner Electrolyte Metab 16:94–100

Bronner F, Stein WD (1992) Modulation of bone calcium-binding sites regulates plasma calcium – an hypothesis. Calcif Tissue Int 50:483–489

Brooks M (1987) Bone blood flow measurement, part 2. Bone Clin Biochem News Rev 4:33–36

Brown EM (1983) Four-parameter model of the sigmoidal relationship between parathyroid hormone release and extracellular calcium concentration in normal and abnormal parathyroid tissue. J Clin Endocrinol Metab 56:572–581

Brown EM, Broadus AE, Brennan MF, Gardner DG, Marx SJ, Spiegel AM, Downs RW Jr, Attie M, Aurbach GD (1979a) Direct comparison in vivo and in vitro of suppressibility of parathyroid function by calcium in primary hyperparathyroidism. J Clin Endocrinol Metab 48:604–610

Brown EM, Gardner DG, Brennan MF, Marx SJ, Spiegel AM, Attie MF, Downs RW Jr, Doppman JL, Aurbach GD (1979b) Calcium-regulated parathyroid hormone release in primary hyperparathyroidism: studies in vitro with dispersed parathyroid cells. Am J Med 66:923–931

Brown EM, Wilson RE, Thatcher JG, Marynick SP (1981) Abnormal calcium-regulated PTH release in normal parathyroid tissue from patients with adenoma. Am J Med 71:565–570

Brown EM, LeBoff MS, Oetting M, Posillico JT, Chen C (1987) Secretory control in normal and abnormal parathyroid tissue. Rec Prog Horm Res 43:337–382

Bushinsky DA (1987) Effects of parathyroid hormone on net proton flux from neonatal mouse calvariae. Am J Physiol 252:F585–F589

Bushinsky DA, Chabala JM, Levi-Setti R (1989) Ion microprobe analysis of mouse calvariae in vitro: evidence for a "bone membrane." Am J Physiol 256: E152–E158

Calvo MS, Eastell R, Offord KP, Bergstralh EJ, Burritt MF (1991) Circadian variation in ionized calcium and intact parathyroid hormone: evidence for sex differences in calcium homeostasis. J Clin Endocrinol Metab 72:69–76

Cantley LK, Ontjes DA, Cooper CW, Thomas CG, Leight GS, Wells SA Jr (1985) Parathyroid hormone secretion from dispersed human hyperparathyroid cells: increased secretion in cells from hyperplastic glands versus adenomas. J Clin Endocrinol Metab 60:1032–1037

Cecchhini AB, Melbin J, Noordergraaf A (1981) Set-point: is it a distinct structural entity in biological control? J Theor Biol 93:387–394

Chambers TJ, Chambers JC, Symonds J et al. (1986) The effect of human calcitonin on cytoplasmic spreading of rat osteoclasts. J Clin Endocrinol Metab 63: 1080–1085

Charkes ND, Brookes M, Makler PPT Jr (1979) Studies of skeletal tracer kinetics: II. Evaluation of a five-compartment model of [^{18}F]fluoride kinetics in rats. J Nucl Med 20:1150–1157

Charles P, Mosekilde L, Taagehoj Jensen F (1986) Primary hyperparathyroidism: evaluated by ^{47}calcium kinetics, calcium balance and serum bone-Gla-protein. Eur J Clin Invest 16:277–283

Conlin PR, Fajtova VT, Mortensen RM, LeBoff MS, Brown EM (1989) Hysteresis in the relationship between serum ionized calcium and intact parathyroid hormone during recovery from induced hyper- and hypocalcemia in normal humans. J Clin Endocrinol Metab 69:593–599

Copp DH (1964) The hormones of the parathyroid glands and calcium homeostasis. In: Frost HM (ed) Bone biodynamics. Little Brown, Boston, pp 409–421

Copp DH (1970) Endocrine regulation of calcium metabolism. Annu Rev Physiol 32:61–86

Copp DH, Shim SS (1963) The homeostatic function of bone as a mineral reservoir. Oral Surg Oral Med Oral Pathol 16:738–744

Copp DH, Moghadan H, Mensen ED, McPherson GD (1961) The parathyroids and calcium homeostasis. In: Greep RO, Talmage RV (eds) The parathyroids. Thomas, Springfield, pp 203–223

Copp DH, Mensen ED, McPherson GD (1965) Regulation of blood calcium. Clin Orthop 17:288–296

Deane N (1966) Kidney and electrolytes. Prentice-Hall, Englewood Cliffs

DeFronzo RA, Goldberg M, Agus ZS (1976) Normal diluting capacity in hyponatremic patients. Ann Intern Med 84:538–542

DeLuca HF (1983) Metabolism and mechanism of action of vitamin D – 1982. In: Peck WA (ed) Bone and mineral research vol 1. Excerpta Medica, Amsterdam, pp 7–73

DeLuca HF, Krisinger J, Darwish H (1990) The vitamin D system: 1990. Kidney Int 38:S2–S8

Dhem A (1964) Ca^{47} in clinical studies of bone physiopathology. In: Medical uses of Ca^{47}: second panel report. International Atomic Energy Agency, Vienna, pp 50–55

Doi Y, Okuda R, Takezawa Y, Shibata S, Moriwaki Y, Wakamatsu N, Shimizu N, Moriyama K, Shimokawa H (1989) Osteonectin inhibiting de novo formation of apatite in the presence of collagen. Calcif Tissue Int 44:200–208

Doty SB, Robinson RA, Schofield B (1976) Morphology of bone and histochemical staining characteristics of bone cells. In: Greep RO, Astwood EB, Aurbach GD (eds) Handbook of physiology, vol VII. American Physiological Society Washington

Dunlay R, Rodriguez M, Felsenfeld AJ, Llach F (1989) Direct inhibitory effect of calcitriol on parathyroid function (sigmoidal curve) in dialysis. Kidney Int 36: 1093–1098

Dziak R, Brand JS (1974) Calcium transport in isolated bone cells: I. Bone cell isolation procedures. J Cell Physiol 84:75–83

Eanes ED (1985) Dynamic aspects of apatite phases of mineralized tissues. In: Butler WT (ed) The chemistry and biology of mineralized tissues. Proceedings of the 2nd international conference on the chemistry and biology of mineralized tissues, Ebsco Media,Birmingham, Alabama, pp 213–220

Edelman IS, James AH, Baden H, Moore FD (1954) Electrolyte composition of bone and the penetration of radiosodium and deuterium oxide into dog and human bone. J Clin Invest 33:127–131

Edmondson JW, Li T-K (1976) The relationship of serum ionized and total calcium in primary hyperparathyroidism. J Lab Clin Med 87:624–629

Eidelman N, Chow LC, Brown WE (1981) Calcium phosphate saturation levels in ultrafiltered serum. Calcif Tissue Int 40:71–78

Engel MB, Catchpole HR (1989) Microprobe analysis of element distribution in bovine extracellular matrices and muscle. Scanning Microsc 3:887–894

Favus MJ (ed) (1990) Primer on the metabolic bone diseases and disorders of mineral metabolism. American Society of Bone and Mineral Research, Kelseyville

Federman M, Nichols G Jr (1974) Bone cell cilia: vestigial or functional organelles? Calcif Tissue Res 17:81–85

Fitzpatrick LA, Leong DA (1990) Individual parathyroid cells are more sensitive to calcium than a parathyroid cell population. Endocrinology 126:1720–1727

Flear CTG, Singh CM (1973) Hyponatraemia and sick cells. Br J Anaesth 45: 976–994

Foldes J, Parfitt AM, Shih M-S, Rao DS, Kleerekoper M (1991) Structural and geometric changes in iliac bone: relationship to normal aging and osteoporosis. J Bone Miner Res 6:759–766

Fox J (1991) Regulation of parathyroid hormone secretion by plasma calcium in aging rats. Am J Physiol 260 (Endocrinol Metab 23):E220–E225

Fox J, Heath H III (1981) The "calcium clamp": effect of constant hypocalcemia on parathyroid hormone secretion. Am J Physiol 240 (Endocrinol Metab 3): E649–E655

Fox J, Offord KP, Heath H III (1981) Episodic secretion of parathyroid hormone in the dog. Am J Physiol 24 (Endocrinol Metab 4):E171–E177

Friedlander MA, Segre GV (1988) Response to parathyroid hormone in normal human kidney donors before and after uninephrectomy. J Clin Endocrinol Metab 114:358–363

Gardin JP, Patron P, Fouqueray B, Prigent A, Paillard M (1988) Maximal PTH secretory rate and set point for calcium in normal subjects and patients with primary hyperparathyroidism. Miner Electrolyte Metab 14:221–228

Gleick J (1988) Chaos: making a new science. Penguin, New York

Glimcher MJ (1984) Recent studies of the mineral phase in bone and its possible linkage to the organic matrix by protein-bound phosphate bonds. Philos Trans R Soc Lond [Biol] 304:479–508

Glimcher MJ (1990) The nature of the mineral component of bone and the mechanism of calcification. In: Avioli LV, Krane SM (eds) Metabolic bone disease and clinically related disorders, 2nd edn. Saunders, Philadelphia, pp 42–56

Goldbeter A, Decroly O (1983) Temporal self-organization in biochemical systems: periodic behavior vs. chaos. Am J Physiol 245:R478–R483

Goulding A, Everitt HE, Cooney JM, Spears GFS (1986) Sodium and osteoporosis. In: Wahlqvist ML, Truswell AS (eds) Recent advances in clinical nutrition, vol 2. Libbey, London, pp 99–108

Grant FD, Conlin PR, Brown EM (1990) Rate and concentration dependence of parathyroid hormone dynamics during stepwise changes in serum ionized calcium in normal humans. J Clin Endocrinol Metab 71:370–378

Green J, Kleeman CR (1991) Role of bone in regulation of systemic acid-base balance. Kidney Int 39:9–26

Groer PG, Marshall JH (1973) Mechanism of calcium exchange at bone surfaces. Calcif Tissue Res 12:175–192

Grubb SA, Edwards G, Talmage RV (1977) Effect of endogenous and infused parathyroid hormone on plasma concentrations of recently administered ^{45}Ca. Calcif Tissue Res 24:209–214

Gylfe E, Akerstrom G, Juhlin C, Klareskog L, Rastad J (1990) Regulation of cytoplasmic Ca^{2+} and hormone release of the parathyroid cell. Horm Cell Regul 210:5–15

Hanley DA, Ayer LM (1986) Calcium-dependent release of carboxyl-terminal fragments of parathyroid hormone by hyperplastic human parathyroid tissue in vitro. J Clin Endocrinol Metab 63:1075–1079

Harms H-M, Kaptaina U, Kulpmann W-R, Brabant G, Hesch R-D (1989) Pulse amplitude and frequency modulation of parathyroid hormone in plasma. J Clin Endocrinol Metab 69:843–851

Harris EK (1981) Statistical aspects of reference values in clinical pathology. Prog Clin Pathol 8:45–66

Harris EK, DeMets DL (1971) Biological and analytic components of variation in long-term studies of serum constituents in normal subjects: V. Estimated biological variations in ionized calcium. Clin Chem 17:983–987

Harris EK, Kanofsky P, Shakarji G, Cotlove E (1970) Biological and analytic components of variation in long-term studies of serum constituents in normal subjects: II. Estimating biological components of variation. Clin Chem 16:1022–1027

Heaney RP (1964) Evaluation and interpretation of calcium-kinetic data in man. Clin Orthop 31:153–183

Heaney RP (1976) Calcium kinetics in plasma: as they apply to the measurements of bone formation and resorption rates. In: Bourne GH (ed) The biochemistry and physiology of bone. Academic, New York, pp 105–133

Heaney RP (1986) Calcium, bone health, and osteoporosis. In: Peck WA (ed) Bone and mineral research vol 4. Elsevier, New York, pp 255–301

Howard JE (1956) Present knowledge of parathyroid function with especial emphasis on its limitations. In: Wolstenholme GEW, O'Connor CM (eds) CIBA Foundation symposium on bone structure and metabolism. Churchill, London, pp 206–221

Hughes WS, Cohen S, Arvan D, Seamonds B (1977) The effect of the alkaline tide on serum-ionized calcium concentration in man. Digestion 15:175–181

Hughes WS, Aurbach GD, Sharp ME, Marx SJ (1984) The effect of the bicarbonate anion on serum ionized calcium concentration in vitro. J Lab Clin Med 103: 93–103

Jaros GG, Guyton AC, Coleman TG (1980) The role of bone in short-term calcium homeostasis: an analog-digital computer simulation. Ann Biomed Eng 8:103–141

Jaros GG, Belonje PC, vanHoorn-Hickman R, Newman E (1984) Transient response of the calcium homeostatic system: effect of calcitonin. Am J Physiol 246 (Regulatory Integrative Comp Physiol 15):R693–R697

Jones SJ, Boyde A (1976) Experimental study of changes in osteoblastic shape induced by calcitonin and parathyroid extract in an organ culture system. Cell Tissue Res 169:449–465

Jung A, Bisaz S, Fleisch H (1973) The binding of pyrophosphate and two diphosphonates by hydroxyapatite crystals. Calcif Tissue Res 11:269–280

Jung A, Bartholdi P, Mermillod B, Reeve J, Neer R (1978) Critical analysis of methods for analysing human calcium kinetics. J Theor Biol 73:131–157

Kaye M, Henderson J (1988) Direct functional assessment of human osteoblasts by radioautography: methodology and application in end stage renal disease. Clin Invest Med 224–233

Kitamura N, Shigeno C, Shiomi K, Lee K, Ohta S, Sone T, Katsushima S, Tadamura E, Kousaka T, Yamamoto I, Dokoh S, Konishi J (1990) Episodic fluctuation in serum intact parathyroid hormone concentration in men. J Clin Endocrinol Metab 70:252–263

Kripke DF, Lavie P, Parker D, Huey L, Deftos LJ (1978) Plasma parathyroid hormone and calcium are related to sleep stage cycles. J Clin Endocrinol Metab 47:1021–1027

Lacroix P (1962) Autoradiographic study of bone with ^{45}Ca. In: McLean FC, Lacroix P, Budy AM (eds) Radioisotopes and bone. Davis, Philadelphia, pp 51–67

Lacroix P (1972) The internal remodeling of bones. In: Bourne GH (ed) The biochemistry and physiology of bone, vol III, 2nd edn. Academic, New York, pp 119–144

Ladenson JH, Bowers GN Jr (1973) Free calcium in serum: II. Rigor of homeostatic control, correlations with total serum calcium, and review of data on patients with disturbed calcium metabolism. Clin Chem 19:575–582

Larsson L, Ohman S (1979) Serum calcium ion activity. Some aspects on methodological differences and intraindividual variation. Clin Biochem 12:138–141

Law WM Jr, Heath H III (1984) Time- and dose-related biphasic effects of synthetic bovine parathyroid hormone fragment 1–34 on urinary cation excretion. J Clin Endocrinol Metab 58:606–608

Lemon GJ, Bassingthwaighte JB, Kelly PJ (1982) Influence of parathyroid state on calcium uptake in bone. Am J Physiol 242:E146–E153

Levine MA, Aurbach GD (1989) Pseudohypoparathyroidism. In: DeGroot LJ (ed) Endocrinology, vol 2. Saunders, Philadelphia, pp 1055–1079

Lipscombe D, Madison DV, Poenie M, Reuter H, Tsien RW, Ysien RY (1988) Imaging of cytosolic Ca^{2+} transients arising from Ca^{2+} stores and Ca^{2+} channels in sympathetic neurons. Neuron 1:355–365

Lloyd HM, Parfitt AM, Jacobi JM, Willgoss DA, Craswell PW, Petrie JJB, Boyle PD (1989) The parathyroid glands in chronic renal failure: a study of their growth and other properties, based on findings in hypercalcemic patients. J Lab Clin Med 114:358–367

LoCascio V, Cominacini L, Adami S, Galvanini G, Davoli A, Scuro LA (1982) Relationship of total and ionized serum calcium circadian variations in normal and hyperparathyroid subjects. Horm Metab Res 14:443–444

Logue FC, Fraser WD, O'Reilly D St J, Cameron DA, Kelly AJ, Beastall GH (1990) The circadian rhythm of intact parathyroid hormone-(1–84): temporal correlation with prolactin secretion in normal men. J Clin Endocrinol Metab 71:1556–1560

Luk SC, Nopajaroonsri C, Simon GT (1974) The ultrastructure of endosteum: a topographic study in young adult rabbits. J Ultrastruct Res 46:165

MacGregor J (1964) Blood-bone equilibrium. In: Frost HM (ed) Bone biodynamics. Little Brown, Boston, pp 409–421

MacGregor J (1966) Some observations on the nature of bone mineral. In: Fleisch H, Blackwood HJJ, Owen M (eds) Calcified tissue. Springer, Berlin Heidelberg New York, pp 138–142

MacGregor J, Brown WE (1965) Blood: bone equilibrium in calcium homeostasis. Nature 205:359–361

Markowitz M, Rotkin L, Rosen JF (1981) Circadian rhythms of blood minerals in humans. Science 213:672–674

Markowitz ME, Arnaud S, Rosen JF, Thorpy M, Laximinarayan S (1988) Temporal interrelationships between the circadian rhythms of serum parathyroid hormone and calcium concentrations. J Clin Endocrinol Metab 67:1068–1073

Marshall DH (1976) Calcium and phosphate kinetics. In: Nordin BEC (ed) Calcium, phosphate and magnesium metabolism. Longman, New York

Marshall JH (1969) Measurements and models of skeletal metabolism. In: Comar CL, Bronner F (eds) Mineral metabolism. Academic, New York, pp 1–122

Marti R, Wild P, Schraner EM, Mueller M, Moor H (1987) Parathyroid ultrastructure after aldehyde fixation, high-pressure freezing, or microwave irradiation. J Histochem Cytochem 35:1415–1424

Massin JP, Vallee G, Savoie JC (1974) Compartmental analysis of calcium kinetics in man: application of a four-compartmental model. Metabolism 23:399–415

Matthews JL (1980) Bone structure and ultrastructure. In: Urist MR (ed) Fundamental and clinical bone physiology. Lippincott, Philadelphia

Matthews JL, Martin JH (1971) Intracellular transport of calcium and its relationship to homeostasis and mineralization – an electron microscope study. Am J Med 50:589–597

Matthews JL, Talmage RV (1981) Influence of parathyroid hormone on bone cell ultrastructure. Clin Orthop 156:27–38

Matthews JL, Talmage RV, Doppelt R (1980) Responses of the osteocyte lining cell complex, the bone cell unit to calcitonin. Metab Bone Dis Rel Res 2: 113–122

Mayer GP, Habener JF, Potts JT Jr (1976) Parathyroid hormone secretion in vivo: demonstration of a calcium-independent, nonsuppressible component of secretion. J Clin Invest 57:678–683

McCance RA (1954) Conference discussion. In: Reifenstein EC (ed) Metabolic interrelations with special reference to calcium. Transactions of the 5th conference. Macy, New York, p 50

McCarthy ID, Hughes SPF (1986) Inhibition of bone cell metabolism increases strontium-85 uptake. Calcif Tissue Int 39:386–389

McElduff A, Lissner D, Wilkinson M, Posen S (1990) Parathyroid hormone sensitivity in primary hyperparathyroidism and idiopathic hypercalciuria: effects on postadenylate cyclase parameters. J Clin Endocrinol Metab 70:1457–1461

McGrath KJ, Heideger WJ, Beach KW (1986) Calcium homeostasis: III. the bone membrane potential and mineral dissolution. Calcif Tissue Int 39:279–283

McLean FC, Budy AM (1964) The mineral of bones and teeth. In: Radiation, isotopes, and bone. Academic, New York, pp 61–77

Melick RA, Baird CW (1967) Changes in plasma calcium after injection of calcium in hypothyroid and hypoparathyroid women. J Clin Endocrinol 27:1303–1308

Melsen F, Mosekilde L, Eriksen EF, Charles P, Steinicke T (1989) In vivo hormonal effects on trabecular bone remodeling, osteoid mineralization, and skeletal turnover. In: Kleerekoper M, Krane SM (eds) Clinical disorders of bone and mineral metabolism. Liebert, New York, pp 73–87

Menanteau J, Neuman WF, Neuman MW (1982) A study of bone proteins which can prevent hydroxyapatite formation. Metab Bone Dis Rel Res 4:157–162

Menton DN, Simmons DJ, Orr BY, Plurad SB (1982) A cellular investment of bone marrow. Anat Rec 203:157–164

Milhaud G (1962) Parameters of calcium kinetics in man. In: Medical uses of Ca^{47}. International Atomic Energy Agency, Vienna, pp 61–62

Miller SC, Jee WSS (1980) The microvascular bed of fatty bone marrow in the adult beagle. Metab Bone Dis Rel Res 2:239–246

Miller SC, Jee WSS (1987) The bone lining cell: a distinct phenotype? Calcif Tissue Int 41:1–5.

Miller SC, Bowman BM, Smith JA, Jee WSS (1980) Characterization of endosteal bone-lining cells from fatty marrow bone sites in adult beagles. Anat Rec 198:163–173

Mioni G, D'Angelo A, Ossi E, Bertaglia E, Marcon G, Maschio G (1971) The renal handling of calcium in normal subjects and in renal disease. Eur J Clin Biol Res 16:881–887

Moore-Ede MC (1986) Physiology of the circadian timing system: predictive versus reactive homeostasis. Am J Physiol 250:R735–R752

Moore-Ede MC, Sulzman FM, Fuller CA (1982) The clocks that time us. Harvard University Press, Cambridge

Moradian-Oldak J, Weiner S, Addadi L, Landis WJ, Traub W (1991) Electron imaging and diffraction study of individual crystals of bone, mineralized tendon and synthetic carbonate apatite. Connect Tissue Res 25:219–228

Morgan B (1973) Osteomalacia, renal osteodystrophy and osteoporosis. Thomas, Springfield

Mundy GR (1989) Calcium homeostasis: hypercalcemia and hypocalcemia. Dunitz, London

Neer RM (1989) Calcium and inorganic phosphate homeostasis. In: DeGroot L (ed) Endocrinology, 2nd edn. Saunders, Philadelphia, pp 927–953

Nellans HN (1990) Intestinal calcium absorption: interplay of paracellular and cellular pathways. Miner Electrolyte Metab 16:101–108

Nemere I, Norman AW (1990) Transcaltachia, vesicular calcium transport, and microtubule-associated calbindin-D_{28K}: emerging views of 1,25-dihydroxyvitamin D_3-mediated intestinal calcium absorption. Miner Electrolyte Metab 16:109–114

Neuman MW (1982) Blood: bone equilibrium. Calcif Tissue Int 34:117–120

Neuman MW, Neuman WF (1980) On the measurement of water compartments, pH, and gradients in calvaria. Calcif Tissue Int 31:135–145

Neuman MW, Imai K, Kawase T, Saito S (1987) The calcium-buffering phase of bone mineral: some clues to its form and formation. J Bone Miner Res 2:171–181

Neuman WF (1969) The milieu interieur of bone: Claude Bernard revisited. Fed Proc 28:1846–1850

Neuman WF (1980) Bone material and calcification mechanisms. In: Urist MR (ed) Fundamental and clinical bone physiology. Lippincott, Philadelphia, pp 83–107

Neuman WF, Bareham BJ (1975) Evidence for the presence of secondary calcium phosphate in bone and its stabilization by acid production. Calcif Tissue Res 18:161–172

Neuman WF, Neuman MW (1958) The chemical dynamics of bone mineral. University of Chicago Press, Chicago

Neuman WF, Neuman MW (1985) Blood: bone calcium homeostasis. Jpn J Oral Biol 27:272–281

Neuman WF, Terepka AR, Canas F, Triffitt JT (1968) The cycling concept of exchange in bone. Calcif Tissue Res 2:262–270

Neuman WF, Brommage R, Myers CR (1977) The measurement of Ca^{2+} effluxes from bone. Calcif Tissue Res 24:113–117

Neuman WF, Neuman MW, Brommage R (1978) Aerobic glycolysis in bone: lactate production and gradients in calvaria. Am J Physiol 234:C41–C50

Neuman WF, Neuman MW, Myers CR (1979) Blood: bone disequilibrium: III. Linkage between cell energetics and Ca fluxes. Am J Physiol 236:C244–C248

Neuman WF, Neuman MW, Diamond AG, Menanteau J, Gibbons WS (1982) Blood: bone disequilibrium: VI. Studies of the solubility characteristics of brushite: apatite mixtures and their stabilization by noncollagenous proteins of bone. Calcif Tissue Int 34:149–157

Nicolis G, Prigogine I (1977) Self organization in nonequilibrium systems. From dissipative structures to order through fluctuations. Wiley, New York

Nordin BEC (1961) Biochemical aspects of parathyroid function and of hyperparathyroidism. In: Sobotka H, Stewart CP (eds) Advances in clinical chemistry, vol 4. Academic, New York, pp 275–320

Nordin BEC (ed) (1988) Calcium in human biology. Springer, Berlin Heidelberg New York

Nordin BEC, Marshall DH, Peacock M, Robertson WG (1975) Plasma calcium homeostasis. In: Talmage RV, Owen M, Parsons JA (eds) Calcium-regulating hormones. Elsevier, New York, pp 239–253

Nussbaum SR, Potts JT Jr (1991) Immunoassays for parathyroid hormone 1–84 in the diagnosis of hyperparathyroidism. J Bone Miner Res 6:S43–S50

Orwoll E, Kane-Johnson N, Cook J, Roberts L, Strasik L, McClung M (1986) Acute parathyroid hormone secretory dynamics: hormone secretion from normal primate and adenomatous human tissue in response to changes in extracellular calcium concentration. J Clin Endocrinol Metab 62:950–955

Owen M, Triffitt JT, Melick RA (1973) Albumin in bone. Ciba Found Symp 11:263–193

Parfitt AM (1969a) Chlorothiazide induced hypercalcemia in juvenile osteoporosis and primary hyperparathyroidism N Engl J Med 281:55–59

Parfitt AM (1969b) Prevention of hypercalcemia (Ca) in vitamin D (D) therapy of hypoparathyroidism. Ann Intern Med 70:64

Parfitt AM (1969c) Study of parathyroid function in man by EDTA infusion. J Clin Endocrinol 29:569–580

Parfitt AM (1969d) A theoretical model of the relationship between parathyroid cell mass and plasma calcium concentration in normal and uremic subjects: an analysis of the concept of autonomy and speculations on the mechanism of parathyroid hyperplasia. Arch Intern Med 124:269–273

Parfitt AM (1972) The spectrum of hypoparathyroidism. J Clin Endocrinol 1972: 152–158

Parfitt AM (1976a) The actions of parathyroid hormone on bone. Relation to bone remodelling and turnover, calcium homeostasis and metabolic bone disease: I. Mechanisms of calcium transfer between blood and bone and their cellular basis. Morphologic and kinetic approaches to bone turnover. Metabolism 25: 809–844

Parfitt AM (1976b) The actions of parathyroid hormone on bone. Relation to bone remodelling and turnover, calcium homeostasis and metabolic bone disease: II. PTH and bone cells: bone turnover and plasma calcium regulation. Metabolism 25:909–955

Parfitt AM (1978) Tubular reabsorption of calcium in pseudohypoparathyroidism. In: Copp DH, Talmage RV (eds) Endocrinology of calcium metabolism. Excerpta Medica, Amsterdam, p 409

Parfitt AM (1979a) Equilibrium and disequilibrium hypercalcemia: new light on an old concept. Metab Bone Dis Rel Res 1:279–293

Parfitt AM (1979b) Target cell resistance in pseudohypoparathyroidism. Single or multiple? In: Norman AW (ed) Vitamin D: basic research and its clinical application. de Gruyter, Berlin, pp 949–950

Parfitt AM (1980) Morphologic basis of bone mineral measurements. Transient and steady state effects of treatment in osteoporosis. Miner Electrolyte Metab 4: 273–287

Parfitt AM (1981) Integration of skeletal and mineral homeostasis. In: DeLuca HF, Frost H, Jee W, Johnston C, Parfitt AM (eds) Osteoporosis: recent advances in pathogenesis and treatment. University Park Press, Baltimore, pp 115–126

Parfitt AM (1982) Hypercalcemic hyperparathyroidism following renal transplantation: differential diagnosis, management, and implications for cell population control in the parathyroid gland. Miner Electrolyte Metab 8:92–119

Parfitt AM (1983) The physiologic and clinical significance of bone histomorphometric data. In: Recker R (ed) Bone histomorphometry. Techniques and interpretations. CRC Press, Boca Raton, pp 143–223

Parfitt AM (1984) The cellular basis of bone remodeling. The quantum concept reexamined in light of recent advances in cell biology of bone. Calcif Tissue Int 36:S37–S45

Parfitt AM (1987) Bone and plasma calcium homeostasis. Bone 8:51–58

Parfitt AM (1988a) The composition, structure and remodeling of bone: a basis for the interpretation of bone mineral measurements. In: Dequeker J, Geusens P, Wahner HW (eds) Bone mineral measurements by photon absorptiometry: methodological problems. Leuven University Press, Leuven, pp 9–28

Parfitt AM (1988b) Idiopathic, surgical and other varieties of parathyroid hormone deficient hypoparathyroidism. In: DeGroot L (ed) Endocrinology, 2nd edn. Saunders, Philadelphia, pp 1049–1064

Parfitt AM (1989) Plasma calcium control at quiescent bone surfaces: a new approach to the homeostatic function of bone lining cells. Bone 10:87–88

Parfitt AM (1990a) Bone-forming cells in clinical conditions. In: Hall BK (ed) Bone: a treatise, vol I. The osteoblast and osteocyte. Telford, Caldwell, pp 351–429

Parfitt AM (1990b) Osteomalacia and related disorders. In: Avioli LV, Krane SM (eds) Metabolic bone disease and clinically related disorders, 2nd edn. Saunders Philadelphia, pp 329–396

Parfitt AM (1990c) Pharmacologic manipulation of bone remodelling and calcium homeostasis. In: Kanis JA (ed) Progress in basic and clinical pharmacology: 4. Calcium metabolism. Karger, Basel, pp 1–27

Parfitt AM (1992) The physiologic and pathogenetic significance of bone histomorphometric data. In: Coe FL, Favus MJ (eds) Disorders of bone and mineral metabolism. Raven, New York, pp 475–489

Parfitt AM, Kleerekoper M (1980a) The divalent ion homeostatic system: physiology and metabolism of calcium, phosphorus, magnesium and bone. In: Maxwell M, Kleeman CR (eds) Clinical disorders of fluid and electrolyte metabolism, 3rd edn. McGraw–Hill, New York, pp 269–398

Parfitt AM, Kleerekoper M (1980b) Clinical disorders of calcium, phosphorus and magnesium metabolism. In: Maxwell M, Kleeman CR (eds) Clinical disorders of fluid and electrolyte metabolism, 3rd edn. McGraw-Hill, New York, pp 947–1152

Parfitt AM, Kleerekoper M, Villanueva AR (1987) Increased bone age: mechanisms and consequences. In: Christiansen C, Johansen C, Riis BJ (eds) Osteoporosis. Osteopress, Copenhagen, pp 301–308

Parfitt AM, Rao DS, Kleerekoper M (1991a) Asymptomatic primary hyperparathyroidism discovered by multi-channel biochemical screening. Clinical course and considerations bearing on the need for surgical intervention. J Bone Miner Res 6:S97–S101

Parfitt AM, Willgoss D, Jacobi J, Lloyd HM (1991b) Cell kinetics in parathyroid adenomas: evidence for decline in rates of cell birth and tumour growth, assuming clonal origin. Clin Endocrinol 35:151–157

Parsons JA (1976) Parathyroid physiology and the skeleton. In: Bourne GH (ed) Biochemistry and physiology of bone, vol IV. Academic, New York

Payne JW, Walser M (1959) Ion association: II. The effects of multivalent ions on the concentration of free calcium ions as measured by the frog heart method. Bull Johns Hopkins Hosp 105:298–310

Payne RB, Carver ME, Morgan DB (1979) Interpretation of serum total calcium: effects of adjustment for albumin concentration on frequency of abnormal values and on detection of change in the individual. J Clin Pathol 32:56–60

Payne RB, Jones DP, Walker AP, Evans RT (1986) Clustering of serum calcium and magnesium concentrations in siblings. Clin Chem 32:349–350

Peacock M, Robertson WG, Nordin BEC (1969) Relation between serum and urinary calcium with particular reference to parathyroid activity. Lancet i:384

Pedersen KO (1972) On the cause and degree of intraindividual serum calcium variability. Scand J Clin Lab Invest 30:191–199

Peterson DR, Heideger WJ, Beach KW (1985) Calcium homeostasis: the effect of parathyroid hormone on bone membrane electrical potential difference. Calcif Tissue Int 37:307–311

Pinto MR, Kelly PJ (1984) Age-related changes in bone in the dog: fluid spaces and their potassium content. J Orthop Res 1:2–7

Ponlot R (1960) Le radiocalcium dans l'étude des os. Arscia, Bruxelles

Posner AS (1988) The mineral of bone. Clin Orthop 200:87–99

Raina V (1972) Normal osteoid tissue. J Clin Pathol 25:229–232

Ramp WK, McNeil RW (1978) Selective stimulation of net calcium efflux from chick embryo tibiae by parathyroid hormone in vitro. Calcif Tissue Res 25:227–232

Rao DS, Parfitt AM, Kleerekoper M, Pumo BS, Frame B (1985) Dissociation between the effects of endogenous parathyroid hormone on cAMP generation and on phosphate reabsorption in hypocalcemia due to vitamin D depletion: an acquired disorder resembling pseudohypoparathyroidism type II. J Clin Endocrinol Metab 61:285–290

Reeve J (1978) The turnover time of calcium in the exchangeable pools of bone in man and the long-term effect of a parathyroid hormone fragment. Clin Endocrinol 8:445–455

Riggs BL, Marshall JH, Jowsey J, Heaney RP, Bassingthwaighte JB (1971) Quantitative ^{45}Ca autoradiography of human bone. J Lab Clin Med 78:585–598

Riggs DS (1963) The mathematical approach to physiological problems. Williams and Wilkins, Baltimore

Riggs DS (1966) A quantitative hypothesis concerning the action of the parathyroid hormone. J Theor Biol 12:364–372

Riggs DS (1970) Control theory and physiologic feedback mechanisms. Williams and Wilkins, Baltimore

Rodan GA, Liberman UA, Paran M, Anbar M (1967) Lack of physicochemical equilibrium between blood and bone calcium in the isolated perfused dog limb. Isr J Med Sci 3:702–713

Rodriguez M, Felsenfeld AJ, Torres A, Pederson L, Llach F (1991) Calcitonin, an important factor in the calcemic response to parathyroid hormone in the rat. Kidney Int 40:219–225

Roelen DL, Frolich M, Papapoulos SE (1989) Renal responsiveness to synthetic human parathyroid hormone 1–38 in healthy subjects. Eur J Clin Invest 19:311–315

Rowland RE (1966) Exchangeable bone calcium. Clin Orthop 49:233–248

Sanderson PH, Marshall F II, Wilson RE (1960) Calcium and phosphorus homeostasis in the parathyroidectomized dog; evaluation by means of ethylenediamine tetraacetate and calcium tolerance tests. J Clin Invest 39:662–670

Scarpace PJ, Neuman WF (1976a) The blood: bone disequilibrium: I. The active accumulation of K^+ into the bone extracellular fluid. Calcif Tissue Res 20:137–149

Scarpace PJ, Neuman WF (1976b) The blood: bone disequilibrium: II. Evidence against the active accumulation of calcium or phosphate into the bone extracellular fluid. Calcif Tissue Res 20:151–158

Schartum S, Nichols G Jr (1961) Calcium metabolism of bone in vitro. Influence of bone cellular metabolism and parathyroid hormone. J Clin Invest 40:2083–2091

Scherft JP (1972) The lamina limitans of the organic matrix of calcified cartilage and bone. J Ultrastruct Res 38:318

Schwarz P, Sorensen HA, Transbol I, McNair P (1990) Induced hypocalcaemia controlled by a citrate clamp technique and the intact parathyroid hormone response obtained. Scand J Clin Lab Invest 50:891–897

Seely EW, LeBoff MS, Brown EM, Chen C, Posillico JT, Hollenberg NK, Williams GH (1989a) The calcium channel blocker Diltiazem lowers serum parathyroid hormone levels in vivo and in vitro. J Clin Endocrinol Metab 68:1007–1012

Seely EW, Moore TJ, LeBoff MS, Brown EM (1989b) A single dose of lithium carbonate acutely elevates intact parathyroid hormone levels in humans. Acta Endocrinol (Copenh) 121:174–176

Segre GV, Harris ST, Neer R, Potts JT Jr (1981) Sigmoidal relationship between plasma parathyroid hormone and calcium concentration in man (abstract). ASBMR:30A

Shannon WA Jr, Roth SI (1974) An ultrastructural study of acid phosphatase activity in normal, adenomatous and hyperplastic (chief cell type) human parathyroid glands. Am J Pathol 77:493–501

Sheikh MS, Schiller LR, Fordtran JS (1990) In vivo intestinal absorption of calcium in humans. Miner Electrolyte Metab 16:130–146

Slatopolsky E, Lopez-Hilker S, Delmez J, Dusso A, Brown A, Martin KJ (1990) The parathyroid-calcitriol axis in health and chronic renal failure. Kidney Int 38:S41–S47

Somerville PJ, Kaye M (1982) Action of phosphorus on calcium release in isolated perfused rat tails. Kidney Int 22:348–354

Staub JF, Tracqui P, Brezillon P, Milhaud G. Perault-Staub AM (1988) Calcium metabolism in the rat: a temporal self-organized model. Am J Physiol 254: R134–R149

Staub JF, Tracqui P, Lausson S, Milhaud G, Perault-Staub AM (1989) A physiological view of in vivo calcium dynamics: the regulation of a nonlinear self-organized system. Bone 10:77–86

Stauffer M, Baylink DJ, Wergedal JE, Rich C (1973) Decreased bone formation, mineralization, and enhanced resorption in calcium-deficient rats. Am J Physiol 225:269–276

Stern PH (1990) Vitamin D and bone. Kidney Int 38:S17–S21

Stote RM, Smith LH, Wilson DM, Dube WJ, Goldsmith RS, Arnaud CD (1972) Hydrochlorothiazide effects on serum calcium and immunoreactive parathyroid hormone concentrations: studies in normal subjects. Ann Intern Med 77: 587–591

Talmage RV, Cooper CW, Park HZ (1970) Regulation of calcium transport in bone by parathyroid hormone. Vitam Horm 28:103–140

Talmage RV, Grubb SA, Norimatsu H, VanderWiel CJ (1980) Evidence for an important physiological role for calcitonin. Proc Natl Acad Sci USA 77:609–613

Talmage RV, Cooper CW, Toverud SU (1983) The physiological significance of calcitonin. In: Peck WA (ed) Bone and mineral research, vol. 1. Excerpta Medica, Amsterdam, pp 74–143

Toffaletti J, Bowers GN Jr (1979) The possible physiologic importance of calcium complexes: an opinion. Clin Chim Acta 97:101–105

Toffaletti J, Cooper DL, Lobaugh B (1991) The response of parathyroid hormone to specific changes in either ionized calcium, ionized magnesium, or protein-bound calcium in humans. Metabolism 40;8:814–818

Tothill P, Hooper G, McCarthy ID, Hughes SPF (1985) The variation with flow-rate of the extraction of bone-seeking tracers in recirculation experiments. Calcif Tissue Int 37:312–317

Triffitt JT, Owen M (1977) Preliminary studies in the binding of plasma albumin to bone tissue. Calcif Tissue Res 23:303–305

Triffitt JT, Owen ME, Ashton BA, Wilson JM (1978) Plasma disappearance of rabbit α_2-HS glycoprotein and its uptake by bone tissue. Calcif Tissue Res 26:155–161

Vander Wiel CJ, Grubb SA , Talmage RV (1978) The presence of lining cells on surfaces of human trabecular bone. Clin Orth Rel Res 134:350–355

Wallfelt C, Gylfe E, Larsson R, Ljunghall S, Rastad J, Akerstrom G (1988) Relationship between external and cytoplasmic calcium concentrations, parathyroid hormone release and weight of parathyroid glands in human hyperparathyroidism. J Endocrin 116:457–464

Waron M, Rich C (1969) Rate of recovery from acute hypocalcemia as a measure of calcium homeostatic efficiency in the dog. Endocrinology 85:1018–1027

Warren HB, Lausen NCC, Segre GV, El-Hajj G, Brown EM (1989) Regulation of calciotropic hormones in vivo in the New Zealand white rabbit. Endocrinology 125:2683–2690

Weiner N (1948) Cybernetics or control and communication in the animal and the machine. Technology Press and Wiley & Sons, New York

Weiner S, Price PA (1986) Disaggregation of bone into crystals. Calcif Tissue Int 39:365–375.

Weiner S, Traub W (1989) Crystal size and organization in bone. Connec Tissue Res 21:259–265

Weisinger JR, Favus MJ, Langman CB, Bushinsky DA (1989) Regulation of 1,25-dihydroxyvitamin D_3 by calcium in the parathyroidectomized, parathyroid hormone-replete rat. J Bone Min Res 4:930–934

Williams GA, Hargis GK, Galloway WB, Henderson WJ (1966) Evidence for thyrocalcitonin in man. Proc Soc Exp Biol Med 122:1273–1279

Wilson P, Kleerekoper M, Lillich R, Parfitt AM (1988) Immunoradiometric assay for intact parathyroid hormone in the diagnosis of hypoparathyroidism. J Bone Min Res 3 (Suppl 1):S131

Wirth DJ, Heideger WJ, Beach KW (1986) Calcium homeostasis II: the sodium-potassium pump. Calcif Tissue Int 38:306–307

Wisser H, Breuer H (1981) Circadian changes of clinical chemical and endocrinological parameters. J Clin Chem Clin Biochem 19:323–337

Yates FE (1982) Outline of a physical theory of physiological systems. Can J Physiol Pharmacol 60:217–248

Yates FE, Garfinkel A, Walter DO, Yates GB (1987) Self-Organizing Systems: the Emergence of Order. Plenum Press, New York

CHAPTER 2
Bone Remodeling and Bone Structure

E.F. Eriksen, A. Vesterby, M. Kassem, F. Melsen, and L. Mosekilde

A. Introduction

Bone remodeling constitutes the lifelong renewal process of bone whereby the mechanical integrity of the skeleton is preserved. It implies the continuous removal of bone (bone resorption) followed by synthesis of new bone matrix and subsequent mineralization (bone formation). Moreover, bone remodeling is an integral part of the calcium homeostatic system together with the kidneys and the gut. The ever ongoing removal of old bone by osteoclastic resorption and subsequent coupled osteoblastic formation of new bone leads to liberation of calcium and matrix constituents to serum.

Disturbances in bone remodeling lead to alterations in bone architecture, removal of structural elements, followed by loss of mechanical competence and fractures. Restoration of bone stucture and mechanical competence can only be achieved if these processes are reversed by treatment regimens creating a positive balance between resorption and formation. Thorough understanding of bone remodeling is therefore very important, not only in relation to clinical decision making, interpretation of bone marker levels in serum, bone mass assessment, or calcium kinetic indices, but also for the design of more effective treatments of metabolic bone diseases.

A unique feature of bone is the fact that remodeling leaves traces behind, traces that can be quantitated using microscopic and stereologic analysis. Moreover, bone lends itself to incorporation of a time marker (Frost 1969). This feature creates the basis for the calculation of rates of activity for the different cell types (Frost 1969; Eriksen et al. 1986). Quantitative bone histology is the only method by which alterations in cellular activity can be separated from changes in cell number. Other techniques of calcium metabolic research (e.g., bone densitometry, assays for biochemical markers in serum, calcium kinetics) only yield data on tissue or organ activity. Consequently these indices are the products of individual cell activity and number of cells.

Bone histomorphometry has yielded important information on bone remodeling in a large variety of metabolic bone diseases. These data have increased our knowledge about the pathogenesis behind these diseases. The most recent treatment regimens for osteoporosis and other metabolic bone diseases with accelerated bone loss are based on selective manipulation of resorptive and formative cell populations. In this setting, bone histomorphometry is mandatory for the evaluation of the effects of a given treatment.

The aim of this review is to update our knowledge of the bone remodeling process. Furthermore, the review will summarize data obtained on hormonal influences on bone remodeling and structural consequences of bone remodeling.

B. Bone Macro- and Microanatomy

The skeleton weighs around 4 kg, and the total volume of bone tissue amounts to 1750 ml, corresponding to a mean total bone calcium content of 1050 g (Parfitt et al. 1983). The skeleton consists of two macroscopically different envelopes: (a) cortical bone, which dominates the long bones of the extremities, and (b) cancellous bone, which dominates in the vertebrae and pelvis. Cortical bone makes up 80% (=1400 ml) of the skeleton and cancellous bone 20% (=350 ml), but, because cancellous bone is metabolically more active, skeletal metabolism is approximately equally distributed between the two envelopes. The two envelopes behave differently and exhibit different responses to metabolic changes and treatment.

When studying bone in polarized light a clear lamellar pattern is visible in both cortical and cancellous bone. It is caused by birefringence due to the arrangement of collagen fibrils in alternating orientations. The lamellae have a constant thickness of $3.2 \mu m$ in normal bone. The mechanism underlying this alternating orientation of fibrils is unknown, but it is obvious that such a "plywood-like" orientation increases the compressive strength of bone. Lamellar thickness exhibits a very low interindividual variance (5%) (Kragstrup et al. 1983a), and thus the lamellae constitute a very convenient yardstick for the analysis of structure thickness and erosion depth in bone.

If bone turnover is very high, disturbed, or during formation of primitive bone the lamellar pattern disappears, "woven bone" is formed. In woven bone the collagen fibrils are laid down in a disorganized manner and the mechanical properties therefore suffer. Formation of woven bone is a problem during fluoride treatment, where the mitogenic activity of osteoblasts may go up to a degree, and where formation of lamellar bone is impossible, but is also seen as a normal phenomenon during intramembraneous bone formation.

I. Cortical Bone

Cortical bone is made up of Haversian systems (cortical osteons), which may branch within the cortex (Fig. 1). They constitute tubular elements consisting of lamellae arranged in a concentric manner around a central (Haversian)

Table 1. Quantitative features of cortical and cancellous bone. (After PARFITT et al. 1983)

Index	Cortical envelope	Cancellous envelope
Fraction of skeleton (%)	80	20
Fraction of skeletal turnover (%)	50	50
Fractional tissue volume (mm^3/mm^3)	0.95	0.20
Surface area to bone volume ratio (mm^2/mm^3)	2.5	20
Total bone volume (mm^3)	1.4×10^6	0.35×10^6
Total internal surface area (mm^2)	3.5×10^6	7.0×10^6
BSU length (mm)	2.5	1.0
Wall thickness (mm)	0.075	0.050
Total number in skeleton	21×10^6	14×10^6

canal containing blood vessels. In a normal skeleton a total of 21×10^6 haversian systems will be found, and the total area available for Haversian remodeling is $3.5\,m^2$ (PARFITT 1983). From the spatial organization of Haversian systems it is obvious that a relatively small surface is covered by cells, in contrast to cancellous bone, where a large surface is covered by cells. This explains the lower metabolic activity of the cortical envelope. Despite making up 80% of the skeleton by volume, only 50% of metabolic activity of bone resides in the cortex (Table 1) (PARFITT 1983). The porosity of cortical bone is usually less than 10% due to either ongoing remodeling or haversian canals of resting osteons (Table 1).

Cortical bone is limited by the periosteum on the outside and the endosteum on the inside. The inner cortical endosteal surface amounts to $0.5\,m^2$ (PARFITT et al. 1983), and exhibits pronounced activity of osteoclasts and osteoblasts. The periosteum is important during growth and fracture repair. During growth the periosteum is important for "modeling" of bone. Modeling is the process whereby bone is reshaped in order to create maximal compressive strength (e.g., in the metaphyseal area of long bones). At the periosteal surface, bone formation exceeds bone resorption, creating a net increase in the outer diameter of the bone with age.

At the endosteum modeling as well as remodeling occurs. The general cellular activity is higher in this area, probably due to the continuous bending and stretching forces operating in this area. At the endosteal surface bone resorption generally exceeds bone formation, resulting in a net expansion of the marrow capacity with age. This endocortical thinning may be especially pronounced during high turnover states (e.g., thyrotoxicosis, around menopause).

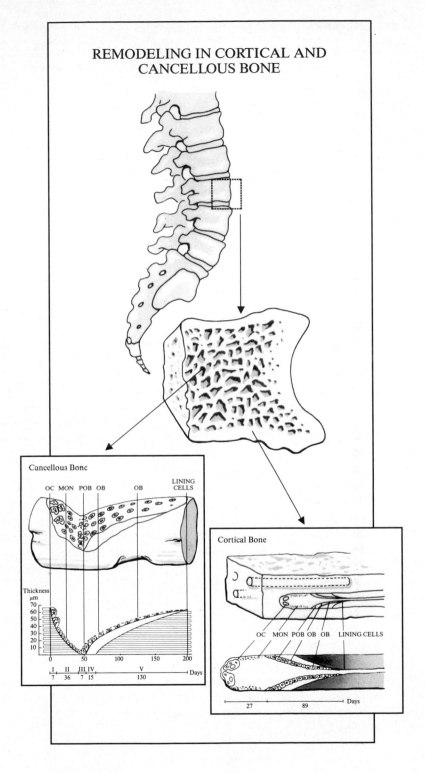

REMODELING IN CORTICAL AND CANCELLOUS BONE

II. Cancellous Bone

Cancellous bone consists of trabeculae with thicknesses ranging from 50 to 400 μm. Trabeculae are interconnected in a honeycomb pattern, maximizing the mechanical properties of the bone. In areas subjected to constant mechanical stress in a certain direction, the cancellous pattern develops in a structure that maximizes adaptation to the given stress pattern (e.g., in the femoral neck area). Trabeculae are made up of semilunar subunits (bone structural units (BSUs), packets, walls, or cancellous bone osteons). The total number of BSUs in cancellous bone has been calculated to be 14×10^6, and the total area of the endosteal surface is about 11 m^2 (PARFITT 1983).

C. Bone Remodeling

Bone remodeling has to be distinguished from bone modeling, which is the process associated with growth of bones in childhood and adolescence (FROST 1964). Bone modeling constitutes primarily processes at the periosteum and endosteum leading to changes in the form of growing bone. During modeling, resorption and formation have no spatial relationship and proceed in an uncoupled fashion. Moreover, the process is continuous and covers a large surface, while remodeling is cyclical and usually covers a small area (PARFITT 1983).

The cells involved in bone remodeling function within the framework of the bone multicellular unit (BMU) or bone remodeling unit (BRU) (FROST 1964; PARFITT 1983) (Fig. 1). The end result of the work of a BMU (or BRU) is a new bone structural unit (BSU). In cortical bone the osteon constitutes a BSU. In trabecular bone the BSU is called trabecular osteon, packet, or wall.

Fig. 1. Remodeling in cancellous and cortical bone. In cortical bone the bone multicellular unit (*BMU*) consists of tunnel (cutting cone) drilled out by advancing osteoclasts (*OC*) followed by mononuclear (*MON*) cells. In younger normal individuals the resorption period lasts around 30 days. Bone formation is initiated by the emergence of preosteoblasts (*POB*) in the *BMU*. Later on preosteoblasts differentiate into osteoblasts (*OB*) that form matrix, which subsequently becomes mineralized and fills out the tunnel except for a central haversian canal (closing cone). The formative period lasts 90 days. The finished new Haversian system constitutes a new cortical bone structural unit (*BSU*).

In cancellous bone the sequence of events is identical, except for the fact that the process takes place on trabecular surfaces. The resorption period lasts about 50 days in younger individuals, and can be subdivided into an osteoclastic period (*I*), mononuclear period (*II*), and preosteoblastic period (*III*). Matrix formation lasts 15 days (*IV*) followed by mineralization for another 130 days (*V*). Thus after a total of around 150 days a new cancellous BSU is formed. (Reproduced with permission from ERIKSEN, Osteoporosis, NOVO-Nordisk A/S, 1992)

The BMU of cortical bone constitutes a cylinder with a cone-shaped top and bottom, the cutting cone, where resorption takes place, and the closing cone, where formation proceeds (Fig. 1). The total BMU in cortical bone is around 400 μm long and 200 μm at the base, and it moves longitudinally through the cortex at a rate of 40 μm/day in dogs (JAWORSKI and LOK 1972). It has been hypothesized that two different types of cortical BMUs exist (PARFITT 1983): (1) one type characterized by lack of longitudinal movement, where remodeling just takes place in situ, and (2) one type with ongoing remodeling as the BMU proceeds through the cortex.

In cancellous bone the BMU can be looked upon as a cortical BMU cut through in the middle (Fig. 1). In three-dimensional terms it constitutes a pancake-like structure (KRAGSTRUP and MELSEN 1983). The cellular changes are similar to those observed in cortical bone (ERIKSEN 1986; AGERBAEK et al. 1991). The vast majority of bone formation in cancellous bone is coupled to bone resorption. Under normal conditions more than 97% of new BSUs are formed on previous resorption sites (HATTNER 1965). Under certain conditions (e.g., growth, Paget disease, fluoride therapy), however, de novo bone formation on quiescent surfaces may occur. In these instances the initial bone formed will have a woven structure.

I. Quantum Concept of Bone Remodeling

According to the quantum concept of Frost, changes in bone mass are caused by an imbalance between the amount of bone resorbed by osteoclasts and the amount of bone formed by osteoblasts (FROST 1964; PARFITT 1979). Bone has to be envisaged as a tissue containing BMUs at discrete locations and at different developmental stages. This arrangement of small subunits constantly turning over bone matrix constituents and mineral creates the basis for the changes in bone mass observed with increasing age and in metabolic bone disease.

The concept of bone remodeling was established from studies on cortical bone (FROST 1964; FROST et al. 1969; JAWORSKI 1971). The concept is based on the hypothesis that every BMU is initiated by the activation of osteoclastic precursors to become osteoclasts and start bone resorption [(A)ctivation-(R)esorption sequence]. The rate by which BMUs are formed is traditionally called the *activation frequency* and, together with the individual cellular function rates at the BMU, it determines tissue level turnover (FROST 1964; ERIKSEN 1986; CHARLES et al. 1987).

While resorption depth and mean wall thickness may only vary by 10%–20% in different diseases, activation frequency may vary by 50%–100%. Thus, in most diseases the activation frequency is the most important regulator of bone turnover and changes in bone mass (PARFITT 1979; ERIKSEN 1986).

II. Coupling Phenomenon

After the termination of bone resorption, bone formation is initiated in the resorption lacuna through "*coupling*" (FROST 1964; PARFITT 1982). The coupling process ensures that the amount of bone removed is laid down again during subsequent formation. The term "coupling" is commonly used indiscriminately with two different meanings attached to it: (a) to indicate the process where resorption is followed by formation ("temporal coupling") and (b) to indicate that the amount of bone resorbed is similar to the amount of bone formed ("quantitative coupling"). The term should only be used when talking about the temporal aspects of the remodeling process. "Imbalance" is the proper expression to use to describe the fact that resorption cavities are either inadequately refilled or cases where formation exceeds resorption (PARFITT 1982; ERIKSEN 1986).

The detailed nature of the activation and coupling mechanism is still unknown, although some growth factors (e.g., lymphokines, IGF-1, TGFβ) and prostaglandins have been invoked (D'SOUZA et al. 1986; PILBEAM and RAISZ 1988). Whether the activation of osteoblasts starts simultaneously with osteoclast recruitment or later during the development of the BMU due to coupling is still unsettled. Mechanical stimulation of bone cells also seems important to the coupling process. Immobilization (in bed or during weightlessness during spaceflight) leads to a pronounced negative bone balance. The same mechanism has also been demonstrated in bone still subject to mechanical stimulation. Using scanning electron microscopic analysis of cancellous bone in normal human vertebrae, MOSEKILDE (1990) demonstrated uncoupling of bone formation in trabeculae that lacked connection to other trabeculae (struts). Trabeculae that were part of an intact network still exhibited normal coupling between resorption and formation. Whether total temporal uncoupling exists is, however, impossible to assess with the current methodology.

D. Evaluation of Bone Remodeling and Structure

Stereology is a discipline which deals with the conversion of two-dimensional observations to three-dimensional information using statistical, mathematical, and geometrical tools. Stereological methods are precise tools for obtaining quantitative information about three-dimensional structures based on observations made on sections. For the information to be accurate, either the structure to be measured or the probe itself (e.g., the test line) must be isotropic (i.e., the structures are randomly oriented in spaces).

In bone which is anisotropic (i.e., some preferential orientation of structures exists) this can be achieved by using anisotropic sections, so-called vertical sections in combination with an anisotropic test system (VESTERBY et al. 1987a,b). Measurements on bone sections using anisotropic test

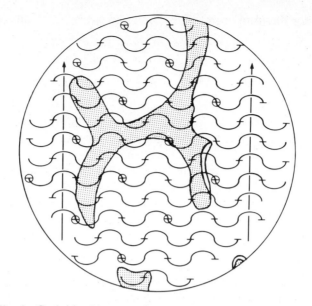

Fig. 2. Cycloid grid system for stereological analysis of bone

systems provide unbiased and therefore valid estimates of bone structural parameters. Furthermore, robust estimates of mean trabecular thickness can be achieved. The anisotropic test system contains test lines with a density which is proportional to the sine of the angle between the test lines and the vertical axis; that is, the density of lines increases with the angle between the vertical axis and the lines (Baddeley et al. 1986). The cycloid is an example of such an anisotropic test system (Fig. 2) (Vesterby et al. 1987). Test systems with numbers at the margin to indicate the correct probability of test lines in relation to the vertical axis are other examples of such anisotropic test systems. Traditionally, points where grid lines cross bone surfaces are called *intersections*.

    Below is summarized how the main indices describing bone remodeling and bone structure are assessed. For a detailed description of the large number of possible histomorphometric indices, please consult Parfitt et al. (1987), Eriksen (1986), and Vesterby et al. (1987b, 1989b).

I. Surface Area Estimates

Estimates of bone surface area [e.g., osteoid covered (OS), labeled (LS), erosion surface area (ES)], and ratio of bone surface area to bone volume (BS/BV) can be obtained with the cycloid test system. The number of intersections between test lines and bone surface area and the number of test points on bone or on bone including marrow space are counted. The conventional formula for the calculation of surface area is used: $S_v = 2 \times I_L$. I is the number of intersections between test lines and bone surfaces and L is the total length of test lines used. These indices provide the basis for the calculation of a wide variety of derived variables (see PARFITT et al. 1987) for detailed analysis of bone structure and remodeling).

E. Evaluation of Bone Resorption

The activity of osteoclasts and other putative resorptive cells is reflected in the amount of bone removed during resorption and the rate by which this process proceeds. The three-dimensional thickness of bone removed during bone resorption is reflected in the index erosion depth (E.De).

I. Cortical Bone

In cortical bone, erosion depth is equivalent to the cross-sectional osteon radius (PIROK et al. 1966; BROULIK et al. 1982). The resorption rate can be calculated from tetracycline-based estimates of the resorption period (RP).

II. Cancellous Bone

COURPRON et al. (1981) devised the first method for the indirect estimation of erosion depth (E.De) by relating mean thickness of interstitial bone to mean trabecular thickness. It has recently been employed by CROUCHER et al. (1989). The method is rather insensitive for assessment of short-term changes in bone resorption, because the thickness estimates are influenced by remodeling that took place before the change of interest occurred.

A more sensitive method, which only measures ongoing resorption, is based on counting the number of lamellae eroded in polarized light (ERIKSEN et al. 1984b). By relating E.De to cell type, the whole resorption sequence can be reconstructed as shown above. The mean depth of completed resorption sites (E.De) is a good index of the amount of bone removed during resorption (CHARLES et al. 1987). From E.De and tetracycline-based values of function periods, a resorption rate can be calculated (ERIKSEN et al. 1984a; CHARLES et al. 1987).

Attempts have been made to delineate the previous surface by curve-fitting procedures (GARRAHAN et al. 1990). The method is based on computer-assisted fitting of spline curves to trabecular surfaces with resorption cavities captured by videocamera-assisted microscopy of bone sections. The method is not correcting for obliquity of the section plane, and, because all cavities regardless of cell type are sampled, the depth estimate will be biased towards too low values. Thus, no direct estimate of bone balance can be calculated from the E.De values obtained with this method.

F. Evaluation of Bone Formation

Osteoblastic activity is reflected in the thicknesses of mineralized and unmineralized bone structures and in the thickness of bone between tetracycline double labels. With a known interval between the administration of tetracycline labels the mineral appositional rate (MAR) is given as: (thickness of bone between labels/labeling interval). The mineralization process is, however, not continuous. Based on systematic tetracycline labeling, on/off periods of mineralization have been demonstrated (Hori et al. 1985). The mechanisms underlying this phenomenon are still unknown. Moreover, a certain period elapses between matrix formation and subsequent matrix mineralization [mineralization lag time (Mlt)]. In order to calculate the correct bone formation period, one therefore has to correct for these phenomena. This is achieved by calculating the adjusted appositional rate (Aj.AR), which is calculated as MAR × [labeled surface area (LS)/osteoid surface area (OS)].

The three-dimensional thickness of bone structures [e.g., trabecular (Tr.Th), cortical (C.Th), lamellar (La.Th), osteoid (O.Th), or interlabel bone thickness] is estimated using test systems with direction numbers and a separate grid with lines and points (Vesterby et al. 1989a). Wall thickness can also be measured by counting lamellae in bone structural units (Steiniche 1989). For further information on tetracycline-based indices please consult Frost (1969), Eriksen (1986), and Parfitt et al. (1987).

I. Cortical Bone

The mean thickness of bone formed in cortical bone is easily calculated as $0.5 \times (D - d)$, where D is the cross-sectional osteon diameter and d the cross-sectional haversian canal diameter. As mentioned above, the duration of the formation period (FP) is easily calculated from tetracycline labels in haversian systems, as wall thickness/Aj.AR (Frost 1969; Eriksen 1986; Parfitt et al. 1987).

II. Cancellous Bone

Mean trabecular bone thickness (Tb.Th) can be calculated from bone surface area and bone volume: [Tb.Th (calculated) = 2 × BV/BS] or it can be measured directly by measuring the length of intercepts in a random direction or measuring the orthogonal intercepts (i.e., intercepts perpendicular to the intersection with a given surface area or cement line) (Kragstrup et al. 1982; Eriksen 1986). Any of the methods can be used as long as it is specified which methods have been used to make comparisons between centers possible. An intraindividual distribution of trabecular thickness can only be assessed from orthogonal intercepts.

The mean thickness of BSUs can also be measured based on area and perimeter, but more precise and less-biased measurements rely on sampling of orthogonal intercepts of completed BSUs (KRAGSTRUP et al. 1983b; ERIKSEN et al. 1984b). Finally, the thickness can also be estimated by the counting of lamellae at randomly distributed intersections.

G. Bone Balance

I. Cortical Bone

In cortical bone a negative balance between resorption and formation will be reflected in an increased diameter of the haversian canal. For obvious reasons no positive balance can be achieved during cortical osteonal remodeling. As described below, normal bone exhibits significant changes in bone balance with age (BROULIK et al. 1982).

II. Cancellous Bone

Bone balance at the BMU level (Dt.BMU) is calculated from mean wall thickness (W.Th) and erosion depth (E.De) as:

DtBMU = WTh-EDe

A positive balance will signal an increase in bone mass and a negative balance loss of bone. The degree of imbalance is correlated to the rate of bone loss for the whole skeleton (ERIKSEN 1986; CHARLES et al. 1987).

III. Calculation of Activation Frequency

The activation frequency (Ac.F) is a measure of the rate by which new remodeling cycles are initiated on the bone surface. It constitutes a major determinant of tissue level bone turnover (BFR/BV), which is the product of Ac.F and BMU-based activity. In cortical bone Ac.F is relatively easy to calculate, because the number of BMUs per unit volume can be counted.

In trabecular bone, however, another approach has to be employed (PARFITT 1983; ERIKSEN et al. 1985d). The duration of the remodeling cycle (remodeling period, RP) is the sum of RsP and FP. The termination of FP is followed by a long period where no remodeling activity occurs on the surface (quiescent period, QP). The total period (RsP + FP + QP) marks the interval from the initiation of one remodeling cycle to the initiation of the next at the same point on the trabecular surface. Thus, AcF, the rate by which new remodeling is initiated, is the reciprocal of the total period, i.e.,

$$Ac.F = 1/(RsP + FP + QP)(time^{-1})$$

IV. Calculation of Tissue Level Indices of Turnover

Volume-based indices describing tissue level bone resorption (BRs.R/BV) and tissue level bone formation (BFR/BV) are easily calculated based on the BMU-derived variables (PARFITT et al. 1983; CHARLES et al. 1987; ERIKSEN et al. 1990). The calculations are based on the product of surface area [active erosion surface area (a.ES) or mineralizing surface area (MS)], rate of activity at the given surface area [erosion rate (ER) or mineral appositional rate (MAR)], and a conversion factor transforming the two-dimensional surface area based indices for resorption or formation into three-dimensional indices, the surface area to volume ratio (BS/BV, the surface area per unit volume).

$$BRs.R/BV = ER \times a.ES \times BS/BV$$

$$BFR/BV = MAR \times MS \times BS/BV$$

The volume-based bone balance is the difference between the volume-referent indices of resorption and formation:

$$Dt.BV/BV = BFR/BV - BRs.R/BV$$

These variables correlate significantly to whole skeletal turnover as assessed by calcium balance and calcium kinetic studies (ARLOT et al. 1984; CHARLES et al. 1987).

H. Indices Pertaining to Cancellous Bone Structure

The mechanical competence of cancellous bone is not only related to the absolute volume of trabecular bone, but also to the integrity of the trabecular network (connectivity). Recently, stereological correct estimators of cancellous bone properties have been devised (BADDELEY et al. 1986; VESTERBY et al. 1987a,b; GUNDERSEN et al. 1988).

I. Trabecular Bone Volume

The fractional volume of trabecular bone is calculated from the number of test points on trabecular bone to number of points on whole bone (trabecular bone and marrow space). Isotrophy of the structure under study is not required.

II. Marrow Space Star Volume

The star volume (GUNDERSEN and JENSEN 1985; VESTERBY et al. 1989b) is a stereological parameter and it can give an estimate of the mean size of an object when seen unobscured from a random point inside the object along

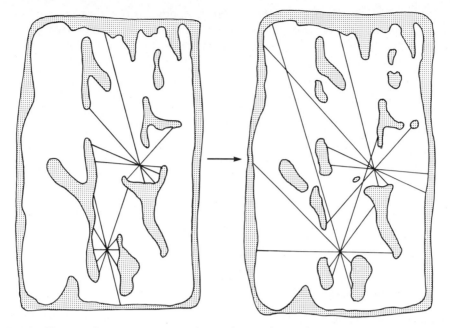

Fig. 3. Changes in marrow star volume due to increasing number of trabecular perforations

straight lines in all possible directions. The star volume can be estimated for all kind of objects including cavities and networks as trabeculae and marrow space (Fig. 3). It is only valid if an unbiased sampling scheme is used.

Marrow Space Star Volume, $V^*_{m.space}$ *(mm³)* is the mean size of the marrow space when seen unobscured from a random point along straight lines in all possible directions. Its mean value is estimated from the length (l_0) of random sine weighted intercepts raised to the power of three through a sufficient number of points (Fig. 3). It is calculated as follows:

$$V^*_{m.space} = \pi/3 \times \bar{l}_0^3.$$

(for iliac crest marrow space the measuring procedure is slightly different (VESTERBY 1990): the length of random intercepts is measured according to the nucleator method from the point (l_m) and the formula is then:

$$V^*_{m.space, iliac\, crest} = 4 \times \pi/3 \times \bar{l}_n^3.$$

The marrow space star volume is an indirect estimate of the connectivity of the trabecular network. A large marrow space star volume indicates a disconnected structure while a low marrow space star volume indicates a tight and connected structure (Fig. 3). It does not, however, tell us anything about the shape, the orientation, or the appearance of the structure. It cannot provide information about the topology of the structure. An estimate of the anisotrophy of the structure under study can be obtained from the volume orientation of surfaces (Odgaard et al. 1990).

The information which is provided by the marrow space star volume can be compared to two-dimensional estimates as trabecular number (mean trabecular plate density, MTPD) and intertrabecular distance (mean trabecular plate separation, MTPS) (Parfitt et al. 1983). The marrow space star volume is, however, a stereological (three-dimensional) parameter and is more sensitive to changes in trabecular bone structure than conventional estimates.

I. The Bone Resorption Sequence

I. Cancellous Bone

Resorption lacunae (Howship lacunae) contain three morphologically very different cell types (Fig. 4): large syncytial osteoclasts, small mononuclear cells containing pyknotic nuclei, and preosteoblasts characterized by large, translucent ovoid nuclei (Baron et al. 1981a,b; Eriksen et al. 1984a).

Osteoclasts are not present during the whole resorptive period. They are primarily seen in early, shallow lacunae. Osteoclasts are mobile and may cover an area two to three times the contact area (Owen 1971; Parfitt 1983), and they generally seem to avoid areas with osteoid. The highest resorption rate is seen during the osteoclastic phase (Eriksen et al. 1984a). As the lacuna deepens osteoclasts are replaced by mononuclear cells, and resorption proceeds. As resorption terminates mononuclear cells are replaced by preosteoblasts (Eriksen et al. 1984) (Fig. 4). This series of events is seen in humans as well as animals like dog or pig (Boyce et al. 1989). Mononuclear cells were first described by Baron et al. (1981b), who thought they represented an inactive reversal phase in between osteoclastic resorption and subsequent osteoblastic formation. Several studies have corroborated that bone resorption still proceeds while mononuclear cells are present (Eriksen et al. 1984a; Eriksen 1986b; Boyce et al. 1989). The detailed nature and function of mononuclear cells are still unsettled. The cells show a positive reaction for tartrate-resistant acid phosphatase (TRAP) like osteoclasts (E.F. Eriksen et al., unpublished data), but whether they just represent cells shed from the osteoclastic syncytium or a separate cell type awaits further studies.

The gradual appearance of morphologically distinct cell types at different depths of the resorption lacuna permits the reconstruction of curves showing time-dependent changes in resorption depth (Eriksen et al. 1984a).

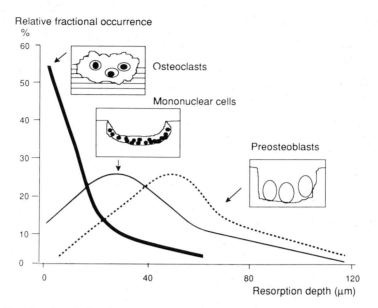

Fig. 4. Depth-related distribution of the three cell types demonstrable in resorption lacunae. Large syncytial osteoclasts occupy the more shallow parts of the lacunae, while small mononuclear cells with pyknotic nuclei are found in the deeper parts. The termination of bone resorption is signaled by the emergence of preosteoblast characterized by large ovoid nuclei

The end points of the curve describing the progression in erosion depth with time are erosion period (EP) and final erosion depth (E.De). E.De is, however, reached as soon as the end of the active erosion period (aEP) (Fig. 5). The interval between the points marking a.EP and EP consequently constitutes a horizontal line (Fig. 5). The points in between are derived from the mean depth below the osteoclasts and mononuclear cells, respectively.

II. Cortical Bone

A similar sequence of events as that reported for cancellous bone has been described for cortical bone (FROST 1964; JAWORSKI 1971; AGERBAEK et al. 1991). The duration of the resorption sequence for this envelope has been calculated to be 30 days (Fig. 1). In cortical bone resorption depth is easier to measure than in trabecular bone. The number of sites per biopsy available for sampling are, however, smaller. The depth is given by the diameter of a resorptive cortical osteon (cutting cone). The final erosion depth is consequently the maximal diameter of any given cortical osteon with preosteblasts in it. The rest of the reconstruction follows the lines outlined above for cancellous bone (AGERBAEK et al. 1991).

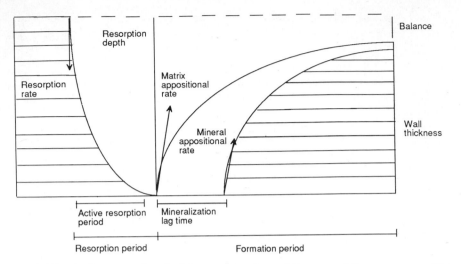

Fig. 5. Key indices associated with reconstruction of the remodeling sequence. The active resorption period ends when preosteoblasts enter the lacuna. The function period of preosteoblasts (5–10 days) added to the active resorption period makes up the total resorption period (*RsP*). Initial osteoblastic matrix formation proceeds for 15–20 days (mineralization lag time) before mineralization ensues. The sum of the mineralization lag time and the mineralization period constitutes the formative period.

The reconstruction of the remodeling sequence enables detailed studies to be performed on resorption rates. Morever, matrix formation rates and mineral appositional rates can be studied separately. Together with the dynamic rate estimates the reconstruction permits calculation of the balance between resorption depth and wall thickness

J. The Bone Formation Sequence

The osteoblast also undergoes characteristic changes in morphology with increasing age of the BMU. These changes were first described by MAROTTI (1977) for cortical osteons. He reported a gradual flattening of the osteoblast accompanied by increasing pyknosis of the nucleus. The same development has been reported for osteoblasts during maturation of BMUs in cancellous bone (PARFITT et al. 1980; ERIKSEN et al. 1984b). Some of the osteoblasts are incorporated into bone as osteocytes, some remain as lining cells covering completed osteons. In trabecular bone the cell number goes down to 70% of initial values, while the reduction is down to 30% of initial values in cortical bone (KIMMEL 1981; PARFITT 1983).

I. Cancellous Bone

The characteristic changes in osteoblast morphology have been the basis for reconstruction of the formative site of cancellous bone (PARFITT et al. 1980).

Osteoblasts were subdivided into three groups: cylindric, cuboidal, and flat, and mean thicknesses of osteoid and calcified matrix below each cell type calculated for each class. In this way a mean curve describing the time-dependent changes in matrix and calcified matrix was constructed. A more detailed reconstruction is, however, possible if the graduation of growth is based on the relative changes in osteoid and calcified matrix (ERIKSEN et al. 1984b).

The formative curve end points are FP and W.Th (Fig. 5). The points in between are calculated from a classification of the fraction osteoid thickness/ wall thickness (O.Th/W.Th) in a sector system. The development of the growth curve is namely characterized by a progressive thinning of osteoid and concurrent thickening of mineralized bone. Thus, the fraction O.Th/W.Th decreases as the trabecular osteon grows, and together with fluorescense measurements introducing the time dimension they form the basis for the construction of curves giving the time-dependent variation in matrix and mineralized bone thickness (Fig. 5). The finished remodeling curve is a very convenient tool for the description of the vast majority of bone histo-morphometric indices pertaining to BMU remodeling and it allows the calculation of curves describing the variation of other histomorphometric indices pertaining to bone formation throughout the formation period (ERIKSEN et al. 1984b; ERIKSEN 1986). The curve is also the only way by which matrix synthesis can be studied separately from matrix mineralization (Fig. 5).

II. Cortical Bone

In cortical bone a similar sequence of events has been described (FROST 1964; JAWORSKI 1971) and reconstructed based on measurements of inner and outer diameters of cortical osteons (Fig. 1). Using this method the formative phase of cortical remodeling has recently been reconstructed by AGERBAEK et al. (1991). The same shape of the growth curve was reported, but the duration for the same age group was somewhat shorter (90 days versus 145 days in cancellous bone) (Fig. 1).

III. The Bone Structural Unit

The end result of bone remodeling is the formation of a new "bone structural unit (BSU)," which in cortical bone constitutes a new haversian system and in cancellous bone a pancake-like structure (packet or wall) filling out the resorption lacuna. Haversian systems are about $2000\,\mu m$ long and have a diameter of $200\,\mu m$ (Table 1). Cancellous bone BSUs have a length of $100\,\mu m$ and a thickness ranging between 40 and $70\,\mu m$ depending on the age of the individual (Table 1).

The thickness of the BSU represents the total work carried out by a group of osteoblasts during one bone formation period (FP). With increasing age the mean thickness of BSUs [mean wall thickness (WTh)] goes down (LIPS et al. 1978; KRAGSTRUP et al. 1983a), probably due to reduced osteoblastic potential with increasing age. It is, however, still unsettled whether wall thickness is determined by the number of osteoblasts recruited at the start of the formation period or the activity of individual osteoblasts. The fact that mitogenic agents like fluoride (FARLEY et al. 1983) and parathyroid hormone (PTH) (NEER et al. 1990) are able to increase bone mass might suggest that an increased number of osteoblasts increases bone mass. On the other hand, thyroid hormones, which also exert mitogenic effects on osteoblasts, reduce mean wall thickness (ERIKSEN et al. 1985b).

The assessment of WTh can be assessed by different stereological methods by digitizing completed BSUs as seen in polarized microscopy (LIPS et al. 1978; KRAGSTRUP et al. 1982). In normal bone or bone subject to long-lasting diseases this approach yields correct results. If, however, assessment of WTh is carried out in order to monitor changes after a given short stimulus to bone (diseases or treatment regimens of short duration), this approach may be erroneous. In this case some of the BSUs sampled may represent bone formation before the given disease or treatment ensued. Here reconstruction of the formative period based on ongoing remodeling may give more correct values. One example of this problem is hyperthyroidism. Due to the relatively short duration of hyperthyroidism, measurements of WTh averaged over the total section will lead to falsely elevated values as discussed above. This is due to the presence of old walls that were formed before the disease started and is shown by the fact that the matrix and mineral growth curves do not converge on the WTh value calulated, but on a lower value (Fig. 6) (ERIKSEN et al. 1985b).

K. Bone Remodeling and Bone Loss

The remodeling process proceeds differently in cortical and cancellous bone. Usually the subcortical area, which is characterized by very high turnover, is considered a third compartment with properties of its own. The turnover generally seems to be higher in this area, and this characteristic probably explains the accelerated bone loss observed at the endocortical domain in high turnover bone disease (e.g., thyrotoxicosis, primary hyperparathyroidism) (PARFITT 1983).

L. Reversible Bone Loss

A *transient, reversible* loss of bone may occur if the number of resorption lacunae suddenly increases (expansion of the remodeling space) (Fig. 6). Due to the A-R-F sequence this will occur before bone formation increases

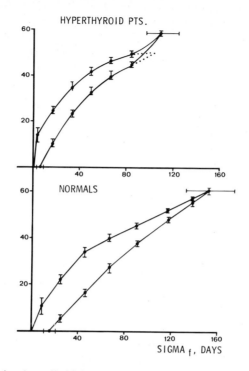

Fig. 6. In thyrotoxicosis wall thickness estimates based on all completed BSUs will provide a biased estimate due to inclusion of walls formed before the start of the disease. A more correct estimate of wall thickness can be obtained by interpolation based on matrix and mineralized bone growth curves (*broken lines*)

and thus lead to an apparent decrease in trabecular bone mass. Once bone formation has caught up, however, bone mass will stabilize at a lower level, provided no net deficit between resorption and formation exists at the individual BMU. The opposite will occur in the case of the activation frequency decreasing (e.g., due to estrogen therapy, bisphosphonate therapy, or alterations in thyroid hormone status), and this reduction of the remodeling space will lead to an apparent increase in bone density (Fig. 7). This may lead to the conclusion that more bone has been formed during treatment. Several authors have demonstrated that changes in remodeling space may be responsible for changes in bone mass ranging between 5% and 10% (FROST 1989; PARFITT 1980; JEROME 1989).

I. Cancellous Bone

Increased bone turnover will increase the number of resorption lacunae per unit volume, and thus increase "porosity" of cancellous bone, but due to the inherent structural properties of cancellous bone the impact will be less obvious than in cortical bone.

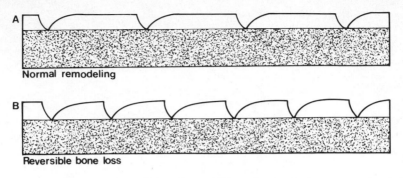

Fig. 7. Normal bone turnover (*A*) and reversible reduction in bone mass due to high turnover and expansion of the remodeling space (i.e., the amount of bone currently turning over) (*B*)

II. Cortical Bone

In cortical bone loss increased remodeling activity leads to increased cortical porosity (e.g., hyperthyroidism or primary hyperparathyroidism). Changes in cortical porosity will be especially obvious if bone mass measurements are performed at sites dominated by cortical bone (e.g., the forearm).

M. Irreversible Bone Loss

Irreversible bone loss may occur in two different ways: (a) through thinning of cortex or trabeculae due to a negative balance per remodeling cycle at each BMU (Fig. 8) or (b) through perforative resorption (Fig. 8). The latter process only plays a role in cancellous bone loss. In cancellous bone the processes are interrelated because thinning of trabeculae predisposes to perforative resorption and thus removal of the structure (REEVE 1986).

I. Cortical Bone

With increasing age and in certain metabolic bone disease, thinning of the cortex due to excessive endosteal resorption occurs (Fig. 8). Another factor is the increase in haversian canal diameter that has been demonstrated with increasing age and in certain metabolic bone disease (BROULIK et al. 1982). This increase will cause increased porosity of the cortex.

II. Cancellous Bone

Due to the huge variation in lacunar depth (ERIKSEN et al. 1984a, 1985a) and fortuitous, simultaneous resorption at two opposite trabecular surfaces,

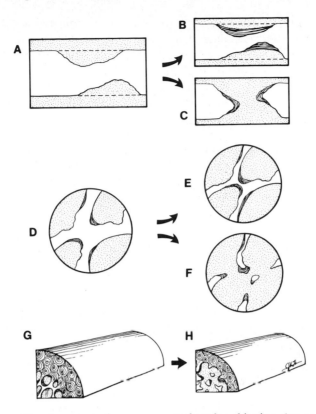

Fig. 8. Irreversible changes in bone mass: trabecular thinning due to incomplete refilling of resorption lacunae ($A \rightarrow B$) or trabecular perforation ($A \rightarrow C$). Corresponding changes at the tissue level are shown in D, E, F. Cortical bone undergoes irreversible bone loss due to thinning of cortex ($G \rightarrow H$). (Reproduced with permission from ERIKSEN et al. 1987)

trabeculae may sometimes undergo perforation, which occurs either through one lacuna penetrating from one side, or two lacunae meeting each other midway through the trabeculum (PARFITT 1984) (Fig. 13). The statistical probability for perforation depends on (PARFITT 1984; ERIKSEN 1986): (a) the activation frequency, (b) the depth of the lacunae, and (c) the thickness of the trabeculae. Every time a trabeculum is perforated, a certain amount of trabecular bone is irreversibly lost. Gradually, plates are converted into a lattice of bars and rods (ARNOLD 1980), some of which in turn may be transsected or completely removed (Fig. 8). All these stages of events have been demonstrated by scanning electron microscopy (DEMPSTER et al. 1986; MOSEKILDE and SOEGAARD 1990).

The predominant affection of bones rich in cancellous bone in high-turnover metabolic bone disease is probably caused by excessive trabecular perforation in this compartment.

An age-related decrease in trabecular plate density (MTPD) and an increase in mean trabecular plate separation (MTPS) have been found (PARFITT 1984; PARISIEN et al. 1988), suggesting that age-related bone loss in iliac crest is also primarily the result of loss of whole structural bone. Similiar suggestions have been made using a computerized model (GARRAHAN et al. 1985) expressing different trabecular two-dimensional, sectional components as nodes, free ends, and struts (COMPSTON et al. 1987, 1989; MELLISH et al. 1989).

In trabecular bone the thickness of bone structural units decreases with advancing age (COURPRON et al. 1981; LIPS et al. 1978). This is, however, associated with a reduction in erosion depth (ERIKSEN et al. 1985a). The reduction in erosion depth, however, outweighs the reduction in mean wall thickness, resulting in a net thinning of trabeculae. Trabecular thickness does not, however, decrease significantly with age (BIRKENHAGER-FRENKL et al. 1986; PARFITT 1983, 1984). This apparent discrepancy is caused by the occurrence of trabecular perforations. Mathematical modeling of the bone loss mechanisms suggests that thin trabeculae are probably removed completely by perforative resorption (REEVE 1986), and this may lead to the lack of change or even increase in trabecular thickness.

The disintegration of trabecular architecture caused by trabecular perforations was primarily observed in whole vertebral bodies in carefully performed inspection studies by Arnold and coworkers (ARNOLD 1968; ARNOLD and WEI 1972; ARNOLD et al. 1966) and others (BROMLEY et al. 1966; ATKINSON 1967; AMSTUTZ and SISSONS 1969; BEDDOE et al. 1976; PESCH et al. 1977). Arnold suggested that the observed changes in bone structure were caused by perforations of trabeculae. This was later supported by others groups using different techniques (PRETEUX et al. 1985; BERGOT et al. 1988; LI. MOSEKILDE 1988).

Estimation of marrow space star volume of iliac crest confirms that bone loss in iliac crest leads to topological changes due to removal of whole bone components (VESTERBY 1990). The age-related structural changes in iliac crest are, however, less pronounced than those in vertebral body, probably reflecting differences in function and loads throughout life.

A recent study by VOGEL et al. (1990) suggests that intertrabecular connectivity was much better in our ancestors. The study was based on 900-year-old skeletons, where age, sex, and sociological status were known. When compared with autopsy data from today, a higher peak bone mass in the older skeletons was found. In the 900-year-old bones trabecular bone volume still decreased with age, but TBV was higher in the lower than in the higher social classes.

III. Bone Turnover and Bone Loss

Several studies have demonstrated that increased bone turnover leads to a negative bone balance and bone loss. In a mixed material of high and low turnover, CHARLES et al. (1985) used a combined calcium balance and calcium kinetics study to investigate the relation between calcium balance (B) and calcium accretion rate (m). When analyzing the regression of m on B they found that the regression line revealed a significant lower slope than the line of identity. Thus, in this material increased turnover led to negative bone balance. The same holds for osteoporotics. In a study on 58 osteoporotics, ERIKSEN et al. (1990) found an increase in negative balance with increased turnover. These findings probably reflect a combination of changes in porosity and the increased risk for trabecular perforations with increased turnover.

N. Implications for Bone Mass Measurements

Due to the differences in architecture and bone remodeling, cortical and cancellous bone have different mechanisms of bone loss, which may lead to different alterations in bone densitometry in different areas of the skeleton dependent on the proportion of cancellous to cortical bone (RIGGS et al. 1981). Changes in turnover not only lead to changes in porosity and absolute bone mass, but also affect the mean bone age. As older bone is more heavily mineralized than younger bone, changes in mean bone age introduce an extra variable (PARFITT 1980; FROST 1989; JEROME 1989). Mathematical modeling based on the histomorphometry data available suggests that bone mass measurements may be out by 40% from "true" bone mass in extreme cases; more commonly, however, the deviation amounts to 5%–15% (PARFITT 1980; FROST 1989). It is important to take these processes into consideration if one is dealing with bone density measurements, otherwise false conclusions may be reached.

When analyzing the changes in bone mass obtained using different treatment regimens, three different patterns stand out (Fig. 9). One variant shows a 5%–10% increase in bone mass after 1 year, then bone mass levels off and ultimately starts to decrease. This initial increase is explained by a lowering of bone turnover leading to an apparent increase in bone mass. Ultimately after 2–3 years, however, the age-dependent bone loss offsets the initial gain and bone mass goes down again. This pattern is seen in some reports on bone mass changes after antiresorptive therapy [estrogen/gestagen (MUNK JENSEN et al. 1988), bisphosphonates (STORM et al. 1990), calcitonin (MARIE et al. 1985)]. Other papers dealing with the effects of antiresorptive therapy describe the same initial gain in bone mass at around 5%–10%, but then bone mass remaining constant (LINDSAY et al. 1980). Provided no change of radiation source in the BMD apparatus or mean bone age occurs, this pattern can only be explained by a certain anabolic effect superceding the age-dependent bone loss. The third pattern shows a gradual increase in bone mass over the treatment period. This development is explained by a pronounced anabolic effect leading to pronounced changes in bone balance,

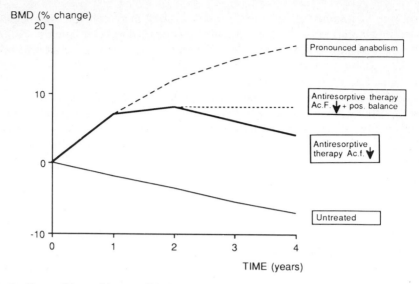

Fig. 9. Reversible and irreversible bone loss and bone measurements. Characteristic patterns for changes in bone mineral density (*BMD*)

and so far has only been reported after treatment with fluoride (Riggs et al. 1990) or parathyroid hormone (Neer et al. 1990).

O. Physiological Ageing Processes in Bone: Differences Between Females and Males

Bone undergoes changes in three-dimensional structure during ageing, and these changes have a profound impact on the physical characteristics of the tissue. These processes start around the age of 25–30 years, where the maximal bone mass (peak bone mass is achieved). In later years new technologies have made the study of these changes possible. These studies have shown that cortical and cancellous bone react differently to the ageing process. Moreover, the pattern of bone loss in the two sexes exhibits significant differences.

When peak bone mass has been reached in normal adults, a steady decline in bone mass sets in around the age of 30 years for both men and women (Courpron et al. 1977; Melsen and Mosekilde 1978).

I. Bone Loss in Cortical Bone

The decrease in bone mass leads to thinning of cortical bone due to tunneling or trabeculation of the endosteal cortical envelope with expansion of the marrow cavity accompanied by some periosteal bone gain (Sedlin et al.

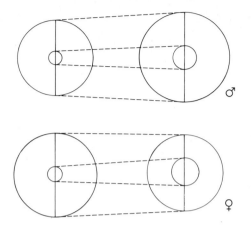

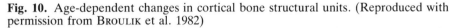

Fig. 10. Age-dependent changes in cortical bone structural units. (Reproduced with permission from BROULIK et al. 1982)

1963; SEDLIN 1964). The mean net loss at the cortical endosteal surface of the metacarpal has been found to be 50 μm/year between the ages of 40 and 70 years in normal female subjects (RIGGS et al. 1981). The mean thickness of the cortical ring of vertebral body also shows an age-related decline (VESTERBY et al. 1991b).

Studies on changes in cortical osteons have demonstrated differences in bone loss mechanisms between the two sexes (BROULIK et al. 1982). Males exhibit an age-dependent increase in resorptive activity leading to an increased osteon diameter. Mean thickness of bone formed in the osteon remained constant with age. Thus, a trend towards a more negative balance between resorption and formation as reflected in an increased haversian canal diameter was detectable (BROULIK et al. 1982) (Fig. 10). Women revealed reduced resorptive activity as reflected in a decrease in osteon diameter with age, but contrary to men, mean thickness of bone went down with age, leading to a pronounced negative balance and increase in haversian canal diameter (Fig. 10) (BROULIK et al. 1982).

II. Bone Loss in Cancellous Bone

The trabecular bone structure of vertebral bodies can be considered a lattice with longitudinal trabeculae supported by horizontally orientated trabeculae. From 20 to 80 years of age a decrease of about 45% in fractional volume of trabecular bone (BV/TV%) is seen (MOSEKILDE and MOSEKILDE 1988), which is accompanied by a decrease in mean thickness of the horizontal trabeculae with no significant changes in mean thickness of vertically orientated trabeculae (LI. MOSEKILDE 1988). An increase in thickness of vertically orientated trabeculae was, however, observed by BERGOT et al. (1988). Furthermore, an increase in the two-dimensional distance between the horizontal trabeculae has been observed for both men and women, which was even slightly greater for women. The age-related increase in distance between the vertical trabeculae do not show sex differences (LI. MOSEKILDE 1988).

Histomorphometry on histological sections from vertebral bodies have confirmed an age-related decrease in mean trabecular bone thickness from 106 μm at 22 years of age to 74 μm at 87 years of age (VESTERBY et al. 1991b). Moreover, a decrease in trabecular star volume was found. More important, however, a pronounced age-related increase in marrow space star volume was demonstrable, which was significantly greater for women than for men (women, 1.93 mm^3/year; men, 1.11 mm^3/year; $2p < 0.02$), demonstrating a clear sex-related difference in the change of trabecular bone structure with a more pronounced destruction of normal trabecular architecture in women than in men with age (Fig. 11) (VESTERBY 1990). These findings corroborate the results reported by AARON et al. (1987) and are consistent with a trend towards a higher erosion depth in perimenopausal women than in men at the same age (ERIKSEN et al. 1985a). This feature of female resorption around menopause combined with the increase in bone turnover is probably the underlying mechanism behind more pronounced disintegration of bone structure in women.

Changes in structure comparable to those observed in the vertebral body have also been described for iliac crest trabecular bone. Little is known about structural changes in the femoral head and column. There is evidence, however, to suggest a different pattern of structural changes (PARFITT et al. 1983). The structural changes seen in the iliac crest are less pronounced than those of the vertebral bodies. The fractional volume of trabecular bone is about 10% higher in the iliac crest. The age-related decrease is, however, parallel to that of the vertebral body and a correlation between the fractional volume of trabecular bone of vertebral body and iliac crest trabecular bone has been demonstrated (MOSEKILDE and MOSEKILDE 1988; MEUNIER et al. 1973a; PØDENPHANT et al. 1986).

Iliac crest trabeculae are thicker than trabeculae in the vertebral body (VESTERBY 1990; PØDENPHANT et al. 1986). Men tend to have thicker trabeculae than women. In general, no age-related changes of mean trabecular thickness are seen either for women or for men (VESTERBY et al. 1989a; PARFITT et al. 1983; AARON et al. 1987; BIRKENHAGER-FRENKL et al. 1988; GARRAHAN et al. 1987). On the contrary, women past 50 years of age show a tendency towards increased mean trabecular thickness just as they exhibit a greater "amount" of thicker trabeculae than younger women (VESTERBY et al. 1989a). This change toward thicker trabeculae in the oldest individuals has also been noted by others (PARFITT et al. 1983; BIRKENHAGER-FRENKL et al. 1988; WAKAMATSU and SISSONS 1969) and the observation is in agreement with the "three-way rule" as proposed by FROST (1990). (This rule predicts a compensatory hypertrophy of remaining trabeculae due to local mechanical loads.)

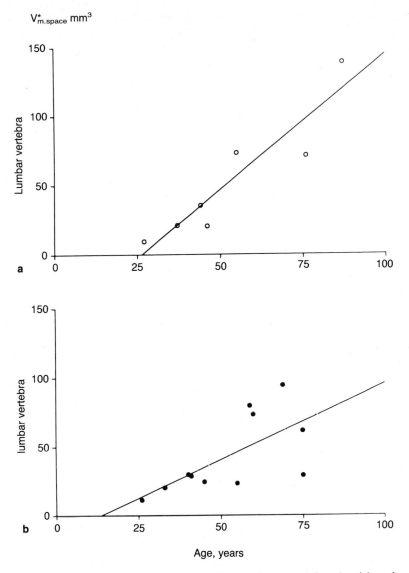

Fig. 11. Changes in marrow star volume with age in normal females (**a**) and males (**b**). Note the more pronounced increase in women

P. Relationship Between Bone Structure and Bone Strength

Several observations suggest that bone strength and fracture risk depend on bone structure (BARTLEY et al. 1966; WEAVER and CHALMERS 1966; BELL et al. 1967; GALANTE et al. 1970; TWOMEY et al. 1983; PARFITT 1987). The compressive strength of the vertebral column and its relationship to bone structural changes has attracted considerable interest due to the increased risk of vertebral fractures in patients with osteoporosis.

I. Cancellous Bone

In vitro studies have demonstrated an age-related decrease in vertebral compressive strength. From the age of 20 to 80 years a 60%–65% decline in load values can thus be seen (MOSEKILDE and MOSEKILDE 1990). There is no sex difference in the rate of decline, but overall men display higher maximum load values than women due to a larger cross-sectional area of vertebral body. The male skeleton is also bigger than the female skeleton.

The compressive strength of vertebral bodies may be a good indicator of vertebral fracture risk, but vertebral body strength cannot be tested in vivo. In normals, however, the average vertebral body compressive strength can be estimated from mechanical tests on iliac crest bone cylinders (MOSEKILDE and MOSEKILDE 1986). It is not yet known whether the same holds for patients with osteoporosis or other metabolic bone diseases.

The age-related decrease in vertebral bone compressive strength is accompanied by a decrease in bone mass. The decline in fractional volume of trabecular bone is 48% from age 20 to 80 years (MOSEKILDE and MOSEKILDE 1988). This reduction is less than the corresponding changes in load values within the same age span, which suggests that structural changes also contribute to the decrease in bone strength seen in normal individuals with age. Moreover, mechanical tests have shown that stress values (= load/area) of whole veretebral bodies are higher than stress values of trabecular bone per se (MOSEKILDE and MOSEKILDE 1986) but with a parallel decline, suggesting that cortical bone becomes of relative greater importance for whole vertebral body strength with age.

The indirect evidence for the importance of vertebral bone structure for vertebral bone strength has recently been corroborated by direct methods (i.e., marrow space star volume measurements) (VESTERBY et al. 1991b). The in vitro strength of the second lumbar vertebra was found related not only to ash density (g/cm^3) and fractional volume of trabecular bone (BV/TV) but also to mean trabecular thickness (Tb.Th), trabecular star volume (V^*_{tr}), marrow space star volume ($V^*_{m.space}$), and mean thickness of the cortical ring of the first lumbar vertebra. Furthermore, multiple regression analysis considering all the measured parameters including the individual's age, sex, height, and weight disclosed that the cortical ring became of primary importance for the compressive strength of the whole vertebral body for normal individuals. Thus, the in vitro compressive strength of the second lumbar vertebra could be predicted from cortical bone, ash density, and surface area with a coefficient of determination (r^2) of 0.92, when the height and sex of the individual were known. The more pronounced disintegration of the trabecular network may therefore not only explain why women have a higher risk of osteoporotic vertebral fractures than men, but also why women are more dependent on cortical bone than men for maintaining the biomechanical competence of vertebral bodies. Further studies on this issue are, however, still needed to confirm this observation primarily to investigate the influence of age on the measured parameters.

The importance of cortical bone for bone strength has previously been proposed by others (ROCKOFF et al. 1967, 1969; MAZESS 1990) based on bone mineral measurements of the spine. Our observations do not confirm the observation of KALENDER et al. (1989), who found that only women lost cortical bone. When choosing regimes for treatment or prevention of osteoporotic vertebral fractures, it may be important to avoid trials which have undesirable effects on cortical bone.

Little is known about structural changes in patients with osteoporosis and metabolic bone diseases. It is well known that patients with osteoporosis on average have lower bone mass compared to age-matched normal individuals (PARFITT et al. 1983; COURPRON et al. 1977), but a great overlap exists. It is therefore important to focus on bone structure and quality of bones. Previously, histomorphometric studies (PARFITT et al. 1983; ARNOLD 1980; KLEEREKOOPER et al. 1985) have indicated that the primary difference between normal individuals and osteoporotic patients is a change of trabecular connectivity with a greater distance between the trabeculae, at least in iliac crest specimens.

Q. Bone Remodeling in Metabolic Bone Disease

The bone loss of most metabolic bone diseases is explained by changes in remodeling leading to changes in bone balance at the BMU and tissue level. It is obvious that the complete study of a given metabolic bone disease should include data on cortical bone remodeling, since cortical bone constitutes 80% of the skeleton. Due to the slower turnover (cortical bone constitutes only 50% of whole skeletal turnover), however, and different architecture the data are more difficult to obtain. The first studies trying to combine data obtained from cortical and cancellous bone have been published (DELMAS et al. 1988; PARFITT et al. 1985). Theoretically they should be better correlated to whole skeletal turnover, and this has also been proven experimentally (DELMAS et al. 1988).

Bone remodeling in metabolic bone diseases is conveniently described by the mean wall thickness as a measure of formative activity, and resorption depth as a measure of resorptive activity, bone balance, and activation frequency. Tissue level bone turnover will be the product of cellular activity and activation frequency, and as described above activation frequency is the most important determinant of tissue level turnover. Finally, the mineralization lag time is given as an index of mineralization defects. Figure 12 shows an example of the use of remodeling curves in the analysis of metabolic

Thickness, μm

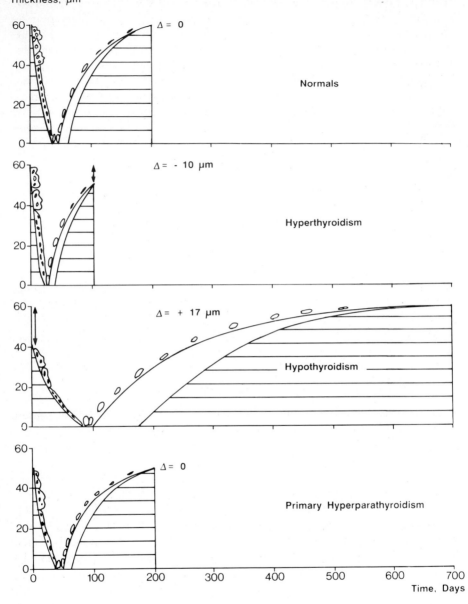

Fig. 12. Reconstruction of the remodeling sequence in different metabolic bone diseases. (Reproduced with permission from ERIKSEN et al. 1989)

Table 2. Bone remodeling of cortical and cancellous bone in different metabolic bone diseases

Disease	W.Th	E.De	Dt.BMU	Mlt	Ac.F
Thyrotoxicosis					
Cancellous	↓	→	Negative	→	↑
Hypothyroidism					
Cancellous	↑	↓	Positive	↑	↓
Cortical	↑	↑	0	?	→
Primary hyperparathyroidism					
Cancellous	↓	↓	0 (negative)	→	↑
Cortical	→	→	0	?	↑
Secondary hyperparathyroidism					
Cancellous	↓	↑	Negative	→(↑)	↑
Acromegaly					
Cancellous	?	?	Positive	→	↑
Cortical	↓	↓	0	?	(↑)
Osteomalacia					
Cancellous	?	?	?	→	↑
Cortical	↓	↓	Positive	↑	↓
Corticosteroid induced osteopenia					
Cancellous	↓	?	Negative	→	↓ ↑
Osteoporosis					
Cancellous	↓	→	Negative	→	(↑)
Cortical	→	→	0	→	→

W.Th, mean wall thickness; E.De, erosion depth; Dt.BMU, balance; Mlt, mineralization lag time; Ac.F, activation frequency.

bone disease. Table 2 represents a summary of our current knowledge about bone remodeling in metabolic bone disease. The data are mainly based on analysis of cancellous bone, but when available, data from cortical bone are given.

I. High and Low Turnover Bone Disease

The combination of a negative balance and increased bone turnover (ADAMS and JOWSEY 1967; MEUNIER et al. 1973b; MELSEN and MOSEKILDE 1977; L. MOSEKILDE et al. 1977a; MOSEKILDE and MELSEN 1978; ERIKSEN et al. 1985b) makes thyrotoxicosis a state of accelerated irreversible bone loss (Fig. 12, Table 2).

The opposite is seen in hypothyroidism, where a significant positive balance is achieved (Fig. 12), but due to the low turnover only small increases in bone turnover occur (ERIKSEN et al. 1985d; ERIKSEN 1986). Mineralization lag time is increased, but this is not caused by a mineralization defect, but rather reflects the profound prolongation of the formative period. In cortical bone both erosion depth and wall thickness are increased and balanced (BROULIK et al. 1982).

Bone turnover is increased in primary hyperparathyroidism (MEUNIER et al. 1972, 1978; MELSEN et al. 1977; ERIKSEN et al. 1986). The wall thickness is reduced (CHARHON et al. 1982; ERIKSEN et al. 1986), but so is resorption depth (ERIKSEN et al. 1986). Bone balance at the level of individual BMUs is therefore preserved, at least in younger individuals (Fig. 12) (ERIKSEN et al. 1986), while a slight negative balance has been demonstrated in older women (CHRISTIANSEN et al. 1990). In cortical bone, erosion depth and wall thickness are similar to those of age-matched normals (BROULIK et al. 1982, Table 2).

Detailed analyses of the bone remodeling sequence in secondary hyperparathyroidism have not been provided yet, but judging from other data available a significant negative balance is present (RAO et al. 1983; SHERRARD et al. 1974; MELSEN and NIELSEN 1977; NILSSON et al. 1985). Due to the extensive tunneling resorption seen in overt secondary hyperparathyroidism, erosion depth has been listed as increased. Secondary hyperparathyroidism is most often seen in association with varying degrees of osteomalacia (SHERRARD et al. 1974; RAO et al. 1983; NILSSON et al. 1985); therefore the mineralization lag time has been listed as being either normal or increased. Recent data by BOYCE et al. (1989) suggest that sufficient levels of vitamin D protect against tunneling resorption in the face of PTH excess. This may explain the beneficial effects of vitamin D supplementation in treatment regimens exploiting the anabolic action of PTH (NEER et al. 1990; REEVE et al. 1985).

No data no wall thickness or resorption depth are currently available from patients with acromegaly, but bone turnover and bone mass have been reported being increased (HALSE et al. 1981). Osteoblastic activity is increased and in cortical bone erosion depth and wall thickness are reduced and balanced (HALSE et al. 1981; BROULIK et al. 1982) (Table 2).

The histological diagnosis of osteomalacia is based on the concurrent presence of two abnormalities: (1) increased mineralization lag time and (2) increased osteoid width (PARFITT et al. 1985a; MELSEN and MOSEKILDE 1980; ERIKSEN et al. 1989). Using only Mlt as the criterion may lead to error in other low turnover stages (e.g., hypothyroidism) and using osteoid width alone may lead to error in high turnover states (e.g., thyrotoxicosis, primary hyperparathyrodism) (ERIKSEN et al. 1989). No data on wall thickness of erosion depth in osteomalcia are currently available. As mentioned above, most osteomalacic states also exhibit bone changes caused by compensatory secondary hyperparathyroidism. In end stage osteomalacia, where the compensation by PTH fails, however, bone turnover is suppressed. Analyses in cortical bone obtained from patients on anticonvulsants have revealed reduced erosion depth and wall thickness, and a positive bone balance (BROULIK et al. 1982) (Table 2).

In long-standing corticosteroid-induced osteopenia a clear reduction of wall thickness has been demonstrated (DEMPSTER et al. 1983) in accordance with the suppression of bone formation (MELSEN and NIELSEN 1977). Bone turnover is decreased (BRESSOT et al. 1979; HODGSON 1990). The acute effects of corticosteroid administration are dominated by secondary hyper-parathyrodism (FINDLING et al. 1982) (Table 2).

II. Bone Remodeling in Osteoporosis

Very few studies have compared bone remodeling in osteoporosis with age- and sex-matched normals. Studies on cortical osteon in osteoporosis revealed no significant changes in osteon diameter or haversian canal diameter when compared with age-matched controls. Thus, for this envelope no negative balance was demonstrable (BROULIK et al. 1982) (Table 2).

ARLOT et al. (1984) demonstrated reduced mean wall thickness in osteoporotics, but could not demonstrate any significant differences with respect to other histomorphometric indices. ERIKSEN et al. (1985c) demonstrated a significant negative bone balance per remodeling cycle in osteoporotics, while STEINICHE et al. (1989) were unable to demonstrate any significant remodeling imbalance. No age-matched material was, however, used as reference in any of the two studies.

In a recent study (ERIKSEN et al. 1990), bone biopsies obtained from 58 osteoporotics were compared with biopsies from 26 age- and sex-matched normals. Mean resorption depth and mean wall thickness were measured in the two groups as well as tetracycline-based indices. Osteoporotics exhibited a slight, although not significant, increase in resorption depth ($p < 0.10$). The activation frequency was also increased, but not significantly so. The most marked difference between the two groups was a pronounced reduction in mean wall thickness in the osteoprotic group ($35\,\mu$m vs. $50\,\mu$m in normals) leading to a pronounced remodeling imbalance (Fig. 13). When bone balance in normals and osteoporotics was compared, osteoporotics in most cases showed values below the line of identity, while all normals exhibited balance values around the line of identity (Fig. 18).

These findings suggest some kind of osteoblastic defect in osteoporotics along the lines proposed by ARLOT et al. (1984). In normals, osteoblasts are able to balance resorptive activity, but in osteoporotics every resorption site is not completely "refilled," which leads to pronounced thinning of trabeculae and eventually removal of the thin trabecular structures by perforative resorption.

R. Final Remarks and Future Perspectives

Osteoporosis is a major public health problem and many programs aim at preventing this disease or aim at reducing risks for future fractures. Fracture risk is generally connected to bone loss and destruction of normal trabecular architecture. Disrupture of normal trabecular connectivity is caused by loss of whole structural bone through a process of osteoclastic perforation of trabeculae. Therapeutic trials and prevention programs are therefore aiming

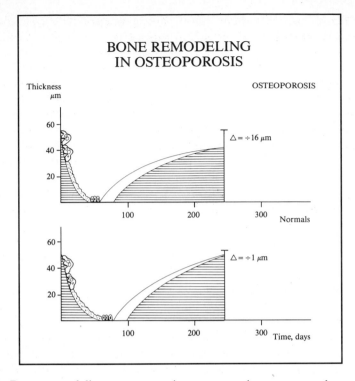

Fig. 13. Bone remodeling sequences in osteoporotic women and age-matched controls. Note the more pronounced negative balance in osteoporotics. (Reconstruction based on data from ERIKSEN et al. 1990). (Reproduced with permission from ERIKSEN, Osteoporosis, NOVO-Nordisk A/S, 1992)

to prevent bone loss and reduce events in the remodeling process which increase the risk of trabecular perforation. With established osteoporosis, attempts have also been made to increase bone mass by increasing bone formation using, e.g., fluoride or parathyroid hormone.

Further research on the regulation of the coupling process and possible ways by which osteoclast-osteoblast interaction may be manipulated holds one of the keys to more successful treatment of osteopenia in the future. FROST (1979) was the first to propose manipulation of the coupling process as a means of increasing bone mass. He introduced the term ADFR (activation-depression-free repeat) to denote a treatment regimen aiming at creating large numbers of individual BMUs each with a possible balance. In practice an increased number of BMUs are created by treatment with an "activator" (mitogenic agents like parathyroid hormone, growth hormone, or thyroid hormone). According to the ARF sequence, however, an increase in the number of BMUs will lead to an initial increase in bone resorption. Therefore, in order to inhibit bone resorption during that phase, a "depressor" of osteoclastic resorption (e.g., bisphosphonates or calcitonin) is given while resorption is thought to proceed (2–4 weeks). The hope was to create a large number of shallow lacunae, which subsequently in theory should undergo "overfilling" during the "free period," where bone formation is thought to proceed without interference. This "overfilling" should then gradually lead to trabecular thickening and increased bone mass.

In the ADFR regimens reported so far, however, the general problem has been the fact that the inhibition of bone resorption also led to a coupled inhibition of bone formation. Moreover, osteoclastic inhibition also led to inhibition of activation. Thus, no definite positive balance has been demonstrable in the ADFR regimens used so far (ALOIA et al. 1987; MARIE et al. 1985; STEINICHE et al. 1991). The increases in bone mass have not exceeded what would be expected from a reduction in activation of new BMUs.

In contrast to the pessimistic results of classical ADFR regimens, cyclic regimens have gained increased recognition as means by which bone mass can be increased. Positive results have been reported for cyclic PTH together with $1,25(OH)_2D_3$ (NEER et al. 1990) and for bisphosphonates (STORM et al. 1990).

Irrespective of what treatment is chosen, a main final goal will be to reduce fracture risk. If this risk can be reduced not only by preventing or increasing bone mass but also by improving trabecular bone structure it is necessary to have tools which can evaluate or demonstrate changes in trabecular bone structure. The stereological parameter the marrow space star volume is the most sensitive tool/parameter in this respect. Unfortunately, noninvasive techniques yielding data on trabecular continuity have not been devised so far.

References

Aaron JE, Makins NB, Sagreiya K (1987) The microanatomy of trabecular bone loss in normal ageing men and women. Clin Orthop 215:260–271

Adams P, Jowsey J (1967) Bone and mineral metabolism in hyperthyroidism: an experimental study. Endocrinology 81:735–740

Agerbæk MO, Eriksen EF, Kragstrup J, Mosekilde L, Melsen F (1991) Reconstruction of the remodeling sequence in normal human cortical bone. Bone Miner 12:101–112

Aloia JF, Vaswani A, Meunier PJ, Edouard CM, Arlot ME, Yeh JK, Cohn SH (1987) Coherence treatment of postmenopausal osteoporosis with growth hormone and calcitonin. Calcif Tissue Int 40:253–259

Amstutz HC, Sissons HA (1969) The structure of vertebral spongiosa. J Bone Joint Surg [Br] 51:540–550

Arlot M, Edouard C, Meunier PJ, Neer R, Reeve J (1984) Impaired osteoblast function in osteoporosis: comparison between calciu balance and dynamic histomorphometry. Br Med J 289:517–520

Arnold JS (1968) External and trabecular morphologic changes in lumbar vertebrae in aging. In: Whedon GD, Cameron JR (eds) Progress in methods of bone mineral measurements. US Department of Health, Education and Welfare, Bethesda, p 370

Arnold JS (1980) Trabecular pattern and shapes in aging and osteoporosis. Metab Bone Dis Rel Res 2S:297–308

Arnold JS, Wei CT (1972) Quantitative morphology of vertebral trabecular bone. In: Stover BJ, Jee WSS (eds) Radiobiology of plutonium. JW, Salt Lake City, p 333

Arnold JS, Bartley MH, Tont SA, Jenkins DP (1966) Skeletal changes in aging and disease. Clin Orthop 49:17–38

Atkinson PJ (1967) Variation in trabecular structure of vertebrae with age. Calcif Tissue Res 1:24–32

Baddeley AJ, Gundersen HJG, Cruz Orive LM (1986) Estimation of surface area from vertical sections. J Microsc 142:259–276

Baron R, Vignery A, Lang R (1981a) Reversal phase and osteopenia: defective coupling between resorption and formation in the pathogenesis of osteoporosis. In DeLuca HF, Frost HM, Jee WSS, Johnston CC, Parfitt AM (eds) Osteoporosis, recent advances in pathogenesis and treatment. University Park Press, Baltimore, p 311

Baron R, Vignery A, Tran Van P (1981b) The significance of lacunar erosion without osteoclasts. Studies in the reversal phase of the remodeling sequence. In: Jee WSS, Parfitt AM (eds) Bone histomorphometry, 3rd international workshop. Armour Montagu, Paris, p 35

Bartley MH, Arnold JS, Haslam RK, Jee WSS (1966) The relationship of bone strength and bone quantity in health, disease, and aging. J Gerontol 21:517–521

Beddoe AH, Darley PJ, Spiers FW (1976) Measurements of trabecular bone structure in man. Phys Med Biol 21:589–607

Bell GH, Dunbar O, Beck JS (1967) Variations in strength of vertebrae with age and their relation to osteoporosis. Calcif Tissue Res 1:75–86

Bergot C, Laval-Jeantet AM, Preteux F, Meunier A (1988) Measurement of anistropic vertebral trabecular bone loss during aging by quantitative image analysis. Calcif Tissue Int 43:143–149

Birkenhaeger-Frenkel DH, Courpron P, Clermont E, Hupscher C, Coutinho MF, Meunier PJ (1986) Trabecular thickness, intertrabecular distance and age related bone loss. Bone 6:402

Birkenhager-Frenkel DH, Courpron P, Hupscher EA, Clermonts E, Coutinho MF, Schmitz PIM, Meunier PJ (1988) Age-related changes in cancellous bone structure. A two-dimensional study in transiliac and iliac crest biopsy sites. Bone Miner 5:197–216

Boyce RW, Eriksen EF, Franks AF, Jankowsky ML, Stokes CL (1989) Effects of intermittent hPTH(1-34) alone or in combination with oral $1,25(OH)_2D_3$ on trabecular bone: 3-D reconstruction of the remodeling site. J Bone Miner Res 4:S276

Bressot C, Meunier PJ, Chapuy MC, Lejeune E, Edouard C, Darby AJ (1979) Histomorphometric profile, pathophysiology and reversibility of corticosteroid induced osteoporosis. Metab Bone Dis Rel Res 1:303–311

Bromley RG, Dockum NL, Arnold JS, Jee WSS (1966) Quantitative histological study of human lumbar vertebrae. J Gerontol 21:537–543

Broulik P, Kragstrup J, Mosekilde L, Melsen F (1982) Osteon cross-sectional size in the iliac crest. Acta Path Microbiol Scand Sect A 90:339–344

Charhon SA, Edouard CM, Arlot M, Meunier PJ (1982) Effects of parathyroid hormone on remodeling of iliac trabecular bone packets in patients with primary hyperparathyroidism. Clin Orthop 162:255–263

Charles P, Poser JW, Mosekilde L, Jensen FT (1985) Estimation of bone turnover evaluated by [47]calcium kinetics. Efficiency of serum bone gamma carboxyglutamic acid containing protein, serum alkaline phosphatase and urinary hydroxyproline excretion. J Clin Invest 76:2254–2258

Charles P, Eriksen EF, Mosekilde L, Melsen F, Jensen FT (1987) Bone turnover evaluated by a combined calcium balance and [47]calcium kinetic study and dynamic histomorphometry. Metabolism 36:1118–1124

Christiansen P, Steiniche T, Mosekilde Le, Hessov I, Melsen F (1990) Primary hyperparathyroidism: changes in trabecular bone remodeling following surgical treatment evaluated by histomorphometric methods. Bone 11:75–80

Compston JE, Mellish RWE, Garrahan NJ (1987) Age-related changes in iliac crest trabecular microanatomic bone structure in man. Bone 8:289–292

Compston JE, Mellish RW, Croucher P, Newcombe R, Garrahan NJ (1989) Structural mechanisms of trabecular bone loss in man. Bone Miner 6:339–350

Courpron P, Meunier P, Bressot C, Giroux JM (1977) Amount of bone in iliac crest biopsy. Significance of the trabecular bone volume. Its value in normal and in pathological conditions. In: Meunier PJ (ed) Bone histomorphometry, 2nd international workshop. Armour Montagu, Paris, p 39

Courpron P, Lepine P, Arlot M, Lips R, Meunier PJ (1981) Mechanisms underlying the reduction with age of the mean wall thickness of the trabecular basic structural unit (BSU) in human iliac bone. In: Jee WSS, Parfitt AM (eds) Bone histomorphometry, 3rd international workshop. Armour Montagu, Paris, p 323

Croucher PI, Mellish RWE, Vedi S, Garrahan NJ, Compston J (1989) The relationship between resorption depth and mean interstitial bone thickness: age related changes in man. Calcif Tissue Int 45:15–19

Delmas PD, Demiaux B, Arlot MA, Edouard C, Malaval L, Meunier PJ (1990) Relationship between bone histomorphometric parameters and biochemical markers of bone turnover. In: Takahashi HE (ed) Bone histomorphometry, Nishimura Niigata, Japan, Smith Gordon, London, p 488

Dempster DW, Arlot MN, Meunier PJ (1983) Mean wall thickness and bone formation periods of trabecular bone packets in corticosteroid induced osteoporosis. Calcif Tissue Int 35:410–415

Dempster DW, Shane E, Horbert W, Lindsay R (1986) A simple method for correlative light and scanning electron microscopy of human iliac crest bone biopsies: qualitative observations in normal and osteoporotic subjects. J Bone Miner Res 1:15–21

D'Souza DM, Ibbotson KJ, Twardzik DR et al. (1986) Transforming growth factor beta (TGF-beta) resorbs bone and is produced by osteoblast like cells. J Bone Miner Res 1:74

Eriksen EF (1986) Normal and pathological remodeling of human trabecular bone: three dimensional reconstruction of the remodeling sequence in normals and in metabolic bone disease. Endocr Rev 7:379–408

Eriksen EF (1992) Osteoporosis. Novo-Nordisk A/S,

Eriksen EF, Melsen F, Mosekilde L (1984a) Reconstruction of the resorptive site in iliac trabecular bone: a kinetic model for bone resorption in 20 normal individuals. Metab Bone Dis Rel Res 5:235–242

Eriksen EF, Gundersen HJG, Melsen F, Mosekilde L (1984b) Reconstruction of the formative site in iliac trabecular bone in 20 normal individuals employing a kinetic model for matrix and mineral apposition. Metab Bone Dis Rel Res 5:243–252

Eriksen EF, Mosekilde L, Melsen F (1985a) Trabecular bone resorption depth decreases with age: differences between normal males and females. Bone 6: 141–146

Eriksen EF, Mosekilde L, Melsen F (1985b) Trabecular bone remodeling and bone balance in hyperthyroidism. Bone 6:421–428

Eriksen EF, Mosekilde L, Melsen F (1985c) Effect of sodium fluoride, calcium phosphate and vitamin D_2 on trabecular bone balance and remodeling in osteoporosis. Bone 6:381–389

Eriksen EF, Mosekilde L, Melsen F (1985d) Kinetics of trabecular bone resorption and formation in hypothyroidism: evidence for a positive balance per remodeling cycle. Bone 7:101–108

Eriksen EF, Mosekilde L, Melsen F (1986) Trabecular bone remodeling and bone balance in primary hyperparathyroidism. Bone 7:213–221

Eriksen EF, Kumar EV, Riggs BL (1987) New developments in medicine, vol 2. Bender, New York, pp 11–23

Eriksen EF, Steiniche T, Mosekilde L, Melsen F (1989) Histomorphometric analysis of bone in metabolic bone disease. Endocrinol Metab Clin North Am 18: 919–954

Eriksen EF, Hodgson SF, Eastell R, Cedel SR, O'Fallon WM, Riggs BL (1990) Cancellous bone remodeling in type I (postmenopausal) osteoporosis: quantitative assessment of rates of formation, resorption and bone loss at tissue and cellular levels. J Bone Miner Res 5:311–319

Farley JR, Wergedal JE, Baylink DJ (1983) Fluoride directly stimulates proliferation and alkaline phosphatase activity of bone forming cells. Science 222:330–332

Findling JW, Adams ND, Leman L (1982) Vitamin D metabolites and parathyroid hromone in Cushing's syndrome: relationship to calcium and phosphorous metabolism. J Clin Endocrinol Metab 54:1034–1044

Frost HM (1964) Dynamics of bone remodeling. In: Frost HM (ed) Bone biodynamics. Little Brown, Boston, pp 315–333

Frost HM (1969) Tetracycline based histological analysis of bone remodeling. Calcif Tissue Res 3:211–237

Frost HM (1979) Treatment of osteoporoses by manipulation of coherent cell populations. Clin Orthop 143:227–244

Frost HM (1989) Some effects of basic multicellular unit-based remodelling on photon absorptiometry of trabecular bone. Bone Miner 7:47–65

Frost HM (1990) Structural adaptation to mechanical usage. Anat Rec 222:403–439

Frost HM, Villanueva AR (1962) Human osteoclastic activity: qualitative histological measurement. Henry Ford Hosp Med Bull 10:229–246

Frost HM, Villanueva AR, Jaworski ZF, Meunier P, Schimizu AG (1969) Evaluation of cellular level Haversian bone resorption in human hyperparathyroid states. Henry Ford Hosp Med J 17:259–266

Galante J, Rostoker W, Ray RD (1970) Physical properties of trabecular bone. Calcif Tissue Res 5:236–246

Garn SM, Rohmann CG, Wagner B, Ascoli W (1967) Continuing bone growth throughout life: a general phenomenon. J Phys Anthropol 26:313–318

Garrahan NJ, Mellish RWE, Compston JE (1985) A new method for the two-dimensional analysis of bone structure in human iliac crest biopsies. J Microsc 142:341–349

Garrahan NJ, Mellish RWE, Vedi S, Compston JE (1987) Measurement of mean trabecular plate thickness by a new computerized method. Bone 8:227–230

Garrahan NJ, Croucher PI, Compston J (1990) A computerized technique for the quantitative assessment of resorption cavities in trabecular bone. Bone 11: 241–245

Gundersen HJG, Jensen EB (1985) Stereological estimation of the volume-weighted mean volume of arbitrary particles observed on random sections. J Microsc 138:127–142

Gundersen HJG, Bagger P, Bendtsen TF, Evans SM, Korbo L, Marcussen N, Moeller A, Nielsen K, Nyengaard JR, Pakkenberg B, Soerensen FB, Vesterby A, West MJ (1988) The new stereologic tools: disector, fractionator and point sampled intercepts and their use in pathological research and diagnosis. APMIS 96:857–881

Halse J, Melsen F, Mosekilde L (1981) Iliac crest bone mass and remodelling in acromegaly. Acta Endocrinol (Copenh) 97:18–22

Hattner R, Epker BN, Frost HM (1965) Kinetics of osteoclasts and their nuclei in evolving secondary haversian systems. J Anat 133:397–402

Hodgson SF (1990) Corticosteroid induced osteoporosis. In: Tiegs RD (ed) Metabolic bone disease, part II. Endocrinology and metabolism clinics of North America. Saunders Philadelphia, p 95

Hori M, Takahashi T, Konno J, Habs T (1985) A classification of in vivo bone labels after double labeling in canine bones. Bone 6:147–154

Jaworski ZFG (1971) Some morphologic and dynamic aspects of remodelling in endosteal-cortical and trabecular surfaces. In: Menczel J, Harell A (eds) Calcified tissue: structural, functional and metabolic aspects. Academic, New York, p 159

Jaworski ZF, Lok E (1972) The rate of osteoclastic bone resorption in haversian remodeling sites of adult dogs rib. Calcif Tissue Res 10:103–108

Jerome CP (1989) Estimation of bone mineral density variation associated with changes in turnover rate. Calcif Tissue Int 44:406–410

Kalender WA, Felsenberg D, Louis O, Lopez P, Klotz E, Osteaux M, Fraga J (1989) Reference values for trabecular and cortical vertebral bone density in single and dual-energy quantitative computed tomography. Eur J Radiol 9: 75–80

Kimmel DB (1981) A light microscopic description of osteoprogenitor cells of remodeling bone in the adult. Metab Bone Dis Rel Res 2S:181–185

Kleerekoper M, Villanueva AR, Staciu J, Sudhaker Rao D, Parfitt AM (1985) The role of the three-dimensional trabecular microstructure in the pathogenesis of vertebral compression fractures. Calcif Tissue Int 37:594–597

Kragstrup J, Melsen F (1983) Three dimensional morphology of trabecular bone osteons reconstructed from serial sections. Metab Bone Dis Rel Res 5:127–131

Kragstrup J, Gundersen HJG, Mosekilde L, Melsen F (1982) Estimation of the three dimensional wall thickness of completed remodeling sites in iliac trabecular bone. Metab Bone Dis Rel Res 4:113–119

Kragstrup J, Melsen F Mosekilde L (1983a) Thickness of lamellae in normal human iliac trabecular bone. Metab Bone Dis Rel Res 4:291–294

Kragstrup J, Melsen F, Mosekilde L (1983b) Thickness of bone formed at remodeling sites in normal iliac trabecular bone: variations with age and sex. Metab Bone Dis Rel Res 5:17–21

Lindsay R, Hart DM, Forrest C, Baird C (1980) Prevention of spinal osteoporosis in oophorectomized women. Lancet ii:1151–1154

Lips P, Courpron P, Meunier PJ (1978) Mean wall thickness of trabecular bone packets. Metab Bone Dis Rel Res 2:13–17

Marie PJ, Rasmussen H, Kuntz D (1985) Treatment of postmenopausal osteoporosis with phosphate and intermittent calcitonin. In: Christiansen C, Arnaud CD, Nordin BEC, Parfitt AM, Peck WA, Riggs BL (eds) Osteoporosis. Aalborg, Denmark, p 549

Marotti G (1977) Decrement in volume of osteoblasts during osteon formation and its effect on the size of corresponding osteocytes. In: Meunier P (ed) Bone histomorphometry. Armour Montagu, Paris, p 385

Mazess RB (1990) Fracture risk: a role for compact bone. Calcif Tissue Int 47: 191–193

Mellish RW, Garrahan NJ, Compston JE (1989) Age-related changes in trabecular width and spacing in human iliac crest biopsies. Bone Miner 6:331–338

Melsen F, Mosekilde L (1977) Morphometric and dynamic studies of bone changes in hyperthyroidism. APMIS 85:141–150

Melsen F, Mosekilde L (1978) Tetracycline double-labeling of iliac trabecular bone in 41 normal adults. Calcif Tissue Res 26:99–102

Melsen F, Mosekilde L (1980) Trabecular bone mineralization lag time determined by tetracycline double labeling in normal and certain pathological conditions. APMIS 88:83–88

Melsen F, Nielsen HE (1977) Osteonecrosis following renal allotransplantation. APMIS 85:99–105

Melsen F, Mosekilde L, Christensen MS (1977) Interrelationships between bone histomorphometry, S-iPTH and calcium-phosphorous metabolism in primary hyperparathyroidism. Calcif Tissue Res 24S:16–22

Meunier P, Vignon G, Bernard J, Edouard C, Courpron P, Porte J (1972) La lecture quantitative de la biopsie osseuse moyenne de diagnostic et d'étude de 106 hyperparathyroidies primitives, secondaires et paraneoplasiques. Rev Rhum Mal Osteoartic 39:635–643

Meunier P, Coupron P, Edouard C, Bernard J, Bringuier J, Vignon G (1973a) Physiological senile involution and pathological rarefaction of bone. Clin Endocrinol Metabol 2:239–256

Meunier P, Bianchi CGS, Edouard C, Bernard JC, Courpron PM, Vignon G (1973b) Bone manifestations in thyrotoxicosis. Orthop Clin North Am 3:745–750

Meunier P, Edouard C, Courpron P (1976) Morphometric analysis of trabecular resorption surfaces in normal iliac bone. In: Jaworski ZFG (ed) Bone histomorphometry. University of Ottawa Press, Ottawa, p 156

Meunier PJ, Bressot C, Edouard CM (1978) Dynamics of bone remodeling in primary hyperparathyroidism. In: Copp DH, Talmage RV (eds) Endocrinology of calcium metabolism. Elsevier, Amsterdam, p 415

Mosekilde L, Melsen F (1978) A tetracycline based histomorphomtric evaluation of bone resorption and bone turnover in hyperthyroidism and hyperparathyroidism. Acta Med Scand 204:97–102

Mosekilde L, Melsen F, Bagger JP (1977a) Bone changes in hyperthyroidism: interrelationships between bone morphometry, thyroid function and calcium phosphorous metabolism. Acta Endocrinol 85:515

Mosekilde L, Christensen MS, Lund B (1977b) The interrelationships between serum 25-hydroxycholecalciferol, serum parathyroid hormone and bone changes in anticonvulsant osteomalacia. Acta Endocrinol 84:559

Mosekilde Li (1988) Age related changes in vertebral trabecular bone architecture assessed by a new method. Bone 9:247–250

Mosekilde Li (1990) Consequence of the remodeling process for vertebral trabecular bone structure: a scanning electron microscopy study. Bone Miner 10:13–35

Mosekilde Li, Mosekilde L (1986) Normal vertebral body size and compressive strength: relations to age and vertebral and iliac trabecular body compressive strength. Bone 7:207–212

Mosekilde Li, Mosekilde L (1988) Iliac crest trabecular bone volume as predictor for vertebral compressive strength, ash density and trabecular bone volume in normal individuals. Bone 9:195–199

Mosekilde Li, Mosekilde L (1990) Sex differences in age-related changes in vertebral body size, density and biomechanical competence in normal individuals. Bone 11:67–73

Mosekilde Li, Soegaard C (1990) Consequences of the remodeling process for vertebral trabecular structure and strength. In: Christiansen C, Overgaard K (eds) Osteoporosis 1990. 3rd international symposium on osteoporosis. Osteopress, Copenhagen, pp 607–609

Munk Jensen N, Pors Nielsen S, Obel EB, Bonne Eriksen P (1988) Reversal of postmenopausal vertebral bone loss by oestrogen and progestagen: a double blind placebo controlled study. Br Med J 296:1150–1152

Neer R, Slovik D, Daly M, Lo C, Potts J, Nussbaum S (1990) Treatment of postmenopausal osteoporosis with daily parathyroid hormone plus calcitriol. Proceedings of the 3rd international symposium on osteoporosis. Osteopress, Copenhagen, pp 1314–1317

Nilsson P, Melsen F, Malmaeus J, Danielson BG, Mosekilde L (1985) Relationships between bone aluminum and bone histomorphometry in patients on maintenance dialysis. Bone 6:21–27

Odgaard A, Jensen EB, Gundersen HJG (1990) Estimation of structural anisotropy based on volume orientation. A new concept. J Microsc 157:149–162

Owen M (1971) Cellular dynamics of bone. In: Bourne GH (ed) The biochemistry and physiology of bone, vol 3, 2nd edn. Academic, New York, p 255

Parfitt AM (1979) Quantum concept of bone remodeling and turnover: implications for the pathogenesis of osteoporosis. Calcif Tissue Int 28:1–7

Parfitt AM (1980) Morphologic basis for bone mineral measurements: transient and steady state effects of treatment in osteoporosis. Miner Electrolyte Metab 4: 273–287

Parfitt AM (1982) The coupling of bone formation to bone resorption: a critical analysis of the concept and of its relevance to the pathogenesis of osteoporosis. Metab Bone Dis Rel Res 4:1–2

Parfitt AM (1983) The physiologic and clinical significance of bone histomorphometric data. In: Recker RR (ed) Bone histomorphometry, techniques and interpretation. CRC Press, Boca Raton, pp 143–223

Parfitt AM (1984) Age related structural changes in trabecular and cortical bone: cellular mechanisms and biomechanical consequences. Calcif Tissue Int 36 [Suppl 1]:123–128

Parfitt AM (1987) Trabecular bone architecture in the pathogenesis and prevention of fracture. Am J Med 82 1B:68–72

Parfitt AM, Villanueva AR, Mathew CHE, Aswani SA (1980) Kinetics of matrix and mineral apposition in osteoporosis and renal osteodystrophy. Relationship to rate of turnover and cell morphology. Metab Bone Dis Rel Res 2S:213–219

Parfitt AM, Mathews CHE, Villanueva AR, Kleerekoper M, Frame B, Rao DS (1983) Relationships between surface, volume, and thickness of iliac trabecular bone in aging and in osteoporosis. J Clin Invest 72:1396–1409

Parfitt AM, Rao DS, Stanciu J, Villanueva AR, Kleerekoper M, Frame B (1985) Irreversible bone loss in osteomalacia. J Clin Invest 76:2403–2412

Parfitt AM, Drezner MK, Glorieux FH, Kanis JA, Malluche HM, Meunier P, Ott SM, Recker RR (1987) Bone histomorphomtry: standardization of nomenclature, symbols and units. J Bone Miner Res 2:595–610

Parisien MV, McMahon D, Pushparaj N, Dempster DW (1988) Trabecular architecture in iliac crest bone biopsies: intra-individual variability in structural parameters and changes with age. Bone 9:289–295

Pesch HJ, Henschke F, Seibold H (1977) Einfluss von Mechanik und Alter auf den Spongiosaumbau in Lendenwirbelkörpern und im Schenkelhals. Eine Strukturanalyse. Virchows Arch [A] 377:27–42

Pilbeam CC, Raisz LG (1988) In vitro inhibition of PTH stimulated prostaglandin E_2 production by 17-beta estradiol. J Bone Miner Res 3:S219

Pirok DJ, Ramser JR, Takahashi H, Vilanueva AT, Frost HM (1966) Normal histological tetracycline and dynamic parameters in human mineralized bone sections. Henry Ford Hosp Med Bull 14:195–218

Pødenphant J, Christiansen C (1988) The value of iliac crest biopsy in spinal osteoporosis. A critical view. In: Christiansen C (ed) Osteoporosis. Aalborg, Denmark, p 735

Pødenphant J, Gotfredsen A, Nilas L, Nørgård H, Brændstrup O (1986) Iliac crest biopsy: representativity for the amount of mineralized bone. Bone 7:427–430

Preteux F, Bergot C, Laval-Jeantet AM (1985) Automatic quantification of vertebral cancellous bone remodeling during aging. Anat Clin 7:203–208

Rao DS, Villanueva AR, Mathews M (1983) Histologic evolution of vitamin D depletion in patients with intestinal malabsorption or dietary deficiency. In: Frame B, Potts JT (eds) Clinical disorders of bone and mineral metabolism. Exerpta Medica, Amsterdam, pp 224–226

Reeve J (1986) A stochastic analysis of iliac trabecular bone dynamics. Clin Orthop 213:264–278

Reeve J, Arlot M, Bernard M, Charhon S, Edouard C, Slovik D, Visman FJ, Meunier PJ (1981) Calcium-47 kinetic measurements of bone turnover compared to bone histomorphometry in osteoporosis: the influence of human parathyroid fragment (hPTH 1-34) therapy. Metab Bone Dis Rel Res 3:23–30

Reeve J, Podbesek TR, Price M (1985) Studies on a "short cycle" ADFR regime using parathyroid peptide hPTH 1-34 in idiopathic osteoporosis and in a dog model. In: Christiansen C, Arnaud CD, Nordin BEC, Parfitt AM, Peck WA, Riggs BL (eds) Osteoporosis. Proceedings of the international symposium on osteoporosis. Osteopress, Copenhagen, p 567

Riggs BL, Wahner HW, Dunn WL, Mazess RB, Offord KP, Melton LJ III (1981) Differential changes in bone mineral density of the appendicular and axial skeleton with aging. J Clin Invest 67:328–335

Riggs BL, Hodgson SF, O'Fallon WM, Chao EYS, Wahner HW, Muhs JM, Cedel SL, Melton LJ III (1990) Effect of fluoride treatment on the fracture rate in postmenopausal women with osteoporosis. N Engl J Med 332:802–809

Rockoff SD, Zettner A, Albright J (1967) Radiographic trabecular quantitation of human lumbar vertebrae in situ: II. Relation to bone quantity, strength and mineral content (preliminary results). Invest Radiol 2:339–352

Rockoff SD, Sweet E, Bleustein J (1969) The relative contribution of trabecular and cortical bone to strength of human lumbar vertebrae. Calcif Tissue Res 3:163–175

Sedlin ED (1964) The ratio of cortical area to total cross section area in rib diaphysis. A quantitative index of osteoporosis. Clin Orthop 36:161–168

Sedlin ED, Frost HM, Villanueva AR (1963) Variations in cross-section area of rib cortex with age. J Gerontol 18:9–13

Sherrard DJ, Baylink DJ, Wergedal JE, Maloney NA (1974) Quantitative histological studies on the pathogenesis of uremic bone disease. J Clin Endocrinol Metab 39:119–136

Steiniche T, Hasling C, Charles P, Eriksen EF, Melsen F, Mosekilde L (1989) A randomized study on the effects of estrogen/gestagen or high dose calcium on trabecular bone remodeling in postmenopausal osteoporosis. Bone 10:313–320

Steiniche T, Hasling C, Charles P, Eriksen EF, Mosekilde L, Melsen F (1991) The effects of ethidronate on trabecular bone remodeling in postmenopausal spinal osteoporosis: A randomized study comparing intermittent treatment and an ADFR regime. Bone 12:155–164

Storm T, Thamsborg G, Steiniche T, Genant HK, Sorensen OH (1990) Effect of intermittent cyclical etidronate therapy on bone mass and fracture rate in women with postmenopausal osteoporosis. N Engl J Med 322:1265–1271

Twomey L, Taylor J, Furniss B (1983) Age changes in the bone density and structure of the lumbar vertebral column. J Anat 136:15–25

Vesterby A (1990) Star volume of marrow space and trabeculae in iliac crest: sampling procedure and correlation to star volume of first lumbar vertebra. Bone 11:149–155

Vesterby A, Kragstrup J, Gundersen HJG, Melsen F (1987a) Unbiased stereological estimation of surface density in bone using vertical sections. Bone 8:13–17

Vesterby A, Gundersen HJG, Melsen F (1987b) Unbiased stereological estimation of osteoid and resorption, fractional surfaces in trabecular bone using vertical sections: sampling efficiency and biological variation. Bone 8:333–337

Vesterby A, Gundersen HJG, Melsen F, Mosekilde L (1989a) Normal postmenopausal women show iliac crest trabecular thickening on vertical sections. Bone 10:333–340

Vesterby A, Gundersen HJG, Melsen F (1989b) Star volume of marrow space and trabeculae of first lumbar vertebra: sampling efficiency and biological variation. Bone 10:7–13

Vesterby A, Gundersen HJG, Melsen F, Mosekilde L (1991a) Marrow space star volume in iliac crest decreases in osteoporotic patients after continuous treatment with fluoride, calcium and vitamin D_2 for five years. Bone 12:33–37

Vesterby A, Mosekilde Li, Gundersen HJG, Melsen F, Mosekilde Le, Holme K, Sørensen L (1991b) Biologically meaningful determinants for the in-vitro strength of lumbar vertebra. Bone 12:219–224

Vogel M, Hahn M, Caselitz P, Woggan J, Pompesius-Kempa P, Delling G (1990) Comparison of trabecular bone structure in man today and an ancient population in Western Germany. In: Takahashi HE (ed) Proceedings of the 5th international workshop on bone histomorphometry. Smith-Gordon, Nishimura, pp 220–223

Wakamatsu E, Sissons HA (1969) The cancellous bone of the iliac crest. Calcif Tissue Res 4:147–161

Weaver JK, Chalmers J (1966) Cancellous bone: its strength and changes with aging and an evaluation of some methods for measuring its mineral content. J Bone Joint Surg [Am] 48:289–299

CHAPTER 3

Biology of the Osteoclast

R. Baron, M. Chakraborty, D. Chatterjee, W. Horne, A. Lomri, and J.-H. Ravesloot

A. Introduction

The osteoclast is the cell responsible for the resorption of the extracellular bone matrix. Under physiological conditions, bone resorption plays an essential role in the homeostasis of both the skeleton and serum calcium. This cellular process is also essential in the growth and remodeling of bone, where it is tightly coupled to the process of bone formation by the osteoblast. It is the integrated functions of these two cell types that lead to the quantitative and qualitative maintenance of the skeleton, to the changes in size and shape of the individual bones during growth, and to bone repair after trauma or fracture. On the other hand, it is the disruption of the coupling between bone resorption and formation that leads to abnormally dense (osteopetrosis and osteosclerosis) or porous bone (osteoporosis). A coupled but high resorption rate characterizes high bone-turnover diseases, such as hyperparathyroidism or Paget's disease, and leads to the disruption of the architecture and function of the skeleton.

The understanding of the cell and molecular biology of the osteoclast has been hampered over the years by the facts that these cells are relatively rare (they cover only 1% of the bone surfaces in the bone of young adults), terminally differentiated (i.e., nonproliferative), firmly attached to mineralized matrices, and quite fragile due to their large size. The development of reliable methods to isolate and culture these cells (Nelson and Bauer 1977; Zambonin-Zallone et al. 1982; Osdoby et al. 1982) or to induce their formation in bone marrow cultures (Testa et al. 1981; Miyaura et al. 1981; Ibbotson et al. 1984; Udagawa et al. 1990), at least to a certain degree of differentiation, has, however, allowed an impressive acceleration of our fundamental understanding of the molecular mechanisms of bone resorption.

Before discussing these mechanisms in greater detail, we will summarize the essential features of the biology of the osteoclast. The osteoclast is a highly motile cell which attaches to, and migrates along, the bone surfaces, mostly comprising the interface between bone and bone marrow (endosteum). It is a multinucleated cell (although mononuclear osteoclasts are also encountered) which is formed by the asynchronous fusion of mononuclear precursors derived from the bone marrow and differentiating within the granulocyte-macrophage lineage. The osteoclast attaches to the mineralized bone matrix that it is going to resorb by forming a tight ring-like zone of adhesion, the sealing zone. This attachment involves the specific interaction between adhesion molecules in the cell's membrane and some bone matrix proteins. The space contained inside this ring of attachment and between the osteoclast and the bone matrix constitutes the bone-resorbing compartment. The osteoclast synthesizes several proteolytic enzymes which are then vectorially transported and secreted into this extracellular bone-resorbing compartment. Simultaneously, the osteoclast lowers the pH of this compartment by extruding protons across its apical membrane (facing the bone matrix). The concerted action of the enzymes and the low pH in the bone-resorbing compartment leads to the extracellular digestion of the mineral and organic phases of the bone matrix. After resorbing to a certain depth, determined by mechanisms that remain to be elucidated, the osteoclast detaches and moves along the bone surface before reattaching and forming another resorption pit. In the process, a certain volume of bone matrix has been removed, only to be replaced, under normal circumstances, by newly formed matrix a few days later. The calcium, phosphate, and other components of the matrix, which have been mobilized during this process, will be either eliminated or reutilized at sites where bone mineralization occurs or else used to maintain the proper ionic concentrations in the extracellular fluids.

From this brief description, it becomes apparent that the osteoclast is a cell that is morphologically and functionally polarized (Fig. 1), with a pole facing the bone matrix and towards which most of the secretion is targeted (the apical pole), and a pole facing the soft tissues in the local micro-environment (bone marrow or periosteum) and which provides mostly regulatory functions (the basolateral pole).

B. Main Morphological Features of the Osteoclast

The osteoclast is usually found singly or in low numbers at one given time and site, characteristically at the interface between soft and calcified tissues in an area where the bone matrix is fully mineralized (Fig. 1). Although this interface includes the periosteum, most of the remodeling activity occurs along the endosteum, i.e., at the interface between the calcified bone matrix and the bone marrow. At the light microscopic (LM) level, the osteoclast is characterized by its size ($50-100\,\mu$m on average), its multinucleation (usually two to ten nuclei), and its presence within a resorptive (Howship's) lacuna along the edge of the calcified matrix-bone marrow interface. The osteoclast is most often found in close apposition to the calcified matrix. The apical area of the cell, closest to the matrix, is characterized by densely stained patches at the periphery (attachment apparatus) and a lightly stained, highly vacuolated, and striated center area corresponding to the ruffled border

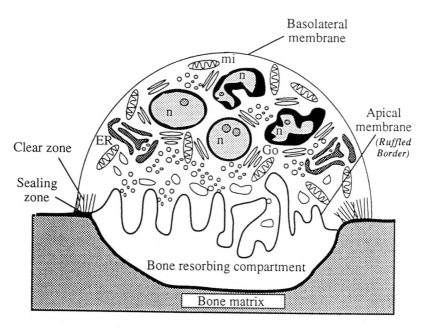

Fig. 1. Morphological characteristics of the osteoclast: See text for detailed explanations. *n*, nuclei; *Go*, Golgi complexes; *mi*, mitochondria; *ER*, endoplasmic reticulum

(Fig. 1). The cytoplasm is usually strongly basophilic, granular, and foamy, with vacuoles of varying sizes located mostly between the nuclei and the rufflcd-border area. The nuclei are characteristically heterogeneous in size, shape, and basophilia, a possible reflection of the asynchronous fusion of mononuclear precursors (NIJWEIDE et al. 1986).

Ultrastructural analysis (HOLTROP and KING 1977; BARON et al. 1985b, 1988) of the osteoclast (Fig. 1) confirms and extends the LM observations. First, the morphological polarity of the cell is evident, with a marked contrast existing between the apical and basolateral domains. The peripheral zone of the apical domain of the plasma membrane of the osteoclast is very closely apposed to the extracellular matrix. This so-called sealing zone (SCHENK et al. 1967) is characterized by a very narrow space (0.2–0.5 nm) between the plasma membrane of the cell and the calcified matrix and by the presence of an organelle-free area in the adjacent cytoplasm, the "clear-zone" (Figs. 1, 2), which is characteristically enriched in contractile proteins (KING and HOLTROP 1975; MARCHISIO et al. 1984). Toward the center of the apical domain, the plasma membrane of the osteoclast develops progressively deeper infoldings, which reach a high degree of geometric complexity. Numerous folds and ampullar spaces are present which, due to the random orientation of the sections through the cells, often appear as "vacuoles" in the cell's cytoplasm. The cytoplasmic side of the membrane forming the

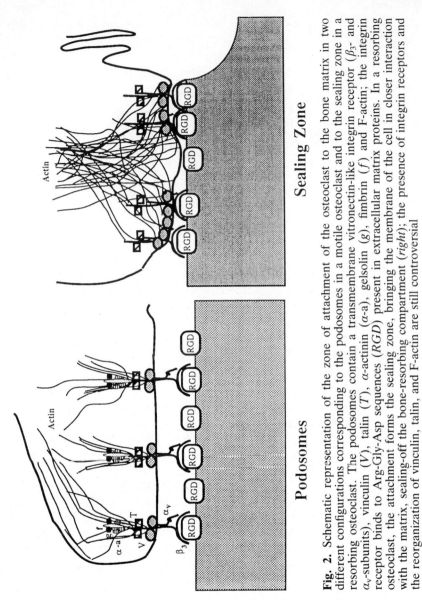

Fig. 2. Schematic representation of the zone of attachment of the osteoclast to the bone matrix in two different configurations corresponding to the podosomes in a motile osteoclast and to the sealing zone in a resorbing osteoclast. The podosomes contain a transmembrane vitronectin-like integrin receptor (β_3- and α_v-subunits), vinculin (V), talin (T), α-actinin (α-a), gelsolin (g), fimbrin (f) and F-actin; the integrin receptor binds to Arg-Gly-Asp sequences (RGD) present in extracellular matrix proteins. In a resorbing osteoclast, the attachment forms the sealing zone, bringing the membrane of the cell in closer interaction with the matrix, sealing-off the bone-resorbing compartment (*right*); the presence of integrin receptors and the reorganization of vinculin, talin, and F-actin are still controversial

ruffled border is lined by small, regularly spaced studs (KALLIO et al. 1971). In contrast, the basolateral domain of the plasma membrane is relatively smooth and is not lined on its cytoplasmic face by any defined structure.

In all species examined so far, one of the most consistent morphological features of the cytoplasmic organization of the osteoclast is the perinuclear distribution of multiple Golgi complexes, which entirely surround each of the cell's nuclei (Fig. 1) (BARON et al. 1985b). All of these Golgi stacks are functionally oriented with the *trans*-side (site of exit of recently synthesized proteins) facing away from the nuclei, as demonstrated by the immuno-localization of sialyl-transferase (BARON et al. 1988). The osteoclast is not, as often thought, poor in rough endoplasmic reticulum: this organelle is quite well developed, but remains limited in extent relative to the large size of the cell. The endoplasmic reticulum is usually concentrated in the basal portion of the cytoplasm of the osteoclast. The perinuclear envelopes, which are in close association with the *cis*-side of the multiple Golgi complexes, are most often found to be actively engaged in the biosynthesis of secretory proteins and enzymes (BARON et al. 1985b, 1988). In addition, the osteoclast is characteristically rich in mitochondria, free polysomes, and coated transport vesicles in the Golgi areas, as well as in multiple vacuolar structures of heterogeneous size and shape, concentrated mostly between the nuclei and the ruffled-border area. As mentioned earlier, many of these vacuoles are pockets of extracellular space cut obliquely through the folds of the plasma membrane.

C. Structure-Function Relationship

The structural features of the osteoclast that have been described above are all the reflection of specific functions (Table 1). The clear zone and the sealing zone are responsible for the attachment of the osteoclast to the bone matrix, the ruffled border corresponds to the area of ion transport and protein secretion, the basolateral membrane is a major site for regulatory influences, the ER and the Golgi complexes are responsible for the synthesis of both secretory and membrane proteins, and the cytoskeleton is involved in the cell's motility, its attachment to bone matrix, and the intracellular transport of membrane vesicles for secretion and membrane trafficking. Mitochondria provide the ATP required for the various energy-dependent systems within the cell, especially the several ion-transporting ATPases, and are a source of CO_2, which is used by carbonic anhydrase to produce protons for the acidification of the bone-resorbing compartment. Finally, abundant free polysomes reflect the fact that the osteoclast, like any other cell, needs to synthesize numerous soluble proteins for its own cytoplasmic use. Since it is the structure-function relationships which are the most important in trying to understand the biology of the osteoclast, we will now describe the various functions that this cell has to perform in order to resorb

Table 1. Structure-function relationships in the osteoclast

Structure	Function
Plasma membrane	
Apical	
Ruffled-border membrane	Ion transport, secretion
Sealing-zone membrane	Attachment, sealing, restriction of membrane domains
Basolateral membrane	Ion transport, regulation (receptors)
Cytoplasmic components	
Cytoskeletal components	Attachment, motility, secretion
Biosynthetic and secretory components (endoplasmic reticulum, Golgi, transport vesicles)	Secretion of proteins required for attachment, for the degradation of the matrix (enzymes), and for cell-cell signaling
Endocytic components	Intracellular degradation
Mitochondria	ATP synthesis, CO_2 generation

bone, adding further details on the morphological organization of the cell as needed.

D. Motility, Attachment, and Establishment of the Bone-Resorbing Compartment

I. Cytoskeletal Organization

All three types of filaments that have been demonstrated in the cytoskeleton of other cells, actin microfilaments, intermediate filaments, and microtubules, are found in osteoclasts. Both the intermediate filaments, composed of vimentin, and microtubules are radially organized in osteoclasts (MARCHISIO et al. 1984; TURKSEN et al. 1988; WARSHAFSKY et al. 1985). Individual cells often exhibit multiple microtubule-organizing centers and there may be a one-to-one correspondence between the microtubule-organizing centers and the nuclei (MATTHEW et al. 1967; MARCHISIO et al. 1984; TURKSEN et al. 1988). Inhibition of microtubule assembly interferes with the cell's functions, possibly because of the role played by microtubules in intracellular translocation of membrane vesicles between the plasma membrane and various intracellular compartments. Disruption of microtubules could interfere with the synthesis, processing, or secretion of hydrolytic enzymes into the resorption compartment or with the translocation of ion pumps or channels to the plasma membrane of the cell, resulting in failure of the cell to efficiently acidify the resorbing compartment (HUNTER et al. 1989; BARON et al. 1990b).

Cytoskeletal structures composed of actin filaments and various actin-binding proteins are involved in osteoclast migration and in adhesion of osteoclasts to bone and other surfaces. Osteoclasts which are migrating across a surface (bone or glass) have a pattern of actin filaments (TURKSEN et al. 1988; ZAMBONIN-ZALLONE et al. 1988; LAKKAKORPI et al. 1989) which is similar to what is seen in other motile cells in culture. While actin filaments are present throughout the cell, the leading edge of the cell, or lamellipodium, which has an irregular, ruffled appearance, contains a prominent network of relatively disorganized actin filaments. Stress fibers, which are commonly seen in, for example, cultured fibroblasts, are seldom observed in osteoclasts. Myosin is also found throughout the cell, but, in contrast to actin, it is more concentrated in the central region of the cell and relatively less abundant in the lamellipodia (WARSHAFSKY et al. 1985; TURKSEN et al. 1988).

II. Attachment Apparatus

1. Clear Zone

The most striking and unique feature of the osteoclast actin cytoskeleton is at the site of cell contact with the substratum. In osteoclasts observed under a variety of conditions, there is a prominent peripheral band of F-actin which contains actin filaments oriented parallel to the plane of the underlying substrate and running around the cell periphery as well as numerous punctate structures where the actin filaments are organized in bundles perpendicular to the plane of the substratum (MARCHISIO et al. 1984, 1987; ZAMBONIN-ZALLONE et al. 1989; LAKKAKORPI and VAANANEN 1991; LAKKAKORPI et al. 1989; KANEHISA et al. 1990; TETI et al. 1991). When osteoclasts are cultured on bone, the band circumscribes the area of active bone resorption (TURKSEN et al. 1988; LAKKAKORPI et al. 1989; KANEHISA et al. 1990) and thus presumably corresponds to the clear zone, where the high density of cytoskeletal elements excludes organelles from the region of the cytoplasm immediately adjacent to the plasma membrane. In electron micrographs, bundles of actin filaments can be observed oriented perpendicular to the bone surface and extending into short cell processes that enter irregularities of the bone surface (KING and HOLTROP 1975; ZAMBONIN-ZALLONE et al. 1988). These bundles of actin filaments apparently correspond to the punctate F-actin structures in isolated osteoclasts cultured on bone slices or on glass. Confocal microscopy has demonstrated that, in actively resorbing osteoclasts, these sites of close cell-substratum contacts may even extend into and across the resorption pits, forming multilacunar resorption areas under the same osteoclast (TAYLOR et al. 1989; LAKKAKORPI and VAANANEN 1991).

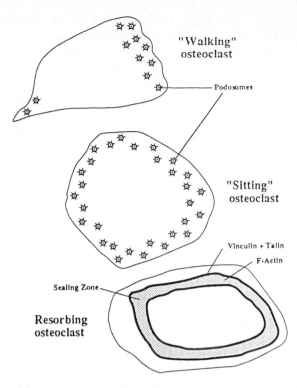

Fig. 3. Schematic representation of three different functional conformations of the attachment apparatus of the osteoclast. (Adapted from Lakkakorpi et al. 1991 and from Kanehisa et al. 1990)

2. Podosomes and the Sealing Zone

The punctate actin structures in the peripheral band, termed "podosomes" (Marchisio et al. 1984; Teti et al. 1991), apparently occur only in cells of monocytic origin (osteoclasts and monocytes) and in cells which have been transformed by the *src*, *fps*, and *abl* oncogenes (Marchisio et al. 1987). In addition to the bundles of actin filaments, the podosomes contain a number of other proteins which have been reported to occur at sites of cell-substratum or cell-cell interaction (see Teti et al. 1991 for review). These include fimbrin, α-actinin, and gelsolin, which are closely associated with the actin filaments in the core of the podosome, as well as vinculin and talin, which appear to form rosette structures surrounding the podosome cores (Marchisio et al. 1984; Teti et al. 1991) (Figs. 2, 3).

In terms of composition and function, podosomes and focal adhesion plaques are clearly related (Teti et al. 1991). There are, however, important functional differences. In contrast to focal adhesion plaques, which are relatively stable and which involve very close association of the cell membrane and the substratum (10–15 nm), podosomes are less tightly associated with the substratum (30 nm) and are highly dynamic, changing size and location and appearing and disappearing with life spans of 2–12 min (KANEHISA et al. 1990; LAKKAKORPI and VAANANEN 1991). It has been suggested that these properties of podosomes may be related to the fact that cells which express podosomes are both highly motile and able to interact with and degrade extracellular matrix proteins (TETI et al. 1991).

As discussed below, this difference in "tightness" of podosomes versus focal adhesion plaques may parallel a functional difference between "attachment points" and a "sealing zone," thereby explaining the apparent reorganization of the attachment apparatus at the time of active resorption by the osteoclast.

Recent observations by ALI et al. (1984), LAKKAKORPI et al. (1989), LAKKAKORPI and VAANANEN (1991), KANEHISA and HEERSCHE (1988), and KANEHISA et al. (1990) provide us with a dynamic view of the attachment of the osteoclast to the bone matrix (Fig. 3). In highly motile ("walking") osteoclasts, few podosomes are observed and seem to be confined to the irregularly shaped leading edge of the cell, or lamellipodium. Upon arrest and attachment, much more numerous podosomes are formed and are organized in a peripheral ring, as described in cells attached on glass. Rapidly thereafter, the seal is established: then the punctate "podosome" structures are either replaced by two concentric rings of vinculin and talin circumscribing a broad central zone of F-actin (KANEHISA et al. 1990; LAKKAKORPI and VAANANEN 1991) or reach such density that they cannot be individually observed when they arrange into two concentric rings. These changes in the organization of the attachment structures could lead to the establishment of a tighter sealing zone by bringing the plasma membrane of the cell closer to the matrix than in the podosome mode. These observations therefore suggest a distinction in time and in specific cell-matrix interactions between the motile cell ("walking"), the cell recently arrested at a future resorbing site ("sitting"), forming a first ring-like structure of punctate attachment sites, and the resorbing cell, with a functionally tight sealing zone (Figs. 2, 3).

3. Role of Integrins

The cytoskeletal complexes described above provide an anchoring structure necessary for stabilizing the interaction of the osteoclast with the bone surface, but, since they are limited to the cytoplasmic side of the plasma membrane, they are not directly responsible for that interaction. This role is filled by integral membrane proteins whose cytoplasmic domains interact with the cytoskeleton while their extracellular domains bind to bone matrix proteins. These transmembrane proteins are members of the integrin family of adhesion molecules, which mediate cell-substratum and cell-cell interactions (HYNES 1987). Integrins are heterodimeric molecular assemblies of an α-subunit and a β-subunit with specific, receptor-like, extracellular binding sites which recognize the Arg-Gly-Asp (RGD) sequence, a motif known to represent the core ligand for all members of the integrin family (Ruoslahti and Pierschbacher 1987). The amino acid sequence surrounding the RGD motif determines which integrin will recognize and bind a specific matrix protein (Ruoslahti and Pierschbacher 1987; Horton and Davies 1989).

Osteoclasts express at least two α-subunits, α_2 and α_v, and at least two β-subunits, β_1 and β_3, implying that multiple integrins may be involved in osteoclast adhesion to the bone matrix. The α_v- and β_3-proteins form a dimer which is closely related, if not identical to the vitronectin receptor (VNR), and is expressed at high levels in osteoclast membranes (Davies et al. 1989). Prior to attachment of the osteoclast to the bone surface, the VNR is distributed over the entire surface of the cell (Neff et al., unpublished). In attached and polarized osteoclasts it is restricted largely to the basolateral membrane (Neff et al., unpublished), although it may be expressed, albeit at a much lower level, in the apical (i.e., ruffled border) membrane (Lakkakorpi et al. 1991). The VNR has been demonstrated in podosomes by immunofluorescence (Zambonin-Zallone et al. 1989), but it has not been detected in the established sealing zone (Neff et al., unpublished; Lakkakorpi et al. 1991), raising the question of whether the integrins are indeed involved in the formation of the sealing zone (Lakkakorpi et al. 1991). These discrepancies could, however, be due to technical difficulties and to the limited access of epitopes that would be present in the tight sealing zone area.

Although the detailed receptor-ligand interactions at the attachment site are only beginning to be elucidated, several RGD-containing matrix proteins have been identified (Teti et al. 1991). Of these, collagen type I, osteopontin, and bone sialoprotein II are the most likely candidates to fill the role of integrin-binding proteins in bone (Teti et al. 1991). Most interestingly, data are now accumulating that suggest that the osteoclast synthesizes and secretes both osteopontin and BSPII, raising the possibility that the osteoclast itself deposits the adhesion molecules required for its attachment to the bone surface and for establishing the sealed-off bone-resorbing compartment.

The important role of integrins in bone resorption, whether it is in the sealing zone, the podosomes, and/or the motility of the osteoclast, is nevertheless well demonstrated. Monoclonal antibodies raised against the osteoclast VNR, originally called the osteoclast functional antigen (OFA) (Davies et al. 1989), inhibit bone resorption and spontaneous lamellipodial motility and induce the retraction of the osteoclast, much like the effect of calcitonin (Chambers et al. 1986). Furthermore, synthetic or natural peptides containing the Arg-Gly-Asp sequence inhibit bone resorption by isolated osteoclasts in culture (Sato et al. 1990). Finally, binding of RGD-containing peptides to osteoclasts induces changes in intracellular calcium and other signal transduction events leading to an activation of the cell (MIYAUCHI et al. 1991). These results indicate that the integrins play an important role in the osteoclast function and, despite the controversy regarding their presence at the sealing zone membrane, most likely mediate the attachment of the osteoclast to the bone surface.

4. Regulation of Bone Resorption and the Attachment Apparatus

Calcitonin, which directly inhibits bone resorption after binding to receptors present on the osteoclast basolateral membrane (NICHOLSON et al. 1986), causes the concurrent loss of the peripheral band of podosomes and other actin filaments and the appearance of a concentration of unorganized actin filaments in the center of the cell with a distribution very similar to that of myosin (WARSHAFSKY et al. 1985; HUNTER et al. 1989; LAKKAKORPI and VAANANEN 1990). Formation of such a centrally located actomyosin network is likely to be functionally related to the calcitonin-induced retraction of the osteoclast (CHAMBERS and MAGNUS 1982) and to the arrested secretion associated with the internalization of the apical membrane (BARON et al. 1990b). In contrast, retinol and retinoic acid, which have been reported to stimulate bone resorption, affect the organization of both microfilaments and microtubules, promoting podosome formation and inducing the reversible depolymerization of microtubules (ZAMBONIN-ZALLONE et al. 1988; OREFFO et al. 1991).

Thus, when osteoclasts are activated or inhibited, rapid and dramatic changes occur in their cytoskeleton and attachment structures, further demonstrating the functional importance of these structures in bone resorption (TETI et al. 1991).

Several of these cytoskeletal changes might be associated with the regulation of the osteoclast's intracellular calcium levels and/or pH (TETI et al. 1991). Inhibition of bone resorption is associated with an elevation of cytoplasmic Ca^{2+} levels after calcitonin treatment (MALGAROLI et al. 1989) and similar cytoskeletal changes are seen when cytoplasmic Ca^{2+} is increased by membrane depolarization, elevating extracellular Ca^{2+} levels or treating osteoclasts with a calcium channel agonist (MIYAUCHI et al. 1990). Reducing intracellular calcium, in contrast, promotes the formation of podosomes (TETI et al. 1989a). Podosome assembly is also induced by decreased cytosolic pH but this effect is mediated via a decreased cytoplasmic Ca^{2+} (TETI et al. 1989a). Furthermore, the binding of RGD-containing matrix proteins to their integrin receptors induces a decrease in intracellular Ca^{2+} and activates bone resorption (MIYAUCHI et al. 1991). One likely candidate for mediating these effects of calcium on actin filament organization is gelsolin, which has been identified in the podosome (MARCHISIO et al. 1987) and is known to affect actin filaments in ways which are differentially activated as Ca^{2+} concentrations increase from nanomolar to micromolar.

Hence, the cytoskeleton and integral membrane receptors of the integrin family play essential roles in osteoclast motility, in the specific attachment on the bone surface, in establishing the seal at the periphery of the extracellular bone-resorbing compartment, and in regulating the activity of the osteoclast. All these are essential components of the integrated function of the osteoclast, i.e., bone resorption, which, as discussed below, also involves the biosynthesis and secretion of several enzymes and the acidification of the bone-resorbing compartment.

E. Proteins Destined for Export: Biosynthetic and Secretory Functions of the Osteoclast

The morphological and cytoskeletal polarity of the osteoclast is only a reflection of the functional polarity of the secretory and transport components of this cell. The osteoclast is actively engaged in the biosynthesis and vectorial secretion of proteolytic enzymes and other proteins.

I. Lysosomal Enzymes

Acid phosphatase and other lysosomal enzymes are found in the secretory pathway. One of the main cytochemical characteristics of the osteoclast is its enrichment in lysosomal enzymes. Ultrastructural studies have shown, however, that this high concentration of lysosomal enzymes in the osteoclast is not due to the presence of phagocytic structures such as secondary lysosomes. Instead, these enzymes are found, for the most part, in elements of the exocytic pathway (BARON et al. 1985b, 1988). Using a variety of techniques to localize multiple enzymes, their presence was demonstrated in the ER, in the Golgi complex, and in numerous transport vesicles of the osteoclast. Thus, localization of arylsulfatase, β-glycerophosphatase, and acid phosphatase by enzyme cytochemistry and localization of β-glucuronidase, cathepsin C, and tartrate-resistant acid phosphatase by immunocytochemistry (BARON et al. 1985b, 1988; ANDERSSON et al. 1986; REINHOLT et al. 1990b) have shown the abundant concentration of these enzymes in the lumen of the ER cisternae, including the perinuclear envelopes, in the cisternae of the Golgi complexes and in very numerous small (50–75 nm), coated vesicles in the Golgi complex areas and throughout the cytoplasm. These latter are particularly abundant between the nuclei and the deep portions of the ruffled-border membrane folds (BARON et al. 1985b, 1988). In addition, some typical secondary lysosomal vacuoles were found, which are also filled with enzymes but are uncoated, are larger, and have a heterogeneous content. These are, however, relatively few and concentrated mostly in the basal portion of the cell, facing the bone marrow compartment. Consequently, this enrichment in lysosomal enzymes does not reflect a high phagocytic activity, but rather a high biosynthetic activity.

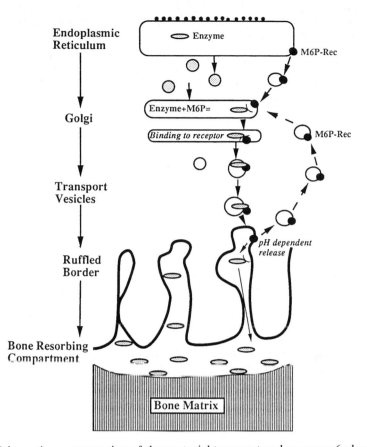

Fig. 4. Schematic representation of the vectorial transport and mannose 6-phosphate and pH-dependent secretion of lysosomal enzymes in the osteoclast (see text for detailed explanations)

The newly synthesized lysosomal enzymes are vectorially secreted into the bone-resorbing compartment (Fig. 4). Although many early studies (VAES 1968, 1988; LUCHT 1971; DOTY and SCHOFIELD 1972), in particular reports of the in vitro correlation between bone resorption and the release of TRAP into the medium (VAES 1968; CHAMBERS et al. 1987), strongly suggested that the osteoclast secreted lysosomal enzymes into the sealed-off extracellular bone-resorbing compartment, this conclusion remained controversial until immunocytochemical studies were possible. Antibodies to TRAP and cathepsin C have, however, allowed the localization of these enzymes in the extracellular bone-resorbing compartment (BARON et al. 1988; ANDERSON et al. 1986; REINHOLT et al. 1990b). The osteoclast is therefore actively engaged in the synthesis of lysosomal enzymes that proceed through the Golgi and are vectorially transported from the *trans*-Golgi region to the ruffled-border apical membrane in coated transport vesicles. These transport vesicles then fuse exclusively with the ruffled border's plasma

membrane and release their content into the bone-resorbing compartment
(Baron et al. 1985b, 1988).

This specific targeting of secretory transport vesicles to the apical domain
of the cell's membrane is accomplished by association with the mannose-6-
phosphate receptor (Baron et al. 1988) (Fig. 4). In most cells, lysosomal
enzymes are sorted out of the main flow of secretory and membrane proteins
at the level of the Golgi apparatus (Kornfeld 1986; Von Figura and
Hasilik 1986) and specifically targeted to late endosomes along the endocytic
pathway (Brown et al. 1986). The newly synthesized enzymes are recognized
by a specific binding protein, the mannose-6-phosphate receptor (Creek and
Sly 1984), which is highly concentrated in membranes of the Golgi compartment (Brown and Farquhar 1984, 1987) and binds mannose-6-phosphate,
which is added to the lysosomal enzymes in the cis-Golgi elements. This
mechanism ensures that the enzymes are sorted out of the flow of other proteins synthesized by the cells. The enzymes remain bound to the mannose-6-
phosphate receptor until they reach an acidified compartment where the low
pH induces their dissociation from the receptor. In this manner, enzymes
are released in the proper compartment, i.e., the late endosome (Brown
et al. 1986).

Despite the fact that the situation is quite different in the osteoclast,
which secretes the newly synthesized enzymes instead of targeting them to
an intracellular organelle, high concentrations of the cation-independent
mannose-6-phosphate receptor are found, localized with lysosomal enzymes
along the exocytic pathway (Baron et al. 1988, 1990b). Both the enzymes
and the mannose 6-phosphate receptors are present in the transport vesicles
and, being in a post-Golgi compartment, the enzymes must be bound to
their receptor during transport towards the ruffled-border. These transport
vesicles then fuse with the ruffled border membrane, probably via specific
interactions, and the enzymes dissociate from their receptors upon exposure
to the low pH in the bone-resorbing compartment. If this process is similar
in the osteoclast and in other cells, the receptors are most likely recycled to
the Golgi for other rounds of transport after delivery.

This could represent the mechanism by which the osteoclast ensures that
the lysosomal enzymes are not secreted towards the surrounding tissues
at the basolateral pole of the cell: a transport vesicle that would reach
the basolateral membrane would not release the enzymes in the microenvironment since at neutral pH the ligands do not dissociate from the
receptors. It is also possible that mannose-6 phosphate receptors present at
the basolateral domain of the cell play a role in recapturing enzymes that
would leak from the resorbing compartment, particularly when the cell
detaches and enters in a motile phase (Baron et al. 1988; Blair et al. 1988).

II. Nature and Specificity of the Secreted Enzymes

The nature and specificity of the enzymes that are secreted by the osteoclast
into the bone-resorbing compartment and which participate in the degrada-

Table 2. Secretory products of the osteoclast

Lysosomal enzymes
   Tartrate-resistant acid phosphatase
   β-Glycerophosphatase
   Arylsulfatase
   β-Glucuronidase
   Cysteine-proteinases (cathepsin B, C, L)

Nonlysosomal enzymes
   Collagenase
   Stromelysin
   Tissue plasminogen activator
   Lysozyme

Other (matrix) proteins
   Bone sialoprotein (BSP)
   Osteopontin
   TGFβ

---

tion of the extracellular matrix, both collagen and noncollagenous proteins, has been the subject of intense discussion over the years (Table 2). Although the best-characterized osteoclast enzyme is the tartrate-resistant acid phosphatase type 5 (HAMMARSTROM et al. 1971), which has been recently cloned and sequenced (EK-RYLANDER et al. 1992), other acid phosphatases as well as aryl-sulfatase, β-glucuronidase, and β-glycerophosphatase have been localized in the osteoclast's biosynthetic pathway (LUCHT 1971; DOTY and SCHOFIELD 1972; BARON et al. 1985b, 1988; ANDERSSON et al. 1986; REINHOLT et al. 1990b). More recently, based upon localization and functional studies, it has become apparent that the osteoclast also synthesizes and secretes several cysteine-proteinases, among which the cathepsins B, L (DELAISSE and VAES 1992; DELAISSE et al. 1991), and C (BARON et al., unpublished) have been specifically identified. The importance of these enzymes is that they are capable of degrading collagen in an acidic environment (DELAISSE et al. 1991; DELAISSE and VAES 1992), such as the one encountered in the bone-resorbing compartment. As such, the presence of these cysteine-proteinases resolved the apparent contradiction between the low pH at the resorbing site and the inability of neutral collagenase to degrade collagen at such a pH in vitro. Furthermore, several recent studies have directly demonstrated the importance of lysosomal cysteine-proteinases in bone resorption since their inhibition led to a decrease in bone resorption (DELAISSE and VAES 1992) and to the accumulation of undigested collagen in the resorbing lacunae (EVERTS et al. 1991).

Although the cathepsins can digest collagen at acidic pH, making collagenase unnecessary, the possibility that this enzyme still plays an important role in bone resorption has been raised by three recent studies. First, and despite the fact that the exact source of the collagenase is not yet firmly established, collagenase has been detected in the bone matrix underlying resorbing osteoclasts (BARON et al. 1990a) and within the cell itself

(Delaisse et al. 1992). Second, inhibition of matrix metalloproteinases also leads to an accumulation of undigested collagen in the bone-resorbing compartment (Everts et al. 1992), an effect similar to inhibiting cysteine-proteinases. Finally, tissue-plasminogen activator (Grills et al. 1990) as well as stromelysin (Delaisse et al. 1992), two enzymes that can activate latent collagenase, have also been found in osteoclasts, further suggesting a role for matrix metalloproteinases in bone resorption. Hence, the osteoclast synthesizes and secretes several classes of enzymes: phosphatases, sulfatases, cysteine-proteinases, and, possibly also, matrix metalloproteinases.

Although the pH optima of the cysteine- and metalloproteinases classes of enzymes in their ability to degrade bone matrix collagen are very different (4.0–5.0 and 7.5 respectively), it is possible to envision a cooperation between the two classes of enzymes during the resorption of bone, particularly because collagenase still has an important activity around pH 6 (Delaisse and Vaes 1992) and stromelysin can still degrade proteoglycans at pH 5. In order to integrate these new data, we have been led to speculate elsewhere, in a collaboration with others (Baron et al. 1990a; Delaisse et al. 1992; Everts et al. 1992), about possible modes in which the two classes of enzymes would cooperate in osteoclastic bone resorption. Besides their direct collagenolytic action, lysosomal cysteine proteinases can generate active collagenase (Eeckhout and Vaes 1977). The actions of the lysosomal acid cysteine proteinases and of collagenase may therefore be exerted sequentially (Baron et al. 1990a). The first phase of the osteoclastic resorption process would involve mainly the cysteine proteinases, degrading the bulk of the collagen as soon as the matrix is demineralized and in the fully sealed-off and acidified bone-resorbing compartment. In contrast, collagenase action would occur at more neutral pH and under two circumstances, i.e., during active bone resorption and after displacement of the cell from its previous resorbing site.

During active osteoclastic bone resorption, the buffering capacity exerted by the solubilized bone salts is likely to cause a gradient of pH extending from the most acid zone, in the immediate vicinity of the ruffled border and its proton pumps, to a more neutral zone, deeper in the resorbing lacuna and towards the interface between mineralized and demineralized matrix. The higher pH in these regions would both favor the activation of procollagenase by the lysosomal cysteine-proteinases, as this process is more efficient around pH 6 than at lower pH (Eeckhout and Vaes 1977), and render the collagenolytic action of collagenase predominant, since cysteine-proteinases are quite inefficient near neutral pH.

Second, as discussed before, the osteoclast moves along the bone surface, successively walking, sitting, resorbing, and walking again (see Fig. 3). The detachment of the cell at the end of a resorptive phase causes the sudden neutralization of the pH of the resorbing compartment, resulting from its opening to outside extracellular fluids. This would immediately prevent further actions of the cysteine proteinases, leaving a fringe of already demineralized but as yet undegraded collagen, as seen at the bottom of resorption pits eroded by isolated osteoclasts (ALI et al. 1984; MURRILLS et al. 1989). The role of collagenase could then be envisioned as removing that collagen fringe at the neutral pH present after displacement of the osteoclast, so as to allow the completion of the resorbing process despite the absence of a sealed-off subosteoclastic acidic microenvironment. Thus, it would then be the cooperative action of a set of acidic- and neutral-pH classes of enzymes that leads to a complete degradation of the extracellular matrix at the resorbing site.

III. Generation of Oxygen-Derived Free Radicals and Synthesis and Secretion of Other Proteins by the Osteoclast

It is becoming increasingly apparent that the osteoclast does not restrict its biosynthetic and secretory activity to making enzymes that are directly involved in bone matrix degradation, albeit most of these secretory products are probably important in bone resorption. As briefly mentioned earlier, there is immunocytochemical and/or in situ hybridization information strongly suggesting that the osteoclast is synthesizing two of the RGD-containing matrix proteins involved in its own adhesion. Both osteopontin, which has been demonstrated at the site of attachment of the osteoclast sealing-zone (REINHOLT et al. 1990a), and BSP have been shown to be synthesized by the osteoclast or potential precursors (MASI et al. 1991). Although these findings can be considered as surprising since these molecules are also, and mostly, synthesized by the osteoblast, they are just another illustration of the fact that many cells synthesize and secrete the proteins that they need to attach on substrates. There is also preliminary evidence suggesting that the osteoclast might produce TGFβ (QI et al. 1991; HOSOI et al. 1991), which the acid environment could activate from its latent form, potentially leading to a local coupling message for the osteoblasts (OREFFO et al. 1989; PFEILSCHIFTER et al. 1990).

In addition to the secretion of enzymes and protons, osteoclasts, like other cells in the monocyte-macrophage lineage, synthesize and secrete lysozyme (HILLIARD et al. 1990), an enzyme involved in the cleavage of certain polysaccharides, and may locally generate oxygen-derived free radicals to resorb bone. It has been shown that superoxide anions, one in a class of oxygen-derived free radicals, are present both intracellularly and under the osteoclast, in the bone-resorbing compartment (GARRETT et al. 1990; KEY et al. 1990). Furthermore, patients with the autosomal recessive form of osteopetrosis show both a defect in superoxide generation by leukocytes and a defect in osteoclastic bone resorption, thereby suggesting that superoxide generation may be involved in normal bone resorption (BEARD et al. 1986). This possibility is further supported by the fact that the generation of free radicals is regulated by agents that regulate bone resorption (GARRETT et al. 1990; KEY et al. 1990) and inhibition of free-radicals generation by superoxide dismutase blocks the stimulation of bone resorption by a number of agents (GARRETT et al. 1990). This hypothesis has been further supported by the fact that an antigen that is highly enriched in the osteoclast plasma membrane and that is recognized by a monoclonal antibody with high specificity for this cell (121F; OURSLER et al. 1985) may be a superoxide dismutase (OURSLER et al. 1989). The exact importance of this pathway in bone resorption remains, however, to be determined.

The motile osteoclast is thus capable of attachment to the bone surface, sealing off an extracellular compartment and secreting into this compartment several enzymes and proteins necessary for bone resorption. The morphological polarity mentioned earlier is therefore paralleled by a functional polarity. Because acidification of the bone-resorbing compartment is required and is also a polarized function of the cell, ionic transport at the basolateral and apical domains of the plasma membrane of the osteoclast has emerged as a major element in the biology of the osteoclast. These processes will be discussed in the following section.

F. Cytosolic and Membrane Proteins: Membrane Composition and Ion Transport

Many proteins made by the osteoclast are, unlike the molecules discussed in the previous section, not destined for export but will remain in the cell's cytosol or be inserted in specific domains of the membrane, such as the numerous integral-membrane proteins involved in ion transport and attachment (proton pumps, Na,K-ATPase, integrins, Ca-ATPase, anion exchangers, etc.).

Acidification of the extracellular bone-resorbing compartment has emerged over the last few years as one of the most important features of the biology of the osteoclast (VAES 1968, 1988; BARON et al. 1985b, 1986; BLAIR et al. 1989; BARON 1989; ARNETT and DEMPSTER 1986), probably determining the requirements for other specific features (sealing zone, enzymes, ruffled-border, etc.). The description of the organization and function of the osteoclast membrane domains needs therefore to be organized around the molecular mechanisms involved in acid secretion by this cell. Briefly, the polarized extrusion of protons across the apical membrane of the osteoclast imposes several ionic and charge constraints on the cell which require several ion-generating and ion-transport systems in the cytosol and in both domains of the plasma membrane (BARON 1989; SIMS et al. 1991). The identification and characterization of these systems has been greatly facilitated by the extended knowledge of the ion transport properties of other cells involved in acid secretion, particularly the kidney tubule intercalated cell and the gastric parietal or oxyntic cell. It had been known for several years that the osteoclast is highly enriched in carbonic anhydrase (GAY and MUELLER 1974), an enzyme which plays an essential role in acid-

Table 3. Antigens present in the plasma membrane of the osteoclast

Antigens that are not restricted to a specific domain	
Antigen 121F (superoxide dismutase)	

Restricted antigens

Basolateral	Apical
Sodium pumps (Na,K-ATPase) $\alpha 1/\beta 1$	LyMbP 100
Bicarbonate/chloride exchanger (AE2)	LEP 100
Vitronectin receptor (α_v/β_3)	Endolyn 78
	Proton pumps

Present but not localized (are in basolateral domain but could be restriced or not)
Na^+/H^+ Antiporter(s)
Calcium ATPase(s)
Calcium channels
Calcium sensor
Potassium channels
Chloride channels
Calcitonin receptors
Integrins with $\beta 1$-subunits

Membrane-associated proteins
Carbonic anhydrase
c-*src*

secreting cells such as the kidney tubule intercalated cell and the gastric mucosa oxyntic cell. In humans, defective CAII is associated with cerebral calcification, tubular acidosis, and osteopetrosis (SLY et al. 1983), providing the first genetic evidence for CAII direct involvement in bone resorption. Similarly, inhibition of carbonic anhydrase activity with acetazolamide blocks the ability of the osteoclast to efficiently resorb bone (MINKIN and JENNINGS 1972; WAITE et al. 1970). As will be discussed later, carbonic anhydrase generates protons and bicarbonate from carbon dioxide and water, providing the cells with protons for acidification at their apical membranes.

I. Apical Membrane and the Process of Acidification

The apical membrane of the osteoclast, or ruffled border, is directly involved in the molecular mechanisms of bone resorption. It is the target for the specific delivery of the newly synthesized secretory enzymes and it is the site of proton extrusion for acidification of the bone-resorbing compartment. The extensive folding of this domain of the plasma membrane is probably due both to the intense vesicular traffic associated with secretion and to the need for increasing the number of proton pumps via an amplification of the apical membrane.

There are several reasons why the apical ruffled-border membrane of the osteoclast could be expected to resemble the limiting membrane of vesicular elements of the endocytic pathway in other cells. First, this membrane limits a compartment that is the extracellular functional equivalent of

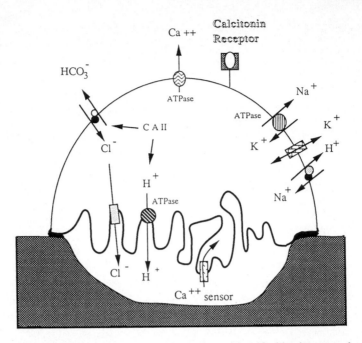

Fig. 5. Major ion transport systems that have been identified in the osteoclast. *Single circles* represent ion-motive ATPases, *double circles* represent ion exchangers, and *rectangles* represent ion channels (see text for detailed explanations)

a lysosome (Baron et al. 1985a and 1985b), with high concentrations of enzymes and a low pH (Mellman et al. 1986). Second, the ruffled-border membrane is the target for delivery of newly synthesized lysosomal enzymes by post-Golgi transport vesicles (Baron et al., 1985b, 1988), as are late endosomes in other cells (Brown et al. 1986). Finally, this membrane is responsible for establishing and maintaining the pH gradient necessary for bone resorption, as are the lysosomal and endosomal membranes for the degradation of internalized material. Immunocytochemical localization of lysosomal and/or endosomal integral membrane proteins has revealed that the ruffled border expresses several endosomal membrane proteins (Baron et al. 1985a,b, 1988), but not the proteins that are normally restricted to mature secondary lysosomes (Baron et al. 1985a). These lysosomal/ endosomal proteins are restricted to the apical domain of the osteoclast's plasma membrane and cannot be demonstrated in the basolateral domain. These observations both established that there is some analogy between endosomal membranes and the ruffled border, and demonstrated that the polarity of the osteoclast that is observed morphologically and in the trafficking of secretory proteins is also present at the level of plasma membrane composition, with certain integral membrane proteins being specifically segregated into one or the other domains of the plasma membrane. It is very likely that the attachment apparatus of the cell plays here a role similar to the tight junctions in epithelial cells in preventing the lateral diffusion of these restricted proteins from one membrane domain to the other. This could explain why the detachment of the osteoclast after calcitonin treatment leads to a loss of membrane polarity (BARON et al. 1990b).

This parallel with endosomes is, however, limited since, as described below, these two membranes differ in other respects: one is intracellular when the other is not, at least in actively resorbing osteoclasts. They also differ in the number and, possibly, the specific nature of the proton pumps.

Proton pumps serve a number of important functions in eukaryotic cells (MELLMAN et al. 1986; FORGAC 1989). In intracellular organelles of the endocytic or exocytic pathways, luminal acidification allows the dissociation of ligands from their receptors, the proteolytic processing of peptides, the entry of viruses into cells (MELLMAN et al. 1986), and the parallel uptake of small molecules into vesicles (HELL et al. 1988; MAYCOX et al. 1988). Proton pumps are also present at the plasma membrane of cells that are specialized in proton secretion, such as the gastric parietal cell, cells lining the distal and collecting kidney tubules (AL-AWQATI 1986), and the osteoclast in bone (BARON et al. 1985b; BLAIR et al. 1989), where they allow acidification of extracellular fluids. During bone resorption, osteoclast-mediated acidification is required for the dissolution of the mineral phase and the enzymatic degradation of the organic phase of the extracellular matrix (BARON et al. 1985b; VAES 1988; BLAIR et al. 1986, 1989).

The H^+ ATPases responsible for acidification in these various cells and organelles are distinguished from each other on the basis of their structure and their sensitivity to various specific inhibitors. The gastric proton pump, which exchanges H^+ for K^+, is composed of one α- (100 kDa) and one β- (55 kDa) subunit. The α-subunit forms a phosphorylated intermediate and, hence, is inhibited by vanadate (AL-AWQATI 1986; NELSON 1991). In contrast, the mitochondrial F0–F1 (F-ATPase) and the vacuolar H^+ ATPase (V-ATPase) (Fig. 6), which share a common evolutionary origin (NELSON and TAIZ 1989), are multisubunit structures (8–10 subunits) with a proton-conducting channel buried in the membrane (F0) and a large cytoplasmic catalytic portion (F1). They are resistant to vanadate and differ in their sensitivity to other specific inhibitors: the V-ATPase is sensitive to N-ethyl maleimide (NEM) and to bafilomycin A1 (BOWMAN et al. 1988) but not to oligomycin, while the reverse is true for the F-ATPase (AL-AWQATI 1986; NELSON 1991).

In an early report, based upon the cross-reactivity of an antibody to a lysosomal membrane protein with the H^+/K^+ ATPase, the possibility that the osteoclast proton pump could be of the P-type was suggested (BARON et al. 1985b). Further studies with antibodies to the gastric proton pump, however, failed to demonstrate its presence in osteoclast membranes (BARON et al., unpublished). More recently, based upon pharmacological and immunochemical data, it has been suggested that the H^+ ATPase present in osteoclast membranes is of the V-type, closely resembling the

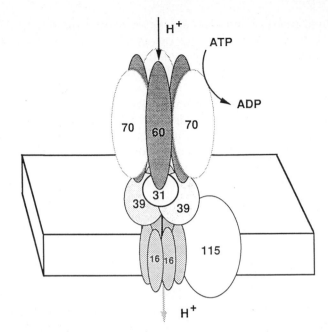

Fig. 6. Schematic representation of the prototype vacuolar H$^+$ ATPase (Adapted from Forgac 1989 and Nelson 1991). The 70- and 60-kDa subunits form the catalytic portion, which binds ATP on the cytoplasmic side of the membrane; the 31- to 39-kDa subunits form the stem, and the 16-kDa subunits form the DCCD-binding proton pore through the membrane; the 100- to 115-kDa subunit is thought to be a regulatory polypeptide (see text for detailed explanations)

pumps present in kidney membranes (Blair et al. 1989; Bekker and Gay 1990a; Vaananen et al. 1990). More specifically, proton transport in inside-out vesicles prepared from osteoclast-enriched cell fractions has been reported to be sensitive to NEM and other V-ATPase inhibitors but not to vanadate or oligomycin. By Western blot, these preparations have been shown to contain the 70-, 60-, and 31-kDa subunits of the V-ATPases (Fig. 6) and cross-reacting antigens have been immunolocalized at the apical ruffled-border membrane of the osteoclast (Blair et al. 1989; Vaananen et al. 1990).

There is, however, evidence in the literature which suggests that there are subtle differences in the properties and structure of mammalian V-ATPases (Forgac 1989; Nelson 1991; Wang and Gluck 1990). The vacuolar proton pumps contained in coated vesicles, endosomes, chromaffin granules, and kidney tubule plasma membranes differ in their subunit composition and it has been suggested that some of these differences may be due to the existence of isoforms of one or more subunit, with only small differences in their apparent molecular weight (Forgac 1989; Wang and Gluck 1990). These observations have led to the hypothesis that variations in isoforms of the multisubunit vacuolar proton pump(s) may constitute the basis for the differential targeting, properties, and regulation of H^+-ATPases present in different organelles in the same cell, in different cells, or in different organs.

In our hands (CHATTERJEE et al. 1992), H^+ transport by inside-out vesicles derived from osteoclast-enriched cell preparations was, unlike other known proton-transport systems, not only sensitive to the V-ATPase inhibitors NEM and bafilomycin A1 but also to the P-ATPase inhibitor vanadate. The ability of osteoclast-derived vesicles to transport protons is about 50-fold higher than that of microsomes from the other cells present in these preparations (CHATTERJEE et al. 1992) and at least twofold greater than that of highly purified endosomes (SCHMID et al. 1989; FUCHS et al. 1989). This very efficient H^+ transport suggests that a high concentration of pumps is present in the osteoclast apical membrane. High-magnification electron microscopy on negatively stained osteoclast microsomes showed the presence of high densities of characteristic ball-and-stalk structures, compatible with the presence of a high number of copies of multisubunit H^+-ATPases (CHATTERJEE et al. 1992), similar to the V-type ATPases observed in kidney tubule apical membranes (D. BROWN et al. 1987).

These results, taken together with several earlier observations (BARON et al. 1985b; ANDERSON et al. 1986; TUUKKANEN and VAANANEN 1986), suggest the possibility that the osteoclast proton pump has properties of both V-type and P-type ATPases. If confirmed, this would make it a novel class of proton transport system.

II. Role of the Basolateral Membrane and Ion Channels in Acidification, Intracellular pH, and Membrane Potential Regulation

The apparently simple process of pumping protons across the ruffled border membrane to acidify the resorption lacuna imposes, in fact, a complex and demanding set of ionic requirements to the cell, essentially designed to maintain the electrochemical balance of the osteoclast during bone resorption. This ionic balancing act requires the coordinated activity of electrogenic ion pumps, ion channels, and electroneutral ion exchangers in order to maintain the cytoplasmic pH and the transmembrane electrical potential within narrow physiological ranges. The two components that are directly involved in the acidification process and dictate the other requirements are the apical electrogenic proton pump itself and carbonic anhydrase II.

Briefly, the protons that the H^+-ATPase transports across the apical membrane are generated in the cytoplasm by the reversible hydration of CO_2 to produce carbonic acid, which ionizes to form protons and HCO_3^-, (GAY and MUELLER 1974; MAREN 1967) (Fig. 5). The generation of bicarbonate and the transfer of the protons out of the cell by the pump alter both the cytoplasmic pH, which becomes more alkaline, and the membrane potential, which becomes hyperpolarized as progressively more positive charges move out across the membrane and negative charges accumulate in the cytosol. Cytoplasmic pH and membrane potential therefore have to be tightly controlled.

Cytoplasmic pH is maintained near neutrality by the action of electroneutral ion exchangers present in the basolateral membrane (Table 3, Fig. 5), probably at a higher number of copies in the osteoclast than in other cell types due to its very active proton transport. Both an acid extruder (the Na^+/H^+ antiporter) and an acid loader (i.e., base extruder, the HCO_3^-/Cl^- exchanger) are present in the osteoclast. When the proton pump is active, the increasing alkalinity in the cytosol activates the HCO_3^-/Cl^- exchanger, which extrudes the excess HCO_3^- in a one-to-one exchange for extracellular Cl^-, preventing the intracellular pH from rising excessively (TETI et al. 1989b; HALL and CHAMBERS 1989; HORNE et al. 1991). If, on the other hand, intracellular pH should fall for some reason, for example if the pump should acutely stop extruding the protons generated by carbonic anhydrase, the Na^+/H^+ antiporter is activated and extrudes protons across the basolateral membrane in exchange for extracellular Na^+ (HALL and CHAMBERS 1990; CHAKRABORTY et al. 1991). It is, in fact, the gradient of Na^+ across the membrane, established by the activity of the sodium pumps found in high numbers in the basolateral membrane of the osteoclast (BARON et al. 1986), which drives the antiporter. These two exchangers therefore keep the intracellular pH within physiologic range but at the cost of an increasing intracellular Cl^- or Na^+ concentration. The activity of the Na^+/K^+ ATPase will allow the sodium which enters the cell to be transported out in a process which exchanges $3Na^+$ for $2K^+$, thereby resulting, like the activity of the proton pump, in hyperpolarizing the membrane.

The hyperpolarization resulting from the activities of the H^+ pump and the Na^+/K^+ ATPase, to which the activity of the Ca^{2+} ATPase also contributes (BEKKER and GAY 1990b), would rapidly reach a level making it nearly impossible to transport any more positively charged ions out of the cell. This would eventually hamper proton generation and electrogenic proton transport, if they were not alleviated by the activity of voltage-sensitive ion channels, which transport positively charged ions into the cell and/or negatively charged ions out of the cell and thus discharge the electrical potential. Two such ionic conductances have been recently described.

First, whole-cell patch-clamp studies have shown that both freshly isolated neonatal rat and embryonic chick osteoclasts possess inwardly rectifying K^+, or G_{ki}, channels (RAVESLOOT et al. 1989a,b; SIMS and DIXON 1989; SIMS et al. 1991). These G_{ki} channels are activated (opened) by a hyperpolarizing E_m. If E_m becomes more negative than the K^+ equilibrium potential (E_k) of $-80\,mV$, K^+ ions flow through G_{ki} channels into the cell, reducing the hyperpolarization. In addition to G_{ki} channels, embryonic chick osteoclasts express two other types of K^+ channels which are both activated by depolarizing E_m values. The first type of channels is present in about 70% of the osteoclasts and is activated transiently when E_m becomes less negative than $-20\,mV$. At those E_m values the channels give rise to outward directed K^+ currents that decrease in time (inactivate). The second type of K^+ channels activates at E_m values more positive than $+30\,mV$ and gives rise to outward K^+ currents in a sustained fashion. As a result of the activity of these K^+ channels, E_m is clamped at values close to E_k. Moreover, G_{ki} channels allow the osteoclast to switch rapidly between this value of E_m and $-15\,mV$ and vice versa (SIMS et al. 1991).

Second, there is evidence for the presence of chloride conductances in osteoclast membranes. Using on-cell and cell-free patch-clamp techniques high-conductance anion channels have been identified in neonatal rat osteoclasts (SCHOPPA et al. 1990; SIMS et al. 1992). A chloride channel with a very high conductance of about $400\,pS$ and voltage sensitivity (opened only at potentials between $-30\,mV$ and $+30\,mV$) was observed (SCHOPPA et al. 1990). Chloride conductances have also been identified in inside out vesicles (BLAIR et al. 1991) and the presence of Cl^- in the acidification buffers is necessary for H^+ transport (BLAIR et al. 1989; BEKKER and GAY 1990a; VAANANEN et al. 1990; CHATTERJEE et al. 1992), but it is not known whether the implied chloride conductance in vesicles corresponds to the conductances that were electrophysiologically characterized. Chloride as well as potassium channels may therefore be present in both the apical and basolateral domains of the plasma membrane of the osteoclast.

It is therefore apparent that the regulation of H^+ transport at the apical surface of the osteoclast is tightly linked to the regulation of intracellular pH and membrane potential, mostly accomplished by exchangers, pumps, and channels present in the basolateral membrane of the cell. These various elements are closely coupled and are also dependent upon the intracellular and extracellular concentrations of various ions, among which calcium is the most prominent.

III. Handling and Regulatory Role of Calcium

There are several obvious reasons for calcium to be of major importance in the regulation of the osteoclast's function. First, the cell's activity is regulated by several calciotropic hormones, whether directly or indirectly, whose main function is the maintenance of calcium homeostasis. Second, the osteoclast is most probably the cell of the body that is exposed to the highest local concentrations of calcium, resulting from the dissolution of hydroxyapatite crystals in the acidic microenvironment of the bone-resorbing compartment. Third, bone resorption being a means by which the organism mobilizes calcium from the skeleton, the calcium that is generated by the action of the osteoclast on bone matrix has to find its way to the extracellular fluids of the body.

Recent studies with isolated osteoclasts have shed some light on these issues. Two groups (ZAIDI 1990; MALGAROLI et al. 1989; MIYAUCHI et al.

1990, 1991) have independently demonstrated that both the incubation of the cells in the presence of calcitonin or in the presence of high extracellular calcium $(2-4\,\text{m}M)$ led to an increase in intracellular calcium concentrations and an inhibition of bone resorption.

Based upon pharmacological studies, the effect of calcitonin on intracellular Ca^{2+} has been attributed mostly to the plasma membrane and intracellular Ca^{2+}-ATPases (MALGAROLI et al. 1989). The basolateral membrane of the osteoclast has indeed been shown to contain high levels of a Ca^{2+}-ATPase, which could play a major role in these movements of Ca^{2+} (BEKKER and GAY 1990b).

Although in whole-cell patch-clamp experiments no Ca^{2+} (or Na^+) channels were found (SIMS and DIXON 1989; RAVESLOOT et al. 1989b), experiments with fluorescent Ca^{2+} dyes indicate that osteoclasts present on glass coverslips, but not on bone, do express voltage-dependent Ca^{2+} channels (MIYAUCHI et al. 1990). In addition, the osteoclast was found to express a novel type of Ca^{2+} channel that opens upon a rise in the extracellular Ca^{2+} concentration (ZAIDI 1990; MIYAUCHI et al. 1990). This "calcium sensor" or calcium-activated calcium channel is strongly reminiscent of the regulatory system found in the principal cells of the parathyroid gland, which themselves respond to elevations in serum calcium by an inhibition of parathyroid hormone secretion (ZAIDI 1990).

Since a rise in the intracellular Ca^{2+} concentration has been shown to inhibit the bone-resorbing activity of osteoclasts (ZAIDI 1990; MIYAUCHI et al. 1990) and to also affect the number and distribution of podosomes (MIYAUCHI et al. 1991), the current hypothesis is that elevations in Ca_i might primarily affect elements of the cytoskeleton and only secondarily the resorbing activity of the cells. This is most interesting in view of the fact that calcitonin, which has been shown to induce an increase in intracellular calcium (MALGAROLI et al. 1989), also disorganizes the cytoskeletal elements involved in the motility, attachment, and secretory organization of the osteoclast (WARSHAFSKY et al. 1985; BARON et al. 1990b; LAKKAKORPI and VAANANEN 1990). Other examples of the involvement of Ca_i in the regulation of osteoclastic activity are provided by platelet-activating factor, which elevates Ca_i and mimicks the other effects of calcitonin (WOOD et al. 1991) and the effects of RGD containing peptides and pH, which decrease Ca_i and activate bone resorption (TETI et al. 1989a; MIYAUCHI et al. 1991).

Taken together, these results (TETI et al. 1991; ZAIDI 1990) have suggested a model (Fig. 7) by which (1) elevations in Ca_i lead to inactivation of the osteoclast and, conversely, activation of the cell is associated with a decrease in Ca_i, (2) elevation of Ca_i may be achieved by ligand-induced (CT, PAF, RGD proteins) or by ion-induced mechanisms (Ca^{2+}, H^+, K^+), and (3) elevation of Ca concentrations in the sealed-off extracellular bone-resorbing compartment would lead to opening of the Ca sensor, elevation of Ca_i, inactivation and detachment of the osteoclast, and, thereby, diffusion of the mobilized extracellular calcium into the extracellular fluids. The osteoclast would then reattach and go through a second cycle of resorbing activity, thereby explaining the cyclic motility of the cell as well as the multilacunar nature of resorption sites in vivo and in vitro.

Since there is clear evidence that the cytoskeleton of the osteoclast can be found in different arrangements (LAKKAKORPI and VAANANEN 1991) (Figs. 2, 3), it is most likely that these correspond to the various steps of the cyclic activity of the osteoclast (TETI et al. 1991; LAKKAKORPI and VAANANEN 1991). It is possible that these various functional conformations also correspond to the two levels of membrane potential measured electrophysiologically (SIMS and DIXON 1989).

G. Conclusion

It appears that the main determinants of the biology of the osteoclast are first its *attachment* to the bone matrix, leading to the formation of the sealed-off bone-resorbing compartment, and, second, the polarized *acidification* of, and *secretion of enzymes* into, this compartment. These determinants constitute today the best-defined targets for therapeutic intervention at the level of the mature cell, to which one can add interventions at the level of the differentiation of this cell type. Other chapters in this volume specifically address the issues of the regulation of bone resorption and the differentiation of the osteoclast lineage. It is, however, germaine to our discussion to emphasize here a few points relevant to these issues.

The mature osteoclast is directly and negatively regulated by calcitonin, for which the cell expresses a high number of receptors in most species (WARSHAWSKY et al. 1980; NICHOLSON et al. 1986). Receptors and/or direct responses to the other peptide or steroid hormones involved in calcium or skeletal metabolism, such as parathyroid hormone or vitamin D_3, have not yet been demonstrated in these cells (CHAMBERS et al. 1985; MERKE et al. 1986), although precursors clearly respond to vitamin D_3 (MIYAURA et al. 1981; ROODMAN et al. 1985; BILLECOCQ et al. 1990b) and, possibly, to PTH. Recent evidence also suggests that the osteoclast expresses receptors for estrogen (OURSLER et al. 1991), possibly linking directly the activity of this cell to postmenopausal osteoporosis. Finally, receptor and nonreceptor tyrosine kinases have been shown to be functionally important in the osteoclast through the observations that bone osteopetrotic mutants express a defective CSF (YOSHIDA et al. 1990; FELIX et al. 1990; WIKTOR-JEDRZEJCZAK et al. 1990) and that knockout of the proto oncogene c-src leads to an osteopetrotic phenotype (SORIANO et al. 1991).

From the point of view of the biology of the osteoclast, while we still know very little about hormone and cytokine receptors in osteoclasts and their effects on bone resorption, it is already known that some of these regulatory events affect the functional determinants described above. Thus, calcitonin affects the cytoskeleton and attachment structures (CHAMBERS and

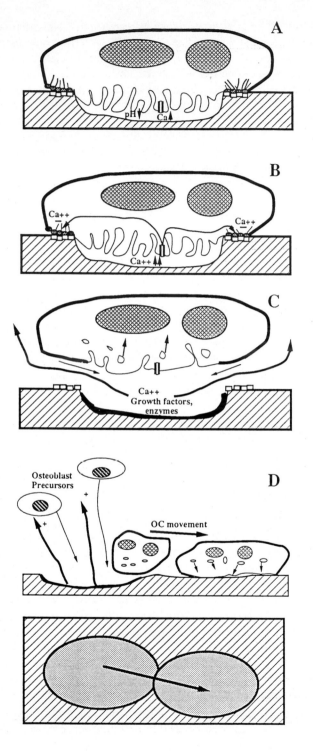

MAGNUS 1982; DEMPSTER et al. 1987; LAKKAKORPI and VAANANEN 1990; WARSHAFSKY et al. 1985), the secretion of enzymes (VAES 1972; BARON et al. 1990b), the motility and volume of the osteoclast (CHAMBERS et al. 1984; CHAMBERS and MAGNUS 1982; CHAMBERS and MOORE 1983) and some ion transport systems (HUNTER et al. 1988; CHAKRABORTY et al. 1991; MALGAROLI et al. 1989). 1,25-Dihydroxyvitamin D_3, which has a profound influence on the differentiation of bone marrow precursors into osteoclasts (MIYAURA et al. 1981; ROODMAN et al. 1985; BILLECOCQ et al. 1990b; TAKAHASHI et al. 1988a,b, 1989), induces the expression of several of the phenotypic and functional markers of the osteoclast: multinucleation and TRAP (MIYAURA et al. 1981; ROODMAN et al. 1985), calcitonin and vitronectin receptors (TAKAHASHI et al. 1988b; BILLECOCQ et al. 1990a), carbonic anhydrase II and one subunit of the sodium pump (BILLECOCQ et al. 1990a,b), and proton pumps (KURIHARA et al. 1990).

Similarly, several natural or synthetic compounds which inhibit bone resorption interfere with these functions and vice versa. Hence, inhibition of attachment with RGD peptides (HORTON and DAVIES 1989; SATO et al. 1990), inhibition of enzymatic degradation with inhibitors of cysteine-proteinases or metalloproteinases (DELAISSE and VAES 1992; EVERTS et al. 1992) or with antibodies to TRAP (ANDERSSON et al. 1991), inhibition of carbonic anhydrase (WAITE et al. 1970), sodium pump (PRALLET et al., unpublished), or proton pump activity (SUNDQUIST et al. 1990), and inhibition of bicarbonate/chloride (HALL and CHAMBERS 1989) or sodium/proton exchange (HALL and CHAMBERS 1990) all lead to an inhibition of bone resorption.

The very facts that all genes are coexpressed during vitamin D_3-induced differentiation and that interference with the activity of any of these gene products, whether pharmacologically or genetically, leads to impaired bone resorption emphasize the functional importance and interdependence of the various components that together define the biology of the osteoclast.

Acknowledgements. The authors work was supported by grants from the National Institutes of Health (NIDR, DE-04724 and NIAMSD, AR-40185 to R.B.) and by Fellowships from the Arthritis Foundation (A.L. and M.C.), the Swebilius Cancer

←──

Fig. 7A–D. Schematic representation of the putative role of a calcium sensor in arresting bone resorption and inducing the detachment and motility of the osteoclast. (Adapted, in part, from TETI et al. 1991 and ZAIDI 1990.) **A** Active resorption increases calcium concentration in resorbing compartment. **B** Calcium sensor in apical membrane opens, increasing intracellular calcium and disrupting the attachment apparatus. **C** The osteoclast detaches, calcium, and other factors and enzymes, are released in the extracellular fluids, and the apical membrane is internalized. **D** The osteoclast (with only basolateral markers) moves and reattaches nearby to form a second lacuna (seen from above *in lower part of figure*); the factors and/or matrix at the former resorption lacuna now recruit locally the osteoblast precursors (coupling)

Research Fund (D.C.), the Brown-Coxe Fund (D.C. and J.H.R.) and the Yale Comprehensive Cancer Center (W.H.). The authors are very grateful to Lynn Neff for her expert technical support and to C. Minkin, A. Teti, A. Zambonin-Zallone, J. Dixon, G. Vaes, and J.M. Delaisse for provinding them with preprints of their most recent reviews on the subjects.

References

Al-Awqati Q (1986) Proton-translocating ATPases. Cell Biol 2:179–199

Ali NN, Boyde A, Jones SJ (1984) Motility and resorption: osteoclastic activity in vitro. Anat Embryol (Berl) 170:51–56

Andersson RE, Woodbury DM, Jee WSS (1986) Humoral and ionic regulation of osteoclast acidity. Calcif Tissue Int 39:252–258

Andersson G, Ek-Rylander B, Hammarstrom LE, Lindskog S, Toverud SU (1986) Immunocytochemical localization of a tartrate-resistant and vanadate-sensitive acid nucleotide tri- and diphosphatase. J Histochem. Cytochem 34:293–298

Andersson G, Ek-Rylander B, Minkin C (1991) Acid phosphatases. In: Rifkin BR, Gay CV (eds) The biology and physiology of the osteoclast. CRC Press, Boca Raton (in press)

Arnett TR, Dempster DW (1986) The effect of pH on bone resorption by rat osteoclasts in vitro. Endocrinology 119:119–124

Baron R (1989) Molecular mechanisms of bone resorption by the osteoclast. Anat Rec 224:317–324

Baron R, Neff L, Lippincott-Schwartz J, Louvard D, Mellman I, Helenius A, Marsh M (1985a) Distribution of lysosomal membrane proteins in the osteoclast and their relationship to acidic compartments. J Cell Biol 101:53a

Baron R, Neff L, Louvard D, Courtoy PJ (1985b) Cell-mediated extracellular acidification and bone resorption: evidence for a low pH in resorbing lacunae and localization of a 100 kD lysosomal membrane protein at the osteoclast ruffled border. J Cell Biol 101:2210–2222.

Baron R, Neff L, Roy C, Boisvert A, Caplan M (1986) Evidence for a high and specific concentration of $(Na^+, K^+)ATPase$ in the plasma membrane of the osteoclast. Cell 46:311–320

Baron R, Neff L, Brown W, Courtoy PJ, Louvard D, Farquhar, MG (1988) Polarized secretion of lysosomal enzymes: co-distribution of cation-independent mannose-6-phosphate receptors and lysosomal enzymes along the osteoclast exocytic pathway. J Cell Biol 106:1863–1872

Baron R, Eeckhout Y, Neff L, Francois-Gillet C, Henriet P, Delaisse JM, Vaes G (1990a) Affinity purified antibodies reveal the presence of (pro)collagenase in the subosteoclastic bone resorbing compartment. J Bone Miner Res 5:S203

Baron R, Neff L, Brown W, Louvard D, Courtoy PJ (1990b) Selective internalization of the apical plasma membrane and rapid redistribution of lysosomal enzymes and mannose 6-phosphate receptors during osteoclast inactivation by calcitonin. J Cell Sci 97:439–447

Beard CJ, Key LL, Newburger PE, Ezekowitz AB, Arceci R, Miller B, Proto P, Ryan T, Anast CS, Simons ER (1986) Neutrophil defect associated with malignant infantile osteopetrosis. J Lab Clin Med 108:498–505

Bekker PJ, Gay CV (1990a) Biochemical characterization of an electrogenic vacuolar proton pump in purified chicken osteoclast plasma membrane vesicles. J Bone Miner Res 5:569–579

Bekker PJ, Gay CV (1990b) Characterization of a calcium ATPase in osteoclast plasma membrane. J Bone Miner Res 5:557–567

Billecocq A, Emanuel J, Jamsa-Kellokumpu S, Prallet B, Levenson R, Baron R (1990a) $1,25(OH)_2D_3$ induces the concomitant expression of the vitronectin receptor, sodium pumps and carbonic anhydrase II in avian bone marrow cells.

In: Cohn DV, Glorieux FH, Martin TJ (eds) Calcium regulation and bone metabolism. Elsevier, Amsterdam, pp 152–156

Billecocq A, Rettig-Emanuel J, Levenson R, Baron R (1990b) 1,25(OH)$_2$D$_3$ regulates the expression of carbonic anhydrase II in non erythroid avian bone marrow cells. Proc Natl Acad Sci USA 87:6470–6474

Blair HC, Kahn AJ, Crouch EC, Jeffrey JJ, Teitelbaum SL (1986) Isolated osteoclasts resorb the organic and inorganic components of bone. J Cell Biol 102:1164–1172

Blair HC, Teitelbaum SL, Schimke PA, Konsek JD, Koziol CM, Schlesinger PH (1988) Receptor-mediated uptake of a mannose-6-phosphate bearing glycoprotein by isolated chicken osteoclasts. J Cell Physiol 137:476–482

Blair HC, Teitelbaum SL, Ghiselli R, Gluck S (1989) Osteoclastic bone resorption by a polarized vacuolar proton pump. Science 245:855–857

Blair HC, Teitelbaum SL, Tan HL, Koziol CM, Schlesinger PH (1991) Passive chloride permeability charge coupled to H$^+$ ATPase of avian osteoclast ruffled membrane. Am J Physiol 260:C1315–C1324

Bowman EJ, Siebers A, Altendorf K (1988) Bafilomycins: a class of inhibitors of membrane ATPases from microorganisms, animal cells, and plant cells. Proc Natl Acad Sci USA 85:7972–7976

Brown D, Gluck S, Hartwig J (1987) Structure of the novel membrane-coating material in proton-secreting epithelial cells and identification as an H$^+$ ATPase. J Cell Biol 105:1637–1648

Brown WJ, Farquhar MG (1984) The mannose-6-phosphate receptor for lysosomal enzymes is concentrated in *cis*-Golgi cisternae. Cell 36:295–307

Brown WJ, Farquhar MG (1987) The distribution of 215 kD mannose-6-phosphate receptors within *cis* (heavy) and *trans* (light) Golgi subfractions varies in different cell types. Proc Natl Acad Sci USA 84:9001–9005

Brown WJ, Goodhouse J, Farquhar MG (1986) Mannose-6-phosphate receptors for lysosomal enzymes cycle between the Golgi complex and endosomes. J Cell Biol 103:1235–1247

Chakraborty M, Su Y, Nathanson M, Rubega-Male A, Slayman C, Baron R (1991) The effects of calcitonin in rat osteoclasts and in a kidney cell line (LLC-PK1) are mediated via an inhibition of the Na$^+$/H$^+$ antiporter. J Bone Miner Res 6:S134

Chambers TJ, Magnus CJ (1982) Calcitonin alters behavior of isolated osteoclasts. J Pathol 136:27–39

Chambers TJ, Moore A (1983) The sensitivity of isolated osteoclasts to morphological transformation by calcitonin. J Clin Endocrinol Metab 57:819–824

Chambers TJ, Athanasou NA, Fuller K (1984) Effect of parathyroid hormone and calcitonin on the cytoplasmic spreading of isolated osteoclasts. J Endocrinol 102:281–286

Chambers TJ, McSheehy PMJ, Thomson BM, Fuller K (1985) The effect of calcium regulating hormones and prostaglandins on bone resorption by osteoclasts disaggregated from neonatal rabbit bones. Endocrinology 116:234–239

Chambers TJ, Fuller K, Darby JA, Pringle JAS, Horton MA (1986) Monoclonal antibodies against osteoclasts inhibit bone resorption in vitro. Bone Miner 1:127–135

Chambers TJ, Fuller K, Darby JA (1987) Hormonal regulation of acid phosphatase release by osteoclasts disaggregated from neonatal rat bone. J Cell Physiol 132:90–96

Chatterjee D, Leit M, Neff L, Chakraborty M, Jamsa-Kellokumpu S, Fuchs R, Baron R (1991) A new and specific type of vacuolar proton pump is present at the osteoclast ruffled-border membrane. J Bone Miner Res 6:S197

Chatterjee D, Chakraborty M, Leit M, Neff L, Jamsa-Kellokumpu S, Fuchs R, Baron R (1992) Sensitivity to vanadate and isoforms of subunits A and B distinguish the osteoblast proton pump from other vascular H$^+$ ATPases. Proc Natl Acad Sci 89:6257–6261

Creek KE, Sly WS (1984) The role of the phosphomannosyl receptor in the transport of acid hydrolases to lysosomes. In: Dingle JT, Dean RT, Sly WS (eds) Lysosomes in biology and pathology. Elsevier, Amsterdam, pp 63–82

Davies J, Warwick J, Totty N, Philp R, Helfrich M, Horton M (1989) The osteoclast functional antigen, implicated in the regulation of bone resorption, is biochemically related to the vitronectin receptor. J Cell Biol 109:1817–1826

Delaisse JM, Vaes G (1992) Mechanism of mineral solubilization and matrix degradation in osteoclastic bone resorption. In: Rifkin BR, Gay CV (eds) The biology and physiology of the osteoclast. CRC Press, Boca Raton (in press)

Delaisse JM, Ledent P, Vaes G (1991) Collagenolytic cysteine proteinases of bone tissue. Biochem J 279:167–174

Delaisse JM, Neff L, Eeckhout Y, Su Y, Vaes G, Baron R (1992) Evidence for the presence of (pro)collagenase in osteoclasts. Bone and Mineral 17 (Suppl):82 (Abstr)

Dempster DW, Murrills RJ, Herbert WR, Arnett TR (1987) Biological activity of chicken calcitonin: effects on neonatal rat and embryonic chicks osteoclasts. J Bone Miner Res 2:443–448

Doty SB, Schofield BH (1972) Electron microscopic localization of hydrolytic enzymes in osteoclasts. Histochem J 4:245–258

Eeckhout Y, Vaes G (1977) Further studies on the activation of procollagenase, the latent precursor of bone collagenase. Effects of lysosomal cathepsin B, plasmin and kallikrein, and spontaneous activation. Biochem J 166:21–31

Ek-Rylander B, Bill P, Norgard M, Nilsson S, Andersson G (1991) Cloning, sequence and developmental expression of a type 5, tartrate-resistant, acid phosphatase of rat bone. J Biol Chem 266:24684–24689

Everts V, Delaisse JM, Korper W, Niehof A, Vaes G, Beertsen W (1992) The degradation of collagen in the bone-resorbing compartment underlying the osteolast involves both cysteine-proteinases and matrix metalloproteinases. J Cell Physiol 150:221–231

Felix R, Cecchini MG, Fleisch H (1990) Macrophage colony stimulating factor restores in vitro bone resorption in the *op/op* osteopetrotic mouse. Endocrinology 127:2592–2594

Forgac M (1989) Structure and function of vacuolar class of ATP-driven proton pumps. Physiol Rev 69:765–796

Fuchs R, Male P, Mellman I (1989) Acidification and ion permeabilities of highly purified rat liver endosomes. J Biol Chem 264:2212–2220

Garrett IR, Boyce BF, Oreffo ROC, Bonewald L, Poser J, Mundy GR (1990) Oxygen-derived free radicals stimulate osteoclastic bone resorption in rodent bone in vitro and in vivo. J Clin Invest 85:632–639

Gay CV, Mueller WJ (1974) Carbonic anhydrase and osteoclasts: localization by labelled inhibitor autoradiography. Science 183:432–434

Grills BL, Gallagher JA, Allan EH, Yumita S, Martin TJ (1990) Identification of plasminogen activator in osteoclasts. J Bone Miner Res 5:499–505

Hall TJ, Chambers TJ (1989) Optimal bone resorption by isolated rat osteoclasts requires chloride/bicarbonate exchange. Calcif Tissue Int 45:378–380

Hall TJ, Chambers TJ (1990) Na^+/H^+ antiporter is the primary proton transport system used by osteoclasts during bone resorption. J Cell Physiol 142:420–424

Hammarstrom LE, Hanker JS, Toverud SU (1971) Cellular differences in acid phosphatase isoenzymes in bone and teeth. Clin Orthop 78:151–167

Hell JW, Maycox PR, Stadler H, Jahn R (1988) Uptake of GABA by rat brain synaptic vesicles isolated by a new procedure. EMBO J 7:3023–3029

Hilliard TJ, Meadows G, Kahn AJ (1990) Lysozyme synthesis in osteoclasts. J Bone Miner Res 5:1217–1222

Holtrop ME, King GJ (1977) The ultrastructure of the osteoclast and its functional implications. Clin Orthop 123:177–196

Horne W, Moya M, Neff L, Chatterjee D, Kellokumpu S, Kopito R, Alper S, Baron R (1991) A band 3-related chloride/bicarbonate exchanger is highly expressed at the basolateral membrane of osteoclasts. J Bone Miner Res 6:S95

Horton MA, Davies J (1989) Perspectives: adhesion receptors in bone. J. Bone Miner Res 4:803–807

Hosoi T, Asaka T, Tomita T, Takeda J, Ouchi Y, Orimo H (1991) Demonstration of local delivery and activation of TGF-beta by osteoclasts in the resorption lacunae. J Bone Miner Res 6:S264

Hunter SJ, Schraer H, Gay CV (1988) Characterization of isolated and cultured chick osteoclasts: the effects of acetazolamide, calcitonin and PTH on acid production. J Bone Miner Res 3:297–303

Hunter SJ, Schraer H, Gay CV (1989) Characterization of the cytoskeleton in isolated chick osteoclasts: effects of calcitonin. J Histochem. Cytochem 37:1529–1537

Hynes RO (1987) Integrins: A family of cell-surface receptors. Cell 48:549–554

Ibbotson KJ, Roodman GD, McManus LM, Mundy GR (1984) Identification and characterization of osteoclast-like cells and their progenitors in cultures of feline marrow mononuclear cells. J Cell Biol 99:471–480

Kallio DM, Garant PR, Minkin C (1971) Evidence of coated membranes in the ruffled border of the osteoclast. J Ultrastruct Res 37:169–177

Kanehisa J, Heersche JNM (1988) Osteoclastic bone resorption: in vitro analysis of the rate of resorption and migration of idividual osteoclasts. Bone 9:73–79

Kanehisa J, Yamanaka T, Doi S, Turksen K, Heersche JNM, Aubin JE, Takeuchi H (1990) A band of F-actin containing podosomes is involved in bone resorption by osteoclasts. Bone 11:287–293

Key LL, Ries WL, Taylor RG, Hays BD, Pitzer BL (1990) Oxygen-derived free radicals in osteoclasts: the specificity and location of the nitroblue tetrazolium reaction. Bone 11:115–119

King GJ, Holtrop ME (1975) Actin-like filaments in bone cells of cultured calvaria as demonstrated by binding to heavy meromyosin. J Cell Biol 66:445–451

Kornfeld S (1986) Trafficking of lysosomal enzymes in normal and disease states. J Clin Invest 77:1–6

Kurihara N, Gluck S, Roodman GD (1990) Sequential expression of phenotype markers for osteoclasts during differentiation of precursors for multinucleated cells formed in long term human marrow cultures. Endocrinology 127:3215–3221

Lakkakorpi P, Vaananen IIK (1990) Calcitonin, PGE2 and dibutyril-cAMP disperse the specific microfilament structure in resorbing osteoclasts. J Histochem Cytochem 38:1487–1493

Lakkakorpi PT, Vaananen HK (1991) Kinetics of the osteoclast cytoskeleton during the resorption cycle in vitro. J Bone Miner Res 6:817–826

Lakkakorpi P, Tuukkanen J, Hentunen T, Jarvelin K, Vaananen K (1989) Organization of osteoclast microfilaments during the attachment to bone surface in vitro. J Bone Miner Res 4:817–825

Lakkakorpi P, Horton MA, Helfrich MH, Karhukorpi E-K, Vaananen HK (1991) Kinetic and confocal microscopic studies of the microfilaments and vitronectin receptor in osteoclasts. J Bone Miner Res 6:S149

Lucht U (1971) Acid phosphatase of osteoclasts demonstrated by electron microscopic histochemistry. Histochemie 28:103–117

Malgaroli A, Meldolesi J, Zambonin-Zallone A, Teti A (1989) Control of cytosolic free calcium in rat and chicken osteoclasts: the role of extracellular calcium and calcitonin. J Biol Chem 264:14342–14347

Marchisio PC, Naldini L, Cirillo D, Primavera MV, Teti A, Zambonin-Zallone A (1984) Cell-substratum interactions of cultured avian osteoclasts is mediated by specific adhesion structures. J Cell Biol 99:1696–1705

Marchisio PC, Cirillo D, Teti A, Zambonin-Zallone A, Tarone G (1987) Rous sarcoma virus transformed fibroblasts and cells of monocytic origin display a peculiar dot-like organization of cytoskeletal proteins involved in microfilament-membrane interactions. Exp Cell Res 169:202–214

Maren TH (1967) Carbonic anhydrase: chemistry, physiology and inhibition. Physiol Rev 47:595–781

Masi L, Brandi ML, Gehron-Robey P, Kerr JM, Young MF, Bernabei PA, Yanagishita M (1991) Bone sialoprotein (BSP) expression in human monoblastic cell line (FLG 29.1). J Bone Miner Res 6:S262

Matthew JL, Martin JH, Race GJ (1967) Giant-cell centriole. Science 155:1423–1424

Maycox PR, Deckwerth T, Hell JW, Jahn R (1988) Glutamate uptake by brain synaptic vesicles: energy dependence of transport and functional reconstitution in proteoliposomes. J Biol Chem 263:15423–15428

Mellman I, Fuchs R, Helenius A (1986) Acidification of the endocytic and exocytic pathway. Annu Rev Biochem 55:663–700

Merke J, Klaus G, Hugel U, Waldherr R, Ritz E (1986) No 1,25-dihydroxyvitamin D3 receptors on osteoclasts of calcium-deficient chicken despite demonstrable receptors on circulating monocytes. J Clin Invest 77:312–314

Minkin C, Jennings JM (1972) Carbonic anhydrase and bone remodeling: sulfonamide inhibition of bone resorption in organ culture. Science 176:1031–1033

Miyauchi A, Hruska KA, Greenfield EM, Duncan R, Alvarez J, Barattolo R, Colucci S, Zambonin-Zallone A, Teitelbaum SL, Teti A (1990) Osteoclast cytosolic calcium, regulated by voltage-gated calcium channels and extracellular calcium, controls podosome assembly and bone resorption, J Cell Biol 111: 2543–2552

Miyauchi A, Alvarez J, Greenfield E, Teti A, Zambonin-Zallone A, Ross FP, Teitelbaum SL, Cheresh D, Hruska K (1991) Matrix protein binding to the osteoclast adhesion integrin mediates a reduction in $[Ca^{2+}]_i$. J Bone Miner Res 6:S96

Miyaura C, Abe E, Kuribayasha T, Tanaka H, Konno K, Nishii Y, Suda T (1981) 1a,25-dihydroxyvitamin D3 induces differentiation of myeloid leukaemia cells. Biochem. Biophys. Res Commun 102:937–943

Murrills RJ, Shane E, Lindsay R, Dempster DW (1989) Bone resorption by isolated human osteoclasts in vitro: effects of calcitonin. J Bone Miner Res 4:259–268

Nelson N (1991) Structure and pharmacology of the proton ATPases. Trends Pharmacol Sci 12:71–75

Nelson RL, Bauer GE (1977) Isolation of osteoclasts by velocity sedimentation at unit gravity. Calcif Tissue Res 22:303–313

Nelson N, Taiz L (1989) The evolution of H^+ ATPases. Trends Biochem Sci 14: 113–116

Nicholson GC, Moseley JM, Sexton PM, Mendelsohn FAO, Martin TJ (1986) Abundant calcitonin receptors in isolated rat osteoclasts. Biochemical and autoradiographic characterization. J Clin Invest 78:355–360

Nijweide PJ, Burger EH, Feyen JH (1986) Cells of bone: proliferation, differentiation and hormonal regulation. Physiol Rev 66:355–360

Oreffo ROC, Mundy GR, Seyedin SM, Bonewald LF (1989) Activation of the bone-derived latent TGF beta complex by isolated osteoclasts. Biochem Biophys Res Commun 158:817–823

Oreffo ROC, Teti A, Francis MJO, Triffitt JT, Carano A, Zambonin-Zallone A (1991) Effect of vitamin A on bone resorption: evidence for a direct stimulation of isolated chicken osteoclasts by retinol and retinoic acid. J Bone Miner Res 3:203–210

Osdoby P, Martini MC, Caplan AI (1982) Isolated osteoclasts and their presumed progenitor cells, the monocyte, in culture. J Exp Zool 224:331–344

Oursler MJ, Bell LV, Clevinger B, Osdoby P (1985) Identification of osteoclast-specific monoclonal antibodies. J Cell Biol 100:1592–1600

Oursler MJ, Li L, Osdoby P (1989) Characterization of an osteoclast membrane protein related to superoxide dismutase. J Bone Miner Res 4:S265

Oursler MJ, Osdoby P, Pyfferoen J, Riggs BL, Spelsberg TC (1991) Avian osteoclasts as estrogen target cells. Proc Natl Acad Sci USA 88:6613–6617

Pfeilschifter J, Bonewald L, Mundy GR (1990) Characterization of the latent transforming growth factor β complex in bone. J Bone Miner Res 5:49–58

Qi DY, Oreffo ROC, Symons GA, DiGiovine FS, Seid J, Duff GW, Russell RGG (1991) TNF-α and TGF-β gene expression in day 14 GM-CFC-derived osteoclasts detected by in situ hybridization. J Bone Mine Res 6:S263

Ravesloot JH, Ypey DL, Nijweide PJ, Buisman HP, Vrijheid-Lammers T (1989a) Three voltage-activated K$^+$ conductances and an ATP activated conductance in freshly isolated embryonic chick osteoclasts. Pfluegers Arch 414:S166–S167

Ravesloot JH, Ypey DL, Vrijheid-Lammers T, Nijweide PJ (1989b) Voltage-activated K$^+$ conductances in freshly isolated embryonic chicken osteoclasts. Proc Natl Acad Sci USA 86:6821–6825

Reinholt FP, Hultenby K, Oldberg A, Heinegard D. (1990a) Osteopontin: a possible anchor of osteoclasts to bone. Proc. Natl Acad Sci USA 87:4473–4475

Reinholt FP, Mengarelli Wildhom S, Ek-Rylander B, Andersson G (1990b) Ultrastructural localization of a tartrate-resistant acid ATPase in bone. J Bone Mine Res 5:1055–1061

Roodman GD, Ibbotson KJ, MacDonald BR, Kuehl TJ, Mundy GR (1985) 1,25-Dihydroxyvitamin D3 causes formation of multinucleated cells with several osteoclast characteristics in cultures of primate marrow. Proc Natl Acad Sci USA 82:8213–8217

Ruoslahti E, Pierschbacher MD (1987) New perspectives in cell adhesion: RGD and integrins. Science 238:491–497

Sato M, Sardana MK, Grasser WA, Garsky VM, Murray JM, Gould RJ (1990) Echistatin is a potent inhibitor of bone resorption in culture. J Cell Biol 111:1713–1723

Schenk R, Spiro D, Wiener J (1967) Cartilage resorption in tibial epiphyseal plate of growing rats. J Cell Biol 34:275–291

Schmid S, Fuchs R, Kielian M, Helenius A, Mellman I (1989) Acidification of endosome subpopulations in wild-type Chinese hamster ovary cells and temperature-sensitive acidification-defective mutants. J Cell Biol 108:1291–1300

Schoppa NE, Su Y, Baron R, Boulpaep EL (1990) Identification of single ion channels in neonatal rat osteoclasts. J Bone Mine Res 5: S204

Sims SM, Dixon SJ (1989) Inwardly rectifying K$^+$ current in osteoclasts. Am J Physiol 256:C1277–C1282

Sims SM, Kelly MEM, Arkett SA, Dixon SJ (1991) Electrophysiology of ostcoclasts. In: Rifkin BR, Gay CV (eds) Biology and physiology of the osteoclast. CRC Press, Boca Raton (in press)

Sims SM, Kelly MEM, Dixon SJ (1991) K$^+$ and Cl$^-$ currents in freshly isolated rat osteoclasts. Eur J Physiol 419:358–370

Sly WS, Hewett-Emmett D, Whyte MP, Yu YS, Tashian RE (1983) Carbonic anhydrase II deficiency identified as the primary defect in the autosomal recessive syndrome of osteopetrosis with renal tubular acidosis and cerebral calcification. Proc Natl Acad Sci USA 80:2752–2756

Soriano P, Montgomery C, Geske R, Bradley A (1991) Targeted disruption of the c-src proto-oncogene leads to osteopetrosis in mice. Cell 64:693–702

Sundquist K, Lakkakorpi P, Wallmark B, Vaananen K (1990) Inhibition of osteoclast proton transport by bafilomycin-A1 abolishes bone resorption. Biochem Biophys Res Commun 168:309–313

Takahashi N, Akatsu T, Sasaki T, Nicholson GC, Mosley JM, Martin TJ, Suda T (1988a) Induction of calcitonin receptors by 1,25-dihydroxyvitamin D3 in osteoclast-like multinucleated cells formed from mouse bone marrow cells. Endocrinology 123:1504–1510

Takahashi N, Yamana H, Yoshiki S, Roodman GD, Mundy GR, Jones SJ, Boyde A, Suda T (1988b) Osteoclast-like cell formation and its regulation by

osteotropic hormones in mouse bone marrow cultures. Endocrinology 122:
1373–1382

Takahashi N, Kukita T, MacDonald BR, Bird A, Mundy GR, McManus LM,
Miller M, Boyde A, Jones SJ, Roodman GD (1989) Osteoclast-like cells
form in long-term human bone marrow but not in peripheral blood cultures.
J Clin Invest 83:543–550

Taylor ML, Boyde A, Jones SJ (1989) The effect of fluoride on the patterns of
adherence of osteoclasts cultured on and resorbing dentine: a 3D assessment of vinculin-labelled cells using confocal microscopy. Anat Embryol
(Berl) 180:427–435

Testa NG, Allen TD, Lajtha LG, Onions D, Jarret O (1981) Generation of
osteoclasts in vitro. J Cell Sci 47:127–137

Teti A, Blair HC, Schlesinger P, Grano M, Zambonin-Zallone A, Kahn AJ,
Teitelbaum SL, Hruska KA (1989a) Extracellular protons acidify osteoclasts,
reduce cytosolic calcium, and promote expression of cell-matrix attachment
structures. J Clin Invest 84:773–780

Teti A, Blair HC, Teitelbaum SL, Kahn AJ, Koziol C, Konsek J, Zambonin-Zallone
A, Schlesinger PH (1989b) Cytoplasmic pH regulation and chloride bicarbonate
exchange in avian osteoclasts. J Clin Invest 83:227–233

Teti A, Marchisio PC, Zambonin-Zallone A (1991) Clear zone in osteoclast function:
role of podosomes in regulation of bone-resorbing activity. Am J Physiol 261:
C1–C7

Turksen K, Kanehisa J, Opas M, Heersche JNM (1988) Adhesion patterns and
cytoskeleton of rabbit osteoclasts on bone slices and glass. J Bone Miner Res
3:389–399

Tuukkanen J, Vaananen HK (1986) Omeprazole, a specific inhibitor of H^+-K^+-
ATPase, inhibits bone resorption in vitro. Calcif Tissue Int 38:123–125

Udagawa N, Takahashi N, Akatsu T, Tranaka H, Sasaki T, Nishihara T, Koga
T, Martin TJ, Suda T (1990) Origin of osteoclasts: mature monocytes and
macrophages are capable of differentiating into osteoclasts under a suitable
microenvironment prepared by bone marrow-derived stromal cells. Proc Natl
Acad Sci USA 87:7260–7264

Vaananen HK, Karhukorpi EK, Sundquist K, Roininen I, Hentunen T, Tuukkanen
J, Lakkakorpi P (1990) Evidence for the presence of a proton pump of the
vacuolar H^+-ATPase type in the ruffled border of osteoclasts. J Cell Biol
111:1305–1311

Vaes G (1968) On the mechanisms of bone resorption: the action of parathyroid
hormone on the excretion and synthesis of lysosomal enzymes and on the
extracellular release of acid by bone cells. J Cell Biol 39:676–697

Vaes G (1972) Inhibitory actions of calcitonin on resorbing bone explants in culture
and on their release of lysosomal hydrolases. J Dent Res 51[Suppl]:362–366

Vaes G (1988) Cellular biology and biochemical mechanism of bone resorption. Clin
Orthop 231:239–271

Von Figura K, Hasilik A (1986) Lysosomal enzymes and their receptors. Annu. Rev
Biochem 55:167–193

Waite LC, Volkert WA, Kenny AD (1970) Inhibition of bone resorption by
acetazolamide in the rat. Endocrinology 87:1129–1139

Wang Z-Q, Gluck S (1990) Isolation and properties of bovine kidney brush border
vacuolar H^+-ATPase. J Biol Chem 265:21957–21965

Warshafsky B, Aubin JE, Heersche JNM (1985) Cytoskeleton rearrangements during calcitonin-induced changes in osteoclast motility in vitro. Bone 6:179–185

Warshawsky H, Goltzman D, Rouleau MF, Bergeron JJM (1980) Direct in vivo
demonstration by radioautography of specific binding sites for calcitonin in
skeletal and renal tissues of the rat. J Cell Biol 85:682–694

Wiktor-Jedrzejczak W, Bartocci A, Ferrante AW, Ahmed-Ansari A, Sell KW,
Pollard JW, Stanley ER (1990) Total absence of CSF 1 in the macrophage
deficient osteopetrotic (op/op) mouse. Proc Natl Acad Sci USA 87:4828–4832

Wood DA, Hapak LK, Sims SM, Dixon SJ (1991) Direct effects of platelet-activating factor on isolated rat osteoclasts. J Biol Chem 266:15369–15376

Yoshida H, Hayashi SI, Kunisada T, Ogawa M, Nishikawa S, Okamura H, Sudo T, Shultz LD, Nishikawa SI (1990) The murine mutation osteopetrosis is in the coding region of the macrophage colony stimulating factor gene. Nature 345: 442–444

Zaidi M (1990) "Calcium receptors" on eukaryotic cells with special reference to the osteoclast. Biosci Rep 10:493–507

Zambonin-Zallone A, Teti A, Primavera MV (1982) Isolated osteoclasts in primary culture: first observations on structure and survival in culture media. Anat Embryol (Berl) 165:405–413

Zambonin-Zallone A, Teti A, Carano A, Marchisio PC (1988) The distribution of podosomes in osteoclasts cultured on bone laminae: effects of retinol. J Bone Miner Res 3:517–523

Zambonin-Zallone A, Teti A, Grano M, Rubinacci A, Abbadini M, Gaboli M, Marchisio PC (1989) Immunocytochemical distribution of extracellular matrix receptors in human osteoclasts: a beta 3 integrin is colocalized with vinculin and talin in the podosomes of osteoclastoma giant cells. Exp Cell Res 182:645–652

CHAPTER 4

Osteoblasts: Differentiation and Function

T.J. MARTIN, D.M. FINDLAY, J.K. HEATH, and K.W. NG

A. Introduction

Cells of the osteoblast lineage occupy a central position in bone metabolism. The formation of a structurally sound skeleton, with its strength and integrity conserved by constant remodeling, and the formation as well as activation of the major bone-resorbing cell, the osteoclast, are the result of direct and indirect influences of osteoblasts.

Bone is a metabolically active organ in which the organizational pattern of the mineral and organic components determines the successful mechanical function of the skeleton. This is achieved by a combination of dense, compact bone and cancellous (trabecular) bone, reinforced at points of stress (GLIMCHER and KRANE 1968; GLIMCHER 1976). The mineral salts of the skeleton contribute about two-thirds of its weight, while the remaining organic matrix consists largely of collagen, with small amounts of proteoglycan, lipid, and several noncollagenous proteins, including osteonectin, osteopontin, osteocalcin (bone gla-protein) and matrix gla-protein. It is the function of osteoblasts to synthesize the organic components of bone and to contribute to the events resulting in its normal mineralization.

The word "osteoblast" has been used traditionally to describe those cells in bone responsible for bone formation. In addition it is now recognized that cells of the osteoblast lineage provide a much wider range of functions. These include an important role as a source of paracrine and autocrine factors (cytokines, growth factors, proteinases), which profoundly influence bone resorption as well as bone formation. Thus we now have a concept of heterogeneity of osteoblast function, which will be considered first before discussing the origin of osteoblasts, their replication and differentiation, and the mechanisms by which they contribute to intercellular communication in bone.

B. Mature Members of the Osteoblast Lineage: Definitions

The view that the osteoblast is concerned primarily with bone formation is reflected in its name. It is quite clear, however, that mature members of the osteoblast lineage have a variety of important functions, determining not only the formation but also the resorption of bone. Mature osteoblasts comprise three main subpopulations: *osteoblasts* synthesizing bone matrix, *lining cells* found along trabeculae and endosteal surfaces, and *osteocytes* in their lacunae, communicating with other osteocytes and cells on the bone surface (Fig. 1).

Osteoblasts are easily recognized histologically as plump, cuboidal, mononuclear cells lying on the matrix which they have synthesized. The gap junctions which connect them to their neighbors and to adjacent bone-lining cells (Doty 1981) provide a mechanism of intercellular communication likely to be important in their function. They also communicate with osteocytes below the bone surface through a network of canalicular connections. The synthesizing osteoblasts have dense peripheral nuclear chromatin and a nucleolus. They have a prominent Golgi apparatus and a basophilic cytoplasm rich in endoplasmic reticulum, reflecting their capacity for protein synthesis. They are rich in alkaline phosphatase and synthesize predominantly type I collagen and certain other proteins including osteonectin, osteocalcin, and bone proteoglycans I (biglycan) and II (decorin). They respond to hormones, such as parathyroid hormone (PTH), 1,25-dihydroxyvitamin D_3, estrogen, growth hormone, and thyroxine. They also respond to a number of growth factors and cytokines which are produced by cells of the osteoblast lineage, although it is not certain to what extent the different

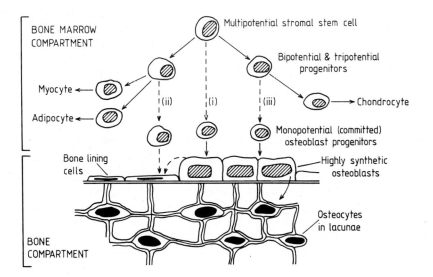

Fig. 1. Hypothetical lineage diagram for the differentiation of cells in the mesenchymal system. Whether committed osteoblast progenitors are derived directly from the multipotential stem cell (*i*) or via tripotential (*ii*) or bipotential (*iii*) intermediate precursor cells is not known. Mature osteoblasts producing organic macromolecules eventually become trapped in their own matrix, forming osteocytes. However, the lineage relationship between osteoblast precursors, bone-lining cells, and the synthesizing osteoblasts is not known (*indicated by dashed lines*)

members of the lineage contribute to their production in bone. Transforming growth factor β (TGFβ), which is stored in bone matrix in large amounts, and insulin-like growth factor-I (IGF-I) are osteoblast products thought to have important paracrine actions in bone.

Bone-lining cells are flattened cells lining the endosteal surfaces and trabeculae (MILLER and JEE 1987). They have little cytoplasm or endoplasmic reticulum, having largely lost their synthetic function, and they have somewhat lessened cytoplasmic basophilia and alkaline phosphatase activity. They possess gap junctions, and also communicate with osteocytes through intercellular processes in canaliculi. The bone-lining cells share some properties with synthetic osteoblasts, including expression of hormone receptors, and probably the ability to produce some growth factors and cytokines. Numerically they are the most abundant of the mature osteoblast populations, and perhaps their main function, to be discussed below, lies in the transmission of intercellular signals within bone.

Osteocytes are osteoblasts which have become trapped behind the advancing mineralization front, and become embedded in lacunae, deep in bone. They are connected with each other, and with surface osteoblasts and bone-lining cells by intercellular processes lying in canaliculi. Although osteocytes do not divide, they are nevertheless active and may contribute to the transport of mineral. They seem to be well situated to sense and respond to changes in physical forces on bone, which could lead them to transmit information to surface cells, programming the latter either to initiate formation or resorption. This is discussed in detail elsewhere in this volume by Lanyon. It is not known whether they synthesize growth factors or cytokines. The long-standing recognition of clear areas around osteocytic lacunae gave rise to the concept of "osteocytic osteolysis" (BELANGER 1969). However, careful ultrastructural analysis has failed to reveal any evidence in support of this (BOYDE and JONES 1987), and it is considered that osteocytes do not contribute to bone matrix destruction or demineralization (PARFITT 1977).

In the adult skeleton, bone is formed in a lamellar arrangement, in which collagen fibers are laid in a parallel and orderly fashion. The lamellar arrangement is essential to the structure of the Haversian system of cortical bone, in which lamellar fibers are arranged concentrically around the central cavity (Haversian canal). From the centre of the Haversian canal there is communication between the osteocytes through small connecting channels (canaliculi). The high degree of organization of bone depends upon the modulated activity of osteoblasts, under the influence of hormones and local factors.

C. Origin of Osteoblasts

Osteoblasts are thought to be derived from pluripotential stem cells present in the stromal fibroblastic system of the bone marrow and in other connective tissues such as the periosteum. Evidence that stromal stem cells differentiate into committed precursor cells which may then give rise to cells of osteogenic, fibroblastic, reticular, or adipocytic character was first obtained by FRIEDENSTEIN (1976), who pioneered the use of diffusion chambers for the study of bone marrow stromal cell differentiation. He showed that bone marrow cells, first grown to confluence in vitro, and then transferred to diffusion chambers and implanted intraperitoneally in rabbits, were able to establish a mixture of tissues including bone. He found that alkaline phosphatase activity was a good marker of cells that had differentiated in an osteogenic direction. Using the same approach, ASHTON et al. (1984) and BAB et al. (1984) found that those bone marrow cells taken from close to the endosteal surface of rabbit femora were more osteogenic than cells taken from the core of the marrow or from the intermediate fraction. Furthermore this distribution was correlated with the colony-forming efficiency of the cells in vitro: stromal fibroblasts from the endosteal surface formed four times as many colonies as the same number of "core" cells. This work confirmed Friedenstein's concept of the CFU-F (colony-forming unit-fibroblastic), which he proposed was a self-renewing multipotential stem cell population. Perhaps his most elegant experiments involved the transplantation of single stromal cell colonies, established first in vitro, under the renal capsule of mice where they formed plaques containing cells of different lineages, including bone and reticular tissue (FRIEDENSTEIN 1981). Furthermore, the host cells in these experiments established hemopoiesis and excavated a marrow cavity, giving the first indication of the ability of stromal cells or osteoblasts to promote osteoclast recruitment from circulating precursors. Direct evidence for involvement of stromal cells or osteoblasts in osteoclast formation has only recently been obtained (TAKAHASHI et al. 1988a; UDAGAWA et al. 1989).

The stromal fibroblast is distinguished by its high content of rough endoplasmic reticulum, microtubules, and microfilaments, consistent with its ability to secrete the macromolecules of the extracellular matrix, particularly collagen. Thus the cell which lies at the origin of the osteoblastic lineage is distinct from that giving rise to osteoclasts, which originate in the hemopoietic system (ASH et al. 1981). Nevertheless it is possible to draw analogies between the two developmental pathways, since in both systems stem cells are able to differentiate into cells of several lineages. In the hemopoietic system it has been possible to delineate the relationship between cells at different stages in the developmental sequence and describe points at which commitment to certain lineages takes place (for review see METCALF 1984). Such a model is thought to apply also to the stromal cell system, and is illustrated in the scheme proposed in Fig. 1, showing the putative relationships between osteoblast precursors, osteoblasts, lining cells, and osteocytes. The identification of intermediate (committed) progenitor cells is still preliminary and relies largely on the studies of Aubin and colleagues (GRIGORIADIS et al. 1988; AUBIN et al. 1990), who have provided most of the information in this regard. They showed that the osteoblast-like cell line, RCJ3.1, which was clonally derived from a fetal rat calvarial population, was capable of differentiating into four distinct tissues of mesenchymal origin: myocytic, chondrocytic, adipocytic, and osteogenic, and that the expression of all these phenotypes was enhanced by dexamethasone. Using repetitive cloning of RCJ3.1 cells, they isolated a number of subclones which exhibited restricted potential to diverge along all these pathways. This has allowed them to propose a series of hierarchical relationships between cells of the stromal cell lineages involving multipotential, tripotential, bipotential, and committed monopotential progenitor cells. It remains uncertain which of these pathways is followed in normal osteoblast development, and this is reflected in the hypothetical pathways proposed in Fig.1.

D. Osteoblast Lineage

Much of the current understanding of the phenotypic properties of osteoblasts has been obtained from studies in rodent cell culture systems, osteogenic sarcoma cell lines, certain stable and transformed cell lines, and organ culture. The observations made in these systems have been extrapolated to adult bone in vivo, and concepts developed of the "osteoblast phenotype." The brief summary of properties of osteoblasts, lining cells, and osteoctyes is expanded in Table 1 into a catalogue of properties associated with this phenotype. It must be emphasized that no single member of the osteoblast lineage would be expected to possess all of these properties. What proportion of them a cell does possess will depend on its state of differentiation, its location in bone and local and humoral influences which all affect gene expression. Clearly, therefore, it is not appropriate to claim that a cell is or is not an osteoblast on the grounds that it expresses, or fails to express, any particular phenotypic property. Throughout this chapter for convenience we will use the generic term, "osteoblast," to cover all mature members of the osteoblast lineage, i.e., osteoblasts, lining cells, and osteocytes. Where appropriate we will draw attention to specific properties of certain of the members.

A major challenge in osteoblast cell biology is to define the pathways of differentiation and to equate each stage with some function in bone. This can be investigated using a model system such as primary bone cell cultures established from calvariae and capable of differentiation in vitro. The osteogenic potential of the population is demonstrated by the formation of nodules which contain multiple layers of cells laying down an organized extracellular matrix consisting predominantly of collagen that subsequently undergoes mineralization (BELLOWS et al. 1986).

According to STEIN et al. (1989), the entire developmental sequence can be divided into three distinct phases. The initial *proliferative phase* (days 0–15) is also characterized by the synthesis of an organized bone-specific

Table 1. Osteoblast phenotypic characteristics

Products	Receptors and/or responses
Alkaline phosphatase	PTH and PTHrP
Type I collagen	Prostanoids
Osteocalcin	$1,25(OH)_2D_3$
Osteoponitin	Retinoids
Osteonectin	EGF and TGFα
Bone proteoglycan I (biglycan)	TNFα
Bone proteoglycan II (decorin)	TNFβ
Thrombospondin	Interleukin-1
Fibronectin	Interleukin-6
Vitronectin	TGFβ
Bone morphogenetic proteins	IGF I
TGFβ	IGF II
Fibroblast growth factors (FGFs)	Bone morphogenetic proteins
IGF I	Glucocorticoids
IGF II	Estrogen
Interleukin-1	LIF
Interleukin-6	Atrial naturetic peptide
TNFα	CGRP
Leukemia inhibitory factor (LIF)	VIP
Colony-stimulating factors, e.g., CSF-1	Growth hormone
Prostanoids	Insulin
Osteoclast-stimulating activity (putative)	
Osteoclast-promoting activity (putative)	

extracellular matrix. The shutdown of proliferation is followed by the phase of *matrix maturation* (days 16–20), which renders the matrix competent for the final phase of *mineralization* (days 20–25). Using genes encoding osteoblast phenotypic characteristics as markers of differentiation, these workers have demonstrated a distinct temporal sequence of gene expression that is functionally related to the developmental phases outlined above. Thus, mRNA for type I procollagen was expressed during the proliferative phase. An enhanced expression of alkaline phosphatase mRNA occurred during the phase of matrix maturation and, later, an increased expression of osteocalcin and osteopontin at the onset of mineralization (OWEN et al. 1990). This is an intriguing working model and one which helps to set goals for studies of hormone and cytokine actions on cells in developing bone. A remarkably similar sequence of expression of osteoblast-specific genes was elegantly demonstrated by in situ hybridization during osteogenic differentiation and new bone formation in mandibular condyles (STRAUSS et al. 1990) and by quantitation of specific mRNAs in developing fetal rat calvariae (YOON et al. 1987).

These are very useful experimental systems in which to study the progression of events during osteoblast differentiation. The developmental sequence demonstrated by these systems, however, also implies that osteoblast differentiation proceeds along a linear path from progenitor cells to fully mature osteoblasts. While this may be a useful concept, there are other possibilities that need to be considered. Studies of osteoblast differentiation in clonal cell lines carried out by several groups (PARTRIDGE et al. 1983; MAJESKA et al. 1980; AUBIN et al. 1982; NG et al. 1988; HEATH et al. 1989) have clearly demonstrated that there is very great heterogeneity among cells of the osteoblast lineage. These clonal cell lines serve as useful models representing osteoblasts at different stages of differentiation, based on the assumption of GREAVES (1986) that clonal cell lines represent cells "arrested" at a particular point in the normal developmental sequence. Such clonal cell lines can be induced to differentiate along a particular pathway when acted upon by factors such as retinoic acid (RA) and TGFβ. By using several different clonal cell lines as models for cells of the same lineage arrested at different stages of differentiation, it is also possible to compare responses to the same factor. With the current information available from these studies, the possibility has to be considered that there is not just one but several "pathways" of osteoblast differentiation and it is the sum total of these different subpopulations that make up what is generally regarded as the "osteoblast phenotype." These studies, complemented by information from osteoblast-rich primary cultures of rodent origin, have provided most of the current understanding of osteoblast differentiation. The scene is now set to identify the state of differentiation of cells in bone by defining their mRNA and protein products by in situ methods, and comparing these states with those which have previously been defined and studied in cultured cell lines.

E. Protein Products of Osteoblasts

Osteoblasts synthesize a collagen-rich matrix which mineralizes to form mature bone. Approximately 90% of the organic matrix of bone is collagen, and almost all of this is type I collagen. Accordingly, type I collagen represents more than 85% of the total collagen expressed by normal or transformed osteoblastic cells in culture. The faithful transcription and translation of type I collagen by osteoblasts is necessary for normal bone formation and, indeed, most of the genetic mutations identified in osteo-genesis imperfecta are located on one of the two structural genes for type I collagen (COLE 1988).

Since type I collagen is present in substantial amounts in tissues which do not mineralize, it seems likely that other osteoblast products influence the mineralization process. A number of non-collagenous proteins of bone have recently been characterized and cloned which potentially fulfil this function, either per se or as a specific mixture unique to a mineralizing extracellular matrix (ECM) (for review see GEHRON ROBEY 1989). For example, osteonectin is a protein capable of high-affinity binding to both hydroxyapatite and collagen, which may facilitate mineralization of type I collagen (TERMINE et al. 1981a,b). More recent data present a less facile picture where osteonectin is also expressed in nonmineralized tissues (HOLLAND et al. 1987), may play a role in suppressing the rate of hydroxy-apatite formation, perhaps allowing crystal growth to proceed in an orderly way (DOI et al. 1989), binds to thrombospondin (CLEZARDIN et al. 1988), a multifunctional component of the ECM of bone, and modulates cell-substratum attachments, as has been shown in endothelial cell culture (SAGE et al. 1989; LANE and SAGE 1990).

Some of the other noncollagenous products of osteoblasts which contribute to the ECM of bone are listed in Table 2. Although in no case has the function of these molecules been determined, clues to their putative function can be obtained by elucidation of their chemical properties deduced from amino acid sequences. In general, the ECM performs a number of functions, including structural support, orientation, and polarization of cells, binding of latent or active cytokines, and direct binding and gene regulation of adjacent cells.

In order to determine ultimately the relative contributions of each of these proteins to a functional mineralizing ECM of bone, the detailed regulation of their production by osteoblasts and pre-osteoblasts requires further study. Information about factors which regulate expression of these substances by osteoblasts (Table 2) is now emerging from cell culture experiments.

It is most likely that, in future, valuable functional information will be obtained from experiments with transgenic animals in which the genes for these molecules are added or deleted.

F. Factors That Influence Osteoblast Differentiation

Many local and systemic factors have been implicated in the regulation of bone formation. While a number of these factors such as IGFs, fibroblast growth factors, platelet-derived growth factor, and epidermal growth factor are potent mitogens, others such as retinoids, TGFβ, bone morphogenetic proteins (BMPs), and 1,25-dihydroxyvitamin D$_3$ have major influences on the differentiation of precursor osteoblasts (CANALIS et al., this volume; MARTIN et al. 1989). These will be discussed in turn below.

The effect of *retinoic acid* (RA) on bone formation has been recognized for several decades (MELLANBY 1944). More recently, it has been implicated as the natural morphogen responsible for pattern formation in developing chick limb buds (THALLER and EICHELE 1987; WAGNER et al. 1990). Osteoblasts are target cells for RA action as evidenced by its ability to inhibit proliferation and confer a more differentiated phenotype on osteoblasts (THEIN and LOTAN 1982; LIVESEY et al. 1985; NG et al. 1985) as well as regulate their gene expression (NG et al. 1989a,b; HEATH et al. 1989, ZHOU et al. 1991).

Table 2. Some noncollagenous proteins in bone matrix

Protein	Possible function	Regulation in osteoblast
Osteonectin	Facilitate mineralization of type I collagen (TERMINE et al. 1981a,b) Suppress rate of hydroxyapatite crystal growth (DOI et al. 1989; ROMBERG et al. 1986) Modulation of cell attachment and detachment (SAGE et al. 1989; LANE and SAGE 1990)	Glucocorticoid[a] (NG et al. 1989b) TGFβ[a] (NODA and RODAN 1987) IGFI[a] (THIEBAUD et al. 1990)
Osteopontin	Cell binding activity (OLDBERG et al. 1986) Osteoclast anchoring activity (REINHOLT et al. 1990) Mineral binding activity (OLDBERG et al. 1986)	1,25(OH)$_2$ vitamin D[a] (PRINCE and BUTLER 1987) TGFβ[a] (NODA et al. 1988b) Retinoic acid[a] (ZHOU et al. 1991) Glucocorticoid[b] (YOON et al. 1987) PTH[b] (NODA and RODAN 1989)
Bone sialoprotein	Cell binding activity (OLDBERG et al. 1988)	Glucocorticoid[a] (OLDBERG et al. 1989) 1,25(OH)$_2$D$_3$[b] (OLDBERG et al. 1989)
Bone proteoglycan I (biglycan)	Function(s) unclear	
Bone proteoglycan II (decorin)	Binding to collagen fibers – regulation of fiber growth (JOHANSSON et al. 1985) Binding/orientation of growth factors (Y. YAMAGUCHI et al. 1990)	
Thrombospondin	Binding and organization of ECM components (MUMBY et al. 1984) Cell attachment (GEHRON ROBEY et al. 1989)	TGFβ[b] (GEHRON ROBEY et al. 1989)
Osteocalcin	Inhibition of mineralization (PRICE et al. 1982) Recruitment of bone cell precursors (MUNDY and POSER 1983)	1,25(OH)$_2$D$_3$[a] (PRICE and BAUKOL 1980) PTH[a] (NODA et al. 1988a) Glucocorticoid[b] (BERESFORD et al. 1984)
Matrix gla-protein	Prevents growth plate mineralization (PRICE et al. 1982)	1,25(OH)$_2$D$_3$[a] (FRASER et al. 1988) RA[a] (ZHOU et al. 1991)

[a] Indicates stimulation.
[b] Indicates inhibition.

Retinoic acid, like steroids and related hormones, exerts its regulatory effects by interacting with receptors that are direct modulators of gene transcription. These nuclear RA receptors (RARs) are members of the steroid/thyroid hormone receptor supergene family by virtue of the presence of a highly conserved DNA-binding domain (EVANS 1988). The RA-RAR complex regulates gene expression by its interaction with RA-responsive elements (RAREs) in the 5' regulatory segments of the target genes. Recent studies have demonstrated the existence of five distinct RA receptors designated αRAR, βRAR, γRAR, RXRα, and RXRβ (BLOMHOFF et al. 1990; KRUST et al. 1989; MANGELSDORF et al. 1990). The almost complete interspecies conservation of the amino acid sequences of the α, β, and γRARs as well as their differential distribution in mouse tissue has raised the strong possibility that each member of the RAR subfamily plays specific roles during development and in the adult animal (ZELENT et al. 1989). UMR 106-06 osteogenic sarcoma cells, pre-osteoblastic UMR 201 cells, and subclones express mRNAs for α, β, and γRARs (ZHOU et al. 1991) and the immortalized pre-osteoblastic cell line, RCT-1, expresses α and γRAR mRNAs (SUVA et al. 1991). Expression of γRAR mRNA is of special interest because of recent reports of specific spatial and temporal distribution of γRAR during embryogenesis (DOLLE et al. 1990, RUBERTE et al. 1990). These in situ hybridization studies showed that the distribution of γRAR transcripts was restricted to areas related to bone and teeth formation and squamous epithelia. These studies imply an important role for γRAR in the transduction of RA signals at the level of gene expression during endochondral bone formation but do not exclude a similar or different role(s) for αRAR or βRAR in osteoblasts.

Transforming growth factor β is the prototype of a family of polypeptides that has varied effects on cell function, differentiation, and proliferation (for reviews, see MASSAGUE 1990; SPORN et al. 1987; SPORN and ROBERTS 1990). TGFβ is highly enriched in bone (HAUSCHKA et al. 1986), where it is synthesized and secreted by osteoblasts (GEHRON ROBEY et al. 1987). The effects of TGFβ are seen in several processes relevant to bone formation, namely, osteoblast proliferation, and differentiation, extracellular matrix synthesis as well as inhibition of matrix degradation (SPORN et al. 1987; CENTRELLA et al. 1987; PFEILSCHIFTER et al. 1987; NODA and RODAN 1987; NODA et al. 1988a; NODA 1989). It has been shown that local injections of TGFβ into the subperiosteal region of newborn rat calvariae or femurs result in localized intramembranous bone formation (MARCELLI et al. 1990; NODA and CAMILLIERE 1989) and chondrogenesis followed by endochondral ossification when the cartilage is replaced by bone (JOYCE et al. 1990). These are very important developments because they make it possible to extrapolate in vitro work on osteoblasts to osteogenesis in vivo.

Urist pioneered the work showing that endochondral bone formation can be stimulated in vivo by bone-derived protein extracts named *bone morphogenetic proteins* (URIST 1965; REDDI and HUGGINS 1972; WANG et al.

1988). A family of BMPs (BMP 1, 2A, 3) was cloned from a human osteosarcoma cDNA libary and each of the three polypeptides expressed was individually capable of inducing cartilage formation in vivo (WOZNEY et al. 1988). BMP 2A (WANG et al. 1990) and a closely homologous protein, BMP 2B (WOZNEY et al. 1988; HAMMONDS et al. 1991), have subsequently been shown to stimulate bone formation after the stage of cartilage formation. The pre-osteoblastic cell line, UMR 201, expresses the mRNAs for BMP 1, BMP 2A, and BMP 3. An increase in the steady state level of BMP 1 mRNA in response to RA in UMR 201 cells (ZHOU et al. 1991) suggests a way in which RA may directly influence endochondral bone formation. While BMP 1 is a novel protein, BMP 2A, BMP 2B, and BMP 3 (also known as osteogenin) and three other recently isolated osteoinductive factors (CELESTE et al. 1990) have all been identified as members of the TGFβ supergene family. Despite these recent advances in the study of osteoblast differentiation and bone formation, knowledge of the mechanism(s) of action of BMPs on osteoblasts is rudimentary. In vitro studies of recombinant human BMP 2B (renamed BMP 4 by CELESTE et al. 1990) have demonstrated its ability to stimulate the proliferation of osteoblast-like cells in culture, and increase their alkaline phosphatase activity and collagen synthesis (HAMMONDS et al. 1991). Osteogenin similarly increased collagen synthesis in primary cultures of osteoblasts and enhanced the responsiveness of these cells to parathyroid hormone (VUKICEVIC et al. 1989). Future studies should consider the regulation of osteoblast differentiation by BMPs acting as autocrine factors. For example, the production of BMPs and their actions upon cells at a very early stage of differentiation may prime them for the cooperative effects of cytokines, growth factors, or hormones (URIST 1989). Evidence for such a mechanism has been demonstrated in experiments where treatment of osteoblast precursors with BMP-2 led to a striking induction of osteocalcin mRNA and protein but only in the presence of 1,25-dihydroxyvitamin D_3 (A. YAMAGUCHI et al. 1991).

1,25-Dihydroxyvitamin D_3 is the most active metabolite of vitamin D and is essential for bone mineralization. Receptors for 1,25-dihydroxyvitamin D_3 are present in osteoblasts (PARTRIDGE et al. 1980; WALTERS et al. 1982) and 1,25-dihydroxyvitamin D_3 alters alkaline phosphatase activity (MANOLAGAS et al. 1981; MAJESKA and RODAN 1982) as well as the expression of matrix proteins such as collagen (HARRISON et al. 1989; CANALIS and LIAN 1985), osteopontin (YOON et al. 1987), osteocalcin (PRICE and BAUKOL 1980), and matrix gla-protein (FRASER et al. 1988) in these cells. Discrepancies related to the effects of 1,25-dihydroxyvitamin D_3 on these parameters in vitro have previously been ascribed to different cell culture systems and conditions. A recent study has clarified these differences. Using primary rat bone cell cultures which were capable of differentiating and forming mineralized nodules in vitro in a developmental sequence as described above, OWEN et al. (1991) showed that 1,25-dihydroxyvitamin D_3 can both positively and negatively regulate expression of osteoblast phenotypic markers such as alkaline phosphatase, type I collagen, osteopontin, matrix gla-protein, and osteocalcin depending on the stage of differentiation as well as the duration of hormone treatment of the osteoblasts in culture. For example, the steady-state levels of collagen and alkaline phosphatase mRNAs in relatively immature osteoblasts were inhibited by 48 h treatment with 1,25-dihydroxyvitamin D_3 during the proliferative phase of culture when the expression of these genes is maximal. However, the same mRNAs were stimulated in mature osteoblasts during the mineralization period at a time when the constitutive expression of these genes was minimal. Similarly, long-term treatment with 1,25-dihydroxyvitamin D_3 produced different results depending on whether it was added during the proliferative or mineralization phases of development. When 1,25-dihydroxyvitamin D_3 was added from day 6 to day 34, subsequent mineralization was inhibited and osteocalcin mRNA was not expressed. On the other hand, treatment initiated at day 20 after the phase of matrix maturation resulted in enhanced osteocalcin mRNA expression.

The regulation of alkaline phosphatase and pro-$\alpha1$(I) collagen gene expression by RA also depends on the stage of differentiation of osteoblasts in culture. In the clonal cell lines, UMR 201 and RCT-1, which represent two models of pre-osteoblasts, alkaline phosphatase mRNA level as well as alkaline phosphate activity were low or undetectable but were markedly stimulated by treatment with RA (NG et al. 1988, 1989a,b; HEATH et al. 1989). In contrast, RA inhibited alkaline phosphatase activity and mRNA levels in UMR 106-06, ROS 17/2.8 osteogenic sarcoma cells and calvarial osteoblasts which have a high constitutive level of expression of this gene (IMAI et al. 1988; NG et al. 1988). A similar observation was made for the control of pro-$\alpha1$(I) collagen mRNA expression by RA which increased steady state levels in UMR 201 and RCT-1 cells but decreased it in UMR 106-06 cells (HEATH et al. 1989; ZHOU et al. 1991). Transcription of the alkaline phosphatase and pro-$\alpha1$(I) collagen genes may be influenced by direct binding of the RA receptor to the promoter elements of these genes, or possibly indirectly through other nuclear factors which are induced by RA. The presence of these unknown factors may in turn be determined by the stage of differentiation of the cells, with the substantial stimulatory effect of RA on alkaline phosphatase expression being evoked in the cells which are at a relatively early stage of differentiation. A recent report has shown that specific combinations of RARs and cell type-specific coregulator proteins may function to integrate the effects of RA on patterns of gene expression within specific cell types during development (GLASS et al. 1990). It is intriguing to speculate that a change in the nature of these coregulators corresponding with a different stage of differentiation of cells within the same lineage may be responsible for altering the response to RA that has been observed.

Hormonal interactions are important in determining cell function. While many factors may influence the expression of phenotypic characteristics, it is important, when trying to understand the processes of differentiation, to distinguish between factors such as RA that may initiate differentiation by transcriptional control and others that could play an important supportive role by modulating the stability of mRNAs. Such a secondary role has been ascribed to tumor necrosis factor a (TNFa) and leukemia inhibitory factor (LIF), which have been shown to interact with RA posttranscriptionally to enhance the steady state levels of alkaline phosphatase mRNA (NG et al. 1989a; ALLAN et al. 1990). This may be an effective mechanism of action for paracrine factors. It might also be noted that, while TNFa enhanced the RA response in the preosteoblastic UMR 201 cells (NG et al. 1989a), it decreased the alkaline phosphatase activity of more mature osteoblasts (BERTOLINI et al. 1986; CANALIS 1987). This provides a further example of a factor having differential effects, depending on the state of differentiation of the target osteoblasts. It has also been demonstrated that dexamethasone and RA have opposing influences on the transcriptional control of osteonectin expression in UMR 201 cells (NG et al. 1989b), thus emphasizing the potential importance of hormonal interactions in the expression of osteoblast characteristics and function.

G. Model of Osteoblast Differentiation

A model of osteoblast differentiation can be proposed that relates the constitutive expression of genes with the stage of differentiation of the osteoblast. This model accommodates the findings on the constitutive and inducible expression of genes in pre-osteoblasts and osteogenic sarcoma cells (ZHOU et al. 1991; A. YAMAGUCHI et al. 1991) with the work of YOON et al. (1987), STEIN et al. (1989), OWEN et al. (1990), and STRAUSS et al. (1990), showing a temporal sequence of expression of genes in osteoblast differentiation. Table 3 indicates the pattern of gene expression proposed in this model of osteoblasts at early, intermediate, and late stages of differentiation.

The significant effect of RA in inducing the genes belonging to the intermediate group highlights the important role played by RA in osteoblast differentiation. It also pinpoints the stage of osteoblast differentiation where RA is most influential. No single differentiating agent, such as RA is

Table 3. Gene expression at stages of differentiation

Early	Intermediate	Late
Pro-$a(1)$I collagen	Osteonectin	Osteocalcin
Growth hormone receptor	Alkaline phosphatase	
Bone sialoprotein	Osteopontin	
Biglycan	Matrix gla-protein	
Bone morphogenetic proteins		
Receptors for retinoic acid		

capable of controlling the entire sequence of differentiation from pre-osteoblasts to fully mature osteoblasts. Hormones and growth factors may act to prime cells to a certain stage of differentiation to enable them to respond to other factors, as exemplified by the effect of BMP-2 to enhance osteoblastic differentiation in preosteoblasts, and inhibit differentiation into myotubes from the same cells (YAMAGUCHI et al. 1991). This concept highlights the need to study the influence of other factors such as TGFβ, the BMPs, 1,25-dihydroxyvitamin D_3, and cytokines and their interactions with each other in the control of osteoblast differentiation.

H. Osteoblast Proliferation

The renewal of the osteoblast population and their replication from pre-cursors are obviously important aspects of osteoblast biology. OWEN et al. (1990) have demonstrated the importance of the proliferation phase in the early stage of osteoblast differentiation. The completion of the synthesis of an organized extracellular matrix marks the end of this phase. Several growth factors of bone such as TGFβ, IGF-I, IGF-II, fibroblast growth factors (acidic and basic), and platelet-derived growth factor are mitogenic for osteoblasts, and their effects are reviewed by CANALIS et al. (Chap. 7, this volume).

Studies in organ and cell culture have identified prostaglandins as promoters of osteoblast replication. In fetal rat calvariae, PGE_2 stimulated periosteal cell replication, and this was followed by a late increase in collagen synthesis (CHYUN and RAISZ 1984). In chicken calvarial cells in culture, PGE_2 stimulated DNA synthesis and replication, as did PTH (FEYEN et al. 1985a,b) through a cyclic AMP-dependent mechanism. In contrast, the predominant effect of PTH and PGE_2 on rat calvarial cells and osteogenic sarcoma cells was an inhibitory one, although stimulation could be seen at low concentrations of PGE_2 or PTH (PARTRIDGE et al. 1985). Prostaglandins are produced in ample amounts by osteoblasts (NOLAN et al. 1983), and it is likely that they are important local regulators of proliferation and other functions. The participation of PTH in local events is unlikely; however, there is evidence for the production in fetal rat bone cultures (BERGMANN et al. 1990) and in human fetal bone (MOSELEY et al. 1991) of PTH-related protein (PTHrP). The possibility that locally produced PTHrP contributes to the control of proliferation is an intriguing one.

I. Hormone Receptors and Responses of Osteoblasts

The actions of hormones and cytokines in bone are discussed in Chaps. 5 and 6 by MUNDY. Here we will consider briefly those effects on osteoblasts which are relevant to our review of the central place of the osteoblast in bone cell biology. With the exception of calcitonin, all of the hormones, cytokines, and growth factors which act upon bone have been shown either to have receptors in osteoblasts, or to elicit responses from osteoblasts or both. The evidence for PTH receptors and direct action on cells of the osteoblast lineage is overwhelming, beginning with the studies of isolated osteoblast populations by LUBEN and COHN (1976), in osteogenic sarcoma cells (MARTIN et al. 1976; MAJESKA et al. 1980; PARTRIDGE et al. 1981), and demonstrated directly by autoradiography in chicken osteoblasts (SILVE et al. 1982). In recent work, PTHrP has also been shown to bind specifically to rat osteoblasts in vitro, and not to osteoclasts (EVELY et al. 1991). In vivo autoradiographic studies have demonstrated PTH receptors on osteoblasts, osteoprogenitor cells, and mononuclear cells of uncertain identity (ROULEAU et al. 1986). There have been two reports purporting to demonstrate specific PTH binding to osteoclasts (RAO et al. 1983; TETI et al. 1991). In the first of these (RAO et al. 1983) antibody against PTH was used to localize PTH in cells after incubation with relatively high concentrations of hormones. No controls for nonspecific binding were possible in these studies. In showing binding of [^{125}I]-labeled bovine PTH (1-84) to chicken osteoclasts, TETI et al. (1991) were unable to show any effect of the hormone on osteoclasts, and limited specificity studies were carried out. PTH action upon osteoblasts is predominantly through activation of adenylate cyclase, with subsequent activation of cyclic AMP-dependent protein kinase (LIVESEY et al. 1982). A number of specific postreceptor events follow this, including stimulation of plasminogen activator activity (ALLAN et al. 1986) and production of collagenase and TIMP (tissue inhibitor of metalloproteinases) (SAKAMOTO et al. 1975; HEATH et al. 1984; PARTRIDGE et al. 1987). Each of these has been shown to be a cyclic AMP-dependent effect of PTH. The demonstration of inositol phosphate metabolism and activation of calcium channels in response to PTH in osteoblast-like cells (FARNDALE et al. 1988; YAMAGUCHI et al. 1987; REID et al. 1987) has yet to be linked precisely to any particular cell response, although it was suggested that it contributes to the full expression of the cyclic AMP-mediated effect of PTH on collagenase release by osteoblasts (CIVITELLI et al. 1989). The actions of PTHrP on osteoblasts are essentially identical to those of PTH. Although receptors for PGE$_2$ have not been demonstrated directly on osteoblasts, the specific actions of PGE$_2$ closely resemble the effects of PTH. Other peptides with initial actions upon osteoblasts very similar to those of PTH and PGE$_2$ are calcitonin gene-related peptide (CGRP), which activates adenylate cyclase in osteoblasts (MICHELANGELI et al. 1989), and vasoactive intestinal peptide (VIP), which also promotes bone resorption (HOHMANN et al. 1983). These two peptides are each located in nerve endings in bone, and are possible neuromodulators of osteoblast function. Receptors for 1,25-dihydroxy-vitamin D$_3$ have been demonstrated in osteoblasts, and, like PTH, 1,25-dihydroxyvitamin D$_3$ inhibits collagen synthesis, stimulates collagenase and plasminogen activator activity, and is a powerful promoter of bone resorption. This will be discussed further in the next section.

One of the most striking hormonal influences on bone in vivo is that of estrogen, withdrawal of which results in substantial bone loss due to increased bone resorption. The action of estrogen on bone has never been adequately explained, but recent evidence has revealed the presence of low numbers of estrogen receptors in osteoblasts (Eriksen et al. 1988; Komm et al. 1988). Furthermore, estrogen treatment of osteoblasts has resulted in increased production of mRNA and protein for IGF-I (Ernst et al. 1989), most likely through a transcriptional effect. Growth hormone has also been shown to have specific receptors on osteoblasts (Barnard et al. 1991), although it has not been shown in these cells that GH causes an increased production of IGF-I. The data with regard to direct estrogen effects on osteoblasts is tantalizing for its suggestion that estrogen may positively influence bone formation. On the other hand, these results have been obtained in cultures of either transformed or neonatal osteoblasts. Estrogen was found to have no detectable effect on parameters of growth or differentiation of osteoblast-rich cell cultures of normal adult human origin (Keeting et al. 1991). These workers point to the lack of evidence for a stimulating effect of estrogen on bone formation in vivo, and propose that the antiresorptive effect of the hormone might be mediated through the osteoblast (lining cell) as will be discussed below.

Several peptide growth factors have receptors on or evoke responses from osteoblasts. Epidermal growth factor (EGF) receptors are located in normal and malignant osteoblasts (Ng et al. 1983a; Shupnik and Tashjian 1982), and EGF treatment results in increased DNA synthesis and cell division (Ng et al. 1983b). Similar effects are produced by TGFα, and both of these peptides are promoters of bone resorption (Tashjian and Levine 1978; Raisz et al. 1980; Ibbotson et al. 1986; Tashjian et al. 1985). Two of the most abundant growth factors in bone are TGFβ and IGF I, both of which act directly on osteoblasts to influence the synthesis of a number of the organic components of bone. These actions are discussed by Canalis et al. (Chap. 7, this volume). In this chapter we will consider the mechanisms through which their production and activation in bone are regulated (see below). Receptors also have been identified for IGF II in osteoblast-like cells (Mohan et al. 1989), and the direct action of PDGF on osteoblasts has been described (Canalis et al., Chap. 7, this volume).

The family of cytokines with actions initially thought to be confined to the immune system contains several members which are produced by osteoblasts and which have substantial actions on bone. Interleukin 1 (IL-1), released from activated monocytes, is a potent bone-resorbing agent (Gowen et al. 1984; Heath et al. 1985) which synergizes with PTH and PGE$_2$ (Dewhurst et al. 1987) and acts directly on osteoblasts (Thomson et al. 1986). The stimulation of bone resorption by the tumor necrosis factors, TNFα and TNFβ, which are cytokines derived from monocytes and lymphocytes respectively, is also mediated by osteoblasts (Thomson et al. 1987). A further cytokine, IL-6, which has a number of activities in combination with IL-1, is produced by osteoblasts and has been found to promote bone resorption (Lowik et al. 1989). Unlike the other cytokines, osteoblast production of IL-6 is promoted by some osteotropic hormones. This will be discussed in Chap. 5 by Mundy. Leukemia inhibitory factor (LIF) has been shown recently to be produced by osteoblasts, to have specific receptors in osteoblasts (Allan et al. 1990), and to promote bone resorption in organ cultures of mouse calvariae (Reid et al. 1990). The latter effect was dependent on prostaglandin synthesis, as shown previously for the resorptive effect of TGFβ in this system. In fetal rat long bones in culture, LIF inhibited resorption (Lorenzo et al. 1990). LIF stimulates DNA synthesis in osteoblasts (Reid et al. 1990), and its effects on the PA-inhibitor system (Allan et al. 1990) are discussed below. In animals bearing tumor cells producing large amounts of LIF, a remarkable increase in trabecular bone formation was observed (Metcalf and Gearing 1989), the significance of which is uncertain at present. A more detailed account of the complex interactions between cytokines is reviewed in Chap. 5 by Mundy.

J. Role of Osteoblasts in Intercellular Communication

There is a long list of hormones and local factors which are capable of promoting bone resorption in vitro and in vivo, and these have been discussed briefly in the preceding section. Activation of resorption in vitro, for example by PTH, PGE_2, 1,25-dihydroxyvitamin D_3, and cytokines, is achieved by the net effect of two mechanisms, the activation of the existing osteoclasts in bone, and the generation of new osteoclasts from precursors. For many years the prevailing view was that resorbing hormones acted directly on cells of the osteoclast lineage. However, with the development during the 1970s of methods of studying the functions of isolated bone cells, evidence began accumulating that the bone-resorbing hormones act directly upon osteoblasts. Even though at that time it was not possible to carry out direct experiments on isolated osteoclasts, nevertheless the patterns of responsiveness of osteoblasts seemed overwhelmingly to favor the idea that bone-resorbing hormones must act first on osteoblasts, most likely lining cells, which would then responsible for the activation of existing osteoclasts, and probably also the generation of new osteoclasts from precursors (Martin et al. 1979; Rodan and Martin 1981). A similar conclusion was reached by Chambers (1980), who argued that, since the osteoclasts were most likely derived from a "wandering" cell, it seemed logical that their activities in bone should be directed by authentic bone cells, and he proposed that osteoblasts should be responsible for this.

I. Osteoclast Activation

Over the next several years evidence was accumulated in support of this hypothesis (Chambers and Fuller 1985; Chambers 1985; Thomson et al.

1986, 1987; EVELY et al. 1991). Osteoclast activation has been studied extensively using cells isolated from newborn rat bone and plated onto thin slices of cortical bone (CHAMBERS 1985). Resorption is quantitated by measuring the areas or numbers of resorption pits produced by osteoclasts in response to treatment with bone-resorbing agents. Highly purified preparations of osteoclasts can be achieved by limiting the period for cell adhesion to 10 min. Osteoclasts become firmly attached in this time while other cells are removed by vigorous washing. Alternatively, deliberate contamination with osteoblasts can be achieved by allowing long settlement periods, or by adding osteoblasts, often osteogenic sarcoma cells. Such experiments show convincingly that the bone-resorbing agents stimulated resorption by a mechanism which required the presence of contaminating osteoblasts. This is true of PTH, 1,25-dihydroxyvitamin D_3 (CHAMBERS 1985), PTHrP (EVELY et al. 1991), TNFα and TNFβ (THOMSON et al. 1987), and IL-1 (THOMSON et al. 1986). Although it was thought for some time that the activation of osteoclasts could be produced by the transfer of medium from osteoblasts stimulated with resorbing agents, this has not been confirmed. It seems more likely now that coculture of osteoblasts and osteoclasts is necessary. Either a labile osteoblast product is responsible or contact between cells is required. It has been suggested that estrogen might produce its inhibitory effect upon resorption by interfering with the osteoblast-osteoclast communication process. Inhibition of osteoclastic resorption by calcitonin, on the other hand, is brought about by a direct action of that hormone upon osteoclasts (NICHOLSON et al. 1986).

The bone-resorbing hormones also cause a shape change to occur in the lining osteoblasts (JONES and BOYDE 1976), which could allow osteoclasts access to the bone surface. This is another factor which could contribute to the role of lining cells in the resorption process. In the final section of this chapter we will discuss the possible involvement of proteinases produced by osteoblasts in the degradation of the organic matrix.

II. Osteoclast Formation

In addition to osteoclast activation, the formation of new osteoclasts is an important part of the response to bone-resorbing hormones. It seems likely that the recruitment of osteoclasts is also an indirect effect, mediated by cells of the osteoblast lineage and perhaps other cells of the marrow stroma. However, this remains a controversial question, and some published data suggest direct effects of bone-resorbing hormones on osteoclast precursors. Osteoclasts are derived from the same hemopoetic stem cell that gives rise to mature blood cells under the influence of several hemopoietic cytokines. Details of these mechanisms are considered in Chap. 5 by Mundy, and the present discussion is confined to the role of osteoblasts.

In generating osteoclasts in cultures of mouse bone marrow, TAKAHASHI et al. (1988b) noted that osteoclast formation took place in close apposition to clusters of osteoblast-like cells, raising the possibility that osteoblasts were contributing to osteoclast formation. The same workers (TAKAHASHI et al. 1988a) showed that cultures of spleen cells could be used as a source of osteoclast precursors provided that the spleen cells were cocultured with osteoblastic cells derived from mouse bone. This ability was not confined to mouse osteoblasts, but certain bone marrow-derived stromal cell lines could also support the formation of osteoclasts in cocultures with spleen cells (UDAGAWA et al. 1989). These experiments drew attention to the fact that the formation of osteoclasts from a pure population of hemopoietic cells requires a contribution by cells of the stromal cell lineage. In more recent work the same group has isolated a clonal line (KS-4) from mouse calvariae possessing properties suggestive of pre-osteoblasts (YAMASHITA et al. 1990), and which is particularly effective at promoting osteoclast formation in coculture with spleen cells. An important finding in these and earlier experiments was that the two cell populations had to be cultured on the same surface; no osteoclasts are formed if they are separated by filters. This implies that cell-cell contact may be necessary for the promotion of osteoclast formation by the osteoblast or stromal cells. The same conclusion was reached in the same group's recent studies of osteoclast formation induced by IL-1 in mouse bone marrow cultures or in cocultures of spleen cells with osteoblasts (AKATSU et al. 1991). Accessory cells (in this case primary osteoblast cultures) were necessary for the IL-1 effect, which required cell contact and was prostaglandin dependent.

On the other hand, two groups support the view that osteoclast development from precursors can in some circumstances be promoted without participation of stromal cells or osteoblasts. HIURA et al. (1991) have been able to stimulate osteoclast formation using conditioned medium from osteoblasts. They explain this difference by the fact that their osteoclast precursors were first enriched by colony formation, and could therefore be maintained in the absence of stromal cells or cell contact as a source of colony-stimulating factors. The data of KURIHARA et al. (1990) demonstrated the formation of multinucleated osteoclast-like cells in human long-term marrow cultures after enrichment of precursors by treatment with colony-stimulating factors. A similar conclusion was reached in studies of osteoclast formation from hemopoietic spleen cells obtained from mice treated with 5-fluorouracil (KURIHARA et al. 1989; HAKEDA et al. 1989).

Thus the need for accessory cells (stromal or committed osteoblasts) to stimulate osteoclast formation is more controversial than is the role of accessory cells in osteoclast activation. On balance we favor the idea that osteoblasts/stromal cells are required, and the ability of osteoblast-like cells and certain marrow stromal cell lines to promote osteoclast formation suggests that this property is likely to occur in cells throughout the osteoblast lineage. The experiments of FRIEDENSTEIN (1981) referred to previously, in which host cells formed marrow in response to primitive cells transplanted under the kidney capsule, is consistent with this concept. One major challenge for studies of osteoblast biology in future is to elucidate the molecular basis of the factor from osteoblasts that supports osteoclast formation. The conceptual diagram (Fig. 2) summarizes these concepts of the regulation of osteoclast formation from stem cells, and their activation in response to circulating and local factors.

III. Coupling of Resorption to Formation

The preceding discussion has concentrated on the ways in which osteoblasts can contribute to the resorption process. It has long been recognized that the processes of resorption and formation are coupled, in that, once resorption has occurred, osteoblasts respond by making more bone matrix. Skeletal remodeling, with its continuous components of formation and resorption, continues throughout life. It is essential that a balance be achieved between resorption and formation, and it has generally been accepted that any change in one of those parameters results in a change in the other. A possible mechanism for the coupling of bone formation and resorption is that resorbing bone produces a factor which influences the rate of osteoblastic activity, and evidence for the existence of such a factor has been produced (HOWARD et al. 1981). From the amount of information available on the production of local activities in bone, it now seems that it is not necessary to postulate the existence of a discrete "coupling factor," but that this coupling process could be mediated by a number of factors.

CANALIS et al. (1989) showed that the bone-resorbing hormone PTH promotes the synthesis of IGF-I by osteoblasts. IGF-I is an important growth factor in bone and promotes the synthesis of type I collagen and other protein components. This interaction could therefore provide a mechanism for the coupling of resorption to formation as discussed by CANALIS et al. (Chap. 7, this volume). Osteoblastic production of IGF-I is promoted also by estrogen (ERNST et al. 1989) and by growth hormone (ERNST and FROESCH 1988). Negative regulation is provided by glucocorticoid, which inhibits IGF-I production (CANALIS et al., Chap. 7, this volume), perhaps thereby contributing to its inhibitory effect on bone formation.

An important component of the physiology of the IGFs is their high affinity for specific binding proteins (IGF BPs) which are found in plasma and other biological fluids, and which can either inhibit or enhance IGF action. In both normal rat osteoblasts (SCHMID et al. 1990) and UMR 106 osteosarcoma cells (TØRRING et al. 1991), PTH has been shown to stimulate IGF BP synthesis and secretion by a cyclic AMP-dependent process. The interaction with BPs is likely to be a major mechanism for controlling the amount of active IGF-I available to stimulate osteoblasts.

The coupling of resorption to formation may also involve activated TGFβ. As will be discussed in the final section of this chapter, PTH and other bone-resorbing hormones increase plasminogen activator (PA)

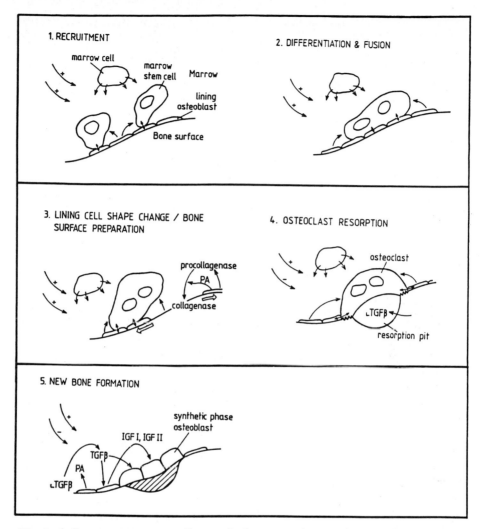

Fig. 2. *1*, Bone marrow stem cells recruited to resorption area under the influence of local (osteoblast- and marrow-derived) circulating factors as well as cell-cell contact signals. *2*, Differentiation of stem cells to preosteoclasts, and fusion to form multinucleated cells in the continued presence of humoral, paracrine factors, and cell adhesion signals. *3*, Lining cell shape change (e.g., caused by PTH) accompanied by preparation of bone surface for osteoclast resorptive activity by activated collagenase. Procollagenase activated by plasmin. Chemotactic factors for osteoclasts released from bone surface. *4*, Bone resorption where osteoclast activity is regulated by local (including cell adhesion signals) and hormonal factors, e.g., stimulated by cytokines, inhibited by calcitonin. *5*, New bone formation influenced by local factors generated by circulating molecules (e.g., PTH) promoting TGFβ activation through PA/plasmin system, and inducing IGF-I and II stimulation of matrix synthesis by active osteoblasts

activity, and the plasmin formed is capable of activating latent TGFβ previously secreted by osteoblasts and stored in the bone matrix. This would therefore provide a mechanism not only for localizing bone formation both spatially and temporally, but also for coupling resorption to formation.

We have considered three major processes where there appears to be transfer of information between osteoblasts and osteoclasts. However, we must also bear in mind that the transfer of information will also take place between cells *within* the osteoblast lineage. In other words, growth factors or cytokines produced by the synthetic osteoblasts, lining cells, or osteocytes could act on each other and also in an autocrine manner.

K. Proteinase Production by Osteoblasts

Proteolysis and increased cellular motility are found at sites of both physiological and pathological tissue remodeling. These processes seem also to be important in bone remodeling, and there is considerable evidence that osteoblasts are largely responsible for the production of proteinases capable of mediating the localized turnover of both unmineralized and demineralized bone matrix. This discussion excludes those enzymes produced by osteoclasts and responsible for direct action upon matrix at acid pH. The proteinases we will consider are the neutral enzymes, collagenase and plasminogen activator (PA) and their inhibitors, all of which can be produced by osteoblasts under the influence of hormones and paracrine factors.

Collagenase is an extremely potent and specific metalloproteinase which acts optimally at neutral pH. The enzyme is released by many connective tissues in culture and was first implicated in bone remodeling by WALKER (1966), who observed that the apparent reversal of osteopetrosis in grey-lethal (gl) mice by PTH was correlated with the presence of "collagenolytic activity" in cell-free extracts of bones taken from PTH-treated gl/gl animals. Since then collagenase has been characterized in the medium of organ cultures of rodent bone (S. SAKAMOTO et al. 1972) and of rodent bone cells (PUZAS and BRAND 1979; S. SAKAMOTO and SAKAMOTO 1984; HEATH et al. 1984; PARTRIDGE et al. 1987). Collagenase is secreted as a proenzyme, which must be activated before it can mediate collagen degradation. There is a wide body of evidence that this is most likely achieved physiologically by the action of plasmin (EECKHOUT and VAES 1977; THOMSON et al. 1989). In addition to regulation of collagenase at the level of its activation, the activity of the active enzyme is also determined by the local levels of the specific inhibitor, TIMP (tissue inhibitor of metalloproteinases), which blocks the activity of collagenase and other members of the metalloproteinase family including stromelysin and gelatinase.

The collagenase of mouse and rabbit bone has been shown by immunohistochemistry to be located within osteoblasts (M. SAKAMOTO and SAKAMOTO 1984; OTSUKA et al. 1984; HEATH and REYNOLDS 1990) and not in osteoclasts (BLAIR et al. 1986). Bone-resorbing agents such as PTH, PGE$_2$, 1,25-dihydroxyvitamin D$_3$, but not IL-1 and EGF, were shown to induce collagenase secretion in primary mouse calvarial osteoblasts and in the rat osteogenic sarcoma-derived cell line UMR 106 (HEATH et al. 1984; PARTRIDGE et al. 1987). Interestingly, PTH also stimulated the secretion of TIMP in these studies, which may provide for a feedback mechanism to limit collagen degradation.

Active collagenase can be extracted directly from rapidly resorbing tissues like the postpartum rat uterus, and its activity, like that of plasmin, is implicated in a wide range of processes including wound healing, cell migration, and angiogenesis. However, the role played by collagenase in bone is not known. Certainly it is unlikely that collagenase could attack mineralized collagen, but involvement in several other steps of the remodeling process has been suggested. In particular, collagenase could catalyze a rate-limiting step in bone resorption if, as has been proposed, the thin layer of unmineralized collagen next to osteoblasts presents a barrier to osteoclastic activity (CHAMBERS et al. 1984; CHAMBERS et al. 1985; CHAMBERS and FULLER 1985). However, this mechanism has not been investigated by in situ methods and it is not known whether, for example, the bone lining cells are able to initiate resorptive activity by producing collagenase. Indeed it has been strongly argued that while such a mechanism might apply to fetal bone, where there is a conspicuous layer of osteoid, it is unlikely to be of significance in adult bone (BOYDE and JONES 1987). In vitro observations have suggested that an alternative function for osteoblast collagenase is to solubilize collagen fibrils once they have been demineralized by osteoclasts. Thus scanning electron micrographs show that recently excavated resorption pits are lined by a network of collagen fibrils, whereas more "mature" Howship's lacunae have smooth linings. As collagenase antisera become more widely available, it will be possible to investigate these hypotheses more directly.

The PA system is tightly regulated in osteoblasts. Several bone-resorbing hormones have been shown to promote PA activity in osteoblast-like cells (HAMILTON et al. 1984, 1985; ALLAN et al. 1986). The effects of PTH and PGE$_2$ were cyclic AMP dependent (ALLAN et al. 1986), whereas other stimulators (e.g., 1,25-dihydroxyvitamin D$_3$) clearly used different second messenger systems. The PA was characterized as being due to tissue-type PA (tPA) (ALLAN et al. 1986) with no evidence at that stage of urokinase type (uPA). We proposed that the significance of PA formation was to activate procollagenase, and allow osteoclastic resorption to proceed (HAMILTON et al. 1985). This concept has been supported by others (PARTRIDGE et al. 1987; THOMSON et al. 1989; PFEILSCHIFTER et al. 1990). The significance of PA control in osteoblasts may be much greater, however. Osteoblasts synthesize TGFβ, which is stored in large amounts in bone matrix in a latent, inactive form (CARRINGTON et al. 1988), capable of activation either by acid or by proteinases, including plasmin (ALLAN et al.

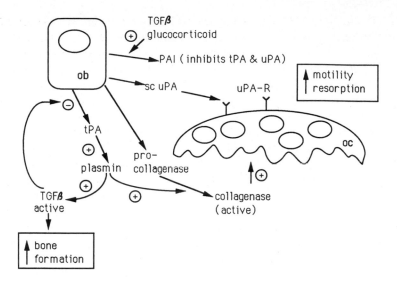

Fig. 3. Some of the possible interactions between osteoblasts (*ob*) and osteoclasts (*oc*) which could be mediated by the components of the PA/plasmin/PAI system. We wish to emphasize the pivotal role of plasmin in determining increases in bone formation through activation of TGFβ, and increases in bone resorption through direct proteolysis including activation of procollagenase. TGFβ and glucocorticoid both enhance production of PAI-1, which inhibits tPA and uPA activity and thereby limits the generation of plasmin. For TGFβ this will provide a feedback mechanism to limit the extent of its own activation and consequently restrict the rate of bone formation. Glucocorticoids, on the other hand, do not enhance bone formation by osteoblasts so the overall effect of glucocorticoid-induced PAI-1 formation is inhibition of TGFβ activation and decreased bone formation

1991). We have proposed that plasmin, generated as a result of PA activation, may be responsible for the local activation of TGFβ, making it available for its stimulatory effects on osteoblast synthesis of collagen and noncollagenous proteins (ALLAN et al. 1990, 1991). Thus, as discussed earlier, this would provide another potent mechanism for coupling bone resorption to formation. The connection with TGFβ is even more significant, given the fact that TGFβ directly inhibits PA activity by enhancing synthesis of the specific PA inhibitor-1 (PAI-1) (ALLAN et al. 1990; PFEILSCHIFTER et al. 1990), through a transcriptional effect (ALLAN et al. 1991). Therefore TGFβ seems to have the capacity to limit the extent of its own activation by regulating the net amount of PA formed under the influence of other stimuli. The many regulated points in these mechanisms make it likely that the control of plasmin generation at local sites in bone is an important aspect of osteoblast function. From data obtained recently, we would also like to propose a further role for the PA enzyme system of osteoblasts. Although in our earlier work we found no evidence for uPA formation by osteoblasts (ALLAN et al. 1986), we have now shown that these cells synthesize uPA mRNA, which is increased substantially by TGFβ (ALLAN et al. 1991) and by PTH, PGE$_2$, and 1,25-dihydroxyvitamin D$_3$ (unpublished). The lack of active uPA in the media from osteoblasts suggests that the cells are producing the single-chain, inactive pro-enzyme, sc uPA. This form is known in other cell systems to bind to specific receptors on adjacent cells, become activated by cleavage to uPA, thereby allowing it to generate plasmin at those sites. This pericellular proteolysis gives rise to cell motility, and the activity is stopped as soon as the appropriate part of the cell reaches PAI-1, which is stored in the matrix, and which specifically inhibits PA activity. Figure 3 illustrates these proposed mechanisms diagrammatically. This general mechanism for uPA action in cell motility would have important implications for osteoblast (and possibly osteoclast) function, and requires further study.

The exquisite control exerted over the formation and activities of collagenase, PAs, and their inhibitors indicate that they are likely to play an important role in osteoblast-mediated bone remodeling.

L. Conclusion

The osteoblast lineage comprises cells with a number of functions in addition to the well recognized role to synthesize the components of the organic matrix of bone and assist in its mineralization. By responding to circulating hormones and to growth factors and cytokines produced by osteoblasts themselves and other cells of marrow, they occupy a central role in a system of cell-cell communication which is essential for normal bone remodeling. This intercellular communication is mediated by products of osteoblasts which are largely uncharacterized, and which act upon osteoclasts and their precursors. Furthermore, there is increasing evidence for the importance of osteoblast-derived proteinases and their inhibitors in these processes.

References

Akatsu T, Takahashi N, Udagawa N, Imamura K, Yamaguchi A, Sato K, Nagata N, Suda T (1991) Role of prostaglandins in interleukin-1-induced bone resorption in mice in vitro. J Bone Miner Res 6:183–190

Allan EH, Hamilton JA, Medcalf RL, Kubota M, Martin TJ (1986) Cyclic AMP-dependent and -independent effects on tissue type plasminogen activator in osteogenic sarcoma cells: evidence from phosphodiesterase inhibition and parathyroid hormone antagonists. Biochim Biophys Acta 888:199–207

Allan EH, Hilton DJ, Brown MA, Evely RS, Yumita S, Metcalf D, Gough NM, Ng KW, Nicola NA, Martin TJ (1990) Osteoblasts display receptors for and responses to leukemia inhibitory factor. J Cell Physiol 145:110–119

Allan EH, Zeheb R, Gelehrter TD, Heaton JH, Fukumoto S, Yee JA, Martin TJ (1991) Transforming growth factor beta stimulates production of urokinase-type plasminogen activator mRNA and plasminogen activator inhibitor-1 mRNA and protein in rat osteoblast-like cells. J Cell Physiol 149:34–43

Ash P, Loutit JF, Townsend KMS (1981) Osteoclasts derive from haematopoietic stem cells according to marker, giant lysosomes of beige mice. Clin Orthop 155:249–258

Ashton BA, Eaglesom CC, Bab I, Owen ME (1984) Distribution of fibroblast colony-forming cells in rabbit bone marrow and assay of their osteogenic potential by an in vivo diffusion chamber method. Calcif Tissue Int 36:83–86

Aubin JE, Heersche JNM, Merrilees, MJ (1982) Isolation of bone cell clones with differences in growth, hormone responses and extracellular matrix production. J Cell Biol 92:452–461

Aubin JE, Heersche JNM, Bellows CG, Grigoriadis AE (1990) Osteoblast lineage analysis in fetal rat calvarial cells. In: Cohn DV, Glorieux FH, Martin TJ (eds) Calcium regulation and bone metabolism. Elsevier, Amsterdam, pp 362–370

Bab I, Ashton BA, Syftestad GT, Owen ME (1984) Assessment of an in vivo diffusion chamber method as a quantitative assay for osteogenesis. Calcif Tissue Int 36:77–82

Barnard R, Ng KW, Martin TJ, Waters MJ (1991) Growth hormone (GH) receptors in clonal osteoblast-like cells mediate a mitogenic response to GH. Endocrinology 128:1459–1464

Belanger LF (1969) Osteocytic osteolysis. Calcif Tissue Res 4:1–12

Bellows CG, Aubin JE, Heersche JNM, Antosa ME (1986) Mineralized nodules formed in vitro from enzymatically released rat calvaria populations. Calcif Tissue Int 38:143–154

Beresford JN, Gallagher JA, Poser JW, Russell RGG (1984) Production of osteocalcin by human bone cells in vitro. Effects of 1,25(OH)$_2$D$_3$, 24, 25(OH)$_2$D$_3$, parathyroid hormone, and glucocorticoids. Metab Bone Dis Rel Res 5:229–234

Bergmann P, Nijs-De Wolf N, Pepersack T, Corvilain J (1990) Release of parathyroid hormone-like peptides by fetal rat long bones in culture. J Bone Miner Res 5:741–746

Bertolini DR, Nedwin GE, Bringman TS, Smith DD, Mundy GR (1986) Stimulation of bone resorption and inhibition of bone formation in vitro by human tumour necrosis factors. Nature 319:516–518

Blair HC, Kahn AJ, Crouch EC, Jeffrey JJ, Teitelbaum SL (1986) Isolated osteoclasts resorb the organic and inorganic components of bone. J Cell Biol 102:1164–1172

Blomhoff R, Green MH, Berg T, Norum KR (1990) Transport and storage of vitamin A. Science 250:399–404

Boyde A, Jones SJ (1987) Early scanning electron microscopic studies of hard tissue resorption: their relation to current concepts reviewed. Scanning Microsc 1:369–381

Canalis E (1987) Effects of tumor necrosis factor on bone formation in vitro. Endocrinology 121:1596–1604

Canalis E, Lian JB (1985) 1,25-Dihydroxyvitamin D$_3$ effects on collagen and DNA synthesis in periosteum and periosteum-free calvaria. Bone 6:457–460

Canalis E, Centrella M, Burch W, McCarthy TL (1989) Insulin-like growth factor I mediates selective anabolic effects of parathyroid hormone in bone cultures. J Clin Invest 83:60–67

Carrington JL, Roberts AB, Flanders KC, Roche NS, Reddi AH (1988) Accumulation, localization, and compartmentation of transforming growth factor-β during endochondral bone development. J Cell Biol 107:1969–1975

Celeste AJ, Iannazzi JA, Taylor RC, Hewick RM, Rosen V, Wang EA, Wozney JM (1990) Identification of transforming growth factor β family members present in bone-inductive protein purified from bovine bone. Proc Natl Acad Sci USA 87:9843–9847

Centrella M, McCarthy TL, Canalis E (1987) Transforming growth factor β is a bifunctional regulator of replication and collagen synthesis in osteoblast-enriched cell cultures from fetal rat bone. J Biol Chem 262:2869–2879

Chambers TJ (1980) The cellular basis of bone resorption. Clin Orthop 151:283–293

Chambers TJ (1985) The pathobiology of the osteoclast. J Clin Pathol 38:241–252

Chambers TJ, Fuller K (1985) Bone cells predispose endosteal surfaces to resorption by exposure of bone mineral to osteoclastic contact. J Cell Sci 76:155–163

Chambers TJ, Thomson BM, Fuller K (1984) Effect of substrate composition on bone resorption by rabbit osteoclasts. J Cell Sci 70:61–71

Chambers TJ, Darby JA, Fuller K (1985) Mammalian collagenase predisposes bone surfaces to osteoclastic resorption. Cell Tissue Res 241:671–678

Chyun YS, Raisz LG (1984) Stimulation of bone formation by prostaglandin E_2. Prostaglandins 27:97–103

Civitelli R, Hruska KA, Jeffrey JJ, Kahn AJ, Avioli LV, Partridge NC (1989) Second messenger signalling in the regulation of collagenase production by osteogenic sarcoma cells. Endocrinology 124:2928–2934

Clezardin P, Malaval L, Ehrensperger AS, Delmas PD, Dechavanne M, McGregor JL (1988) Complex formation of human thrombospondin with osteonectin. Eur J Biochem 175:275–284

Cole WG (1988) Osteogenesis Imperfecta. Baillieres Clin Endocrinol Metab 2:243–265

Dewhurst FE, Ago JM, Peros WJ, Stashenko P (1987) Synergism between parathyroid hormone and interleukin 1 in stimulating bone resorption in organ culture. J Bone Miner Res 2:127–134

Doi Y, Okuda Y, Takegawa Y, Shibata S, Moniraki Y, Wakamatsu N, Shimizu N, Moriyama K, Shimokawa H (1989) Osteonectin inhibiting de novo formation of apatite in the presence of collagen. Calcif Tissue Int 44:200–208

Dolle P, Ruberte E, Kastner P, Petkovich M, Stoner CM, Gudas LJ, Chambon P (1990) Differential expression of genes encoding a, β and γ retinoic acid receptors and CRABP in the developing limbs of the mouse. Nature 342:702–705

Doty SB (1981) Morphological evidence of gap junctions between cells. Calcif Tissue Int 33:509–512

Eeckhout Y, Vaes G (1977) Further studies on the activation of procollagenase, the latent precursor of bone collagenase. Effects of lysosomal cathepsin B, plasmin and kallikrein, and spontaneous activation. Biochem J 166:21–31

Eriksen EF, Colvard DS, Berg NJ, Graham ML, Mann KG, Spelsberg TC, Riggs BL (1988) Evidence of estrogen receptors in normal human osteoblast-like cells. Science 241:84–87

Ernst M, Froesch ER (1988) Growth hormone dependent stimulation of osteoblast-like cells in serum-free cultures via local synthesis of insulin-like growth factor-I. Biochem Biophys Res Commun 151:142–147

Ernst M, Heath JK, Rodan GA (1989) Estradiol effects on proliferation, messenger RNA for collagen and insulin-like growth factor-1, and parathyroid hormone-responsive adenylate cyclase activity in osteoblastic cells from calvariae and long bones. Endocrinology 125:825–833

Evans RM (1988) The steroid and thyroid hormone receptor superfamily. Science 240:889–895

Evely RS, Bonomo A, Schneider H-G, Moseley JM, Gallagher JA, Martin TJ (1991) Structural requirements for the action of parathyroid hormone-related protein (PTHrP) on bone resorption by isolated osteoclasts. J Bone Miner Res 6:85–94

Farndale RW, Sandy JS, Atkinson SJ, Pennington SR, Meghji S, Meikle MC (1988) Parathyroid hormone and prostaglandin E_2 stimulate both inositol phosphates and cyclic AMP accumulation in mouse osteoblast cultures. Biochem J 252:263–268

Feyen JHM, DiBon A, van der Plas A, Lowik CWGM, Nijweide PJ (1985a) Effects of exogenous prostanoids on the proliferation of osteoblast-like cells in vitro. Prostaglandins 30:827–840

Feyen JHM, van der Plas A, Nijweide PJ (1985b) A direct effect of parathyroid hormone on the proliferation of osteoblast-like cells, a possible involvement of cyclic AMP. Biochem Biophys Res Commun 129:918–925

Fraser JD, Otawara Y, Price PA (1988) 1,25-Dihydroxyvitamin D_3 stimulates the synthesis of matrix γ-carboxyglutamic acid protein by osteosarcoma cells: mutually exclusive expression of vitamin K-dependent bone proteins by clonal osteoblastic cell lines. J Biol Chem 263:911–916

Friedenstein AJ (1976) Precursor cells of mechanocytes. Int Rev Cytol 47:327–355

Friedenstein AJ (1981) Stromal mechanisms of bone marrow: cloning in vitro and retransplantation in vivo. Haematol Bluttransfus 25:19–29

Gehron Robey P (1989) The biochemistry of bone. Endocrinol Metab Clin North Am 18:859–902

Gehron Robey P, Young MF, Flanders KC, Roche NS, Kondaiah P, Reddi AH, Termine JD, Sporn MB, Roberts AB (1987) Osteoblasts synthesize and respond to transforming growth factor-β (TGFβ) in vitro. J Cell Biol 105:457–463

Gehron Robey P, Young MF, Fisher LW, McClair TD (1989) Thrombospondin is an osteoblast-derived component of mineralized extracellular matrix. J Cell Biol 108:719–727

Glass CK, Devary OR, Rosenfeld MG (1990) Multiple cell type-specific proteins differentially regulate target sequence recognition by the a retinoic acid receptor. Cell 63:729–738

Glimcher MJ (1976) Composition, structure and organization of bone and other mineralized tissues and the mechanism of calcification. In: Aubach GD (ed) Handbook of physiology, endocrinology, parathyroid gland, section 7, vol 7. American Physiological Society, Washington, pp 25–48

Glimcher MJ, Krane SM (1968) The organization and structure of bone and the mechanism of calcification. In: Ramachandran GN, Goudl BS (eds) A treatise on collagen. Biology of collagens, vol 2B. Academic, New York, pp 68–91

Gowen M, Wood DD, Ihrie EJ, McGuire MKB, Russell RGG (1984) An interleukin 1 like factor stimulates bone resorption in vitro. Nature 306:378–380

Greaves MF (1986) Differentiation-linked leukemogenesis in lymphocytes. Science 234:697–704

Grigoriadis, AE, Heersche JNM, Aubin JE (1988) Differentiation of muscle, fat, cartilage, and bone from progenitor cells present in a bone-derived clonal cell population: effect of dexamethasone. J Cell Biol 106:2139–2151

Hakeda Y, Huira K, Sato T, Okazaki R, Matsumoto T, Ogata E, Ishitani R, Kumegawa M (1989) Existence of parathyroid hormone binding sites on murine hemopoietic blast cells. Biochem Biophys Res Commun 163:1481–1486

Hamilton JA, Lingelbach SR, Partridge NC, Martin TJ (1984) Stimulation of plasminogen activator release in osteoblast-like cells by bone-resorbing hormones. Biochem Biophys Res Commun 122:230–236

Hamilton JA, Lingelbach SR, Partridge NC, Martin TJ (1985) Regulation of plasminogen activator production by bone resorbing hormones in normal and malignant osteoblasts. Endocrinology 116:2186–2191

Hammonds RG Jr, Schwall R, Dudley A, Berkemeier L, Lai C, Lee J, Cunningham N, Reddi AH, Wood WI, Mason AJ (1991) Bone-inducing activity of mature BMP-2b produced from a hybrid BMP-2a/2b precursor. Mol Endocrinol 4:149–155

Harrison JR, Petersen DN, Lichtler AC, Mador AT, Rowe DW, Kream BE (1989) 1,25-Dihydroxyvitamin D_3 inhibits transcription of type-1 collagen genes in the rat osteosarcoma cell line ROS 17/2.8. Endocrinology 125:327–333

Hauschka PV, Maurakos AE, Lafrati MD, Doleman SE, Klagsbaun M (1986) Growth factors in bone matrix: isolation of multiple types by affinity chromatography on heparin-sepharose. J Biol Chem 261:12665–12674

Heath JK, Reynolds JJ (1990) Bone cell physiology and in vitro techniques in its investigation. In: Stephenson JC (ed) New techniques in metabolic bone disease. Butterworth, London, pp 21–39

Heath JK, Atkinson SJ, Meikle MC, Reynolds JJ (1984) Mouse osteoblasts synthesize collagenase in response to bone resorbing agents. Biochim Biophys Acta 802:151–154

Heath JK, Saklatvala J, Meikle MC, Atkinson SJ, Reynolds JJ (1985) Pig interleukin 1 (catabolin) is a potent stimulator of bone resorption in vitro. Calcif Tissue Int 37:95–97

Heath JK, Rodan SB, Yoon K, Rodan GA (1989) Rat calvarial cell lines immortalized with SV-40 Large T antigen: constitutive and retinoic acid-inducible expression of osteoblastic features. Endocrinology 124:3060–3068

Hiura K, Sumitani K, Kawata T, Higashino K, Okawa M, Sato T, Hakeda Y, Kumagawa M (1991) Mouse osteoblastic cells (MC3T3-E1) at different stages of differentiation have opposite effects on osteoclastic cell formation. Endocrinology 128:1630–1637

Hohmann EL, Levine L, Tashjian AH Jr (1983) Vasoactive intestinal peptide stimulates bone resorption via a cyclic adenosine $3'-5'$: monophosphate-dependent mechanism. Endocrinology 112:1233–1240

Holland PW, Harper SJ, McVey JH, Hogan BLM (1987) In vivo expression of mRNA for the Ca^{++} binding protein SPARC (osteonectin) revealed by in situ hybridization. J Cell Biol 105:473–482

Howard GA, Bottemiller BL, Turner RT, Rader JI, Baylink DJ (1981) Parathyroid hormone stimulates bone formation and resorption in organ culture: evidence for a coupling mechanism. Proc Natl Acad Sci USA 78:3204–3208

Ibbotson KJ, Harrod J, Gowen M, D'Souza S, Smitt DD, Winkler ME, Derynck R, Mundy GR (1986) Human recombinant transforming growth factor a stimulates bone resorption and inhibits formation in vitro. Proc Natl Acad Sci USA 83:2228–2232

Imai Y, Rodan SB, Rodan GA (1988) Effects of retinoic acid on alkaline phosphatase messenger ribonucleic acid, catecholamine receptors and G proteins in ROS 17/2.8 cells. Endocrinology 122:456–463

Johanson S, Hedman K, Kjellen et al. (1985) Structure and interactions of proteoglycans in the extracellular matrix produced by cultured human fibroblasts. Biochem J 232:161–168

Jones SJ, Boyde A (1976) Experimental study of changes in osteoblast shape induced by calcitonin and parathyroid extract in an organ culture system. Cell Tissue Res 169:449–465

Joyce ME, Roberts AB, Sporn MB, Bolander ME (1990) Transforming growth factor-β and the initiation of chondrogenesis and osteogenesis in the rat femur. J Cell Biol 110:2195–2207

Keeting PE, Scott RE, Colvard DS, Han IK, Spelsberg TC, Riggs BC (1991) Lack of a direct effect of estrogen on proliferation and differentiation of normal human osteoblast-like cells. J Bone Miner Res 6:297–304

Komm BS, Terpening CM, Benz DJ, Graeme EA, O'Malley BW, Haussler MR (1988) Estrogen binding receptor mRNA, and biologic response in osteoblast-like osteosarcoma cells. Science 241:81–84

Krust A, Kastner P, Petkovich M, Zelent A, Chambon P (1989) A third human retinoic acid receptor, hRARγ. Proc Natl Acad Sci USA 86:8819–8823

Kurihara N, Suda T, Muira Y, Nakauchi H, Kodama H, Hiura K, Hakeda Y, Kumegawa M (1989) Generation of osteoclasts from isolated hemopoietic progenitor cells. Blood 74:1295–1302

Kurihara N, Chenu C, Miller M, Civin C, Roodman GD (1990) Identification of committed mononuclear precursors for osteoclast-like cells formed in long term human marrow cultures. Endocrinology 126:2733–2741

Lane TF, Sage EH (1990) Functional mapping of SPARC: peptides from two distinct Ca^{++} binding sites modulate cell shape. J Cell Biol 111:3065–3076

Livesey SA, Kemp BE, Re CA, Partridge NC, Martin TJ (1982) Selective hormonal activation of cyclic AMP-dependent protein kinase isoenzymes in normal and malignant osteoblasts. J Biol Chem 257:14989–14998

Livesey SA, Ng KW, Collier GR, Kubota M, Steiner AL, Martin TJ (1985) Effects of retinoids on cellular content and human parathyroid hormone activation of cyclic adenosine 3':5'-monophosphate-dependent protein kinase isoenzymes in clonal rat osteogenic sarcoma cells. Cancer Res 45:5734–5740

Lorenzo JA, Sousa SL, Leaky CL (1990) Leukemia inhibitory factor (LIF) inhibits basal bone resorption in fetal rat long bone cultures. Cytokines 2:266–271

Lowik CWGM, Van der Pluijm G, Hoekman K, Aarden L, Bijvoet OLM, Papapoulos S (1989) Parathyroid hormone (PTH) and PTH-like protein stimulate interleukin-6 production by osteogenic cells: a possible role of interleukin-6 in osteoclastogenesis. Biochem Biophys Res Commun 162:1546–1550

Luben RA, Cohn DV (1976) Effects of parathormone and calcitonin on citrate and hyaluronate metabolism in cultured bone. Endocrinology 98:413–419

Majeska RJ, Rodan GA (1982) The effect of $1,25(OH)_2D_3$ on alkaline phosphatase in osteoblastic osteosarcoma cells. J Biol Chem 257:3362–3365

Majeska RJ, Rodan SB, Rodan GA (1980) Parathyroid hormone-responsive clonal lines from rat osteosarcoma. Endocrinology 107:1494–1503

Mangelsdorf DJ, Ong ES, Dyck JA, Evans RM (1990) Nuclear receptor that identifies a novel retinoic acid response pathway. Nature 345:224–229

Manolagas SC, Burton DW, Deftos LJ (1981) 1,25-Dihydroxyvitamin D_3 stimulates the alkaline phosphatase activity of osteoblast-like cells. J Biol Chem 256:7115–7117

Marcelli C, Yates AJ, Mundy GR (1990) In vivo effects of human recombinant transforming growth factor β on bone turnover in normal mice. J Bone Miner Res 5:1087–1096

Martin TJ, Ingleton PM, Underwood JCE, Melick RA, Michelangeli VP, Hunt NH (1976) Parathyroid hormone responsive adenylate cyclase in an induced transplantable osteogenic sarcoma in the rat. Nature 260:436–438

Martin TJ, Partridge NC, Greaves M, Atkins D, Ibbotson KJ (1979) Prostaglandin effects on bone and role in cancer hypercalcemia. In: MacIntyre I, Szelke M (eds) Molecular endocrinology. Elsevier, Amsterdam, pp 251–264

Martin TJ, Ng KW, Suda T (1989) Bone cell physiology. Endocrinol Metab Clin North Am 18:833–858

Massague J (1990) The transforming growth factor-β family. Annu Rev Cell Biol 6:597–641

Mellanby E (1944) Croonian lecture. Nutrition in relation to bone growth and nervous system. Proc R Soc Lond [Biol] 132:28–46

Metcalf D (1984) The heamopoietic colony stimulating factors. Elsevier, Amsterdam

Metcalf D, Gearing DP (1989) A fatal syndrome in mice engrafted with cells producing high levels of leukemia inhibitory factor (LIF). Proc Natl Acad Sci USA 86:5948–5952

Michelangeli VP, Fletcher AE, Allan EH, Nicholson GC, Martin TJ (1989) Effects of calcitonin gene-related peptide on cyclic AMP formation in chicken, rat and mouse bone cells. J Bone Miner Res 4:262–272

Miller SC, Jee WSS (1987) The bone lining cell: a distinct phenotype? Calcif Tissue Int 41:1–5

Mohan S, Linkhart T, Rosenfeld R, Baylink D (1989) Characterization of the receptor for insulin-like growth factor II in bone cells. J Cell Physiol 140:169–176

Moseley JM, Hayman JA, Danks JA, Alcorn D, Grill V, Southby J, Horton MA (1991) Immunohistochemical detection of parathyroid hormone-related protein (PTHrP) in human fetal epithelia. J Clin Endocrinol Metab 73:478–484

Mumby SM, Raugi GJ, Bornstein P (1984) Interactions of thrombospondin with extracellular matrix protein: selective binding to type V collagen. J Cell Biol 98:646–652

Mundy GR, Poser JW (1983) Chemotactic activity of the gamma-carboxyglutamic acid containing protein of bone. Calcif Tissue Int 35:164–168

Ng KW, Partridge NC, Niall H, Martin TJ (1983a) Epidermal growth factor receptors in clonal lines of a rat osteogenic sarcoma and in osteoblast-rich rat bone cells. Calcif Tissue Int 35:298–303

Ng KW, Partridge NC, Niall H, Martin TJ (1983b) Stimulation of DNA synthesis by epidermal growth factor in osteoblast-like cells. Calcif Tissue Int 35:624–628

Ng KW, Livesey SA, Collier F, Gummer PR, Martin TJ (1985) Effect of retinoids on the growth, ultrastructure, and cytoskeletal structures of malignant rat osteoblasts. Cancer Res 45:5106–5113

Ng KW, Gummer PA, Michelangeli VP, Bateman JF, Mascara T, Cole WG, Martin TJ (1988) Regulation of alkaline phosphatase expression in a neonatal rat clonal calvarial cell strain by retinoic acid. J Bone Miner Res 3:53–61

Ng KW, Hudson PJ, Power BE, Manji SS, Gummer PR, Martin TJ (1989a) Retinoic acid and tumour necrosis factor-α act in concert to control the level of alkaline phosphatase mRNA. J Mol Endocrinol 3:57–64

Ng KW, Manji SS, Young MF, Findlay DM (1989b) Opposing influences of glucocorticoid and retinoic acid on transcriptional control in preosteoblasts. Mol Endocrinol 3:2079–2085

Nicholson, GC, Moseley JM, Sexton PM, Mendelsohn FAO, Martin TJ (1986) Abundant calcitonin receptors in isolated rat osteoclasts. Biochemical and autoradiographic characterization. J Clin Invest 78:355–360

Noda M (1989) Transcriptional regulation of osteocalcin production by transforming growth factor-β in rat osteoblast-like cells. Endocrinology 124:612–619

Noda M, Camilliere MJ (1989) In vivo stimulation of bone formation by transforming growth factor β. Endocrinology 124:2991–2994

Noda M, Rodan GA (1987) Type β transforming growth factor (TGFβ) regulation of alkaline phosphatase expression and other phenotype-related mRNA's in osteoblastic rat osteosarcoma cells. J Cell Physiol 133:426–434

Noda M, Rodan GA (1989) Transcriptional regulation of osteopontin production in rat osteoblast-like cells by parathyroid hormone. J Cell Biol 108:713–718

Noda M, Yoon K, Rodan GA (1988a) Cyclic AMP-mediated stabilization of osteocalcin mRNA in rat osteoblast-like cells treated with parathyroid hormone. J Biol Chem 263:18574–18577

Noda M, Yoon K, Prince CW, Butler WT, Rodan GA (1988b) Transcriptional regulation of osteopontin production in rat osteosarcoma cells by type β transforming growth factor. J Biol Chem 263:13916–13921

Nolan RD, Partridge NC, Godfrey HM, Martin TJ (1983) Cyclo-oxygenase products of arachidonic acid metabolism in rat osteoblasts in culture. Calcif Tissue Int 35:294–297

Oldberg A, Fraizen A, Heinegard D (1986) Cloning and sequence analysis of rat bone sialoprotein (osteopontin) cDNA reveals an Arg-Gly-Asp cell-binding sequence. Proc Natl Acad Sci USA 83:8819–8823

Oldberg A, Fraizen A, Heinegard D, Pierschbacher M, Ruoslahti E (1988) Identification of a bone sialoprotein receptor in osteosarcoma cells. J Biol Chem 263:19433–19436

Oldberg A, Jiskog-Hed B, Axelsson S, Heinegard D (1989) Regulation of bone sialoprotein mRNA by steroid hormones. J Cell Biol 109:3183–3186

Otsuka K, Sodek J, Limeback H (1984) Synthesis of collagenase and collagenase inhibitors by osteoblast-like cells in culture. Eur J Biochem 145:123–129

Owen TA, Aronow M, Shalhoub V, Barone LM, Wilming L, Tassinari MS, Kennedy MB, Pockwinse S, Lian JB, Stein GS (1990) Progressive development of the rat osteoblast phenotype in vitro: reciprocal relationships in expression of genes associated with osteoblast proliferation and differentiation during formation of the bone extracellular matrix. J Cell Physiol 143:420–430

Owen TA, Aronow MS, Barone LM, Bettencourt B, Stein GS, Lian JB (1991) Pleiotropic effects of vitamin D on osteoblast gene expression are related to the proliferative and differentiated state of the bone cell phenotype: dependency upon basal levels of gene expression, duration of exposure and bone matrix competency in normal rat osteoblast cultures. Endocrinology 128:1496–1504

Parfitt AM (1977) The cellular basis of bone turnover and bone loss. Clin Orthop 127:236–247

Partridge NC, Frampton RJ, Eisman JA, Michelangeli VP, Elms E, Bradley TR, Martin TJ (1980) Receptors for 1,25(OH)$_2$ vitamin D$_3$ enriched in cloned osteoblast-like rat osteogenic sarcoma cells. FEBS Lett 115:139–141

Partridge NC, Alcorn D, Michelangeli VP, Kemp BE, Ryan GB, Martin TJ (1981) Functional properties of hormonally responsive cultured normal and malignant rat osteoblastic cells. Endocrinology 108:213–219

Partridge NC, Alcorn D, Michelangeli VP, Ryan G, Martin TJ (1983) Morphological and biochemical characterization of four clonal osteogenic sarcoma cell lines of rat origin. Cancer Res 43:4388–4394

Partridge NC, Opie AL, Opie RT, Martin TJ (1985) inhibitory effects of parathyroid hormone on growth of osteogenic sarcoma cells. Calcif Tissue Int 37:519–525

Partridge NC, Jeffrey JJ, Ehlich LS, Teitelbaum SL, Fliszar C, Welgus HG, Kahn AJ (1987) Hormonal regulation of the production of collagenase and a collagenase inhibitor activity by rat osteogenic sarcoma cells. Endocrinology 120:1956–1962

Pfeilschifter J, D'Souza SM, Mundy GR (1987) Effects of transforming growth factor-β on osteoblastic osteosarcoma cells. Endocrinology 121:212–219

Pfeilschifter J, Erdmann J, Schmidt W, Naumann A, Minne HW, Ziegler R (1990) Differential regulation of plasminogen activator and plasminogen activator inhibitor by osteotropic factors in primary cultures of mature osteoblasts and osteoblast precursors. Endocrinology 126:703–711

Price PA, Baukol SA (1980) 1,25-Dihydroxyvitamin D$_3$ increases synthesis of the vitamin K-dependent bone protein by osteosarcoma cells. J Biol Chem 255:11660–11663

Price PA, Williamson MK, Haba T, Dell RB, Jee WSS (1982) Excessive mineralization with growth plate closure in rats on chronic warfarin treatment. Proc Natl Acad Sci USA 79:7734–7738

Prince CW, Butler WT (1987) 1,25-Dihydroxyvitamin D$_3$ regulates the biosynthesis of osteopontin, a bone-derived cell attachment protein, in clonal osteoblast-like osteosarcoma cells. Coll Relat Res 7:305–315

Puzas JE, Brand JS (1979) Parathyroid hormone stimulation of collagenase secretion by isolated bone cells. Endocrinology 104:559–569

Raisz LG, Simmons HA, Sandberg AL, Canalis E (1980) Direct stimulation of bone resorption by epidermal growth factor. Endocrinology 107:207–212

Rao LG, Murray TM, Heersche JNM (1983) Immunohistochemical demonstration of parathyroid hormone binding to specific cell types in fixed rat bone tissues. Endocrinology 113:805–810

Reddi AH, Huggins C (1972) Biochemical sequences in the transformation of normal fibroblasts in adolescent rats. Proc Natl Acad Sci USA 69:1601–1605

Reid IR, Civitelli R, Halstead LR, Avioli LV, Hruska KA (1987) Parathyroid hormone acutely elevates intracellular calcium in osteoblast-like cells. Am J Physiol 253:E45–E54

Reid IR, Lowe C, Cornish J, Skinner SJM, Hilton DJ, Wilson TA, Gearing DP, Martin TJ (1990) Leukemia inhibitory factor: a novel bone-active cytokine. Endocrinology 126:1416–1419

Reinhold FP, Hultenby K, Oldberg A, Heinegard D (1990) Osteopontin – a possible anchor of osteoclasts to bone. Proc Natl Acad Sci USA 87:4473–4475

Rodan GA, Martin TJ (1981) Role of osteoblasts in hormonal control of bone resorption – a hypothesis. Calcif Tissue Int 33:349–351

Romberg RN, Werness PG, Riggs BL, Mann KG (1986) Inhibition of hydroxyapatite crystal growth by bone-specific and other calcium-binding proteins. Biochemistry 25:1176–1180

Rouleau MF, Warshawsky H, Goltzman D (1986) Parathyroid hormone binding in vivo to renal, hepatic and skeletal tissues of the rat using an autoradiographic approach. Endocrinology 118:919–928

Ruberte E, Dolle P, Krust A, Zelent A, Morris-Kay G, Chambon P (1990) Specific spatial and temporal distribution of retinoic acid receptor gamma transcripts during mouse embryogenesis. Development 108:213–222

Sage EH, Vernon RB, Funk SE, Everitt EA, Angello J (1989) SPARC, a secreted protein associated with cellular proliferation, inhibits cell spreading in vitro and exhibits Ca^{++}-dependent binding to the extracellular matrix. J Cell Biol 109:341–356

Sakamoto M, Sakamoto S (1984) Immunocytohemical localization of collagenase in isolated mouse bone cells. Biomed Res 5:29–38

Sakamoto S, Sakamoto M (1984) Isolation and characterization of collagenase synthesized by mouse bone cells in culture. Biomed Res 5:39–46

Sakamoto S, Goldhaber P, Glimcher MJ (1972) The further purification and characterization of mouse bone collagenase. Calcif Tissue Res 10:142–151

Sakamoto S, Sakamoto M, Goldhaber P, Glimcher MJ (1975) Collagenase and bone resorption: isolation of collagenase from culture medium containing serum after stimulation of bone resorption by addition of parathyroid extract. Biochem Biophys Res Commun 63:172–178

Schmid C, Schapfer I, Boni-Schnetzler M, Mary J-L, Schivander J, Zapf J, Froesch ER (1990) PTH and cAMP stimulate the expression of the growth hormone (GH)-dependent insulin-like growth factor binding protein (IGFBP-3) by rat osteoblasts in vitro. In: Christiansen C, Overgaard K (eds) Osteoporosis 1990, København, Denmark, pp 264–273

Shupnik MA, Tashjian AH Jr (1982) Epidermal growth factor and phorbol ester actions on human osteosarcoma cells. J Biol Chem 257:12161–12164

Silve CM, Hradek GT, Jones AL, Arnaud CD (1982) Parathyroid hormone receptor in intact embryonic chicken bone: characterization and cellular location. J Cell Biol 94:379–386

Sporn MB, Roberts AB (1990) TGFβ: problems and prospects. Cell Regul 1:875–882

Sporn MB, Roberts AB, Wakefield LM (1987) Some recent advances in the chemistry and biology of transforming growth factor-β. J Cell Biol 105:1039–1044

Stein GS, Lian JB, Gerstenfeld LG, Shalhoub V, Aronow M, Owen T, Markose E (1989) The onset and progression of osteoblast differentiation is functionally related to cellular proliferation. Connect Tissue Res 20:3–13

Strauss PG, Closs EI, Schmidt J, Erfle V (1990) Gene expression during osteogenic differentiation in mandibular condyles in vitro. J Cell Biol 110:1369–1377

Suva LJ, Ernst M, Rodan GA (1991) Retinoic acid increases zif268 early gene expression in rat preosteoblastic cells. Mol Cell Biol 11:2503–2510

Takahashi N, Akatsu T, Udagawa N, Sasaki T, Yamaguchi A, Moseley JM, Martin TJ, Suda T (1988a) Osteoblastic cells are involved in osteoclast formation. Endocrinology 123:2600–2602

Takahashi N, Akatsu T, Sasaki T, Nicholson GC, Moseley JM, Martin TJ, Suda T (1988b) Induction of calcitonin receptors by 1–25 dihydroxyvitamin D_3 in osteoclast-like multinucleated cells formed from mouse bone marrow cells. Endocrinology 123:1504–1510

Tashjian AH Jr, Levine L (1978) Epidermal growth factor stimulates prostaglandin production and bone resorption in cultured mouse calvaria. Biochem Biophys Res Commun 85:966–971

Tashjian AH Jr, Voelkel EF, Lazzaro M, Singer FR, Roberts AB, Derynck R, Winlker ME, Levine L (1985) α and β transforming growth factors stimulate prostaglandin production and bone resorption in cultured mouse calvaria. Proc Natl Acad Sci USA 82:4535–4538

Termine JD, Belcourt AB, Conn KM, Kleinman HK (1981a) Mineral and collagen-binding proteins of fetal calf bone. J Biol Chem 256:10403–10408

Termine JD, Kleinman HK, Whitson SW, Conn KM, McGarvey ML, Martin GR (1981b) Osteonectin, a bone-specific protein linking mineral to collagen. Cell 26:99–105

Teti A, Rizzoli R, Zambonin-Zallone A (1991) Parathyroid hormone binding to cultured avian osteoclasts. Biochem Biophys Res Commun 174:1217–1222

Thaller C, Eichele G (1987) Identification and spatial distribution of retinoids in the developing chick limb bud. Nature 327:625–628

Thein R, Lotan R (1982) Sensitivity of cultured human osteosarcoma and chondrosarcoma cells to retinoic acid. Cancer Res 42:4771–4775

Thiebaud D, Ng KW, Findlay DM, Harker M, Martin TJ (1990) Insulin like growth factor I regulates mRNA levels of osteonectin and pro-α, (I) collagen in clonal preosteoblastic calvarial cells. J Bone Miner Res 5:761–767

Thomson BM, Saklatvala J, Chambers TJ (1986) Osteoblasts mediate interleukin 1 responsiveness of bone resorption by rat osteoclasts. J Exp Med 164:104–112

Thomson BM, Mundy GR, Chambers TJ (1987) Tumour necrosis factors α and β induce osteoblastic cells to stimulate osteoclastic bone resorption. J Immunol 138:775–779

Thomson BM, Atkinson SJ, McGarrity AM, Hembry RM, Reynolds JJ, Meikle MC (1989) Type I collagen degradation by mouse calvarial osteoblasts stimulated with 1,25-dihydroxyvitamin D_3: evidence for a plasminogen-plasmin-metalloproteinase activation cascade. Biochim Biophys Acta 1014:125–132

Tørring O, Firek AF, Heath J, Conover CA (1991) Parathyroid hormone and parathyroid hormone-related peptide stimulate insulin-like growth factor-binding protein secretion by rat osteoblast like cells through an adenosine 3′, 5′-monophosphate-dependent mechanism. Endocrinology 128:1006–1014

Udagawa N, Takahashi N, Akatsu T, Sasaki T, Yamaguchi A, Kodama H, Martin TJ, Suda T (1989) The bone marrow-derived stromal cell lines MC3T3-G2/PA6 and ST2 support osteoclast-like cell differentiation in co-cultures with mouse spleen cells. Endocrinology 125:1805–1813

Urist MR (1965) Bone formation by autoinduction. Science 150:893–899

Urist MR (1989) Bone morphogenetic protein, bone regeneration, heterotopic ossification and the bone-bone-marrow consortium. In: Peck WA (ed) Bone and Mineral Research Volume 6. Elsevier, Amsterdam, pp 57–112

Vukicevic S, Luyten FP, Reddi AH (1989) Stimulation of the expression of osteogenic and chondrogenic phenotypes in vitro by osteogenin. Proc Natl Acad Sci USA 86:8793–8797

Wagner M, Thaller C, Jessell T, Eichele G (1990) Polarizing activity and retinoid synthesis in the floor plate of the neural tube. Nature 345:819–822

Walker DG (1966) Elevated bone collagenolytic activity and hyperplasia of parafollicular light cells of the thyroid in parathormone-treated grey-lethal mice. Z Zellforsch 72:100–124

Walters MR, Rosen DM, Norman AW, Luben RA (1982) 1,25-Dihydroxyvitamin D_3 receptors in an established bone cell line. J Biol Chem 257:7481–7484

Wang EA, Rosen V, Cordes P, Hewick RM, Kriz RW, Luxenberg DP, Sibley BS, Wozney JM (1988) Purification and characterization of other distinct bone-inducing factors. Proc Natl Acad Sci USA 85:9484–9488

Wang EA, Rosen V, D'Alessandro JS, Banduy M, Cordes P, Harada T, Israel DI, Hewick RM, Kerns KM, LaPan P, Luxenberg DP, McQuaid D, Moutsatsos IK, Nove J, Wozney JM (1990) Recombinant human bone morphogenetic protein induces bone formation. Proc Natl Acad Sci USA 87:2220–2224

Wozney JM, Rosen V, Celeste AJ, Mitsock LM, Whitters MJ, Kriz RW, Hewick RM, Wang EA (1988) Novel regulators of bone formation: molecular clones and activities. Science 242:1528–1534

Yamaguchi A, Katagiri T, Ikeda T, Wozney JM, Rosen V, Wang EA, Kahn AJ, Suda T, Yoshiki S (1991) Recombinant human bone morphogenetic protein-2 stimulates osteoblast maturation and inhibits myogenic differentiation in vitro. J Cell Biol 113:681–687

Yamaguchi DT, Hahn TJ, Iida-Klein A, Kleeman CR, Muallem S (1987) Parathyroid hormone-activated calcium channels in an osteoblast-like clonal osteosarcoma cell line. J Biol Chem 262:7711–7721

Yamaguchi Y, Mann DM, Ruoslahti E (1990) Negative regulation of transformation growth factor-β by the proteoglycan decorin. Nature 346:281–284

Yamashita T, Asano K, Takahashi N, Akatsu T, Udagawa N, Sasaki T, Martin TJ, Suda T (1990) Cloning of an osteoblastic cell line involved in the formation of osteoclast-like cells. J Cell Physiol 145:587–595

Yoon K, Buenaga R, Rodan GA (1987) Tissue specificity and developmental expression of rat osteopontin. Biochem Biophys Res Commun 148:1129–1136

Zelent A, Krust A, Petkovich M, Kastner P, Chambon P (1989) Cloning of murine retinoic acid receptor α and β cDNA's and of a novel third receptor γ predominantly expressed in skin. Nature 339:714–717

Zhou H, Hammonds RG Jr, Findlay DM, Fuller PJ, Martin TJ, Ng KW (1991) Retinoic acid-induced gene expression in malignant, non-transformed and immortalized osteoblasts. J Bone Miner Res 6:767–775

CHAPTER 5

Cytokines of Bone

G.R. MUNDY

A. Introduction

In recent years, it has become increasingly obvious that the cellular events involved in bone remodeling are likely modulated by a group of local factors. These local factors, or osteotropic cytokines, have extremely potent effects on bone cells in both in vitro and in vivo systems.

Many of the effects of bone active cytokines on bone cells appear to be overlapping and are seemingly redundant. Thus, interleukin-1 (IL-1), tumor necrosis factor (TNF), and lymphotoxin seem to have essentially identical effects on bone resorption. As more is understood of the complex mechanisms involved in osteoclastic resorption, then the physiologic role of each of these factors should become apparent.

Cytokine regulation of bone remodeling is more likely to be important for trabecular bone than for cortical bone. In contrast to the bone cells in haversian systems, the remodeling cells on the endosteal surfaces of trabecular bone are in much closer proximity to the cells in the marrow cavity, which in turn are likely sources of cytokines such as IL-1 and TNF. Thus, cytokines may be more important for regulation of bone remodeling at these sites than for events in cortical bone. The cells in haversian systems may be more influenced by systemic hormones such as PTH. In primary hyperparathyroidism, cortical bone seems to be preferentially affected. However, in osteoporosis, and particularly in postmenopausal osteoporosis associated with estrogen deficiency, bone loss in trabecular bone is more prominent than loss of cortical bone.

B. Nature of the Osteotropic Cytokines

Many of the potent osteotropic cytokines are familiar growth regulatory peptides which have important regulatory roles in many other essential organ processes such as embryogenesis, angiogenesis, tumorigenesis, wound healing, and immune responses. Thus, factors such as IL-1, TNF, interleukin-6 (IL-6), and transforming growth factor β (TGFβ) all have multiple effects which are independent of those on bone cells. However, in addition to these factors which have multiple target organs, there may also be other cytokines which have specific, or at least relatively specific, effects on bone. Thus, some of the growth regulatory factors in the extended TGFβ family which are found in bone such as the bone morphogenetic proteins appear to be relatively specific for bone cells or their precursors. It is highly that additional bone-specific peptides will be identified. To date, most observations have been made on factors identified in other systems. With improvements in assays for measuring bone-active factors, it appears highly likely that additional factors with specific effects on bone cells will be recognized.

C. Cell Source of the Osteotropic Cytokines

Most of the osteotropic cytokines are clearly products of immune cells. Thus, cytokines such as IL-1, TNF, lymphotoxin, and IL-6 are well-known products of the monocyte-macrophage series. Since these cells are abundant in the neighborhood of bone remodeling units on trabecular bone surfaces, it is hardly surprising that the importance of these cells are likely sources of the bone active cytokines has been emphasized. However, these cells are not the only potential sources for osteotropic cytokines. Stromal cells and bone cells produce IL-1, TNF, IL-6, and leukemia inhibitory factor. Several groups have shown independently that bone cells may be sources of essentially all of the bone-resorbing cytokines (GOWEN et al. 1990). It is still unclear whether bone cell production of cytokines is regulated in a physiologically important manner. Although enhanced production has been shown by lipopolysaccharide, the physiological relevance of this observation is not yet clear. Cytokine production by bone cells may be enhanced by other cytokines. For example, IL-6 and LIF production may be enhanced by IL-1 and TNF. Production of these cytokines may be inhibited by estrogens (GIRASOLE et al. 1990) and glucocorticoids (M. GOWEN, personal communication).

Cytokines may be responsible for the complex molecular mechanisms involved in osteoclast activation. Mature osteoclasts are activated to resorb bone when they are in intimate contact with bone-lining cells. The molecular mechanisms have not been clearly identified, but likely involve both soluble factors and cell-cell contact. Stromal cells or bone-lining cells adjacent to osteoclasts interact with the bone-resorbing cell and presumably transmit the resorbing stimulus.

D. Interactions Between Systemic Factors and Cytokines

Synergism has been shown between PTH or PTH-rP and IL-1α in vivo to cause hypercalcemia (K. SATO et al. 1989) and in vitro to cause bone resorption (DEWHRIST et al. 1987). Similarly, there may be a complicated relationship between PTH and TGFα and PTH and IL-1 and TGFβ. TGFα, EGF, IL-1, and TNF inhibit the capacity of PTH (and presumably PTH-rP) to cause increases in adenylate cyclase activity in boen and renal tubular cells (GUTIERREZ et al. 1987), whereas TGFβ enhances PTH-mediated adenylate cyclase activity (GUTIERREZ et al. 1990). Whether these responses have biological significance is not entirely clear, although recent work by PIZURKI et al. (1990) has shown that the effects of PTH-rP and PTH on renal phosphate transport may be enhanced by TGFα.

E. Interactions Between Cytokines

The cytokines of bone appear at first sight to have overlapping or redundant effects. Thus, TNF and IL-1 seem to have essentially identical effects on osteoclast formation, differentiation, and activation. However, it is difficult from the information available to discern which of these effects are direct and which are indirect. For example, each of these factors may under appropriate circumstances induce the other. It is possible that there are subtle differences in their modes of action which still remain to be determined.

The effects of the cytokines are also interwoven in other complex ways. For example, TNF effects on bone may be inhibited partially by antibodies to the IL-1 80-kDa receptor, or the 80-kDa IL-1 receptor antagonist. Similarly, the effects of IL-1 on bone may be markedly enhanced by IL-6, and IL-6 antibodies may block these effects. These complicated interactions between cytokines indicate that in vitro studies which examine the effects of single cytokines administered exogenously do not necessarily measure the single effects of these cytokines alone.

F. Diseases Associated with Abnormal Cytokine Production

The hypothesis that local factors are primarily responsible for bone remodeling has been strengthened by recent data which directly implicate the requirement of at least one of these cytokines for normal osteoclastic bone resorption. In mice with the *op/op* variant of osteopetrosis, there is a defect in the coding region for the colony-stimulating factor (CSF) of the macrophage series (CSF-M), with decreased CSF-M production. The mice do not form functional osteoclasts. As a result, these mice do not form marrow cavities properly and they develop the disease osteopetrosis. The disease can be reversed by treatment with CSF-M (FELIX et al. 1990). This is the first direct evidence that defective production of a specific cytokine can produce a bone disease.

Osteopetrosis is not the only disease in which osteotropic cytokines have been implicated. Other examples are osteoporosis, malignant disease, and chronic inflammatory diseases. In osteoporosis, it has been shown that peripheral blood monocytes from patients with this disease constitutively produce the cytokines IL-1 and TNF in increased amounts compared with those of normal individuals (PACIFICI et al. 1987, 1989). The production of these cytokines has been linked with a high turnover form of osteoporosis. Moreover, in postmenopausal women, production of cytokines such as IL-1 by monocytes from the peripheral blood can be decreased by treatment with estrogens. The assumption here is that the peripheral blood cells which produce these osteotropic cytokines are representative of cells in the marrow microenvironment.

In myeloma, the cytokines lymphotoxin, IL-1β, and IL-6 have all been implicated in the bone destruction and hypercalcemia (GARRETT et al. 1987; KAWANO et al. 1989; COZZOLINO et al. 1989). Long-term cultures of human myeloma cells constitutively express lymphotoxin (GARRETT et al. 1987). Mixed cell cultures of myeloma cells and other marrow cells produce IL-1β. IL-6 is an important growth factor in myeloma and its level in the circulation correlates with the tumor bulk. In patients with plasma cell leukemia, there may be high circulating levels of IL-6 (KLEIN et al. 1989; BATAILLE et al. 1989). Recently, we have found that IL-6 causes hypercalcemia and increased bone resorption in vivo (BLACK et al. 1990).

Cytokines such as IL-1α have also been implicated in the bone destruction and hypercalcemia associated with solid tumors (K. SATO et al. 1989; FRIED et al. 1989). For example, a number of squamous cell carcinomas have now been associated with increased IL-1α production. Sometimes this is produced in conjunction with other factors such as parathyroid hormone-related protein and together these factors may act synergistically to increase the serum calcium (K. SATO et al. 1989). Cytokines may also be involved in the bone destruction associated with chronic inflammatory diseases such as rheumatoid arthritis and periodontal disease. The inflamed gingiva or synovia in these diseases may produce increased amounts of IL-1, TNF, and IL-6 and all of these cytokines may contribute to the increased localized osteolytic bone destruction which is associated with these states.

G. Interleukin-1

Interleukin-1α (IL-1α) and interleukin-1β(IL-1β) are powerful and potent bone-resorbing cytokines. GOWEN et al. (1983) first showed that natural human purified IL-1 resorbed bone. This preparation probably contained predominantly IL-1β. HEATH et al. (1985) showed that porcine IL-1 could also resorb bone and then GOWEN and MUNDY (1986) showed that recombinant human IL-1α and IL-1β were potent bone-resorbing factors of identical potency and effects. These experiments were performed using neonatal mouse calvariae. Similar results were found using fetal rat long bones. IL-1 resorbs bone in concentrations as low as $10^{-11} M$. These data suggest that IL-1 may be one of the major components of the bone-resorbing activity present in activated leukocyte culture supernatants.

DEWHIRST et al. (1985) settled this issue using fetal rat long bone organ cultures to purify bone-resorbing activity in activated leukocyte culture supernatants stimulated by phytohemagglutinin. They identified interleukin-β by N-terminal amino acid sequence. However, this group were aware before their experiment that IL-1 was present in the leukocyte culture supernatants and they may have overlooked other activities which were also present. Since other cytokines such as IL-1α, TNF, and lymphotoxin certainly must have been present in their starting media, they almost certainly did. LORENZO et al. (1987) found that bone-resorbing activity present in leukocyte culture supernatants could be inhibited with neutralizing antibodies to IL-1β. Again, this does not mean that Il-1β is the only cytokine in activated leukocyte culture supernatants that resorbs bone. If bone-resorbing activity is due to the combined or synergistic effects of several factors working in concert, abrogation of any one of these factors may completely neutralize biological activity. It has subsequently been shown that synergistic interactions between IL-1 and other cytokines do indeed occur (see earlier).

The issue of synergism between IL-1 and other cytokines and systemic hormones may be very important for determining the effects of these factors on bone cells both in physiological and pathological situations. STASHENKO et al. (1987) showed that IL-1 was synergistic with parathyroid hormone in organ cultures of fetal rat long bones. SABATINI et al. (1987) found that the effects of IL-1 on bone resorption were potentiated by TNF and transforming growth factor α (TGFα). K. SATO et al. (1989) found that IL-1α and parathyroid hormone-related protein (PTH-rP) produced synergistic effects on plasma calcium in rats when each was given by injection. More recently, we have found that IL-1α and IL-1β may have produced synergistic effects on bone when given with IL-6 (BLACK et al. 1990). Similar data have been shown in fetal rodent bone cultures by ISHIMI et al. (1990). Since IL-1 is almost always exposed to bone cells in the presence of circulating factors such as parathyroid hormone or other locally produced cytokines, these interactions are clearly important for determining the effects of IL-1 on bone resorption both in physiological and pathological circumstances.

Recently, it has become clear that interactions between IL-1 and other cytokines may be very important for IL-1 to exert maximal effects. For example, IL-1 is known to stimulate expression and secretion of IL-6 in bone cells and in calvarial organ cultures (FEYEN et al. 1989; LOWIK et al. 1989). We have found that neutralizing antibodies to IL-6 block the effects of IL-1 to stimulate bone resorption in organ culture (BLACK et al. 1990).

Interleukin-1 probably exerts its effects on bone-resorbing cells in several ways. It is clearly a growth regulatory factor for osteoclast precursors and stimulates proliferation of precursor cells. When added to human marrow cell cultures, it stimulates the formation of 23C6-positive multinucleated cells. IL-1 promotes proliferation of committed precursors and subsequent differentiation (PFEILSCHIFTER et al. 1989). However, it not only promotes differentiation of committed precursors to form mature multi-nucleated cells, but also probably acts indirectly on the mature cell to stimulate bone resorption (THOMSON et al. 1986). Its effects on mature osteoclasts may be at least in part indirect, and mediated through other cells such as bone-lining cells. The precise molecular mechanisms by which it causes osteoclasts to resorb bone are unknown.

The effects of IL-1 on osteoclastic bone resorption appear to be mediated through the 80-kDa receptor. There are two receptors for IL-1, a 60-kDa receptor which is present on monocytes and macrophages and an 80-kDa receptor which is present on athymic fibroblasts and T lymphocytes (CARTER et al. 1990; BENNJAMIN et al. 1989; HANNUM et al. 1990; H. EISENBERG et al. 1989). We have used antibodies to the 80-kDa receptor and shown that these antibodies block the capacity of IL-1 to stimulate osteoclastic bone resorption. Also, more recently, we have used a naturally occurring IL-1 receptor antagonist which blocks the 80-kDa receptor and have shown that this receptor antagonist inhibits the capacity of IL-1 to stimulate osteoclastic bone resorption (GARRETT et al. 1990a). SECKINGER et al. (1990) have also shown that this antagonist blocks IL-1-mediated bone resorption in organ culture.

Interleukin-1 causes enhanced osteoclastic bone resorption in vivo as well as in vitro. SABATINI et al. (1988) showed that 3-day infusions of IL-1 caused hypercalcemia and increased osteoclastic bone resorption (Fig. 1). BOYCE et al. (1989a) showed that IL-1 given by daily injection for 3 days caused hypercalcemia and increased bone resorption, which lasted for 7–10 days. In these experiments, IL-1 was given subcutaneously over the calvaria and changes in bone were noted locally in calvarial bone adjacent to the site of injection, on the other side of the calvaria, and in the vertebrae. The changes which occurred locally were associated with a marked inflammatory

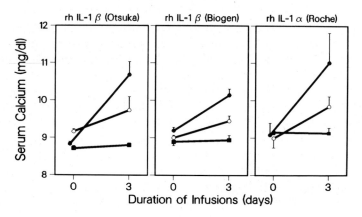

Fig. 1. Effects of a 3-day subcutaneous infusion of recombinant human IL-1α via the Alzet osmotic minipump in normal mice (from SABATINI et al. 1988). There was a parallel marked increase in osteoclastic bone resorption

response (Fig. 2). This inflammatory response was impaired if the mice were given indomethacin in doses which inhibit prostaglandin synthesis. There was no inflammatory response in distant bones and there was no effect on the bone resorption at distant sites when indomethacin was administered. These data suggest that IL-1 probably acts locally by increasing prostaglandin synthesis initially, but also by effects which are independent of prostaglandins or prostaglandin synthesis.

In other experiments, BOYCE et al. (1989b) followed carefully the changes in plasma calcium occurring immediately after injections of IL-1. Surprisingly, there was a transient fall in plasma-ionized calcium which occurred for a period of about 6h followed by a more prolonged hypercalcemic response (Fig. 3). This transient fall occurred even in mice which were already hypercalcemic. The reasons responsible for this fall are not known but may involve rapid calcium fluxes. They could be blocked by indomethacin. The transient fall of ionized calcium seen in mice given bolus injections of IL-1 may be responsible for the transient hypocalcemia which is sometimes seen with sepsis. IL-1 may be produced in a pulsatile manner or as a bolus in patients with sepsis, and this may be at least part of the explanation of hypocalcemia which occurs in those circumstances.

Interleukin 1α has been implicated in the bone resorption and hypercalcemia which occurs in malignant disease. K. SATO et al. (1989) and FRIED

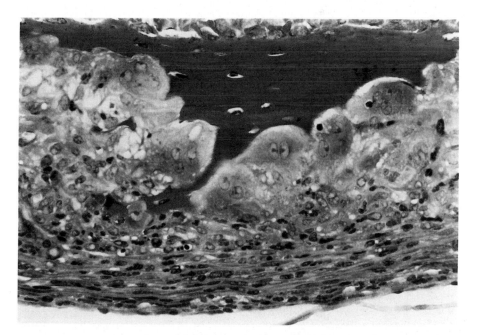

Fig. 2. Effects of injections of recombinant human IL-1α for 3 days on quantitative bone histomorphometry in calvariae of normal mice (from BOYCE et al. 1989a)

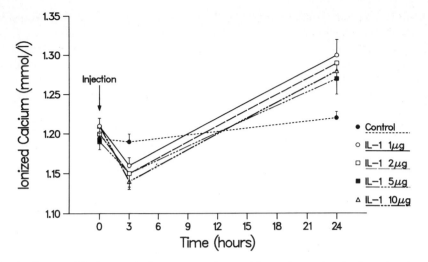

Fig. 3. Sequential changes in bone resorption and bone formation in the calvariae of mice in response to IL-1 (from Boyce et al. 1989a)

et al. (1989) have shown that IL-1α is produced by some solid tumors. Tumors in which IL-1α has been demonstrated have been squamous cell carcinoma, and in some of these the tumors have also been shown to produce parathyroid hormone-related protein (PTH-rP). It is likely in these circumstances that other cytokines such as IL-6 are produced in conjunction with IL-1. IL-1β has been implicated in the bone destruction and hypercalcemia which occurs in myeloma. This has been discussed earlier. IL-1β is not produced by cultured human myeloma cells in established culture (Garrett et al. 1987). However, IL-1β appears to be produced by freshly isolated marrow cells from patients with myeloma, possibly from the contaminating non-neoplastic host mononuclear cells (Kawano et al. 1989; Cozzolino et al. 1989).

Interleukin-1 has also been linked to the bone destruction which occurs in chronic inflammatory diseases such as rheumatoid arthritis and periodontal disease. In these conditions, accumulations of chronic inflammatory cells occur in the gingiva or synovia respectively and lead to adjacent bone destruction, at least part and maybe all of which is osteoclastic. In these circumstances, IL-1 is present in the synovial fluid. It is likely that it exerts its effects in conjunction with other cytokines such as TNF and IL-6.

Recently, there have been separate bodies of evidence suggesting a role for cytokines such as IL-1 in patients with osteoporosis. Pacifici et al. (1987, 1989) have shown that, in some patients with osteoporosis, unseparated peripheral blood mononuclear cells produce IL-1 constitutively in increased amounts compared with corresponding controls. They have linked this production of IL-1 with high bone turnover states. They have also shown that this increase of constitutively produced IL-1 can be inhibited in post-menopausal patients by treatment of the patients with estrogen replacement therapy. It appears that IL-1 is not the only cytokine involved in the situation. The same group has found that TNF and GM-CSF also seem to be produced in increased amounts constitutively by monocytes in osteoporotic subjects.

It is possible that IL-1 could be involved in the mechanism of action of estrogens on bone. Estrogens apparently inhibit bone resorption by indirect means. Recently, it has been shown that estrogens may impair the production of cytokines and IL-6 which is induced by IL-1 in bone cells (GIRASOLE et al. 1990). The bone cells which have been shown to have this property are both freshly isolated human bone cells and osteosarcoma cells. Thus, these osteotropic cytokines may be normal regulators of bone turnover. Removal of estrogens may lead to increased production of these cytokines by bone cells, which in turn could lead to increased bone resorption. Increased production of these cytokines could presumably be suppressed by treatment with estrogens.

Lesions in these granuloma which include osteoclastic bone resorption occurring adjacent to abnormal cells which have been shown to produce increased amounts of IL-1 may be the pathophysiological mechanism responsible for the bone destruction which occurs in this and similar conditions such as histiocytic granuloma (BOYCE et al. 1989a).

Interleukin-1 has complex and apparently paradoxical effects on bone formation which will require much further study. Continued presence of IL-1 causes inhibition of bone formation in vivo. Similar responses are seen in vitro (CANALIS 1986; SMITH et al. 1987). IL-1 appears to stimulate proliferation of early cells in the osteoblast lineage but to inhibit differentiated function. In contrast, transient exposure to IL-1 followed by withdrawal may lead to a formative response, particularly if it is given in low doses. Possibly the mechanism responsible is that IL-1 causes proliferation of bone cells as has been described by a number of workers including CANALIS (1986), GOWEN et al. (1985), and SMITH et al. (1987). Following withdrawal, perhaps some of these proliferating cells may differentiate down the osteoblast lineage. BOYCE et al. (1989a) performed an experiment in vivo in which he gave IL-1 intermittently for 3 days and then examined bones histologically in the mice during the following 4 weeks. The phase of osteoclastic bone resorption lasted for about a period of 7–10 days but this was followed by disappearance of the osteoclasts and a phase of intense new bone formation (Fig. 4). Not surprisingly, the new bone was of woven nature. The lesions in bone occurred in patches, and at some sites in the calvarial bones, which was the site examined, the bone which was resorbed was completely replaced over a period of 28 days by newly formed bone.

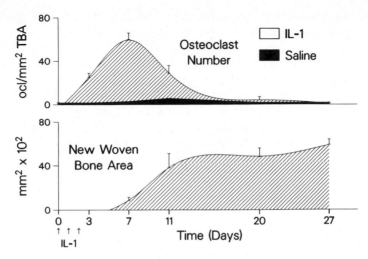

Fig. 4. Effects of injections of recombinant human IL-1α on calcium homeostasis in normal mice. There is initial hypocalcemia followed by more prolonged hypercalcemia (Boyce et al. 1989b)

H. Interleukin-1 Receptor Antagonist

Recently, a cytokine related to the IL-1 family but which has no IL-1 effects has been identified (Carter et al. 1990; Hannum et al. 1990; S.P. Eisenberg et al. 1990; Arend et al. 1989). This cytokine interferes with some of the biological effects of IL-1 by binding to one of the IL-1 receptors. IL-1 has two receptors, an 80-kDa high-affinity receptor which is present on T lymphocytes and fibroblasts, and mediates the effects of the IL-1 molecules on these cells, and a separate 40-kDa receptor which is present on pre-B cells, bone marrow granulocytes, and macrophages. This cytokine, which is a naturally occurring endogenous IL-1 receptor antagonist, competes with IL-1 of binding to the 80-kDa receptor. It has identical effects on bone in vitro to those of antibodies to the IL-1 80-kDa receptor (Garrett et al. 1990a). The protein has been purified and the gene molecularly cloned and expressed (Carter et al. 1990; Hannum et al. 1990; S.P. Eisenberg et al. 1990). It has similar affinity for the 80-kDa receptor as IL-1. It has 26% homology with IL-1β and 19% with IL-1α. The gene has very similar organization to the IL-1 genes and this peptide is almost certainly part of the IL-1 family. It has a molecular weight of 17 kDa and 152 amino acids. It is a secreted protein with a well-defined signal sequence. It is produced by monocytes but it is clearly under separate regulatory control (Arend et al. 1989). We have examined the effects of this IL-1 receptor antagonist on bone resorption in vitro and on plasma-ionized calcium in vivo. It has no discernable effect on plasma-ionized calcium. However, it does inhibit the effects of IL-1 to increase plasma-ionized calcium (GARRETT et al. 1990b). This indicates that the effects of IL-1 on bone resorption are mediated through the 80-kDa receptor. We and others (SECKINGER et al. 1990) have also examined the effects of the IL-1 receptor antagonist on bone resorption in vitro. IL-1 receptor antagonists block the effects of both IL-1α and IL-1β on bone resorption in organ cultures. It partially inhibits TNF and lymphotoxin, but has no effects on bone resorption which is stimulated by parathyroid hormone or 1,25 dihydroxyvitamin D. It must be given in relatively large doses to produce this effect, so whether this will be a useful therapeutic agent remains to be determined (GARRETT et al. 1990a). However, these data clearly demonstrate the important interactions which exist between the various cytokines during bone resorption which is mediated by these factors.

I. Tumor Necrosis Factor and Lymphotoxin

Lymphotoxin and TNF are two closely related cytokines which have equivalent effects on bone. They are multifunctional cytokines which are produced by activated lymphocytes and lymphoid cell lines or activated monocytes or macrophages respectively. Although they have separate single copy genes, they share the same receptor mechanism. Both molecules have identical overlapping biological effects, particularly on tumor cells, where they may either enhance or inhibit cell proliferation. Their predominant effect on bone is the stimulation of osteoclastic bone resorption (BERTOLINI et al. 1986). This effect was first shown in fetal rat long bones and was later confirmed in neonatal mouse calvariae (TASHJIAN et al. 1987). Their effects on bone organ cultures and particularly in murine calvariae, appear to be mediated through prostaglandin synthesis, since they can be blocked by inhibitors of prostaglandin synthesis. It is difficult to separate the effects of these molecules from those of IL-1 because they seem to overlap, although the effects of lymphotoxin and TNF may be more dependent on prostaglandin synthesis than those of IL-1.

It is likely that there are important interactions which occur between TNF and other cytokines on the bone resorption apparatus. As already mentioned, TNF has overlapping effects with those of IL-1. However, these effects may not be precisely the same, since Boyce and coworkers believe that the pattern of osteoclast stimulation seen in vivo with TNF is different from that seen with IL-1 (JOHNSON et al. 1989; BOYCE et al. 1989a). It has been shown on many occasions that TNF can induce IL-1 production, and ROODMAN et al. (1987) found that, in long-term marrow cultures, addition of TNF led to IL-1 generation in the conditioned media, and that in part the effects of TNF could be inhibited by using neutralizing antibodies to IL-1. More recently, we have found evidence that several other cytokines may be involved in mediating TNF effects on bone. In part, the effects of TNF on bone to cause resorption and on calcium homeostasis to cause hyper-calcemia can be inhibited partially by the use of the recently described IL-1 receptor antagonist (BLACK et al. 1990; GARRETT et al. 1990a). These data suggest that availability of the 80-kDa IL-1 receptor is required for TNF to exert its biological effects on bone resorption and calcium homeostasis. More recently, we have found that neutralizing antibodies to IL-6 can inhibit the effects of TNF on bone (GARRETT et al. 1990a). These effects have yet to be confirmed in vivo. However, all of these data indicate that there are complex interactions which occur between cytokines when bone resorption is stimulated.

Tumor necrosis factor also affects cells with the osteoblast phenotype (BERTOLINI et al. 1986). In osteosarcoma cells it inhibits differentiated function and stimulates cell proliferation (SMITH et al. 1987). TNF inhibits synthesis of collagenase-digestible protein but stimulates cell proliferation in organ cultures of fetal rat calvariae (BERTOLINI et al. 1986). It may also influence the effects of other factors on osteoblastic cells. For example, it impairs the cyclic AMP response to PTH in cells with the osteoblast phenotype. The effects of TNF on cells with the osteoblastic phenotype may be markedly enhanced by treatment of the cells with retinoic acid (NG et al. 1989).

Lymphotoxin and TNF also cause hypercalcemia and increased bone resorption in vivo. This was first shown with repeated injections of TNF in mice and by infusions of lymphotoxin in mice [TASHJIAN et al. 1987, 1987 (TNF); GARRETT et al. 1987]. It was later confirmed using Chinese hamster ovarian (CHO) cells which were transfected with the human TNF gene (JOHNSON et al. 1989). These tumor cells were inoculated into nude mice and the effects of the tumor cell products in vivo on bone morphology and calcium homeostasis were determined. There was a marked increase on osteoclastic bone resorption and hypercalcemia occurring in mice bearing CHO tumors transfected with TNF and stably expressing this cytokine, whereas there was no such change in mice carrying CHO tumors carrying the empty vector (JOHNSON et al. 1989).

Production of TNF in some tumor models may be responsible for paraneoplastic syndromes, such as cachexia, hypercalcemia, and leuko-cytosis. This has been most convincingly shown in a squamous cell carcinoma of the jaw which was inoculated in nude mice (YONEDA et al. 1991a,b,c). In tumor-bearing nude mice, this tumor was associated with these paraneo-plastic syndromes. These syndromes could be abrogated by inoculation of mice with neutralizing antibodies to TNF, or by removal of the spleen, which depleted the mice of host immune cells. TNF was not produced by the tumor cells. These mice had circulating TNF concentrations which were fourfold increased above normal (YONEDA et al. 1991b). Further studies showed that splenic peripheral blood and marrow mononuclear cells from normal animals released TNF when exposed to conditioned media harvested from this tumor. A soluble factor with a molecular weight of 40 kDa which is responsible for stimulating TNF production has been identified in this conditioned medium.

A similar mechanism has been demonstrated in several other tumor models. In the rat Leydig cell tumor which is associated with cachexia, hypercalcemia, and leukocytosis, tumor cell conditioned medium stimulates TNF production by host immune cells (SABATINI et al. 1990a). In the A375 melanoma, which is also associated with cachexia, we found also that the tumor produced a factor which stimulated TNF production. In this case, we identified the factor as GM-CSF (SABATINI et al. 1990b).

Lymphotoxin may play an important pathophysiological role in myeloma. In this situation, production of lymphotoxin by cultured neoplastic cells has been demonstrated and part of the bone-resorbing activity produced by cultures of myeloma cells in vitro can be blocked or abrogated by neutralizing antibodies to lymphotoxin (GARRETT et al. 1987). This may not be the only mechanism by which osteoclasts are stimulated in myeloma, since production of other cytokines such as IL-6 and IL-1 by other cells may also be important. TNF is also likely involved in the localized bone destruction which occurs in chronic inflammatory diseases such as rheumatoid arthritis and periodontal disease, where it accumulates in conjunction with other cytokines such as IL-6 and IL-1 in the inflammatory fluids.

J. Interleukin-6

This multifunctional cytokine is a growth factor for B cells and pre-B cells. It is likely a paracrine growth factor in myeloma (KLEIN et al. 1989; BATAILLE et al. 1989). These latter workers have found that circulating concentrations of this factor are increased in patients with myeloma and particularly in those with very markedly increased tumor cell burdens such as occur in plasma cell leukemia. IL-6 is related closely in function to other cytokines IL-1, TNF, and G-CSF. Each of these cytokines has overlapping functions, although each also has novel additional functions (for review, see AKIRA et al. 1990).

Interleukin-6 appears to have no effects on bone-resorbing activity in fetal rat long bone or in neonatal mouse calvarial assays. However, LOWIK et al. (1989) showed that it could stimulate bone resorption in cultures of fetal murine metacarpal bones and ISHIMI et al. (1990) found that it stimulated bone resorption in cultures of fetal murine calvariae. It is possible that these cultures contain more primitive cells. KUKITA et al. (1990) have shown that IL-6 causes increased formation of multinucleated cells with the osteoclast phenotype in long-term human marrow cultures. All of these results are consistent with the notion that IL-6 has an effect predominantly on cells early in the osteoclast lineage. Thus, it may be active in fetal murine cultures because these bones contain more precursors than the neonatal mouse calvariae or fetal rat long bones.

Although IL-6 is often considered as a stromal cell product, in fact it is produced by many cells. FEYEN et al. (1989) first showed that it could be produced by bone cells in culture as well as by organ cultures of bone which were treated with parathyroid hormone, IL-1, 1,25 dihydroxyvitamin D3, and TNF. This work has been confirmed by a number of other groups (LOWIK et al. 1989; ISHIMI et al. 1990). However, production of IL-6 by bone cultures and bone cells seems to be greater when the stimulus is a cytokine such as IL-1 or TNF than systemic hormones such as parathyroid hormones (I.R. GARRETT and K. BLACK, personal communication). The fact that its production by bone cells and by bone cultures may be regulated by cyto-tropic hormones suggests that IL-6 may play an important physiological role in bone cell metabolism. Recently, GIRASOLE et al. (1990) have sug-gested that IL-6 production by bone cells can be inhibited by estrogens, although this could not be confirmed by others (M. GOWEN, personal communication).

We have administered IL-6 by single or multiple bolus injections and found no effect on plasma calcium. However, more recently we have used Chinese hamster ovarian cells (CHO cells) which were transfected with the cDNA for murine IL-6 (BLACK et al. 1991). These cells stably express this cytokine and can be carried as tumors in nude mice. We injected nude mice with these tumors and injected other nude mice with CHO tumors which had not been transfected with IL-6, and which serve as controls for these experiments. The mice carrying tumors bearing CHO cells expressing IL-6 developed hypercalcemia.

Interleukin-6 may be involved in many of the cytokine-mediated bone resorptive states. However, its major role may be in myeloma. In this situation, it is clearly produced in the circulation as a paracrine growth factor (KLEIN et al. 1989; BATAILLE et al. 1989). We and others have found that, although it is a powerful bone-resorbing factor in its own right, it can also markedly potentiate the bone-resorbing effects of other cytokines such as IL-1 and TNF. Under these circumstances, production of these bone-resorbing cytokines by the myeloma cells or host cells in the marrow may be markedly enhanced by the circulating IL-6 concentrations.

One other pathological situation where IL-6 may be important is in Paget's disease of bone. In Paget's disease, the osteoclasts are large and multinucleated. The number of nuclei in affected cells is clearly greater than the nuclear numbers in non-Pagetic osteoclasts. Working on the hypothesis that IL-6 may be responsible for this increased osteoclast formation and multinuclearity, KURIHARA et al. (1990) examined marrow plasma and serum from patients with Paget's disease. They found increased IL-6 in the marrow plasma but not in the peripheral blood serum. They then examined pro-duction of IL-6 by multinucleated cells formed in long-term Pagetic marrow cultures. IL-6 production by these cells was clearly increased. At least part of the source for IL-6 may have been the osteoclasts themselves, since they identified IL-6 in the cells by in situ hybridization and by immunohistochemistry. IL-6 therefore may play a pathophysiologic role in the abnormality in osteoclast function which occurs in Paget's disease. Whether this is an epiphenomenon occurring as a consequence of viral disease or whether this is an important proximal event in the pathophysiology of Paget's disease remains to be determined.

K. Gamma-Interferon

Gamma-interferon is a multifunctional cytokine which in most biological systems has similar effects to TNF and IL-1 and seems to work in conjunction or synergistically with these cytokines. It has been extensively studied for its potential cytotoxic effects. However, γ-interferon opposes the effects of IL-1 and TNF on the bone resorption apparatus (GOWEN et al. 1986; GOWEN and MUNDY 1986). GOWEN et al. (1986) reported that γ-interferon appeared to be more effective in inhibiting bone resorption due to IL-1 and TNF than in inhibiting bone resorption due to systemic factors such as parathyroid hormone and 1,25 dihydroxyvitamin D. At higher concentrations, γ-interferon may inhibit bone resorption independent of the mediator. There have been conflicting reports on its effects on prostaglandin synthesis, but in our hands this does not seem to be an important factor in its inhibitory effects on bone resorption. TAKAHASHI et al. (1986) found that γ-interferon inhibited formation of cells with osteoclast characteristics in long-term human marrow cultures. Surprisingly, these workers found using autoradiography that there was a greater effect on cell differentiation than on proliferation of osteoclast precursors. γ-Interferon appears to have no discernable effects on isolated osteoclasts in vitro.

Gamma-interferon has not been tested extensively in in vivo studies, but in one report 5 days treatment with murine γ-interferon returned serum calcium to normal in nude mice bearing a human squamous cell carcinoma associated with hypercalcemia (SATOH et al. 1990). γ-Interferon has different effects on osteoblasts to IL-1 and TNF. It inhibits thymidine incorporation although it also inhibits differentiated function (SMITH et al. 1987). In organ cultures of fetal rat calvariae, it has additive effects with those of TNF to inhibit collagen synthesis (SMITH et al. 1987). γ-Interferon is produced in relatively large amounts by the myeloma cells. This may be one explanation for the observation that myeloma cells may be smaller and contain less nuclei than the osteoclast stimulated by other types of neoplastic cells (C. MARCELLI, personal communication).

L. β_2-Microglobulin

β_2-Microglobulin is a peptide believed for many years to play an important role in cell-mediated immune responses. The importance of this role has recently been cast in doubt by experiments showing that transgenic mice which fail to express β_2-microglobulin due to homologous recombination experiments have no major defects in immune response mechanisms. Its role in bone cell metabolism was first suggested by CANALIS and coworkers (1987a). These investigators reported that the growth factor activity for bone cells identified in conditioned media harvested from organ cultures of fetal rat calvaria was identical to β_2-microglobulin. Their evidence was based on purification and on Western blotting using antibodies to β_2-microglobulin. However, JENNINGS et al. (1989) believe that the β_2-microglobulin identified in their bone matrix preparations is not a bone cell mitogen, and that the mitogenic effects observed by other groups were due to contaminating TGFβ. In further studies, CENTRELLA et al. (1989) showed that β_2-microglobulin preparations enhanced the production and effects of insulin-like growth factor-1 (IGF-1) on bone cells. Synthesis of IGF-1 was increased, and β_2-microglobulin increased IGF-1 binding to target bone cells.

One of the interesting facets for potential roles of β_2-microglobulin in bone is that it is an important prognostic factor in myeloma (DURIE 1984). There is a positive correlation between the myeloma cell mass and the serum β_2-microglobulin level. Whether this has any pathophysiologic significance for the bone lesions in myeloma has not been investigated.

M. Osteoclastpoietic Factor

Since osteoclasts have a similar hematopoietic stem cell precursor as the formed elements of the blood, and the formed elements of the blood are derived from stem cell precursors under the direction of specific growth regulatory factors known as CSFs, it has always seemed likely that there may be a growth regulatory factor for osteoclasts akin to the CSFs. We have searched for such a factor. In this search, we examined a human tumor, a squamous cell carcinoma of the maxilla. This tumor has proved to be a useful source of other CSFs. It produces colony-stimulating factor-G (CSF-G), colony-stimulating factor-GM (CSF-GM), and colony-stimulating factor-M (CSF-M). When this tumor was inoculated into nude mice, mice developed leukocytosis. They also had hypercalcemia. The reason for believing that this tumor would be a good source of a similar factor for osteoclasts was that animals carrying this tumor have a marked increase in osteoclast activity on endosteal bone surfaces, and the animals develop hypercalcemia in the absence of production of other known tumor-derived bone-resorbing factors such as parathyroid hormone-related protein. We tested conditioned media harvested from these tumor cells and found they stimulated formation of cells with the osteoclast phenotype in three culture systems, long-term human marrow cultures, murine marrow cultures, and HL-60 cells (YONEDA et al. 1990, 1991d). The human cells and characteristics of the osteoclast phenotype as determined by multinuclearity, staining with tartrate-resistant acid phosphatase and 23C6 antibodies, and responsivity to calcitonin. The multinucleated murine marrow cells stained positively with tartrate-resistant acid phosphatase and formed resorption pits on calcified matrices. The HL-60 cells had the osteoclast phenotype as determined by the capacity to form resorption pits on calcified matrices, presence of calcitonin receptors, presence of tartrate resistant acid phosphatase and staining with 23C6 antibodies, and responsivity to calcitonin. This osteoclastpoietic factor appears not to be any of the known CSFs as determined by its molecular size (it is smaller) and by retention of activation after incubation with neutralizing antibodies. It is a relatively small peptide and its isolation and identification is of interest. It will also be important to determine whether it is produced by stromal cells or activated leukocytes, whether it is involved in human diseases such as osteopetrosis, and whether it has an important role in normal bone turnover.

N. Colony-Stimulating Factors

The osteoclast almost certainly shares a common precursor with the formed elements of the blood. Since there are growth regulatory factors (CSFs) for these cell lineages which act as proliferative factors on progenitors in each of these lineages, and frequently have overlapping effects on other lineages, it is not surprising that these factors should also have effects on osteoclast formation. Many of the reports of the effects of CSFs on bone resorption are conflicting, which probably reflects the proportion of different cell types in the model system studied and the timing with which CSFs are added. This has certainly been the experience reported by N. TAKAHASHI et al. (personal communication) and MacDONALD et al. (1986). Conflicting reports have arisen particularly over the effects of CSF-M and CSF-GM on these marrow cultures (VAN DER WIJNGAERT et al. 1987; HAGENAARS et al. 1989; SHINAR et al. 1990). However, it is now clear that, depending on the starting population of cells, these factors may direct cells down the osteoclast lineage or down other lineages. N. TAKAHASHI (personal communication) has shown the importance of the timing of the addition of CSF-M and 1,25 dihydroxy-vitamin D for whether monocytes or osteoclasts would be formed from marrow cells in long-term culture. If CSF-M and 1,25 dihydroxyvitamin D were added together, then monocytes were formed preferentially. However, when 1,25 dihydroxyvitamin D and CSF-M were added sequentially, then osteoclasts were formed. The importance of CSF-M for normal osteoclast formation has recently been shown convincingly by the demonstration that one variant of murine osteopetrosis, the *op/op* mouse, has deficient production of CSF-M by stromal cells and by immune cells. In these animals, there is a defect in the coding region of CSF-M (YOSHIDA et al. 1990). Recently, FELIX et al. (1990) and KODAMA et al. (1991) have shown independently that the bone-resorbing abnormalities in this model can be reversed by administration of CSF-M. It is still not clear whether CSF-M is acting directly on the bone resorption apparatus, or whether it is inducing the production of other cytokines which are in turn responsible for mediating the effects of CSF-M on osteoclasts. However, these experiments do indicate that CSF-M is necessary for normal osteoclast formation and marrow cavity development. CSF-M and CSF-GM have been shown by MacDonald et al. (1986) to stimulate the formation of cells with osteoclast characteristics in culture.

It has been interesting to note that there are now a number of human and animal tumors associated with granulocytosis in which increased production of CSFs are involved. In many of these tumors, hypercalcemia associated with increased bone resorption occurs. This has been noted particularly by authors in Japan (K. Sato et al. 1979, 1986; Toya et al. 1981; Kondo et al. 1983; Yoneda et al. 1985, 1986) and particularly in squamous cell carcinomas of the head and neck. Nude mice carrying these tumors may develop similar leukocytosis-hypercalcemia syndromes. This paraneoplastic leukocytosis-hypercalcemia syndrome occurs more frequently together than would be expected by chance occurrences (Yoneda et al. 1991a). In one study of 225 patients with oral malignancies, 10 patients had hypercalcemia, 11 patients had leukocytosis, and 4 had both syndromes together. The occurrence of the two paraneoplastic syndromes in the same patient was far greater than could have been expected by chance (Yoneda et al. 1991a). In one human tumor studied extensively by Yoneda et al. (1991b), the granulocytosis, hypercalcemia, and leukocytosis could be abrogated by splenectomy as well as by excision of the tumor from the nude mice. This tumor was shown to produce CSF-G, CSF-M, CSF-GM, and IL-6 in culture (Yoneda et al. 1991b,c).

It is possible that CSFs could produce their effects on osteoclast formation indirectly. For example, early studies showed that CSF activity stimulates IL-1 production (Moore et al. 1980) and CSF activity stimulated prostaglandin synthesis (Kurland et al. 1979). Recently, Sabatini et al. (1990b) showed that the A375 human tumor causes cachexia in nude mice. This cachexia is associated with increased plasma TNF. TNF in this model is not produced by the tumor cells. Sabatini et al. (1990b) purified the tumor factor responsible for increasing TNF production by normal host immune cells in the mice and identified GM-CSF as the tumor-derived mediator. In a similar model, the MH-85 human squamous cell carcinoma, increased TNF production by host immune cells was caused not only by GM-CSF, but also by a second tumor-derived TNF-inducing factor produced by the tumor cells (Yoneda et al. 1991b).

O. Leukemia-Inhibitory Factor (Differentiation-Inducing Factor)

Leukemia inhibitory factor (LIF) is a glycoprotein which was purified from a T-lymphocyte cell line by its capacity to stimulate differentiation of myeloid cells to mature monocytes (METCALF and GEARING 1987). This glycoprotein appears to be identical to a cytokine which was purified from mouse L29 cells and Ehrlich's ascites tumor cells (TOMIDA et al. 1984; ICHIKAWA 1970). This activity was originally called differentiation-inducing factor and was examined for its effects on bone resorption in organ cultures of neonatal mouse calvariae by ABE et al. (1986), who found that this factor stimulated bone resorption in this culture system, and also increased the formation of cells with the osteoclast phenotype in murine marrow cultures (ABE et al. 1988). Moreover, this factor was shown to be produced by the osteoblastic cell line MC3T3-E1 (ABE et al. 1988).

More recently, REID et al. (1990) confirmed that the recombinant molecule also stimulated osteoclastic bone resorption in organ cultures of neonatal mouse calvaria. Osteoblasts respond to it by increased proliferation (REID et al. 1990). METCALF and GEARING (1987) showed that mice carrying cells transfected stably with LIF and expressing it in large amounts showed excess bone formation, although the bone changes were not described in detail. S.C. MANOLAGAS has suggested that production of LIF by cells with the osteoblast phenotype can be inhibited by estrogens (personal communication).

Little is yet known about the effects of this factor on bone in vivo. METCALF and GEARING (1987) reported that cells transfected with this factor to stably produce it and then inoculated into mice developed bone abnormalities associated with mild increases in plasma calcium.

P. Prostaglandins and Other Arachidonic Acid Metabolites

A number of arachidonic acid metabolites have long been implicated as modulators of bone cell function. Since these nonpeptide factors are produced by immune cells, marrow cells, and bone cells in the bone microenvironment, it is probably reasonable to consider them as potential local mediators of bone cell function. Prostaglandins of the E series were first identified by KLEIN and RAISZ (1970) as stimulators of osteoclastic bone resorption. These workers had noted that parathyroid hormone increased the cyclic AMP content of bone organ cultures, and, since prostaglandins of the E series have a similar effect, they tested their effects to stimulate the resorption of bone. They found that prostaglandins were slow-acting but powerful mediators of osteoclastic bone resorption in this organ culture system. Prostaglandins of the E series produced similar effects in cultures of neonatal mouse calvariae. Prostaglandins of the E series also enhance multinucleate cell formation in long-term marrow cultures, although the effects are different in man and mouse (CHENU et al. 1990; AKATSU et al. 1989). Following the observations that prostaglandins of the E series stimulate bone resorption, workers then showed that bone resorption could also be stimulated by less stable precursors of prostaglandins of the E series, including endoperoxides (TASHJIAN et al. 1977; RAISZ et al. 1977). Later, it was shown that prostaglandins of the E series caused transient contraction of osteoclast cell membranes, a phenomenon which has been associated with inhibition of bone resorption (CHAMBERS and ALI 1983). However, it is likely that this effect is not long-lasting and the overall effect of prostaglandins on bone resorption is stimulatory. Whether prostaglandins of the E series have a systemic effect or not is unknown but unlikely. Infusions of prostaglandins of the E series into the aorta have caused mild elevations in the serum calcium, but only when large doses have been administered (FRANKLIN and TASHJIAN 1975).

It is more likely that prostaglandins of the E series are important as local modulators of bone resorption. It has been recognized for many years that other factors which stimulate bone resorption may do so by generating prostaglandins in the microenvironment of bone-resorbing cells. This was first noted with complement-sufficient serum (RAISZ et al. 1974), and later verified in mouse calvariae for a number of growth factors including epidermal growth factor and the transforming growth factors (TASHJIAN et al. 1978, 1985). However, the effect of growth factors on the generation of prostaglandin synthesis in bone organ cultures depends on the bone organ culture system employed. Thus, prostaglandin generation is more common in neonatal mouse calvariae than it is in fetal rat long bones. In fetal rat long bones, growth factors such as the transforming growth factors and epidermal growth factor stimulate bone resorption by a non-prostaglandin-dependent mechanism (RAISZ et al. 1980; IBBOTSON et al. 1985, 1986). Partial explanation for this is provided by the experiments of LERNER (1987) and GARRETT and MUNDY (1989). These workers found that, in neonatal mouse calvariae, freshly explanted calvariae produced large quantities of prostaglandins of the E series. When a peptide cytokine or growth factor was then added to the culture system, the generation of E series prostaglandins was maintained rather than further stimulated (GARRETT and MUNDY 1989). In further clarification of the potential role of prostaglandins of the E series on the effects of cytokines on bone resorption, BOYCE et al. (1989a,b) performed in vivo experiments in normal intact mice which were injected or infused with recombinant human interleukin-1α. These workers found that part of the effect of interleukin-1 on bone resorption was mediated by prostaglandins and in part was independent of prostaglandin synthesis, by using indomethacin as a blocker of prostaglandin synthesis. They found that the local inflammatory effects of the peptide cytokine on bone resorption appeared to be prostaglandin related but the long-distance or systemic effects were prostaglandin unrelated. Moreover, these workers found that a transient hypocalcemic effect of interleukin-1 was inhibited by indomethacin, suggesting it was dependent on prostaglandin synthesis, whereas the sustained hypercalcemic effect of interleukin-1 occurred independent of indomethacin therapy (BOYCE et al. 1989b).

Prostaglandins of the E series have effects not just on bone resorption but also on bone formation. Although they have been shown to have biphasic effects on bone-forming cells in vitro (CHYUN and RAISZ 1984), in vivo it appears their effects are clearly associated with an increase in periosteal bone formation (JEE 1985, 1987).

Prostaglandins have been implicated in a number of disease states. They were initially implicated in the hypercalcemia of malignancy. TASHJIAN et al. (1972) provided evidence that they may be important in the hypercalcemia associated with two animal models of the hypercalcemia of malignancy, the HSDM-1 mouse fibrosarcoma and the VX-2 rabbit carcinosarcoma. In both of these models, cultured tumor cells produced prostaglandins of the E series and hypercalcemia was abrogated by treatment of the animals with indomethacin. This led to a spate of case reports of the use of indomethacin in the treatment of hypercalcemia of malignancy and a more prolonged study by SEYBERTH et al. (1975), who showed increased urinary excretion of a stable metabolite of prostaglandins of the E series in a number of patients with the humoral hypercalcemia of malignancy. These patients also apparently responded to indomethacin. About the same time, there were a number of reports of the potential role of prostaglandins of the E series in the osteolytic bone destruction associated with metastatic breast cancer. POWLES et al. (1976) and BENNETT et al. (1975) showed that freshly isolated breast cancer cells contained relatively large amounts of prostaglandins of the E series and caused bone resorption when cocultured with organ cultures of neonatal mouse calvariae. However, in a follow-up study, POWLES et al. (1982) could find no evidence that treatment of patients with metastatic breast cancer with indomethacin had any beneficial effect on osteolytic bone destruction. Moreover, indomethacin is usually ineffective in the treatment of humoral hypercalcemia of malignancy (MUNDY et al. 1983). VALENTIN et al. (1985) used cultured human breast cancer cells to show that production of prostaglandins by these cells was markedly enhanced when the cells were treated with estrogens or antiestrogens. This increase in prostaglandin production was associated with an increase in bone-resorbing activity, and may account for the hypercalcemic fare which occurs in some patients with metastatic breast cancer treated with estrogens or antiestrogens.

Prostaglandins of the E series have not been linked just with the humoral hypercalcemia of malignancy but also with a number of chronic inflammatory conditions including periodontal disease and rheumatoid arthritis. They are clearly present in inflammatory fluids in increased amounts and may play a role in these circumstances.

There have also been recent reports that other arachidonic acid metabolites may influence osteoclast activity. Arachidonic acid can be metabolized by an alternative enzyme system, the 5-lipoxygenase pathway, to produce a number of leukotriene compounds. Although some workers have reported that these are very effective stimulators of bone resorption in neonatal mouse calvariae (MEGHI et al. 1988; EL ATTAR and LIN 1983; EL ATTAR et al. 1986), others have found less convincing effects. Since these compounds are also found in inflammatory fluids, they have been linked to the localized bone loss associated with inflammatory conditions such as periodontal disease and rheumatoid arthritis (EL ATTAR et al. 1986; EL ATTAR and LIN 1983; DAVIDSON et al. 1983).

Q. Transforming Growth Factor β

Transforming growth factor β is an unusual growth regulatory factor which is produced by most proliferating cells and has receptors on most cells in the body. It represents a family of peptides with similar structure which are highly conserved. It appears to have unusual but very powerful effects on bone cells. Its effects on bone have also been discussed in this volume by CANALIS (see Chap. 7).

R. Bone Morphogenetic Proteins

Bone morphogenetic proteins belong to the extended TGFβ family. They are discussed in more detail in the accompanying chapter by WOZNEY and ROSEN (see Chap. 20). They have a limited homology to TGFβ but a fairly close homology to each other.

S. Other Bone-Derived Growth Factors

There will also be no detailed description of the effects of other local bone-derived growth factors on bone cells in this section, since this should be covered in more detail in the chapter by CANALIS (see Chap. 7). Nevertheless, it is clear that in addition to TGFβ and the BMPs (covered by WOZNEY and ROSEN in Chap. 20) a number of other growth factors generated in bone may be important in the bone remodeling process. These growth factors include insulin-like growth factor-1 (IGF-1), insulin-like growth factor II (IGF-II), acidic and basic fibroblast growth factors, and platelet-derived growth factors. IGF-1 enhances bone cell proliferation and also increases collagen synthesis in fetal rat calvarial organ cultures (CENTRELLA and CANALIS 1985). It appears likely to these bone organ cultures that the effects of parathyroid hormone to stimulate collagen synthesis following transient exposure are due to IGF-1 (CANALIS et al. 1989a,b). Similarly, IGF-II is also present in bone and is released in bone when bones are resorbed. HAUSCHKA et al. (1986) and Baylink and colleagues (HOWARD et al. 1981; MOHAN et al. 1988) have identified a mitogenic activity in bone extracts which appears to be IGF-II. Platelet-derived growth factor also has powerful proliferative effects on bone cells and is present in the bone matrix. It is also expressed by bone cells and osteosarcoma cells (GRAVES et al. 1984a,b). Recently, GRAVES has shown its effects to act in bone cells in a paracrine or autocrine manner (GRAVES et al. 1989). Fibroblast growth factors are also present in demineralized bone matrix and have proliferative effects on bone cells. Fibroblast growth factor may also stimulate expression of TGFβ in cultures of rat bone cells (RODAN et al. 1987; GLOBUS et al. 1988; CANALIS et al. 1987b, 1988).

References

Abe E, Tanaka H, Ishimi Y, Chisato M, Hayashi T, Nagasawa H, Tomida M, Yamaguchi Y, Hozumi M, Suda T (1986) Differentiation-inducing factor purified from conditioned medium of mitogen-treated spleen cell cultures stimulates bone resorption. Proc Natl Acad Sci USA 83:5958–5962

Abe E, Ishimi Y, Takahashi N, Akatsu T, Ozawa H, Yamana H, Yoshiki S, Suda T (1988) A differentiation-inducing factor produced by the osteoblastic cell line MC3T3-E1 stimulates bone resorption by promoting osteoclast formation. J Bone Miner Res 3:635–645

Akatsu T, Takahashi N, Debari K, Morita I, Murota S, Nagata N, Takatani O, Suda T (1989) Prostaglandins promote osteoclast like cell formation by a mechanism involving cyclic adenosine 3',5'-monophosphate in mouse bone marrow cell cultures. J Bone Miner Res 4:29–35

Akira S, Hirano T, Taga T, Kishimoto T (1990) Biology of multifunctional cytokines: IL-6 and related molecules (IL-1 and TNF). FASEB J 4:2860–2867

Arend WP, Joslin FG, Thompson RC, Hannum CH (1989) An IL-1 inhibitor from human monocytes. Production and characterization of biologic properties. J Immunol 15:1851 1858

Bataille R, Jourdan M, Zhang XG, Klein B (1989) Serum levels of interleukin-6, a potent myeloma cell growth factor, as a reflect of disease severity in plasma cell dyscrasias. J Clin Invest 84:2008–2011

Benjamin WR, Tare NS, Hayes TJ, Becker JM, Anderson TD (1989) Regulation of hemopoiesis in myelosuppressed mice by human recombinant IL-1 alpha. J Immunol 142:792–799

Bennett A, McDonald AM, Simpson JS, Stanford IF (1975) Breast cancer, prostaglandins, and bone metastases. Lancet i:1218–1220

Bertolini DR, Nedwin GE, Bringman TS, Mundy GR (1986) Stimulation of bone resorption and inhibition of bone formation in vitro by human tumour necrosis factor. Nature 319:516–518

Black K, Mundy GR, Garrett IR (1990) Interleukin-6 causes hypercalcemia in vivo, and enhances the bone resorbing potency of interleukin-1 and tumor necrosis factor by two orders of magnitude in vitro. J Bone Miner Res 5 [Suppl 2]:787

Black K, Garrett IR, Mundy GR (1991) Chinese hamster ovarian cells transfected with the murine interleukin-6 gene cause hypercalcemia as well as cachexia, leukocytosis and thrombocytosis in tumor-bearing nude mice. Endocrinology 128:2657–2659

Boyce BR, Aufdemorte TB, Garrett IR, Yates AJP, Mundy GR (1989a) Effects of interleukin-1 on bone turnover in normal mice. Endocrinology 125:1142–1150

Boyce BR, Yates AJP, Mundy GR (1989b) Bolus injections of recombinant human interleukin-1 cause transient hypocalcemia in normal mice. Endocrinology 125:2780–2783

Canalis E (1986) Interleukin-1 has independent effects on deoxyribonucleic acid and collagen synthesis in cultures of rat calvariae. Endocrinology 118:74–81

Canalis E, McCarthy T, Centrella M (1987a) A bone-derived growth factor isolated from rat calvariae is beta 2 microglobulin. Endocrinology 121:1198–1200

Canalis E, Lorenzo J, Burgess WH, Maciag T (1987b) Effects of endothelial cell growth factor on bone remodeling in vitro. J Clin Invest 79:52–58

Canalis E, Centrella M, McCarthy T (1988) Effects of basic fibroblast growth factor on bone formation in vitro. J Clin Invest 81:1572–1577

Canalis E, Centrella M, Burch W, McCarthy TL (1989a) Insulin-like growth factor I mediates selective anabolic effects of parathyroid hormone in bone cultures. J Clin Invest 83:60–65

Canalis E, McCarthy T, Centrella M (1989b) Growth factors and the regulation of bone remodeling. J Clin Invest 81:277–281

Carter DB, Deibel MR Jr, Dunn CJ, Tomich CSC, Laborde AL, Slightom JL, Berger AE, Bienkowski MJ, Sun FF, McEwan RN, Harris PKW, Yem AW, Waszak GA, Ghosay JG, Sieu LC, Hardee MM, Zurcher-Neely HA, Reardon IM, Heinrikson RL, Truesdell SE, Shelly JA, Eessalu TE, Taylor BM, Tracey DE (1990) Purification, cloning, expression and biological characterization of an interleukin-1 receptor antagonist protein. Nature 344:633–638

Centrella M, Canalis E (1985) Local regulators of skeletal growth: a perspective. Endocr Rev 6:544–551

Centrella M, McCarthy TL, Canalis E (1989) Beta-2-microglobulin enhances insulin-like growth factor I receptor levels and synthesis. J Biol Chem 264:18268–18271

Chambers TJ, Ali NN (1983) Inhibition of osteoclastic motility by prostaglandins I2, E1, E2 and 6-oxoE1. J Pathol 139:383–397

Chenu C, Kukita T, Mundy GR, Roodman GD (1990) Prostaglandins E2 inhibits formation of osteoclast-like cells in long-term human marrow cultures but is not a mediator of the inhibitory effects of transforming growth factor β. J Bone Miner Res 5:677–681

Chyun YS, Raisz LG (1984) Stimulation of bone formation by prostaglandin E2. Prostaglandins 27:97–103

Cozzolino F, Torcia M, Aldinucci D, Rubartelli A, Miliani A, Shaw AR, Lansdorp PM, Diguglielmo R (1989) Production of interleukin-1 by bone marrow myeloma cells. Blood 74:387–390

Davidson EM, Rae SA, Smith MJ (1983) Leukotriene B_4, a mediator of inflammation present in synovial fluid in rheumatoid arthritis. Ann Rheum Dis 42:677–679

Dewhirst FE, Stashenko PP, Mole JE, Tsurumachi T (1985) Purification and partial sequence of human osteoclast-activating factor: identity with interleukin-1 beta. J Immunol 135:2562–2568

Dewhirst FE, Ago JM, Peros WJ, Stashenko P (1987) Synergism between parathyroid hormone and interleukin-1 in stimulating bone resorption in organ culture. J Bone Miner Res 2:127–134

Durie BGM (1984) Recent advances in multiple myeloma and the related monoclonal gammopathies. In: Fairbanks VF (ed) Current hematology, vol 3. Wiley, New York, 239–285

Eisenberg H, Pallotta J, Sacks B, Brickman AS (1989) Parathyroid localization, 3-dimensional modeling, and percutaneous ablation techniques. Endocrinol Metab Clin North Am 18:659–700

Eisenberg SP, Evans RJ, Arend WP, Verderber E, Brewer MT, Hannum CH, Thompson RC (1990) Primary structure and functional expression from complementary DNA of a human interleukin-1 receptor antagonist. Nature 343:341–346

El Attar TMA, Lin HS (1983) Relative conversion of arachidonic acid through lipoxygenase and cyclo-oxygenase pathways by homogenates of diseased periodontal tissues. J Oral Pathol 12:7–10

El Attar TMA, Lin HS, Killoy WJ, Vanderhoek JY, Goodson JM (1986) Hydroxy fatty acids and prostaglandin formation in diseased human periodontal pocket tissue. J Periodont Res 21:169–176

Felix R, Cecchini MG, Fleisch H (1990) Macrophage colony stimulating factor restores in vivo bone resorption in the *op/op* osteopetrotic mouse. Endocrinology 127:2592–2594

Feyen JHM, Elford P, Dipadova FE, Trechsel U (1989) Interleukin-6 is produced by bone and modulated by parathyroid hormone. J Bone Miner Res 4:633–638

Franklin RB, Tashjian AH (1975) Intravenous infusion of prostaglandin E2 raises plasma calcium concentration in the rat. Endocrinology 97:240–243

Fried RM, Voelkel EF, Rice RH, Levine L, Gaffney EV, Tashjian AH (1989) Two squamous cell carcinomas not associated with humoral hypercalcemia produce a potent bone resorption-stimulating factor which is interleukin-1 alpha. Endocrinology 125:742–751

Garrett IR, Mundy GR (1989) Relationship between interleukin-1 and prostaglandins in resorbing neonatal calvariae. J Bone Miner Res 4:789–794

Garrett IR, Durie BGM, Nedwin GE, Gillespie A, Bringman T, Sabatini M, Bertolini DR, Mundy GR (1987) Production of the bone resorbing cytokine lymphotoxin by cultured human myeloma cells. N Engl J Med 317:526–532

Garrett IR, Black KS, Mundy GR (1990a) Interactions between interleukin-6 and interleukin-1 in osteoclastic bone resorption in neonatal mouse calvariae. Calcif Tissue Int 46 [Suppl 2]:140

Garrett IR, Boyce BF, Oreffo ROC, Bonewald L, Poser J, Mundy GR (1990b) Oxygen-derived free radicals stimulate osteoclastic bone resorption in rodent bone in vitro and in vivo. J Clin Invest 85:632–639

Girasole G, Sakagami Y, Hustmyer FG, Yu XP, Derrigs HG, Boswell S, Peacock M, Boder G, Manolagas SC (1990) 17-β estradiol inhibits cytokine induced IL-6 production by bone marrow stromal cells and osteoblasts. J Bone Miner Res 5 [Suppl 2]:795

Globus RK, Patterson-Buckendahl P, Gospodarowicz D (1988) Regulation of bovine bone cell proliferation by fibroblast growth factor and transforming growth factor beta. Endocrinology 123:98–105

Gowen M, Mundy GR (1986) Actions of recombinant interleukin-1, interleukin-2 and interferon gamma on bone resorption in vitro. J Immunol 136:2478–2482

Gowen M, Meikle MC, Reynolds JJ (1983) Stimulation of bone resorption in vitro by a nonprostanoid factor released by human monocytes in culture. Biochim Biophys Acta 762:471–474

Gowen M, Wood DD, Russell RG (1985) Stimulation of the proliferation of human bone cells in vitro by human monocyte products with interleukin-1 activity. J Clin Invest 75:1223–1229

Gowen M, Nedwin G, Mundy GR (1986) Preferential inhibition of cytokine stimulated bone resorption by recombinant interferon gamma. J Bone Miner Res 1:469–474

Gowen M, Chapman K, Littlewood A, Hughes D, Evans D, Russell G (1990) Production of tumor necrosis factor by human osteoblasts is modulated by other cytokines, but not by osteotropic hormones. Endocrinology 126:1250–1255

Graves DT, Antoniades HN, Williams SR, Owen AJ (1984a) Evidence for functional platelet-derived growth factor receptors on MG-63 human osteosarcoma cells. Cancer Res 44:2966–2970

Graves DT, Owen AJ, Barth RK, Tempst P, Winoto A, Fors L, Hood LE, Antoniades HN (1984b) Detection of c-sis transcripts and synthesis of PDGF-like proteins by human osteosarcoma cells. Science 226:972–997

Graves DT, Valentin-Opran A, Delgado R, Valente AJ, Mundy GR, Piche J (1989) The potential role of platelet-derived growth factors as an autocrine or paracrine factor for human bone cells. Connect Tissue Res 23:209–218

Gutierrez GE, Mundy GR, Derynck R, Hewlett KL, Katz MS (1987) Inhibition of parathyroid hormone-responsive adenylate cyclase in clonal osteoblast-like cells by transforming growth factor alpha and epidermal growth factor. J Biol Chem 262:15845–15850

Gutierrez GE, Mundy GR, Manning DR, Hewlett EL, Katz MS (1990) Transforming growth factor β enhances parathyroid hormone stimulation of adenylate cyclase in clonal osteoblast-like cells. J Cell Physiol 144:438–447

Hagenaars CE, van der Kraan AAM, Kawilarangde EWM, Visser JWM, Nijweide PJ (1989) Osteoclast formation from cloned pluripotent hemopoietic stem cells. Bone Miner 6:179–189

Hannum CH, Wilcox CJ, Arend WP, Joslin FG, Dripps DJ, Heimdal PL, Armes LG, Sommer A, Eisenberg SP, Thompson RC (1990) Interleukin-1 receptor antagonist activity of a human interleukin-1 inhibitor. Nature 343:336–340

Hauschka PV, Mavrakos AE, Iafrati MD, Doleman SE, Klagsbrun M (1986) Growth factors in bone matrix. J Biol Chem 261:12665–12674

Heath JK, Saklatvala J, Meikle MC, Atkinson SJ, Reynolds JJ (1985) Pig interleukin-1 (catabolin) is a potent stimulator of bone resorption in vitro. Calcif Tissue Int 37:95–97

Howard GA, Bottemiller BL, Turner RT, Rader JI, Baylink DJ (1981) Parathyroid hormone stimulates bone formation and resorption in organ culture: evidence for a coupling mechanism. Proc Natl Acad Sci USA 78:3204–3208

Ibbotson KJ, Twardzik DR, D'Souza SM, Hargreaves WR, Todaro GJ, Mundy GR (1985) Stimulation of bone resorption in vitro by synthetic transforming growth factor-alpha. Science 228:1007–1009

Ibbotson KJ, Harrod J, Gowen M, D'Souza S, Smith DD, Mundy GR (1986) Human recombinant transforming growth factor alpha stimulates bone resorption and inhibits formation in vitro. Proc Natl Acad Sci USA 83:2228–2232

Ichikawa Y (1970) Further studies on the differentiation of a cell line of myeloid leukemia. J Cell Physiol 76:175–184

Ishimi Y, Miyaura C, Jin CH, Akatsu T, Abe T, Nakamura Y, Yamaguchi A, Yoshiki S, Matsuda T, Hirano T, Kishimoto T, Suda T (1990) IL-6 is produced by osteoblasts and induces bone resorption. J Immunol 145:3297–3303

Jee WS, Ueno K, Deng YP, Woodbury DM (1985) The effects of prostaglandin E2 in growing rats: increased metaphyseal hard tissue and cortico-endosteal bone formation. Calcif Tissue Int 37:148–157

Jee WS, Ueno K, Kimmel DB, Woodbury DM, Price P, Woodbury LA (1987) The role of bone cells in increasing metaphyseal hard tissue in rapidly growing rats treated with prostaglandin E2. Bone 8:171–178

Jennings JC, Mohan S, Baylink DJ (1989) Beta 2-microglobulin is not a bone cell mitogen. Endocrinology 125:404–409

Johnson RA, Boyce BF, Mundy GR, Roodman GD (1989) Tumors producing human TNF induce hypercalcemia and osteoclastic bone resorption in nude mice. Endocrinology 124:1424–1427

Kawano M, Tanaka H, Ishikawa H, Nobuyoshi M, Iwato K, Asaoku H, Tanabe O, Kuramoto A (1989) Interleukin-1 accelerates autocrine growth of myeloma cells through interleukin-6 in human myeloma. Blood 73:2145–2148

Klein DC, Raisz LG (1970) Prostaglandins: stimulation of bone resorption in tissue culture. Endocrinology 86:1436–1440

Klein B, Zhang XG, Jourdan M, Bataille R (1989) Cytokines involved in human multiple myeloma. Monoclonal. Gammapathies II 12:55–59

Kodama H, Yamasaki A, Nose M, Niida S, Ohgame Y, Abe M, Kumegawa M, Suda T (1991) Congenital osteoclast deficiency in osteopetrotic (op/op) mice is cured by injections of macrophage colony-stimulating factor. J Exp Med 173:269–272

Kondo Y, Sato K, Ohkawa H, Ueyama Y, Okabe T, Sato N, Asano S, Mori M, Ohsawa N, Kosaka K (1983) Association of hypercalcemia with tumors producing colony-stimulating factor(s). Cancer Res 43:2368–2374

Kukita A, Bonewald L, Rosen D, Seyedin S, Mundy GR, Roodman GD (1990) Osteoinductive factor inhibits formation of human osteoclast-like cells. Proc Natl Acad Sci USA 87:3023–3026

Kurihara N, Bertolini D, Suda T, Akiyama Y, Roodman GD (1990) IL-6 stimulates osteoclast-like multinucleated cell formation in long term human marrow cultures by inducing IL-1 release. J Immunol 144:4226–4230

Kurland JI, Pelus LM, Ralph P, Bockman RS, Moore MA (1979) Induction of prostaglandin E synthesis in normal and neoplastic macrophages: role for colony-stimulating factor(s) distinct from effects on myeloid progenitor cell proliferation. Proc Natl Acad Sci USA 76:2326–2330

Lerner UH (1987) Modifications of the mouse calvarial technique improve the responsiveness to stimulators of bone resorption. J Bone Miner Res 2:375–383

Lorenzo JA, Sousa SL, Alander C, Raisz LG, Dinarello CA (1987) Comparison of the bone resorbing activity in the supernatants from phytohemagglutinin stimulated human peripheral blood mononuclear cells with that of cytokines through the use of an antiserum to interleukin-1. Endocrinology 121:1164–1170

Lowik CWGM, Vanderpluijm G, Bloys H, Hoekman K, Bijvoet OLM, Aarden LA, Papapoulos SE (1989) Parathyroid hormone (PTH) and PTH-like protein (Plp) stimulate interleukin-6 production by osteogenic cells – a possible role of interleukin-6 in osteoclastogenesis. Biochem Biophys Res Commun 162:1546–1552

MacDonald BR, Mundy GR, Clark S, Wang EA, Kuehl TJ, Stanley ER, Roodman GD (1986) Effects of human recombinant CSF-GM and highly purified CSF-1 on the formation of multinucleated cells with osteoclast characteristics in long term bone marrow cultures. J Bone Miner Res 1:227–233

Marcelli C, Yates AJP, Mundy GR (1990) In vivo effects of human recombinant transforming growth factor beta on bone turnover in normal mice. J Bone Miner Res 5:1087–1096

Meghji S, Sandy J, Scutt AM, Harvey W, Harris M (1988) Stimulation of bone resorption by lipoxygenase metabolites of arachidonic acid. Prostaglandins 36:139–149

Metcalf D, Gearing DP (1987) Fatal syndrome in mice engrafted with cells producing high levels of the leukemia inhibitory factor. Proc Natl Acad Sci USA 86:5948–5952

Mohan S, Jennings JC, Linkhart TA, Baylink DJ (1988) Primary structure of human skeletal growth factor: homology with human insulin-like growth factor-II. Biochim Biophys Acta 966:44–55

Moore RN, Oppenheim JJ, Farrar JJ, Carter CS, Waheed A, Shadduck RK (1980) Production of lymphocyte-activating factor (Interleukin-1) by macrophages activated with colony-stimulating factors. J Immunol 125:1302–1305

Mundy GR, Wilkinson R, Heath DA (1983) Comparative study of available medical therapy for hypercalcemia of malignancy. Am J Med 74:421–432

Ng KW, Hudson PJ, Power BE, Manji SS, Gummer PR, Martin TJ (1989) Retinoic acid and tumour necrosis factor-alpha act in concert to control the level of alkaline phosphatase mRNA. J Mol Endocrinol 3:57–64

Pacifici R, Rifas L, Teitelbaum S, Slatopolsky E, McCracken R, Bergfeld M, Lee W, Avioli LV, Peck WA (1987) Spontaneous release of interleukin-1 from human blood monocytes reflects bone formation in idiopathic osteoporosis. Proc Natl Acad Sci USA 84:4616–4620

Pacifici R, Rifas L, McCracken R, Vered I, McMurty C, Avioli L, Peck WA (1989) Ovarian steroid treatment blocks a postmenopausal increase in blood monocyte interleukin-1 release. Proc Natl Acad Sci USA 86:2398–2402

Pfeilschifter J, Mundy GR, Roodman GD (1989) Interleukin-1 and tumor necrosis factor stimulate the formation of human osteoclast-like cells in vitro. J Bone Miner Res 4:113–118

Pizurki L, Rizzoli R, Bonjour JP (1990) Inhibition by (D-Trp12, Tyr34) bPTH (7-34) amide of PTH and PTHrP effects on Pi transport in renal cells. Am J Physiol 259:F389–392

Powles TJ, Dowsett M, Easty GC, Easty DM, Neville AM (1976) Breast cancer osteolysis, bone metastases, and anti-osteolytic effect of aspirin. Lancet i:608–610

Powles TJ, Muindi J, Coombes RC (1982) Mechanisms for development of bone metastases and effects of anti-inflammatory drugs. In: Powles TJ, Bockman RS,

Honn KV, Ramwell P (eds) Prostaglandins and related lipids, vol 2. Liss, New York, pp 541–553

Raisz LG, Sandberg AL, Goodson JM, Simmons HA, Mergenhagen SE (1974) Complement-dependent stimulation of prostaglandin synthesis and bone resorption. Science 185:789–791

Raisz LG, Dietrich JW, Simmons HA, Seyberth HW, Hubbard WN, Oates JA (1977) Effects of prostaglandin endoperoxides and metabolites and bone resorption in vitro. Nature 267:532–535

Raisz LG, Simmons HA, Sandberg AL, Canalis E (1980) Direct stimulation of bone resorption by epidermal growth factor. Endocrinology 107:270–273

Reid LR, Lowe C, Cornish J, Skinner SJM, Hilton DJ, Willson TA, Gearing DP, Martin TJ (1990) Leukemia inhibitor factor – a novel bone-active cytokine. Endocrinology 126:1416–1420

Rodan SB, Wesolowski G, Thomas K, Rodan GA (1987) Growth stimulation of rat calvaria osteoblastic cells by acidic fibroblast growth factor. Endocrinology 121:1917–1923

Roodman GD, Takahashi N, Bird A, Mundy GR (1987) Tumor necrosis factor α (TNF) stimulates formation of osteoclast-like cell (OCL) in long term human marrow cultures by stimulating production of interleukin-1 (IL-1). Clin Res 35:515A

Sabatini M, Garrett IR, Mundy GR (1987) TNF potentiates the effects of interleukin-1 on bone resorption in vitro. J Bone Miner Res 2:34

Sabatini M, Boyce B, Aufdemorte T, Bonewald L, Mundy GR (1988) Infusions of recombinant human interleukin-1 alpha and beta cause hypercalcemia in normal mice. Proc Natl Acad Sci USA 85:5235–5239

Sabatini M, Yates AJ, Garrett R, Chavez J Dunn J, Bonewald L, Mundy GR (1990a) Increased production of tumor necrosis factor by normal immune cells in a model of the humoral hypercalcemia of malignancy. Lab Invest 63: 676–681

Sabatini M, Chavez J, Mundy GR, Bonewald LF (1990b) Stimulation of tumor necrosis factor release from monocytic cells by the A375 human melanoma via granulocyte-macrophage colony stimulating factor. Cancer Res 50:2673–2678

Sato K, Mimura H, Han DC, Kariuchi T, Ueyama Y, Ohkawa H, Okabe T, Kondo Y, Ohsawa N, Tsushima T, Shizume K (1986) Production of bone-resorbing activity and colony-stimulating activity in vivo and in vitro by a human squamous cell carcinoma associated with hypercalcemia and leukocytosis. J Clin Invest 78:145–154

Sato K, Fujii Y, Kasono K, Ozawa M, Imamura H, Kanaji Y, Kurosawa H, Tsushima T, Shizume K (1989) Parathyroid hormone-related protein and interleukin-1α synergistically stimulate bone resorption in vitro and increase the serum calcium concentration in mice in vivo. Endocrinology 124:2172–2178

Sato N, Asano S, Ueyama Y, Mori M, Okabe T, Kondo Y, Ohsawa N, Kosaka K (1979) Granulocytosis and colony-stimulating activity (CSA) produced by a human squamous cell carcinoma. Cancer 43:605–610

Satoh T, Sato K, Shizume K, Yamazaki K, Demura H (1990) Repeated injection of mouse interferon-gamma (IFn-γ) decreases serum calcium concentration in tumor-bearing hypercalcemic nude mice. J Bone Miner Res 5 [Suppl]:484

Seckinger P, Klein-Nulend J, Alander C, Thompson RC, Dayer JM, Raisz LG (1990) Natural and recombinant human IL-1 receptor antagonists block the effects of IL-1 on bone resorption and prostaglandin production. J Immunol 145:4181–4184

Seyberth HW, Segre GV, Morgan JL, Sweetman BJ, Potts JT, Oates JA (1975) Prostaglandins as mediators of hypercalcemia associated with certain types of cancer. N Engl J Med 293:1278–1283

Shinar DM, Sato M, Rodan GA (1990) The effects of hemopoietic growth factors on the generation of osteoclast-like cells in mouse bone marrow cultures. Endocrinology 126:1728–1735

Smith D, Gowen M, Mundy GR (1987) Effects of interferon gamma and other cytokines on collagen synthesis in fetal rat bone cultures. Endocrinology 120:2494–2499

Stashenko P, Dewhirst FE, Peros WJ, Kent RL, Ago JM (1987) Synergistic interactions between interleukin-1, tumor necrosis factor, and lymphotoxin in bone resorption. J Immunol 138:1464–1468

Takahashi N, Mundy GR, Roodman GD (1986) Recombinant human gamma interferon inhibits formation of human osteoclast like cells. J Immunol 137:3541–3549

Tashjian AH, Voelkel EF, Levine L, Goldhaber P, (1972) Evidence that the bone resorption-stimulating factor produced by mouse fibrosarcoma cells is prostaglandin E2: a new model for the hypercalcemia of cancer. J Exp Med 136:1329–1343

Tashjian AH, Rice JE, Sides K (1977) Biological activities of prostaglandin analogues and metabolites on bone in organ culture. Nature 266:645–647

Tashjian AH, Wright DR, Ivey JL, Pont A (1978) Calcitonin binding sites in bone: relationships to biological response and "escape". Recent Prog Horm Res 34:285–334

Tashjian AH, Voelkel EF, Lazzaro M, Singer FR, Roberts AB, Derynck R, Winkler ME, Levine L (1985) Alpha and beta transforming growth factors stimulate prostaglandin production and bone resorption in cultured mouse calvaria. Proc Natl Acad Sci USA 82:4535–4538

Tashjian AH, Voelkel EF, Lazzaro M, Goad D, Bosma T, Levine L (1987) Tumor necrosis factor α (cachectin) stimulates bone resorption in mouse calvaria via a prostaglandin-mediated mechanism. Endocrinology 120:2029–2036

Thomson BM, Saklatvala J, Chambers TJ (1986) Osteoblasts mediate interleukin-1 stimulation of bone resorption by rat osteoclasts. J Exp Med 164:104–112

Tomida M, Yamamoto-Yamaguchi Y, Hozumi M (1984) Purification of a factor inducing differentiation of mouse myeloid leukemic M1 cells from conditioned medium of mouse fibroblast L929 cells. J Biol Chem 259:10978–10982

Toya M, Kuroda M, Obuchi M, Ikawa T, Habu K, Ichikawa T (1981) A case report of the maxillary cancer associated with marked leukocytosis and hypercalcemia. J Otolaryngol Jpn 84:1554–1562

Valentin A, Eilon G, Saez S, Mundy GR (1985) Estrogens and anti-estrogens stimulate release of bone resorbing activity by cultured human breast cancer cells. J Clin Invest 75:726–731

Van der Wijngaert FP, Tas MC, van der Meer JWM, Burger EH (1987) Growth of osteoclast precursor-like cells from whole mouse bone marrow: Inhibitory effect of CSF-1. Bone Miner 3:97–110

Yoneda T, Bessho M, Nishikawa N, Matusumoto K, Sakuda M (1985) Pathogenesis of hypercalcemia and leukocytosis in a patient with tongue cancer. Jpn J Oral Surg 31:1917–1924

Yoneda T, Nishikawa N, Nishimura R, Kato I, Sakuda M (1989) Three cases of oral squamous cancer associated with leukocytosis, hypercalcemia or both. Oral Surg 68:604–611

Yoneda T, Mundy GR, Roodman GD (1990) Induction of differentiation of the human promyelocytic HL-60 cells into cells with the osteoclast phenotype. In: Cohn DV, Glorieux FH, Martin TJ (eds) Calcium regulation and bone metabolism. Basic and clinical aspects, vol 10. Excerpta Medica, Amsterdam, pp 425–429

Yoneda T, Nishimura R, Kato I, Ohmae M, Takita M, Sakuda M (1991a) Frequency of the hypercalcemia-leukocytosis syndrome in oral malignancies. Cancer 51:2438–2443

Yoneda T, Alsina MM, Chavez JB, Bonewald L, Nishimura R, Mundy GR (1991b) Evidence that splenic cytokines play a pathogenetic role in the paraneoplastic syndromes of cachexia, hypercalcemia and leukocytosis in a human tumor in nude mice. J Clin Invest 87:977–985

Yoneda Y, Aufdemorte TB, Nishimura R, Nishikawa N, Sakuda M, Alsina MM, Chavez JB, Mundy GR (1991c) Occurrence of hypercalcemia and leukocytosis with cachexia in a human squamous cell carcinoma of the maxilla in athymic nude mice. A novel experimental model of three concomitant paraneoplastic syndromes. J Clin Oncol 9:468–477
Yoneda T, Kato I, Bonewald LF, Chisoku H, Burgess WH, Mundy GR (1991d) A novel osteoclastpoietic peptide: purification and characterization. J Bone Miner Res 6 [Suppl 1]:454
Yoshida H, Hayashi SI, Kunisada T, Ogawa M, Nishikawa S, Okamura H, Sudo T, Shultz LD, Nishikawa SI (1990) The murine mutation osteopetrosis is in the coding region of the macrophage colony stimulating factor gene. Nature 345:442–444

CHAPTER 6

Hormonal Factors Which Regulate Bone Resorption

G.R. MUNDY

A. Introduction

The activity of bone cells is controlled by circulating systemic factors and by locally produced factors or cytokines. This distinction is not absolute, since some cytokines may circulate when produced in large amounts. The production of the three major systemic factors (parathyroid hormone, calcitonin, and 1,25-dihydroxyvitamin D) is regulated by extracellular fluid calcium, and their primary role in maintenance of calcium homeostasis rather than control of bone cell function. Nevertheless, to maintain calcium homeostasis, bone cell function may be altered. In this chapter, the effects of these systemic factors on bone cell activity will be reviewed.

B. Parathyroid Hormone

It has been known for 70 years that parathyroid hormone (PTH) affects bone cell function, may alter bone remodeling, and causes bone loss. It is now apparent that PTH acts on both bone-resorbing cells and bone-forming cells. Its overall effects may depend on whether it is administered continuously or intermittently. When administered continuously, it increases osteoclastic bone resorption and suppresses bone formation. However, when administered in low doses intermittently, its major effect is stimulation of bone formation, a response which has been called the anabolic effect of PTH.

In recent years there has been a very great increase in our understanding of the synthesis and secretion of parathyroid hormone, the domains in the hormone necessary for binding and activation of the PTH receptor, and very recently molecular cloning of the receptor itself. These exciting advances are reviewed in Chap. 15.

I. Effects of PTH on Bone Resorption

For many years it has been known that PTH stimulates osteoclasts to resorb bone. This was first shown in vivo by BARNICOT (1948), who found that, when parathyroid glands were grafted into subcutaneous tissue adjacent to the calvariae of rodents, there was a marked increase in adjacent osteoclast activity. This confirmed clinical observations which had been made by Albright and others over the preceding 30 years. These workers had noted that, in patients with primary hyperparathyroidism, there was a profound loss of bone associated with increased osteoclastic bone resorption (the bone disease referred to in those times as "osteitis fibrosa cystica"). In the last 30 years, much information has been accumulated on the effects of PTH on cells in the osteoclast lineage. The organ culture experiments of GAILLARD (1961) and RAISZ (1965) using fetal rat long bones showed that there was a marked response in these organ cultures to PTH, indicating an increase in osteoclast activity with degradation of the bone matrix and release of bone mineral. In these systems, PTH was effective at concentrations of 10^{-7}–10^{-9} M (Fig. 1). This is clearly a much greater concentration than the concentrations of PTH that bone cells are likely to be exposed to. However, PTH is a very sticky molecule and it is not clear in these organ culture systems whether the effective concentration of PTH that the bone cells in the organ culture are exposed to may be much lower than those actually added to the tissue culture dishes. The effects of PTH in these organ culture systems show a number of specific characteristics. One of the first described RAISZ et al. (1972a) was the phenomenon of "induction." By this term, RAISZ meant that parathyroid hormone caused a prolonged resorptive response in the bones following a brief 4- to 6-h exposure. He later contrasted this response to other agents such as prostaglandins of the E series and 1,25-dihydroxyvitamin D, which required more prolonged incubation in the bone cultures to stimulate resorption. In light of present knowledge, it is possible that agents which induce induction can do so by activating mature

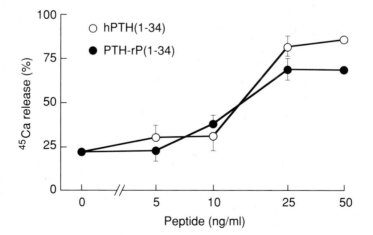

Fig. 1. Effects of a human PTH 1-34 on bone resorption in fetal rat long bones as measured by release of previously incorporated ^{45}Ca. In this experiment, PTH is compared with synthetic human PTH-rP 1:34 (from YATES et al. 1988)

osteoclasts to resorb bone, whereas the agents which are less effective at causing induction are those agents which probably exert their major effects to increase the formation of new osteoclasts. The resorption of bone in vitro was associated with the production of lysosomal enzymes which appeared in the organ culture media. This was first demonstrated by VAES (1968) and confirmed by EILON and RAISZ (1978). As well as lysosomal enzymes, collagenase appeared in the organ culture media. The bones also responded to PTH with an increase in synthesis and turnover of hyaluronic acid (LUBEN et al. 1974), which may be responsible for facilitating cell movement over the bone surface or possibly in the removal of mineral from the bone matrix.

In the in vivo situation, bone cells are never exposed to PTH alone. Other local and systemic hormones are always present to interact with PTH in its effects on target cells. In vitro studies have demonstrated that the effects of PTH on osteoclastic bone resorption may be modulated by other factors. GARABEDIAN et al. (1974) showed that PTH and 1,25-dihydroxyvitamin D may work in concert on bone to increase the serum calcium concentration. This may be particularly important because PTH stimulates the production of 1,25-dihydroxyvitamin D by the renal tubules and in states such as primary hyperparathyroidism bone cells are likely exposed to a combination of both of these hormones. There is evidence that the effects of PTH on renal tubular cells are enhanced by 1,25-dihydroxyvitamin D (YAMAMOTO et al. 1984). RAISZ (1970) described a synergistic effect of PTH and the vitamin D metabolites on bone resorption in organ cultures, although STERN et al. (1983) could not confirm these results. PTH may work in concert with other factors to stimulate bone resorption. For example, STASHENKO et al. (1987) have shown that it can work in concert with interleukin-1 to stimulate bone resorption and SATO et al. (1989) have shown that PTH and interleukin-1α have synergistic effects on serum calcium in vivo. Similarly, PTH, transforming growth factor α, and epidermal growth factor have synergistic effects on bone resorption in vitro (LORENZO and QUINTIN 1984; SABATINI et al. 1990) and more recently we have found that transforming growth factor α can act synergistically with PTH-rP on bone resorption (see later) (YATES et al. 1991). The effects of PTH on osteoclastic bone resorption in organ culture can be inhibited by calcitonin (RAISZ and NIEMANN 1967), cortisol (RAISZ et al. 1972b), and neutral phosphate (RAISZ and NIEMANN 1969; BRAND and RAISZ 1972). However, the effects of calcitonin are shortlasting and cortisol does not inhibit PTH-stimulated bone resorption unless the concentrations of glucocorticoid are high (STRUMPF et al. 1978). There are some histologic features of osteoclasts stimulated with PTH which are worthy of note. PTH causes an increase in the number of osteoclasts and these cells show increased volume of the ruffled borders, which is the specialized portion of the plasma membrane which is adjacent to the bone surface and across which mineral is resorbed and matrix is degraded (HOLTROP et al. 1974). These responses in osteoclasts occur quite rapidly, with a change in the size of the ruffled border being noted within 1 h of exposure of bone cells to PTH.

Parathyroid hormone probably acts at multiple steps in the osteoclast lineage. It clearly stimulates the mature multinucleated osteoclast to form a ruffled border and resorb bone, but in addition also has effects on earlier cells in the osteoclast lineage. It is surprising that, although a lot of information is currently available on the biochemical and morphologic events which are associated with PTH-mediated bone resorption, the precise molecular mechanisms by which PTH exerts its effects on cells in the osteoclast lineage is still not known. Nevertheless, although we do not understand the molecular mechanism of osteoclast activation by PTH, in vitro studies have clarified our understanding of the cellular mechanisms by which PTH increases bone resorption.

Current evidence suggests that PTH acts on precursor cells in the osteoclast lineage to increase the formation of new osteoclasts. These observations come from different types of experiments. The data of Roodman and colleagues (IBBOTSON et al. 1984; KURIHARA et al. 1991) using marrow cell cultures shows that PTH acts on marrow mononuclear cells to increase the formation of cells with osteoclast characteristics, such as cross-reactivity with 23C6 monoclonal antibodies which preferentially recognize the osteoclast vitronectin receptor, capacity to form resorption lacunae on bone matrices, and presence of the osteoclast proton pump and calcitonin receptors. Although in earlier experiments it seemed possible that these effects could be mediated indirectly through other cells, more recently KURIHARA et al. (1991) have reported that PTH stimulates colony-forming units of the granulocyte-macrophage type (CFU-GM). The CFU-GM-derived cells were plucked from methyl cellulose and grown in liquid culture to form multinucleated cells which stain positively with 23C6 monoclonal antibody in low concentrations. This property has been shown to correlate positively with other osteoclast characteristics such as the presence of the osteoclast vacuolar proton pump and calcitonin receptors (KURIHARA et al. 1991). Staining with 23C6 monoclonal antibodies is not specific for the osteoclast, but these antibodies will not cross-react with macrophages or macrophage polykaryons at the concentrations used in these experiments. These authors refer to the starting cells in the colonies they pluck from methyl cellulose as "early precursors." These early precursors still have other potentials because some of them form 23C6-negative polykaryons. "Late precursors" (defined as these colonies cultured for a further 2 weeks with 1,25-dihydroxyvitamin D) are unipotent and form only 23C6-positive multinucleated cells. Late precursors do not apparently respond to PTH, suggesting that the effects of PTH at this stage are mediated indirectly. These results show that PTH is acting directly on the cells in the colonies which are devoid of osteoblasts or stromal cells to stimulate their differentiation. However, it does not exclude the possibility that PTH could also have additional indirect effects to stimulate osteoclast precursor proliferation and differentiation. HAKEDA et al. (1989) have also shown in a different system that PTH can act directly on mononuclear cells presumably in the osteoclast lineage. They showed binding of PTH to hematopoietic blast cells supported by granulocyte-macrophage colony-stimulating factor (GM-CSF) and found that PTH stimulated these cells to form multinucleated giant cells. These data suggest that PTH acts to stimulate osteoclast formation, but does not act on mononuclear late precursors. In organ culture systems, LORENZO et al. (1983) showed that the resorbing effects of PTH on bone were not dependent on cell proliferation, suggesting that PTH does not act on proliferating cells in the osteoclast lineage. When organ cultures were incubated with hydroxyurea, bone resorption was unaffected. These data are not necessarily in conflict with the cell culture experiments of KURIHARA et al. (1991) and HAKEDA et al. (1989), although the cell culture studies do suggest that PTH does affect cells capable of proliferation.

Parathyroid hormone also stimulates mature osteoclasts to resorb bone. Current data suggest that this effect is indirect. McSHEEHY and CHAMBERS (1986) showed that when freshly dispersed osteoclasts isolated from rat bone surfaces were cultured on bovine bone, resorption lacunae were not formed unless cells with the osteoblast phenotype were added. This experiment has been confirmed by other groups since. Earlier, JONES and BOYDE (1978) noted that the initial response of cells on a bone surface to PTH was retraction of cells in the osteoblast lineage, allowing osteoclasts to insinuate pseudopodia containing ruffled borders through the retracted area to the bone surface. RODAN and MARTIN (1981) pointed out soon after that agents which stimulate osteoclastic bone resorption such as PTH and prostaglandins of the E series stimulate adenylate cyclase activity in cells with the osteoblast phenotype, and that the potency of these factors on osteoblast-like cells is correlated very closely with their potency as bone resorption factors. They suggested that PTH may stimulate osteoclastic bone resorption by interacting with cells in the osteoblast lineage. This led to additional changes and subsequent bone resorption.

The question over whether PTH also has direct effects on osteoclasts has been reopened recently with a report by TETI et al. (1991). These controversial results will require confirmation.

Recently, ROULEAU and coworkers (1988) have used autoradiography to demonstrate in rat bones a possible target cell for PTH. They suggest this cell is an elliptical cell which may be a cell in the osteoblast lineage, but does not appear morphologically to be a mature osteoblast. This cell is seen in the intertrabecular spaces of the metaphyseal region in rat long bones. Whether this is the target cell for PTH-mediated bone resorption is not possible to tell. MITCHELL et al. (1990) studied PTH receptors on the rat osteosarcoma cell line UMR-106. They found three morphologically distinct cell types in subconfluent cultures. One of these cell types appeared morphologically similar to the cells seen in the rat metaphysis, and had the most abundant PTH binding.

The mechanisms by which cells of the osteoblast phenotype communicate with osteoclasts to stimulate bone resorption are still not known. This may involve the production of soluble mediators, or it may involve cell interactions. For example, it is possible that cells in the osteoblast lineage could form gated channels through cell interactions with osteoclasts and that information representing the bone-resorbing signal could be transferred in that manner. Further work is needed in this area.

For some years, it has been suggested that osteoblasts may prepare the bone surface for osteoclastic bone resorption by producing proteolytic enzymes. Investigators who have favored this hypothesis include Teitelbaum and Kahn (1980), Sakamoto and Sakamoto (1982), and Chambers (1985). Sakamoto and Sakamoto (1982) first suggested that collagenase expression in bone is restricted to the osteoblasts. They used immunocytochemical methods. Chambers suggested that osteoblasts release collagenase which prepares the bone surface for later osteoclastic resorption in response to PTH. This concept suggested that the surface of bone would then be more readily degraded by proteolytic enzymes. Hamilton et al. (1985) showed that cells in the osteoblast lineage released plasminogen activator when exposed to PTH and suggested that this enzymatic cascade may be responsible for similar events, possibly by activating latent collagenase or by having a direct proteolytic effect on the proteins of the exposed bone surface. Heersche (1978) had earlier proposed that macrophage production of collagenase may be important in the resorption process and he suggested that collagenase produced by macrophages may work in concert with osteoclast-derived lysosomal enzymes. Perry et al. (1984) suggested that PTH causes collagenase release by immune cells rather than by osteoblasts. However, Jones et al. (1985) feel that there is no evidence for a role of collagenase produced by the osteoblasts from their studies using scanning electron microscopy. They claim that bone surfaces show no evidence of removal of osteoid tissue around osteoblasts, and also indicate that they see no evidence that mineralizing surfaces require exposure to osteoblasts prior to resorption. Although this is a controversial area, current methodology does not allow it to be clarified definitively.

In states of hyperparathyroidism, there may be increased numbers of mononuclear cells in the osteoclast lineage present in the marrow. In a patient with hyperparathyroidism and osteitis fibrosa cystica (MacDonald et al. 1986), there was a marked increase in the formation of cells with features of the osteoclast phenotype over 3 weeks of culture compared with similarly treated cultures from normal individuals. This observation suggests that, in patients with primary or secondary hyperparathyroidism, there are increased numbers of mononuclear cells in the osteoclast lineage present in the bone marrow. Although it could be argued that 1,25-dihydroxyvitamin D is responsible for this effect, similar findings are found in patients with secondary hyperparathyroidism and renal failure where 1,25-dihydroxyvitamin D concentrations are low. In vivo, states of primary and secondary hyperparathyroidism are associated with an unusual form of bone disease associated with subperiosteal osteoclastic resorption. It appears that osteoclast precursors in the periosteum are activated and resorb adjacent bone. This does not occur in other types of bone disease for reasons which are not clear. Why cells at this site should be particularly sensitive to PTH (*which* is presumably the mediator of this effect) remains unclear.

II. Effects of PTH on Bone Formation

It is clear that PTH has direct effects on cells in the osteoblast lineage. In fact, PTH responsiveness has been used as one of the criteria for cells with the osteoblast phenotype. PTH acts directly on osteosarcoma cells as well as on freshly isolated rodent and human osteoblasts. Responsiveness to PTH includes an increase in adenylate cyclase activity, changes in rates of proliferation, and changes in synthesis of alkaline phosphatase and type-I collagen.

In organ cultures of fetal rat calvariae, PTH causes decreased synthesis of type-I collagen (DIETRICH et al. 1967a). It can also oppose the stimulatory effects of insulin-like growth factor 1 (IGF-1) on type-I collagen synthesis (RAISZ et al. 1990). In small doses, PTH causes the production of stimulatory activity in conditioned media harvested from fetal rat calvarial organ cultures. CANALIS et al. (1989) has shown that this activity can be ascribed to IGF-1, since it is blocked by neutralizing antibodies. However, IGF-1 is not the only growth factor released by bone cultures in response to PTH. When organ cultures of neonatal mouse calvariae are stimulated to resorb by PTH (or other bone-resorbing hormones), active transforming growth factor β (TGFβ) appears in the conditioned media (PFEILSCHIFTER and MUNDY 1987). Since TGFβ is a powerful bone stimulatory factor, it appears likely that it is also important in the anabolic effect of PTH.

For some years, it has been thought that PTH may stimulate bone resorption by an effect on osteocytes to increase the volume of osteocytic lacunae. This was observed particularly in patients with primary hyperparathyroidism. However, in recent years BOYDE (1981) has thrown doubt on this concept. Using scanning electron microscopy, Boyde has been unable to show any evidence for osteocytic osteolysis. Criteria for resorption in this system consists of the appearance of exposed collagen fibrils in the lacunar bed. This has not been shown. Boyde ascribes the increase in size of osteocytic lacunae in primary hyperparathyroidism to an artifact of preparation of woven bone sections.

III. Signal Transduction Mechanisms for PTH in Bone Cells

There are several signal transduction mechanisms for PTH. Whether these work independently in bone cells or have differing importance for bone-resorbing or bone-forming cells is difficult to cell. One of the problems is that the target cell for PTH-mediated bone resorption has not been identified.

It has long been known that PTH stimulates adenylate cyclase activity in bone and kidney cells which is regulated by a guanine nucleotide binding protein (G protein). This is accompanied by an increase in intracellular cyclic AMP with activation of protein kinase A followed by intracellular protein phosphorylation. Generation of cyclic AMP has been used as a marker for PTH biological effects in vivo in the diagnosis of primary hyperparathyroidism, since cyclic AMP diffuses from renal tubular cells into the tubule luman and appears in the urine. It is also used as a marker for biological activity of PTH-rP in patients with the humoral hypercalcemia of malignancy.

The relationship between the effects of PTH to stimulate cyclic AMP generation in bone cells and bone resorption has remained nuclear and is still difficult to discern (PECK 1979). Bone resorption is associated with an increase in cyclic AMP in bone organ cultures. However, the same effects are seen with calcitonin, which produces the opposite biological effect to PTH since it inhibits osteoclastic bone resorption. The situation has not been clarified with the use of cyclic AMP analogs, which tend to give biphasic effects in organ culture systems. The most likely explanation is that PTH acts on different cells in bone to calcitonin, which directly acts on osteoclasts.

Recently, an alternative messenger system for PTH has been described in both bone cells and renal tubular cells. The effects of PTH on both bone cells and renal tubular cells is associated with an increase in intracellular calcium. This increased intracellular calcium has multiple sources, although it is clear that one of these sources is via the generation of inositol 1,4,5 triphosphate (IP3), and at least part of the increased intracellular calcium is due to IP3-mediated intracellular events. This increase in IP3 occurs secondary to activation of phospholipase C, also regulated by a G protein. This leads to polyphosphoinositide hydrolysis and the generation of IP3. The activation of phospholipase C is also associated with increased 1,2-diacylglycerol generation and activation of protein kinase C. It is still not known which of the biological effects of PTH are mediated through this signal transduction mechanism. The recent cloning of the receptor for PTH may help to clarify this situation. This topic has recently been reviewed by DUNLAY et al. (1990).

IV. Effects of PTH on Bone Turnover

Parathyroid hormone enhances bone turnover or remodeling in vivo. This has long been noted in clinical conditions associated with hyperparathyroidism, including primary hyperparathyroidism and hyperparathyroidism which occurs secondary to hypocalcemia. The mechanisms by which PTH stimulates bone-forming cells in vivo remain unclear. The observation described above that PTH has an inhibitory effect on osteoblastic cells in vitro suggests that the in vivo response of PTH to stimulate bone formation must be indirectly mediated. It appears most likely that the direct effects are over-ridden by the generation of coupling factors which are formed in bone as a consequence of the PTH stimulus, as first suggested by the work of HOWARD and colleagues (1981). The recent in vitro observations of CANALIS et al. (1989) have led to the suggestion that the effects of PTH to stimulate bone formation in vivo may be related to local generation of insulin-like growth factor 1 (IGF-1), which is responsible for this stimulatory effect. However, these data may have been overinterpreted. Other growth factors are also generated by bone in response to PTH. The most important of these may be TGFβ, which is probably an even more powerful stimulator of bone formation than IGF-1. In the embryonic rat calvarial organ culture system which Canalis used to measure effects of potential bone growth stimulants, TGFβ does not have a prominent effect. However, TGFβ clearly has power-ful effects on osteoblastic bone formation in vivo (see Chap. 7). There are almost certainly a number of growth factors generated locally by bone in response to PTH, including not only IGF-1 and TGFβ but possibly others such as IGF-II, the BMPs, PDGF, and the heparin-binding fibroblast growth factors.

There is another observation which may have clinical relevance but is still not explained. This observation is that PTH when administered in low doses in vivo produces an anabolic or stimulatory effect on bone-forming cells. This has been noted in humans and in rodents (PARSONS and POTTS 1972; TAM et al. 1982; KALU et al. 1970; GUNNESS-HEY and HOCK 1984). This is in contrast to the resorptive or catabolic effect which is seen when PTH is administered in larger doses. These observations have been used by Neer, Reeve, and colleagues (REEVE et al. 1980, 1989; SLOVIK et al. 1986) as a rationale for using PTH in low doses intermittently as a form of therapy in patients with osteoporosis associated with low bone turnover. Whether this anabolic effect is again indirect and mediated through IGF-1, TGFβ, or other growth factors is unknown. The recent observations of HARMS et al. (1989) and KITAMURA et al. (1990) may be relevant. These workers showed that, in normal individuals, PTH is released in pulsatile spikes of 6–8/h. These observations were made possible by the advent of better assays for measuring PTH, namely immunoradiometric and immunochemi-columinescent assays. Measuring PTH secretion every 2 min enabled them to show the pulsatility of normal PTH secretion. These spikes of PTH secretion occurred independent of changes in extracellular fluid calcium. Their physiologic significance is unclear. However, numerous in vitro and in vivo studies have demonstrated that the effects of intermittent PTH are different from those of continuous PTH. For example, intermittent PTH causes an anabolic effect on bone formation not seen with continuous PTH. As further evidence of the potential importance of these studies, in a preliminary study HARMS et al. (1989) showed that PTH pulsatility was reduced in several patients with osteoporosis. Since low-dose PTH given intermittently has been advocated as a treatment which can promote bone formation, this intermittent pulsatile effect of PTH on the skeleton may have pathophysiologic significance.

V. Effects of PTH on Calcium Homeostasis

Although PTH is probably the major regulator of extracellular fluid calcium homeostasis (Fig. 2), and clearly affects bone remodeling cells, it is not likely that PTH-mediated changes in bone remodeling cells are important in the maintenance of extracellular fluid calcium homeostasis. It is more likely that PTH exerts its major effects on calcium homeostasis via its capacity to increase renal tubular calcium reabsorption in the distal tubules of the kidney. Increases in the rates of bone turnover which are greater than

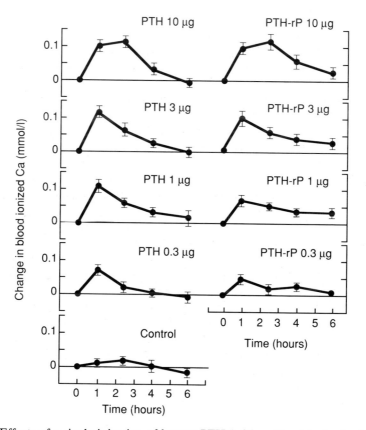

Fig. 2. Effects of a single injection of human PTH 1:34 on blood-ionized calcium in normal mice. There is a rapid rise in blood-ionized calcium which returns to baseline over the following 6h. In this experiment, the effect of the single subcutaneous injection of PTH was compared with synthetic human PTH-rP 1:34. The effects were essentially identical (from YATES et al. 1988)

those seen in primary hyperparathyroidism occur in Paget's disease and thyrotoxicosis, although in these circumstances hypercalcemia is unusual. It is also likely that bone-lining cells play a role in maintenance of extracellular fluid calcium which has still not been clearly delineated. PARFITT (1976a,b, 1979, 1987, 1989, see Chap. 1) has produced convincing evidence of this concept on a number of occasions. Although it is unknown whether PTH may regulate fluxes of calcium between the bone fluid and the extracellular fluid across this bone-lining layer, it is clear that these cells are responsive to PTH and such mechanisms are likely.

Parathyroid hormone synthesis and secretion are controlled by extracellular fluid calcium concentrations through a long negative feedback loop. Suppression of PTH released from the parathyroid glands occurs when the total serum calcium is greater than 11.5 mg/dl. Maximum PTH secretion occurs when the total serum calcium is 7.5 mg/dl. Outside the range of 7.5–11.5 mg/dl, there is no change in PTH secretion. It is likely that PTH responds to rapid changes in extracellular fluid calcium concentrations with immediate effects, whereas the other major calciotropic hormone, 1,25-dihydroxyvitamin D, is a more long-term regulator of extracellular fluid calcium. 1,25-Dihydroxyvitamin D is formed through several hydroxylation steps in the liver and kidney and is slower in production than release of the peptide PTH from the parathyroid glands, which is essentially instantaneous.

With increased entry of calcium into the extracellular fluid (for example, from increased bone destruction), PTH secretion will be suppressed, albeit not maximally. The homeostatic response to the increase in extracellular fluid calcium will be an increase in the amount of calcium filtered by the glomerulus, associated with decreased renal tubular calcium reabsorption. Suppression of PTH release is responsible for the decrease in renal tubular calcium reabsorption. There may also be a decrease in bone turnover, although the effects of a decrease in bone turnover caused by parathyroid gland suppression on calcium homeostasis is unlikely to be of major importance. There may be also an alteration of exchange of calcium between the bone fluid and the extracellular fluid, although these fluxes have not been thoroughly studied and are not well understood.

In summary, the effects of PTH on bone-forming and bone-resorbing cells are complex. Although much information is known regarding expression of PTH in the parathyroid cell and regulation of PTH synthesis and secretion, there is still much to be learned about the mechanisms by which PTH stimulates osteoclasts and osteoblasts and the relationship between these effects and maintenance of normal bone volume and control of calcium homeostasis.

C. 1,25-Dihydroxyvitamin D

The active vitamin D metabolites have complex effects on calcium homeostasis (Fig. 3). 1,25-Dihydroxyvitamin D and 25-hydroxyvitamin D promote

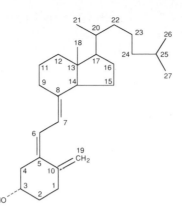

Fig. 3. Structure of vitamin D_3 (cholecalciferol). Cholecalciferol is formed in the skin by irradiation of 7-dihydrocholesterol. Ergocalciferol is formed by irradiation of ergosterol, which is derived from plants and is ingested in the diet. Ergocalciferol (vitamin D_2) differs from cholecalciferol (vitamin D_3) by having a double bond between the C22 and 23 positions and a methyl group at C24. Dihydrotachysterol does not have a double bond between C10 and C19. This results in rotation of the ring so that the hydroxyl group at C3 corresponds to the C1 position, and dihydrotachysterol does not require renal hydroxylation for activity

the absorption of calcium and phosphate from the gastrointestinal tract (Fig. 4). The active vitamin D metabolites also stimulate osteoclastic bone resorption both in vitro and in vivo. In addition to these effects, the active vitamin D metabolites have a complex relationship with PTH. They probably work in concert with PTH on its target organs, on bone cells, and in renal tubules, but also influence PTH secretion. 1,25-Dihydroxyvitamin D suppresses PTH secretion by parathyroid glands directly (SLATAPOLSKY et al. 1984) and indirectly by increasing serum calcium concentrations. In the absence of vitamin D, there is a failure of mineralization of the nonmineralized bone matrix, which is also called osteoid tissue. This leads to the histologic picture of rickets in children or osteomalacia in adults. The primary function of the active metabolites may be to provide an adequate supply of minerals at the bone-forming site for the adequate mineralization of newly formed bone matrix.

I. Vitamin D Receptor

The receptor for vitamin D has now been identified and characterized. The receptor is a 3.8S nuclear protein of approximately 55000 daltons (HAUSSLER et al. 1987, 1988; McDONNELL et al. 1988). When the receptor binds to 1,25-dihydroxyvitamin D, there is a conformational change in the complex which facilitates binding to specific DNA sites. The receptor protein is homologous to the *verb*-A oncogene, and belongs to the super-

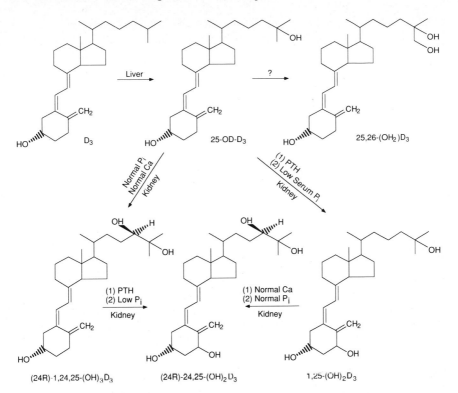

Fig. 4. Formation of the active metabolites of vitamin D from parent vitamin D compounds, and regulation of metabolic pathways responsible for their production

family of steroid hormone receptors which includes the estrogen receptor, the glucocorticoid receptor, the progesterone receptor, the androgen receptor, the thyroid hormone receptor, and the retinoic acid receptors (EVANS 1988). These receptors are not only homologous in their amino acid composition, but are also likely to have similar conformations. The region of the receptor that binds to DNA to lead to gene expression is known as the zinc finger. In these regions of the receptor, the amino acids form a finger-like structure which is stabilized by zinc which binds to four cysteines at the base of each protrusion. The finger-like region is stabilized by this zinc bridging the base. These zinc fingers are thought to mediate DNA binding, although it is not known exactly how this occurs. These regions of the vitamin D receptor have important implications for the disease known alternatively as vitamin D-resistant rickets or hereditary resistance to 1,25-dihydroxyvitamin D. In this condition, HUGHES and colleagues (1988) have discovered point mutations in the zinc finger regions of the receptor in different kindreds. Different point mutations are present in different families. The receptors do not bind to DNA normally and the consequence is resistance to 1,25-dihydroxyvitamin D. The children develop the syndrome of rickets with high circulating concentrations of 1,25-dihydroxyvitamin D.

II. Effects of 1,25-Dihydroxyvitamin D on Osteoclasts

The active metabolites of vitamin D were first shown to resorb bone in vitro by Raisz et al. (1972c). Subsequent in vivo studies indicated that 1,25-dihydroxyvitamin D works synergistically with PTH to stimulate bone resorption and increase the serum calcium (Garabedian et al. 1974). Synergistic interactions between PTH and 1,25-dihydroxyvitamin D on bone resorption in organ cultures have been difficult to show, although there have been some suggestions that synergism may occur (Raisz 1970). 25-Hydroxyvitamin D and 1,25-dihydroxyvitamin D are not the only bone-resorbing vitamin D metabolites. 19 nor,10 keto-25 hydroxyvitamin D has also been shown to stimulate bone resorption in organ culture (Stern 1980; Stern et al. 1985). The effects of 1,25-dihydroxyvitamin D on osteoclastic bone resorption are different from those of other known bone-resorbing factors. The vitamin D metabolites have a relatively slow onset of action on osteoclastic bone resorption and have a very shallow dose-response curve. They are extremely potent stimulators of bone resorption. They are so potent that this organ culture assay has been used as a bioassay for 1,25-dihydroxyvitamin D. Exposure of bone cultures to 1,25-dinydroxyvitamin D is associated with an increase both in osteoclast number and activity with an increase in ruffled border size as well as volume of the clear zones.

Mature osteoclasts do not appear to have receptors for 1,25-dihydroxyvitamin D (Merke et al. 1986). Since it is likely that 1,25-dihydroxyvitamin D exerts its influence on mature osteoclasts as well as earlier cells in the osteoclast lineage, the effects on mature osteoclasts are presumably indirectly mediated through other cells (McSheehy and Chambers 1987). However, the major effects of 1,25-dihydroxyvitamin D on osteoclastic bone resorption may be to stimulate the fusion or differentiation of committed osteoclast progenitors to form mature cells. There is considerable evidence that 1,25-dihydroxyvitamin D has novel effects as a differentiation agent. It stimulates the fusion of cells in the monocyte-macrophage lineage (Abe et al. 1981; Roodman et al. 1985), and can act as a factor which causes differentiation of human leukemic cells into more mature cells (Miyaura et al. 1982; Reitsma et al. 1983; Dodd et al. 1983). Vitamin D metabolites also stimulate the differentiation of epidermal cells (Hosomi et al. 1983) and have been suggested as a therapy in psoriasis (Morimoto et al. 1986). In baboon and human marrow cell cultures, 1,25-dihydroxyvitamin D promotes the fusion of committed progenitors to form multinucleated cells. Some of these multinucleated cells have characteristics of osteoclasts and some have characteristics of macrophage polykaryons (Ibbotson et al. 1984; Roodman et al. 1985). 1,25-Dihydroxyvitamin D has no influence on the proliferation of mononuclear cells in these studies (ROODMAN et al. 1985). In more recent studies, YONEDA et al. (1991) have shown that, upon exposure to 1,25-dihydroxyvitamin D and tumor cell products which promote osteoclast differentiation, HL-60 cells which have the capability of forming monocytes, granulocytes, or eosinophils can be induced to differentiate along the osteoclast lineage. These observations on the effects of 1,25-dihydroxyvitamin D as a factor which promotes osteoclast differentiation were utilized by KEY et al. (1984), who treated an infant with malignant osteopetrosis with 1,25-dihydroxyvitamin D. In this disorder, there is a failure to form competent osteoclasts. Following 3 months of therapy with 1,25-dihydroxyvitamin D, bone histology revealed active osteoclasts and bone resorption.

1,25-Dihydroxyvitamin D also has additional effects on bone cells which may be indirect. It has an important immunoregulatory role (for review, see MANOLAGAS et al. 1985). 1,25-Dihydroxyvitamin D influences and modulates cytokine production by normal immune cells. For example, it has been shown that 1,25-dihydroxyvitamin D impairs interleukin-2 production by phytohemagglutinin-stimulated peripheral blood lymphocytes (TSOUKAS et al. 1984). This impairs mitogenesis in the cells, but this effect can be reversed by the addition of exogenous interleukin-2 to the cultures (RIGBY et al. 1984). 1,25-Dihydroxyvitamin D can increase interleukin-1 and procathepsin D production from the monocytic cell line U937 (AMENTO et al. 1984). 1,25-Dihydroxyvitamin D receptors are present in activated T lymphocytes (PROVVEDINI et al. 1983) and under certain circumstances may be produced by immune cells (FETCHICK et al. 1986). It is difficult to dissect the relative importance of these indirect effects on osteoclastic bone resorption, but many of these cytokines are such potent regulators of osteoclast function that they may be important.

Recently, there have been some interesting reports of novel biological activity ascribed to a metabolite of the vitamin D endocrine system. This metabolite, the 23(S)25(R)-1,25-dihydroxyvitamin D_3-lactone, inhibits osteoclastic bone resorption caused by 1,25-dihydroxyvitamin D, but also inhibits bone resorption which has been stimulated by PTH and interleukin-1. These observations have been made in bone organ cultures and cultures of marrow mononuclear cells which form cells with osteoclast characteristics over time (ISHIZUKA et al. 1984, 1985, 1986, 1987, 1988; KIYOKI et al. 1985; KURIHARA et al. 1989, 1990). These data suggest that the lactone metabolite is not interfering with 1,25-dihydroxyvitamin D effects by acting as a competitive antagonist for binding to the 1,25-dihydroxyvitamin D receptor, since the effects of PTH and interleukin-1 on bone resorption are not likely to be dependent on this receptor. The lactone is present in serum in concentrations of $4 \times 10^{-10} M$. No other known vitamin D metabolite has this activity. Although some investigators believe that this metabolite is not formed under physiological conditions and is not naturally occurring, nevertheless it is a potential therapeutic as an inhibitor of bone resorption.

III. Effects of Vitamin D Metabolites on Cells of the Osteoblast Lineage

Absence of vitamin D leads to failure of mineralization of newly formed bone. These effects are probably indirect and caused by inadequate supply of calcium and phosphate at the mineralization site (Underwood et al. 1984). Thus, it appears clear that 1,25-dihydroxyvitamin D is necessary for adequate supply of mineral at new sites of bone formation. However, 1,25-dihydroxyvitamin D also has what appears to be unique effects on osteoblasts. In organ cultures of fetal rat calvariae, it inhibits bone collagen synthesis. In cell culture studies, it promotes the production of the bone Gla protein (osteocalcin) which is used as a marker of cells in the osteoblast lineage (Price and Baukol 1980). 1,25-Dihydroxyvitamin D also influences alkaline phosphatase content in cells of the osteoblast phenotype (Manolagas et al. 1981; Rodan and Rodan 1984). It may also influence the responsiveness of cells in the osteoblast lineage to PTH as measured by their cyclic AMP responses. For example, in the presence of 1,25-dihydroxyvitamin D, cyclic AMP responses may be blunted (Catherwood 1985; Kubota et al. 1985). Thus, 1,25-dihydroxyvitamin D may act as an important differentiation factor for cells in the osteoblast lineage, and is clearly required not just for the formation of normal bone matrix but also for mineralization of normal bone matrix.

D. Calcitonin

Although calcitonin has been identified for 30 years, and its effects on bone cells in vitro have been clearly delineated, we still know little of its physiological role in calcium homeostasis or of its importance in the bone remodeling process. Friedman et al. (1968) demonstrated that calcitonin inhibits osteoclastic bone resorption in cultures of fetal rat long bones. Its inhibitory effects on osteoclastic bone resorption are independent of the stimulus. Its effects on osteoclasts are mediated by cyclic AMP. At the ultrastructural level, calcitonin decreases the size of the ruffled border and clear zone of the osteoclast within minutes (Holtrop and Raisz 1979). Other evidence suggests that calcitonin inhibits the formation of fresh osteoclasts from precursors and causes dissolution of preformed osteoclasts into mononuclear cells (Baron and Vignery 1976). When isolated osteoclasts are studied on bone surfaces, calcitonin causes a striking change with a decrease in cell motility and retraction of the plasma membrane. Chambers and Moore (1983), Chambers and Ali (1983) and Ali and Chambers (1983) have related this to inhibition of bone resorption, although it is not clear that there is a direct relationship between this effect and bone resorption or that such responses occur where osteoclasts are actively resorbing bone in vivo.

The effects of calcitonin on osteoclastic bone resorption are short lived (Wener et al. 1972). This was first demonstrated in organ culture, where it was observed that calcitonin inhibited PTH-stimulated bone resorption transiently, but then in the continued presence of calcitonin bone resorption recurred. Similar effects were seen in vivo when calcitonin was administered. This loss of responsiveness of osteoclasts to calcitonin in its continued presence is referred to as the "escape" phenomenon. It has now been observed numerous times in patients with primary hyperparathyroidism or hypercalcemia of malignancy who have been treated with calcitonin (Au 1975; BINSTOCK and MUNDY 1980). The molecular mechanism for the escape phenomenon has never been demonstrated clearly. However, TASHJIAN et al. (1978) showed downregulation of calcitonin receptors on bone cells (presumably osteoclasts) in the continued presence of calcitonin using an organ culture system. The disadvantages of this study were that a mixed cell population was used. Recently, it has been found that HL-60 cells can be induced to differentiate into multinucleated cells which resorb bone and express calcitonin receptors in response to a factor present in tumor-conditioned media which promotes osteoclast formation (YONEDA et al. 1991). The multinucleated cells express calcitonin receptors with similar number and binding affinity as those on freshly isolated rodent osteoclasts. Addition of cortisol to these cells led to an increase in receptor binding and number. A parallel phenomenon may be responsible for the capacity of glucocorticoids to prevent the escape phenomenon in vivo and in bone organ cultures. Another possible explanation for the escape phenomenon is that, in the presence of calcitonin, a second population of osteoclasts emerges which is nonresponsive to calcitonin (KRIEGER and TASHJIAN 1981). Not all osteoclasts are responsive to calcitonin. For example, in many circumstances, it appears likely that chicken osteoclasts do not contain calcitonin receptors (NICHOLSON et al. 1987).

The calcitonin escape phenomenon can be prevented. WENER et al. (1972) showed that in organ cultures the simultaneous addition of corticosteroids with calcitonin rendered bones responsive to calcitonin for more prolonged periods (Fig. 5). Later, Au (1975) reported a patient with parathyroid carcinoma who did not respond satisfactorily to either corticosteroids alone or to calcitonin alone but the combination of both agents rendered the patient normocalcemic. This was confirmed in a larger series of patients by BINSTOCK and MUNDY (1980). Osteoclast responsiveness to calcitonin seems to vary in different conditions. Osteoclasts are probably least responsive to calcitonin when treated with PTH and most responsive when they are activated by cytokines such as interleukin-1 or tumor necrosis factor. The reasons for these differences are unclear. However, they can also be seen in disease states. For example, the osteoclasts in Paget's disease are exquisitely sensitive to calcitonin (or at least in most cases). In contrast, osteoclasts activated by PTH in hyperparathyroidism are usually unresponsive or minimally responsive to calcitonin.

This transient effect of calcitonin on osteoclastic bone resorption is exemplified by patients with medullary carcinoma of the thyroid. These patients have markedly increased circulating concentrations of bioactive

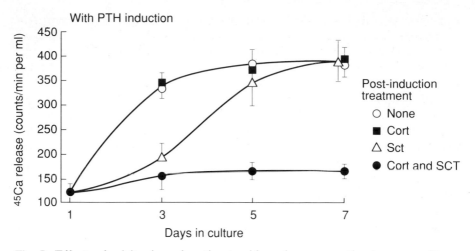

Fig. 5. Effects of calcitonin and corticosteroids on bone resorption in organ culture. Bone resorption is inhibited only transiently by calcitonin, but this escape from inhibition in the continued presence of calcitonin is blocked if the bones are treated with cortisol at the same time as calcitonin (from RAISZ et al. 1972c)

calcitonin. In fact, when serum from patients with medullary carcinoma is applied directly to organ cultures of bone, bone resorption is inhibited. However, these same patients show no disturbance of calcium homeostasis. This can only be explained by the presence of downregulation of osteoclasts by the high circulating levels of calcitonin tonically released by the tumors.

Since calcitonin has only a transient effect to inhibit osteoclastic bone resorption, there has been considerable speculation whether it has an important role in the maintenance of calcium homeostasis. Currently, the most popular concept for its teleological role is that it may inhibit bone resorption transiently at times when bone turnover is not required for maintenance of extracellular calcium homeostasis. For example, following a calcium-rich meal, calcium is absorbed from the gut and there is no need for active bone turnover to provide an adequate supply of extracellular fluid calcium. Since calcitonin synthesis and secretion by thyroid parafollicular cells can be stimulated by calcium as well as by gut hormones such as gastrin, both of which are presumably increased following a calcium-rich meal, this explanation does have attraction.

Receptors for calcitonin have been identified on osteoclasts, on renal tubular cells, and on a number of tumor cell lines including cells with the osteoclast phenotype (NICHOLSON et al. 1986; MARX et al. 1973; FINDLAY et al. 1983; GUTIERREZ et al. 1984; FORREST et al. 1985). They are also present on placental cells and, recently, the calcitonin receptor gene has been cloned and expressed (S. GOLDRING, personal communication).

Calcitonin is a product of a very complex gene. A number of other proteins are expressed by this gene, the most important of which may be the calcitonin gene-related peptide (CGRP). The calcitonin gene undergoes alternative tissue-specific splicing (for review, see HENDY and O'RIORDAN 1984; FISCHER, this volume). In the thyroid gland, the major product of this gene is calcitonin. However, in the brain, the major product is a related protein called the calcitonin gene-related peptide, which is not related to calcitonin structurally. This peptide has neuromuscular and vascular effects (ROSENFELD et al. 1983). CGRP inhibits bone resorption in vitro (D'SOUZA et al. 1986; Roos et al. 1986). Although it has similar effects to calcitonin in organ culture systems, it is certainly much less potent. It has also been shown to lower the serum calcium in vivo (TIPPINS et al. 1984; STRUTHERS et al. 1985). Its effects in the rabbit are much more dramatic than its effects in other species. It has never been clear whether calcitonin has any demonstrable effect on bone-forming cells. In the hands of most investigators, no consistent effect on bone formation has been described. However, FARLEY et al. (1988) have suggested that calcitonin can stimulate proliferation of cells. Surprisingly, some workers have demonstrated that procalcitonin has a stimulatory effect on cells with the osteoblast phenotype (BURNS et al. 1989). Whether this can be validated by other workers or shown to cause an effect on bone formation in vivo, or whether procalcitonin is actually secreted, remains to be documented.

E. Amylin

Recently, a factor has been purified from the pancreatic beta cell which has been implicated in the pathophysiology of pancreatic amyloid and possibly plays an etiological role in type-2 diabetes mellitus. This factor is known as islet-associated polypeptide (IAPP) or amylin. Several groups have shown in preliminary studies that amylin can inhibit the capacity of isolated osteoclasts to resorb bone (ZAIDI et al. 1990; KOOPMANS et al. 1990). The effects on osteoclasts appear to be different from those of calcitonin or CGRP, and amylin was less potent than calcitonin. Amylin bears about 50% homology at the amino acid level to CGRP. We have tested amylin for its effects on osteoclastic bone resorption in fetal rat long bones but have not been able to show an effect. This is clearly an interesting factor. Whether it has an important physiological role in calcium homeostasis has yet to be demonstrated.

F. Cortisol

Glucocorticoids have complex effects on calcium homeostasis and bone cell biology. Cortisol inhibits calcium absorption from the gut (KIMBERG et al. 1971), probably directly by an effect on gut endothelium, but also indirectly by effects on vitamin D metabolism and PTH secretion. Whether there is a direct effect of glucocorticoids on vitamin D metabolism has been controversial.

Glucocorticoids clearly have complex effects on bone cell function. Glucocorticoids are inhibitors of osteoclast formation and differentiation. In organ culture systems, glucocorticoids in pharmacologic doses inhibit bone resorption (Raisz et al. 1972a). They are more effective at inhibiting bone resorption mediated by cytokines such as interleukin-1 than they are against PTH effects (Strumpf et al. 1978). They have been fairly ineffective at lowering the serum calcium in the majority of patients with the hypercalcemia of malignancy and are usually ineffective as therapeutic agents in patients with primary hyperparathyroidism (Mundy and Martin 1982). However, they do effectively lower the serum calcium in patients with diseases such as sarcoidosis or vitamin D intoxication, where the major pathogenetic reason for hypercalcemia is increased calcium absorption from the gut. The most convincing evidence suggests that the major effect of glucocorticoids on the gut is a direct effect on the epithelium, and not an indirect effect mediated by effects to impair hydroxylation mechanisms required to convert vitamin D to biologically active metabolites (Mundy and Roodman 1987). When glucocorticoids are added to cultures of marrow cells, cells with the osteoclast phenotype do not form (Suda et al. 1983). Glucocorticoids may have differing effects on mature osteoclasts. Teitelbaum et al. (1981) showed that cortisol stimulated macrophages directly to cause release of lysosomal enzymes and enhance mineral release from bone particles. More recently, Reid et al. (1986) found that, in neonatal mouse calvariae, glucocorticoids could actually enhance the bone-resorbing effects of PTH.

Glucocorticoids also have complex effects on cells with the osteoblast lineage. In organ cultures of fetal rat calvariae, glucocorticoids have biphasic effects. At high concentrations they stimulate bone collagen synthesis, but at low concentrations when used for long periods bone collagen synthesis is inhibited (Dietrich et al. 1979b). Calcitonin and cortisol may influence the effects of other factors in cells with the osteoblast phenotype. In particular, glucocorticoids promote differentiation of these cells to express alkaline phosphatase. In vivo, the major effects on cells of the osteoblast phenotype are probably to inhibit differentiation of osteoblast precursors and differentiated function in mature cells. In pharmacologic doses, glucocorticoid therapy is always associated with osteoporosis and the characteristic feature of this osteoporosis is impaired osteoblast function and decreased bone formation.

G. Thyroid Hormones

Thyroid hormones have important effects on bone turnover, although there is no evidence that their production is feedback regulated by effects they may have no calcium homeostasis or bone remodeling. However, in states of thyroid hormone deficiency, rates of bone turnover are markedly suppressed (Mosekilde and Melsen 1978) and in thyrotoxicosis rates of bone formation are enhanced. Hypercalcemia occurs occasionally in patients with hyperthyroidism. Although the frequency has been debated, when careful measurements of serum-ionized calcium are made it will be found commonly (BAXTER and BONDY 1966; FARNSWORTH and DOBYNS 1974; FRITZEL et al. 1967; BURMAN et al. 1976). However, it is rare that hypercalcemia is a finding of clinical importance in patients with hyperthyroidism. The morphologic picture in the bone suggests a picture resembling that of primary hyperparathyroidism and osteitis fibrosa cystica (FOLLIS 1953). However, MEUNIER (1972) and PARFITT et al. (1976b) have suggested that the morphologic features of hyperthyroidism are different from those of primary hyperparathyroidism. In hyperthyroidism, there is absence of the irregularly woven bone which is seen in patients with primary hyperparathyroidism and the increases in osteoclastic resorption in thyrotoxicosis are less obvious.

In elderly patients with thyrotoxicosis, osteopenia is frequent. In fact, the picture may be readily confused with that of osteoporosis in the postmenopausal years. KRANE et al. (1956) showed by calcium balance studies and ^{45}Ca calcium kinetic studies that there was a marked increase in bone turnover associated with both increased bone resorption and increased bone formation. In most patients, serum alkaline phosphatase is increased, indicating increased osteoblast activity and serum urine hydroxyproline is also increased. These latter findings may be due not just to increased bone turnover but to increased collagen degradation in general (KIVIRIKKO et al. 1965; POSEN et al. 1977; ASKENASI et al. 1975). The mechanism by which hyperthyroidism is associated with increased osteoclastic bone resorption is probably related to a direct effect of thyroid hormones on osteoclasts. In organ cultures of fetal rat long bones, the thyroid hormones thyroxine and triiodothyronine have been shown to stimulate osteoclastic bone resorption (MUNDY et al. 1976). The effects of thyroid hormones in this system are similar to those of PTH, although thyroid hormones are slower acting than parathyroid hormone and are less powerful bone resorbers. Thyroid hormone has not been examined for its effects in other types of bone-resorbing systems such as isolated osteoclasts or marrow cell cultures, although it would be interesting to know how it affects these in vitro systems. The effects of thyroid hormone on fetal rat long bones can be inhibited by agents such as cortisol, phosphate, and propranolol, all of which have been used in the treatment of thyrotoxic hypercalcemia (DIETRICH et al. 1979b; RUDE et al. 1976).

H. Estrogens

Estrogens clearly inhibit the increase in bone resorption associated with the post-menopausal period. This has been suspected for 50 years and it has long been recognized that bone loss associated with osteoporosis is most common in postmenopausal females (ALBRIGHT 1940). The rapid loss of bone which occurs immediately after ovarian failure was demonstrated by

Heaney using calcium kinetics continued with calcium balance studies (Heaney et al. 1977, 1978a, 1978b), and by Lindsay et al. (1980) using cortical bone thickness in the metacarpal bone and has been confirmed many times since with more sophisticated techniques for measuring bone mass or bone mineral density (Slemenda et al. 1987; Riggs et al. 1981). The use of biochemical markers of bone resorption and bone formation (urine hydroxyproline, serum bone Gla protein, serum alkaline phosphatase, tartrate-resistant acid phosphatase activity) indicates that bone turnover is increased initially following estrogen withdrawal, and that bone resorption is relatively greater than bone formation. The increase in bone resorption associated with estrogen deficiency means an increase in number of activation sites which in turn provide more available surfaces for later bone formation, but also means increased depth of resorption cavities. The rapid phase of bone loss lasts for about 10 years after the onset of ovarian failure or ablation. Both cortical and trabecular bone are involved. However, losses are more apparent in the vertebrae and the appendicular skeleton than in the femoral neck, suggesting that the major effect is on trabecular bone (Stevenson et al. 1989). This rapid loss of bone following menopause can be prevented or inhibited by treatment with estrogens (Lindsay et al. 1976, 1978, 1980; Christiansen et al. 1980, 1981; Recker et al. 1977; Horsman et al. 1977; Riis et al. 1987). Similar effects are observed in animals following ovarian ablation, although the duration of the rapid phase of bone loss may be much shorter. Treatment with estrogens prevents this rapid loss, and estrogen treatment is now recognized as the most valuable single measure in the prevention of postmenopausal bone loss. It has been suggested that estrogen therapy may lead to an increase in bone mass, although whether this merely indicates an insufficient treatment period for remodeling sites to readjust to the inhibition of bone resorption is not known.

   Although estrogens have such profound effects on bone cells, and particularly on osteoclastic bone resorption, their mechanism of action remains a mystery. They seem to have no discernable direct effects in any of the commonly used in vitro bone resorption systems. Since the effects of estrogen on bone resorption appear to be indirect, for many years investigators have looked for estrogen-mediated effects on the systemic calciotropic hormones PTH, 1,25-dihydroxyvitamin D, and calcitonin. Estrogens may decrease PTH secretion, but they may have more important effects on opposing peripheral actions of PTH on its target organs (Heaney 1965; Riggs and Melton 1990). Estrogens increase calcitonin synthesis and secretion (Stevenson et al. 1983; Greenberg et al. 1990) and also increase 1,25-dihydroxyvitamin D concentrations, which may be the mechanism by which they increase calcium absorption from the gut. However, it appears unlikely that these effects are significant for the inhibitory effects of estrogen on bone resorption.

   It was not appreciated until just a few years ago that there are estrogen receptors in bone cells, albeit in small numbers. The receptors are present in cells of the osteoblast lineage (Komm et al. 1988; Erikssen et al. 1988). Recently, there has been a preliminary report that there may also be estrogen receptors in osteoclasts (Oursler et al. 1990). The latter finding notwithstanding, investigators have tried recently to link the presence of estrogen receptors in cells with the osteoblast phenotype with inhibition of osteoclastic bone resorption. A number of indirect mechanisms have been suggested. Estrogens have been shown to enhance expression of growth factors by osteoblastic cells, including transforming growth β (TGFβ) and insulin-like growth factor I (IGF-I). Since TGFβ has been shown to inhibit osteoclastic bone resorption in some in vitro systems (Chenu et al. 1988; Pfeilschifter et al. 1988), inhibiting production of TGFβ might lead to increased bone resorption (and decreased bone formation). IGF-I has no known effects on bone resorption. The other possibility, not exclusive of the TGFβ notion, is that not only cells of the immune system, but also cells of the osteoblast lineage release cytokines, and there is now convincing evidence that cytokine production by these cells may be inhibited by estrogens. For example, Girasole et al. (1990) have shown that estrogens inhibit IL-6, TNF, and LIF production by osteoblastic cells. Pacifici et al. (1987, 1989) have shown enhanced production of the cytokines IL-1, TNF, and GM-CSF by cultured peripheral blood monocytes in some patients with high-turnover osteoporosis. In postmenopausal patients treated with estrogens, this effect may be reversed so that peripheral blood cells harvested from these patients produce less cytokines in vitro. Another mechanism which has been proposed is that estrogens affect prostaglandin production by bone cells. Raisz and colleagues have shown that 17β-estradiol, testosterone, and dihydrotestosterone inhibit prostaglandin production in bone organ cultures. Since prostaglandins are important local stimulators of bone resorption, decreased prostaglandin production could lead to impaired local bone resorption. Whether these phenomena represent the mechanism by which the estrogen effects on bone cell function are mediated will require further study.

Androgens probably affect osteoclastic bone resorption in a similar manner to estrogens. Males who are hypogonadal or castrated have decreased bone mass associated with increased bone resorption. Androgens probably have similar effects to decrease the rate of bone loss in hypogonadal men as estrogens do in recently hypogonadal women.

In addition to their effects on bone resorption, estrogens may also have effects on bone formation. In women undergoing rapid bone loss associated with the postmenopausal period or oophorectomy, estrogen withdrawal leads to an increase in the number of activation sites for bone resorption which upon estrogen replacement therapy provide new surfaces where bone formation can take place due to the coupling phenomenon. Thus there may be a transient increase in bone formation for several years following estrogen replacement therapy. However, it is also possible that there may be a more prolonged effect of estrogens to stimulate bone formation directly.

Low doses of estrogen increase skeletal growth in children, and it is clear that there is a marked increase in endosteal bone formation in rodents and birds treated with estrogens. Estrogen has now been shown to enhance expression of TGFβ and IGF-1 in cells with the osteoblast phenotype (Komm et al. 1988; Erikssen et al. 1988; Gray et al. 1989), so although the major effect of estrogen may be to inhibit osteoclastic bone resorption, it may also have an additional effect to stimulate bone formation. It is possible that androgens, which have long been used as a therapy for osteoporosis, could have similar effects.

References

Abe E, Miyaura C, Sakagami H, Takida M, Konno K, Yamazaki T, Yoshiki S, Suda T (1981) Differentiation of mouse myeloid leukemia cells induced by 1 alpha, 25-dihydroxyvitamin D3. Proc Natl Acad Sci USA 78:4990–4994

Albright F, Bloomberg F, Smith PH (1940) Postmenopausal osteoporosis. Trans Assoc Am Physicians 55:298–305

Ali NN, Chambers TJ (1983) The effect of prostaglandin I_2 and ca-carba-PGI_2 on the motility of isolated osteoclasts. Prostaglandins 25:603–614

Amento EP, Bhalla AK, Kurnick JT, Kradin RL, Clemens TL, Holick SA, Holick MR, Krane SM (1984) 1-Alpha 25-dihydroxyvitamin D3 induces maturation of the human monocyte cell line U937, and, in association with a factor from human T lymphocytes, augments production of the monokine, mononuclear cell factor. J Clin Invest 73:731–739

Askensai R, Demeester-Mirkine N (1975) Urinary excretion of hydroxylysyl glycosides and thyroid function. J Clin Endocrinol Metab 40:342–346

Au WYW (1975) Calcitonin treatment of hypercalcemia due to parathyroid carcinoma: synergistic effect of prednisone on long term treatment of hypercalcemia. Arch Intern Med 135:1594–1597

Barnicot NA (1948) The local action of the parathyroid and other tissues on the bone in intracerebral grafts. J Anat 82:233–248

Baron R, Vignery A (1976) Changes in the osteoclastic pools and the osteoclast nuclei balance after a single injection of salmon calcitonin in the adult rat. In: Meunier PJ (ed) Bone histomorphometry. Armour Montagu, Paris, p 147

Baxter JD, Bondy PK (1966) Hypercalcemia of thyrotoxicosis. Ann Intern Med 65:429–442

Binstock ML, Mundy GR (1980) Effect of calcitonin and glucocorticoids in combination in malignant hypercalcemia. Ann Intern Med 93:269–272

Boyde A (1981) Electron microscopy of the mineralizing front. In: Jee WS, Parfitt AM (eds) Bone histomorphometry. 3rd international workshop. Société Nouvelle de Publications Médicales et Dentaires, Paris, pp 69–78

Brand JS, Raisz LG (1972) Effects of thyrocalcitonin and phosphate ion on the parathyroid hormone stimulated resorption of bone. Endocrinology 90:479–487

Burman KD, Monchik JM, Earll JM, Wartofsky L (1976) Ionized and total serum calcium and parathyroid hormone in hyperthyroidism. Ann Intern Med 84:668–671

Burns DM, Forstrom JM, Friday KE, Howard GA, Roos BA (1989) Procalcitonin's amino-terminal cleavage peptide is a bone-cell mitogen. Proc Natl Acad Sci USA 86:9519–9523

Canalis E, Centrella M, Burch W, McCarthy TL (1989) Insulin-like growth factor I mediates selective anabolic effects of parathyroid hormone in bone cultures. J Clin Invest 83:60–65

Catherwood BD (1985) 1,25-Dihydroxycholecalciferol and glucocorticosteroid regulation of adenylate cyclase in an osteoblast-like cells line. J Biol Chem 260:736–743

Chambers TJ (1985) The pathobiology of the osteoclast. J Clin Pathol 38:241–252

Chambers TJ, Ali HN (1983) Inhibition of osteoclastic motility by prostaglandins I_2, E_1 E_2 and 6-oxoE_1. J Pathol 139:383–397

Chambers TJ, Moore A (1983) The sensitivity of isolated osteoclasts to morphological transformation by calcitonin. J Clin Endocrinol Metab 57:819–824

Chenu C, Pfeilschifter J, Mundy GR, Roodman GD (1988) Transforming growth factor β inhibits formation of osteoclast-like cells in long-term human marrow cultures. Proc Natl Acad Sci USA 85:5683–5687

Christiansen C, Christiensen MS, McNair P, Hagen C, Stocklund KE, Transbol I (1980) Prevention of early postmenopausal bone loss: controlled 2-year study in 315 normal females. Eur J Clin Invest 10:273–279

Christiansen C, Christensen MS, Transbol I (1981) Bone mass in postmenopausal women after withdrawal of oestrogen/gestagen replacement therapy. Lancet i:459–461

Dietrich JW, Canalis EM, Maina DM, Raisz LG (1976a) Hormonal control of bone collagen synthesis in vitro: effects of parathyroid hormone and calcitonin. Endocrinology 98:943–949

Dietrich JW, Canalis EM, Maina DM, Raisz LG (1976b) Dual effect of glucocorticoids on bone collagen synthesis. Pharmacology 18:234–230

Dietrich JW, Canalis EM, Maina DM, Raisz LG (1979a) Effects of glucocorticoids on fetal rat bone collagen synthesis in vitro. Endocrinology 104:715–721

Dietrich JW, Mundy GR, Raisz LG (1979b) Inhibition of bone resorption in tissue culture by membrane-stabilizing drugs. Endocrinology 104:1644–1648

Dodd RC, Cohen MS, Newman SL, Gray TK (1983) Vitamin D metabolites change the phenotype of monoblastic U937 cells. Proc Natl Acad Sci USA 80:7538–7541

D'Souza SM, MacIntyre I, Girgis SI, Mundy GR (1986) Human synthetic calcitonin-gene related peptide inhibits bone resorption in vitro. Endocrinology 119:58–61

Dunlay R, Civitelli R, Miyauchi A, Dobre CV, Gupta A, Goligorsky M, Hruska K (1990) Parathyroid hormone receptor coupling to phospholipase C is an alternate pathway of signal transduction in the bone and kidney. In: Cohn DV, Glorieux FH, Martin TJ (eds) Calcium regulation and bone metabolism, vol 10. Excerpta Medica, Amsterdam, pp 24–32

Eilon G, Raisz LG (1978) Comparison of the effects of stimulators and inhibitors of resorption on the release of lysosomal enzymes and radioactive calcium from fetal bone in organ culture. Endocrinology 103:1969–1975

Erikssen EF, Colvard DS, Berg NJ (1988) Evidence of estrogen receptors in normal human osteoblast-like cells. Science 241:84–86

Evans RM (1988) The steroid and thyroid hormone receptor superfamily. Science 240:889–895

Farley JR, Tarbaux NM, Hall SL, Linkhart TA, Baylink DJ (1988) The anti-bone resorptive agent calcitonin also acts in vitro to directly increase bone formation and bone cell proliferation. Endocrinology 123:159–167

Farnsworth AW, Dobyns BM (1974) Hypercalcemia and thyrotoxicosis. Med J Aust 2:782–784

Fetchick DA, Bertolini DR, Sarin P, Weintraub ST, Mundy GR, Dunn JF (1986) Production of 1,25 dihydroxyvitamin D by human T-cell lymphotrophic virus-I transformed lymphocytes. J Clin Invest 78:592–596

Findlay DM, Michelangeli VP, Orlowski RC, Martin TJ (1983) Biological activities and receptor interactions of des-Leu[16] Salmon and des-Phe[16] human calcitonin. Endocrinology 112:1288–1291

Follis RH (1953) Skeletal changes associated with hyperthyroidism. Bull Johns Hopkins Hosp 92:405–421

Forrest SM, Ng KW, Findlay DM, Michelangeli VP, Livesey SA, Partridge NC, Zajac JD, Martin TJ (1985) Characterization of an osteoblast-like clonal cell line which responds to both parathyroid hormone and calcitonin. Calcif Tissue Int 37:51–56

Friedman J, Au WYW, Raisz LG (1968) Responses of fetal rat bone to thyrocalcitonin in tissue culture. Endocrinology 82:149–156

Fritzel D, Malleson A, Marks V (1967) Plasma levels of ionized calcium and magnesium in thyroid disease. Lancet 1:1360–1361

Gaillard PJ (1961) Parathyroid and bone tissue in culture. In: Greep RO, Talmage RV (eds) The parathyroids. Thomas, Springfield, p 20

Garabedian M, Tanaka Y, Holick MF, DeLuca HF (1974) Response of intestinal calcium transport and bone calcium mobilization to 1,25-dihydroxyvitamin D3 in thyroparathyroidectomised rats. Endocrinology 94:1022–1027

Girasole G, Wang JM, Pedrazzoni M, Pioli G, Balotta C, Passeri M, Lazzarin A, Ridolfo A, Mantovani A (1990) Augmentation of monocyte chemotaxis by 1 alpha, 25-dihydroxyvitamin D3. Stimulation of defective migration of AIDS patiens. J Immunol 145:2459–2464

Gray TK, Mohan S, Linkhart TA, Baylink DJ (1989) Estradiol stimulates in vitro the secretion of insulin-like growth factors by the clonal osteoblastic cell line, UMR-106. Biochem Biophys Res Commun 158:407–412

Greenberg C, Kirkreja SC, Bowser EN, Hargis GK, Henderson WT, Williams GA (1990) Effect of estradiol and progesterone on calcium secretion. Endocrinology 118:2594–2598

Gunness-Hey M, Hock JM (1984) Increased trabecular bone mass in rats treated with human synthetic parathyroid hormone. Metab Bone Dis Rel Res 5:177–181

Gutierrez GE, Mundy GR, Katz MS (1984) Adenylate cyclase of osteoblast-like cells from rat osteosarcoma is stimulated by calcitonin as well as parathyroid hormone. Endocrinology 115:2342–2346

Hakeda Y, Hiura K, Sato T, Okazaki R, Matsumoto T, Ogata E, Ishitani R, Kumegawa M (1989) Existence of parathyroid hormone binding sites on murine hemopoietic blast cells. Biochem Biophys Res Commun 163:1481–1486

Hamilton JA, Lingelbach S, Partridge NC, Martin TJ (1985) Regulation of plasminogen activator production by bone-resorbing hormones in normal and malignant osteoblasts. Endocrinology 116:2186–2191

Harms HM, Kaptaina U, Kulpmann WR, Brabant G, Hesch RD (1989) Pulse amplitude and frequency modulation of parathyroid hormone in plasma. J Clin Endocrinol Metab 69:843–851

Haussler MR, Mangelsdorf DJ, Komm BS (1987) Molecular biology of the vitamin D hormone. In: Cohn DV, Martin TJ, Meunier PJ (eds) Calcium regulation and bone metabolism, vol 9. Excerpta Medica, Amsterdam, pp 465–474

Haussler MR, Mangelsdorf DJ, Komm BS, Terpening CM, Yamaoka K, Allegretto EA, Baker AR, Shine J, McDonnell DP, Hughes M (1988) Molecular biology of the vitamin D hormone. Recent Prog Horm Res 44:263–305

Heaney RP (1965) A unified concept of osteoporosis. Am J Med 39:377–380

Heaney RP, Recker RR, Saville PD (1977) Calcium balance and calcium requirements in middle-aged women. Am J Clin Nutr 30:1603–1611

Heaney RP, Becker RR, Saville PD (1978a) Menopausal changes in calcium balance performance. J Lab Clin Med 92:953–963

Heaney RP, Becker RR, Saville PD (1978b) Menopausal changes in bone remodeling. J Lab Clin Med 92:964–970

Heersche JNM (1978) Mechanism of osteoclastic bone resorption. A new hypothesis. Calcif Tissue Res 26:81–84

Hendy GN, O'Riordan JLH (1984) The genes that control calcium homeostasis. Clin Endocrinol 21:465–470

Holtrop ME, Raisz LG (1979) Comparison of the effects of 1,25 dihydroxycholecalciferol, prostaglandin E2, and osteoclast activating factor with parathyroid hormone on the ultrastructure of osteoclast cultured long bones of rats. Calcif Tissue Int 29:201–206

Holtrop ME, Raisz LG, Simmons HA (1974) The effects of parathyroid hormone, colchicine and calcitonin on the ultrastructure and the activity of osteoclasts in organ culture. J Cell Biol 60:346–355

Horsman A, Gallagher JC, Simpson M, Nordin BEC (1977) Prospective trial of estrogen and calcium in postmenopausal women. Br Med J ii:789–792

Hosomi J, Hosoi J, Abe E, Suda T, Kuroki T (1983) Regulation of terminal differentiation of cultured mouse epidermal cells by 1α,25-dihydroxyvitamin D3. Endocrinology 3:1950–1957

Howard GA, Bottemiller BL, Turner RT, Rader JI, Baylink DJ (1981) Parathyroid hormone stimulates bone formation and resorption in organ culture: evidence a coupling mechanism. Proc Natl Acad Sci USA 78:3204–3208

Hughes MR, Malloy PJ, Kieback DG, Kesterson RA, Pike JW, Feldman D, O'Malley BW (1988) Point mutations in the human vitamin D receptor gene associated with hypocalcemic rickets. Science 242:1702–1705

Ibbotson KJ, Roodman GD, McManus LM, Mundy GR (1984) Identification and characterization of osteoclast-like cells and their progenitors in cultures of feline marrow mononuclear cells. J Cell Biol 99:471–480

Ishizuka S, Norman AW (1986) The difference of biological activity among four diastereoisomers of 1α,25-dihydroxyvitamin D_3-26, 23-lactone. J Steroid Biochem 25:505–510

Ishizuka S, Norman AW (1987) Metabolic pathways from 1α,25-dihydroxyvitamin D_3 to 1α,25-dihydroxyvitamin D_3-26, 23-lactone. J Biol Chem 262:7165–7170

Ishizuka S, Ishimoto S, Norman AW (1984) Biological activity assessment of 1α,25-dihydroxyvitamin D_3-26, 23-lactone in the rat. J Steroid Biochem 20:611–616

Ishizuka S, Oshida J, Tsuruta H, Norman AW (1985a) The steriochemical configuration of the natural 1α,25-dihydroxyvitamin D_3-26, 23-lactone. Arch Biochem Biophys 242:82–89

Ishizuka S, Kiyoki M, Orimo H (1985b) Biological activity and characteristics of 1α, 25(OH)$_2$D$_3$-26, 23-lactone. In: Norman AW, Schaefer K, Grigoleit HG, Herrath DV (eds) Vitamin D: chemical, biochemical and clinical update. de Gruyter, Berlin, pp 402–403

Ishizuka S, Kurihara N, Hakeda Y, Maeda N, Ikeda K, Kumegawa M, Norman AW (1988) 1α,25-Dihydroxyvitamin D_3 [1α,25-(OH)$_2$D$_3$]-26,23-lactone inhibits 1,25-(OH)$_2$D$_3$-mediated fusion of mouse bone marrow mononuclear cells. Endocrinology 123:781–786

Jones SJ, Boyde A (1978) Scanning electron microscopy of bone cells in culture. In: Copp DH, Talmage RV (eds) Endocrinology of calcium metabolism. Excerpta Medica, Amsterdam, p 97

Jones SJ, Boyde A, Ali NN, Maconnachie E (1985) A review of bone cell and substratum interactions. Scanning Microsc 7:5–24

Kalu DN, Doyle FH, Pennock J, Doyle FH, Foster GV (1970) Parathyroid hormone and experimental osteosclerosis. Lancet 1:1363–1366

Key L, Carnes D, Cole S, Holtrop M, Bar-Shavit Z, Shapiro F, Arceci R, Steinberg J, Gundberg C, Kahn A, Teitelbaum S, Anast C (1984) Treatment of congenital osteopetrosis with high dose calcitriol. N Engl J Med 310:410–415

Kimberg DV, Baerg RD, Gershon E, Graudusius RT (1971) Effect of cortisone treatment on the active transport of calcium by the small intestine. J Clin Invest 50:1309–1321

Kitamura N, Shigeno C, Shiomi K, Lee KC, Ohta S, Sone T, Katsushima S, Tadamura E, Kousaka T, Yamamoto I, Dokoh S, Konishi J (1990) Episodic fluctuation in serum intact parathyroid hormone concentration in men. J Clin Endocrinol Metab 70:252–263

Kivirikko KT, Laitinen O, Lamberg BA (1965) Value of urine and serum hydroxyproline in the diagnosis of thyroid disease. J Clin Endocrinol Metab 25:1347–1352

Kiyoki M, Kurihara N, Ishizuka S, Ishii S, Hakeda Y, Kumegawa M, Norman AW (1985) The unique action for bone metabolism of 1α, 26-23-lactone. Biochem Biophys Res Commun 127:693–698

Komm BS, Terpening CM, Benz DJ (1988) Estrogen binding, receptor mRNA, and biologic response in osteoblast-like osteosarcoma cells. Science 241:81–84

Koopmans SJ, Krans HMJ, van der Pluim G, Lowik C (1990) Pancreatic amylin induces hypocalcemia and antagonizes insulin action on carbohydrate metabolism in the rat. J Bone Miner Res 5 [Suppl]:477

Krane SM, Brownell GL, Skanbury JB, Corrigon H (1956) The effect of thyroid disease on calcium metabolism in man. J Clin Invest 35:874–887

Krieger NS, Tashjian AH (1981) Inhibition of ouabain of parathyroid hormone stimulated bone resorption. J Pharmacol Exp Ther 217:586–591

Kubota M, Ng KW, Martin TJ (1985) Effect of 1,25 dihydroxyvitamin D3 on cyclic AMP responses to hormones in clonal osteogenic sarcoma cells. Biochem J 231:11–17

Kurihara N, Ishizuka S, Kumegawa M, Mundy GR, Roodman GR (1989) 23(S) 25(R)-1,25(OH)$_2$D$_3$-26,23-lactone, (1,25D-lactone) which is present in normal serum is an inhibitor of osteoclast-like cells (OCL) formation in human bone marrow cultures. Clin Res 37:454A

Kurihara N, Chenu C, Miller M, Civin C, Roodman GD (1990) Identification of committed mononuclear precursors for osteoclast-like cells formed in long term human marrow cultures. Endocrinology 126:2733–2741

Kurihara N, Civin C, Roodman GD (1991) Osteotropic factor responsiveness of highly purified populations of early and late precursors for human multinucleated cells expressing the osteoclast phenotype. J Bone Miner Res 6:257–261

Lindsay R, Aitken JM, Anderson JB, Hart DMM, MacDonald EB, Clarke AC (1976) Long-term prevention of postmenopausal osteoporosis by oestrogen. Lancet i:1038–1040

Lindsay R, Hart DM, Purdie D, Ferguson MM, Clark AS, Kraszewski A (1978) Comparative effects of oestrogen and a progestogen on bone loss in postmenopausal women. Clin Sci 54:193–195

Lindsay R, Hart DM, Forrest G, Baird C (1980) Prevention of spinal osteoporosis in oophorectomised women. Lancet ii:1151–1154

Lorenzo JA, Quinton J (1984) Epidermal growth factor enhances the resorptive response to parathyroid hormone. Calcif Tissue Int 36:465

Lorenzo JA, Raisz LG, Hock JM (1983) DNA synthesis is not necessary for osteoclastic responses to parathyroid hormone in cultured fetal rat long bones. J Clin Invest 72:1924–1929

Luben RA, Goggins JF, Raisz LG (1974) Stimulation by parathyroid hormone of bone hyaluronate synthesis in organ culture. Endocrinology 94:737–745

MacDonald BR, Mundy GR, Clark S, Wang EA, Kuehl TJ, Stanley ER, Roodman GD (1986) Effects of human recombinant CSF-GM and highly purified CSF-1 on the formation of multinucleated cells with osteoclast characteristics in long term bone marrow cultures. J Bone Miner Res 1:227–233

Manolagas SC, Burton DW, Deftos LJ (1981) 1,25-Dihydroxyvitamin D3 stimulates the alkaline phosphatase activity of osteoblast-like cells. J Biol Chem 256:7115–7117

Manolagas SC, Provvedini DM, Tsoukas C (1985) Interactions of 1,25 dihydroxyvitamin D3 and the immune system. Mol Cell Endocrinol 43:113–122

Marx SJ, Woodard C, Aurbach GD, Glossmann H, Keutmann HT (1973) Renal receptors for calcitonin: binding and degradation of hormone. J Biol Chem 248:4797–4802

McDonnell DP, Pike JW, O'Malley BW (1988) The vitamin D receptor: a primitive steroid receptor related to thyroid hormone receptor. J Steroid Biochem 30:41–46

McSheehy PMJ, Chambers TJ (1986) Osteoblastic cells mediate osteoclastic responsiveness to parathyroid hormone. Endocrinology 118:824–828

McSheehy PMJ, Chambers TJ (1987) 1,25 Dihydroxyvitamin D3 stimulates rat osteoblastic cells to release a soluble factor that increases osteoclastic bone resorption. J Clin Invest 80:425–429

Merke J, Klaus G, Hugel U, Waldherr R, Ritz E (1986) No 1,25 dihydroxyvitamin D3 receptors on osteoclasts of calcium-deficient chicken despite demonstrable receptors on circulating monocytes. J Clin Invest 77:312–314

Meunier PJ, Bianchi GGS, Edouard CM, Bernard JC, Courpron P, Vignon GE (1972) Bony manifestations of thyrotoxicosis. Orthop Clin North Am 3:745–774

Mitchell J, Rouleau MF, Goltzman D (1990) Biochemical and morphological characterization of parathyroid hormone receptor binding to the rat osteosarcoma cell line UMR-106. Endocrinology 126:2327–2335

Miyaura C, Abe E, Nomura H, Hishii Y, Suda T (1982) 1 Alpha, 25-dihydroxyvitamin D3 suppresses proliferation of murine granulocyte-macrophage progenitor cells (CFU-C). Biochem Biophys Res Commun 108:1728–1733

Morimoto S, Onishi T, Imanaka S, Yukawa H, Kozuka T, Kitano Y, Yoshikawa K, Kumahara Y (1986) Topical administration of 1,25 dihydroxyvitamin D3 for psoriasis: report of five cases. Calcif Tissue Int 38:119–122

Mosekilde L, Melsen F (1978) Morphometric and dynamic studies of bone changes in hypothyroidism. Acta Pathol Microbiol Scand 86:56–62

Mundy GR, Martin TJ (1982) The hypercalcemia of malignancy: pathogenesis and management. Metabolism 31:1247–1277

Mundy GR, Roodman GD (1987) Osteoclast ontogeny and function. In: Peck WA (ed) Bone and mineral research, vol V. Elsevier, Amsterdam, pp 209–280

Mundy GR, Shapiro JL, Bandelin JC, Canalis EM, Raisz LG (1976) Direct stimulation of bone resorption by thyroid hormones. J Clin Invest 58:529–534

Nicholson GC, Moseley JM, Sexton PM, Mendelsohn FAO, Martin TJ (1986) Abundant calcitonin receptors in isolated rat osteoclasts. Biochemical and autoradiographic characterization. J Clin Invest 78:355–360

Nicholson GC, Moseley JM, Sexton PM, Martin TJ (1987) Chicken osteoclasts do not possess calcitonin receptors. J Bone Miner Res 2:53–59

Oursler MJ, Pyfferoen J, Osdoby P, Riggs BL, Spelsberg TC (1990) Osteoclasts express mRNA for estrogen receptor. J Bone Miner Res 5:517

Pacifici R, Rifas L, Teitelbaum S, Slatopolsky E, McCracken R, Bergfeld M, Lee W, Avioli LV, Peck WA (1987) Spontaneous release of interleukin-1 from human blood monocytes reflects bone formation in idiopathic osteoporosis. Proc Natl Acad Sci USA 84:4616–4620

Pacifici R, Rifas L, McCracken R, Vered I, McMurty C, Avioli L, Peck WA (1989) Ovarian steroid treatment blocks a postmenopausal increase in blood monocyte interleukin-1 release. Proc Natl Acad Sci USA 86:2398–2402

Parfitt AM (1976a) The actions of parathyroid hormone on bone: relation to bone remodeling and turnover, calcium homeostasis, and metabolic bone disease: I. Mechanisms of calcium transfer between blood and bone and their cellular basis: morphological and kinetic approaches to bone turnover. Metabolism 25:809–844

Parfitt AM (1976b) The actions of parathyroid hormone on bone. Relation to bone remodeling and turnover, calcium homeostasis and metabolic bone disease: II. PTH and bone cells: bone turnover and plasma calcium regulation. Metabolism 25:909–955

Parfitt AM (1979) Equilibrium and disequilibrium hypercalcemia: new light on an old concept. Metab Bone Dis Relat Res 1:279–293

Parfitt AM (1987) Bone and plasma calcium homeostasis. Bone 1:51–58

Parfitt AM (1989) Plasma calcium control at quiescent bone surfaces: a new approach to the homeostatic function of bone lining cells. Bone 10:87–88

Parsons JA, Potts JT (1972) Physiology and chemistry of parathyroid hormone. Clin Endocrinol Metab 1:33–78

Peck WA (1979) Cyclic AMP as a second messenger in the skeletal actions of parathyroid hormone: a decade-old hypothesis. Calcif Tissue Int 29:1–4

Perry HM, Dunn J, Chappel JC, Kahn AJ, Teitelbaum SL (1984) Partial characterization of a parathyroid hormone stimulated osteoblast produced resorptive factor. Calcif Tissue Int 36:468

Pfeilschifter J, Mundy GR (1987) Modulation of transforming growth factor beta activity in bone cultures by osteotropic hormones. Proc Natl Acad Sci USA 84:2024–2028

Pfeilschifter JP, Seyedin S, Mundy GR (1988) Transforming growth factor β inhibits bone resorption in fetal rat long bone cultures. J Clin Invest 82:680–685

Posen S, Cornish C, Kleerekoper M (1977) Alkaline phosphatase and metabolic bone disorders. In: Avioli LV, Krane SM Metabolic bone disease, vol 1. Academic, New York, p 142

Price PA, Baukol SA (1980) 1,25-Dihydroxyvitamin D3 increases synthesis of the vitamin K-dependent bone protein by osteosarcoma cells. J Biol Chem 255:11660–11663

Provvedini DM, Tsoukas CD, Deftos LJ, Manolagas SC (1983) 1,25 Dihydroxyvitamin D3 receptors in human leukocytes. Science 221:1181–1183

Raisz LG (1965) Bone resorption in tissue culture. Factors influencing the response to parathyroid hormone. J Clin Invest 44:103–116

Raisz LG (1970) Physiologic and pharmacologic regulation of bone resorption. N Eng J Med 282:909–916

Raisz LG, Niemann I (1967) Early effects of parathyroid hormone and thyrocalcitonin on bone in organ culture. Nature 214:486–487

Raisz LG, Niemann I (1969) Effects of phosphate, calcium and magnesium on bone resorption and hormonal responses in tissue culture. Endocrinology 85:446–452

Raisz LG, Trummel CL, Simmons H (1972a) Induction of bone resorption in tissue culture: prolonged response after brief exposure to parathyroid hormone or 25-hydroxycholecalciferol. Endocrinology 90:744–751

Raisz LG, Trummel CL, Wener JA, Simmons H (1972b) Effect of glucocorticoids on bone resorption in tissue culture. Endocrinology 90:961–967

Raisz LG, Trummel CL, Holick MF, DeLuca HF (1972c) 1,25 Dihydroxy-cholecalciferol: a potent stimulator of bone resorption in tissue culture. Science 175:768–769

Raisz LG, Simmons HA, Vargas SJ, Kemp BE, Martin TJ (1990) Comparison of the effects of amino-terminal synthetic parathyroid hormone-related peptide (PTH-rP) of malignancy and parathyroid hormone on resorption of cultured fetal rat long bones. Calcif Tissue Int 46:233–238

Recker RR, Saville PD, Heaney RP (1977) The effect of estrogens and calcium carbonate on bone loss in postmenopausal women. Ann Intern Med 87:649–655

Reeve J, Meunier PJ, Parsons JA, Bernat M, Bijvoet OLM, Courpron P, Edouard C, Klenerman L, Neer RM, Renier JC, Slovik D, Vismans FJFE, Potts JT (1980) Anabolic effect of human parathyroid hormone fragment on trabecular bone in involutional osteoporosis: a multicentre trial. Br Med J 280:1340–1344

Reeve J, Davies U, Arlot M, Bradbeer JN, Green JR, Hesp R, Edouard C, Hulme P, Podbesek RD, Katz D, Zanelli JM, Meunier PJ (1989) Parathyroid peptide (hPTH 1-34) in the treatment of osteoporosis. In: Kleerekoper M, Krane SM (eds) Clinical disorders of bone and mineral metabolism. Liebert, New York, pp 621–627

Reid IR, Katz JM, Ibbertson HK, Gray DH (1986) The APD, on bone resorption in neonatal mouse calvaria. Calcif Tissue Int 38:38–43

Reitsma PH, Rothbert PG, Astria SM, Trial J, Bar-Shavit Z, Hall A, Teitelbaum SL, Kahn AJ (1983) Regulation of *myc* gene expression in HL-50 leukaemia cells by a vitamin D metabolite. Nature 306:492–494

Rigby WFC, Stacy T, Fanger MW (1984) Inhibition of T lymphocyte mitogenesis by 1,25 dihydroxyvitamin D3 (Calcitriol). J Clin Invest 74:1451–1455

Riggs BL, Melton LJ (1990) Clinical review 8 – clinical heterogeneity of involutional osteoporosis – implications for preventive therapy. J Clin Endocrinol Metab 70:1229–1232

Riggs BL, Wahner HW, Dunn WL, Mazess RB, Offord KP, Melton LJ (1981) Differential changes in bone mineral density of the appendicular and axial skeleton with aging: relationship to spinal osteoporosis. J Clin Invest 67:328–335

Riggs BL, Hodgson SF, O'Fallon WM, Chao EYS, Wahner HW, Muhs JM, Cedel SL, Melton LJ (1990) Effect of fluoride treatment on the fracture rate in postmenopausal women with osteoporosis. N Engl J Med 322:802–809

Riis BJ, Thomsen K, Strom V, Christiansen C (1987) The effect of percutaneous estradiol and natural progesterone on postmenopausal bone loss. Am J Obstet Gynecol 156:61–65

Rodan GA, Martin TJ (1981) Role of osteoblasts in hormonal control of bone resorption – a hypothesis. Calcif Tissue Int 33:349–351

Rodan GA, Rodan SB (1984) Expression of the osteoblastic phenotype. In: Peck WA (ed) Bone and mineral research, vol 2. Elsevier, Amsterdam, p 244

Roodman GD, Ibbotson KJ, MacDonald BR, Kuehl TJ, Mundy GR (1985) 1,25 Dihydroxyvitamin D3 causes formation of multinucleated cells with several osteoclast characteristics in cultures of primate marrow. Proc Natl Acad Sci USA 82:8213–8217

Roos BA, Fisher JA, Pignat W, Alander CB, Raisz LG (1986) Evaluation of the in vivo and in vitro calcium regulating actions of noncalcitonin peptides produced via calcitonin gene expression. Endocrinology 118:46–51

Rosenfeld MG, Mermod JJ, Amara SG, Swanson LW, Sawchenko PE, Rivier J, Vale WW, Evans RW (1983) Production of a novel neuropeptide encoded by the calcitonin gene via tissue-specific RNA processing. Nature 304:129–135

Rouleau MF, Mitchell J, Goltzman D (1988) In vivo distribution of parathyroid hormone receptors in bone: evidence that a predominant osseous target cell is not the mature osteoblast. Endocrinology 123:187–191

Rude RK, Oldham SB, Singer FR, Nicholoff JT (1976) Treatment of thyrotoxic hypercalcemia with propranolol. N Engl J Med 294:431–433

Sabatini M, Yates AJ, Garrett R, Chavez J, Dunn J, Bonewald L, Mundy GR (1990) Increased production of tumor necrosis factor by normal immune cells in a model of the humoral hypercalcemia of malignancy. Lab Invest 63:676–681

Sakamoto S, Sakamoto M (1982) Biochemical and immunohistochemical studies on collagenase in resorbing bone in tissue culture. A novel hypothesis for the mechanism of bone resorption. J Periodont Res 17:523–526

Sato K, Fujii Y, Kasono K, Ozawa M, Imamura H, Kanaji Y, Kurosawa H, Tsushima T, Shizume K (1989) Parathyroid hormone-related protein and interleukin-1α synergistically stimulate bone resorption in vitro and increase the serum calcium concentration in mice in vivo. Endocrinology 124:2172–2178

Slatopolsky E, Weerts C, Thielan J, Horst R, Harter H, Martin KJ (1984) Marked suppression of secondary hyperparathyroidism by intravenous administration of 1,25 dihydroxycholecalciferol in uremic patients. J Clin Invest 74:2136–2143

Slemenda C, Hui SL, Longcope C, Johnston CC (1987) Sex steroids and bone mass: a study of changes about the time of the menopause. J Clin Invest 80:1261–1269

Slovik DM, Rosenthal DI, Doppelt SH, Potts JT, Campbell JA, Neer RM (1986) Restoration of spinal bone in osteoporotic men by treatment with human parathyroid hormone (1-34) and 1,25-dihydroxyvitamin D. J Bone Miner Res 1:377–381

Stashenko P, Dewhirst FE, Peros WJ, Kent RL, Ago JM (1987) Synergistic interactions between interleukin-1, tumor necrosis factor, and lymphotoxin in bone resorption. J Immunol 138:1464–1468

Stern PH (1980) The vitamin-D and bone. Pharmacol Rev 32:47–80

Stern PH, Halloran BP, DeLuca HF, Hefley TJ (1983) Responsiveness of vitamin D deficient fetal rat limb bones to parathyroid hormone in culture. Am J Physiol 244:E421

Stern PH, Horst RL, Gardner R, Napoli JL (1985) 10-Keto or 25-hydroxy substitution confer equivalent in vitro bone resorbing activity to vitamin D3. Arch Biochem Biophys 236:555–558

Stevenson JC, Abeyasekera G, Hillyard CJ (1983) Regulation of calcium-regulating hormones by exogenous sex steroids in early postmenopause. Eur J Clin Invest 13:481–487

Stevenson JC, Lee B, Devenport M, Cust MP, Ganger KF (1989) Determinants of bone density in normal women: risk factors for future osteoporosis? Br Med J 298:924–928

Strumpf M, Kowalski MA, Mundy GR (1978) Effects of glucocorticoids on osteoclast-activating factor. J Lab Clin Med 92:772–778

Struthers AD, Brown MJ, Beecham JL, Morris HR, Maclntyre I, Stevenson JC (1985) The acute effect of human calcitonin-gene related peptide in man. J Endocrinol 104 [Suppl]:225

Suda T, Testa NG, Allen TD (1983) Effects of hydrocortisone on osteoclasts generated in cat bone marrow cultures. Calcif Tissue Int 35:82–86

Tam CS, Heersche JNM, Murray TM, Parsons JA (1982) Parathyroid hormone stimulates the bone apposition rate independently of its resorptive action: differential effects of intermittent and continuous administration. Endocrinology 110:506–512

Tashjian AJ, Wright DR, Ivey JL, Pont A (1978) Calcitonin binding sites in bone: relationships to biological response and escape. Recent Prog Hormon Res 34:285–334

Teitelbaum SL, Kahn AJ (1980) Mononuclear phagocytes, osteoclasts and bone resorption. Miner Electrolyte Metab 3:2–9

Teitelbaum SL, Malone JD, Kahn AJ (1981) Glucocorticoid enhancement of bone resorption by rat peritoneal macrophages in vitro. Endocrinology 108:795–799

Teti A, Rizzoli R, Zambonin-Zallone A (1991) Parathyroid hormone binding to cultured avian osteoclasts. Biochem Biophys Res Commun 174:1217–1222

Tippins JR, Morris HR, Panico M, Etienne T, Bevis P, Girgis S, Maclntyre I, Azria M, Attingner M (1984) The myotropic and plasma calcium modulating effects of calcitonin gene-related peptide (CGRP). Neuropeptides 4:425–434

Tsoukas CD, Provvedini DM, Manolagas SC (1984) 1,25 Dihydroxyvitamin D3: a novel immunoregulatory hormone. Science 224:1438–1440

Underwood JL, DeLuca HF (1984) Vitamin D is not directly necessary for bone growth and mineralization. Am J Physiol 246:E493–E498

Vaes G (1968) On the mechanism of bone resorption. The action of parathyroid hormone on the excretion and synthesis on the lysosomal enzymes and on the extracellular release of acid by bone cells. J Cell Biol 39:676–697

Wener JA, Gorton SJ, Raisz LG (1972) Escape from inhibition of resorption in cultures of fetal bone treated with calcitonin and parathyroid hormone. Endocrinology 90:752–759

Yamamoto M, Kawanobe Y, Takahashi H, Shimazawa E, Kimura S, Ogata E (1984) Vitamin D deficiency and renal calcium transport in the rat. J Clin Invest 74:507–513

Yates AJP, Gutierrez GE, Smolens P, Travis PS, Katz MS, Aufdemorte TB, Boyce BF, Hymer TK, Poser JW, Mundy GR (1988) Effects of a synthetic peptide of a parathyroid hormone-related protein on calcium homeostasis, renal tubular calcium reabsorption and bone metabolism. J Clin Invest 81:932–938

Yates AJP, Oreffo ROC, Mayor K, Mundy GR (1991) Inhibition of bone resorption by inorganic phosphate is mediated both by reduced osteoclast formation and by impaired activity of mature osteoclasts. J Bone Miner Res 6:473–468

Yoneda T, Alsina MM, Garcia JL, Mundy GR (1991) Differentiation of HL-60 cells into cells with the osteoclast phenotype. Endocrinology 129:683–689

Zaidi M, Moonga BS, Ghatei MA, Gilbey S, Wimalawansa SJ, Bloom SR, MacIntyre I, Datta HK (1990) Amylin: a new bone-conserving hormone from the pancreas: in vivo and in vitro studies on potency and mode of action. J Bone Miner Res 5 [Suppl]:9

CHAPTER 7

Factors That Regulate Bone Formation

E. Canalis, T.L. McCarthy, and M. Centrella

A. Introduction

Bone formation and bone resorption, the two major processes of bone remodeling, are regulated by defined agents and mechanisms. The formation of new bone consists of the production of a new bone matrix by the osteoblast, and its mineralization by, as yet, poorly understood mechanisms. Since the formation of new bone is primarily a function of the osteoblast, agents that regulate bone formation can act by either increasing or decreasing the replication of cells of the osteoblastic lineage or modifying the differentiated function of the osteoblast.

Bone formation is controlled by systemic hormones and by local factors. For the most part, the local regulators of bone formation are growth factors which act directly on cells of the osteoblastic lineage. Growth factors are polypeptides with important effects on cell function. Certain growth factors are present in the circulation and may function as systemic agents, but for the most part they are synthesized by specific tissues in which they act as local regulators of cell metabolism. These local factors may affect their cell of origin or different cells and they are respectively termed autocrine or paracrine factors (James and Bradshaw 1984; Canalis et al. 1989b).

While systemic hormones are likely to have direct effects on bone formation, frequently their actions are mediated by local growth factors. Systemic hormones can regulate growth factor activity at four different levels: (1) synthesis, (2) activation, (3) receptor binding, and (4) binding proteins. They can modify the synthesis of a local growth factor, activate factors which are synthesized in an inactive form, regulate the binding of growth factors to their target cell receptors or modify the synthesis of their binding proteins. By any of these four mechanisms, singly or in combination, a systemic hormone can alter the activity of a growth factor, which itself can mediate selected effects of a hormone in a specific tissue. The production of a growth factor is not unique to any tissue. It has been postulated that a major role of the systemic hormones is to provide target-tissue specificity for a growth factor. This is done by modulating the factors present in tissues expressing receptors for the systemic hormone. For example, insulin-like growth factor I is synthesized by a variety of tissues (Lund et al. 1986), but its synthesis is regulated by different hormones in different tissues. In skeletal cells, its synthesis is primarily enhanced by parathyroid hormone, in the liver and cartilage by growth hormone, and in endometrial cells by estradiol-17β (McCARTHY et al. 1989a; MATHEWS et al. 1988; ISAKSSON et al. 1985; SIMMEN et al. 1990). It is apparent therefore that, while the same growth factor is synthesized by a variety of cells, it can be finely modulated by a hormone for which a cell has specific receptors. It is important to note that a hormone may regulate local growth factor activity at more than one level (Fig. 1), and while much attention has been paid to the regulation of the synthesis or activation of local factors, their actions can be significantly modified by alternate means. Recent work revealed that another critical step at which growth factor activity may be regulated is through alterations in receptor binding. These could result from changes in receptor number or affinity (CENTRELLA et al. 1988). Binding proteins also play a role in growth factor function since they can act by storing the factor, or by modifying its half-life, its biological activity, and its ability to bind to a target cell receptor (BINOUX et al. 1986). Skeletal cells have been shown to synthesize a number of "classic" growth factors. In addition, skeletal cells synthesize cytokines and other factors important in the induction of new bone, which will be discussed in Chaps. 5 by MUNDY and 21 by WOZEY of this book. The present chapter will address the more "classic" growth factors synthnsized by skeletal cells. They are platelet-derived growth factor (PDGF) AA, insulin-like growth factors (IGFs) I and II, transforming growth factor β_1 and β_2 (TGFβ_1 and β_2, fibroblast growth factors (FGFs), heparin-binding growth factors (HBGFs) 1 and 2, cytokines (interleukin-6, colony-stimulating factors, tumor necrosis factor α), and eosteoinductive factors. (GRAVES et al. 1989; McCARTHY et al. 1989a; CENTRELLA and CANALIS 1985; GLOBUS et al. 1989). Initial observations indicate that PDGF and FGF have mitogenic activity for cells of thc osteoblastic lineage, whereas IGF and TGFβ affect the replicatiun and differentiated function of the osteoblast (CANALIS et al. 1989b). It is currently not entirely clear why bone cells synthesize a variety of growth factors with similar biological

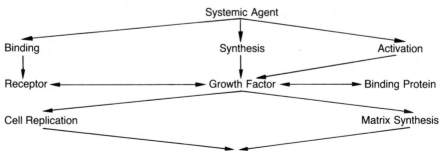

Fig. 1. Schematic representation of the hormonal regulation of skeletal growth factors

activities, and it is likely that they have important interactions among themselves.

B. Platelet-Derived Growth Factor

Platelet-derived growth factor is a polypetide with an approximate molecular mass (M_r) of 30000 (HELDIN and WESTERMARK 1987). PDGF was initially isolated from platelets and was subsequently found to be synthesized by a variety of normal and malignant cells including those present in skeletal tissue (GRAVES et al. 1984, 1989; HELDIN and WESTERMARK 1987; BETSHOLTZ et al. 1986; HELDIN et al. 1986). PDGF is a dimer which is the product of two genes, *PDGF-A* and *PDGF-B* (HELDIN and WESTERMARK 1987; BETSHOLTZ et al. 1986; DOOLITTLE et al. 1983; COLLINS et al. 1985). Therefore, three forms of mature PDGF exist, and A-chain homodimer, a B-chain homodimer, and an A- and B-chain heterodimer, and they are termed PDGF AA, BB, and AB. The A and B chains of PDGF contain significant amino acid sequence homology and the various PDGF isoforms share many biological activities (HELDIN and WESTERMARK 1987; BETSHOLTZ et al. 1986; BECKMANN et al. 1988; SIEGBAHN et al. 1990). In most culture systems tested, PDGF BB seems to be the form that has the greatest biological activity.

Platelets and serum are rich in PDGF AB and PDGF BB, and in certain species, such as the rat, the major circulating form of PDGF is the BB homodimer (BOWEN-POPE et al. 1989). Malignant cells, including osteosarcoma cell lines, have been shown to express both PDGF A and B transcripts (BETSHOLTZ et al. 1986; GRAVES et al. 1984). In contrast, normal bone cells from humans and rodents express only PDGF A mRNA (GRAVES et al. 1989; CENTRELLA et al. 1990d). This would suggest that PDGF BB acts primarily as a systemic agent and that it could also play a role in malignant cell function. The possible role of PDGF BB in the biology of malignancy is further supported by its effects on malignant transformation and by the fact that the *PDGF B* gene is a product of the c-*sis* proto-oncogene, which is homologous to the transforming region of the simian sarcoma virus, v-*sis* (COLLINS et al. 1985). While information about the regulation of PDGF synthesis by skeletal cells is not available, the fact that PDGF AA is the isoform expressed by normal bone cells leads us to believe that it acts as a local regulator of normal bone cell function.

It is possible that the synthesis of PDGF in skeletal cells is modified by agents similar to those found to regulate PDGF synthesis in other cell systems. For instance, PDGF AA synthesis in nonskeletal cells is enhanced by interleukin 1, tumor necrosis factor α, TGFβ, and acidic FGF, although it is not known if any of these agents regulate skeletal PDGF AA synthesis (RAINES et al. 1989; GAY and WINKLES 1990; KAVANAUGH et al. 1988). PDGF AA has been shown to mediate the effects of other agents on cell metabolism. For example, PDGF AA mediates the effects of interleukin 1 on endothelial cell replication and of TGFβ on smooth muscle cell replication, and similarly PDGF AA may mediate the effects of other agents on bone cell function (Raines et al. 1989; Majack et al. 1990). PDGF BB is not expressed in uninduced normal bone cells and is considered to act as a systemic factor (Centrella et al. 1990d). However, it is possible that selected agents under specific conditions might induce the synthesis of PDGF BB in bone cells, and as such it could also play a role in the local regulation of bone formation.

Studies performed in our laboratory have revealed that PDGF AA, BB, and AB stimulate DNA synthesis and cell replication in calvarial cultures as well as in cultures of osteoblast-enriched cells (Centrella et al. 1989a, 1990a; Canalis et al. 1989c). PDGF increases bone collagen synthesis and this effect is secondary to its stimulatory effect on cell replication. In addition, PDGF enhances matrix apposition rates in cultured bones (Pfeilschifter et al. 1990b). PDGF BB has more potent effects on bone cell replication than PDGF AA, and PDGF AB has an intermediate effect (Centrella et al. 1990a). These results are similar to those described in nonskeletal cell systems. In addition to its effect on bone formation, PDGF has been reported to increase bone resorption and collagen degradation (Tashjian et al. 1982; Canalis et al. 1989c). The mechanism for this effect is not known, and studies on the effects of PDGF on bone resorption were carried out with somewhat impure preparations of the polypeptide.

Molecular studies have revealed the existence of two PDGF receptor genes, which encode two receptor subunits (Yarden et al. 1986; Lee et al. 1990), known as the α- and the β-subunit. PDGF binds to one or both subunits and forms a complex as part of the receptor activation process. It is important to note that, while PDGF BB can bind to either the α- or the β-PDGF receptor subunit, PDGF AA binds primarily to the α-subunit (Heldin et al. 1988; Seifert et al. 1989). Data on PDGF receptors in osteoblasts are still inconclusive, although studies using labeled PDGF BB have revealed at least one PDGF receptor with an M_r of 185 000 and a K_d of 0.4–0.7 nanomolar (Centrella et al. 1989a). Receptor studies performed with radiolabeled PDGF AA have indicated that this isoform binds to bone cells with an approximate K_d of 4 nM (Centrella et al. 1990a).

While little is known about the regulation of PDGF synthesis by bone cells, it is now clear that the activity of PDGF in bone cells can be modified by alterations in the binding to its receptors. This is more apparent with the PDGF AA than with the BB isoform, and agents that modulate PDGF AA binding have been shown to modify the biological activity of this PDGF isoform. For instance, interleukin 1 induces a dose-related stimulation of PDGF AA binding to osteoblastic cells, with a twofold increase in apparent PDGF AA binding sites (Centrella et al. 1990d). As a consequence of this effect, interleukin 1 enhances the effect of PDGF AA on bone cell mitogenesis to essentially the same extent as that of PDGF BB. TGFβ in skeletal and nonskeletal cell systems was shown to decrease the binding of

PDGF to its cell receptor (CENTRELLA et al. 1990d; BRYCKAERT et al. 1988). So far, most of the results obtained indicate a regulation of PDGF AA binding, whereas initial studies suggest that the binding of PDGF BB to its osteoblastic cell receptor is not modified by other agents. The significance of the differential regulation of the binding of the two PDGF isoforms is not clear. These studies indicate that some local skeletal growth factors are not only modulated at the level of synthesis, but also at the level of receptor-binding. This information is critical to our understanding of growth factor action. Even though the concentrations of a growth factor may remain constant, alterations in receptor binding can result in substantial changes in biological activity and can in this way mediate the effects of systemic agents. Currently, there is no information about the existence of specific PDGF-binding proteins in bone, and they do not appear to play a role in the regulation of PDGF activity.

In summary, recent observations demonstrate that bone synthesizes PDGF AA and serum contains PDGF BB and AB. PDGF has significant effects on bone cell replication and as a consequence on bone collagen synthesis. PDGF AA appears to act primarily as a local regulator of bone cell metabolism while PDGF BB is likely to act as a systemic agent. While little is known about the regulation of PDGF AA synthesis, there is evidence to indicate modulation of PDGF AA activity at the level of receptor binding. PDGF BB might be critical in wound healing or fracture repair, since it is released after platelet aggregation. It may also play an entirely different role in bone cell physiology than that of PDGF AA.

C. Heparin-Binding Growth Factors

Heparin-binding growth factors are members of a family of seven related heparin-binding proteins (BURGESS and MACIAG 1989). Acidic fibroblast growth factor (aFGF) and basic fibroblast growth factor (bFGF) are the two better known forms of HBGFs and were the first to be purified, sequenced, and cloned (BURGESS et al. 1985; ESCH et al. 1985; GIMENEZ-GALLEGO et al. 1985). Acidic and basic FGFs are polypeptides with an M_r of 16000 to 17000. These two growth factors are products of different genes, but, like other members of the heparin-binding growth factor family, they have significant homology in their amino acid sequence, and similar mitogenic activity for a number of cell systems (BURGESS et al. 1985; ESCH et al. 1985; GIMENEZ-GALLEGO et al. 1985). FGFs are best known for their potent angiogenic activities, which are secondary to their effects on chemotaxis and replication of endothelial cells. Initially HBGFs were isolated from the central nervous system, but subsequent work revealed that they are synthesized by a variety of cell systems, including normal and tumor cells (KLAGSBRUN et al. 1986).

Bone matrix is a source of FGFs, and bovine skeletal cells, expressing the osteoblastic phenotype, secrete basic as well as acidic FGF (GLOBUS et al. 1989). It is conceivable that other cells present in the skeletal tissue synthesize FGF. One possibility could include endothelial cells, which are a known source of basic FGF (VLODAVSKY et al. 1987). While FGFs are synthesized by cells present in the skeletal tissue, little is known about the regulation of their synthesis in this tissue. Sequence analysis indicates that the genes for FGFs do not encode a leader peptide, suggesting that these proteins are not released from cells through classic secretory processes (ABRAHAM et al. 1986). It is possible that FGFs exit their cell of origin after cell membrane disruption or after cell death, and are then stored in the extracellular matrix. Therefore, FGF activity may be regulated at the level of activation of stored factor and not of synthesis. At the present time, information about the synthesis, activation, and release of FGFs from skeletal tissue is not available, and additional work is needed in this area of study.

Fibroblast growth factors have been shown to be mitogenic for a number of normal and tumor cells, including cells of bone (CANALIS et al. 1987, 1988a; McCARTHY et al. 1989b). Acidic and basic FGF cause a dose-dependent stimulation of DNA synthesis and cell replication in cultures of intact calvariae and isolated osteoblastic cells. As a consequence of this mitogenic effect, both forms of FGF enhance collagen and noncollagen protein synthesis in bone cultures. In bone cells, as in other cell systems, FGFs interact with heparin, which enhances the effect of aFGF on bone cell replication. This effect is either due to a stabilization of the structure of aFGF by heparin or is due to an enhancement of the binding of aFGF to its bone cell receptor (SCHREIBER et al. 1985). Several forms of FGF receptors have been identified and cloned, some of which belong to the immuno-globulin superfamily of proteins, a finding that also applies to the receptors of other growth factors (JOHNSON et al. 1990). There is no published infor-mation on the characterization and expression of the FGF receptor in cells of the osteoblast lineage. Furthermore, there is no information indicating whether the binding of either basic or acidic FGF to their osteoblast receptors is regulated by hormones or other growth factors. Further studies are needed to determine if any agents modify the biological actions of FGF in bone by altering the binding of FGF to its receptors.

While FGFs have mitogenic activities in a variety of cell systems, their specific role in bone cell physiology is presently unclear. The effects of FGFs on endothelial cell replication would indicate that they are important in revascularization and tissue repair (MONTESANO et al. 1986). These actions, in association with their effects on bone cell replication, would suggest a role in wound healing and fracture repair. Topical administration of FGFs could be useful in the therapy of these two processes (LYNCH et al. 1989). Since FGFs are also mitogens for chondrocytes, they may be relevant in cartilage repair. Prostatic tissue has been shown to synthesize bFGF, and this factor could play a role in the formation of new bone observed subsequent to bone metastases by carcinoma of the prostate (STORY et al. 1987).

In summary, FGFs or HBGFs have significant effects on bone cell replication, but their specific function in bone cell biology and their role as therapeutic agents needs further study.

D. Insulin-Like Growth Factors and Their Binding Proteins

Insulin-like growth factors (IGFs) are polypeptides with an M_r of 7500 (DAUGHADAY and ROTWEIN 1989). There are two forms of IGF – IGF I, initially termed somatomedin-C, and IGF II, initially termed multiplication-stimulating activity. The two forms of IGF are encoded by different genes, but have significant amino acid sequence homology and share many biological activities (RINDERKNECHT and HUMBEL 1976). IGF I appears to be the principal regulator of growth.

While both forms of IGF are present in the systemic circulation, they are also synthesized by multiple tissues where they likely act as local regulators of cell function. The major source of systemic IGF I is the liver, and the synthesis of liver-derived IGF I is mostly under growth hormone control (MATHEWS et al. 1988). The role of systemic IGF I is not entirely clear since most tissues synthesize this growth factor. Systemic IGF I likely contributes to the general regulation of cell growth in various tissues and cell systems, and may be important in the maintenance of a basal level of IGF I. The locally produced IGF I is also under hormonal control and may be more crucial to the function of IGF I as a regulator of specific cell functions in defined tissue systems. The hormones modifying the synthesis of the local IGF I are different in various tissues. For instance, endometrial IGF I is under estradiol-17β control, whereas cartilage IGF I is under growth hormone control (SIMMEN et al. 1990; ISAKSSON et al. 1985). This differential regulation of IGF I synthesis by various hormones allows for the targeting of IGF I to a specific tissue, whose cells contain receptors for the hormone that regulates IGF I. In the skeletal tissue, IGF I and IGF II are among the most prevalent growth factors (CANALIS et al. 1988b; FROLICK et al. 1988). Their concentrations vary between 1 and 3 nM in bone cultures. Experiments using Northern blot analysis have confirmed that IGF I and II are synthesized by most cell types present in skeletal tissue including bone fibroblasts and osteoblasts (MCCARTHY et al. 1990b). Therefore, IGFs may act either as paracrine or autocrine regulators of bone formation. Parathyroid hormone is one of the most potent stimulators of IGF I synthesis by skeletal cells (MCCARTHY et al. 1989a). The effect of parathyroid hormone in bone cells is secondary to changes in cyclic AMP concentrations, and is independent of its effects on intracellular calcium (MCCARTHY et al. 1990b). Like parathyroid hormone, other agents that enhance cyclic AMP production by bone cells also increase IGF I synthesis. These agents include the parathyroid hormone related peptide as well as prostaglandin E_2 (CANALIS et al. 1990; MCCARTHY et al. 1990d). In addition to agents that modify cyclic AMP production, other mechanisms appear to contribute to the regulation of IGF I synthesis in bone cells. Hormones without an effect on cyclic AMP, such as growth hormone and estradiol-17, also increase IGF I transcripts in bone cells (McCARTHY et al. 1989a; ERNST et al. 1989). It is important to point out, however, that the effect of growth hormone is minor in comparison to parathyroid hormone and that estradiol-17β increases IGF I transcripts but not polypeptide levels. The only hormone currently known to inhibit skeletal IGF I synthesis is cortisol (McCARTHY et al. 1990c).

Less is known about the modulation of IGF II synthesis by bone cells, although it appears that IGF II production in skeletal as well as nonskeletal cell systems is not under strict hormonal control. Agents found to enhance IGF I production in bone cell cultures, such as those shown to induce cAMP, were without effect on IGF II mRNA expression and polypeptide levels (McCARTHY et al. 1990b).

Insulin-like growth factor I has important actions on bone formation and can mediate positive or negative effects of hormones in bone metabolism. For example, parathyroid hormone enhances not only skeletal IGF I production, but, when calvariae in culture are transiently exposed to parathyroid hormone, it causes an increase in bone collagen synthesis which is mediated by IGF I (CANALIS et al. 1989d). These results, indicating that IGF I mediates selected anabolic effects of parathyroid hormone on bone, are critical to the understanding of the function of this hormone in bone metabolism. In vivo studies have confirmed an anabolic effect for parathyroid hormone on bone formation, which was lost in hypophysectomized animals and was restored by growth hormone treatment (HOCK and FONSECA 1990). This would support a role also for growth hormone in bone formation, possibly through the generation of IGF I. Although growth hormone does not stimulate bone formation directly, its anabolic role has been further documented in amenorrheic nonhuman primates, in which it had an effect in the maintenance of bone mass (MANN et al. 1990). Intermittent parathyroid hormone administration has been used for the treatment of osteoporosis with some success (SLOVIK et al. 1986) and its combination with growth hormone should be considered in light of the current body of experimental data. IGF I could also be relevant to the pathogenesis of metabolic bone disease. Glucocorticoids, for example, decrease IGF I synthesis and oppose the effects of IGF I on bone formation (McCARTHY et al. 1990c). This would suggest that the decrease in IGF I synthesis might contribute to the inhibitory effect of glucocorticoids on bone formation.

Insulin-like growth factor I and IGF II have similar effects on bone formation. However, IGF I is effective at doses that are four to seven times lower than those required for IGF II (McCARTHY et al. 1989c). Both forms of IGF increase preosteoblastic cell replication and have an independent stimulatory effect on osteoblastic collagen synthesis. The stimulatory effect on collagen synthesis is regulated at the transcriptional level since IGF I and II increase type I collagen transcript levels in osteoblast-enriched cultures.

IGF I also increases bone matrix apposition rates, confirming its effect on bone formation (HOCK et al. 1988). In addition, both forms of IGF have been shown to decrease collagen degradation in calvarial cultures (McCARTHY et al. 1989c). This action is not selective to bone cultures since IGFs have also been shown to decrease proteoglycan degradation in cartilage cultures (LUYTEN et al. 1988). The mechanism of this effect is not clear, although IGF I and II could decrease the production of collagen-degrading enzymes or increase the production of collagenase inhibitors. Through these three main actions – an increase in bone cell populations, an increase in osteo-blastic collagen synthesis, and a decrease in collagen degradation – IGF I and II play a major function in the maintenance of bone mass.

Osteoblastic cultures express both the IGF type 1 and type 2 receptors (CENTRELLA et al. 1990b). It is not known which receptor mediates the anabolic effects of IGF on bone. It is possible that in bone cells, as in other cell systems, the type 1 receptor mediates the effects of IGF I and II on bone formation. Because the IGF type 2 receptor is the mannose-6-phosphate receptor, which is associated with lysosomal enzymes, it is possible that it plays a role in matrix degradation (MACDONALD et al. 1988). Hormones have been shown to modify the binding of IGF to its bone cell receptor and through this mechanism they can regulate IGF effects on bone cell metabolism. 1,25-Dihydroxyvitamin D_3 enhances the binding of IGF I, whereas cortisol decreases the binding of IGF II to bone cells (KUROSE et al. 1990; McCARTHY et al. 1990a).

Insulin-like growth factor I is probably one of the most important regulators of bone mass because it is synthesized by bone cells and it is present in substantial concentrations in bone tissue. Furthermore, its synthesis and binding are regulated and it has major effects on bone formation. The amount of clinical information regarding the role of IGF I in metabolic bone disease is quite limited. Recent studies have revealed that there is a good correlation between serum levels of IGF I and physical activity, and physical exercise increases the expression of IGF I mRNA in muscle (POEHLMAN and COPELAND 1990; DEVOL et al. 1990). Changes in muscle mass are usually associated with changes in bone mass, and these studies may be relevant to the increase in skeletal mass observed after exercise.

From a therapeutic point of view it is impractical to infuse IGF I in patients with metabolic bone disease because it would have nonspecific effects in a variety of nonskeletal tissues in addition to bone. Furthermore, its administration could result in serious side effects. The acute infusion of IGF I to humans and rats causes hypoglycemia because, like insulin, it increases the transport of glucose into cells (GULER et al. 1987; JACOB et al. 1989). A logical approach to the use of IGF I for the treatment of osteoporosis would be the modification of the local skeletal IGF I activity. This can be done by agents that enhance either the synthesis of IGF I or the binding of IGF I to its osteoblastic receptor. For example, one could use agents like parathyroid hormone and its analogues to enhance cyclic AMP production in bone cells so that IGF I production is selectively increased within the skeletal tissue.

Insulin-like growth factors, like many hormones and growth factors, have specific binding proteins (BINOUX et al. 1986). The IGF-binding proteins (IGF-BP) are present in the systemic circulation and are synthesized by most of the tissues that produce IGF. There are four IGF-BPs that have been identified and fully characterized. These comprise IGF-BP 1, originally isolated from amniotic fluid and placental tissue, IGF-BP 2, initially isolated from rat liver cell cultures, IGF-BP 3, a major systemic form of IGF-BP, and IGF-BP 4, initially isolated from osteosarcoma cell cultures. The role of IGF-BPs in cell metabolism seems complex; IGF-BPs can bind IGF and in doing so they may prevent its biological actions, or may increase its half-life. In addition, IGF-BPs appear important modulators of IGF binding to its cell receptor. While bone cultures have been shown to contain, and likely synthesize, IGF-BPs, with the exception of IGF-BP 4, they have not been fully characterized (CANALIS et al. 1989a; MOHAN et al. 1989). It is possible that bone cells synthesize the other three forms of IGF-BPs, and work is currently underway to answer this question. IGF-BP 4 has an M_r of 24000–26000, binds preferentially to IGF II, and prevents its biological actions (MOHAN et al. 1989). The other IGF-BPs bind IGF I and II, but their actions on bone cell function have not been reported. The synthesis of IGF-BPs in nonskeletal tissues is under hormonal control. For instance, the synthesis of IGF-BP 1 is increased by glucocorticoids and that of IGF-BP 3 is under growth hormone control (ORLOWSKI et al. 1990; BAXTER and MARTIN 1986). However, little is known about the regulation of IGF-BP synthesis in bone tissue. It is likely that agents that modify the synthesis of IGF-BPs will play a major role in the modulation of IGF actions since IGF-BPs modify the effects of this growth factor.

In addition to IGF-BPs, skeletal IGF interacts with other local growth factors and with β_2-Microglobulin. Work performed in our laboratory revealed that β_2-microglobulin has similar effects on bone cell function as those described for IGF I, and β_2-microglobulin acts at least in part by enhancing the binding of IGF I to its bone cell receptor (CENTRELLA et al. 1989b). β_2-microglobulin and IGF I are synergistic for some of their effects on osteoblastic cell function. While β_2-microglobulin does not appear to be a growth factor in the classic sense, it seems to play an important role in bone cell function through the regulation of IGF binding.

In summary, IGF I and II have important effects on bone formation and are likely to play a major role as physiological regulators of skeletal metabolism, in the maintenance of bone mass, and indirectly in the therapy of metabolic bone disease.

E. Transforming Growth Factor Beta

Transforming growth factors are polypeptides that have been isolated from a variety of normal and malignant tissues (BARNARD et al. 1990). TGFs were initially identified because of their ability to transform the growth of non-neoplastic indicator cells into a pattern resembling the growth of malignant cells. Initially, two TGFs were identified, TGFα and TGFβ. TGFα is a relatively small polypeptide with significant amino acid sequence homology with epidermal growth factor (MARQUARDT et al. 1984). TGFα is not synthesized by bone cells, but because it stimulates bone resorption it might play a role in the development of hypercalcemia of selected forms of malignancy (IBBOTSON et al. 1985).

Transforming growth factor β is a polypeptide with an M_r of 25000 (BARNARD et al. 1990), which is synthesized by skeletal cells and is one of the most prevalent growth factors present in the bone matrix (CENTRELLA and CANALIS 1985; SEYEDIN et al. 1986). TGFβ was initially defined by its biological actions and the first form to be sequenced was TGFβ_1 (DERYNCK et al. 1985). Over the past several years a number of members of the TGFβ family have been reported. At the present time at least five classic TGFβ isoforms have been identified as well as a number of polypeptides which share significant amino acid sequence homology with TGFβ and form the TGFβ superfamily of polypeptides. Among these, there is a group of osteo-inductive growth factors or bone morphogenetic proteins (WOZNEY et al. 1988). These factors induce the formation of new bone and will be discussed in Chap. XXI of this book. Other members of the TGFβ superfamily include activin and inhibin, and activin and TGFβ have similar stimulatory effects on bone formation (CENTRELLA et al. 1991).

The TGFβ isoforms known to be synthesized by bone cells are TGFβ_1 and β_2. In general, TGFβ_1, β_2, and β_3 have similar biological activities although their potencies vary according to the cell systems where they are tested (TEN DIJKE et al. 1990; GRAYCAR et al. 1989). Information about the regulation of TGFβ synthesis by skeletal cells is somewhat limited. TGFβ is synthesized as a large precursor and binding protein complex (MIYAZONO et al. 1988). As part of this complex, TGFβ is inactive but its half-life is substantially prolonged (WAKEFIELD et al. 1990). A major step in the regulation of TGFβ is its conversion into a biologically active peptide and this is accomplished by transient alkalinization or acidification or by proteolytic cleavage. Parathyroid hormone induces the production of plasminogen activator in bone, which in turn activates TGFβ and makes it available to target cells (PFEILSCHIFTER et al. 1990a). The activation of TGFβ may have significant implications not only in the regulation of the polypeptide, but also in the development of therapeutic maneuvers. Agents that activate TGFβ in a specific tissue could be used to target its anabolic effects.

Transforming growth factor β_1 has been shown to have important actions on bone cell function. It has been studied extensively in skeletal and nonskeletal tissues although other isoforms of TGFβ appear to have similar effects. In normal bone cultures, TGFβ has been shown to stimulate pre-osteoblastic cell replication and stimulate osteoblastic collagen synthesis (CENTRELLA et al. 1987; HOCK et al. 1990). The effects of TGFβ result in an increase in matrix apposition rates as determined by bone histomorphometry and autoradiographic analysis (HOCK et al. 1990). The actions of TGFβ in vitro correlate with in vivo studies in which the topical administration of TGFβ results in an icrease in bone formation (NODA and CAMILLIERE 1989; JOYCE et al. 1990b). TGFβ has complex effects on bone resorption. Although initial work revealed that TGFβ stimulated bone resorption due to an increase in prostaglandin synthesis, recent observations have indicated that TGFβ has biphasic effects on osteoclast cell formation which are dependent on the dose employed and system studied (CHENU et al. 1988; SHINAR and RODAN 1990). An inhibitory effect on bone catabolism in association with an anabolic effect on bone would be similar to the effects described for IGF. Since these two factors also appear to be the most prevalent in bone tissue, their actions could have major relevance to the preservation of bone mass.

Bone cells have three discrete TGFβ receptors that, with the factor, form a complex with an M_r of 65000, 80000, and 250000 (CENTRELLA et al. 1988). It appears that the TGFβ receptors with an M_r of 65000 and 80000 are crucial for the transduction of its effects (LAIHO et al. 1990). The effects of TGFβ on bone cell function can be regulated by altering the binding of the growth factor to its receptors (CENTRELLA et al. 1990c). Treatment with glucocorticoids opposes the effects of TGFβ on DNA and collagen synthesis in bone cells and the mechanism of this action seems to be related to a shifting of TGFβ binding away from active receptors with an M_r of 65000 and 80000 and towards the complex with an M_r of 250000 (CENTRELLA et al. 1990c). The modification of TGFβ binding by glucocorticoids may have important implications in the development of glucocorticoid-induced osteopenia. These changes in association with a decrease in IGF II binding to bone cells and an inhibition of skeletal IGF I synthesis could explain in part the market inhibitory effects of these steroids on bone formation.

In addition to its direct effect on bone cell function, TGFβ has important interactions with other growth factors. TGFβ mRNA is increased by FGF, whereas TGFβ decreases PDGF AA binding to its bone cell receptor (NODA and VOGEL 1989; CENTRELLA et al. 1990). TGFβ might regulate the synthesis or binding of other skeletal growth factors, although additional work will be required to clarify the various interactions among these growth factors.

While TGFβ is produced by bone cells and is stored in the bone matrix in significant quantities, it is also present in blood platelets from which it is likely released during platelet aggregation. Therefore, in addition to its role as a local regulator of bone cell function, TGFβ might play a role as a systemic agent. Because TGFβ would be released primarily during platelet aggregation it could participate in the process of wound healing and fracture repair. In fact, TGFβ has been shown to initiate and regulate critical events during fracture repair (JOYCE et al. 1990a). Furthermore, cells within the fracture callus have been shown to express TGFβ mRNA, and this factor may be induced and act at the local level during fracture healing.

In summary, either as a systemic or as a local agent, TGFβ has important in vitro and in vivo effects on bone formation, and it is likely to be a major regulator of bone remodeling.

In conclusion, bone formation is a complex process regulated by systemic and local agents. Initially, work focused on the regulation of bone formation by hormones and systemic agents; recently, much of our attention has turned to the local regulators of skeletal growth. These agents can be modulated at a variety of levels and have critical effects on bone cell replication and differentiated function. It is likely that through the regulation of the local factors we will target their activities to bone tissue and devise new therapeutic alternatives for metabolic bone disease, osteoporosis, and fracture repair.

Acknowledgments. This work was supported by grants from the National Institutes of Health AR21707, AR39201, and DK42424 and a grant from the National Osteoporosis Foundation. The authors thank Miss Beverly Faulds for expert secretarial assistance.

References

Abraham JA, Whang JL, Tumolo A, Mergia A, Friedman J, Gospodarowicz D, Fiddes JC (1986) Human basic fibroblast growth factors: nucleotide sequence and genomic organization. EMBO J 5:2523–2528

Barnard JA, Lyons RM, Moses HL (1990) The cell biology of transforming growth factor β. Biochim Biophys Acta 1032:79–87

Baxter RC, Martin JL (1986) Radioimmunoassay of growth hormone-dependent insulin-like growth factor binding protein in human plasma. J Clin Invest 78:1504–1512

Beckmann MP, Betsholtz C, Heldin CH, Westermark B, DiMarco E, DiFiore PP, Robbins KC, Aaronson SA (1988) Comparison of biological properties and transforming potential of human PDGF-A and PDGF-B chains. Science 241:1346–1349

Betsholtz C, Johnsson A, Heldin CH, Westermark B, Lind P, Urdea MS, Eddy R, Shows TB, Philpott K, Mellor AL, Knott TJ, Scott J (1986) cDNA sequence and chromosomal localization of human platelet-derived growth factor A-chain and its expression in tumour cell lines. Nature 320:695–699

Binoux M, Hossenlopp S, Hardouin D, Seurin D, Lassarre C, Gourmelen M (1986) Somatomedin (insulin-like growth factor)-binding proteins. Molecular forms and regulation. Horm Res 24:141–151

Bowen-Pope DF, Hart CE, Seifert RA (1989) Sera and conditioned media contain different isoforms of platelet-derived growth factor (PDGF) which bind to different classes of PDGF receptor. J Biol Chem 264:2502–2508

Bryckaert MC, Lindroth M, Lonn A, Tobelem G, Wasteson A (1988) Transforming growth factor (TGFβ) decreases the proliferation of human bone marrow fibroblasts by inhibiting the platelet-derived growth factor (PDGF) binding. Exp Cell Res 179:311–321

Burgess WH, Maciag T (1989) The heparin-binding (fibroblast) growth factor family of proteins. Annu Rev Biochem 58:575–606

Burgess WH, Wehlman T, Firesel R, Johnson WV, Maciag T (1985) Multiple forms of endothelial cell growth factor. J Biol Chem 260:11389–11392

Canalis E, Lorenzo J, Burgess WH, Maciag T (1987) Effects of endothelial cell growth factor on bone remodeling in vitro. J Clin Invest 79:52–58

Canalis E, Centrella M, McCarthy T (1988a) Effects of basic fibroblast growth factor on bone formation in vitro. J Clin Invest 81:1572–1577

Canalis E, McCarthy T, Centrella M (1988b) Isolation and characterization of insulin-like growth factor I (Somatomedin C) from cultures of fetal rat calvariae. Endocrinology 122:22–27

Canalis E, Centrella M, McCarthy TL (1989a) Role of insulin-like growth factor I and II on skeletal remodeling. In: Raizada MK (ed) Molecular and cellular aspects of insulin and IGF I/II: implications for the central nervous system. pp 459–466

Canalis E, McCarthy T, Centrella M (1989b) The role of growth factors in skeletal remodeling. Endocrinol Metab Clin North Am 18:903–918

Canalis E, McCarthy TL, Centrella M (1989c) Effects of platelet-derived growth factor on bone formation in vitro. J Cell Physiol 140:530–537

Canalis E, Centrella M, Burch W, McCarthy T (1989d) Insulin-like growth factor I mediates selective anabolic effects of parathyroid hormone in bone cultures. J Clin Invest 83:60–65

Canalis E, McCarthy TL, Centrella M (1990) Differential effects of continuous and transient treatment with parathyroid hormone related peptide (PTHrp) on bone collagen synthesis. Endocrinology 126:1806–1812

Centrella M, Canalis E (1985) Transforming and nontransforming growth factors are present in medium conditioned by fetal rat calvariae. Proc Natl Acad Sci USA 82:7335–7339

Centrella M, McCarthy TL, Canalis E (1987) Transforming growth factor beta is a bifunctional regulator of replication and collagen synthesis in osteoblast-enriched cell cultures from fetal rat bone. J Biol Chem 262:2869–2874

Centrella M, McCarthy TL, Canalis E (1988) Parathyroid hormone modulates transforming growth factor β activity and binding in osteoblast-enriched cell cultures from fetal rat parietal bone. Proc Natl Acad Sci USA 85:5889–5893

Centrella M, McCarthy TL, Canalis E (1989a) Platelet-derived growth factor enhances deoxyribonucleic acid and collagen synthesis in osteoblast-enriched cultures from fetal rat parietal bone. Endocrinology 125:13–19

Centrella M, McCarthy TL, Canalis E (1989b) β_2-Microglobulin enhances insulin-like growth factor I receptor levels and synthesis in bone cell cultures. J Biol Chem 264:18268–18271

Centrella M, McCarthy TL, Canalis E (1990a) Relative effects of hetero- and homodimeric isoforms of platelet-derived growth factors in fetal rat bone cells. In: Cohn DV, Glorieux FH, Martin TJ (eds) Calcium regulation and bone metabolism: 10. Basic and clinical aspects. Elsevier, Amsterdam, pp 324–329

Centrella M, McCarthy TL, Canalis E (1990b) Receptors for insulin-like growth factors I and II in osteoblast-enriched cultures from fetal rat bone. Endocrinology 126:39–44

Centrella M, McCarthy TL, Canalis E (1990c) Glucocorticoid control of transforming growth factor β (TGFβ) binding and effects in osteoblast-enriched cultures from fetal rat bone. J Bone Miner Res 5 [Suppl 2]:S211

Centrella M, McCarthy TL, Ladd C, Canalis E (1990d) Expression of platelet-derived growth factor (PDGF) and regulation of PDGF binding are both isoform specific in osteoblast-enriched cultures from fetal rat bone. J Bone Miner Res 5 [Suppl 2]:S86

Centrella M, McCarthy TL, Canalis E (1991) Activin-A binding and biochemical effects in osteoblast-enriched cultures from fetal rat parietal bone. Mol Cell Biol 11:250–258

Chenu C, Pfeilschifter J, Mundy GR, Roodman GD (1988) Transforming growth factor β inhibits formation of osteoclast-like cells in long-term human marrow cultures. Proc Natl Acad Sci USA 85:5683–5687

Collins T, Ginsburg D, Boss JM, Orkin SH, Pober JS (1985) Cultured human endothelial cells express platelet-derived growth factor B chain: cDNA cloning and structural analysis. Nature 316:748–750

Daughaday WH, Rotwein P (1989) Insulin-like growth factors I and II. Peptide, messenger ribonucleic acid and gene structures, serum, and tissue concentrations. Endocr Rev 10:68–91

Derynck R, Jarrett JA, Chen EY, Eaton DH, Bell JR, Assoian RK, Roberts AB, Sporn MB, Goeddel DV (1985) Human transforming growth factor-β complementary DNA sequence and expression in normal and transformed cells. Nature 316:701–705

DeVol DL, Rotwein P, Sadow JL, Novakofski J, Bechtel PJ (1990) Activation of insulin-like growth factor gene expression during work-induced skeletal muscle growth. Am J Physiol 259:E89–E95

Doolittle RF, Hunkapiller MW, Hood LE, Devare SG, Robbins KC, Aaronson SA, Antoniades HN (1983) Simian sarcoma virus *onc* gene, v-*sis* is derived from the gene (or genes) encoding a platelet-derived growth factor. Science 221: 275–277

Ernst M, Heath JK, Rodan GA (1989) Estradiol effects on proliferation, messenger ribonucleic acid for collagen and insulin-like growth factor-I, and parathyroid hormone-stimulated adenylate cyclase activity in osteoblastic cells from calvariae and long bones. Endocrinology 125:825–833

Esch F, Baird A, Ling N, Ueno N, Hill F, Denoroy L, Klepper R, Gospodarowicz D, Bohlen P, Guillemin R (1985) Primary structure of bovine pituitary basic fibroblast growth factor (FGF) and comparison with the amino-terminal sequence of bovine brain acidic FGF. Proc Natl Acad Sci USA 82:6507–6511

Frolik CA, Ellis LF, Williams DC (1988) Isolation and characterization of insulin-like growth factor-II from human bone. Biochem Biophys Res Commun 151:1011–1018

Gay CG, Winkles JA (1990) Heparin-binding growth factor-1 stimulation of human endothelial cells induces platelet-derived growth factor A-chain gene expression. J Biol Chem 265:3284–3292

Gimenez-Gallego G, Rodkey J, Bennett C, Rios-Candelore M, DiSalvo J, Thomas K (1985) Brain-derived acidic fibroblast growth factor: complete amino acid sequence and homologies. Science 230:1385–1388

Globus RK, Plouet J, Gospodarowicz D (1989) Cultured bovine bone cells synthesize basic fibroblast growth factor and store it in their extracellular matrix. Endocrinology 124:1539–1547

Graves DT, Owen AJ, Barth RK, Tempst P, Winoto A, Fors L, Hood LE, Antoniades HN (1984) Detection of c-*sis* transcripts and synthesis of PDGF-like proteins by human osteosarcoma cells. Science 226:972–974

Graves DT, Valentin-Opran A, Delgado R, Valente AJ, Mundy G, Piche J (1989) The potential role of platelet-derived growth factor as an autocrine or paracrine factor for human bone cells. Connect Tissue Res 23:209–218

Graycar JL, Miller DA, Arrick BA, Lyons RM, Moses HL, Derynck R (1989) Human transforming growth factor-beta 3: recombinant expression, purification, and biological activities in comparison with transforming growth factors-beta 1 and -beta 2. Mol Endocrinol 3:1977–1986

Guler HP, Froesch R, Zapf J (1987) Short term metabolic effects of recombinant human insulin-like growth factor I in healthy adults. N Engl J Med 317:137–140

Heldin CH, Westermark B (1987) PDGF-like growth factors in autocrine stimulation of growth. J Cell Physiol 5:31–34

Heldin CH, Johnsson H, Wennergren A, Wernstedt S, Betsholtz C, Westermark B (1986) A human osteosarcoma cell line secretes a growth factor structurally related to a homodimer of PDGF A-chains. Nature 319:511–514

Heldin H, Backstrom G, Ostman A, Hammacher A, Ronnstrand L, Rubin K, Nister M, Westermark B (1988) Binding of different dimeric forms of PDGF to human fibroblasts: evidence for two separate receptor types. EMBO J 7:1387–1393

Hock JM, Fonseca J (1990) Anabolic effect of human synthetic parathyroid hormone-(1-34) depends on growth hormone. Endocrinology 127:1804–1810

Hock JM, Centrella M, Canalis E (1988) Insulin-like growth factor I (IGF-I) has independent effects on bone matrix formation and cell replication. Endocrinology 122:254–260

Hock JM, Canalis E, Centrella M (1990) Transforming growth factor beta (TGF-Beta-1) stimulates bone matrix apposition and bone cell replication in cultured fetal rat calvariae. Endocrinology 126:421–426

Ibbotson KJ, Twardzik DR, D'Souza SM, Hargreaves WR, Todaro GJ, Mundy GR (1985) Stimulation of bone resorption in vitro by synthetic transforming growth factor alpha. Science 228:1007–1009

Isaksson OG, Eden S, Jansson JO (1985) Mode of action of pituitary growth hormone on target cells. Annu Rev Physiol 47:483–499

Jacob R, Barrett E, Plewe G, Fagin KD, Sherwin RS (1989) Acute effects of insulin-like growth factor I on glucose and amino acid metabolism in the awake fasted rat. Comparison with insulin. J Clin Invest 83:1717–1723

James R, Bradshaw RA (1984) Polypeptide growth factors. Annu Rev Biochem 53:259–292

Johnson DE, Lee PL, Lu J, Williams LT (1990) Diverse forms of a receptor for acidic and basic fibroblast growth factors. Mol Cell Biol 10:4728–4736

Joyce ME, Jingushi S, Bolander ME (1990a) Transforming growth factor-β in the regulation of fracture repair. Orthop Clin North Am 21:199–209

Joyce ME, Roberts AB, Sporn MB, Bolander ME (1990b) Transforming growth factor-β and the initiation of chondrogenesis and osteogenesis in the rat femur. J Cell Biol 110:2195–2207

Kavanaugh WM, Harsh GR, Starksen NF, Rocco CM, Williams LT (1988) Transcriptional regulation of the A and B chain genes of platelet derived growth factor in microvascular endothelial cells. J Biol Chem 263:8470–8472

Klagsbrun M, Sasse J, Sullivan R, Smith JA (1986) Human tumor cells synthesize an endothelial cell growth factor that is structurally related to basic fibroblast growth factor. Proc Natl Acad Sci USA 83:2448–2452

Kurose H, Yamaoka K, Okada S, Nakajima S, Seino Y (1990) 1,25-Dihydroxyvitamin D3 [1.25-(OH)2D3] increases insulin-like growth factor I (IGF-I) receptors in clonal osteoblastic cells. Study on interaction of IGF-I and 1.25-(OH)2D3. Endocrinology 126:2088–2094

Laiho M, Weis FMB, Massague J (1990) Concomitant loss of transforming growth factor (TGF)-β receptor types I and II in TGF-β-resistant cell mutants implicates both receptor types in signal transduction. J Biol Chem 265:18518–18524

Lee KH, Bowen-Pope DF, Reed RR (1990) Isolation and characterization of the α platelet-derived growth factor receptor from rat olfactory epithelium. Mol Cell Biol 10:2237–2246

Lund PK, Moats-Staats BM, Hynes MA, Simmons JG, Jansen M, D'Ercole AJ, Van Wyk JJ (1986) Somatomedin/insulin-like growth factor-I and insulin-like growth factor-II mRNAs in rat fetal and adult tissues. J Biol Chem 261:14539–14544

Luyten FP, Hascall VC, Nissley PS, Morales TI, Reddi AH (1988) Insulin-like growth factors maintain steady state metabolism of proteoglycans in bovine articular cartilage explants. Arch Biochem Biophys 267:416–425

Lynch SE, Colvin RB, Antoniades HN (1989) Growth factors in wound healing. Single and synergistic effects on partial thickness porcine skin wounds. J Clin Invest 84:640–646

MacDonald RG, Pfeffer SR, Coussens L, Tepper MA, Brocklebank CM, Mole JE, Anderson JK, Chen E, Czech MP, Ullrich A (1988) A single receptor binds both insulin-like growth factor II and mannose-6-phosphate. Science 239:1134–1137

Majack RA, Majesky MW, Goodman LV (1990) Role of PDGF-A expression in the control of vascular smooth muscle cell growth by transforming growth factor-β. J Cell Biol 111:239–247

Mann DR, Orr TE, Rudman CG, Gould KG (1990) Effect of growth hormone supplementation on bone loss in GnRH agonist-treated female monkeys. J Bone Miner Res 5 [Suppl 2]:S139

Marquardt H, Hunkapiller MW, Hood LE, Todaro GJ (1984) Rat transforming growth factor type 1: structure and relation to epidermal growth factor. Science 223:1079–1082

Mathews LS, Hammer RE, Brinster RL, Palmiter RD (1988) Expression of insulin-like growth factor I in transgenic mice with elevated levels of growth hormone is correlated with growth. Endocrinology 123:433–437

McCarthy TL, Centrella M, Canalis E (1989a) Parathyroid hormone enhances the transcript and polypeptide levels of insulin-like growth factor I in osteoblast-enriched cultures from fetal rat bone. Endocrinology 124:1247–1253

MCarthy TL, Centrella M, Canalis E (1989b) Effects of fibroblast growth factors on deoxyribonucleic acid and collagen synthesis in rat parietal bone cells. Endocrinology 125:2118–2126

McCarthy TL, Centrella M, Canalis E (1989c) Regulatory effects of insulin-like growth factor I and II on bone collagen synthesis in rat calvarial cultures. Endocrinology 124:301–309

McCarthy TL, Canalis E, Centrella M (1990a) Cortisol differentially modulates insulin-like growth factor I and II binding on osteoblast-enriched fetal rat bone cells. J Bone Miner Res 5 [Suppl 2]:S138

McCarthy TL, Centrella M, Canalis E (1990b) Cyclic AMP induces insulin-like growth factor I synthesis in osteoblast-enriched cultures. J Biol Chem 265:15353–15356

McCarthy TL, Centrella M, Canalis E (1990c) Cortisol inhibits the synthesis of insulin-like growth factor I in skeletal cells. Endocrinology 126:1569–1575

McCarthy TL, Centrella M, Raisz LG, Canalis E (1990d) Prostaglandin E$_2$ stimulates insulin-like growth factor I synthesis in osteoblast-enriched cultures from fetal rat bone. J Bone Miner Res 5 [Suppl 2]:S86

Miyazono K, Hellman U, Wernstedt C, Heldin CH (1988) Latent high molecular weight complex of transforming growth factor-β1: purification from human platelets and structural characterization. J Biol Chem 263:6407–6415

Mohan S, Bautista CM, Wergedal J, Baylink DJ (1989) Isolation of an inhibitory insulin-like growth factor (IGF) binding protein from bone cell-conditioned medium: a potential local regulator of IGF action. Proc Natl Acad Sci USA 86:8338–8342

Montesano R, Vassalli JD, Baird A, Guillemin R, Orci L (1986) Basic fibroblast growth factor induces angiogenesis in vitro. Proc Natl Acad Sci USA 83:7297–7301

Noda M, Camilliere JJ (1989) In vivo stimulation of bone formation by transforming growth factor β. Endocrinology 124:2991–2994

Noda M, Vogel R (1989) Transcriptional regulation of transforming growth factor β (TGFβ) gene expression in osteoblast-like cells by fibroblast growth factor (FGF). J Bone Miner Res 4:S326

Orlowski CC, Ooi GT, Rechler MM (1990) Dexamethasone stimulates transcription of the insulin-like growth factor-binding protein-1 gene in H4-II-E rat hepatoma cells. Endocrinology 4:1592–1599

Pfeilschifter J, Erdmann J, Schmidt W, Naumann A, Minne HW, Ziegler R (1990a) Differential regulation of plasminogen activator and plasminogen activator inhibitor by osteotropic factors in primary cultures of mature osteoblasts and osteoblast precursors. Endocrinology 126:703–711

Pfeilschifter J, Oechsner M, Naumann A, Gronwald, RGK, Minne HW, Ziegler R (1990b) Stimulation of bone matrix apposition in vitro by local growth factors: a comparison between insulin-like growth factor I, platelet-derived growth factor, and transforming growth factor. Endocrinology 127:69–75

Poehlman ET, Copeland KC (1990) Influence of physical activity on insulin-like growth factor I in healthy younger and older men. J Clin Endocrinol Metab 71:1468–1473

Raines EW, Dower SK, Ross R (1989) Interleukin-1 mitogenic activity for fibroblasts and smooth muscle cells is due to PDGF-AA. Science 243:393–396

Rinderknecht E, Humbel RE (1976) Amino-terminal sequences of two polypeptides from human serum with nonsuppressible insulin-like and cell-growth-promoting activities: evidence for structural homology with insulin B chain. Proc Natl Acad Sci USA 73:4379–4381

Schreiber AB, Kenney J, Kowalski WJ, Friesel R, Mehlman T, Maciag T (1985) Interaction of endothelial cell growth factor with heparin: characterization by receptor and antibody recognition. Proc Natl Acad Sci USA 82:6138–6142

Seifert RA, Hart CE, Phillips PE, Forstrom JW, Ross R, Murray MJ, Bowen-Pope DF (1989) Two different subunits associate to create isoform-specific platelet-derived growth factor receptors. J Biol Chem 264:8771–8778

Seyedin SM, Thompson AY, Bentz H, Rosen DM, McPherson JM, Conti A, Siegel NR, Galluppi GR, Piez KA (1986) Cartilage-inducing factor-A. Apparent indentity to transforming growth factor-beta. J Biol Chem 261:5693–5696

Shinar DM, Rodan GA (1990) Biphasic effects of transforming growth factor-β on the production of osteoclast-like cells in mouse bone marrow cultures: the role of prostaglandins in the generation of these cells. Endocrinology 126:3153–3158

Siegbahn A, Hammacher A, Westermark B, Heldin CH (1990) Differential effects of the various isoforms of platelet-derived growth factor on chemotaxis of fibroblasts, monocytes, and granulocytes. J Clin Invest 85:916–920

Simmen RCM, Simmen FA, Hofig A, Farmer SJ, Bazer FW (1990) Hormonal regulation of insulin-like growth factor gene expression in pig uterus. Endocrinology 127:2166–2174

Slovik DM, Rosenthal DI, Doppelt SH, Potts JT, Daly MA, Campbell JA, Neer RM (1986) Restoration of spinal bone in osteoporotic men by treatment with human parathyroid hormone (1-34) and 1,25-dihydroxyvitamin D. J Bone Miner Res 1:377–381

Story MT, Sasse J, Jacobs SC, Lawson RK (1987) Prostatic growth factor: purification and structural relationship to basic fibroblast growth factor. Biochemistry 26:3843–3849

Tashjian AH, Hohmann EL, Antoniades HN, Levine L (1982) Platelet-derived growth factor stimulates bone resorption via a prostaglandin-mediated mechanism. Endocrinology 111:118–124

ten Dijke P, Iwata KK, Goddard C, Pieler C, Canalis E, McCarthy TL, Centrella M (1990) Recombinant transforming growth factor type β3: biological activities and receptor binding properties in isolated bone cells. Mol Cell Biol 10:4473–4479

Vlodavsky I, Fridman R, Sullivan R, Sasse J, Klagsbrun M (1987) Aortic endothelial cells synthesize basic fibroblast growth factor which remains cell associated and platelet-derived growth factor-like protein which is secreted. J Cell Physiol 131:402–408

Wakefield LM, Winokur TS, Hollands RS, Christopherson K, Levinson AD, Sporn MB (1990) Recombinant latent transforming growth factor β1 has a longer plasma half-life in rats than active transforming growth factor β1, and a different tissue distribution. J Clin Invest 86:1976–1984

Wozney JM, Rosen V, Celeste AJ, Mitsock LM, Whitters MJ, Kriz RW, Hewick RM, Wang EA (1988) Novel regulators of bone formation: molecular clones and activities. Science 242:1528–1534

Yarden J, Escobedo JA, Kuang WJ, Yang-Feng TL, Daniel TO, Tremble PM, Chen EY, Ando ME, Harkins RN, Francke U, Fried VA, Ullrich A, Williams LT (1986) Structure of the receptor for platelet-derived growth factor helps define a family of closely related growth factor receptors. Nature 323:226–232

CHAPTER 8

Mineralization

H.C. ANDERSON and D.C. MORRIS

A. Introduction

The critical role of cells in biologic mineralization is becoming more and more evident. The following observations point to cells as the most important controlling factor in the initiation and propagation of mineral: (1) During development, cell-derived inductive signals direct skeletal cells to enter pathways of differentiation characteristic of mineralizing tissues. (2) Skeletal cells secrete the extracellular matrix into which mineral is selectively deposited. (3) Differentiated skeletal cells generate matrix vesicles (MVs) which are slectively placed in the matrix to serve as initial sites for mineral deposition and to control the distribution of mineral. (4) Cells control the composition of the matrix, thereby promoting or inhibiting mineral deposition. (5) Cells control the ionic and chemical milieu in which mineralization occurs.

Only a few years ago mineralization was visualized as being primarily a physicochemical phenomenon in which mineral nucleation is achieved by extracellular, nonliving chemical structure(s) in the matrix (e.g., collagen tertiary structure) that serve as templates upon which the first mineral crystals are formed. Initial crystals can then serve as nuclei for further mineral propagation. In this view both initiation and propagation are controlled by nonliving chemical factors residing in the matrix. In recent years, however, the prevailing opinion has shifted to a view that envisions cells as being more importantly involved in mineral initiation (through matrix vesicles) while mineral propagation remains primarily extracellular and physicochemical. Nevertheless, there is an increasing awareness that mineral propagation is also regulated by cells by creating the matrix and ionic milieu in which mineralization may or may not progress.

The objective of this review is to illuminate the critical role of skeletal cells in both the initiation and propagation of the calcification mechanism.

B. Direct Cellular Control of Mineralization Through Matrix Vesicles

Matrix vesicles are tiny ($0.1-0.2\,\mu$m in diameter), extracellular, membrane-invested particles that are selectively clustered at sites of incipient mineralization in the matrix of growth plate cartilage (H.C. ANDERSON 1969; BONUCCI 1970), developing bone (ANDERSON and REYNOLDS 1973), induced bone (H.C. ANDERSON 1976), fracture callus (SCHENK et al. 1970), predentine (BERNARD 1972; EISENMAN and GLICK 1972; OZAWA and NAJIMA 1972; SISCA and PROVENZA 1972; SLAVKIN et al. 1972), and tendon (ARSENAULT et al. 1991; LANDIS 1987). The first crystallites of hydroxyapatite mineral are seen within matrix vesicles, often in association with the inner surface of the vesicle membrane (Fig. 1). Vesicles near the mineralization front accumulate increasing numbers of hydroxyapatite (HA) crystallites (Fig. 1), and begin to show penetration of the vesicle membrane by rigid crystal profiles. Such images of early mineral deposition within matrix vesicles are seen even with the most advanced techniques of tissue preparation including frozen sectioning (ALI et al. 1977; GAY et al. 1978) and anhydrous freeze-

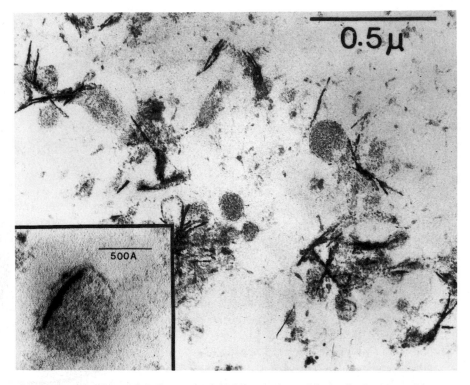

Fig. 1. *Insert at lower left* shows a calcifying matrix vesicle in the hypertrophic zone of rat growth plate. The first electron microscopically observable crystalline apatite mineral is seen as a needle-like, electron-dense precipitate within the matrix vesicle, often in apposition to the inner leaflet of the vesicle membrane. (Reprinted from ANDERSON et al. 1984). Subsequent deposition of apatite needles occurs at the surfaces of matrix vesicles to form radial clusters of mineral, as shown *at right*. The clusters grow by crystal proliferation and eventually fuse to form contiguous mineral. (Reprinted from ANDERSON 1969)

substitution (MORRIS et al. 1983; OZAWA and YAMAMOTO 1983). For a summary see H.C. ANDERSON (1989).

As extravesicular mineral propagation occurs, the matrix vesicles become engulfed in electron-dense apatite deposits and can no longer be seen except with decalcification. Removal of Ca with EDTA shows persistent, but fragmented membranes of matrix vesicles entombed in heavy mineral deposits (H.C. ANDERSON 1969) (Fig. 2). The concealment of matrix vesicles by mineral deposits explains morphometric data (REINHOLT and WERNERSON 1988) showing a decline in the number of vesicles in the calcifying zone of growth plate cartilage. The concealment of matrix vesicles at an advanced stage of calcification in no way precludes an association between MVs and HA during initial stages of mineralization.

Matrix vesicles are essentially exocytosed pieces of skeletal cells, bounded by a biologically active membrane and containing a selected array of enzymes, proteins, and lipids that can interact to initiate mineralization. Skeletal MVs are, for the most part, shed from the cortex of chondrocytes, osteoblasts, and odontoblasts by a budding process that does not require cell death or disintegration. Since budding is the predominant mode of MV

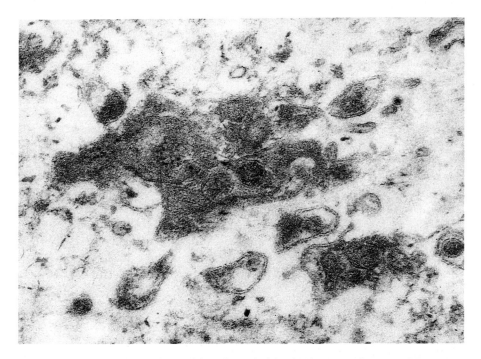

Fig. 2. Remnants of matrix vesicles, bounded by broken membranes with typical bilayers, are visible in EDTA- decalcified cartilage at the epiphyseal-metaphyseal junction of mouse growth plate. (Reprinted from ANDERSON 1969) Electron micrograph, ×80 000

biogenesis (AKISAKA and GAY 1985a; AKISAKA et al. 1986, 1988; BORG et al. 1981; CECIL and ANDERSON 1978; WUTHIER et al. 1978), it is therefore evident that molecules present at the exposed surfaces of vesicles will correspond to those of the exterior surface of the mother cell. The fact that the MV membrane is "right-side-out" with respect to the cell membrane has been confirmed in freeze-fracture and freeze-etch studies that can determine the "sidedness" of the asymmetric unit membranes of cells and vesicles (CECIL and ANDERSON 1978; WUTHIER et al. 1978). The process of vesiculation and vesicles release is a common phenomenon in nature, and often is related to a time in the cell cycle, postmitosis. This phenomenon has been compared to "apoptosis" (KARDOS and HUBBARD 1982), the process of programmed cell death which is often preceded by vesiculation. The analogy with apoptosis fits cell behavior of the growth plate where maturing chondrocytes of the upper hypertrophic zone apparently give rise to MVs before undergoing marked hypertrophy, hydropic degeneration, and ultimately cell death at the base of the growth plate (FARNUM and WILSMAN 1989). However, osteoblasts and odontoblasts appear not to undergo programmed cell death after vesiculation, so apoptosis would not appear to be a necessary fate for all vesiculating cells.

One feature common to MV biogenesis in all skeletal tissues is the polarized nature of the vesiculation process: only the lateral surfaces of growth plate chondrocytes appear to give rise to MVs in growth plate (RALPHS and ALI 1986); only mineral-facing surfaces of osteoblasts release MVs (AKISAKA et al. 1986; PALUMBO 1986); and only the apical surfaces of pre-odontoblasts generate dentinal MVs (BERNARD 1972; EISENMAN and GLICK 1972; SISCA and PROVENZA 1972; SLAVKIN et al. 1972). This form of cellular polarization is reminiscent of the polarization of renal tubular epithelium in which the apical and basolateral membranes are specialized for certain specific functions such as secretion or anchorage by virtue of their relative local enrichment of functional molecules. An example would be the exclusive localization of Na^+K^+ ATPase of the sodium pump to the basolateral membrane of the renal tubular cell (KASHGARIAN et al. 1985). The ability of skeletal cells to polarize their vesiculating membrane implies an ability to endow the MV precursor membrane with a selected, nonrandom array of proteins, lipids, etc., which could be especially conducive to mineralization. An example of such molecular sorting may be reflected in the selective enrichment of acidic phospholipids (with Ca^{2+}-binding ability) in MVs over that seen in plasma membranes of mother chondrocytes (PERESS et al. 1974; WUTHIER 1975). Also, the inventory of major proteins is different in MVs than in chondrocyte plasma membranes, there being fewer major proteins and a different spectrum of major molecular weights in MVs versus cell membranes (BOHN et al. 1985; MUHLRAD et al. 1983; STEIN et al. 1981). The basic conclusion to be drawn from evidence of cell polarity in MV biogenesis is that the cells *can* control the molecular composition of budded membranes, and probably do so in order to achieve an optimal level of calcifying activity at a cell-determined, nonrandom site in the matrix.

C. Mechanism of Matrix Vesicle Calcification

Matrix vesicles are avid calcifiers. This has been amply demonstrated in various in vitro test systems devised to assess the calcifiability of MVs. Matrix vesicles can be experimentally calcified in vitro in tissue slices of growth plate (H.C. ANDERSON et al. 1975; ANDERSON and SAJDERA 1976; ANDERSON and HSU 1978), in isolated preparations of matrix vesicles obtained by differential centrifugation of collagenase-liquified growth plate (ALI et al. 1970; ALI and EVANS 1973; HSU and ANDERSON 1977), or after MV release from cultures of chondrocytes (H.C. ANDERSON et al. 1990; GLASER and CONRAD 1981; GOLUB et al. 1983; WUTHIER et al. 1985) or osteoblasts (STECHSCHULTE et al. 1991). Calcium-depositing activity of MVs can be quantified by measuring the amount of ^{45}Ca deposited when any of the MV preparations listed above are incubated in a calcifying solution containing physiologic levels of Ca^{2+} and PO_4^{3-} plus, usually, a phosphate ester such as ATP, AMP, or β-glycerophosphate (βGP) (ALI and EVANS 1973; HSU and ANDERSON 1977; ANDERSON and HSU 1978). Rachitic growth plate, in which calcification has been arrested by deprivation of dietary phosphate, is a particularly abundant source of precalcified matrix vesicles with all calcifying mechanisms intact. These MVs are merely awaiting the availability of an adequate physiologic ionic environment in which to initiate productive calcification (H.C. ANDERSON et al. 1975; JOHNSON et al. 1989; SIMON et al. 1973). Although matrix vesicles residing in tissue slices of rachitic cartilage can initiate calcification without the addition of any phosphate donor molecule (H.C. ANDERSON et al. 1975; ANDERSON and HSU 1978), it has been shown repeatedly that isolated MVs usually require the addition of modest amounts of ATP (ALI and EVANS 1973; HSU and ANDERSON 1978) or AMP (MURPHREE et al. 1982) in the incubation mixture in order to initiate the calcification cascade. Even though MV calcification in cartilage tissue slices is self-sustaining in the absence of βGP, it is nevertheless greatly enhanced by providing βGP (ANDERSON and HSU 1978; BELLOWS et al. 1991). One explanation of MV calcification being dependent upon the availability of an ester phosphate in the incubation medium is that ester phosphate is utilized as a substrate for phosphatases known to be concentrated in the membrane of the matrix vesicle, including ATPase, alkaline phosphatase (ALP), inorganic pyrophosphatase (PPiase), and nucleoside triphosphate pyrophosphatase (NTPPase).

I. Role of Alkaline Phosphatase

There is a great deal of evidence indicating an important role for matrix vesicle ALP and related enzymes in the normal mineralization of cartilage and bone. Some of the evidence is as follows. Chick bone matrix vesicle pyrophosphatase activity was required for the calcification of embryonic long-bone rudiments in organ culture (ANDERSON and REYNOLDS 1973). Inhibitors of vesicle alkaline phosphatase activity such as heat, beryllium,

levamisole, and EHDP also inhibited calcification of matrix vesicles in tissue
slices of rachitic rat growth plate cartilage (Anderson and Sajdera 1976;
Fallon et al. 1980), and the heat inactivation curve for isolated matrix
vesicle alkaline pyrophosphatase exactly paralleled the pattern of inhibition
of calcification in growth plate tissue slices (H.C. Anderson 1985). The
removal of phosphatase substrates such as ATP and AMP from calcifying
solutions prevented calcification in isolated matrix vesicles (see above), and,
although solubilized ALP alone was not capable of initiating ^{45}CaPO$_4$
deposition, our studies have shown that, when phosphatase is incorporated
into the membranes of reconstituted vesicles, calcium deposition is restored
(Hsu et al. 1978; Hsu and Anderson 1978). Recent studies by Bellows et
al. (1991) in micromass cultures of isolated bone cells have implicated
matrix vesicles in the initiation of this form of in vitro calcification, and have
shown that levamisole, an inhibitor of ALP, can effectively arrest the early
calcification process, and that the process is greatly enhanced by addition of
β-GP, a well-known substrate for ALP. Cytochemistry shows that concentrated ALP, Ca-ATPase, and pyrophosphatase activity resides in the
membranes of matrix vesicles adjacent to hypertrophic chondrocytes
(Akisaka and Gay 1985b, 1986; H.C. Anderson et al. 1970; Matsuzawa
and Anderson 1971; Morris et al. 1986; Lewinson et al. 1982), to periosteal
osteoblasts (Bernard 1978) and to odontoblasts (Larsson 1973; Ozawa and
Najima 1972; Takano et al. 1986). It is believed that a terminal portion of
the ALP molecule attaches to phosphatidylinositol of the cell membrane
(Fedde et al. 1988; Low 1987; Register et al. 1986) and that most of the
ALP molecule projects from the outer surface of the chondrocyte and MV
membrane (Fedde et al. 1988; Randall et al. 1989; Register et al. 1986).
ALP activation occurs just before the onset of matrix vesicle mineralization
(Akisaka and Gay 1985b, 1986; Matsuzawa and Anderson 1971) and may
well be the triggering event of the calcification cascade (Fig. 4). Following
initiation of mineralization there is a decrease in Ca^{2+}-ATPase and ALP in
vesicle membranes (Akisaka and Gay 1985b; Matsuzawa and Anderson
1971; Genge et al. 1988).

II. Role of Lipids

Evidence is strong for the involovement of lipids in MV calcification.
Isolated matrix vesicles were shown to be very enriched in acidic phospholipids (Peress et al. 1974; Wuthier 1975). Such lipids may serve as a
nonenergy-requiring calcium trap during mineralization (Cotmore et al.
1971; Peress et al. 1974; Wuthier 1968, 1975; Yaari and Shapiro 1982). In
fact, vesicles contain calcium-phosphate-phospholipid complexes (Boskey
and Posner 1977; Boskey et al. 1980; Wuthier and Gore 1977) which
together with membrane-associated proteolipids are capable of initiating
mineral in vitro (Boyan-Salyers and Boskey 1980; Boyan 1985; Ennever et
al. 1977, 1978), and have been found in significant quantities in bone

(ENNEVER et al. 1977) and in calcifying oral bacteria (BOYAN-SALYERS and BOSKEY 1980; BOYAN 1985; ENNEVER et al. 1978). The latter bacteria are associated with dental plaque and calculus formation. As mentioned above, acidic Ca-binding phospholipids, particularly phosphatidyl serine (PS), are concentrated in the MV membrane, and PS has been shown to be localized at the inner leaflet of the MV membrane (MAJESKA et al. 1979), where the first crystals of hydroxyapatite appear (Figs. 1, 3). Thus, Ca-binding phospholipids are strategically placed to serve as a calcium localizer, close to the site of ALP enzymatic activity.

III. Constitutive Proteins of Matrix Vesicles

Until recently, most proteins of the MV membrane or sap had escaped identification. Only the phosphatases, ALP, PPiase, and NTPPase were

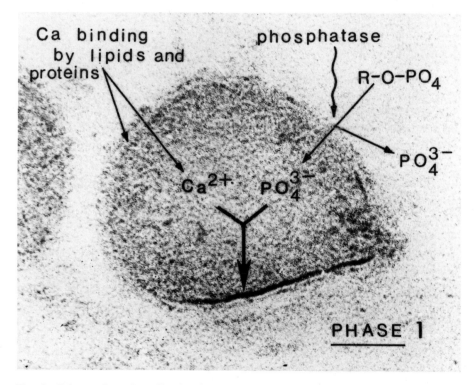

Fig. 3. Scheme for mineralization in matrix vesicles. During phase, 1 intravesicular calcium concentration is increased by its affinity for lipids and Ca-binding proteins of the vesicle membrane interior. Phosphatase (e.g., alkaline phosphatase, pyrophosphatase, or adenosine triphosphatase) at the vesicle membrane acts upon ester phosphate of matrix or vesicle fluid to produce a local increase in PO_4 in the vicinity of the vesicle membrane. The intravesicular ionic product $[Ca^{2+}] \times [PO_{3-}^4]$ is thereby raised, resulting in initial deposition of $CaPO_4$ near the membrane. (Reprinted from ANDERSON 1978)

identified with certainty. However, recent studies have confirmed the presence in isolated MVs of the following calcium-binding proteins: calpactin (GENGE et al. 1989; MORRIS et al. 1990b), calbindin (BALMAIN et al. 1989), type X collagen (HABUCHI et al. 1985; MORRIS et al. 1991; WU et al. 1989, 1991a), and anchorin C-II (annexin V) (GENGE et al. 1990; MORRIS et al. 1991; WU et al. 1991a). The latter belongs to a family of phospholipid-dependent calcium-binders known as the annexins (CRUMPTON and DEDMAN 1990). Calpactin II (annexin I) and anchorin CII (annexin V) have been identified in both chick and rat matrix vesicles (GENGE et al. 1989, 1990; MORRIS et al. 1991). In the case of annexin V, a recent paper indicates that this protein is intimately associated with the formation of calcium channels across acidic phospholipid bilayer membranes (ROJAS et al. 1990). Given that matrix vesicles are involved in the initial nucleation of calcium phosphate, the presence of this protein delineates a mechanism by which calcium could enter vesicles in a regulated manner. These calcium-binding proteins provide an additional calcium attracting force into MVs.

Other proteins which have been identified in isolated MVs include actin (MUHLRAD et al. 1983; MORRIS et al. 1990b), lactate dehydrogenase (OHASHI-TAKAUSHI et al. 1990), the proteoglycan link protein, and the hyaluronic acid-binding region of proteoglycan (WU et al. 1991b). It has also recently been shown that MVs contain carbonic anhydrase (MORRIS et al. 1990b; STECHSCHULTE et al. 1992). The latter may be linked to a proton-transporting mechanism, as discussed below in the section on "the ionic milieu at calcification sites."

IV. Biphasic Hypothesis of Mineralization-Crystal Initiation Phase

Given all of the above facts now known about MV structure and composition, a biphasic mineralization mechanism is envisioned (Figs. 3, 4). Phase I is the period during which the first mineral is formed, primarily along the inner leaflet of the MV membrane (Fig. 3). Ca^{2+} is attracted to the MV by the aforementioned calcium-binding phospholipids and by the various calcium-binding proteins (calpactin, calbindin, type X collagen). Earlier evidence suggests that calpactin would normally be concentrated beneath the membrane while calbindin would be expected to be dissolved in the vesicle sap. A local increase in PO_4^{3-} (either bound or unbound) is accomplished by phosphatase, including ALP, residing in the vesicle membrane. Phosphatase activity increases as MVs approach the mineralization front (MATSUZAWA and ANDERSON 1971).

The exact role of ALP in promoting calcification is probably as much debated now as it was when the enzyme was first shown by Robison in the 1920s to be associated with mineralization (ROBISON 1923). Proposed mechanisms of ALP action include: (1) hydrolysis of ester phosphate in the ECF or vesicle sap to yield orthophosphate for incorporation into nascent $CaPO_4$ mineral; (2) translocation of PO_4 from a donor molecule, e.g., nucleoside

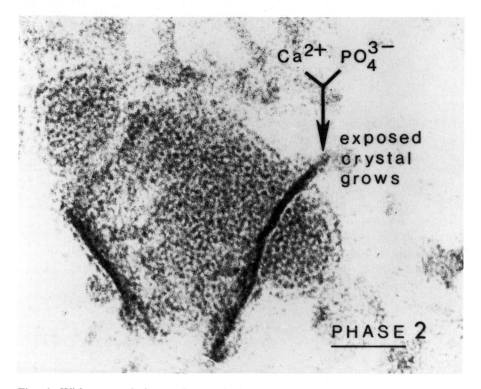

Fig. 4. With accumulation and growth, intravesicular crystals are exposed to the extravesicular environment. Phase 2 begins with exposure of preformed apatite crystals to extravesicular fluid, which in normal animals is supersaturated with respect to apatite, enabling further crystal proliferation to take place. Matrix vesicles pictured are in rat growth plate cartilage. (Reprinted from ANDERSON 1978)

triphosphate in ECF or vesicle sap to a receptor molecule, e.g., nascent $CaPO_4$ mineral, by phosphotransferase activity (ARSENIS et al. 1976); (3) hydrolysis of pyrophosphate (PPi), a known inhibitor of apatite crystal growth, into two orthophosphate (Pi) molecules which, in turn, can be utilized in the formation of nascent mineral (ANDERSON and REYNOLDS 1973), and (4) the ALP of MVs, which has been shown to bind to type II and X collagen (WU et al. 1991a), and is located mostly on the outer surface of the MV membrane, may create a bridge or "nexus" across which mineral propagation can occur from initial mineralization sites in MVs to secondary mineralization sites in adjacent collagen. Other MV phosphatases that can regulate mineralization are Ca^{2+}/Mg^{2+}-ATPase, known to be associated with an outwardly directed Ca^{2+} pump and shown recently to vanish from the MV just prior to the appearance of mineral (AKISAKA and GAY 1985b), and nucleoside triphosphate pyrophosphohydrolase (NTPPase), which cleaves ATP to AMP plus PPi. PPi is known to have a dual action: (1) promoting the very first stages of mineralization in MVs through its hydrolysis by ALP, thus providing PO_4 for nascent mineral formation (Anderson and Reynolds 1973) and (2) inhibiting mineral propagation by a crystal-poisoning effect, after initial mineral has formed (Fleisch and Bisaz 1962; Francis et al. 1969). Thus phase I of mineralization is accomplished by a complex interaction between calcium-binding molecules and phosphate-metabolizing enzymes residing in or near the MV membrane. The membrane provides a protected microenvironment in which Ca^{2+} and PO_4^{3-} can be concentrated, localized, and interacted to form the first, rather unstable, nuclei of mineral (Sauer and Wuthier 1988). Once thesse nuclei are transformed into HA, a protective microenvironment is no longer required and actually serves as an impediment to mineral propagation. At this point crystals penetrate the MV membrane (Anderson 1969; Eanes and Hailer 1985).

V. Biphasic Hypothesis of Mineralization-Crystal Growth Phase

Phase II commences with exposure of preformed mineral to the ECF surrounding MVs (Fig. 4). In the absence of apatite, cartilage fluid contains insufficient Ca and PO_4 to initiate mineral deposition, but when presented with preformed apatite from MVs, active crystal proliferation is anticipated, given levels of Ca^{2+} and PO_4^{3-} which are normal for cartilage fluid (Howell et al. 1968; Wuthier 1977).

Figure 4 indicates that rigid HA crystals actually penetrate or perforate the vesicle lipid bilayer. A good deal of electron microscopic evidence suggests that such a perforation occurs. Recently, this supposition has been strengthened by the experimental work of Eanes and Hailer (1985) in which HA is induced to form and to accumulate within artificially produced liposomes. In Eanes' experimental model, the intravesicular HA crystals ultimately perforate their investing liposomal membranes. Exposure of HA to the extraliposomal fluid leads to a rapid proliferation of extravesicular HA, both in vivo and in vitro.

The rate of phase 2 calcification is controlled by matrix components which can accelerate or retard mineral propagation (see Table 1). Seed crystals, provided by matrix vesicles, serve as templates for new crystal proliferation in what is essentially a physicochemical process. The rate of

Table 1. Molecules governing rate of mineral proliferation

Promoters	Inhibitors
Physiologic Ca^{2+} and PO_4^{3-}	Low Ca^{2+} and PO_4^{3-} in ECF
Collagen proteins	Ca-binding matrix
	(osteocalcin, bone sialoprotein)
Ester phosphate: ATP, AMP, βGP	Polyphosphates and PPi
(substrates for MV phosphatases)	

HA nucleation is governed by extracellular factors, for example sufficient Ca^{2+} and PO_4^{3-}, as continuously supplied in the normal ECF by homeostatic mechanisms, supports HA crystal proliferation. Collagen serves as a substratum into which mineral is deposited (ARSENAULT 1989; DUDLEY and SPIRO 1961; GLIMCHER 1954), providing a favorable environment for HA nucleation and propagation after mineralization has entered the extravesicular phase. Ester phosphates in the ECF such as ATP or PPi may be hydrolyzed at the surfaces of MVs where phosphatases are concentrated, thus providing a localized enrichment of Pi for HA crystal nucleation and proliferation. Abnormally low serum and ECF levels of Ca^{2+} and/or PO_4^{3-} in rickets (BOSKEY and TIMCHAK 1989; HOWELL et al. 1968; JOHNSON et al. 1989; YOSHIKAWA et al. 1985) tend to slow the rate of mineral proliferation. Also numerous calcium-binding proteins of the matrix have been shown to inhibit crystal proliferation in vitro. These include aggregated proteoglycans (CAMPO and ROMANO 1986; CHEN et al. 1984; CUERVO et al. 1973; DZIEWAITKOWSKI and MAJZNERSKI 1985; NEMETHCSOKA and SARKOZI 1982; SHIMIZU et al. 1991), bone Gla-protein, known as "osteocalcin" (BOSKEY et al. 1985; BOSKEY 1989; MENANTEAU et al. 1982; PRICE et al. 1976; ROMBERG et al. 1986), phosphoproteins (DESTENO and FEAGIN 1975; FUJISAWA et al. 1987; MENANTEAU et al. 1982), osteonectin (MENANTEAU et al. 1982; ROMBERG et al. 1986), and the α-2HS-glycoprotein of bone (TRIFFIT 1987). Although most studies indicate an inhibitory effect, some recent work by LINDE and LUSSI (1989) shows that if phosphoprotein, proteoglycan, or bone Gla protein are immobilized onto Sepharose beads they can actually promote HA nucleation from a physiological calcifying solution (but when in solution these same proteins inhibit apatite propagation). The effect of proteoglycans and noncollagenous matrix proteins is discussed below in Sect. E.II.

It is widely agreed that pyrophosphate and related bisphosphonates and polyphosphates can impede in vitro mineral propagation, presumably by coating preformed crystals and thus preventing their ability to nucleate new crystals (FLEISCH and BISAZ 1962; FRANCIS et al. 1969; LARSSON 1974; REGISTER and WUTHIER 1985; RUSSELL et al. 1973; SCHENK et al. 1973; TERMINE and CONN 1976). The observation that PPi is a crystal poison (FRANCIS et al. 1969) led to the development of the bisphosphonate analogs of PPi such as ethane-1-hydroxy-1, 1-diphosphonate (EHDP or etidronate) which have similar mineral inhibiting properties, but cannot be hydrolyzed and inactivated by ALP or related enzymes (FRANCIS et al. 1969; RUSSELL et al. 1973).

For obvious reasons, it is very important to the host animal to confine and direct the mineralization process toward biologically useful deposition only. Therefore only certain strategically located cells are able to initiate mineralization through the elaboration and selective placement of active matrix vesicles. When it is uncontrolled, mineralization contributes materially to the morbidity associated with important calcific diseases such as atherosclerosis, arteriosclerosis, heart valve calcifications, arthritis, cataracts, and tympanosclerosis leading to deafness (H.C. ANDERSON 1983, 1988).

Phase 2 of progressive mineralization does not rely upon the intermediation of matrix vesicles. In fact, when the matrix becomes heavily mineralized, residual matrix vesicles are buried, fragmented, and essentially destroyed by the encroachment of proliferating mineral crystals (Fig. 2) (H.C. ANDERSON 1969; REINHOLT and WERNERSON 1988). Thus matrix vesicle numbers decline in the zone of provisional calcification of the growth plate, and have not been identified in the matrix of fully mineralized bone.

D. Indirect Cellular Control of Mineralization

Not only do cells directly influence the site, rate, and type of mineralization through the synthesis and strategic placement of MVs, but they also regulate mineralization indirectly through morphogens (BMP), hormones (PTH, growth hormone, and 1,25-dihydroxyvitamin D_3), cytokines (TGFβ and FGF), the selective synthesis of matrix molecules (collagens, proteoglycans, noncollagenous calcium-binding proteins), and the regulation of the ionic milieu.

I. Effect of Bone Morphogens on the Calcification Mechanism

A morphogen is defined here as an autocrine or paracrine factor which is diffusible over short distances and initiates a specific pattern of differentiation by a population of previously undifferentiated target cells in the vicinity of the morphogen-producing cell. In bone, the classic morphogen is bone morphogenetic protein (BMP) (URIST and STRATES 1970). BMP or BMP-like morphogenetic activity resides in a variety of bone-inducing cells (H.C. ANDERSON 1990) including the apical epidermal ridge of developing limb bud (LYONS et al. 1990), bone cells (LYONS et al. 1990; TAKAOKA et al. 1982, 1989), and amniotic cells (H.C. ANDERSON et al. 1964; LYONS et al. 1990). The target cells for BMP are undifferentiated mesenchymal cells of the central limb bud (LYONS et al. 1990), pre-odontoblastic cells of the tooth bud (LYONS et al. 1990), and osteoblastic precursor cells of the bone marrow stoma (OWEN et al. 1987; TRIFFIT 1989), periosteum (TRIFFIT 1989), and skeletal muscle (HUGGINS 1931; SMITH and TRIFFIT 1986). The latter three sources of osteoprogenitor cells all contribute to the callus that reunites the broken ends of a fractured bone. In all of these situations the morphogenetic influence of BMP or related morphogens is essential in order to direct undifferentiated mesenchymal cells to become phenotypic skeletal cells. One of the most characteristic features of this pathway of osseous differentiation is the synthesis and secretion of a calcifiable matrix of cartilage, osteoid or predentin. Without the guiding influence of inducer cells secreting a morphogen, these undifferentiated mesenchymal cells of bone, cartilage, and tooth could never produce a calcifiable matrix with MVs and phosphatase.

II. Role of Growth Factors in Mineralization

A confusing picture exists at the moment with regard to the possible role(s) for the various known cytokines in promoting skeletal differentiation and calcification. Opposing effects have been reported for several cytokines depending upon which cultured skeletal cell type was chosen as the test subject. Nevertheless, it seems likely that certain cytokines are involved at least in promoting the proliferation of mesenchymal cells that are committed to a pathway of skeletal differentiation. Transforming growth factor-β (TGFβ) is present in very high quantities in bone (SEYEDIN et al. 1986). It has been shown to both promote and inhibit cell division and differentiation of immature skeletal cells (ANTOSZ et al. 1989; MUNDY and BONEWALD 1990; ROBEY et al. 1987; ROZIER et al. 1989). When placed near the periosteum it stimulates not only periosteal cell division but also the accumulation of new bone from osteoblastic cells (HOCK et al. 1990; JOYCE et al. 1990; MARCELLI et al. 1990). As the picture of how these cytokines work in vivo becomes more clear, some of them will likely be shown to regulate cell division and differentiation of osteoprogenitor cells. A change in numbers of cells programmed to make a calcifiable matrix can have an important, cell-mediated effect on the economy or balance of skeletal tissues.

III. Hormones That Affect Calcification

Although many hormones affect the growth and metabolism of skeletal cells, and through them calcification, the regulatory effects of growth hormone (GH), parathyroid hormone (PTH), and 1,25-OH$_2$ vitamin D$_3$ (1,25-OH$_2$D$_3$) are probably best understood.

Growth hormone (GH) is known to promote bone growth by stimulating the growth plate. However, an increased growth rate is thought not to be brought about by the direct effect of GH on cells of the growth plate and metaphysis, but rather through the formation of somatomedins which in turn stimulate the synthesis of cartilage matrix (NILSSON et al. 1987; VANWYK et al. 1974). In recent years it has been determined that somatomedins B and C are the same as epidermal growth factor and insulin-like growth factor I (IGF I) respectively (HELDIN et al. 1981; KLAPPER et al. 1983) and that a third somatomedin known as "multiplication-stimulating activity" (MSA) is the same as IGF II (MARQUARDT and TODARO 1981). The two IGFs have overlapping activities, with both being capable of stimulating both the growth of chondrocytes and the phenotypic expression of chondrocytes (LUYTEN et al. 1988) and osteoblasts (VAN WYK 1988).

Parathyroid hormone is known to have an anabolic effect upon bone cells, increasing their numbers, increasing the amount of osteoid secretion available for calcification, and increasing the osteoblast ALP activity. The latter finds its way into MVs as well as into the circulation (GUNNESS-HEY and HOCK 1984; HOCK et al. 1987; PARSONS 1976; PLIAM et al. 1982). PTH also exerts a second influence on mineralization by increasing Ca^{2+} levels in the ECF. PTH raises serum Ca^{2+} by promoting bone resorption with the release of stored Ca^{2+} and by promoting Ca^{2+} absorption from the gut (by stimulating the synthesis of $1,25\text{-}OH_2D_3$). Although PTH reduces serum PO_4^{3-} levels by increasing the renal excretion of PO_4 (PARSONS 1976), the concomitant increase in serum Ca^{2+} ion brought about by PTH usually exceeds the decrease in PO_4^{3-}, thus rendering the serum and ECF somewhat more saturated with regard to these two ions. Metastatic calcification is a frequent clinical complication of a PTH-induced elevation of $[Ca^{2+}] \times [PO_4^{3-}]$. There is also a marked increase in the number of renal stones generated by patients with hyperparathyroidism, as well as frequent pathological calcification seen in lung, stomach, and kidney.

IV. Pathological Calcification

It is not the intent of this review to discuss the mechanism of pathological calcification to any depth; however, suffice it to say at this point that virtually all forms of pathological calcification (both metastatic and dystrophic types) begin with an initial deposition of $CaPO_4$ mineral within or upon membrane-bounded subcellular particles. Dystrophic calcification occurs when ischemic or devitalized cells can no longer exclude Ca^{2+} from their cytoplasm. Thus cytosolic Ca accumulates resulting in $CaPO_4$ deposits in the mitochondria (H.C. ANDERSON 1983; JENNINGS et al. 1975). A little later in the agonal struggle of ischemic cells, vesiculation of the plasma membrane occurs, followed by overt cell rupture with dispersal of membrane vesicles into the extracellular space. The latter vesicles also initiate calcification (H.C. ANDERSON 1985, 1988). In metastatic calcification (as opposed to dystrophic calcification discussed above), high ECF Ca^{2+} promotes the entry of abnormal amounts of Ca^{2+} into the cytosol. At first mitochondria sequester massive amounts of $CaPO_4$. Then the damaged cell disrupts, as in dystrophic calcification, with dispersal of calcifiable vesicular cell debris into the ECF. The following generalizations can be made about pathological calcification: (1) the form of $CaPO_4$ mineral that accumulates at the microscopic site of initial calcification is almost always HA regardless of the tissue involved; (2) intracellular pathological calcification begins in mitochondria; (3) extracellular pathological calcification begins in exfoliated membranous vesicles which may calcify by a mechanism analogous to that of matrix vesicles of normal skeletal tissue (MORRIS et al. 1990c; TANIMURA et al. 1983); (4) in virtually every instance of pathological calcification, mineral deposition is initiated by the action of a biological membrane; and (5) the rate of pathological calcification will be governed by the availability of Ca^{2+} and PO_4^{3-} in the ECF, which in turn is manifestly affected by serum levels of PTH.

V. Vitamin D

We have chosen to discuss the calcification effects of only one of the metabolically active analogs of vitamin D, $1,25\text{-}OH_2D_3$, because this form of the vitamin is the most completely studied with regard to mineralizing systems. $1,25\text{-}OH_2D_3$ can promote mineralization in several different ways. First, as discussed above, $1,25\text{-}OH_2D_3$ is the most potent form of vitamin D for promoting absorption of Ca^{2+} from the gut (DeLuca 1985; Lawson et al. 1971). As indicated above, the unopposed effect of $1,25\text{-}OH_2D_3$ is to increase serum and ECF levels of Ca^{2+}, through Ca^{2+} absorption, thus raising the ion product of $[Ca^{2+}] \times [PO_4^{3-}]$ and favoring the deposition of $CaPO_4$ mineral in bones and soft tissues. In chickens, a failure of calcification can be caused by a deficiency of vitamin D alone (Boyde and Shapiro 1987; Crenshaw et al. 1974; Dickson et al. 1984; Jande and Dickson 1980) in which case serum Ca^{2+} falls, creating reduced $[Ca^{2+}] \times [PO_4^{3-}]$. In rats, lowering the serum PO_4^{3-} is the most effective way to induce rickets (Yendt and Howard 1955).

The question of whether $1,25\text{-}OH_2D_3$ has a direct effect upon bone has been debated for a long time. However, recent evidence indicates that $1,25\text{-}OH_2D_3$ can promote the differentiation (Tsonis 1991) and calcification of growth plate cartilage by augmenting ALP expression in cartilage cells and matrix vesicles (Boyan et al. 1988; Franceschi and Young 1990). $1,25\text{-}OH_2D_3$ is presumed to operate by activation of intranuclear receptors in cartilage and bone cells (Fine et al. 1985; Narbaitz et al. 1983; Tsonis 1991). After activation, increased expression of ALP results from an increased transcription of message for ALP (Franceschi and Young 1990). The fact that $1,25\text{-}OH_2D_3$ exposure can also increase ALP activity in isolated matrix vesicles (Boyan et al. 1988) implies a direct effect of the hormone upon ALP of the MV membrane since no nuclear receptors or signal transduction mechanism would be available to $1,25\text{-}OH_2D_3$ at the MV level.

E. Cellular Regulation of the Composition and Mineralizing Potential of Matrix

I. Collagen

Collagen, type I, is the predominant form of collagen in mineralizing matrix of bone, tendon, and dentin, and it has been known for a long time that type I collagen can and does calcify during mineralization (Acenzi et al. 1965; Dudley and Spiro 1961). During calcification, type I collagen fibrils are infiltrated by deposits of plate-like HA with the long axis of the crystallites rotating with respect to the long axis of the collagen fibril (Arsenault 1989). It has been suggested that the pattern of deposition of

HA crystallites is in register with the 640 Å major banding repeat in type I collagen (Dudley and Spiro 1961; Glimcher 1954; Robinson and Watson 1952); however, recent work by Arsenault in mineralizing turkey tendon raises doubt about this hypothesis (Arsenault 1989, 1991). His findings suggest a significant lack of conformity between the "hole zone" of the axial repeat of quarter-staggered collagen molecules, and the distribution of HA crystallites within collagen fibrils. Nevertheless, it is clear that collagen type I is a preferential site for the growth of HA crystals during progressive mineralization of bone matrix. It is also clear that cells in general do not secrete type I collagen in order to initiate mineralization at selected sites, since type I collagen is the most common form of collagen throughout the body, and it usually does not mineralize. This points up the permissive rather than initiating role of collagen in the mineralization mechanism, and it should be noted that collagen has never been found to be an active nucleator of HA in vitro.

The same permissive function in mineralization seems to be exhibited by the type II collagen which predominates in cartilage. Electron microscopy of growth plate has shown convincingly that HA deposition begins within matrix vesicles, then continues at the surfaces of matrix vesicles and finally spreads to involve adjacent type II collagen fibrils (Fig. 1) (Akisaka et al. 1988; H.C. Anderson 1969; Gay et al. 1978; Morris et al. 1983). The nature of the molecular bridge or nexus between MVs and the adjacent cartilage matrix has been studied recently. Wuthier and colleagues have shown that there is a binding affinity between ALP, which resides mostly at the outer surfaces of MVs, and type II collagen (Wu et al. 1989). Furthermore, significant binding affinities have been demonstrated between calpactin and anchorin CII, both membrane-associated proteins of MVs, and collagens type I, II, and X (Wu et al. 1991a). Morris et al. have shown by EM immunocytochemistry that both anchorin CII and collagen type X can be identified in the vicinity of the MV membrane surface, thus supporting the suggestion that MVs are bonded to the matrix by the interaction of these molecules (Morris et al. 1991).

Poole and colleagues have proposed a calcification-promoting activity for the C-propeptide fraction of type II collagen (Hinek et al. 1987; Poole et al. 1984), which was initially designated "chondrocalcin," because it was found to be associated with mineral deposits by light and electron microscopic immunocytochemistry. However, the C-propeptide is known to be a Ca-binding peptide, and so it was never quite certain whether it initiated mineral or whether it was simply adsorbed to $CaPO_4$ mineral after HA deposition had begun. As with other forms of collagen, no convincing data have been put forward to indicate that the C-propeptide can initiate calcification from a physiologic calcium phosphate solution. One wonders whether the C-propeptide might be found to inhibit in vitro calcification after the fashion of other Ca-binding proteins of skeletal matrix such as osteocalcin (Boskey et al. 1985; Boskey 1989).

Type X collagen is a low molecular weight nonfibrillar peptide found almost exclusively in the hypertrophic and calcifying cartilage matrix of the growth plate (GIBSON et al. 1986; REGINATO et al. 1986; SCHMID and LINSENMAYER 1985; SOLURSH et al. 1986). Immunocytochemistry indicated that type X collagen is especially concentrated in MVs (HABUCHI et al. 1985). The only evidence to date that type X collagen may promote calcification has been circumstantial, i.e., the selective binding of type X into hypertrophic matrix which ultimately will calcify. To our knowledge, purified type X has never been shown to initiate or accelerate HA deposition from a calcifying solution. Recent studies have confirmed the presence of significant quantities of type X in fractions of isolated growth plate MVs (MORRIS et al. 1991; WU et al. 1989). Immunogold studies using an antimammalian type X antibody to localize type X in growth plate by electron microscopy show it is distributed rather diffusely throughout the matrix of hypertrophic cartilage, and that, although apparently not concentrated within MVs, type X is at least in contact with the MV membrane in vivo, and could serve as a bridging molecule to promote the spread of mineral into the matrix (MORRIS et al. 1991).

II. Proteoglycans and Noncollagenous Proteins of Matrix

Whether proteoglycans of cartilage and bone matrix promote or inhibit mineralization is a debate which began in the 1950s when Sobel put forward his hypothesis that calcification requires mucoprotein as a "calcium concentrating mechanism" (SOBEL et al. 1960), and continues up to the present (BUCKWALTER 1987; CAMPO and ROMANO 1986; CAMPO and BETZ 1987; CHEN et al. 1984; CUERVO et al. 1973; HUNTER 1987; NEMETHCZOKA and SARKOZI 1982; POOLE et al. 1982; SHIMIZU et al. 1991). Some facts appear to be well established including the following: (1) acidic proteoglycans tend to inhibit in vitro mineralization (CAMPO and BETZ 1987; CHEN et al. 1984; CUERVO et al. 1973; DZIEWAITKOWSKI and MAJZNERSKI 1985; NEMETHCSOKA and SARKOZI 1982) and the inhibitory effect is related to the degree of proteoglycan aggregation (CAMPO and ROMANO 1986; CHEN et al. 1984; CUERVO et al. 1973; FRANZEN et al. 1982; LOHMANDER and HJERPE 1975). (2) Proteoglycans of the growth plate become less aggregated as they approach the mineralization front (BUCKWALTER 1987; CAMPO and ROMANO 1986; FRANZEN et al. 1982; LOHMANDER and HJERPE 1975). The assertion that there is an overall decrease in proteoglycan content at the mineralization front (HIRSCHMAN and DZIEWAITKOWSKI 1966) is still debated (BUCKWALTER 1987; POOLE et al. 1982). A consensus view of how proteoglycans function in mineralization might be construed as follows. Proteoglycans, in general, retard mineral propagation in areas of matrix that do not normally calcify such as the upper growth plate. Conversely, an inherently low content of large proteoglycan aggregates as in osteoid of newly formed bone would promote the more rapid calcification of bone. In growth plate regions destined for calcification, the cellular release of proteases from hypertrophic and/or degenerating chondrocytes partially degrades proteoglycans (Shimizu et al. 1991) to smaller aggregates with fewer glycosaminoglycan residues (Lohmander and Hjerpe 1975; Shimizu et al. 1991), thus locally reducing their calcification-inhibiting effect without necessarily altering the total concentration of proteoglycan sulfate. Finally, at sites of active mineralization where local ECF concentrations of Ca^{2+} are high, further proteoglycan removal may be accomplished by calcium ion, since the latter is known to be a good solvent for proteoglycans (Anderson and Sajdera 1971; Sajdera and Hascall 1969). In this scenario, cartilage cells and bone cells would initially prevent mineralization by secreting mineral-inhibiting proteoglycans for assimilation into the upper growth plate matrix. Later these same cells would promote mineralization at desired sites in the lower growth plate by the selective local release of proteoglycan-degrading enzymes (C.C. Brown et al. 1989; Ehrlich et al. 1985; Granda and Posner 1971; Shimizu et al. 1991).

Noncollagenous proteins of the matrix that may regulate mineral propagation have been discussed briefly above. Most of these proteins are calcium binding and the balance of evidence suggests that when adsorbed to mineral deposits they do not promote mineralization, and often are inhibitory to the growth of mineral. The list of these proteins is growing and includes the following: bone gla-protein (osteocalcin) (Hauschka et al. 1975; Price et al. 1976), matrix gla-protein (Price and Williamson 1985), osteonectin (SPARC protein) (Bolander et al. 1988; Termine et al. 1981), osteopontin and related sialoproteins (Butler 1989; Reinholt et al. 1990; Triffit 1987; Young et al. 1990), phosphoproteins including phosphophoryn (Glimcher 1989; Veis and Perry 1967), α_2-HS-glycoprotein (Triffit 1987), the acidic glycoprotein (BAG-75) recently described by Gorski et al. (1990), thrombospondin (Robey et al. 1989), and chondronectin (Varner et al. 1986). The specific metabolic role(s) of these proteins remain unclear. Studies of animals which are severely deficient in bone gla-protein indicate no defect in the calcification mechanism (Lian et al. 1984; Price and Nishimoto 1980). This is not necessarily the case for the other proteins cited above, but it does point up the fact that a role in mineralization has been suggested for all of them, but never convincingly documented for any of them. It has been suggested by Price and Sloper (1983) that osteocalcin's function may be to oppose net calcium loss from the bone surfaces under-going resorption. One may speculate that bone gla-protein functions as a mineral stabilizer, inhibiting both the accretion of new HA crystals and the resorption of existing mineral.

III. Control of Angiogenesis

Angiogenesis factor(s) that promote the ingrowth of capillaries into the mineralizing growth plate may play an important role in regulating the ionic composition of the ECF at the calcification front. An increased presence of

FGF, a known angiogenic factor, in the lower hypertrophic zone matrix has been revealed by immunocytochemistry (JINGUISHI et al. 1989). Recent work of R.A. BROWN et al. (1987) and McFARLAND et al. (1990) shows that chondrocytes at the base of the growth plate elaborate a nonprotein endothelial cell stimulating factor (ESAF) of low molecular weight that promotes the ingrowth of metaphyseal capillaries through the activation of procollagenase. Stimulating the ingrowth of capillaries into the mineralization front by elaboration of ESAF is yet another way that cartilage cells can regulate mineralization in their immediate environment. Mineralization would be promoted by: (1) ESAF-stimulated collagenolytic activity releasing collagen-anchored Ca-binding proteoglycans and thus reducing the diffusion barrier to Ca^{2+} and PO_4^{3-} from approaching capillaries; and (2) by stimulating capillary ingrowth into the mineralization front, thus narrowing the distance across which Ca^{2+} and PO_4^{3-} must diffuse in order to participate in mineral formation.

IV. Cellular Regulation of the Ionic Milieu at Calcification Sites

The rate of mineral formation is critically related to the regulation of phosphate levels in the ECF. HOWELL et al. (1968) and WUTHIER (1977) have found that cartilage matrix fluid levels of unbound, ultrafiltrable inorganic Ca and PO_4 in growth plate ECF are metastable with respect to $CaPO_4$ mineral, meaning that at these concentrations (and the slightly alkaline pH known to be present) spontaneous precipitation of $CaPO_4$ would not normally occur, but if nuclei of HA are added to such a metastable solution they will seed HA crystal formation as long as Ca and Pi are constantly supplied (as by the blood stream).

The mechanism by which cells maintain $[Ca^{2+}] \times [PO_4^{3-}]$ metastability in cartilage and bone ECF is not fully understood; however, it is known that a significant source of intracellular and extracellular inorganic phosphate (Pi) is derived from the breakdown of ATP and other nucleoside triphosphates. A key enzyme in this metabolic pathway is nucleoside triphosphate pyrophosphatase (NTPPase), which catalyzes the hydrolysis of ATP to AMP and pyrophosphate (PPi) (HSU 1983; SIEGEL et al. 1983). This process occurs intracellularly in mitochondria and also at the cell surface of chondrocytes and matrix vesicles (CASWELL and RUSSELL 1985). Probably not much PPi accumulates at the mineralization front because it is quickly broken down to orthophosphate (Pi) by ecto-alkaline phosphatase and/or inorganic pyrophosphatase. The latter two phosphatases are concentrated at the membrane surfaces of chondrocytes and matrix vesicles near the mineralization front, and may actually represent the activity of only one enzyme, ALP, which is capable of hydrolyzing PPi as well as other ester phosphates (such as β-GP). The latter substrate is commonly used in vitro to demonstrate ALP activity. PPi formation and catabolism is as follows.

$$
\begin{array}{c}
\text{ATP} \\
\text{CTP} \\
\text{GTP} \\
\text{UTP}
\end{array}
\xrightarrow{\text{NTPPase}}
\begin{array}{c}
\text{AMP} \\
\text{CMP} \\
\text{GMP} \\
\text{UMP}
\end{array}
+ \text{PPi} \xrightarrow{\text{ALP}} 2\text{Pi}
$$

Through this mechanism cells can raise the local ECF concentration of Pi thus increasing the likelihood of its incorporation into nascent CaPO$_4$ mineral which is growing in the adjacent matrix. (For a recent review of interactivity of ALP and NTPPase at the cell surface see CASWELL et al. 1991.)

Pyrophosphate seems to have a dual role in mineralization. During initial stages of mineralization in matrix vesicles of developing chick bone the addition of micromolar (physiologic) quantities of PPi stimulate mineralization (ANDERSON and REYNOLDS 1973; FLEISCH et al. 1966). However, after crystal initiation, during the mineral propagation phase, PPi at somewhat higher concentrations retards mineral propagation (ANDERSON and REYNOLDS 1973; FLEISCH et al. 1966) presumably by coating preformed crystals and thus preventing their growth in the extracellular space (FRANCIS et al. 1969; FLEISCH and BISAZ 1962). By hydrolyzing PPi, ALP at the MV surface promotes mineralization in two ways: (1) by providing a supply of Pi for crystal initiation and (2) by preventing "crystal poisoning" as caused by PPi which can retard crystal growth. It should be recognized that, in addition to PPi being supplied by cells at the mineralization front, it is also supplied in constant micromolar amounts in the blood and ECF. This homeostatically regulated, constant low-level supply of PPi throughout the body is believed to reflect a universal degradative pathway for ATP. Through the circulation of PPi, MVs involved in initiating mineralization are provided a limitless supply of PPi, available at precisely the micromolar concentration that has been shown in vitro to augment mineral initiation.

What other phosphate ester substrates would be available to cells and matrix vesicles for utilization in mineralization? In cells, the ATP level is probably high, i.e., in the millimolar range, but this is not where mineralization begins. It is speculated that the failure to hydrolyze significant quantities of ATP to PPi and thence to Pi may be partially due to the outward orientation of NTPPase and ALP at the cell and vesicle membrane which would make intracellular substrate inaccessible to these ectoenzymes (CASWELL et al. 1991; FEDDE et al. 1988). Another factor which might retard intracellular mineralization would be the high cytosolic concentration of ATP and PPi, both of which are known to coat apatite crystals and thereby inhibit crystal propagation.

The level of ATP and/or other nucleosides in the ECF of calcifying cartilage is approximately 1–2 mM, which is approximately ten times serum levels (HOWELL et al. 1968; WUTHIER 1977). The level of ATP in the sap of MVs is unknown, but could reflect high intracellular levels since the MVs appear to bud from the surfaces of skeletal cells (AKISAKA and GAY 1985a;

CECIL ANDERSON 1978; WUTHIER et al. 1978) and presumably would carry cytosolic levels of ATP into the matrix. The "leakiness" of MV membranes for ATP and other nucleosides is unknown. If the MVs were sufficiently leaky, they might lower internal ATP to levels that would permit intra-vesicular calcification, while at the same time releasing ATP to be used as substrate for phosphatases producing PPi and Pi at the surfaces of MVs. Control of ATP leakiness is another way that cells can indirectly influence the calcification rate through matrix vesicles.

V. Control of pH

Control of pH is yet another mechanism by which cells and MVs can regulate their local milieu to favor or inhibit calcification. The distribution and relative activity of carbonic anhydrase (CAH) is important in this regard. Hypertrophic chondrocytes of the growth plate and isolated matrix vesicles are known to be very enriched in carbonic anhydrase II (MORRIS et al. 1990b; STECHSCHULTE et al. 1992), an isoenzyme of CAH that vigorously catalyzes the reaction:

$$CO_2 + H_2O \xrightarrow{\text{CAH}} H_2CO_3 \rightarrow H^+ + HCO_3^-$$

in which the dissociation of carbonic acid (H_2CO_3) to H^+ + HCO_3^- is nonenzymatic.

Two forms of CAH-II exist: one is soluble and distributed diffusely throughout the cytosol; the second is concentrated under the plasma membrane (R.E. ANDERSON et al. 1982; GAY and MULLER 1974; GAY et al. 1974, 1982, 1984; VAANANEN 1984). In chick osteoclasts, whose bone resorptive activities include the extracellular release of protons (H^+) to dissolve HA at sites of bone resorption, CAH is concentrated just under the membrane of the ruffled border (R.E. ANDERSON et al. 1982; GAY et al. 1984), where its activity may be coupled with a proton-exporting mechanism (proton pump) that is located at the ruffled border (BARON 1989; VAANANEN 1984; VAANANEN et al. 1988, 1990).

It is probably safe to assume that MV CAH resides in the vesicle sap under the MV membrane. Whether CAH has an important function in MV mineralization remains to be documented. Nevertheless, it is interesting to speculate on how CAH might function in proton transport at the initial mineralization site just under the MV membrane. One set of speculations relates to the chemical steps in HA formation: during the hydroxylation of a unit cell of HA, two hydroxyls are incorporated into each HA molecule and two H^+ ions released. The resulting acid formation must somehow be neutralized or dissipated in order to stabilize the HA structure, since HA is highly soluble even in weak acid. The buffering capacity of the MV sap is unknown but could be regulated by CAH. It is conceivable that CAH could be linked to an outwardly directed proton transport mechanism excluding

H^+ ions from the internum of the vesicle during the critical early stages of nascent HA formation. CAH is known to promote calcium carbonate mineral formation in invertebrates, and in avian egg shell formation (Gay et al. 1974; Giraud 1977; Isenburg et al. 1963; Kingsley and Watanabe 1987), but its role in $CaPO_4$ mineralization remains to be clarified. Given the increased activity of CAH at the mineralization front in growth plate (Gay et al. 1982; Vaananen 1984) and its presence in MVs we feel it is likely that CAH will be found to play a role in cell-mediated calcification.

References

Acenzi A, Bonucci E, Bocciarelli DS (1965) An electron microscope study of osteon calcification. J Ultrastruct Res 12:287–303

Akisaka T, Gay CV (1985a) The plasma membrane and matrix vesicles of mouse growth plate chondrocytes during differentiation as revealed in freeze-fracture replicas. Am J Anat 173:269–286

Akisaka T, Gay CV (1985b) Ultrastructural localization of calcium-activated adenosine tri-phosphatase (Ca^{2+}-ATPase) in growth plate cartilage. J Histochem Cytochem 33:925–932

Akisaka T, Gay CV (1986) Ultrastructural demonstration of p-nitrophenyl phosphatase (p-NPPase) activity in the epiphyseal growth plate. Acta Histochem Cytochem 19:21–29

Akisaka T, Subita GP, Shiginaga Y (1986) Ultrastructural observations on chick bone processed by quick freezing and freeze-substitution. Cell Tissue Res 247:469–475

Akisaka T, Kawaguchi H, Subita GP, Shigenaga Y, Gay CV (1988) Ultrastructure of matrix vesicles in chick growth plate as revealed by quick freezing and freeze-substition. Calcif Tissue Int 42:383–393

Ali SY, Evans L (1973) The uptake of [^{45}Ca] calcium ions by matrix vesicles isolated from calcifying cartilage. Biochem J 134:647–650

Ali SY, Sajdera SW, Anderson HC (1970) Isolation and characterization of calcifying matrix vesicles from epiphyseal cartilage. Proc Natl Acad Sci USA 67:1513–1520

Ali SY, Gray JC, Wisby A, Phillips M (1977) Preparation of thin cryosections for electron probe analysis of calcifying cartilage. J Microsc 111:65–76

Anderson HC (1969) Vesicles associated with calcification in the matrix of epiphyseal cartilage. J Cell Biol 41:59–72

Anderson HC (1976) Osteogenetic epithelial – mesenchymal cell interactions. Clin Orthop 119:211–224

Anderson HC (1978) Introduction to the second conference on matrix vesicle calcification. Metab Bone Dis Rel Res 1:83–88

Anderson HC (1983) Calcific diseases: a concept. Arch Pathol Lab Med 107:341–348

Anderson HC (1985) Matrix vesicle calcification: review and update. In: Peck WA (ed) Bone and mineral research, vol 2. Elsevier, New York, pp 109–149

Anderson HC (1988) Mechanisms of pathologic calcification. Rheum Clin North Am 14:303–319

Anderson HC (1989) Mechanism of mineral formation in bone. Lab Invest 60:320–330

Anderson HC (1990) The role of cells versus matrix in bone induction. Connect Tiss Res 24:3–12

Anderson HC, Hsu HHT (1978) A new method to measure ^{45}Ca accumulation by matrix vesicles in slices of rachitic growth plate cartilage. Metab Bone Dis Rel Res 1:193–198

Anderson HC, Reynolds JJ (1973) Pyrophosphate stimulation of initial mineralization in cultured embryonic bones. Fine structure of matrix vesicles and their role in mineralization. Dev Biol 34:211–227

Anderson HC, Sajdera SW (1971) Fine structure of bovine nasal cartilage. Extraction as a technique to study proteoglycans and collagen in cartilage matrix. J Cell Biol 49:650–663

Anderson HC, Sajdera SW (1976) Calcification of rachitic cartilage to study matrix vesicle function. Fed Proc 35:148–153

Anderson HC, Merker PC, Fogh J (1964) Formation of tumors containing bone after intramuscular injection of transformed human amnion cells (FL) into cortisone-treated mice. Am J Pathol 44:507–519

Anderson HC, Matsuzawa T, Sajdera SW, Ali SY (1970) Membranous particles in calcifying cartilage matrix. Trans N Y Acad Sci (Series II) 32:619–630

Anderson HC, Cecil R, Sajdera SW (1975) Calcification of rachitic rat cartilage in vitro by extracellular matrix vesicles. Am J Pathol 79:237–255

Anderson HC, Stechschulte DJ Jr, Collins E, Jacobs D, Morris DC, Hsu HHT, Redford P, Zeiger J (1990) Matrix vesicle biogenesis in vitro by rachitic and normal rat chondrocytes. Am J Pathol 136:391–398

Anderson HC, Kanabe S, Vaananan HK, Oppliger I, Morris DC, Bohn WW, Hsu HHT (1984) Phosphatases and matrix vesicle calcification. In: Cohn DV, Potts JT, Fujita T (eds) Endocrine control of bone and calcium metabolism. Elsevier, Amsterdam, pp 410–413

Anderson RE, Schraer H, Gay CV (1982) Ultrastructural immunocytochemical localization of carbonic anhydrase in normal and calcitonin-treated chick osteoclasts. Anat Rec 204:9–20

Antosz ME, Bellows CG, Aubin JE (1989) Effects of transforming growth factor β and epidermal growth factor on cell proliferation and the formation of bone nodules in isolated fetal rat calvaria cells. J Cell Physiol 140:386–395

Arsenault AL (1989) A comparative electron microscopic study of apatite cyrstals in collagen fibrils of rat bone, dentin and calcified turkey leg tendons. Bone Miner 6:165–177

Arsenault AL (1991) Vectorial sequence of mineralization in the turkey leg tendon determined by electron microscopic imaging. Calcif Tissue Int 48:46–55

Arsenis C, Hackett MH, Huang S-M (1976) Resolution specificity and transphosphorylase activity of calcifying cartilage alkaline phosphatases. Calcif Tissue Res 20:159–171

Balmain N, Holton P, Cuisinier-Gleizes P, Mathieu H (1989) Immunoreactive calbindin-D9K localization in matrix vesicle initiated calcification in rat epiphyseal cartilage: an immunoelectron microscopic study. J Bone Miner Res 4:565–575

Baron R (1989) Molecular mechanisms of bone resorption by the osteoclast. Anat Rec 224:317–324

Bellows CG, Aubin JE, Heersch JNM (1991) Initiation and progression of mineralization of bone nodules formed in vitro: the role of alkaline phosphatase and organic phosphate. Bone Miner 14:27–40

Bernard GW (1972) Ultrastructural observations of initial calcification in dentin and enamel. J Ultrastruct Res 41:1–17

Bernard GW (1978) Ultrastructural localization of alkaline phosphatase in initial intramembranous ossification. Clin Orthop 135:218–225

Bohn WW, Stein RM, Hsu HHT, Morris DC, Anderson HC (1984) Isolation of a plasma membrane-enriched fraction from collagenase suspended rachitic rat growth plate chondrocytes. J Orthop Res 1:319–324

Bolander ME, Young MF, Fisher LW, Yamada Y, Termine JD (1988) Osteonectin cDNA sequence reveals potential binding regions for calcium and hydroxyapatite and shows homologies with both a basement membrane protein (SPARC) and a serine proteinase inhibitor (OVOMUCOID). Proc Natl Acad Sci USA 85:2919–2923

Bonucci E (1970) Fine structure and histochemistry of calcifying globules in epiphyseal cartilage. Z Zellforsch and Mikrosk Anat 103:192–217

Borg TF, Runyon R, Wuthier RE (1981) A freeze-fracture study of avian epiphyseal cartilage differentiation. Anat Rec 199:449–457

Boskey AL (1989) Non collagenous matrix proteins and their role in mineralization. Bone Miner 6:111–123

Boskey AL, Posner AS (1977) In vitro nucleation of hydroxyapatite by a bone calcium-phospholipid-phosphate complex. Calcif Tissue Res 22 [Suppl]:197–201

Boskey AL, Timchak DM (1989) Phospholipid changes in the bones of the vitamin-D deficient phosphate deficient, immature rat. Metab Bone Dis Rel Res 5:81–85

Boskey AL, Posner AS, Lane JM, Goldberg MR, Cordella DM (1980) Distribution of lipids associated with mincralization in the bovine epiphyseal growth plate. Arch Biochem Biophys 199:305–311

Boskey AL, Wians FH Jr, Hauschka PV (1985) The effect of osteocalcin on in vitro lipid induced hydroxyapatite formation and seeded hydroxyapatite growth. Calcif Tissue Int 37:57–62

Boyan BD (1985) Proteoplipid-dependent calcificiation. In: Butter WT (ed) The chemistry and biology of mineralized tissue. EBSCO Media, Birmingham, pp 125–131

Boyan BD, Schwartz Z, Carnes DL, Ramirez V (1988) The effects of vitamin D metabolites on the plasma and matrix vesicle membranes of growth and resting cartilage cells in vitro. Endocrinology 122:2851–2860

Boyan-Salyers BD, Boskey AL (1980) Relationship between proteolipids and calcium-phospholipid-phosphate complexes in Bacterionema matruchotii calcification. Calcif Tissue Int 30:167–174

Boyde A, Shapiro IM (1987) Morphological observations concerning the pattern of mineralization of the normal and the rachitic chick growth cartilage. Anat Embryol (Berl) 175:457–466

Brown CC, Hembry RM, Reynolds JJ (1989) Immunolocalization of metalloproteinases and their inhibitor in the rabbit growth plate. J Bone Joint Surg [Am] 71:580–593

Brown RA, Taylor C, McLaughlin B, McFarland CD, Weiss JB, Ali SY (1987) Epiphyseal growth plate cartilage and chrondrocytes in mineralizing cultures produce a low molecular mass, angiogenic procollagenase activator. Bone Miner 3:143–158

Buckwalter JA (1987) Changes in proteoglycan aggregates during cartilage mineralization. Calcif Tissue Int 41:228–236

Butler WT (1989) The nature and significance of osteopontin. Connect Tissue Res 23:123–136

Campo RD, Betz RR (1987) Loss of proteoglycans during decalcification of fresh metaphysis with disodium ethylenediaminetetraacetate (EDTH). Calcif Tissue Int 41:52–55

Campo RD, Romano JE (1986) Changes in cartilage proteoglycans associated with calcification. Calcif Tissue Int 39:175–184

Caswell Am, Russell RGG (1985) Identification of ectonucleoside triphosphate pyrophosphatase in human articular chondrocytes in monolayer culture. Biochim Biophys Acta 847:40–47

Caswell AM, Whyte MP, Russell RGG (1991) Hypophosphatasia and the extracellular metabolism of inorganic pyrophosphate: clinical and laboratory aspects. Crit Rev Clin Lab Sci 28:175–232

Cecil RNA, Anderson HC (1978) Freeze-fracture studies of matrix vesicle calcification in epiphyseal growth plate. Metab Bone Dis Rel Res 1:89–97

Chen CC, Boskey AL, Rosenberg L (1984) The inhibitory effect of cartilage proteoglycans on hydroxapatite growth. Calcif Tissue Int 36:285–290

Cotmore JM, Nichols G Jr, Wuthier RE (1971) Phospholipid-calcium phosphate complex: enhanced calcium migration in the presence of phosphate. Science 172:1339–1341

Crenshaw MA, Ramp WK, Gonnerman WA, Toverud SU (1974) Effects of dietary vitamin D levels on the in vitro mineralization of chick metaphysis. Proc Soc Exp Biol Med 146:488–493

Crumpton MJ, Dedman JR (1990) Protein terminology tangle. Nature 345:212

Cuervo LA, Pita JC, Howell DS (1973) Inhibition of calcium phosphate mineral growth by proteoglycan aggregate fractions in a synthetic lymph. Calcif Tissue Res 13:1–10

DeLuca HF (1985) The vitamin D-calcium axis-1983. In: Rubin RP, Weiss GB, Putney JW Jr (eds) Calcium in biological systems. Plenum, New York, pp 491–511

Desteno CV, Feagin FF (1975) Effect of matrix bound phosphate and fluoride on mineralization of dentin. Calcif Tissue Int 17:151–159

Dickson IA, Hall AK, Jande SS (1984) The influence of dihydroxylated vitamin D metabolites on bone formation in the chick. Calcif Tissue Int 36:114–122

Dudley HR, Spiro D (1961) The fine structure of bone cells. J Biophys Biochem Cytol 11:627–649

Dziewaitkowski DD, Majznerski LL (1985) Role of proteoglycans in endochondral ossification: inhibition of calcification. Calcif Tissue Int 37:560–564

Eanes Ed, Hailer AW (1985) Liposome-mediated calcium phosphate formation in metastable solutions. Calcif Tissue Int 37:390–394

Ehrlich MG, Tebor GB, Armstrong AL, Mankin HJ (1985) Comparative study of neutral proteoglycanase activity by growth plate zone. J Orthop Res 3: 269–276

Eisenman DR, Glick PL (1972) Ultrastructure of initial crystal formation in dentin. J Ultrastruct Res 41:18–28

Ennever J, Boyan-Salyers B, Riggan LJ (1977) Proteolipid and bone matrix calcification. J Dent Res 56:967–970

Ennever J, Riggan LJ, Vogel JJ, Boyan-Salyers B (1978) Characterization of Bacterionema matruchotii calcification nucleator. J Dent Res 51:637–642

Fallon MD, Whyte MP, Teitlebaum SL (1980) Stereospecific inhibition of alkaline-phosphatase by L-tetramisole prevents in vitro cartilage calcification. Lab Invest 43:489–494

Farnum GE, Wilsman NJ (1989) Cellular turnover at the chondro-osseous junction of growth plate cartilage: analysis by serial sections at the light microscopic level. J Orthop Res 7:654–666

Fedde KN, Lane CC, Whyte MP (1988) Alkaline phosphatase is an ectoenzyme that acts on micro-molar concentrations of natural substrates at physiologic pH in human osteosarcoma (SAOS-2) cells. Arch Biochem Biophys 264:400–409

Fine N, Binderman I, Somjen D, Earon Y, Edelstein S, Weisman Y (1985) Angioradiographic localization of 24R, 25-dihydroxy vitamin D3 in epiphyseal cartilage. Bone 6:99–104

Fleisch H, Bisaz S (1962) Mechanism of calcification: Inhibitory role of pyrophosphate. Nature 195:911

Fleisch H, Straumann F, Schenk R, Bisaz S, Allgower M (1966) Effect of condensed phosphates on calcification of chick embryo femurs in tissue culture. Am J Physiol 211:821–825

Franceschi RT, Young J (1990) Regulation of alkaline phosphatase by 1,25-didydroxy-vitamin D3 and ascorbic acid in bone derived cells. J Bone Miner Res 5:1157–1167

Francis MD, Russel RGG, Fleisch H (1969) Diphosphonates inhibit formation of calcium phosphate crystals in vitro and pathological calcification in vivo. Science 165:1264–1266

Franzen A, Heinegaard D, Reiland S, Olsson S-E (1982) Proteoglycans and calcification of cartilage in the femoral head epiphysis of the immature rat. J Bone Joint Surg [Am] 64:600–609

Fujisawa R, Kuboki Y, Sasaki S (1987) Effects of dentin phosphoryn on precipitation of calcium phosphate in gel in vitro. Calcif Tissue Int 41:44–47

Gay CV, Muller WJ (1974) Carbonic anhydrase and osteoclasts: localization by labeled inhibitor autoradiography. Science 183:432–434

Gay CV, Faleski EJ, Schraer H, Schraer R (1974) Localization of carbonic anhydrase in avian gastric mucosa, shell gland and bone by immuno-histochemistry. J Histochem Cytochem 22:819–825

Gay CV, Schraer H, Hargest TE Jr (1978) Ultrastructure of matrix vesicles and mineral in unfixed embryonic bone. Metab Bone Dis Rel Res 1:105–108

Gay CV, Anderson RE, Schraer H, Howell DS (1982) Identification of carbonic anhydrase in chick growth plate cartilage. J Histochem Cytochem 30:391–394

Gay CV, Schraer H, Anderson RE, Hanmin C (1984) Current studies on the location and function of carbonic anhydrase in osteoclasts. Ann NY Acad Sci 429:473–478

Genge BR, Sauer GR, Wu LNY, McClean FM, Wuthier RE (1988) Correlation between loss of alkaline phosphatase activity and accumulation of calcium during matrix vesicle mediated mineralization. J Biol Chem 263:118513–18519, 1988

Genge BR, Wu LNY, Wuthier RE (1989) Identification of phospholipid-dependent calcium-binding proteins as constituents of matrix vesicles. J Biol Chem 264:10917–10921

Genge BR, Wu LNY, Wuthier RE (1990) Differential fractionation of matrix vesicle proteins. Further characterization of the acidic phospholipid-dependent Ca^{2+}-binding proteins. J Biol Chem 288:4703–4710

Gibson GJ, Bearman CH, Flint MH (1986) The immunoperoxidase localization of type X collagen in chick cartilage and lung. Collagen Res Rel 6:163–184

Giraud MM (1977) Carbonic anhydrase and integument calcification in crab *Carcinus maenas* Linne (original title in French). Comp Rend Acad Sci D 284/6:453–456

Glaser JH, Conrad EH (1981) Formation of matrix vesicles by cultured chick embryo chondrocytes. J Biol Chem 256:12607–12611

Glimcher MJ (1954) Molecular biology of mineralized tissues with particular reference to bone. Rev Mod Phys 31:359–393

Glimcher MJ (1989) Mechanism of calcification: role of collagen fibrils and collagen-phosphoprotein complexes in vitro and in vivo. Anat Rec 224:139–153

Golub EE, Schattschneider SC, Berthold P, Burke A, Shapiro IM (1983) Induction of chondrocyte vesiculation in vitro. J Biol Chem 258:616–621

Gorski JP, Griffin D, Dudley G, Stanford C, Thomas R, Huang C, Lai E, Karr B, Solursh M (1990) Bone acidic glycoprotein-75 is a major synthetic product of osteoblastic cells and localized as 75 and/or 50-kDa forms in mineralized phases of bone and growth plate and in serum. J Biol Chem 265:14956–14963

Granda JL, Posner AS (1971) Distribution of four hydrolases in the epiphyseal plate. Clin Orthop 74:269–272

Gunness-Hey M, Hock JM (1984) Increased trabecular low mass in rats treated with human synthetic parathyroid hormone. Metab Bone Dis Rel Res 5:177–181

Habuchi H, Conrad HE, Glaser JH (1985) Coordinate regulation of collagen and alkaline phosphatase levels in chick embryo chondrocytes. J Biol Chem 260:13029–13032

Hauschka PV, Lian JB, Gallop PM (1975) Direct identification of the calcium-binding amino acid, δ-carboxyglutamic acid, in mineralized tissue. Proc Natl Acad Sci USA 72:3925–3929

Heldin CH, Wasteson A, Fryklund L, Westermark B (1981) Somatomedin B: mitogenic activity derived from contaminant epidermal growth factor. Science 213:1122–1123

Hinek A, Reiner A, Poole AR (1987) The calcification of cartilage matrix in chondrocyte culture: studies of the c-propeptide of Type II collagen (chondrocalcin). J Cell Biol 104:1435–1441

Hirschman A, Dziewaitkowski DD (1966) Protein-polysaccharide loss during endochondral ossification. Immunochemical evidence. Science 154:393–395

Hock JM, Hummert JR, Boyce R, Fonseca J, Raisz LG (1987) Resorption is not essential for the stimulation of bone growth by HPTH-(1–34) in rats in vivo. J Bone Miner Res 4:449–458

Hock JM, Canalis E, Centrella M (1990) Transforming growth factor beta stimulates bone matrix apposition and bone cell replication in cultured fetal rat calvariae. Endocrinology 126:421–426

Howell DS, Pita JC, Marquez JF, Madruga JE (1968) Partition of calcium phosphate and protein in the fluid phase aspirated at calcifying sites in epiphyseal cartilage. J Clin Invest 47:1121–1132

Hsu HHT (1983) Purification and partial characterization of ATP-pyrophosphohydrolase from fetal bovine epiphyseal cartilage. J Biol Chem 258:3463–3464

Hsu HHT, Anderson HC (1977) A simple and defined method to study calcification by isolated matrix vesicles. Effect of ATP and vesicle phosphatase. Biochem Biophys Acta 500:162–172

Hsu HHT, Anderson HC (1978) Calcification of isolated matrix vesicles and reconstituted vesicles from fetal bovine cartilage. Proc Natl Acad Sci USA 75:3805–3808

Hsu HHT, Cecil RNA, Anderson HC (1978) The role of adenosine triphosphatase, phospholipids and vesicular structure in the calcification of isolated and reconstituted matrix vesicles. Metab Bone Dis Rel Res 1:169–172

Huggins CB (1931) The formation of bone under the influence of epithelium of the urinary tract. Arch Surg 22:377–408

Hunter GK (1987) An ion-exchange mechanism of cartilage calcification. Connect Tiss Res 16:111–120

Isenburg HD, Lavine LS, Weissfullner H (1963) The suppression of mineralization in a coccolithophorid by an inhibitor of carbonic anhydrase. J Protozool 10:477–9

Jande SS, Dickson I (1980) Comparative histological study of the effects of high calcium diet and vitamin D supplements on epiphyseal plates of vitamin-D-deficient chicks. Acta Anat 108:463–468

Jennings RB, Ganote CE, Reimer KA (1975) Ischemic tissue injury. Am J Pathol 81:179–198

Jinguishi S, Joyce M, Roberts A, Sporn M, Muniz O, Howell D, Dean D, Ryan U, Bolander M (1989) Distribution of acidic fibroblast growth factor, basic fibroblast growth factor and transforming growth factor $\beta 1$ in rat growth plate. J Bone Miner Res 4:5325

Johnson TJ, Morris DC, Anderson HC (1989) Matrix vesicles and calcification of rachitic rat osteoid. J Exp Pathol 4:123–132

Joyce ME, Roberts AB, Sporn MB, Bolander ME (1990) Transforming growth factor-β and the initiation of chondrogenesis and osteogenesis in the rat femur. Clin Res 38:407A

Kardos TB, Hubbard MJ (1982) Are matrix vesicles apoptotic bodies? In: Dixon AD, Sarnat BG (eds) Factors and mechanisms influencing bone growth. Liss, New York, pp 45–60

Kashgarian M, Biemesderfer D, Caplan M, Forbush B (1985) Monoclonal antibody to (Na^+, K^+) ATPase: immunocytochemical localization along nephron segments. Kidney Int 28:899–913

Klapper DG, Svoboda ME, VanWyk JJ (1983) Sequence analysis of somatomedin C: confirmation of identity with insulin-like growth factor-1. Endocrinology 112:2215–2217

Kingsley RJ, Watanabe N (1987) Role of carbonic anhydrase in calcification in the Gorgonian *Leptogorgia virgulata*. J Exp Zool 241:171–180

Landis WJ (1987) A study of calcification in the leg tendons from the domestic turkey. J Ultrastr Mol Str Res 94:217–238

Larsson A (1973) Studies on dentinogenesis in the rat. Ultrastructural observations on early dentin formation with special reference to "dentinal globules" and alkaline phosphatase activity. A Anat Entwickl Gesch 142:103–115

Larsson AK (1974) The short-term effects of high doses of ethylene-1-hydroxy-1, 1-diphosphonate upon early dentin formation. Calcif Tissue Res 16:109–127

Lawson DE, Fraser DR, Kodicek E, Morris HR, Williams DH (1971) Identification of 1,25-dihydroxycholecalciferol, a new kidney hormone controlling calcium metabolism. Nature 230:228–230

Lewinson D, Toister Z, Silbermann M (1982) Quantitative and distributional changes in the activity of alkaline phosphatase during the maturation of cartilage. J Histochem Cytochem 30:261–269

Lian JB, Tassinari M, Glowacki J (1984) Resorption of implanted bone prepared from normal and warfarin-treated rats. J Clin Invest 73:1223–1226

Linde A, Lussi A (1989) Mineral induction by polyanionic dentin and bone proteins at physiologic ionic conditions. Connect Tissue Res 21:197–203

Lohmander A, Hjerpe A (1975) Proteoglycans of mineralizing rib and epiphyseal cartilage. Biochem Biophys Acta 404:93–109

Low MG (1987) Biochemistry of the glycosyl-phosphatidylinositol membrane protein anchors. Biochem J 244:1–13

Luyten FP, Hascall VC, Nissley SP (1988) Insulin-like growth factors maintain steady state metabolism of proteoglycans in bovine articular cartilage. Arch Biochem Biophys 267:416–425

Lyons KM, Pelton RW, Hogan BLB (1990) Organogenesis and pattern formation in the mouse: RNA distribution patterns suggest a role for bone morphogenetic protein-2A (BMP-2A). Development 109:833–844

Majeska R, Holwerda DL, Wuthier RE (1979) Localization of phosphatidyl serine in isolated chick epiphyseal cartilage matrix vesicles with trinitrobenzensulfonate. Calcif Tissue Int 27:41–46

Marcelli C, Yates AJ, Mundy GR (1990) In vivo effects of human recombinant transforming growth factor β on bone turnover in normal mice. J Bone Miner Res 5:1087–1096

Marquardt H, Todaro GJ (1981) Purification and primary structure of a polypeptide with multiplication-stimulating activity from rat liver cell cultures: homology with human insulin-like growth factor-2. J Biol Chem 256:6859–6865

Matsuzawa T, Anderson HC (1971) Phosphatases of epiphyseal cartilage studied by electron microscopic cytochemical methods. J Histochem Cytochem 19:801–808

McFarland CD, Brown RA, McLaughlin B, Ali SY, Weiss JB (1990) Production of endothelial cell stimulating angiogenesis factor (ESAF) by chondrocytes during in vitro cartilage calcification. Bone Miner 11:319–333

Menanteau J, Neuman WF, Neuman MW (1982) A study of bone proteins which can prevent hydroxyapatite formation. Metab Bone Dis Rel Res 4:157–162

Morris DC, Vaananen HK, Anderson HC (1983) Matrix vesicle calcification in rat epiphyseal growth plate cartilage prepared anhydrously for electron microscopy. Metab Bone Dis Rel Res 5:131–137

Morris DC, Vaananen HK, Munoz P, Anderson HC (1986) Light and electron microscopic immunolocalization of alkaline phosphatase in bovine growth plate cartilage. In: Ali SY (ed) Cell mediated calcification and matrix vesicles. Elsevier, Amsterdam, pp 21–26

Morris DC, Randall JC, Stechschulte DJ Jr, Zeiger S, Mansur DB, Anderson HC (1990a) Enzyme cytochemical localization of alkaline phosphatase in cultures of chondrocytes derived from normal and rachitic rats. Bone 11:345–352

Morris DC, Moylan P, Levine D, Stechschulte DJ Jr, Anderson HC (1990b) Imunochemical and immunocytochemical identification of matrix vesicle proteins. J Bone Miner Res 5:S231

Morris DC, Stechschulte DJ Jr, Moylan P, Hermreck A, Anderson HC (1990c) Isolation of matrix vesicles from atherosclerotic plaques. Proc Hugh Lofland conference on art wall metabolism, May 23–26

Morris DC, Moylan P, Stechschulte DJ Jr, Anderson HC (1991) Immunochemical and immunocytochemical identification of anchorin CII and type X collagen in rat matrix vesicles. J Bone Miner Res 6 [Suppl 1]:S97

Muhlrad A, Setton A, Sela J, Bab I, Deutsch D (1983) Biochemical characterization of matrix vesicles from bone and cartilage. Metab Bone Dis Rel Res 5:93–99

Mundy GR, Bonewald LF (1990) Role of TGF-beta in bone remodeling. Ann NY Acad Sci 593:91–97

Murphree S, Hsu HHT, Anderson HC (1982) In vitro formation of crystalline apatite by matrix vesicles isolated from rachitic rat epiphyseal cartilage. Calcif Tissue Int 34:S62–S68

Narbaitz R, Stumpf WE, Sar M, Huange S, DeLuca HF (1983) Autoradiographic localization of target cells for 1δ,25-dihydroxy-vitamin D3 in bones from fetal rats. Calcif Tissue Int 35:177–182

Nemethcsoka M, Sarkozi A (1981) The effect of proteoglycans of cartilage and oversulfated polysaccharides on the development of calcium-hydroxy-apatite (CHA) crystal formation in vitro. Acta Biol Hung 33:407–417

Nilsson A, Isgaard J, Lindahl A (1987) Effects of unilateral arterial infusion of GH and IGF-1 on tibial longitudinal bone growth in hypophysectionized rats. Calcif Tissue Int 40:91–96

Ohashi-Takeuchi H, Yamada N, Hosokawa R, Noguchi T (1990) Vesicles with lactate dehydrogenease and alkaline phosphatase present in resting zone of epiphyscal cartilage. Biochem J 266:309–312

Owen ME, Cave J, Joyner CJ (1987) Clonal analysis in vitro of osteogenic differentiation of marrow CFU-F. J Cell Sci 87:731–738

Ozawa II, Najima T (1972) Ultrastructure and cytochemistry of matrix vesicles in developing cartilage and tooth germ. In: 4th international congress on histochemistry and cytochemistry, Kyoto, pp 311–312

Ozawa H, Yamamoto T (1983) An application of energy-dispersive X-ray microanalysis for the study of biological calcification. J Histochem Cytochem 31:210–213

Palumbo C (1986) A three dimensional ultrastructural study of osteoid-osteocytes in the tibia of chick embryos. Cell Tissue Res 246:125–131

Parsons, JA (1976) Parathyroid physiology and the skeleton. In: Bourne GH (ed) Biochemistry and physiology of bone, vol IV, Academic Press, New York, pp 159–226

Peress NS, Anderson HC, Sajdera SW (1974) The lipids of matrix vesicles from bovine fetal epiphyseal cartilage. Calcif Tissue Res 14:275–281

Pliam NB, Nyiredy KO, Arnaud CD (1982) Parathyroid hormone receptors in avian bone cells. Proc Natl Acad Sci USA 79:2061–2063

Poole RA, Pidoux I, Rosenberg L (1982) Role of proteoglycans in endochondral ossification: immunofluorescent localization of link protein and proteoglycan monomer in bovine fetal epiphyseal growth plate. J Cell Biol 92:249–260

Poole AR, Pidoux I, Reiner H, Choi H, Rosenberg LC (1984) Association of an extracellular protein (Chondrocalcin) with the calcification of cartilage in endochondral bone formation. J Cell Biol 98:54–65.

Price PA, Nishimoto SK (1980) Radioimmunoassay of the vitamin-K dependent protein of bone and its discovery in plasma. Proc Natl Acad Sci USA 77:2234–2238

Price PA, Sloper SA (1983) Concurrent warfarin treatment further reduces bone mineral levels in 1,25-dihydroxyvitamin D3-treated rats. J Biol Chem 258:6004–6007

Price PA, Williamson MK (1985) Primary structure of bovine matrix Gla protein, a new vitamin-K dependent bone protein. J Biol Chem 260:14971–14975

Price PA, Otsuka AS, Poser JP, Kristaponis J, Raman N (1976) Characterization of a γ-carboxyglutamic acid-containing protein from bone. Proc Natl Acad Sci USA 73:1447–1451

Ralphs JR, Ali SY (1986) Histochemical localization of alkaline phosphatase in rabbit ulnar growth plate. In: Ali SY (ed) Cell mediated calcification and matrix vesicles. Elsevier, Amsterdam, pp 69–74

Randall JC, Morris DC, Zeiger S, Masuhara K, Tsuda T, Anderson HC (1989) Presence and activity of alkaline phosphatase in two human osteosarcoma cell lines. J Histochem Cytochem 37:1069–1074

Reginato Am, Lash JW, Jimenez SA (1986) Biosynthetic expression of type X collagen in embryonic chick sternum cartilage during development. J Biol Chem 261:2897–2904

Register TC, Wuthier RE (1985) Effect of pyrophosphate and two diphosphonates on ^{45}Ca and ^{32}Pi uptake and mineralization by matrix vesicle-enriched fractions and by hydroxyapatite. Bone 6:307–312

Register TC, McClean FM, Low MG, Wuthier RE (1986) Roles of alkaline phosphatase and labile internal mineral in matrix vesicle-mediated calcification. Effect of selective release of membrane-bound alkaline phosphatase and treatment with isoosmotic pH 6 buffer. J Biol Chem 261:9354–9360

Reinholt FP, Wernerson A (1988) Septal distribution and the relationship of matrix vesicle size to cartilage mineralization. Bone Miner 4:63–71

Reinholt FP, Hultenby K, Oldberg A, Hienegard D (1990) Osteopontin – a possible anchor of osteoclasts to bone. Proc Natl Acad Sci USA 87:4473–4475

Robey PG, Young MF, Flanders KC, Roche NS, Kondaiah P, Reddi AH, Termine JD, Sporn MB, Roberts AB (1987) Osteoblasts synthesize and respond to transforming growth factor type-β (TGF-β) in vitro. J Cell Biol 105:457–463

Robey P, Young M, Fisher L, McClain T (1989) Thrombospondin is an osteoblast-derived component of mineralized extracellular matrix. J Cell Biol 108:719–727

Robinson RA, Watson ML (1952) Collagen-crystal relationships in bone as seen in the electron microscope. Anat Rec 114:383

Robison R (1923) The possible significance of hexose phosphoric esters in ossification. Biochem J 17:286–293

Rojas E, Pollard HB, Haigler HT, Parra C, Burns Al (1990) Calcium-activated endonexin II forms calcium channels across acidic phospholipid bilayer membranes. J Biol Chem 265:21207–21215

Romberg RW, Werness PG, Riggs BL, Mann KB (1986) Inhibition of hydroxyapatite crystal growth by bone-specific and other calcium-binding proteins. Biochemistry 25:1176–1180

Rozier RN, O'Keefe RJ, Crabb ID, Puzas JE (1989) Transforming growth factor beta; an autocrine regulator of chondrocytes. Connect Tissue Res 20:295–301

Russell RGG, Kislig AM, Casey PA, Fleisch H, Thornton J, Schenk R, Williams DA (1973) Effect of diphosphonates and calcitonin on the chemistry and quantitative histology of rat bone. Calcif Tissue Res 11:179–195

Sajdera SW, Hascall VC (1969) Protein polysaccharide complex from bovine nasal cartilage. A comparison of low and high shear extraction procedures. J Biol Chem 244:77–87

Sauer GR, Wuthier RE (1988) Fourier transform infrared characterization of mineral phases formed during induction of mineralization by collagenase-released matrix vesicles in vitro. J Biol Chem 263:13718–13724

Schenk RK, Miller J, Zinkernagel R, Willenegger H (1970). Ultrastructure of normal and abnormal bone repair. Calcif Tissue Res 4 [Suppl]:110–111

Schenk R, Merz WA, Muhlbauer R, Russell RGG, Fleisch H (1973) Effect of ethane-1-hydroxy-1, 1-diphosphonate (EHDP) and dichloromethylene diphosphonate (Cl$_2$-MDP) on the calcification and resorption of cartilage and bone in the tibial epiphysis and metaphysis of rats. Calcif Tissue Res 11:196–214

Schmid TM, Linsenmayer TF (1985) Immunolocalization of short chain cartilage collagen (Type X) in avian tissues. J Cell Biol 100:598–605

Seyedin SM, Thompson Ay, Bentz H, Rosen DM, McPherson JM, Conti A, Siegel NR, Gallupi GR, Piez KA (1986) Cartilage-inducing factor-A apparent identity to transforming growth factor-β. J Biol Chem 261:5693–5695

Shimizu K, Hanamoto T, Hamakubu T, Lee WJ, Suzuki K, Nakagawa Y, Murachi T, Yamamuro T (1991) Immunohistochemical and biochemical demonstration of calcium-dependent cysteine proteinase (CALPAIN) in calcifying cartilage of rats. J Orthop Res 9:26–36

Siegel SA, Hummel CF, Carty RP (1983) The role of nucleoside triphosphate pyrophosphohydrolase in in vitro nucleoside triphosphate-dependent matrix vesicle calcification. J Biol Chem 25814:8601–8607

Simon DR, Berman I, Howell DS (1973) Relationship of extracellular matrix vesicles to calcification in normal and healing rachitic epiphyseal cartilage. Anat Rec 176:167–180

Sisca RF, Provenza DV (1972) Initial dentin formation in human decidious teeth. An electron microscopic study. Calcif Tissue Res 9:1–16

Slavkin HC, Bringas P Jr, Croissant R, Bavetta LA (1972) Epithelial-mesenchymal interactions during odontogenesis: II. Intercellular matrix vesicles. Mech Ageing Dev 1:139–161

Smith R, Triffit JT (1986) Bones in muscles: the problems of soft tissue ossification. Q J Med (New Series) 61:985–990

Sobel AE, Laurence PA, Burger M (1960) Nuclei formation and cyrstal growth in mineralizing tissues. Trans NY Acad Sci 22:233–241

Solursh M, Jensen KL, Reiter RS, Schmid TM, Linsenmayer TF (1986) Environmental regulation of type X collagen production by cultured limb mesenchyme, mesectoderm and sternal chondrocytes. Dev Biol 117:90–101

Stechschulte DJ Jr, Morris DC, Silverton SF, Anderson HC, Vaananen HK (1992) Presence and specific concentration of carbonic anhydrase in rat matrix vesicles. Bone and Mineral 17:187–192

Stechschulte DJ Jr, Morris DC, Croughan WS, Davis L, Anderson HC (1991b) Isolation and in vitro calcification of matrix vesicles derived from fetal rat calvariae. J Bone Miner Res 6 [Suppl 1]:S98

Stein RM, Hsu HHT, Anderson HC (1981) Protein profiles of isolated fetal calf and rachitic rat matrix vesicles by polyacrylamide gel electrophoresis. In: Ascenzi A, Bonucci E, de Bernard B (eds) Proceedings of the 3rd international conference on matrix vesicles. Wichtig, Milano, pp 117–122

Takano Y, Ozawa H, Crenshaw MA (1986) Ca-ATPase and ALPase activities at the initial calcification sites of dentin and enamel in rat incision. Calcif Tissue Res 243:91–99

Takaoka K, Yoshikawa H, Shimizu M, Ono K, Amitani K, Nakata Y (1982) Partial purification of bone-inducing substances from a murine osteosarcoma. Clin Orthop 164:265–270

Takaoka K, Yoshikawa H, Masuhara K, Sugamoto K, Tsuda T, Aoki Y, Ono K, Sakamoto Y (1989) Establishment of a cell line producing human bone morphogenetic protein from a human osteosarcoma. Clin Orthop 244:258–264

Tanimura A, McGregor DH, Anderson HC (1983) Matrix vesicles in atherosclerotic calcification. Proc Soc Exp Biol Med 172:173–177

Termine JD, Conn KM (1976) Inhibition of apatite formation by phosphorylated metabolites and macromolecules. Calcif Tissue Res 22:149–157

Termine JD, Kleinman HK, Whitson WS, Conn KM, McGarvey ML, Martin GR (1981) Osteonectin, a bone specific protein linking mineral to collagen. Cell 26:99–105

Triffit JT (1987) The special proteins of bone tissue. Clin Sci 72:399–408

Triffit JT (1989) Initiation and enhancement of bone formation. A Review. Acta Orthop Scand 58:673–684

Tsonis P (1991) 1,25-Dihydroxyvitamin D_3 stimulates chondrogenesis of the chick limb bud mesenchymal cells. Dev Biol 143:130–134

Urist MR, Strates BS (1970) Bone morphogenetic protein. J Dent Res 50:1392–1406

Vaananen HK (1984) Immunohistochemical localization of carbonic anhydrase isoenzymes I and II in human bone, cartilage and giant cell tumor. Histochemistry 81:485–487

Vaananen HK, Hentunen T, Lakkakorpi P, Parvinen EK, Sundquist K, Tuukkanen J (1988) Mechanism of osteoclast mediated bone resorption. Ann Chir Gynaecol 77:193–196

Vaananen HK, Karhukorpi EK, Sundquist K, Wallmark B, Roininen I, Hentunen T, Tuurkanen J, Lakkakorpi P (1990) Evidence for the presence of a proton pump of the vacuolar $H^+ATPase$ type in ruffled borders of osteoclasts. J Cell Biol 111:1305–1311

Van Wyk JJ (1988) The different roles of IGF-1 and IGF-2 in growth and differentiation. In: Imura K (ed) Progress in endocrinology 1988. Elsevier, Amsterdam, pp 947–955

Van Wyk JJ, Underwood LE, Hintz RE, Clemmons DR, Voima J, Weaver RP (1974) The somatomedins: a family of insulin-like growth factors under growth hormone control. Recent Prog Horm Res 30:259–318

Varner HH, Horn VJ, Martin GR Hewitt AT (1986) Chondronectin interactions with proteoglycan. Arch Biochem Biophys 244:824–830

Veis A, Perry A (1967) The phosphoprotein of dentin matrix. Biochemistry 6:2409–2416

Wu LNY, Sauer GR, Genge BR, Wuthier RE (1989) Induction of mineral deposition by primary cultures of chicken growth plate chondrocytes in ascorbate containing media – evidence of an association between matrix vesicles and collagen. J Biol Chem 264:21346–21355

Wu LNY, Genge BR, Lloyd GC, Wuthier RE (1991a) Collagen binding proteins in collagenase-released matrix vesicles from cartilage. J Biol Chem 266:1195–1203

Wu LNY, Genge BR, Wuthier RE (1991b) Association between proteoglycans and matrix vesicles in the extracellular matrix of growth plate cartilage. J Biol Chem 266:1187–1194

Wuthier RE (1968) Lipids of mineralizing epiphyseal tissues in the bovine fetus. J Lipid Res 9:68–78

Wuthier RE (1975) Lipid composition of isolated cartilage cells, membranes and matrix vesicles. Biochim Biophys Acta 409:128–143

Wuthier RE (1977) Electrolytes of isolated epiphyseal chondrocytes matrix vesicles and extracellular fluid. Calcif Tissue Res 23:125–133

Wuthier RE, Gore ST (1977) Partition of inorganic ions and phospholipids in isolated cell membrane and matrix vesicle fractions: evidence for Ca-Pi-acidic phospholipid complexes. Calcif Tissue Res 24:163–171

Wuthier RE, Linder RE, Warner GP, Gore ST, Borg TK (1978) Non-enzymatic isolation of matrix vesicles: characterization and initial studies on ^{45}Ca and ^{32}P-orthophosphate metabolism. Metab Bone Dis Rel Res 1:125–136

Wuthier RE, Chin JE, Hale JR, Register TC, Hale LV, Ishikawa Y (1985) Isolation and characterization of calcium-accumulating matrix vesicles from chondrocytes of chick epiphyseal growth plate cartilage in primary culture. J Biol Chem 260:15972–15979

Yaari A, Shapiro IM (1982) Effect of phosphate on phosphatidyl serine-mediated calcium transport. Calcif Tissue Int 34:43–48

Yendt ER, Howard JE (1955) Studies on the mode of action of citrate therapy in rickets. Bull Johns Hopkins Hosp 96:101–115

Yoshikawa H, Masuhara K, Takaoka K, Ono K, Tanaka H, Seino Y (1985) Abnormal bone formation induced by osteosarcoma-derived bone-inducing substance in the x-linked hypophosphatemic mouse. Bone 6:235–239

Young MF, Kerr JM, Termine JD, Wewer UM, Wang MG, McBride OW, Fisher LW (1990) cDNA cloning, mRNA distribution and heterogeneity, chromosomal location and RFLP analysis of human osteopontin. Genomics 7:491–502

CHAPTER 9

Pathogenesis of Osteoporosis

L.G. RAISZ and K.C. SHOUKRI

A. Introduction

There has been a remarkable increase in research on osteoporosis during the last 2 decades. Clinical studies have characterized the primary osteoporotic syndromes and have resulted in a new classification (RIGGS and MELTON 1986). Laboratory studies have demonstrated many local factors which regulate bone metabolism, and this has led to the concept that local as well as systemic factors are important in pathogenesis (RAISZ 1988). The mechanisms of secondary forms of osteoporosis have been explored. Nevertheless, there is still considerable controversy concerning pathogenesis, and there are many gaps in our knowledge. There has also been confusion concerning terminology. For the purpose of this chapter we will define "primary osteoporosis" as the condition in which there is a decrease in bone mass and strength leading to an increased frequency of fracture and which is not due to an associated disorder. The term "secondary osteoporosis" will be used for those patients with certain specific diseases or drug therapies which can cause bone loss and fractures. The term "osteopenia" will be used to describe conditions in which decreased bone mass has been found without a clear-cut association with fractures. While this usage avoids the problem of deciding whether or not there is a "fracture threshold," it does not resolve it. There is as yet no agreement as to whether one can make a diagnosis of osteoporosis before fracture occurs, yet it seems obvious that the disease must have been present just prior to as well as after the fracture.

This chapter will emphasize data in humans, in relevant animal models, and in vitro which indicate possible pathogenetic mechanisms. However, it is important to acknowledge that at present the fundamental pathogenetic mechanisms of osteoporosis in any of its forms are not fully understood. Hence we will also attempt to point out important gaps in our knowledge and suggest possible ways of filling these gaps.

B. Primary Osteoporosis

Several different classifications of primary osteoporosis have been proposed. The simplest classification might be based on the site of a fracture associated with diminished bone mass and strength – that is, osteoporosis with: (1) Colles' fracture of the distal radius, (2) vertebral compression fractures, (3) fracture of the neck or greater trochanter of the femur, or (4) fractures at other sites. Indeed, there is evidence for some degree of selective bone loss at the fracture site in osteoporotic patients (Riggs et al. 1981; Ruegsegger et al. 1984; Johnston et al. 1985). Attempts have been made to classify osteoporosis based on bone turnover, that is separating patients who have high rates of resorption and formation from those in whom the rates are low (Eriksen et al. 1990). However, the most widely used classification has been that of type I, or postmenopausal osteoporosis, and type II, or senile osteoporosis (Johnston et al. 1985; Riggs and Melton 1986). The basis for this classification is that it is possible to group patients clinically into those who have a relatively early onset after menopause and predominantly vertebral crush fractures and those who have predominantly hip fractures with the highest incidence in much older patients. The nonspecific term "type I" is preferred over "postmenopausal" because vertebral crush fractures can occur in men and premenopausal women. The term "type II" is preferred to "senile" osteoporosis because, while the highest rate of hip fractures certainly occurs in older individuals, the frequency begins to increase much earlier, even before the menopause (Brody et al. 1984). There are a number of rare forms of primary osteoporosis. Juvenile osteoporosis occurs in pre-adolescent and adolescent children, appears to be self-limited, and may be associated with accelerated linear growth with delay in the consolidation of bone mass during the prepubertal and pubertal phases of rapid growth (Smith 1980; Hoekman et al. 1985). Regional migratory osteoporosis (Lakharpal et al. 1987) and osteoporosis associated with pregnancy have been described (Smith et al. 1985). Little is known of the pathogenesis of these unusual forms and they will not be discussed further.

The fact that the majority of patients with vertebral crush fracture syndrome are postmenopausal women has focused attention on the role of the loss of ovarian hormones as the major pathogenetic factor. However, all women lose ovarian hormones at the menopause, while only a small proportion develop vertebral compression. Considerable attention has been paid to this group of early vertebral crush fracture patients because they have a disorder which is often progressive and debilitating.

The decrease in bone mass and strength in osteoporosis may be due to:

1. Low Peak Bone Mass

It has been postulated that the patients at highest risk for fracture either have not achieved an adequate peak bone mass early in life or have lost bone premenopausally. There are no longitudinal studies which would allow us to choose between these alternatives. However, there clearly are racial and genetic determinants of bone mass and strength which can affect fracture incidence (Evans et al. 1988; Seeman et al. 1989; Bauer 1988;

KELLY et al. 1991; LUCKEY et al. 1989; MEIER et al. 1991; POCOCK et al. 1987).

2. Rapid Bone Loss

Whatever the bone mass at menopause, there is a wide variation in the rates of bone loss thereafter (HEANEY et al. 1978). The limited data available suggest that the rapid losers have high rates of bone resorption. Bone formation may increase in these individuals, but not sufficiently to compensate for the rapid rates of loss (CHRISTIANSEN et al. 1987; RIGGS and MELTON 1986; ERIKSEN et al. 1990). Thus rapid loss is associated with "high turnover." On the other hand, vertebral crush fractures are also found in patients who show "low turnover" on biopsy with relatively little osteoclastic or osteoblastic activity. It is possible that high turnover was present in these individuals at an earlier time. However, the possibility that decreased bone formation without accelerated resorption is largely responsible for the pathogenesis of vertebral crush fractures in some type I osteoporotic patients has not been ruled out. Almost nothing is known about the contribution of changes in bone quality to osteoporosis. There is evidence that cell viability is decreased in femoral neck fractures (EVENTOV et al. 1991) and age-related changes in cell replication could be responsible for the age-related decrease in the mean wall thickness of products of new bone (DEMPSTER 1989).

The epidemiology of osteoporosis has contributed to our concepts of pathogenesis. Osteoporotic fractures, particularly Colles' fracture but also hip fracture, show a relatively early increase in frequency, beginning before the menopause (RIGGS and MELTON 1986; MELTON et al. 1989; BRODY et al. 1984). The increase in incidence of vertebral crush fractures is both menopause and age related, but there may be a distinction between the severe, progressive compression fracture syndrome occurring in a small population early after menopause and the wedge fractures occurring in a large number of women and some men later in life. Indeed, the latter may not represent a true osteoporotic syndrome. In contrast to these patterns, which are consistent with a pathogenetic mechanism that is independent of age, the incidence of hip fracture shows an exponential pattern of increasing rate with age. This pattern has been called "Gompertzian," based on Benjamin Gompertz's early description of the exponential increase in mortality with age (MELTON 1990). Thus the concept has arisen that like stroke, which is thought to be the result of cumulative multifactorial damage due to hypertension and vascular disease with age, the incidence of hip fracture is the cumulative result of age-related bone loss, increasing fragility of bone, weakness and atrophy of surrounding tissues, and an increased frequency of falls.

Comparison of patients with vertebral and hip fractures (types I, II) shows differences, not only in age, but in the distribution of bone loss and in certain metabolic parameters. Thus hip fracture patients have lower cortical bone mass, lower serum calcium concentration, and higher parathyroid hormone levels than patients with vertebral fractures (Johnston et al. 1985). However, some of this difference may be age-related, and there is substantial overlap in all these parameters. Moreover, hip and vertebral fractures often occur in the same patient.

I. Calcium-Regulating Hormones

1. Parathyroid Hormone

The role of parathyroid hormone (PTH) in the pathogenesis of osteoporosis remains controversial. The fact that PTH increases with age has now been established using immunoassays for the intact hormone as well as bioassays (Forero et al. 1987; Young et al. 1987). This increase has been considered to be a form of secondary hyperparathyroidism due to calcium deficiency. This is probably due to: (1) decreased dietary intake, (2) impaired intestinal absorption, and (3) decreased ability to synthesize 1,25-dihydroxyvitamin D [1,25(OH)$_2$D]. On the other hand, PTH levels are not elevated in vertebral crush fracture patients. Slightly decreased levels have been reported in some series, and recent studies have shown that the PTH response to a hypocalcemic stimulus may be blunted. Thus, phosphate loading, which reduces serum-ionized calcium, produces a smaller increase in PTH in crush fracture patients than in age-matched controls. 1,25(OH)$_2$D levels decreased in the patients presumably due to the effect of the phosphate, while in the controls there is an increase, presumably due to the increase in PTH (Silverberg et al. 1989a).

While PTH clearly stimulates bone resorption, its effects on bone formation are more complex. PTH has a direct inhibitory effect on collagen synthesis in cell and organ culture (Kream et al. 1990; Raisz and Kream 1983; Podbesek et al. 1983; Hori et al. 1988), but when given intermittently it can increase bone formation in organ culture and trabecular bone mass in experimental animals (Hock and Fonseca 1990; Liu et al. 1991) as well as in osteoporotic patients (Hodsman et al. 1991; Slovik et al. 1986). In primary hyperparathyroidism (see below), trabecular bone volume of iliac crest biopsies is actually higher than in age-matched controls, while cortical bone thickness is much reduced (Silverberg et al. 1989b; Parisien et al. 1990). The anabolic effect of PTH has been attributed to an effect on growth factors. In vitro, there is evidence for stimulation of Insulin Growth Factor 1 (IGF-1) production (Canalis et al. 1989) and of activation of Transforming Growth Factor β (TGFβ) (Pfeilschifter and Mundy 1987). It is possible that these responses differ in cortical and cancellous bone, but there are as yet no data on this point.

All of these data support a pathogenetic role for PTH in age-related cortical bone loss and hence in type II osteoporotic fractures. Whether the decrease in PTH in type I osteoporosis is pathogenetic is less clear. Lack of an intermittent PTH response to a low calcium stimulus could contribute to trabecular bone loss. Alternatively, the decreased PTH response could be the result of chronic suppression of the parathyroid glands. This could occur if local factors were responsible for increased bone resorption in these patients and decreased the need for PTH to maintain serum calcium levels. This alternative is supported by studies which show a decreased amplitude and frequency of pulsatile secretion of PTH in osteoporotic patients (HARMS et al. 1989).

2. 1,25-Dihydroxyvitamin D

Low levels of vitamin D metabolites have been reported in patients with hip (LIPS et al. 1987) or vertebral fractures in whom bone biopsies do not show osteomalacia, but only osteoporosis, as well as in patients with low vertebral bone mass (VILLAREAL et al. 1991; MAWER et al. 1991). Decreased $1,25(OH)_2D$ levels might be explained by an impaired PTH response (SILVERBERG et al. 1989a), but when 25 hydroxyvitamin D levels are also decreased, this suggests that either exposure to the sun or dietary vitamin D sources are diminished or that hepatic synthesis is impaired. However, most studies show only a small proportion of patients with low vitamin D levels, and there is no clear correlation between the severity of bone disease and the level of any vitamin D metabolite.

One reason for considering the vitamin D hormone system to be less important in the pathogenesis of osteoporosis has been the failure to demonstrate consistent improvement in osteoporotic patients with vitamin D therapy (OTT and CHESTNUT 1989). However, some studies have shown an increase in bone mass with vitamin D metabolites (ALOIA et al. 1988) as well as an increase in osteocalcin in response to $1,25(OH)_2D$ stimulation in osteoporotic patients (DUDA et al. 1987). Any attempt to evaluate the role of vitamin D is complicated by our limited understanding of its effects on bone. $1,25(OH)_2D$ can clearly increase intestinal calcium absorption and support bone mineralization at low physiologic concentrations, but it stimulates bone resorption at high concentrations (RAISZ 1990). The effects on bone formation are less clear. A direct inhibitory effect on collagen synthesis can be observed at high concentrations, both in vivo and in vitro. Lower concentrations of $1,25(OH)_2D$ can increase the production of one bone protein, osteocalcin and may be anabolic. Data from experimental animals are not consistent, partly because it is so difficult to separate effects on the intestine from effects on bone.

3. Calcitonin

When calcitonin was first discovered and shown to be a potent inhibitor of bone resorption, it seemed logical to expect that deficiency of this hormone would result in bone loss and that treatment with calcitonin would be highly effective in osteoporosis. However, careful clinical studies have not shown calcitonin deficiency in patients with vertebral crush fractures (Tiegs et al. 1985). Treatment with large doses of calcitonin can increase bone mass, especially in patients with high bone turnover, but the therapeutic doses are pharmacologic, not physiologic (Civitelli et al. 1988). There may be a role for other products of the calcitonin gene. Both the alternative gene product, calcitonin gene-related peptide, and the N-propeptide of calcitonin have been reported to affect bone cells, but there are no clinical data on these proteins (Burns et al. 1989).

II. Systemic Hormones

1. Sex Hormones

Recent studies on the action of sex hormones on bone have provided us with important new insight into the possible pathogenetic mechanisms in osteoporosis. Estrogen has been studied most extensively, but the effects of androgen deficiency have been found to resemble the changes seen with estrogen deficiency in both animal and human studies.

Estrogen withdrawal is associated with a rapid increase in bone resorption (Stepan et al. 1989). Based on biochemical measurements of bone markers, the highest rates of resorption are associated with more rapid bone loss (Christiansen et al. 1987). The increase in bone resorption is sustained for up to 15 years in estrogen-deficient women, although the rates may be higher during the first few years of estrogen deficiency (Riggs et al. 1981). The absolute rates of formation are also increased in estrogen deficiency, presumably because of the increase in the number of bone remodeling sites. However, the net effect of estrogen deficiency is continued bone loss, indicating that the bone formation response is insufficient to maintain bone mass (Heaney et al. 1978). Thus there is "uncoupling" of the bone remodeling cycle.

Although effects of estrogen on calcium-regulating hormones have been described, many studies show changes in bone turnover after sex hormone withdrawal or treatment which are independent of changes in PTH, $1,25(OH)_2D$, or calcitonin. The finding of receptors for sex hormones in bone cells makes it likely that they act directly. While the specific cell types and stages that have estrogen receptors in vivo have not been defined, most positive studies have been on cells of the osteoblast lineage (Eriksen et al. 1988; Komm et al. 1988). How these receptors mediate changes in bone formation and resorption is less clear. There is evidence that sex hormones can act by altering the production of local factors. Estrogens and androgens have been shown to inhibit the production of prostaglandins by bone. Bone excised from oophorectomized rats produces more Prostaglandin E_2 (PGE_2) than from sham operated animals and pretreatment with estradiol inhibits that production (Feyen and Raisz 1987). In organ culture estradiol can inhibit prostaglandin production, particularly when it is stimulated by PTH (Pilbeam et al. 1989). Since prostaglandins are powerful stimulators of bone resorption, it is possible that the increase in resorption that occurs with estrogen withdrawal is due to increased production of this local mediator; however, these organ culture studies have also suggested that inhibition of bone resorption by estradiol can be independent of prostaglandin production since it occurs in the presence of the cyclooxygenase inhibitor indomethacin. Effects of estrogens on growth factors, particularly insulin-like growth factor (IGF-1) and transforming growth factor β (TGFβ), have been reported in cell cultures (ERNST et al. 1990). Effects on IGF-1 synthesis and release as well as increases in mRNA levels have been reported in different experiments. IGF-1 binding proteins may also be increased by estrogen treatment. The effect on TGFβ may be to activate this factor rather than increase its synthesis.

Estrogen treatment can reduce production of Interleukin-1 (IL-1) by peripheral macrophages, which could be a mechanism for decreased bone resorption (PACIFICI et al. 1989). Other investigators have failed to show any difference in cytokine production by peripheral blood mononuclear cells in osteoporotic subjects when compared to normal controls (ZARABEITIA et al. 1991; STOCK et al. 1989). In addition, the effect of estrogen on IL-1-producing cells adjacent to bone is not known. Indeed, it is possible that any increase in IL-1 production by peripheral macrophages in estrogen deficiency is an effect of increased resorption rather than a cause. Fragments of collagen, such as might be released during resorption, have recently been shown to activate macrophages and increase their production of IL-1 and other cytokines (PACIFICI et al. 1991).

Androgens are clearly important in maintaining bone mass in men and may play a role in women as well. In some studies the decrease in bone mass in postmenopausal women has shown a better correlation with androgen levels than with estrogen levels, which are uniformly low (BUCHANAN et al. 1988; LONGCOPE et al. 1985). The mechanism of androgen effects on bone is not well understood. Androgen deficiency is associated with increased bone resorption and prostaglandins may also play a part here since testosterone and dehydrotestosterone treatment can reduce prostaglandin production by bone in organ culture (PILBEAM and RAISZ 1990). Androgens may also stimulate bone growth factor production. Finally, there might be an indirect androgen effect on bone, due to increased muscle mass and strength.

Progestins as well as estrogens decrease at the menopause, but there is little clinical evidence that this plays an important pathogenetic role in bone loss. Estrogen alone can prevent bone loss in oophorectomized women. Women with short luteal phases or anovulatory cycles presumably secrete less progesterone and have been found to have low bone mass, but a causal association has not been demonstrated (PRIOR et al. 1990).

2. Other Systemic Hormones

While glucocorticoids can clearly produce secondary osteoporosis (see below), there is little evidence that changes in glucocorticoid production are important in primary osteoporosis. There are clinical studies which suggest that growth hormone might play a role in bone loss. Certainly, growth hormone secretion tends to decrease with age, and this is probably responsible for the age-related decrease in circulating IGF-1 (Rudman et al. 1981). When vertebral crush fracture patients were compared with age-matched controls, IGF-1 levels were not different (Bennett et al. 1984). However, growth hormone can also stimulate IGF-1 production directly in skeletal tissue (McCarthy et al. 1989), which would not be reflected in circulating IGF-1 levels. Circulating IGF-1 could play a role in some forms of secondary osteoporosis, particularly that associated with malnutrition.

Insulin is clearly important for skeletal growth. In cell and organ culture, insulin has a selective stimulatory effect on osteoblastic collagen synthesis (Raisz and Kream 1983). There is evidence that patients with insulin-dependent diabetes have lower bone mass and an increased frequency of fractures (Auwerx et al. 1988; Bouillon 1991). Insulin deficiency is not ordinarily considered a major pathogenetic factor in primary osteoporosis, but resistance to the anabolic effect of insulin could play a role.

Thyroid hormones may also play a role in bone metabolism since they can stimulate resorption in organ culture by prostaglandin-dependent and prostaglandin-independent mechanisms (Klaushofer et al. 1989; Mundy et al. 1976). Moreover, specific receptors which bind triiodothyronine have been identified in bone tissues (Krieger et al. 1988).

III. Local Factors

There are a number of clinical features of osteoporosis, particularly vertebral crush fracture syndrome, which are better explained by local rather than systemic pathogenetic mechanisms. The fact that a few patients with this syndrome are premenopausal women or men suggests that there may be specific pathogenetic factors other than estrogen deficiency. Thus the mechanisms may differ from the complex, multifactorial, age-related loss of bone mass and strength which leads to hip fracture in older patients. Moreover, patients with vertebral crush fractures often show localized loss of bone in the vertebral bodies, with relative preservation of bone mass in other portions of the skeleton. The trabecular and cortico-endosteal portions of bone adjacent to the marrow appear to be more affected than other sites (Brown et al. 1987). This might suggest that the pathogenetic factors are derived from hematopoietic cells, but it is also possible that the extensive stromal network in the marrow and the pre-osteoblasts and pre-osteoclasts are directly involved. There is a long list of factors produced by bone cells and adjacent hematopoietic cells which might play a pathogenetic role. These are discussed in detail elsewhere in this volume. We will focus on the possible roles of four groups of compounds, the interleukins and related cytokines, prostaglandins and other eicosanoids, IGFs, and the TGFβ family.

1. Interleukins

Interleukin 1α and β, as well as tumor necrosis factor α and β (TNFα and TNFβ), are potent stimulators of bone resorption and inhibitors of bone formation. While there is as yet no direct evidence that IL-1 or related compounds are responsible for the bone loss that leads to vertebral crush fractures, there are many reasons for exploring this possibility. IL-1 and TNα production are increased in peripheral blood macrophage cultures from vertebral crush fracture patients (PACIFICI et al. 1987), including men and premenopausal women as well as postmenopausal women, although, as noted above, this may be an effect rather than a cause of bone loss. The observation that IL-1 and TNFβ are responsible for increased bone resorption in multiple myeloma and that this disease can produce an accelerated vertebral crush fracture syndrome that closely mimics primary osteoporosis makes a role for these cytokines at least plausible (KAWANO et al. 1989). Another reason for believing that lymphoid cells may be involved in pathogenesis is the finding that the ratio of OK4 ("helper") cells to OK8 ("suppressor") cells is increased in osteoporotic patients compared to age-matched controls (ROSEN et al. 1990; IMAI et al. 1990).

2. Prostaglandins

Prostaglandins, particularly of the E series, are potent multifunctional regulators of bone cell function (RAISZ and MARTIN 1983). There is increasing evidence that endogenous prostaglandins play a role in the local regulation of bone metabolism. Prostaglandin production in bone is regulated by mechanical forces, systemic hormones, and local growth factors. Increased prostaglandin production may be responsible for the increase in bone resorption that occurs with immobilization (THOMPSON and RODAN 1988). Bones from oophorectomized rats make more PGE_2 than bones from sham operated controls, and pretreatment with estrogen reverses this (FEYEN and RAISZ 1987). Moreover, the bone loss due to estrogen deficiency in rats can be partially reversed by treatment with a nonsteroidal anti-inflammatory agent, which inhibits prostaglandin production (LANE et al. 1990). Estrogen also decreases PGE_2 production in bone organ cultures (PILBEAM et al. 1989).

It is difficult to assign a specific role for prostaglandins in the pathogenesis of osteoporosis because of their complex biphasic effects (RAISZ and FALL 1990). PGE_2 and related compounds can both stimulate and inhibit bone resorption and bone formation. There is a direct inhibitory effect on osteoclasts which is transient; its physiologic role is uncertain. With prolonged treatment there is stimulation of osteoclastic bone resorption involving the recruitment of new osteoclasts. This is almost certainly important in bone loss associated with inflammation and immobilization and could play a role in osteoporosis. PGE_2 can directly inhibit collagen synthesis by osteoblasts, but the major effect of PGE_2 infusions or injections in animal studies has been to increase bone formation (Jee et al. 1985). The mechanism of this anabolic effect is not clear. It can be demonstrated in organ cultures, particularly when bone formation is inhibited by gluco-corticoids. A role for IGF-1 in the anabolic response to PGE_2 has been suggested because glucocorticoids inhibit and PGE_2 stimulates IGF-1 production in bone cell cultures (McCarthy et al. 1990, 1991). We need to know more about both the effects and production of PGE_2 in human bone to relate these observations to the pathogenesis of primary osteoporosis.

3. Growth Factors

Many growth factors have been identified in extracts of bone matrix and in the medium of cultured bone cells (Canalis et al. 1991). These factors are generally found to consist of families of related proteins, and new members of some families are being identified at such a rapid rate that the ultimate number of growth factors is hard to predict. The major families which have been shown to act on bone cells are: (1) insulin-like growth factors, (2) TGFβ and related peptides, (3) fibroblast growth factors, (4) platelet-derived growth factors, and (5) epidermal growth factors/TGFα. While all are mitogenic, they differ in their effect on the differentiation and the function of osteoblasts.

Insulin growth factors (IGFs) I and II are potent pleiotypic stimulators of both replication and differentiation of cells of the osteoblast lineage. They are produced by bone, and their production is highly regulated (Canalis et al. 1991). A decrease in local or systemic IGF production could be important in the age-related decrease in osteoblast function, which is represented histologically by an age-related decrease in the width of packets of new bone formed during remodeling. IGF I production in bone is inhibited by glucocorticoids, and this could be responsible for the even greater decrease in the width of new packets seen in glucocorticoid-induced osteoporosis (Dempster 1989). IGF I production in bone can be stimulated by growth hormone, PTH, PGE_2 and possibly also sex hormones (McCarthy et al. 1989; Canalis et al. 1989; Linkhart and Keffer 1991; McCarthy et al. 1991). Thus, a defect in the local production of IGFs or their regula-tion could be important in the pathogenesis of impaired bone formation in osteoporosis. A special difficulty in assessing the role of IGFs is that bone also produces binding proteins which can either inhibit or enhance their action. The production of the binding proteins in bone cells is also regulated (Chen et al. 1991), sometimes in parallel to the effects on the IGFs themselves.

Transforming growth factor β and a family of related peptides, which have been called bone morphogenetic proteins (BMP) or osteogenins, have been extracted from bone and are potent mitogens. Active TGFβ can also inhibit bone resorption and increase bone cell differentiation. Regulation of TGFβ may be accomplished more by activation than by altering the amount synthesized. Indeed, the TGFβ and BMP in bone may be present largely in a latent, matrix-bound form. All the potent bone resorbers can release active TGFβ from bone in organ culture (PFEILSCHIFTER and MUNDY 1987). This active form could then both inhibit further resorption and initiate the replication and differentiation of osteoblast precursors. Thus TGFβ is a prime candidate for the role of a "coupling factor." However, we do not know whether the major source is resorbed matrix or cellular secretion. If TGFβ and BMPs are simply released and activated during resorption, it is hard to see how they could be involved in the pathogenesis of osteoporosis, but if cellular production is critical, then a deficiency could be pathogenetic because resorption would be prolonged and formation delayed.

While the other growth factors such as platelet-derived growth factor, fibroblast growth factor, and epidermal growth factor may turn out to be important in the pathogenesis of osteoporosis, there is as yet little to suggest such a role (CANALIS et al. 1991). These factors are present in bone and in adjacent marrow cells and are probably released during injury and repair. They could play a role in the healing, or lack of healing, of osteoporotic fractures.

IV. Calcium and Other Nutrients

One of the most controversial aspects of osteoporosis research has been the debate over whether calcium deficiency is an important pathogenetic factor (AVIOLI and HEANEY 1991). Certainly, calcium deficiency in childhood and adolescence could affect peak bone mass. That this may lead to an increase in fracture incidence later in life is suggested by an epidemiologic analysis of hip fractures comparing two regions in Yugoslavia. In one region the habitual intake of calcium was about 900 mg/day and in the other it was 600 mg/day. Although both groups had similar rates of bone loss with age, the high calcium group had a higher peak bone mass and fewer hip fractures after age 60 years (MATKOVIC et al. 1979). However, these regions may also have differed in the intake of other nutrients and in life-style. Analysis of all the available data does suggest that calcium has some effect on both bone mass and fracture incidence (CUMMING 1990). The strongest argument against a major role for calcium is the fact that many populations which have low calcium intakes do not have a high incidence of osteoporotic fractures. This could be explained by genetic differences in their bone mass and strength as well as differences in physical activity or other aspects of diet. Calcium supplementation certainly does not abrogate age-related bone loss, but may slow the rate of loss, particularly in the appendicular skeleton. Moreover, in one study postmenopausal women with very low calcium intakes were shown to have lower rates of bone loss when they increased their calcium intake (DAWSON-HUGHES et al. 1990).

Other nutrients may play a role in reaching peak bone mass and in preventing or causing further bone loss. High protein intakes have been implicated as a cause of bone loss because they cause hypercalciuria (Heaney and Recker 1982). However, in balance studies using natural sources of protein, there is no evidence for more negative balance with increased protein intake. Moreover, there is not as clear an epidemiologic association between protein intake and the incidence of osteoporotic fractures as there is for protein intake and renal stones. Ascorbic acid deficiency can cause osteoporosis (Tsunenari et al. 1991), but this does not appear to be a factor in primary osteoporosis. Deficiencies of trace elements such as boron (F.H. Nielson et al. 1987) and copper (T. Wilson et al. 1981) have been implicated in bone loss, but the evidence is limited.

There is generally a positive correlation between body weight and bone density (Ribot et al. 1988; Liel et al. 1988). The basis for this correlation is not fully understood. Increased weight is probably associated with increased muscle mass, and this would result in increased mechanical force on the skeleton. In postmenopausal women, the increase in weight is associated with an increase in body fat, which in turn increases the conversion of adrenal androgen to estrone by aromatization, and this could increase bone mass. Finally, it is possible that genetic determinants influence body weight and bone mass in the same direction (Seeman et al. 1989).

V. Physical Activity and Life-style

Although the skeleton is formed on a cartilage template which is determined genetically, both the amount and form of the bones can subsequently be modified by mechanical forces (Dalsky et al. 1988). Studies on complete immobilization in animals suggest that about half of the mass of an individual bone can be lost if it is no longer subjected to mechanical force (Thompson and Rodan 1988). Increases in bone mass as great as 15%–25% have been demonstrated in bones subjected to increased stress.

While these effects could certainly be relevant to immobilization-induced osteoporosis, their role in primary osteoporosis is less clear. Epidemiologic studies suggest that an increase in the incidence of hip fracture may be related to the increase in the use of automobiles, elevators, and other forms of transportation available to our aging population and their more sedentary life-style and hence the decrease in walking, stair climbing, and other physical activities (Gardsell et al. 1991). By the same token, increased physical activity is believed to help prevent osteoporosis. Vigorous weight-bearing exercise has been shown to increase vertebral bone mass in postmenopausal women (Dalsky et al. 1988). Exercise may not be entirely beneficial to bone, however. Intense exercise in women may produce hypothalamically mediated amenorrhea. This in turn may lead to decreased sex hormone production and bone loss (Marcus et al. 1988). Thus, the fact that mechanical forces can influence bone metabolism is well established, but the mechanisms are poorly understood. There are a number of observations pointing to a role for prostaglandins in mediating the effects of mechanical forces, but other local mediators could play a role (EL HAJ et al. 1990).

Several other life-style factors have been associated with decreased bone mass. Probably the most consistent of these is cigarette smoking. Women who smoke cigarettes generally have a lower bone mass at all ages (MAZESS and BARDEN 1991). This may be because smoking decreases estrogen levels by increasing metabolic degradation (MICHNOVICZ et al. 1986; CASSIDENTI et al. 1991). Smoking may also have effects on nutrition or may have direct effects on bone (FANG et al. 1991). There is also some evidence that relatively modest alcohol intakes may be associated with decreased bone mass, although this is not consistent (BIKLE et al. 1990; CHAPPARD et al. 1991). Finally, caffeine intake has been implicated as a cause of bone loss, perhaps by increasing urinary calcium excretion, but recent epidemiologic studies do not show any association between low bone mass and high caffeine intakes (MASSEY 1991).

VI. Alternative Hypotheses

Two alternative hypostheses for the pathogenesis of osteoporosis are presented in Fig. 1. Hypothesis A, which we have labeled "type I,' focuses on the role of local factors which regulate resorption and formation. Bone loss arises because of an excess of local resorption stimulators or a deficiency of bone growth factors which is aggravated by sex hormone deficiency. This scheme could explain the relatively low PTH response and decreased vitamin D activation in patients with vertebral crush fracture syndrome. Hypothesis B, labeled "type II," focuses on cellular aging, calcium deficiency, and secondary hyperparathyroidism. These can interact with sex hormone deficiency to increase bone resorption and limit bone formation. This combination is likely to occur in older men and women and thus could be considered most appropriate to explain type II osteoporosis. However, the contribution of sex hormone deficiency in men has not been adequately evaluated. These hypotheses are presented mainly to provide a framework for future investigators. Some of the possible experimental approaches that might support or refute these are mentioned at the conclusion of this chapter.

C. Secondary Osteoporosis

There are a number of forms of osteoporosis which we term "secondary" because they are associated with specific diseases or ascribed to the effects of pharmacologic agents. Clinically, the distinction between primary and secondary osteoporosis is not always clear cut. For example, hyperthyroidism or excessive thyroid hormone replacement is likely to aggravate osteoporosis, but has not been shown to cause osteoporosis in the absence

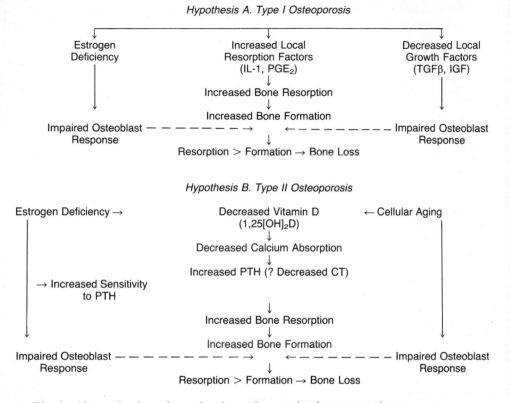

Fig. 1. Alternative hypotheses for the pathogenesis of osteoporosis

of other risk factors. Even glucocorticoid-induced osteoporosis, which is the most common and severe form of secondary osteoporosis, leads to fractures most often in postmenopausal women who are at higher risk for primary osteoporosis. The major forms of secondary osteoporosis are listed in Table 1. We will only touch briefly on those forms for which there is minimal information on pathogenesis.

I. Glucocorticoid-Induced Osteoporosis

Probably the most common form of secondary osteoporosis is that induced by glucocorticoids. Endogenous glucocorticoid excess due to Cushing's syndrome is relatively rare. However, osteoporosis can be the presenting manifestation of Cushing's disease (Ross and Linch 1982) both in children and adults. Exogenous glucocorticoids are a more common cause of osteoporosis because they are administered to large numbers of patients with chronic inflammatory disorders. Many of these patients are more susceptible to osteoporosis because their illness itself causes bone loss. In rheumatoid

Table 1. Causes of secondary osteoporosis

A. Endocrine causes
   1. Hyperparathyroidism
   2. Cushing's syndrome
   3. Hypogonadism
   4. Hyperthyroidism
   5. Prolactinoma
   6. Diabetes mellitus
   7. Acromegaly
   8. Pregnancy and lactation
B. Bone marrow disorders
   1. Plasma cell dyscrasias: multiple myeloma and macroglobulinemia
   2. Systemic mastocytosis
   3. Leukemias
   4. Lymphomas
   5. Chronic anemias: sickle cell disease and thalassemia minor
   6. Lipidoses: Gaucher's disease
   7. Myeloproliferative disorders: polycythemia rubra vera
C. Connective tissue disorders
   1. Osteogenesis imperfecta
   2. Ehlers-Danlos syndrome
   3. Marfan's syndrome
   4. Homocystinuria
   5. Menke's syndrome
   6. Scurvy
D. Drug induced
   1. Corticosteroids
   2. Heparin
   3. Anticonvulsants
   4. Methotrexate, cyclosporin A
   5. GnRH agonist or antagonist therapy
   6. Aluminum-containing antacids
E. Immobilization
F. Renal disease
   1. Chronic renal failure
   2. Renal tubular acidosis
G. Nutritional and gastrointestinal
   1. Malabsorption
   2. Prolonged total parenteral nutrition
   3. Postgastrectomy
   4. Hepatobiliary disease
   5. Chronic hypophosphatemia
H. Miscellaneous
   1. Familial dysautonomia (Riley-Day disease)
   2. Reflex sympathetic dystrophy

arthritis and hepatic disease, inflammatory and nutritional factors are likely to aggravate bone loss. Physical activity is limited in most patients on glucocorticoid therapy and thus can contribute to bone loss.

The incidence and severity of glucocorticoid-induced osteoporosis appears to depend on the total amount and/or duration of steroid therapy. It can occur in patients treated with relatively low doses. However, patients on low-dose long-term steroids (<8 mg prednisone or its equivalent per day) appear to lose bone less rapidly than those on a higher maintenance dose (De Deuxchaisnes et al. 1984; Reid and Heap 1990). The incidence of fractures is highest in the group that we expect to be most susceptible, that is, Caucasian postmenopausal women. Nevertheless, with glucocorticoid, excess osteoporotic fractures can occur in both sexes, all races and at all ages. Vertebral and rib fractures are particularly common, but appendicular fractures are also seen. Another skeletal complication of prolonged glucocorticoid therapy is aseptic necrosis, particularly of the head of the femur or humerus. While this lesion is not directly due to osteoporosis, it is possible that the weakness of the underlying bone does contribute to the progression or severity of aseptic necrosis.

Glucocorticoid-induced osteoporosis is the result of a combination of systemic effects on mineral metabolism and local effects on bone. Inhibition of calcium absorption appears to be due to a direct effect on the intestine rather than an alteration in vitamin D activation. The intestinal response to vitamin D metabolites is diminished with glucocorticoid treatment, perhaps due to a change in $1,25(OH)_2D$ receptors (Morris et al. 1990). Impairment of calcium absorption can be overcome by using pharmacologic doses of vitamin D either in the form of $25(OH)D$ or $1,25(OH)_2D$ (Colette et al. 1987). The impairment of calcium absorption can lead to secondary hyperparathyroidism, which is considered the major factor responsible for increased bone resorption in glucocorticoid-treated patients (Morris et al. 1990). Studies with different glucocorticoid analogs used therapeutically have shown differences in the effect on calcium absorption and differences in the initial rates of bone loss. This may be due to differences in metabolism and distribution. For example, deflazacort, a glucocorticoid which when taken orally must be deacetylated in the liver before it can act on cells, appears to cause less early bone loss than prednisone or prednisolone which could act directly on the intestinal epithelium when given orally (Gennari et al. 1984).

There are other indirect effects of glucocorticoids which could contribute to bone loss, although these are probably less important than impairment of calcium absorption. Patients on glucocorticoids often have increased calcium and phosphorus excretion in the urine. The mechanisms of these renal effects are not known. Glucocorticoids can inhibit growth hormone secretion and at high concentrations also inhibit gonadotropin secretion, which can decrease sex hormone production (Sakakura et al. 1975; Luton et al. 1977; Hsueh and Erickson 1978; Doer and Pirke 1976; Schaison et al. 1978; MacAdams et al. 1986). Exogenous glucocorticoids will reduce ACTH secretion and decrease the production of adrenal androgens, which are a major source of estrone in postmenopausal women, through aromatization in adipose tissue (Crilly et al. 1978). Finally, the muscle weakness that occurs with glucocorticoid excess could contribute to bone loss through a decrease in mechanical stress (Askari et al. 1976).

Even if glucocorticoids had none of the indirect effects outlined above, we would still expect to see substantial bone loss because of their powerful direct effects on bone. Inhibition of bone formation is probably more important than stimulation of bone resorption. Indeed, some studies suggest that bone resorption is not increased unless there is marked secondary hyperparathyroidism. Studies on the direct effects of glucocorticoids on bone resorption have yielded conflicting results. Prolonged glucocorticoid treatment in organ culture usually results in a decrease in bone resorption, probably due to a decrease in the replication and differentiation of osteoclast precursors (DIETRICH et al. 1979; DEMPSTER 1989). In short-term organ culture studies at low doses and in studies with macrophage-induced resorption of bone particles, glucocorticoids have been found to increase resorption (GRONOWICZ et al. 1990). This effect can occur with physiologic concentrations and may be transient. Glucocorticoids clearly can have an inhibitory effect on bone resorption in response to some stimuli, particularly IL-1. Glucocorticoids could also reduce the resorptive response to agents which act by stimulating endogenous prostaglandin production. They do not inhibit resorption stimulated by PTH or $1,25(OH)_2D$, except at very high concentrations (RAISZ et al. 1972).

The major effect of glucocorticoids is to inhibit bone formation both in vitro and in vivo. In organ culture, there is a paradoxical biphasic effect. At physiologic concentrations, glucocorticoids can transiently increase collagen synthesis by osteoblasts. Moreover, relatively low concentrations of glucocorticoids can enhance the differentiation of osteoblastic cells in culture and increase their ability to produce mineralizing nodules. However, the long-term effect of glucocorticoids in organ culture is to inhibit collagen synthesis (CHYUN et al. 1984; CANALIS 1983). This appears to follow inhibition of the replication of osteoblast precursors. However, decreased collagen synthesis cannot be explained on the basis of decreased replication since glucocorticoids can inhibit collagen synthesis even in the presence of inhibitors of DNA synthesis such as aphidicolin. Thus glucocorticoids must also inhibit differentiation of pre-osteoblasts. These effects could be due to a decrease in the production or activation of local growth factors. Glucocorticoids can decrease IGF I production by bone cells, both in cell and organ culture, and addition of IGF I can overcome glucocorticoid inhibition (McCARTHY et al. 1990). PGE_2 can also reverse the glucocorticoid effect (RAISZ and FALL 1990), but IGF I may still be the common denominator, since there is a close correlation between the increase in collagen synthesis with PGE_2 and the increase in IGF I production in glucocorticoid-treated organ cultures. Glucocorticoids may also decrease the activity of TGFβ either by direct inhibition of synthesis or by inhibiting enzymes, such as plasminogen activator, which are necessary to convert this factor from the latent to the active form. In vivo rapid decreases in osteocalcin levels in response to corticosteroids have been observed which suggest a rapid inhibitory effect on osteoblast function (N.K. NIELSEN et al. 1988).

II. Hyperparathyroidism

The classical severe bone disease of hyperparathyroidism (HPT), osteitis fibrosa cystica, is now rarely seen clinically in primary HPT, although it is seen in some patients with renal failure and severe secondary HPT. On the other hand, patients with mild primary HPT in whom symptoms are minimal do have some bone disease when studied by histomorphometric analysis of iliac crest bone biopsies (Parisien et al. 1990). The skeletal abnormalities are different from those observed in severe cases, and cystic lesions are rare. The major features of the bone disease are a generalized increase in bone turnover with a marked increase in the amount of bone surface undergoing active remodeling, both resorption and formation. Trabecular bone volume is usually well preserved and may even be increased above that expected for age, but cortical thickness is decreased in these biopsies. This selective effect on cortical bone has been confirmed by bone densitometry, which shows that almost half the patients have a reduced cortical bone mass of the radius, more than two standard deviations below that expected for age, while only one-sixth have a similar degree of reduction in lumbar bone density (Silverberg et al. 1989b). From these results, one might expect a greater incidence of appendicular fractures and no increase in vertebral crush fractures in hyperparathyroid patients. Some studies bear this out (R.J. Wilson et al. 1988), while others suggest that vertebral as well as appendicular fractures are increased, but the epidemiologic data are far from adequate (Peacock 1991).

Since primary HPT is most common in postmenopausal women, it could represent an aggravating factor for the development of osteoporosis in this population. Nevertheless, PTH excess cannot be demonstrated in patients with vertebral crush fractures (Silverberg 1989a). Bone loss may not be progressive. One recent study suggested that most of the bone loss occurred early in the course of the disease and that bone mass was subsequently stable (Rao et al. 1988). Whatever the mechanisms, decreased bone mass is considered an indication for neck exploration and an attempt at surgical cure in patients with HPT.

III. Hyperthyroidism

There is ample evidence, both in vitro and in vivo, that excess thyroid hormone can increase bone resorption (Baran and Braverman 1991). In vivo, this is associated with an increased bone turnover, but the formation response may not be adequate and as a result bone mass may decrease. Bone loss has been observed in hypothyroid patients treated with thyroid hormone replacement. This has been particularly striking in studies in which a mixture of thyroxin (T_4) and triiodothyronine (T_3) were used. It is possible that the addition of T_3, which produces high serum concentrations for a short period, has a particularly adverse effect on bone (Coindre et al. 1986).

Even when T_4 is used for replacement, the doses are often excessive as evidenced by a reduction in thyroid-stimulating hormone (TSH) to below normal values, and this may contribute to bone loss (GREENSPAN et al. 1991). In patients who have hypothyroidism due to destruction of thyroid tissue, calcitonin deficiency might also play a role in the adverse response to hormone replacement (BODY and HEATH 1987). However, some investigators have failed to detect any bone loss in patients treated with thyroid replacement including those with suppressed TSH (TOH and BROWN 1990). Neither endogenous nor exogenous hyperthyroidism has been associated with an increase in osteoporotic fractures in epidemiologic studies. However, in many clinical series a large proportion of patients with vertebral crush fractures are found to be on thyroid hormone replacement therapy.

IV. Hypogonadism

The mechanisms by which loss of estrogen and androgen result in bone loss have already been discussed. Clinically, there are many different forms of hypogonadism which can be associated with osteoporosis. Bone loss is regularly observed in almost all forms of hypogonadism, but these are not enough epidemiologic data to determine the incidence of fractures in most of these conditions. Nevertheless, osteoporotic fractures have been reported in patients with anorexia nervosa (RIGOTTI et al. 1984, 1991; CROSBY et al. 1985), athletic amenorrhea (MARCUS et al. 1988), and Turner's (BEALS 1973) and Kallmann's syndromes. Amenorrhea in women with polycystic ovary syndrome or late onset adrenal hyperplasia is not associated with a decreased bone mass, presumably because there is no decrease in estrogen, or if there is it is compensated by an increase in androgen production from the adrenal or ovary. Patients with prolactinoma often have amenorrhea and may have a reduction in bone mass, but this has not been clearly associated with fractures (SCHLECHTE et al. 1987). Finally, as noted above, women with anovulatory cycles and short luteal phases may have a reduction in bone mass (PRIOR et al. 1990). While this has been ascribed to a decrease in progesterone secretion, a change in estrogen production has not been ruled out. Patients with endometriosis have also been reported to have low bone mass but this has not been confirmed in other studies (COMITE et al. 1989; LANE et al. 1991a,b; DODIN et al. 1991). Estrogen production may not be decreased in these patients, and the loss of bone has been attributed to a possible increase in inflammatory mediators such as IL-1, which have been found in the peritoneal cavity.

V. Nutritional and Gastrointestinal Disorders

In the past, the most common form of bone disease in nutritional and gastrointestinal disorders was considered to be osteomalacia due to deficiency or malabsorption of vitamin D and calcium. Recent bone biopsy studies on patients with malnutrition and gastrointestinal disorders have shown osteoporosis without impairment of mineralization as the predominant lesion. In western countries, alcoholism (BIKLE et al. 1990), chronic liver disease (DIAMOND et al. 1990), inflammatory bowel disease (COMPSTON et al. 1987), and parenteral nutrition (SHIKE et al. 1986) have all been associated with osteoporosis. While low levels of 25(OH)D are sometimes encountered in these patients, other biochemical changes associated with osteomalacia such as hypocalcemia, hypophosphatemia, and increased bone alkaline phosphatase are less common. Many factors may contribute to low bone mass in these individuals. Alcoholism and liver disease are associated with diminished testosterone levels in men, and alcoholics may have increased glucocorticoid secretion (alcoholic pseudo-Cushing's disease). Failure of hepatocellular function as well as protein deficiency and poor caloric intake may result in diminished production of IGF I (UNTERMAN et al. 1985). Whether the low albumin levels in chronic liver disease have any effect on bone is not clear, although albumin is deposited in bone matrix and may play some role in bone formation. Alcoholism is associated with an increased incidence of hip fractures which could be due to more frequent traumatic events as well as effects on bone (FELSON et al. 1988).

Decreased bone mass has been documented in both protein calorie malnutrition (marasmus) and protein deficiency (kwashiorkor). Here, again, growth factor production may be diminished and glucocorticoid secretion increased. Other factors such as low calcium and phosphorus intake and associated inflammatory disorders with increased IL I and TNFα (cachectin) production could contribute to bone loss. Total parenteral nutrition is also associated with metabolic bone disease in which aluminum deposition and hypercalciuria could play a role, but additional nutritional factors may also be involved (HURLEY and McMAHON 1990; KLEIN and COBURN 1991).

VI. Renal Disease

The most common metabolic bone diseases in patients with chronic renal failure are (1) osteitis fibrosa, associated with secondary hyperparathyroidism, (2) osteomalacia, associated with impaired vitamin D activation, and (3) aluminum osteodystrophy, associated with alumium toxicity from antacids or aluminum-containing dialysis fluid. Osteoporosis has also been described in patients with chronic renal failure, but is not common. A more definite association between osteoporosis and renal disease has been observed with tubular disorders. In renal hypercalciuria due to impaired tubular reabsorption, the high rate of urinary calcium excretion is associated with decreased bone mass (SAKHAEE et al. 1985). Indeed, a recent study suggests that a renal calcium leak is a general feature of osteoporosis (NORDIN et al. 1991). A role for renal calcium loss in the pathogenesis of osteoporosis is also supported by the finding that hypertensive patients treated with thiazide diuretics, which reduce urine calcium secretion, have a higher bone mass and a lower incidence of fractures than age-matched hypertensive patients on other drugs (FELSON et al. 1991; LACROIX et al. 1990). It is possible that thiazides have a direct effect on the skeleton, since they are related to carbonic anhydrase inhibitors, which can decrease bone resorption by reducing osteoclast hydrogen ion production. Renal tubular acidosis in children is most often associated with rickets and osteomalacia, but some older patients may show osteoporosis. Acquired renal tubular acidosis can occur in chronic renal disease, particularly pyelonephritis, and is a potential but probably rare cause of osteoporosis.

VII. Multiple Myeloma and Other Hematologic Disorders

Multiple myeloma is not always listed among secondary forms of osteoporosis because the clinical picture is usually one of localized lytic bone lesions. However, multiple myeloma can present as vertebral crush fracture syndrome. In these patients the myeloma cells are presumably widespread through the vertebral marrow and produce diffuse osteolysis and vertebral collapse. There may or may not be isolated lytic lesions in other bones. Early studies on multiple myeloma showed that the osteolytic activity was due to an "osteoclast activating factor" (OAF) released by the myeloma cells, similar to the OAF released by phytohemagglutinin or antigen-stimulated human mononuclear cell cultures. The latter OAF has been identified as IL I. However, TNFα and TNFβ are also forms of OAF. OAF from normal cells was recently identified as IL I, while OAF from myeloma cells could be either TNFβ (lymphotoxin) (GARRETT et al. 1987) or IL I (KAWANO et al. 1989). These findings give support to a possible role of cytokines in the pathogenesis of primary osteoporosis as discussed above. Other lymphoproliferative disorders can produce osteolysis, but usually do not present with a typical osteoporotic syndrome. Some lymphomas and leukemias have been found to produce the PTH-related peptide of malignancy or to convert 25(OH)D to the active hormonal form, 1,25(OH)$_2$D, rather than produce cytokines. Nevertheless some patients with lymphoblastic leukemia do present with vertebral fractures (COHN et al. 1987; RIBEIRO et al. 1988).

In addition to lymphoproliferative disorders, bone loss is characteristic of the hemolytic anemias in which there is marked bone marrow hyperplasia (RAISZ 1981). Children with homozygous β-thalassemia have significant cortical thinning and an increased tendency to fracture. In these patients PTH levels are decreased, and it seems likely that the hyperplastic marrow produces bone-resorbing factors (ZAMBONI et al. 1986; POOTRAKUL et al. 1981). These might be cytokines or prostaglandins, but have not yet been identified. Decreased bone density has been described in hemochromatosis (DIAMOND et al. 1989), polycythemia rubra vera (JACOBS and GOODMAN 1990), and sickle cell hemoglobinopathy (OZOH et al. 1990), possibly because of increased production of cytokines by bone marrow cells.

VIII. Mast Cells and Heparin

Systemic mastocytosis has been associated with osteoporosis and some studies have suggested that there is an increased number of mast cells in the marrow area adjacent to bone in patients with primary osteoporosis (Chines et al. 1991; Cundy et al. 1987). Mast cells have many products which might mediate bone loss. The major prostaglandin produced by mast cells is PGD_2, which is not a potent bone resorber but could have local effects. Another product of mast cells is heparin. Its role in osteoporosis is supported by clinical observations that patients on prolonged high-dose heparin therapy can develop osteoporosis (Ginsberg et al. 1990). Heparin was found to increase PTH response and also to be a direct stimulator of bone resorption in mouse calvarial cultures (Goldhaber 1965). In long-bone organ cultures, heparin had no direct stimulatory effect, but did interact with fibroblast growth factors (FGFs). Both acidic and basic FGF could stimulate bone resorption, but the effect of acidic FGF was weak and markedly enhanced by addition of heparin, while the dose response curve for basic FGF was shifted to the left so that lower doses could stimulate bone resorption in the presence of heparin (Simmons and Raisz 1991). Heparin has also been shown to inhibit collagen synthesis in cultured calvaria (Hurley et al. 1990a,b). This effect of heparin appears to be independent of its anticoagulant activity and is seen with the purified low molecular weight preparation in current clinical use. Whether there are specific heparin receptors on osteoblasts and osteoclasts is not known; however, the concentrations of heparin required to stimulate bone resorption or inhibit bone formation are relatively high (5–125 μg/ml). Some recent clinical evidence from patients who are receiving heparin during pregnancy to prevent the complications of autoimmune disease as well as thromboembolic disorders suggests that bone loss can occur under these circumstances and thus could contribute to the risk of osteoporosis (Ginsberg et al. 1990).

IX. Osteogenesis Imperfecta

Osteogenesis imperfecta is a heterogeneous genetic disorder associated with increased fractures. In its most severe form multiple fractures occur in utero and the disorder is lethal. In milder forms there may be an increase in fractures in childhood which then cease after puberty, with a subsequent increase in women after the menopause (Paterson et al. 1984). In the mild form of osteogenesis imperfecta (so-called type I) the defect is usually associated with a decrease in collagen gene expression and a decrease in bone density in the young adults even after they have stopped having multiple fractures (Kurtz 1985). A recent report described a patient with vertebral compression fractures who had a defect in the gene for α_2 (I) procollagen (CPL1A2), as this defect was also found in other members of the family and associated with increased fractures (Spotila et al. 1991).

While the clinical picture of these patients with osteogenesis imperfecta differs from that seen in most forms of primary and secondary osteoporosis, it is possible that subtle defects in the genes for collagen or other bone matrix proteins are responsible for bone fragility in other patients in whom the diagnosis of osteoporosis is made. However, it is difficult to explain the typical high turnover forms of osteoporosis in which excessive resorption is the major pathogenetic mechanism on the basis of a genetic defect in matrix unless this genetic defect results in an increased susceptibility of the bone to destruction by osteoclasts.

X. Miscellaneous Therapeutic Agents

Other than glucocorticoids, there are no drugs which have been clearly demonstrated to produce osteoporosis. However, there are a number of pharmacologic agents which might have such an effect. The bone disease associated with phenytoin (diphenlhydantoin) and other drugs used in epilepsy such as carbamazepine (LAMBERG-ALLARDT 1990) has been called "anticonvulsant osteomalacia," but patients on these drugs sometimes show a clinical picture of decreased bone mass without the biochemical or morphological findings of osteomalacia (GOTFREDSEN 1986). Anticonvulsants have multiple direct and indirect actions which could reduce bone mass. Early studies focused on the reduction in 25(OH)D levels, probably associated with an alteration in vitamin D metabolism in the liver as well as diminished dietary intake and inadequate sunlight exposure. These effects have been observed with other anticonvulsants such as phenylbarbital and carbamazepine, but not with sodium valproate. Phenytoin has been found to affect bone directly in organ culture at relatively high concentrations, inhibiting both resorption and formation. The relevance of this to clinical changes in bone metabolism has not been established. Slowing of bone accretion in children and decreased bone mass in adult epileptics may be related to anticonvulsants, but could also be due to physical inactivity, inadequate nutrition, and abnormalities of motor development. This, in turn, is likely to lead to an increased incidence of fractures.

It seems likely that the agents used in cancer chemotherapy and immunosuppression can lead to osteoporosis. In addition to suppressing ovarian function with chemotherapy, they are potent inhibitors of cell replication which are likely to diminish bone remodeling.

Immunosuppressive agents used in transplantation may have powerful effects on bone. In vitro, cyclosporin A was found to inhibit bone resorption, but in vivo studies are inconsistent (ORCEL et al. 1989, 1991; SCHLOSBERG et al. 1989). Although some decrease in bone resorption has been reported in animals, an increase in resorption has also been observed (MOVSOWITZ et al. 1989). It is possible that this is related to an increase in the synthesis of $1,25(OH)_2D$ (STEIN et al. 1991). If this is the case, one might expect that after renal transplantation, when the capacity to synthesize $1,25(OH)_2D$ is restored, a further increase in production due to cyclosporin could be responsible for accelerated bone resorption and bone loss.

D. Conclusion

In this chapter we have summarized our current, limited understanding of the pathogenesis of primary and secondary osteoporosis. We have suggested that excessive production or response to local resorptive factors or decreased production or response to local growth factors is important in the pathogenesis of primary osteoporosis, but this view is not yet supported by direct evidence. Obtaining such direct evidence presents formidable difficulties. Local regulators are produced in relatively small amounts, and production may be site-specific. To assess variations in production at the level of gene transcription, it will be necessary to use such methods as the polymerase chain reaction to amplify mRNA levels for the protein factors themselves or for the enzymes which produce nonprotein factors. To determine which cells are involved, it will also be necessary to localize the factors by in situ hybridization of mRNA or immunocytochemistry. These techniques are currently being developed, but have not yet been applied to a comparison of osteoporotic and normal bone. If the major pathogenetic mechanism is a change in response to these factors rather than their production, the problem will be even more difficult. Receptors for the local factors will have to be identified and quantitated. Signal transduction mechanisms for some factors have not yet been identified and this must also be explored further.

These new applications of the techniques of molecular and cellular biology to metabolic bone disease are exciting prospects for the future. Meanwhile, our improved ability to assess bone resorption and bone formation by noninvasive biochemical methods and the improved precision of measures of bone mass at multiple sites will also contribute to our understanding of pathogenesis, particularly in assessing the relative importance of changes in resorption and formation. These studies will also help us to refine our therapeutic approach. Unfortunately, while we have agents which clearly can inhibit bone resorption, there is as yet no reliable method for increasing bone formation in a structurally effective manner. Fluoride, which does stimulate bone formation, may produce weaker bone since fracture incidence can increase (RIGGS et al. 1990). However, as knowledge of the regulation of osteoblast function increases, more physiologic stimulation of bone formation may become feasible. Thus we can expect more effective approaches to therapy, not only from improved understanding of the pathogenesis, but from improved understanding of the alterations in bone metabolism in osteoporosis.

References

Aloia JF, Vaswani A, Yeh JK, Ellis K, Yasumura S, Cohn SH (1988) Calcitriol in the treatment of postmenopausal osteoporosis. Am J Med 84:401–408

Askari A, Vignos PJ Jr, Moskowitz RW (1976) Steroid myopathy in connective tissue disease. Am J Med 61:485–492

Auwerx J, Dequeker J, Bouillon R, Geusens P, Nijs J (1988) Mineral metabolism and bone mass at peripheral and axial skeleton in diabetes mellitus. Diabetes 37:8–12

Avioli LV, Heaney RP (1991) Calcium intake and bone health. Calcif Tissue Int 48:221–223

Baran DT, Braverman LE (1991) Thyroid hormones and bone mass. J Clin Endocrinol Metab 72:1182–1183

Bauer RL (1988) Ethnic differences in hip fracture – a reduced incidence in Mexican-Americans. Am J Epidemiol 127:145–149

Beals RK (1973) Orthopedic aspects of the XO (Turner's) syndrome. Clin Orthop 97:19–34

Bennett AE, Wahner HW, Riggs BL, Hintz RL (1984) Insulin-like growth factors I and II: aging and bone density in women. J Clin Endocrinol Metab 59:701–704

Bikle D, Stessin A, Halloran B, Steinbach L, Recker RR (1990) Alcohol-induced bone disease. Osteoporosis 3:1544–1551

Body JJ, Heath H III (1987) Estimates of circulating monomeric calcitonin: physiological studies in normal and thyroidectomized man. J Clin Endocrinol Metab 57:897–903

Bouillon R (1991) Diabetic bone disease. Calcif Tissue Int 49:155–160

Brody JA, Farmer ME, White LR (1984) Absence of menopausal effect on hip fracture occurrence in white females. Am J Public Health 74:1397–1398

Brown JP, Delmas PD, Arlot M, Meunier PJ (1987) Active bone turnover of the cortico-endosteal envelope in postmenopausal osteoporosis. J Clin Endocrinol Metab 64:954 959

Buchanan JR, Myers C, Lloyd T et al. (1988) Determinants of peak trabecular bone density in women: the role of androgen, estrogen and exercise. J Bone Miner Res 3:673–680

Burns DM, Birnbaum RS, Roos BA (1989) A neuroendocrine peptide derived from the amino-terminal half of rat procalcitonin. Mol Endocrinol 3:140–147

Canalis E (1983) Effect of glucocorticoids on type I collagen synthesis, alkaline phosphatase activity, and deoxyribonucleic acid content in cultured rat calvariae. Endocrinology 112:931–939

Canalis E, Centrella M, Burch W et al. (1989) Insulin-like growth factor-1 mediates selective anabolic effects of parathyroid hormone in bone culture. J Clin Invest 83:60–65

Canalis E, McCarthy TL, Centrella M (1991) Growth factors and cytokines in bone cell metabolism. Annu Rev Med 42:17–24

Cassidenti DL, Vijod AG, Vijod MA, Stanczyk FZ, Lobo RA (1990) Short-term effects of smoking on the pharmacokinetic profiles of micronized estradiol in postmenopausal women. Am J Obstet Gynecol 163:1953–1960

Chappard D, Plantard B, Petitjean M, Alexandre C, Riffat G (1991) Alcoholic cirrhosis and osteoporosis in men – a light and scanning electron microscopy study. J Stud Alcohol 52:269–274

Chen TL, Chang LY, Bates RL, Perlman AJ (1991) Dexamethasone and 1,25-dihydroxyvitamin D_3 modulation of insulin-like growth factor-binding proteins in rat osteoblast-like cell cultures. Endocrinology 128:73–80

Chines A, Pacifici R, Avioli LV, Teitelbaum SL, Korenblat PE (1991) Systemic mastocytosis presenting as osteoporosis – a clinical and histomorphometric study. J Clin Endocrinol Metab 72:140–144

Christiansen C, Riis BJ, Rodbro P (1987) Prediction of rapid bone loss in postmenopausal women. Lancet I:1105–1108

Chyun YS, Kream BE, Raisz LG (1984) Cortisol decreases bone formation by inhibiting periosteal cell proliferation. Endocrinology 114:477–480

Civitelli R, Gonnelli S, Zacchei F, Bigazzi S, Vattimo A, Avioli LV, Genarri C (1988) Bone turnover in postmenopausal osteoporosis. Effect of calcitonin treatment. J Clin Invest 82:1268–1274

Cohn SL, Morgan ER, Mallette LE (1987) The spectrum of metabolic bone diseases in lymphoblastic leukemia. Cancer 59:346–350

Coindre JM, David JP, Riviere L, Goussot JF, Roger P, de Mascarel A, Meunier PJ (1986) Bone loss in hypothyroidism with hormone replacement. Arch Intern Med 146:48–53

Colette C, Monnier L, Pares Herbute N, Blotman F, Mirouze J (1987) Calcium absorption in corticoid treated subjects: effects on a single oral dose of calcitriol. Horm Metab Res 19:335–338

Comite F, Delman M, Hutchinson-Williams K, DeCherney AH, Jensen P (1989) Reduced bone mass in reproductive-aged women with endometriosis. J Clin Endocrinol Metab 69:837–842

Compston JE, Judd D, Crawley EO, Evans WD, Evans C, Church HA, Reid EM, Rhodes J (1987) Osteoporosis in patients with inflammatory bowel disease. Gut 28:410–415

Crilly RG, Cawood M, Marshall DH, Nordin BE (1978) Hormonal status in normal, osteoporotic, and corticosteroid-treated postmenopausal women. J R Soc Med 71:733–736

Crosby LO, Kaplan FK, Portschak MJ (1985) Effect of anorexia nervosa on bone morphometry in young women. Clin Orthop 201:271–277

Cumming RG (1990) Calcium intake and bone mass: a quantitative review of the evidence. Calcif Tissue Int 47:194–201

Cundy T, Beneton MNC, Darby AJ, Marshall WJ, Kanis JA (1987) Osteopenia in systemic mastocytosis: natural history and responses to treatment with inhibitors of bone resorption. Bone 8:149–156

Dalsky GP, Stock KS, Ehsani AA, Slatopolsky E, Lee WC, Birge SJ (1988) Weight-bearing exercise training and lumbar bone mineral content in postmenopausal women. Ann Intern Med 108:824–828

Dawson-Hughes B, Dallal GE, Krall EA, Sadowski L, Sahyoun N, Tannenbaum S (1990) A controlled trial of the effect of calcium supplementation on bone density in postmenopausal women. N Engl J Med 323:878–883

de Deuxchaisncs CN, Devogelaer JP, Esselinckx W, Bouchez B, Depresseux G, Romboot-Lindemans C, Huaux JP (1984) The effect of low dosage glucocorticoids on bone mass in rheumatoid arthritis: a cross sectional and longitudinal study using single photon absorptiometry. Adv Exp Med Biol 171:210–239

Dempster DW (1989) Perspectives: bone histomorphometry in glucocorticoid-induced osteoporosis. J Bone Miner Res 4:137–141

Diamond T, Stiel D, Posen S (1989) Osteoporosis in hemochromatosis: iron excess, gonadal deficiency or other factors? Ann Intern Med 110:430–436

Diamond T, Stiel D, Lunzer M, Wilkinson M, Roche J, Posen S (1990) Osteoporosis and skeletal fractures in chronic liver disease. Gut 31:82–87

Dietrich JW, Canalis EM, Maina DM, Raisz LG (1979) Effect of glucocorticoids on fetal rat bone collagen synthesis in vitro. Endocrinology 104:715–721

Dodin S, Lemay A, Maheux R, Dumont M, Turcot-Lemay L (1991) Bone mass in endometriosis patients treated with GnRH agonist implant or danazol. Obstet Gynecol 77:410–415

Doer P, Pirke KM (1976) Cortisol-induced suppression of plasma testosterone in normal adult males. J Clin Endocrinol Metab 43:622–629

Duda RJ, Kumar R, Nelson KI, Zinsmeister AR, Mann KG, Riggs BL (1987) 1,25-Dihydroxyvitamin-D stimulation test for osteoblast function in normal and osteoporotic postmenopausal women. J Clin Invest 79:1249–1253

El Haj AJ, Minter SL, Rawlinson SCF, Suswillo R, Lanyon LE (1990) Cellular responses to mechanical loading in vitro. J Bone Miner Res 5:923–932

Eriksen EF, Colvard DS, Berg NJ, Graham ML, Mann KG, Spelsberg TC, Riggs BL (1988) Evidence of estrogen receptors in normal human osteoblast-like cells. Science 241:84–86

Eriksen EF, Hodgson SF, Eastell R, Cedel SL, O'Fallon WM, Riggs BL (1990) Cancellous bone remodelling in type I (postmenopausal) osteoporosis: quantitative assessment of rates of formation, resorption, and bone loss at tissue and cellular levels. J Bone Miner Res 5:311–319

Ernst M, Schmid C, Froesch RE, Heath JK, Rodan GA (1990) Evidence for a direct effect of estrogen on bone cells in vitro. J Steroid Biochem 34:279–284

Evans RA, Marel GM, Lancaster EK, Kos S, Evans M, Wong SYP (1988) Bone mass is low in relatives of osteoporotic patients. Ann Intern Med 109:870–873

Eventov I, Frisch B, Cohen Z, Hammel I (1991) Osteopenia, hematopoiesis, and bone remodeling in the iliac crest and femoral biopsies – a prospective study of 102 cases of femoral neck fractures. Bone 12:1–6

Fang MA, Frost PJ, Iidaklein A, Hahn TJ (1991) Effects of nicotine on cellular function in UMR 106-01 osteoblast-like cells. Bone 12:283

Felson DT, Kiel DP, Anderson JJ, Kannel WB (1988) Alcohol consumption and hip fractures – the Framingham study. Am J Epidemiol 128:1102–1110

Felson DT, Sloutskis D, Anderson JJ, Anthony JM, Kiel DP (1991) Thiazide diuretics and the risk of hip fracture – results from the Framingham study. JAMA 265:370–373

Feyen JHM, Raisz LG (1987) Prostaglandin production by calvariae from sham operated and oophorectomized rats: effect of 17β-estradiol in vivo. Endocrinology 121:819–821

Forero MS, Klein RF, Nissenson RA, Nelson K, Heath H III, Arnaud CS, Riggs BL (1987) Effects of age on circulating immunoreactive and bioactive parathyroid hormone levels in women. J Bone Miner Res 2:363–366

Gardsell P, Johnell O, Nilsson BE, Sernbo I (1991) Bone mass in an urban and a rural population – a comparative, population-based study in Southern Sweden. J Bone Miner Res 6:67–76

Garrett RI, Durie BGM, Nedwin GE, Gillespie A, Bringman T, Sabatini M, Bertolini DR, Mundy GR (1987) Production of lymphotoxin a bone-resorbing cytokine, by cultured human myeloma cells. N Engl J Med 317:526–532

Gennari C, Imbimbo B, Montagnani M, Bernini M, Nardi P, Avioli LV (1984) Effects of prednisone and deflazacort on mineral metabolism and parathyroid hormone activity in humans. Calcif Tissue Int 36:245–252

Ginsberg JS, Kowalchuk G, Hirsh J, Brill-Edwards P, Burrows R, Coates G, Webber C (1990) Heparin effect on bone density. Thromb Haemost 64:286–289

Goldhaber P (1965) Heparin enhancement of factors stimulating bone resorption in tissue culture. Science 147:407–408

Gotfredsen A, Borg J, Nilas L, Tjellesen L, Christiansen C (1986) Representativity of regional to total bone mineral in healthy subjects and "anticonvulsive treated" epileptic patients. Measurements by single and dual photon absorptiometry. Europ J Clin Invest 16:198–203

Greenspan SL, Greenspan FS, Resnick NM, Block JE, Friedlander AL, Genant HK (1991) Skeletal integrity in premenopausal and postmenopausal women receiving long-term L-thyroxine on bone density. Am J Med 91:5–14

Gronowicz G, McCarthy MB, Raisz LG (1990) Glucocorticoids stimulate resorption in fetal rat parietal bones in vitro. J Bone Miner Res 5:1223–1230

Harms H-M, Kataina U, Kulpmann W-R, Brabant G, Hesch R-D (1989) Pulse amplitude and frequency modulation of parathyroid hormone in plasma. J Clin Endocrinol Metab 69:842

Heaney RP, Recker RR (1982) Effects of nitrogen phosphorus and caffeine on calcium balance in women. J Lab Clin Med 99:46–55

Heaney RP, Recker RR, Saville PD (1978) Menopausal changes in bone remodeling. J Lab Clin Med 92:964–970

Hock JM, Fonseca J (1990) Anabolic effect of human synthetic parathyroid hormone (1–34) depends on growth hormone. Endocrinology 127/4:1804–1810

Hodsman AB, Steer BM, Fraher LJ, Drost DJ (1991) Bone densitometric and histomorphometric responses to sequential human parathyroid hormone (1–38) and salmon calcitonin in osteoporotic patients. Bone Miner 14:67–83

Hoekman K, Papapoulos SE, Peters ACB et al. (1985) Characteristics and bisphosphonate treatment of a patient with juvenile osteoporosis. J Clin Endocrinol Metab 61:952–956

Hori M, Uzawa T, Morita K, Noda T, Takahashi H, Inoue J (1988) Effect of human parathyroid hormone (PTH (1–34)) on experimental osteopenia of rats induced by ovariectomy. Bone Miner 3:193–199

Hsueh AJ, Erickson GF (1978) Glucocorticoid inhibition of FSH induced estrogen production in cultured rat granulosa cells. Steroids 32:639–648

Hurley DL, McMahon MM (1990) Long-term parenteral nutrition and metabolic bone disease. Endocrinol Metab Clin North Am 19:113–132

Hurley MM, Kream BE, Raisz LG (1990a) Effects of heparin on bone formation in cultured fetal rat calvaria. Calcif Tissue Int 48:183–188

Hurley MM, Kream BE, Raisz LG (1990b) Structural determinants of the capacity of heparin to inhibit collagen synthesis in 21-day fetal rat calvariae. J Bone Miner Res 5:1127–1134

Imai Y, Tsunerari T, Fukase M, Fujita T (1990) Quantitative bone histomorphometry and circulating T lymphocyte subsets in postmenopausal osteoporosis. J Bone Miner Res 5:393–400

Jacobs P, Goodman H (1990) Lytic bone lesions in polycythaemia rubra vera. Europ J Haematol 45:275–277

Jee WSS, Ueno K, Deng YP, Woodbury DM (1985) The effects of prostaglandin E_2 in growing rats: increased metaphyseal hard tissue and corticoendosteal bone formation. Calcif Tissue Int 37:148–157

Johnston CC, Norton J, Khairi MRA, Kernek C, Edouard C, Arlot M, Meunier PJ (1985) Heterogeneity of fracture syndromes in postmenopausal women. J Clin Endocrinol Metab 61:551–556

Kawano M, Yamamoto I, Iwato K, Tanaka H, Asaoku H, Tanabe O, Ishikawa H, Nobuyoshi M, Ohomoto Y, Hirai Y, Kuramoto A (1989) Interleukin-1-beta rather than lymphotoxin as the major bone resorbing activity in human multiple myeloma. Blood 73:1646–1649

Kelly PJ, Hopper JL, Macaskill GT, Pocock NA, Sambrook PN, Eisman JA (1991) Genetic factors in bone turnover, J Clin Endocrinol Metab 72:808–813

Klaushofer K, Hoffman O, Gleispach H, Hans-Jorg L, Czerwenka E, Koller K, Peterlik M (1989) Bone-resorbing activity of thyroid hormones is related to prostaglandin production in cultured neonatal mouse calvaria. J Bone Miner Res 4:305–312

Klein GL, Coburn JW (1991) Parenteral nutrition – effect on bone and mineral homeostasis. Annu Rev Nutr 11:93–120

Komm MBS, Terpening CM, Benz DJ, Graeme KA, Gallegos A, Korc M, Greene GL, O'Malley BW, Haussler MR (1988) Estrogen binding, receptor mRNA and biologic response in osteoblast-like osteosarcoma cells. Science 241:81–84

Kream BE, Petersen DN, Raisz LG (1990) Parathyroid hormone blocks the stimulatory effect of insulin-like growth factor-I on collagen synthesis in cultured 21-day fetal rat calvariae. Bone 11:411–415

Krieger NA, Stappanbeck TS, Stern PH (1988) Characterization of specific thyroid hormone receptors in bone. J Bone Miner Res 3:473–478

Kurtz D, Morrish K, Shapiro J (1985) Vertebral bone mineral content in osteogenesis imperfecta. Calcif Tissue Int 37:14–18

LaCroix AZ, Wienpahl J, White LR, Wallace RB, Scherr PA, George LK, Cornoni-Huntley J, Ostfeld AM (1990) Thiazide diuretic agents and the incidence of hip fracture. N Engl J Med 322:286–290

Lakharpal S, Ginsburg WW, Luthra HS, Hunder GC (1987) Transient osteoporosis: a study of 56 cases and a review of the literature. Ann Intern Med 106:444–450

Lamberg-Allardt C, Wilska M, Saraste KL, Gronlund T (1990) Vitamin D status of ambulatory and nonambulatory mentally retarded children with and without carbamazepine treatment. Ann Nutr Metab 34:216–220

Lane N, Coble T, Kimmel DB (1990) Effect of naproxen on cancellous bone in ovariectomized rats. J Bone Miner Res 5:1029–1036

Lane N, Baptista J, Orwoll E (1991a) Bone mineral density of the lumbar spine in women with endometriosis. Fertil Steril 55:537–543

Lane N, Baptista J, Snow-Harter C (1991b) Bone mineral density of the lumbar spine in endometriosis: subjects compared to an age-similar control population. J Clin Endocrinol Metab 72:510–514

Liel Y, Edwards J, Shary J et al. (1988) Effects of race and body habitus on bone mineral density of the radius, hip and spine in premenopausal women. J Clin Endocrinol Metab 66:1247–1250

Linkhardt TA, Keffer MJ (1991) Differential regulation of insulin-like growth factor-I (IGF-I) and IGF-II release from cultured neonatal mouse calvaria by parathyroid hormone, transforming growth factor beta, and 1,25-dihydroxy-vitamin D_3. Endocrinology 128:1511–1518

Lips P, Van Ginkel FC, Jongen MJM, Rubertus F, Van der Vjigh WJF, Netelenbos JC (1987) Determinants of vitamin D status in patients with hip fracture and in elderly control subjects. Am J Clin Nutr 46:1005–1010

Liu CC, Kalu DN, Salerno E, Echon R, Hollis BW, Rau M (1991) Pre-existing bone loss associated with ovariectomy in rats is reversed by parathyroid hormone. J Bone Miner Res 6:1071–1080

Longcope C, Baker RS, Hui SL, Johnston CC Jr (1985) Androgen and estrogen dynamics in women with vertebral crush fractures. Maturitas 6:309–318

Luckey MM, Meier DE, Mandeli JP, DaCosta MC, Hubbard ML, Goldsmith SJ (1989) Radial and vertebral bone density in white and black women: evidence for racial differences in premenopausal bone homeostasis. J Clin Endocrinol Metab 69:762–770

Luton JP, Thieblot P, Valcke JC, Mahoudeau JA, Bricaire H (1977) Reversible gonadotropin deficiency in male Cushing's disease. J Clin Endocrinol Metab 45:488–497

MacAdams MR, White RH, Chipps BE (1986) Reduction of serum testosterone levels during chronic glucocorticoid therapy. Ann Intern Med 104:648–651

Marcus R, Cann C, Madorg P et al. (1988) Menstrual function and bone mass in elite women distance runners. Ann Intern Med 102:158–163

Massey LK (1991) Perspectives: caffeine and bone: directions of research. J Bone Miner Res 6:1149–1151

Matkovic V, Kostial K, Simonovic I, Buzina R, Brodarec A, Nordin BEC (1979) Bone status and fracture rates in two regions of Yugoslavia. Am J Clin Nutr 32:540–549

Mawer EB, Arlot ME, Reeve J, Green JR, Dattani J, Edouard C, Meunier PJ (1991) The relationship between serum vitamin-D concentrations and in vivo tetracycline labeling of osteoid in crush fracture osteoporosis. Calcif Tissue Int 48:78–81

Mazess RB, Barden HS (1991) Bone density in premenopausal women – effects of age, dietary intake, physical activity, smoking and birth control pills. Am J Clin Nutr 53:132–142

McCarthy TL, Centrella M, Canalis E (1989) Parathyroid hormone enhances the transcript and polypeptide levels of insulin-like growth factor I in osteoblast-enriched cultures from fetal rat bone. Endocrinology 124:1247–1253

McCarthy TL, Centrella M, Canalis E (1990) Cortisol inhibits the synthesis of insulin-like growth factor-I in skeletal cells. Endocrinology 126:1569–1575

McCarthy TL, Centrella M, Raisz LG, Canalis E (1991) Prostaglandin E_2 stimulates insulin-like growth factor I synthesis in osteoblast-enriched cultures from fetal rat bone. Endocrinology 128:2895–2900

Meier DE, Luckey MM, Wallenstein S, Clemens TL, Orwoll ES, Waslien CI (1991) Calcium, vitamin D and parathyroid hormone status in young white and black women: association with racial differences in bone mass. J Clin Endocrinol Metab 72:703–710

Melton LJ, III (1990) A "Gompertzian" view of osteoporosis. Calcif Tissue Int 46:285–286

Melton LJ, Kan SH, Frye MA et al. (1989) Epidemiology of vertebral fractures in women. Am J Epidemiol 129:1000–1011

Michnovicz JJ, Hershcopf RJ, Naganuma H et al. (1986) Increased 2-hydroxylation of estradiol as a possible mechanism for the anti-estrogenic effect of cigarette smoking. N Engl J Med 315:1305–1309

Morris HA, Need AG, O'Loughlin PD, Horowitz M, Bridges A, Nordin BEC (1990) Malabsorption of calcium in corticosteroid-induced osteoporosis. Calcif Tissue Int 46:305–308

Movsowitz C, Epstein S, Ismail F et al. (1989) Cyclosporin A in the oophorectomized rat: unexpected severe bone resorption. J Bone Miner Res 4:393–398

Mundy GR, Shapiro JL, Bandelin JG, Canalis EM, Raisz LG (1976) Direct stimulation of bone resorption by thyroid hormones. J Clin Invest 58:529–534

Nielson FH, Hunt CD, Mullen LM, Hunt JR (1987) Effect of dietary boron on mineral, estrogen, and testosterone metabolism in postmenopausal women. FASEB J 1:394–397

Nielsen HK, Charles P, Moskilde L (1988) The effect of single oral doses of prednisone on the circadian rhythm of serum osteocalcin in normal subjects. J Clin Endocrinol Metab 67:1025–1030

Nordin BEC, Need AG, Morris HA, Horowitz M, Robertson WG (1991) Evidence for a renal calcium leak in postmenopausal women. J Clin Endocrinol Metab 72:401–407

Orcel P, Bielakoff J, Modrowski D (1989) Cyclosporin A induces in vivo inhibition of resorption and stimulation of formation in rat bone. J Bone Miner Res 4:387–391

Orcel P, Denne MA, DeVernejoul MC (1991) Cyclosporin-A in vitro decreases bone resorption, osteoclast formation, and the fusion of cells of the monocyte macrophage lineage. Endocrinology 128:1638–1646

Ott SM, Chestnut CH III (1989) Calcitriol treatment is not effective in postmenopausal osteoporosis. Ann Intern Med 110:267–274

Ozoh JO, Onuigbo MAC, Nwankwo N, Ukabam SO, Umerah BC, Emeruwa CC (1990) Vanishing of vertebra in a patient with sickle cell haemoglobinopathy. Br Med J 301:1368–1369

Pacifici R, Rifas L, Teitelbaum S, Slatopolsky E, McCracken R, Bergfeld M, Lee W, Avioli LV, Peck WA (1987) Spontaneous release of interleukin 1 from human blood monocytes reflects bone formation in idiopathic osteoporosis. Proc Natl Acad Sci USA 84:4616–4620

Pacifici R, Rifas L, McCracken R et al. (1989) Ovarian steroid treatment blocks a postmenopausal increase in blood monocyte interleukin-1 release. Proc Natl Acad Sci USA 86:2398–2402

Pacifici R, Carano A, Santoro SA, Rifas L, Jeffrey JJ, Malone JD, McCracken R, Avioli LV (1991) Bone matrix constituents stimulate interleukin-1 release from human blood mononuclear cells. J Clin Invest 87:221–228

Parisien M, Silverberg SJ, Shane E, de la Cruz L, Lindsay R (1990) The histomorphometry of bone in primary hyperparathyroidism: preservation of cancellous bone structure. J Clin Endocrinol Metab 70:930–938

Paterson CR, McAllion S, Stellman JL (1984) Osteogenesis imperfecta after the menopause. N Engl J Med 310:1694–1696

Peacock M (1991) Interpretation of bone mass determinations as they relate to fracture: implications for asymptomatic primary hyperparathyroidism. J Bone Miner Res 6:S77

Pfeilschifter J, Mundy GR (1987) Modulation of type β transforming growth factor activity in bone cultures by osteotropic hormones. Proc Natl Acad Sci USA 84:2024–2028

Pilbeam CC, Raisz LG (1990) Effects of androgens on parathyroid hormone and interleukin-1-stimulated prostaglandin production in cultured neonatal mouse calvariae. J Bone Miner Res 5:1183–1188

Pilbeam CC, Klein-Nulend J, Raisz LG (1989) Inhibition by 17β-estradiol of PTH stimulated resorption and prostaglandin production in cultured neonatal mouse calvariae. Biochem Biophys Res Commun 163:1319–1324

Pocock NA, Eisman JA, Hopper JL, Yeates MG, Sambrook PN, Eberl S (1987) Genetic determinants of bone mass in adults. J Clin Invest 80:706–710

Podbesek RD, Edouard C, Meunier PJ et al. (1983) Effects of two treatment regimens with synthetic human parathyroid fragment on bone formation and the tissue balance of trabecular bone in greyhounds. Endocrinology 112:1000–1006

Pootrakul P, Hungsprenges S, Fucharoen S, Baylink D, Thompson E, English E, Lee M, Burnell J, Finch C (1981) Relation between erythropoiesis and bone metabolism in thalassemia. N Engl J Med 304:1470–1472

Prior JC, Vigna YM, Schechter MT, Burgess AE (1990) Spinal bone loss and ovulatory disturbances. N Engl J Med 323:1221–1227

Raisz LG (1981) What marrow does to bone. N Engl J Med 304:1485–1486

Raisz LG (1988) Local and systemic factors in the pathogenesis of osteoporosis. N Engl J Med 318:818–828

Raisz LG (1990) Recent advances in bone cell biology: interactions of vitamin D with other local and systemic factors. Bone Miner 9:191–197

Raisz LG, Fall PM (1990) Biphasic effects of prostaglandin E_2 on bone formation in cultured fetal rat calvariae: interaction with cortisol. Endocrinology 126:1654–1659

Raisz LG, Kream BE (1983) Regulation of bone formation, part 2. N Engl J Med 309:83–89

Raisz LG, Martin TJ (1983) Prostaglandins in bone and mineral metabolism. In: Peck WA (ed) Bone and mineral research, vol 2, Elsevier, Amsterdam, p 286

Raisz LG, Trummel CL, Wener JA, Simmons HA (1972) Effect of glucocorticoids on bone resorption in tissue culture. Endocrinology 90:961–967

Rao DS, Wilson RJ, Kleerekoper M et al. (1988) Lack of biochemical progression or continuation of accelerated bone loss in mild asymptomatic primary hyperparathyroidism: evidence for biphasic disease course. J Clin Endocrinol Metab 67:1294–1298

Reid IR, Heap SW (1990) Determinants of vertebral mineral density in patients receiving long-term glucocorticoid therapy. Arch Intern Med 150:2545–2548

Ribeiro RC, Pui CH, Schell MJ (1988) Vertebral compression fracture as a presenting feature of acute lymphoblastic leukemia in children. Cancer 61:589–592

Ribot C, Tremollieres F, Pouilles JM et al. (1988) Obesity and postmenopausal bone loss: the influence of obesity on vertebral density and bone turnover in postmenopausal women. Bone 8:327–331

Riggs BL, Melton LJ III (1986) Involutional osteoporosis. N Engl J Med 314:1676–1686

Riggs BL, Wahner HW, Dunn WL, Mazess RB, Offord KP, Melton LJ III (1981) Differential changes in BMD of the appendicular and axial skeleton with aging: relationship to spinal osteoporosis. J Clin Invest 67:328–334

Riggs BL, Hodgson SF, O'Fallon WM, Chao EY, Wahner HW, Muhs JM, Cedel SL, Melton LJ III (1990) Effect of fluoride treatment on fracture rate in postmenopausal women with osteoporosis. N Engl J Med 322:802–809

Rigotti NA, Nussbaum SR, Herzog DB et al. (1984) Osteoporosis in women with anorexia nervosa. N Engl J Med 311:1601–1606

Rigotti NA, Neer RM, Skates ST, Herzog DB, Nussbaum SR (1991) The clinical course of osteoporosis in anorexia nervosa. A longitudinal study of cortical bone mass. JAMA 265:1133–1138

Rosen CJ, Usiskin K, Owens M, Barlascini CO, Belsky M, Adler RA (1990) T lymphocyte surface antigen markers in osteoporosis. J Bone Miner Res 5:851–856

Ross EJ, Linch DC (1982) Cushing's syndrome – killing disease: discriminatory value of signs and symptoms aiding early diagnosis. Lancet 2:646–649

Rudman D, Kutner MH, Rogers CM, Lubin MF, Fleming GA, Bain RP (1981) Impaired growth hormone secretion in the adult population: relation to age and adiposity. J Clin Invest 67:1361–1369

Ruegsegger P, Dambacher MA, Ruegsegger E, Fischer JA, Anliker M (1984) Bone loss in premenopausal and postmenopausal women: a cross-sectional and longitudinal study using QCT. J Bone Joint Surg [Am] 66:1015–1023

Sakakura M, Takebe K, Nakagawa S (1975) Inhibition of LH secretion induced by synthetic LRH by long-term treatment with glucocorticoids in human subjects. J Clin Endocrinol Metab 40:776–790

Sakhaee K, Nicar MJ, Glass K, Pak CYC (1985) Postmenopausal osteoporosis as a manifestation of renal hypercalciuria with secondary hyperparathyroidism. J Clin Endocrinol 61:368–373

Schaison G, Durand F, Mowszowicz J (1978) Effect of glucocorticoids on plasma testosterone in men. Acta Endocrinol 89:126–131

Schlechte J, El-Khoury G, Kathol M, Walker L (1987) Forearm and vertebral bone mineral in treated and untreated hyperprolactinemic amenorrhea. J Clin Endocrinol Metab 64:1021–1026

Schlosberg M, Movsowitz C, Epstein S et al. (1989) The effect of cyclosporin A administration and its withdrawal on bone mineral metabolism in the rat. Endocrinology 124:2179–2184

Seeman E, Hopper JL, Bach LA Cooper ME, Parkinson E, McKay J, Jerums G (1989) Reduced bone mass in daughters of women with osteoporosis. N Engl J Med 320:554–558

Shike M, Shils ME, Heller A, Alcock N, Vigorita V, Brockman R, Holick MF, Lane J, Flombaum C (1986) Bone disease in prolonged parenteral nutrition: osteopenia without mineralization defect. Am J Clin Nutr 44:89–98

Silverberg SJ, Shane E, de la Cruz L et al. (1989a) Abnormalities in parathyroid hormone secretion and 1,25 dihydroxyvitamin D_3 formation in women with osteoporosis. N Engl J Med 320:277–281

Silverberg SJ, Shane E, de la Cruz L et al. (1989b) Skeletal disease in primary hyperparathyroidism. J Bone Miner Res 4:283–291

Simmons HA, Raisz LG (1991) Effects of acidic and basic fibroblast growth factor and heparin on resorption of cultured fetal rat long bones. J Bone Miner Res 6:1301–1305

Slovik DM, Rosenthal DI, Doppelt SH, Potts JT Jr, Daly MA, Campbell JA, Neer RM (1986) Restoration of spinal bone in osteoporotic men by treatment with human parathyroid hormone (1–34) and 1,25-dihydroxyvitamin D. J Bone Miner Res 1:377–381

Smith R (1980) Idiopathic osteoporosis in the young. J Bone Joint Surg [Br] 62:417–427

Smith R, Stevenson JC, Winearls CG, Woods CG, Wordsworth BP (1985) Osteoporosis of pregnancy. Lancet I/8439:1178–1180

Spotila LD, Constantinou CD, Sereda L, Ganguly A, Riggs BL, Prockop DJ (1991) Mutation in a gene for type I procollagen (COL1A2) in a woman with postmenopausal osteoporosis: evidence for phenotypic genotypic overlap with mild osteogenesis imperfecta. Proc Natl Acad Sci USA 88:5423–5427

Stein B, Halloran BP, Reinhardt T, Engstrom GW, Bales CW, Drezner MK, Currie KL, Takizawa M et al. (1991) Cyclosporin-A increases synthesis of 1,25-dihydroxyvitamin D_3 in the rat and mouse. Endocrinology 128:1369–1373

Stepan JJ, Pospichal J, Schreiber V, Kanka J, Mensik J, Presl J, Pacovsky V (1989) The application of plasma tartrate-resistant acid phosphatase to assess changes in bone resorption in response to artificial menopause and its treatment with estrogen or norethisterone. Calcif Tissue Int 45:273–280

Stock JL, Coderre JA, McDonald B et al. (1989) Effects of estrogen in vivo and in vitro on spontaneous interleukin-1 release by monocytes from postmenopausal women. J Clin Endocrinol Metab 68:364–368

Thompson DD, Rodan GA (1988) Indomethacin inhibition of tenotomy-induced bone resorption in rats. J Bone Miner Res 3:409–414

Tiegs RD, Body JJ, Wahner HW, Barta J, Riggs BL, Heath H III (1985) Calcitonin secretion in postmenopausal osteoporosis. N Engl J Med 312:1097–1100.

Toh SH, Brown PH (1990) Bone mineral content in hypothyroid male patients with hormone replacement: a 3-year study. J Bone Miner Res 5:463–468

Tsunenari T, Fukase M, Fujita T (1991) Bone histomorphometric analysis for the cause of osteopenia in vitamin-C-deficient rat (ODS rat). Calcif Tissue Int 48:18–27

Unterman TG, Vazquez RM, Slas AJ, Martyn PA, Phillips LS (1985) Nutrition and somatomedin: XIII. Usefulness of somatomedin-C in nutritional assessment. Am J Med 78:228–234

Villareal DT, Civitelli R, Chines A, Avioli LV (1991) Subclinical vitamin D deficiency in postmenopausal women with low vertebral bone mass. J Clin Endocrinol Metab 72:628–634

Wilson RJ, Rao DS, Ellis B, Kleerekoper M, Parfitt AM (1988) Mild asymptomatic hyperparathyroidism is not a risk factor for vertebral fractures. Ann Intern Med 109:959–962

Wilson T, Katz JM, Gray DH (1981) Inhibition of active bone resorption by copper. Calcif Tissue Int 33:35–39

Young G, Marcus R, Minkoff JR, Kim LY, Segre GV (1987) Age-related rise in parathyroid hormone in man: the use of intact and midmolecule antisera to distinguish hormone secretion from retention. J Bone Miner Res 2:367–374

Zamboni G, Marradi P, Tagliaro F, Dorizzi R, Tato L (1986) Parathyroid hormone, calcitonin and vitamin-D metabolites in beta-thalassaemia major. Eur J Pediatr 145:133–136

Zarabeitia MT, Riancho JA, Amado JA, Napal J, Gonzales-Macias J (1991) Cytokine production by peripheral blood cells in postmenopausal osteoporosis. Bone Miner 14:161–167

CHAPTER 10
Vitamin D Metabolism

J.A. EISMAN

A. Overview

A decade or so ago the concept of vitamin D metabolism was deceptively simple. The vitamin was produced in the skin (vitamin D_3, cholecalciferol) under the influence of the ultraviolet component of sunlight or was derived from some food sources (largely vitamin D_2, ergocalciferol). These vitamins D were equally potent in man so the term vitamin D was commonly used. This vitamin, bound to a serum vitamin D binding protein (DBP), was transferred in the blood to the liver, where it was converted to 25-hydroxyvitamin D (see Fig. 1). This metabolite also bound to the DBP was carried in blood to the kidney, which was the sole site of a further 1a-hydroxylation to produce the active hormonal form, 1,25-dihydroxyvitamin D. The form of this hormone derived from vitamin D_3 has been given the trivial name of calcitriol. However, clinically this was sometimes used to imply both 1,25-dihydroxycholecalciferol and 1,25-dihydroxyergocalciferol. The 24-hydroxylation pathway, which also existed in the kidney, was seen as an alternate to 1-hydroxylation and of uncertain significance. The hormone was considered to act like other steroidal hormones through a receptor but it had not been cloned and its structure was unknown. Despite this gap it was "clear" that the receptor existed in the vitamin D target organs, primarily bone and gut, and presumably not elsewhere. The two major controversies of the time related to 24-hydroxylation (was it the first step in a degradation pathway or did it confer unique functions) and receptor localization (did receptor reside in the nucleus or cytosol prior to activation).

In a few short years the picture has become much more complex and much more interesting. The physiology has been clarified with evidence of direct 1,25-dihydroxyvitamin D (calcitriol) feedback on the parathyroid gland. The 1-hydroxylation has been shown to occur outside the kidney in several normal (and abnormal) tissues and physiological situations. Many tissues, including malignant cells, have been shown to be responsive to calcitriol with both physiological and pathological implications. The 24-hydroxylation pathway has been defined in almost all vitamin D responsive tissues with its exposure to the active hormone a hallmark of a normal response. Nevertheless the significance of this pathway is still debated. The 1,25-dihydroxyvitamin D (calcitriol) receptor (VDR) has been cloned from

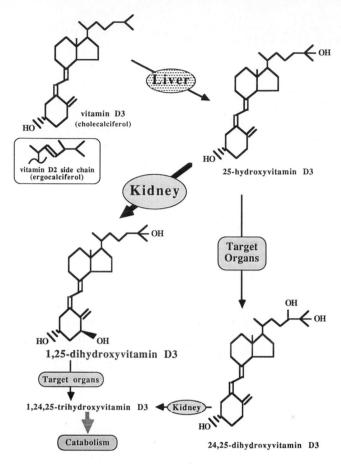

Fig. 1. Vitamin D$_3$ metabolism from 25-hydroxyvitamin D$_3$ to di- and trihydroxylated metabolites and catabolism

several species including man and many vitamin D resistance disorders characterized at this level. Most recently the DNA element required for activation by vitamin D, the so-called vitamin D responsive element (VDRE), has been identified in the osteocalcin gene from several species, although the element required for downregulation has yet to be identified. The involvement of calcitriol outside the classical calcium homeostatic system in the regulation of cellular replication and function has opened an entirely new area of vitamin D research. It has led to renewed pharmaceutical interest with the development of nonhypercalcemic analogues which retain cellular regulatory activities. This chapter will attempt to summarize the older data and present the newer advances on that background.

B. Dermal Production of Vitamin D₃ and Dietary Sources of Vitamin D

I. Substrate and Chemistry

The production of vitamin D in the skin under the influence of ultraviolet light is one of the oldest pieces of information in the physiology of vitamin D. Although the substrate for synthesis of vitamin D₃, 7-dehydrocholesterol, is derived from cholesterol enzymatically, the UV light-induced changes in 7-dehydrocholesterol do not depend upon any enzymatic or cofactor function: They can take place as readily in the test tube as in the skin. Indeed the skin may hamper the reaction, particularly pigmented skin, which may absorb some of the UV rays and effectively compete for this energy form. It has been assumed for decades that this would be the case to explain the high risk of vitamin D deficiency syndromes in peoples with more pigmented skin moving into climates with relatively low incident light. However, only recently have the various steps been elucidated and the effect of skin color been demonstrated (see below). The role of vitamin D binding protein (DBP) in removing the vitamin from the skin and thus shifting the reaction equilibria from the various pre-vitamins and over-irradiation products into vitamin D provides an intriguing story.

Cholesterol is initially converted to 7-dehydrocholesterol in the dermis. In this situation it is susceptible to UV-B light (Fig. 2). This results in

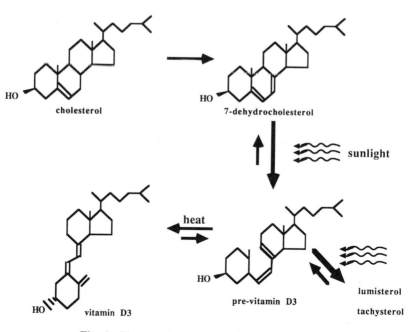

Fig. 2. Photobiology of vitamin D₃ in the skin

cleavage of the 9,10 carbon-carbon bond of the B ring and the production of a series of radiation and overradiation products, which are in equilibrium with pre-vitamin D_3 and each other. The pre-vitamin D_3 rearranges to form vitamin D_3 by a nonenzymatic but energy-dependent process. Interestingly, vitamin D_3 has a much greater affinity for serum vitamin D binding protein than any of the other compounds in this equilibrium mixture. This allows its selective removal from the dermis, which results in reequilibration of these reaction products and formation of more vitamin D_3. Despite this selective mechanism there are no enzymatic steps in vitamin D_3 formation apart from the dehydrogenation of cholesterol to yield the substrate.

II. Ultraviolet Light and Skin Pigmentation

The section of the ultraviolet light involved is the UV-B region, which approximately corresponds to the region responsible for sun burn. It is perhaps not surprising then that skin pigmentation, which protects against this adverse effect of sunlight, may also reduce the vitamin synthetic effect of sunlight. Holick and coworkers (Holick et al. 1980, 1981) have shown that skin pigmentation in United States blacks compared with whites may have a dual effect on vitamin D metabolism. It not only increases the UV dose required to produce a "minimal erythematous reaction" but also it decreases the vitamin D synthetic response from a given erythematous dose. It seems likely that other skin pigmentations will have similar effects (Clemens et al. 1982; Bell et al. 1985a; Reasner et al. 1990). This mechanism may be an important contributor to vitamin D deficiency syndromes in ethnic groups, characterized by pigmented skin, living in regions of limited sunlight exposure. The mechanism of the lesser vitamin D response to a dose of UV light, which produces an equivalent erythematous response, is unclear. It may be secondary to the pigment effect or could potentially relate to the clearance mechanism by the serum DBP (see below). Clearly the reduced vitamin D response would be a protective mechanism against vitamin D toxicity with evolutionary value in climes close to the equator. In earlier times this mechanism may have contributed with dietary mechanisms to the high prevalence of rickets/osteomalacia in ethnic Indians in the United Kingdom and other groups with limited vitamin D intake and/or sunlight exposure (Ellis et al. 1977; Ellis and Cooke 1978; Bachrach et al. 1979; Robertson et al. 1982). In many contries osteomalacia remains a risk for the elderly, in whom diet may be poor and sunlight exposure may be limited due to life-style and clothing choices (Lester et al. 1977; Francis et al. 1983; Pettifor et al. 1978). Among some ethnic groups women, who are traditionally heavily dressed, are at increased risk of vitamin D deficiency even in countries with moderate sunlight availability. If their babies are well swaddled and breast feeding is prolonged, the baby will be at increased risk of rickets. The availability of vitamin D supplements for children and adults and the supplementation of foods in many countries has minimized this potential problem.

III. Dietary Sources of Vitamin D

Approximately half of all vitamin D is considered to come from dietary sources. This figure has been obtained from studies on seasonal variations in serum 25-hydroxyvitamin D levels (HADDAD and HAHN 1973; McLAUGHLIN et al. 1974; ARNAUD et al. 1977; STRYD et al. 1979). The major dietary sources are from high-fat foods including eggs, some cheese, liver, and oily fish (Table 1). In the United States milk is fortified with vitamin D, so that dairy produce is an important dietary source of both calcium and vitamin D. However, in the United Kingdom, Europe, and Asia-Pacific regions this is not usually the case.

Absorption of dietary sources of vitamin D depends upon normal fat absorption. There is some evidence for an enterohepatic or entero-enteric circulation of vitamin D and its metabolites (ARNAUD et al. 1975). Malabsorption would therefore interfere not only with absorption of dietary vitamin D but also with this potential salvage pathway. Thus in any situation where fat absorption is compromised, vitamin D deficiency becomes a potential problem (Table 2). Thus any hepatic or pancreatic disease puts vitamin D absorption at risk, while any disorder of the bowel including celiac syndrome may limit absorption. The presence of normal vitamin D sources within fatty components of the diet exaggerates this effect. One strategy for overcoming this problem in clinical situations may be to use vitamin D supplements in the fasted state.

Table 1. Dietary sources of vitamin D

Source	IU/100 g
Dairy produce	
Cow's milk	0.5–4
Hard cheese	80–100
Butter, cream	30
Margarine	320
Eggs, 200–350	
Liver (lamb, calf, chicken)	20–50
Sea fish	
Oily	
Canned	230–500
Fresh	650–900
Shrimp – canned	105
Eel	
Fresh	5,000
Smoked	6,400
Cod liver oil	8,600

Approximate contents derived from Geigy Scientific Tables (1981), vol 1. Ciba-Geigy, Basle, pp 242–260.

Table 2. Causes of rickets/osteomalacia

1. Simple vitamin D deficiency
    Inadequate dietary intake
    Limited sunlight exposure
2. Intestinal fat malabsorption
    Intestinal malabsorption
    Cholestasis
    Pancreatic malabsorption
3. Liver disease
    Hepatic enzyme induction
4. Renal 1-hydroxylase defects
    Hypoparathyroidism
    Chronic renal failure
    Fanconi syndrome – inherited and acquired
    Vitamin D resistant rickets type I
5. Target organ insensitivity
6. Hypophosphatemic rickets/osteomalacia
7. Acidosis-related rickets/osteomalacia
8. Others
    Oncogenous osteomalacia
    Hypophosphatasia

C. Serum Vitamin D Binding Protein

I. Ethnic Differences

Serum vitamin D binding protein (DBP) was known for decades as a serum protein (group-specific component) of unknown function. Its genetics had been well studied and it was known to have different genotypes in different ethnic groups. Interestingly, there are major differences between the genotypes in black and white racial groups. It is not clear whether these genotypes correspond to different phenotypes of vitamin D_3 affinity. If one or other genotype resulted in a higher or lower affinity for vitamin D_3 this, by altering the removal rate of vitamin D_3 from the skin, could alter the overall skin synthesis of vitamin D_3 (see above). However, as DBP is relatively undersaturated, moderate changes in DBP capacity would not alter removal of vitamin D_3 from the dermis. Thus the overall significance of DBP to vitamin D metabolism and function remains unclear.

II. Binding Affinities and Function

The hierarchy of binding affinities of DBP with respect to vitamin D_3 metabolites is 25-hydroxyvitamin D > vitamin D > 1,25-dihydroxyvitamin D (Bouillon et al. 1978, 1980). As a result of this hierarchy and its large capacity, the serum DBP acts as a very effective carrier protein and "sink" for 25-hydroxyvitamin D. It has high capacity for vitamin D but carries 1,25-dihydroxyvitamin D less effectively. Thus about 10% of 1,25-

dihydroxyvitamin D and only 1% of 25-hydroxyvitamin D are unbound in serum (BOUILLON et al. 1981). These affinity and capacity characteristics set the free (effective) levels of these and other vitamin D metabolites in the circulation. There has been some discussion whether the DBP has any role in facilitating transport of vitamin D metabolites across cell membranes into or out of cells (VANBAELEN et al. 1977, 1980). However, the half-life of DBP in serum is quite different from that of 25-hydroxyvitamin D, making it unlikely that it functions primarily in this role (HADDAD et al. 1988). As DBP is relatively undersaturated, only marked deficiencies might be expected to effect its functions. An interesting example of such a situation is the nephrotic syndrome, where renal protein losses result in very low DBP levels. However, it is not clear that even this extreme depletion results in significant pathology. The possibility of some other as yet unknown function exists and the overall significance of DBP to vitamin D metabolism and function remains unclear.

D. Hepatic 25-Hydroxylation

I. Microsomal 25-Hydroxylase

The next step in the activation of vitamin D is its 25-hydroxylation in the liver (BLUNT et al. 1968). The enzyme which mediates the oxidation reaction is a microsomal P450 (BHATTACHARYYA and DELUCA 1973). Some earlier data indicated that the reaction may be regulated but these data are also consistent with saturation of an enzyme system rather than regulation per se (PONCHON et al. 1969; TUCKER et al. 1973; BHATTACHARYYA and DELUCA 1973; SHEPARD and DELUCA 1980). Thus this step appears not to be regulated and to be very robust. It operates fairly normally even in situations of quite severe liver damage (LUND et al. 1977). This robustness and the ability of this enzyme to oxidize cholesterol suggest some similarity to hepatic detoxification enzymes (USUI et al. 1990). However, one situation in which its function does appear to be limiting is in infants with marked prematurity. In this situation vitamin D replacement may be less effective than 25-hydroxyvitamin D therapy although more recent studies suggest that calcium supplementation per se may be most effective (KOO 1988; CARPENTER 1989).

II. Vitamin D Catabolism

An interesting variation on this hepatic role is the possible induction by parathyroid hormone of vitamin D catabolism and biliary excretion, possibly through 1,25-dihydroxyvitamin D (CLEMENTS et al. 1987a,b). This somewhat surprising result indicates that hyperparathyroidism secondary to vitamin D deficiency may in fact exacerbate the deficiency by "consuming" existing vitamin D stores. This mechanism may explain the relatively acute onset of deficiency symptoms in situations where the deficiency has been chronic. It may also help explain why fat malabsorption or poor sunlight exposure alone can lead to vitamin D deficiency states. This mechanism, which appears not to be a simple increase in transit of vitamin D through the activation pathway, is as yet unexplained. Another interesting aspect of hepatic vitamin D metabolism is the induction of degradation enzymes in individuals treated with certain drugs, including alcohol and barbiturates (Dent et al. 1970; Stamp et al. 1972; Hahn et al. 1972, 1977; Christiansen et al. 1983; Laitinen et al. 1990). This pathway appears not to be specific but rather a common degradation pathway. Enzyme inducers, such as barbiturates, have been used in the therapy of vitamin D toxicity due to excessive vitamin D intake. However, in normal individuals this effect does not influence vitamin D status (Wark et al. 1979). It is not clear whether this pathway is related to or distinct from the usual vitamin D metabolic pathways. Moreover, these findings raise the possibility that the hepatic microsomal hydroxylase activity is not specific to vitamin D metabolism and the 25-hydroxylation of vitamin D but rather is a nonspecific oxidative detoxification enzyme in the liver. This function in detoxification would be quite consistent with the marked resistance of this pathway to hepatic injury in the adult and its occasional inadequacy in the premature infant.

III. 25-Hydroxyvitamin D Bioactivity

The 25-hydroxylated vitamin D metabolites are more bioactive than their parent vitamin D. However, they are still approximately three orders of magnitude less active than their subsequent 1-hydroxylated metabolites. Nevertheless in conditions of extreme vitamin D overloading, the 25-hydroxyvitamin D metabolites may act in the subsequent functional pathways without the need for that activation step. The serum vitamin D binding protein may act in a protective role in this situation by binding a relatively high proportion (99%) of the serum 25-hydroxyvitamin D. The combination of an inherently lower biological activity and a proportionally lower serum free level can render 25-hydroxyvitamin D biologically inactive in vivo despite levels 500- to 1000-fold higher than those of the subsequent 1-hydroxylated metabolites. These considerations notwithstanding, some studies suggest that serum 25-hydroxyvitamin D may contribute to the basal level of vitamin D action in man (Eastwood and DeWardener 1979).

E. Renal 1-Hydroxylation

I. Proximal Tubule Mitochondrial P450

The identification of the function of the kidney in 1-hydroxylation was one of the major advances in understanding of the vitamin D function in animals and man (DeLuca 1975, 1978a,b, 1979). The central role of the kidney in the activation step and the nature of that activation was demonstrated in an elegant series of experiments using double-labeled vitamin D (Fraser and Kodicek 1970; Gray et al. 1971; Holick et al. 1971; Lawson et al. 1971; Haussler et al. 1971). It was another decade before extrarenal synthesis of 1,25-dihydroxyvitamin D was demonstrated (see below) and the role of such synthesis in vivo is still not entirely clear. In those initial studies the whole kidney was identified as the functional organ. This concept fitted extremely well with the observations of vitamin D deficiency-like syndromes in end stage renal failure. Although in the early 1970s it seemed clear that a simple loss of vitamin D activation would explain renal osteodystrophy, subsequent studies have shown a much more complex situation. Secondary hyperparathyroidism does relate to inefficiency of the vitamin D activation mechanism. However, the osteomalacic changes are quite unresponsive to replacement therapy and seem to be due largely to heavy metal accumulation at the bone-forming surface (for review see Eisman 1988).

In subsequent studies the site of 1-hydroxylation has been fairly clearly localized to the proximal tubule. However, there may be subtle differences between species in this localization. The localization of 25-hydroxyvitamin D 1-hydroxylase activity along the nephron became possible with the use of microdissection techniques. In elegant studies of isolated teased nephron segments from the rabbit and rat kidney, virtually all the activity resides in the proximal convoluted tubule with some activity in the straight cortical portion proximal to the loop of Henle (Kawashima et al. 1981, 1982; Kawashima and Kurikawa 1983). The localization at the subcellular level is more certain (Gray et al. 1972; Paulson and DeLuca 1985). The enzyme is a mitochondrial P450 complex, including an iron-sulfur protein as part of a tripartite functional unit. This complex transfers molecular (singlet) oxygen onto the 25-hydroxyvitamin D substrate in the highly specific 1-a configuration (Ghazarian et al. 1973, 1974; Ghazarian and DeLuca 1974; Pedersen et al. 1976). It is remarkable that the 1-b isomer of 1,25-dihydroxyvitamin D has less than 1/1000th the activity of the biologically active metabolite (Paaren et al. 1977). The specific components of this complex have been purified and shown to function in reconstitution experiments. Although it has been difficult to obtain sufficient material for full sequencing and gene isolation to proceed, work is now very close to identifying the 1-hydroxylase at the gene level. This will enhance studies of its tissue localization and of the regulation of its activity in intact cells and in vivo. The 24- and 26-hydroxylases have been more amenable to study in part due to the larger amount of material that is produced in most target tissues. The genes for the 24-hydroxylase have now been cloned by Okuda and his coworkers (Ohyama et al. 1991). There is interesting preliminary evidence for variants of both of these hydroxylases with different tissue distributions and possibly distinct regulatory mechanisms.

II. Regulation of Renal 1-Hydroxylation

The most powerful regulator of vitamin D activation in the kidney was shown to be parathyroid hormone and the active product 1,25-dihydroxy-vitamin D itself (BOYLE et al. 1971; OMDAHL et al. 1972; GARABEDIAN et al. 1972; RASMUSSEN et al. 1972; FRASER and KODICEK 1973; LARKINS et al. 1973, 1974a,b; HENRY et al. 1974; JONES et al. 1976). However, their precise mechanisms remain somewhat unclear. It has been difficult to demonstrate the parathyroid effect in intact, isolated renal cell systems. Part of this difficulty may relate to instability of the system and a need to induce de novo synthesis of the mitochondrial enzymes. However, it is still formally possible that this effect is in part indirect, requiring some other in vivo component of the response, including changes in calcium and phosphate in vivo. It is clear that calcium and phosphate do exert specific effects on the renal 1-hydroxylase in vivo (HUGHES et al. 1975; BAXTER and DeLuca 1976). Part of these effects are independent of parathyroid hormone (LARKINS et al. 1973; SUDA et al. 1973; TRECHSEL et al. 1980; SPANOS et al. 1981). However, the precise molecular mechanisms of these effects are not clear. Parathyroid hormone can change intracellular calcium as well as cyclic AMP levels. It is not clear whether the effects on the 1-hydroxylase activity are mediated through changes in the amount of enzyme level or in activity of preexisting enzyme. Even changes in actual enzyme level could be due to changes in the level of gene transcription, mRNA translation, or post-translational changes. The effect of 1,25-dihydroxyvitamin D on its own production is inhibitory, consistent with a product inhibition feedback loop (TANAKA and DeLuca 1974, 1984). However, the mechanisms have not been established and may be mediated through inhibition of de novo enzyme synthesis rather than changes in activity of existing enzyme. Irrespective of the mechanism it is a very potent inhibition, such that it is difficult to demonstrate any 1-hydroxylase activity in kidneys isolated from vitamin D replete animals.

Calcium is both a direct and an indirect regulator of renal 1-hydroxylase activity (BIKLE and RASMUSSEN 1975, 1978). Its indirect effect through regulation of parathyroid hormone is the more potent of the two effects. As the serum calcium level falls the parathyroid hormone level rises and this potently increases renal 1-hydroxylase activity. In the opposite situation of a high serum calcium the fall in parathyroid hormone levels effectively suppresses the renal 1-hydroxylase activity. These effects have also been shown in man (BILEZIKIAN et al. 1978; EISMAN et al. 1979a; EISMAN 1983b; EISMAN et al. 1976; PRINCE et al. 1983). In several careful studies a direct calcium effect has also been shown to exist. This operates in the same direction as its indirect effect through parathyroid hormone. Under certain circumstances, e.g., primary hyperparathyroidism, the presence of these two pathways may contribute to the relatively modest increases in serum 1,25-dihydroxyvitamin D levels. Phosphate is also a regulator of renal

1-hydroxylase activity, increasing effective activity when phosphate levels are low and decreasing it when they are high. The mechanisms of these ionic effects are far from clear at either a cellular or subcellular level. Serum levels of these ions may directly effect the proximal tubular cells in the kidney. Alternately transport of these ions across the tubular cells from tubular lumen to blood may alter tubule cell function. Irrespective of whether one or both of these primary mechanisms operate, both could alter intracellular levels of ionized calcium and this may be the final mediator at the mitochondrion. Certainly there is strong evidence for a direct effect of these ions on renal mitochondrial function in vitro. However, it is not clear that this mechanism is relevant in the intact living cell. These mechanisms require further investigation. Molecular biological studies along these lines should answer some of these questions.

Apart from the obvious effects of calcium phosphate and parathyroid hormone, renal 1-hydroxylase activity is regulated by a variety of other hormonal factors. The more important of these hormones include estrogen, growth hormone, prolactin, and insulin (SPANOS and MACINTYRE 1977; BOASS et al. 1977; CASTILLO et al. 1977; FONTAINE et al. 1978). Although the situation is complex, the positive effects of these agents are most likely indirect. For example estrogen therapy increases hepatic production of vitamin D binding protein. Over time after initiation of estrogen therapy, the total serum 1,25-dihydroxyvitamin D levels rise but the free level remains relatively constant. Similarly during pregnancy and lactation, serum 1,25-dihydroxyvitamin D levels rise considerably. However, again much of the increase can be accounted for as due to increased serum binding and not real increases in free levels. The effects of growth hormone, prolactin, and insulin may reflect some common growth factor mediator. Irrespective of their mechanisms, these hormones do have a trophic effect on the renal 1-hydroxylase.

III. Pathophysiology of Renal 1-Hydroxylation

The central role of the kidney in the activation of 25-hydroxyvitamin D to 1,25-dihydroxyvitamin D led to the discovery of this hormonal function. Moreover, the many forms of bone disease seen in situations of renal impairment led naturally to this concept. In fact there are a wide range of renal diseases which present with disorders of bone and calcium homeostasis. The common but conceptually simple situation of renal failure fits precisely with the concepts of regulation outlined above. However, there are many different disorders which affect the renal 1-hydroxylase activity, quite specifically in some instances.

The most unique and specific disorder in this regard is the isolated 1-hydroxylase deficiency of vitamin D resistant rickets type I (VDRR I), which in an affected child is characterized by rickets (FRASER et al. 1973; FRASER and SCRIVER 1976). Renal function is otherwise normal or at least can be returned to normal with replacement of active vitamin D_3, 1,25-dihydroxyvitamin D_3 (calcitriol). Replacement in this situation at normal synthesis rates completely corrects the disorder, indicating the extreme specificity of the lesion in the 1-hydroxylase enzyme. Replacement of calcitriol equivalent to normal production rates is 0.25–2.0 mg/day in adults or 15 ng/kg per day in children (Scriver et al. 1978; Rosen et al. 1977; Chesney et al. 1978, 1983; Delvin et al. 1981; Zelikovic and Chesney 1989). Another relatively specific disturbance of calcium homeostasis in which an insensitive renal 1-hydroxylase plays a role is pseudohypoparathyroidism (Drezner et al. 1973). Here, however, the lesion resides in the parathyroid hormone receptor or in postreceptor events in kidney and/or bone. Nevertheless, there is inefficient induction of the 1-hydroxylase, and therapy with calcitriol at replacement levels reverses the clinical disorder.

The Fanconi syndrome of tubular damage may affect 1-hydroxylase activity as part of the overall tubular dysfunction. This syndrome can thus alter calcium homeostasis irrespective of the fundamental cause of the renal damage. Renal tubular acidosis is another interesting problem in this regard. There has been considerable discussion as to whether the acidosis alters bone directly or whether there is another effect directly on the 1-hydroxylase (Kawashima et al. 1982; Chesney et al. 1984). Some studies indicate that the renal 1-hydroxylase is essentially unaffected by acidosis within a physiologically viable range. However, other studies suggest that there may be a specific effect of the acidosis itself on the kidney. The primary renal lesion causing the acidosis may also affect 1-hydroxylase activity. However, in the absence of such a direct effect, it seems likely that the effect of the acidosis on bone per se is more important than any secondary renal action.

F. Extrarenal 1-Hydroxylation

Some years after the demonstration of the "exclusive" production of 1,25-dihydroxyvitamin D in the kidney, information began to accumulate suggesting alternate tissue sources under some circumstances. The most compelling early evidence was for production from sarcoid tissue and this was shown to result in significant and detectable circulating levels of 1,25-dihydroxyvitamin D in anephric individuals with active sarcoidosis (Bell et al. 1979; Barbour et al. 1981; Lambert et al. 1982). Initially it was considered likely that the apparent 1,25-dihydroxyvitamin D in serum was another vitamin D metabolite which coeluted from separation columns with authentic 1,25-dihydroxyvitamin D and happened to be detectable in or interfere with the competitive binding assay. However, more and different separation steps were used, making a chance coelution increasingly unlikely. This work was confirmed with in vitro studies using macrophages from sarcoid subjects and the material was shown to dilute in parallel with authentic 1,25-dihydroxyvitamin D_3. It eventually became clear that authentic 1,25-dihydroxyvitamin D was being produced under these circumstances and indeed could be produced by normal activated macrophages (MASON et al. 1984; ADAMS et al. 1983, 1985; REICHEL et al. 1987).

I. Physiological Extrarenal 1-Hydroxylation

In due course a variety of other tissues were shown to produce 1,25-dihydroxyvitamin D in vitro in confirmation of in vivo evidence for extrarenal production of 1,25-dihydroxyvitamin D. These included particularly normal macrophages (KOEFFLER et al. 1985a; REICHEL et al. 1987; DUSSO et al. 1991), keratinocytes (BIKLE et al. 1986a,b; PILLAI et al. 1988a,b), bone cells (TURNER et al. 1980, 1983; HOWARD et al. 1981), and placental tissue (WEISMAN et al. 1979; GRAY et al. 1979; Y. TANAKA et al. 1979b). There is also evidence of production of 1,25-dihydroxyvitamin D by embryonic and other dedifferentiated cells (PUZAS et al. 1983; FRANKEL et al. 1983). The biological significance of these extrarenal sources of 1,25-dihydroxyvitamin D remains somewhat uncertain. There is good evidence for local functions of 1,25-dihydroxyvitamin D on other cell types in these tissues. So the most likely role is a paracrine one effecting replication and differentiation of certain cell types within those tissues. Thus in dermal and hematopoietic production, it seems unlikely that these sources contribute significantly to normal circulating levels of 1,25-dihydroxyvitamin D. Placental production could have such a role; however, some workers do not find such activity (HOLLIS et al. 1989). Placentally produced 1,25-dihydroxyvitamin D could be destined for functions within the maternal biological system and have a specific role in fetal biology replacing the 1-hydroxylase function of the developing fetal kidneys. The potential impact of parathyroid hormone-related peptide, which is also produced by the placenta and effects maternofetal calcium transfer therein, remains to be evaluated. Indeed the regulation of 1,25-dihydroxyvitamin D production in these extrarenal tissues remains enigmatic. Thus some data suggest that macrophage 1-hydroxylase is resistant to repression by 1,25-dihydroxyvitamin D itself, whereas renal 1-hydroxylase is exquisitely sensitive to inhibition by 1,25-dihydroxyvitamin D.

II. Pathological Extrarenal 1-Hydroxylation

As mentioned above it was initially in sarcoidosis that extrarenal 1-hydroxylation was demonstrated. This mechanism explained the long-observed event of hypercalcemia, which was often a major problem in terms of morbidity and even eventual mortality from sarcoidosis. It also explained the recognized vitamin D sensitivity in sarcoidosis. Initially it was considered this phenomenon represented an unusual aberration with no physiological relevance. However, it soon became apparent that this mechanism could be observed in other granulomatous diseases including tuberculosis (GKONOS et al. 1984; BELL et al. 1985b; CADRANEL et al. 1988). In certain hematological malignancies a similar mechanism may obtain, but tumorous production of parathyroid hormone-related peptide may be the more common mechanism for hypercalcemia in these situations.

G. Renal and Target Tissue 24-Hydroxylation

The biological function of 24-hydroxylated vitamin D metabolites has been the center of considerable discussion and debate for some time and there are two schools of thought (BOYLE et al. 1973; ORNOY et al. 1978; KANIS et al. 1978; CORVOL et al. 1978; NORMAN et al. 1980; KUMAR et al. 1982). On the one hand there is evidence particularly in the avian species of specific functions for 24,25-dihydroxyvitamin D not fulfilled by 1,25-dihydroxyvitamin D. There is some evidence in certain human inborn errors of vitamin D metabolism of a similar role. On the other hand the 24-hydroxylated metabolites are considered to be the first step in the vitamin D catabolic pathway without any unique or specific effect in normal man (HOLICK et al. 1972b, 1973; CASTILLO et al. 1978; MALLUCHE et al. 1980; HARVEY et al. 1989). In the latter view all the "specific" functions can be explained by dose and biological half-life effects in vivo, e.g., in egg hatchability (HENRY and NORMAN 1978; SUNDE et al. 1978). This debate is unlikely to be resolved in the near future. One problem for the "specific" function view is that it has not been possible to demonstrate specific receptors for 24,25-dihydroxyvitamin D. Moreover, it is clear that 24-hydroxylation can be the first step in catabolic pathways. However, a receptor may have merely eluded detection and the role of 24-hydroxylation in catabolism does not preclude a specific role under some circumstances. Also 24-hydroxylase activity is one of the earliest biological responses that can be detected in vitamin D target tissues in vitro and as such is nearly ubiquitous. Thus it is virtually impossible to construct a biological study using naturally occurring vitamin D compounds that could exclude 24-hydroxylated compounds playing some role. The "catabolic" function view is supported by studies using side-chain modified analogues of 1,25-dihydroxyvitamin D which are not susceptible to 24-hydroxylation (Y. TANAKA et al. 1979a). However, adjacent carbon atoms in the side chain could be hydroxylated introducing psuedo-24-hydroxy functionality.

I. Renal 24-Hydroxylation

In the early studies of renal vitamin D metabolism, it became apparent that there were two major alternative metabolites: 1,25-dihydroxyvitamin D and 24,25-dihydroxyvitamin D. It has been shown clearly that circulating levels of 1,25-dihydroxyvitamin D effectively suppress renal 1-hydroxylase activity and increase 24-hydroxylase activity (OMDAHL et al. 1972; FRASER and KODICEK 1973; TANAKA and DELUCA 1974; LARKINS et al. 1974a,b; HENRY et al. 1974; HUGHES et al. 1975; Y. TANAKA et al. 1975; BAXTER and DELUCA 1976). Calcium and phosphate levels may also influence the 24-hydroxylase but in the opposite direction to their effects on the 1-hydroxylase. In part it is this precise counterregulation of the 24-hydroxylase which has led to the concept of it having a specific and unique function. A complication to the assessment of these roles is the fact that any 25-hydroxylated vitamin D analogue is subject to 24-hydroxylation including 1,25-dihydroxyvitamin D itself. Thus a family of 24-hydroxylated compounds exists and any one of these could have its own specific function and could be produced by more than one pathway. Thus the trihydroxylated metabolite, 1,24,25-trihydroxyvitamin D, could be generated by the 1-hydroxylation of 24,25-dihydroxyvitamin D or the 24-hydroxylation of 1,25-dihydroxyvitamin D. Circulating levels of this metabolite have not been measured extensively and its role remains uncertain.

II. Target Tissue 24-Hydroxylation

Although 24-hydroxylation was originally recognized in the kidney (KNUTSON and DELUCA 1974; Y. TANAKA et al. 1975), it is now recognized as one of the initial responses in target tissues (KUMAR et al. 1976, 1978, 1979). In fact it has been accepted as a marker of 1,25-dihydroxyvitamin D responsive cells in vitro and in vivo (EISMAN et al. 1984; SHER et al. 1985a,b). The 24-hydroxylation appears to be similar to the 1-hydroxylase, incorporating elemental oxygen via a mitochondrial P450 (MADHOK et al. 1977). However, it is a distinct enzyme from the 1-hydroxylase and, because of the greater level of enzyme produced, is much closer to being completely identified than the 1-hydroxylase itself. The regulation of the 24-hydroxylase in target tissues, as in the kidney, is most closely related to exposure to 1,25-dihydroxyvitamin D. It is not known whether 24-hydroxylase activity is regulated by calcium and phosphate in nonrenal target tissues.

III. Catabolic Versus Unique Functions of 24,25-Dihydroxyvitamin D

The different schools of thought about the biological significance of 24-hydroxylated metabolites have yet to resolve this question. Since 24,25-dihydroxyvitamin D can be 1-hydroxylated to 1,24,25-trihydroxyvitamin D in vivo (HARNDEN et al. 1976; KUMAR et al. 1976, 1978), it is difficult to exclude the effect of such a metabolite in in vivo studies. For example, in birds hatchability of eggs is dependent upon vitamin D. Interestingly, 1,25-dihydroxyvitamin D is an inadequate replacement for vitamin D in this activity, whereas 24,25-dihydroxyvitamin D is effective (SUNDE et al. 1978; ORNOY et al. 1978). This result has been adduced as evidence for a unique effect of 24,25-dihydroxyvitamin D. However, this interpretation has been criticized on the bases that different dose levels of 1,25-dihydroxyvitamin D and 24,25-dihydroxyvitamin D were used, that these vitamin D metabolites have different biological half-lives, and that production of 1,24,25-trihydroxyvitamin D in vivo could have mediated the effects. Other studies have used chemically modified vitamin D metabolites with fluorinated side-chain carbon atoms to render them resistant to 24-hydroxylation. The fact that these side-chain modified analogues appear to have full biological activity has been interpreted as showing that absence of 24-hydroxylation dose not result in loss of any activity (Y. TANAKA et al. 1979a). However, this interpretation has been criticized on the basis that other side-chain carbon atoms can be hydroxylated and these could act as psuedo-24-hydroxy groups. Given the complexity of vitamin D metabolism, this argument remains difficult to resolve.

H. Vitamin D Catabolism

The predominant mechanism for catabolism of vitamin D is through side-chain oxidation and cleavage (KUMAR and DeLUCA 1976, 1977). A series of oxidized metabolites of 1,25-dihydroxyvitamin D has been identified involving hydroxylation at the 23 and 24 carbons with cyclization of the side chain to produce the 26-23 lactone and cleavage to produce appropriate 23-carboxylic acids (see Fig. 3). Comparable pathways appear to exist for those metabolites which lack the la-hydroxyl group (HARNDEN et al. 1976; HORST 1979; ESVELT and DeLUCA 1981; Y. TANAKA et al. 1981; NAPOLI et al.

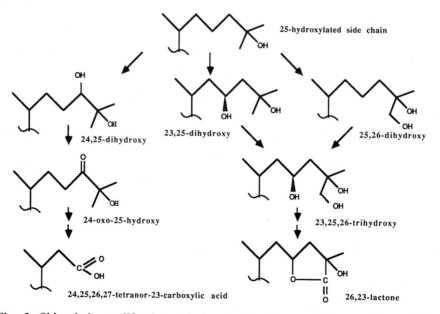

Fig. 3. Side chain modifications of vitamin D with respect to putative catabolic pathways

1982). The precise sequence of some of these steps is undefined, e.g., it is not clear whether the 26-23-lactone can yield the 23-carboxylic acid, which for 1,25-dihydroxyvitamin D has the trivial name of calcitroic acid. Most of these side-chain hydroxylation, cyclization, and cleavage steps have been identified in target tissues. Recent studies have shown that parathyroid hormone may increase the activity of the catabolic pathways. This novel work by Fraser and coworkers (CLEMENTS et al. 1987a,b) has shown increased metabolic clearance rates from serum of vitamin D and its metabolites in animals with increased parathyroid hormone levels. The effect is not explained by changes in calcium and/or phosphate levels and does not appear to be explained by increased "consumption" by passage along the activation pathways. Rather the data are more consistent with an overall increase in the catabolic pathways. The physiological or pathological significance of this mechanism is uncertain.

An interesting aspect of the catabolic pathways is the possibility of hepatic clearance of vitamin D metabolites conjugated with bile acids in the bile (LITWILLER et al. 1982). It is not clear whether these compounds may be reabsorbed from the intestine in an entero-enteric circulation. As these compounds have generally been modified at the side chain and thus have diminished biological activity, it seems unlikely that they would make any further major contribution to calcium homeostasis. On the other hand, in fat malabsorption, the vitamin D deficiency seems out of proportion to the approximately equal contributions of dietary sources and skin-produced vitamin D_3 to overall vitamin D stores. This discrepancy would be consistent with the existence of some entero-enteric circulation.

The regulation of these catabolic pathways has not been studied. However, these pathways are of high capacity and it seems likely that earlier steps, i.e., the sequential hydroxylation of the side chain, are rate-limiting. Potential functions of these catabolic metabolites remain controversial. None has been clearly shown to have unique functions at this time. However, studies continue to suggest that 24-hydroxylated metabolites and even metabolites further advanced along the "catabolic" pathways, e.g., the 26,23-lactone, may have distinct physiological roles. It is not clear whether these metabolites have specific, unique functions or whether the apparent differences are due to different biological half-lives as has been suggested previously.

I. Target Tissues

I. Bone and Calcium Related

The major organs and tissues involved in bone and calcium homeostasis are the intestine, bone, kidney, and parahyroid glands. The presence of specific receptor for 1,25-dihydroxyvitamin D has been described in each of these tissues. Indeed the receptor was initially described and extensively studied in chicken duodenum and the action of 1,25-dihydroxyvitamin D first well characterized (Boyle et al. 1972; Tsai et al. 1972; Tsai and Norman 1973; Brumbauge et al. 1974; DeLuca 1978a,b; Norman 1990). It was from this source that the receptor was eventually cloned (McDonnell et al. 1987), allowing the human receptor to be cloned shortly thereafter (Baker et al. 1988; Burmester et al. 1988). In the small intestine vitamin D is necessary for normal calcium and phosphate transport and supports epithelial growth and replication. In the vitamin D deficient animal the villi of the small intestine are flattened and the tissue is generally atrophic. In various in vivo and in vitro experiments the role of 1,25-dihydroxyvitamin D has been clearly shown as being able to support normal growth and function of the villi and to stimulate active calcium transport (reviewed by Wasserman and Fullmer 1989 and Suda et al. 1990). The ability of 1,25-dihydroxyvitamin D to stimulate calcium transport has been used in various models, e.g., the everted gut sac, to examine the biological activity of vitamin D metabolites and analogues. The actual mechanisms of the calcium transport effect remain uncertain, although there is induction of various proteins including calcium-binding protein (calbindin-28K) (Sonnenberg et al. 1984; Bishop et al. 1985; Rhoten et al. 1985). Although calbindin has been extensively studied and cloned (Hunziker et al. 1983; Theofan et al. 1986; Minghetti et al. 1988), this protein seems unable to explain the calcium transport effect. Some studies, which have shown very rapid responses in calcium transport as early as a few minutes after exposure to 1,25-dihydroxyvitamin D, suggest nongenomic effects (see below). However, while the majority of the response could be explained by genomic actions, the precise mechanism remains unknown.

In bone a wide range of effects has been described (Tanaka and DeLuca 1971; Raisz et al. 1972; Holick et al. 1972b; Balsan et al. 1986); for recent review see Raisz (1990). 1,25-Dihydroxyvitamin D acts primarily on cells of the osteoblast lineage to change their function and to change the activity of osteoclasts via some as yet undefined osteoblast-osteoclast signal (Wong et al. 1977; Holtrop and Raisz 1979; McSheehy and Chambers 1987; Sato et al. 1991). 1,25-Dihydroxyvitamin D also acts to recruit osteo-clasts from the monocyte-macrophage lineage of cells (Huh et al. 1987; Kurihara et al. 1989) but does not act directly upon the osteoclasts per se. In the osteoblast cells, 1,25-dihydroxyvitamin D changes the synthesis of alkaline phosphatase, osteocalcin, and matrix g-glutamic acid-containing protein and type I collagen (Raisz et al. 1978; Beresford et al. 1986; Rowe and Kream 1982; Yoon et al. 1987, 1988). Synthesis of the first three of these proteins is induced by 1,25-dihydroxyvitamin D while that of the last, type I collagen, is inhibited. The dose response of osteocalcin to 1,25-dihydroxyvitamin D was shown to have a half-maximal dose of approximately $10^{-10} M$, close to the circulating physiological concentration of 1,25-dihydroxyvitamin D (Price and Baukol 1980). The DNA element required for these genomic effects mediated through the vitamin D receptor has now been identified for the inductive effects (MORRISON et al. 1989; KERNER et al. 1989; DEMAY et al. 1989, 1990; LIAN et al. 1989); however, that for the repressive actions has not been identified to date. Thus the role of 1,25-dihydroxyvitamin D in bone appears to be via modulation of the normal interaction ("coupling") between osteoblast and osteoclast function. The additional action of recruitment of osteoclasts presumably explains the effect of toxic levels of vitamin D resulting in hypercalcemia rather than hyperostosis.

The role of vitamin D in the kidney is still uncertain. It certainly has a role in the repression of 1-hydroxylase and induction of 24-hydroxylase activity. However, despite many studies it is not clear whether it has any other specific effects on calcium and phosphate handling. Some studies suggest that 1,25-dihydroxyvitamin D plays a permissive role for regulation of phosphate handling by parathyroid hormone. The 1,25-dihydroxyvitamin D receptor is localized to regions of the kidney where calcium transport occurs but this is also close to where the hydroxylase activities are found. Induction of 24-hydroxylase activity in other target tissues seems to be one of the first responses to 1,25-dihydroxyvitamin D. In the kidney the 24-hydroxylase induction is also an early event and as in other tissues its significance is unclear.

The parathyroid glands are clearly important in calcium homeostasis and parathyroid hormone is the major inducer of 1-hydroxylase activity. It is perhaps not surprising then that there would be some feedback of 1,25-dihydroxyvitamin D onto parathyroid hormone synthesis and secretion. This negative feedback effect has now been shown to occur independent of any indirect effects through changes in calcium and phosphate homeostasis (HENRY and NORMAN 1975; SILVER et al. 1986; RUSSELL et al. 1986).

II. Hematopoietic Cells

In the late 1970s it became apparent that a variety of tissues were targets of 1,25-dihydroxyvitamin D action. The demonstration by Eisman and coworkers (EISMAN et al. 1979b, 1980, 1981, 1983c; FRAMPTON et al. 1982, 1983) of specific high-affinity receptors in human breast cancer cells started a decade of research into 1,25-dihydroxyvitamin D actions in many tissues, which did not fit into the classical model of calcium homeostasis. These studies included evidence of effect on cancer cell replication in vitro and xenograft growth in vivo (FRAMPTON et al. 1982, 1983; EISMAN et al. 1987). Subsequently one of the most productive of those areas has been in cells of the hematopoietic lineage in vitro (ABE et al. 1981, 1986; BAR-SHAVIT et al. 1981, 1983; DODD et al. 1983; MCCARTHY et al. 1983; MANGELSDORF et al. 1984; TANAKA et al. 1982; KOEFFLER et al. 1984, 1985b; MIYAURA et al. 1989) and in vivo (HONMA et al. 1983) as reviewed (TSOUKAS et al. 1984; SUDA 1989; REICHEL et al. 1989). At the time of this work the connection with osteoclast biology was not fully appreciated. However, with the recognition that 1,25-dihydroxyvitamin D particularly affected the monocyte-macrophage lineage and with developments in bone cell biology, the central role of 1,25-dihydroxyvitamin D in the recruitment and differentiation of osteoclast precursors could be studied more easily in vitro. In this role 1,25-dihydroxy-vitamin D interacts with many other hormones particularly the retinoids. This regulation is quite complex as macrophages are able to produce 1,25-dihydroxyvitamin D normally in vitro and may do so in vivo (see above). The production of 1,25-dihydroxyvitamin D by macrophages was demonstrated initially in sarcoidosis, but normal macrophages can produce 1,25-dihydroxyvitamin D under certain conditions (KOEFFLER et al. 1985a; HOSOI et al. 1985; REICHEL et al. 1987, 1989; DUSSO et al. 1991). This production of and response to 1,25-dihydroxyvitamin D within the same cell lineage suggests a paracrine role for 1,25-dihydroxyvitamin D. It is not clear whether circulating levels of 1,25-dihydroxyvitamin D play any role in the normal regulation of these hematopoietic cells or whether there is any overall role for 1,25-dihydroxyvitamin D in the replication and differentiation of hematopoietic cells other than those destined to enter an osteoclast precursor pool.

Cells of the hematopoietic lineage have provided useful models of vitamin D action and of interactions between peptide and steroidal regulators of bone cell biology. This approach is discussed in more detail in Chap. 3.

III. Skin and Skin Appendages

With respect to the skin and its appendages, vitamin D receptors were demonstrated in melanoma cells (COLSTON et al. 1981; FRAMPTON et al. 1982) and subsequently in melanocytes as well as keratinocytes (CLEMENS et al. 1983; HOSOMI et al. 1983; HOLICK et al. 1987; HOLICK 1988; PILLAI et al. 1988a,b). Moreover 1,25-dihydroxyvitamin D production has been shown in keratinocytes and melanocytes (FRANKEL et al. 1983; BIKLE et al. 1986a,b; HOLICK et al. 1987; HOLICK 1988; PILLAI et al. 1988a,b). Thus in the skin there are responses to 1,25-dihydroxyvitamin D (e.g., SMITH et al. 1986; HODGINS and MURAD 1986; REGNIER and DARMON 1991), consistent with a paracrine function for locally produced 1,25-dihydroxyvitamin D, similar to that in the hematopoietic system. The presence of this mechanism in the skin, which is also the site of vitamin D formation, raises the question as to whether 1,25-dihydroxyvitamin D has any function in the regulation of the photosynthesis of vitamin D_3. A logical mechanism could be through the effects of 1,25-dihydroxyvitamin D on melanocyte function (RANSOM et al. 1988). The sense of this interaction is that in the presence of high circulating 1,25-dihydroxyvitamin D levels the level of skin pigmentation would be increased. Although this might be expected to limit vitamin D photosynthesis, it could also limit the overirradiation of the previtamin D_3 in the skin. This could enhance the overall generation of vitamin D at a time when demand for this substrate for 1,25-dihydroxyvitamin D production was increased. However, it is not clear whether this mechanism has any major role in vivo.

Another interesting connection for the skin and vitamin D function is in vitamin-resistant rickets type II. In this clinical condition there is a deficiency or aberrant function of the vitamin D receptor with associated symptoms and signs of rickets and hypocalcemia (CLEMENS et al. 1983). This clinical situation is resistant to replacement doses of 1,25-dihydroxyvitamin D but in some cases responds to supraphysiological doses (BROOKS et al. 1978; EIL et al. 1981; FELDMAN et al. 1982; LIBERMAN et al. 1983; PIKE et al. 1984). There is a subset of children with a more severe form and effectively complete resistance to 1,25-dihydroxyvitamin D even at doses some 100-fold above replacement. In these children there is also complete alopecia, suggesting a functional role of the 1,25-dihydroxyvitamin D paracrine system in the regulation of dermal appendages such as the hair follicle. However, in most other forms of vitamin D deficiency (or excess) there are no clinically obvious changes in hair growth. Thus it may be that a severe deficiency is required or that, in the vitamin D resistant rickets type II, there is an associated but unrelated abnormality in the hair follicle per se.

IV. Reproduction and Endocrine Glands

Vitamin D receptors and/or responses have now been described in many endocrine tissues and other tissues involved in reproduction. These include the hypothalamus, thyroid, pancreas, adrenal, ovary, oviduct (COTY 1980), testis (WALTERS 1984), placenta, and breast cells and tissues (see reviews EISMAN 1983c; WALTERS 1985; HAUSSLER 1986; HAUSSLER et al. 1988). The role in these various tissues is still largely conjectural. In the pancreas there is an effect on insulin secretion, raising the possibility that 1,25-dihydroxyvitamin D plays a permissive role for hormone secretion in various of these tissues. This could be a direct role or could be through some effect on membrane calcium transport and intracellular calcium shifts.

The reproductive aspects are interesting in their own right. The placenta is both a site of action of 1,25-dihydroxyvitamin D and may be a site of its production (Y. TANAKA et al. 1979b; WEISMAN et al. 1979; HOLLIS et al. 1989). Whether locally produced 1,25-dihydroxyvitamin D acts in the placenta or contributes to fetal and maternal circulating 1,25-dihydroxyvitamin D levels normally is being investigated. Interestingly 1,25-dihydroxyvitamin D may regulate pituitary secretion of prolactin (WARK and TASHJIAN 1983). Pregnancy in a woman with 1-hydroxylase deficiency provides a useful model to examine this question. Here the placental tissue, which is of fetal origin, would not necessarily share the mother's genetic defect in the 1-hydroxylase and apparently placenta-derived 1,25-dihydroxyvitamin D does appear in the maternal circulation. Nevertheless, the possibility of paracrine actions of placental 1,25-dihydroxyvitamin D on the placenta and uterus and of local actions within the fetus deserve further investigation.

V. Other Tissues

Vitamin D receptors and/or responses have now been described in a wide range of tissues. In fact it may now be more appropriate to define tissues or cells where 1,25-dihydroxyvitamin D receptors have been conclusively shown to be absent. This list is shrinking as more sophisticated techniques are used. In some tissues receptor have not been found in differentiated cells but have been found in immature precursor cells (see for reviews EISMAN 1983c, 1988; WALTERS 1985; HAUSSLER 1986; HAUSSLER et al. 1988). One example of this situation is the osteoclast, which has already been discussed above. Another tissue is skeletal muscle (BOLAND 1986), where receptors have been identified in myoblasts but not mature skeletal muscle cells. Moreover, other types of differentiated muscle, e.g., cardiac muscle, not only have receptors but respond to 1,25-dihydroxyvitamin D functionally (WALTERS et al. 1986). Hepatic tissue is another tissue, which had been used as a standard negative control but in which 1,25-dihydroxyvitamin D receptors have been defined using nuclear extracts to diminish the high "background" due to the proteins produced by the liver and present in large amounts in routine homogenates. Another technique which has been particularly useful for defining the presence of receptors has been intact cell binding in cultured cells (SHER et al. 1981, 1985a,b). This approach was originally used to demonstrate the presence of receptors in human breast cancer cells in culture and has now been widely used for other tissues (EISMAN et al. 1986a,b). Its particular advantage is that it examines the receptor in the biologically relevant situation of a living cell albeit in culture. It is much less subject to swamping by other binding proteins or to degradation of receptor in broken cell preparations. Irrespective of the methods used it is becoming clear now that 1,25-dihydroxyvitamin D receptors are expressed in most if not all tissues and cell types and particularly in immature undifferentiated tissues.

J. Vitamin D Receptor

I. Functional Role

Specific high-affinity 1,25-dihydroxyvitamin D receptor was first defined in the chick intestine. The chick had been used because of the relative ease of establishing a model of vitamin D deficiency and rickets in various avian species compared with rodent models, which are relatively resistant to the development of rickets even in the presence of vitamin D deficiency. Moreover, in the rat serum vitamin D binding protein obscured specific binding of

1,25-dihydroxyvitamin D, just as it had "inhibited" 1-hydroxylase activity in rat kidney studies. The evidence for a specific receptor in the intestine predated demonstration of the renal activation of 25-hydroxyvitamin D by 1-hydroxylation. Subsequent studies defined the receptor to be a protein approximately 60 kDa in size and to sediment at between 3.2 and 3.7 S in sucrose density gradients. The affinity of the receptor was initially thought to be relatively low with K_d of about $10^{-10} M$. However, with the availability of progressively higher specific activity of the $[^3H]$-1,25-dihydroxyvitamin D, the affinity was realized to be higher, with K_ds of $1-2 \times 10^{-11} M$ being described (EISMAN and DELUCA 1977, 1978). The specificity of the receptor was shown to be quite remarkable, with the immediate precursor of 1,25-dihydroxyvitamin D, i.e., 25-hydroxyvitamin d, having 500- to 1000-fold lower affinity for the receptor isolated from chick intestine or a variety of other tissues including human breast cancer cells (see Table 3). The parent vitamin D had about six orders of magnitude lower affinity for the receptor. 24-Hydroxylation reduced binding affinity of any metabolite by about 10-fold, e.g., 1,24,25-trihydroxyvitamin D had 10- to 15-fold lower affinity for the receptor than 1,25-dihydroxyvitamin D itself. A variety of other steroidal hormones including estrogens, antiestrogens, androgens, gluco-corticoids, mineralocorticoids, and progestins had virtually no ability to compete for bindings to the receptor in vitro. For a time there was considerable discussion about the precise size of the receptor and about its subcellular localization in the occupied and unoccupied states. The debate about size became somewhat irrelevant after the cloning of the 1,25-dihydroxyvitamin D receptor. With respect to the intracellular localizaton of the occupied receptor, it is clear that it does have affinity for various nuclear components. There are biochemical and immunoblotting data which suggest that the unoccupied receptor may reside primarily in the nucleus (WALTERS et al. 1980, 1981; KING and GREENE 1984), and there are other data which do not support this view (SHER et al. 1981, 1985a). However, the concept that unoccupied steroid hormone receptors equilibrate between the cytosol and the nucleus has made the latter debate moot. Apart from glucocorticoid

Table 3. Relative affinity of some naturally occurring vitamin D metabolites for the vitamin D receptor. (Modified from EISMAN and DELUCA 1977, 1978; EISMAN et al. 1979b; EISMAN 1983a,b, 1988)

1,25-Dihydroxyvitamin D_3	1.0
1,25-Dihydroxyvitamin D_2	0.8–1.0
1,24,25-Dihydroxyvitamin D_3	0.07
1a-Dihydroxyvitamin D_3	0.005
25-Dihydroxyvitamin D_3	0.002
24,25-Dihydroxyvitamin D_3	0.0003
25,26-Dihydroxyvitamin D_3	0.0003
Vitamin D_3	0.000001

receptors which appear to have a specific cytosolic binding protein (heat shock proteins 90, hsp 90), the equilibrium hypothesis is probably applicable generally.

II. End Organ Resistance

Important models of the mechanism of vitamin D action were found in the "experiments of nature" of vitamin D resistant rickets. These inborn errors of metabolism result in rickets with severe hypocalcemia. In type I vitamin D resistant rickets the defect lies in the renal 1-hydroxylase. The clinical picture bears some similarities to pseudohypoparathyroidism with high serum PTH and low serum 1,25-dihydroxyvitamin D levels. However, the serum phosphate levels are high in pseudohypoparathyroidism and relatively low in vitamin D resistant rickets type I. In type II vitamin D resistant rickets the mechanism is quite distinct although the clinical picture is similar to type I VDRR (EIL et al. 1981; ADAMS et al. 1982; FELDMAN et al. 1982; LIBERMAN et al. 1983; PIKE et al. 1984). One severe form of type II vitamin D resistant rickets is associated with complete alopecia (see above). Therapy to correct serum calcium levels has no obvious effect on the alopecia and the mechanism of this abnormality in hair growth is unknown. In type II vitamin D resistant rickets the major abnormality is in the receptor with functional defects ranging from complete or relative deficiency of receptor to apparently aberrant function. Families and individuals with these disorders have been carefully investigated by various groups. In some cases receptor appears to be almost completely absent while in others the level is much reduced below levels seen in normal target tissues. More commonly there is abnormal 1,25-dihydroxyvitamin D binding or normal 1,25-dihydroxyvitamin D but failure of nuclear localization of occupied receptor. In some cases the precise mechanism remains uncertain. However, in each case the "experiment of nature" provides some insight into the structure-function requirements of the 1,25-dihydroxyvitamin D receptor. Molecular biological studies have been invaluable in the further examination of these receptor abnormalities.

III. Molecular Biology

The study of structure-function relationships in the 1,25-dihydroxyvitamin D receptor received a major boost when the avian duodenal 1,25-dihydroxy-vitamin D receptor was cloned (McDONNELL et al. 1987). The human and rat receptors were cloned shortly after that (BAKER et al. 1988; BURMESTER et al. 1988), opening the way to study of the disorder of signal transduction in natural (vitamin D resistant rickets type II) or synthetic mutants of the 1,25-dihydroxyvitamin D receptor. The receptor was found to be a member of the steroid hormone-retinoid-thyroid hormone receptor superfamily (see review HAUSSLER et al. 1988). The domain structure is highly conserved between members of this family, particularly the DNA-binding and ligand-binding regions with the intervening "hinge" region. There is strong homology between members of the superfamily at the DNA and particularly the amino acid sequence levels and all are zinc finger proteins. However, the 1,25-dihydroxyvitamin D receptor would appear to have diverged from the other members relatively early in evolutionary terms. Although it is a zinc finger protein, it has a relatively short C-terminal region but otherwise is very similar to the other family members. Elegant studies using site-directed mutagenesis have established the functional importance of individual amino acids in the structure of the zinc fingers. The naturally occurring mutants in vitamin D resistant rickets type II mainly appear to involve the zinc finger regions, which explains the predominance of poor DNA localization as the apparent mechanism in functional studies in this condition. Cloning of the 1,25-dihydroxyvitamin D receptor gene has also opened the way to expression and preparation of large amounts of the receptor for physico-chemical studies (SONE et al. 1991). Crystallization of the receptor seems likely in the near future and this will provide further insight into the ligand- and DNA-binding regions. Receptor produced in this way is being used for gel-shift and DNAase foot-printing studies to confirm vitamin D responsive elements identified from transcriptional studies in 1,25-dihydroxyvitamin D responsive genes.

IV. Vitamin D Response Element in Responsive Genes

The molecular mechanism of action of 1,25-dihydroxyvitamin D was the target of considerable interest from the time that its steroid hormone action mechanism became apparent. Work in this area lagged until the 1,25-dihydroxyvitamin D receptor was cloned, although the eventual definition of the responsive element did not depend in any way upon the cloning of the receptor gene. The tool, which opened the way to determining a vitamin D responsive element, was the cloning of the rat osteocalcin gene. This gene has the advantage that it is relatively small and its expression is upregulated in vivo and in vitro in certain bone-derived cells. Several groups (MORRISON et al. 1989; KERNER et al. 1989; DEMAY et al. 1989; LIAN et al. 1989) working in the rat and human genes identified the region of the vitamin D responsive element and despite some initial confusion the nucleus of the region appears to be a doubly palindromic structure with considerable overall homology to other steroid hormone responsive elements (see Fig. 4). At the time of the identification it was noted (MORRISON et al. 1989) that certain adjacent regions are essential for induction to take place. Multiple repeats of the same region may overcome this requirement but the molecular physiology is consistent with several different proteins binding to the DNA secondary to binding of the 1,25-dihydroxyvitamin D receptor. Work currently underway with gel shift and DNAase footprinting is producing results consistent with this concept.

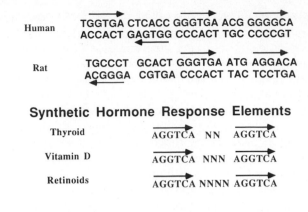

Fig. 4. Vitamin D responsive element in the human osteocalcin gene promoter showing homology to other steroid hormone receptor responsive elements. (Modified from MORRISON et al. 1989)

There is a repressive effect of 1,25-dihydroxyvitamin D on several different genes including the collagen type I genes (LICHTLER et al. 1989). The responsive element for this negative effect (nVDRE) has not been identified at present. The genes which are repressed by 1,25-dihydroxyvitamin D do not appear to have regions homologous to the positive vitamin D reponsive element. The mechanism of this effect therefore may not be a direct effect but rather may be mediated through the induction of a repressor. In this regard there is the clear model of induction of one gene, osteocalcin, and repression of another, collagen type I, within the same cell type, the osteoblast. The physiological significance of these effects, in which one gene is induced while another is repressed in cells of the same lineage, deserves and is receiving considerable further research effort.

K. Genomic and Nongenomic Effects

The mechanism of action of 1,25-dihydroxyvitamin D involves genomic effects, which are considered to be the principal if not the only pathway. One of the earliest demonstrations of an apparently genomic effect is the regulation of the c-*myc* oncogene in leukemic cells by 1,25-dihydroxyvitamin D (REITSMA et al. 1983; KUROKI et al. 1983; MIYAURA et al. 1985). 1,25-Dihydroxyvitamin D was able to completely suppress expression of this oncogene as long as it was present in the medium bathing the cells. However, despite the evidence for genomic mechanisms of action for 1,25-dihydroxy-vitamin D in vivo and in vitro, there are some effects which suggest somewhat different pathways. At times there has been some confusion about the distinctions between nongenomic and nonreceptor mediated effects and between mechanisms of action and defining changes in gene transcription. In some cases inhibitors of gene transcription or protein synthesis have not been effective in blocking 1,25-dihydroxyvitamin D responses. This has led to the concept that such effects much be non-genomic, despite the fact that these inhibitors are incompletely effective in certain in vivo systems. Moreover, as mechanisms of 1,25-dihydroxyvitamin D response are further understood, certain proteins and enzymes have been recognized as fulfilling essential roles and appropriate genetic mechanisms have been defined. Nevertheless there are some situations where non-genomic mechanisms would appear to be acting. Even here there is still evidence of marked specificity between vitamin D metabolites. At the present time this specificity is still most consistent with a receptor-mediated effect albeit acting through a nongenomic mechanism. Changes in calcium transport, in polyamine and phosphoinosotide metabolism, and in mem-brane fluidity have been noted.

The marked rapidity of certain responses suggests that nongenomic effects may be operative. For example, intestinal calcium transport can respond to 1,25-dihydroxyvitamin D within minutes in vitamin D replete animals, suggesting that there may be nongenomic effects, although priming by prior exposure to 1,25-dihydroxyvitamin D is required. With increasing knowledge genomic effects are being better defined but potential non-genomic effects may be closely interlinked with such effects. For example, 1,25-dihydroxyvitamin D-occupied receptor may alter the stability or func-tion of certain cytosolic or membrane proteins and thus alter their effective activity. Such an effect would be nongenomic, potentially very rapid, but still involve receptor in providing the observed sensitivity and specificity. This area of research is complicated by potential multiple mechanisms of action through several second messenger systems operating in tandem or concert.

Polyamine turnover in the intestine is an interesting example of such possible multiple effects of 1,25-dihydroxyvitamin D in cell function. 1,25-Dihydroxyvitamin D alters cell turnover and growth (SPIELVOGEL et al. 1972) as well as other functions, such as calcium transport. 1,25-Dihydroxyvitamin D alters polyamine turnover through induction of spermidine N^1-acetyl-transferase and ornithine decarboxylase (SHINKI et al. 1985, 1986, 1989; STEEVES and LAWSON 1985). The net effect of this action is to increase levels of putrescine in cells. This is via a dual action of increasing conversion of ornithine to putrescine and of enhanced recycling of spermidine (derived from putrescine) back to putrescine via N^1-acetylspermidine. In some studies in vitamin D deficient animals, putrescine administration was able to increase intestinal cell replication and villus length towards that seen in normal vitamin D replete animals. This treatment was also able to restore calcium transport which had been decreased by blockers of putrescine synthesis in vivo (Suda et al. 1990). Despite these multiple types of effects, they are still quite consistent with genomic effects of action of 1,25-dihydroxyvitamin D.

Calcium transport in the intestine and 1,25-dihydroxyvitamin D effects in the kidney have been linked to the transcriptional regulation of a calcium-binding protein, calbindin D. Although expression of intestinal calbindin-D_{28K} is regulated by 1,25-dihydroxyvitamin D, there has been some uncertainty as to whether it is expressed rapidly enough to explain the most rapid increases in calcium transport across intestinal cells (see reviews Berdal et al. 1989; Wasserman and Fullmer 1989; Wasserman et al. 1990). This calbindin is expressed in several other tissues (Sonnenberg et al. 1984; Rhoten et al. 1985) including kidney and bone, and in pancreas as well as other endocrine tissues (for review see Christakos et al. 1989). It is expressed in brain tissue but in this tissue is unresponsive to 1,25-dihydroxyvitamin D induction. Calbindin-D_{28K} is a member of a family of proteins, including myosin light-chain kinase and calmodulin, with a high affinity for calcium ($10^{-8}-10^{-6}M$) and an unusual secondary structural motif called an "E-F hand." Calbindin has been suggested to function in calcium transport as a calcium "sink" near the apical membrane which could also deliver calcium to a higher affinity calcium pump at the basolateral membrane (Kretsinger et al. 1982). It is still not certain whether the synthesis of calbindin is regulated by 1,25-dihydroxyvitamin D at the gene level or if it is induced secondary to increased intracellular calcium levels. There is also evidence in the intestine for a calmodulin-mediated calcium transport pathway. This mechanism appears to use preformed calmodulin as the calcium-binding arm of an induced transport pathway. The 105 K_{Da} protein involved in this localization of calmodulin to adjacent to the enterocyte brush border (Bikle and Munson 1985) may be induced by 1,25-dihydroxyvitamin D and as such may complement the effect of enhanced expression of calbindin-D_{28K}.

In osteoblasts, type I collagen and the bone-specific protein osteocalcin are regulated by 1,25-dihydroxyvitamin D. Interestingly these two genes are regulated in opposite directions, i.e., the collagen gene is repressed while the osteocalcin gene is induced. The significance of these actions in the regulation of normal bone turnover, formation, and resorption is not known. However, these genes have provided valuable models to study 1,25-dihydroxyvitamin D action at the molecular level. In fact it was in human and rat versions of the osteocalcin gene (Morrison et al. 1989; Kerner et al. 1989; Demay et al. 1989; Lian et al. 1989) that the vitamin D responsive element was first identified (see above).

The very rapid response defined in intestinal calcium transport (Nemere and Szego 1981; Nemere et al. 1984) still does suggest nongenomic actions with possible candidates including changes in membrane fluidity (Brasitus et al. 1986) and membrane-related calcium shift (FARACH-CARSON et al. 1991). Changes in cyclic AMP and cyclic GMP have been reported but this area has not been well studied (see review, WASSERMAN and FULLMER 1989). The mechanisms of such rapid potentially nongenomic responses require further study. It should be emphasized that "nongenomic" in this context does not imply lack of specificity but rather suggests an alternate non-transcriptional pathway of receptor-mediated regulation. It remains to be seen whether 1,25-dihydroxyvitamin D receptor subtypes will be found to explain such different pathways.

L. Summary

The current concept of vitamin D is of at least two functional systems; one intimately involved in bone and calcium homeostasis and the other a more fundamental role in the regulation of cellular differentiation and function in most if not all tissues in the body. The former role is a refined version of the concept of the entire range of vitamin metabolism and function of little more than a decade ago. The latter role provides a rationale for local production of 1,25-dihydroxyvitamin D and introduces concepts of 1,25-dihydroxyvitamin D as an important mediator of previously unthought of autocrine and paracrine functions. Studies of the mechanisms of the regulation of the 1-hydroxylase will be aided when the 1-hydroxylase gene has been cloned. This seems imminent now that the 24- and 26-hydroxylase genes have been cloned. The biological significance of 24-hydroxylation remains unresolved.

   The bone and calcium homeostasis concept of vitamin D metabolism and function includes dermal production of vitamin D_3 and its activation by hepatic and renal activation as well as its subsequent catabolism predominantly through side-chain modification and cleavage. The cloning of the intracellular 1,25-dihydroxyvitamin D receptor and its molecular mechanism of action at the gene level has been the focus of much research recently. The molecular mechanisms involved in mediating 1,25-dihydroxyvitamin D actions in responsive tissues are the prime target for much current research.

   The second more fundamental role focuses both on extrarenal production of 1,25-dihydroxyvitamin D and on 1,25-dihydroxyvitamin D functions in tissues not classically involved in bone or calcium homeostasis. The roles in malignant cells, which opened this area, are gradually being seen as amplifications of normal physiological mechanisms rather than pathological markers of malignancy per se. These areas are providing fertile ground for further investigations of 1,25-dihydroxyvitamin D function. The role of 1,25-dihydroxyvitamin D in relation to hematopoietic cells, skin and appendages, and various endocrine and reproductive tissues are clear examples of such areas.

In both these areas it needs to be determined whether nongenomic actions of 1,25-dihydroxyvitamin D do in fact exist and if so whether 1,25-dihydroxyvitamin D receptor mediates these actions. Research in relation to potential nongenomic effects in other steroidal hormone systems may shed light on this area. The vitamin D system has become much more complex and much more interesting over the last decade. Advances in molecular biology are helping to unravel some of the enigmas in vitamin D metabolism and function. Vitamin D research will continue to provide a fertile ground for the efforts of a wide range of research scientists, including physiologists, biochemists, and cell and molecular biologists.

Acknowledgments. Thanks are due to Ms. Kay Cooper and Ms. Kylie Eisman for invaluable assistance with the bibliography.

References

Abe E, Miyaura C, Sakagami H, Takeda M, Konno K, Yamazaki T, Yoshiki S, Suda T (1981) Differentiation of mouse myeloid leukemia cells induced by 1,25-dihydroxyvitamin D_3. Proc Natl Acad Sci USA 78:4990–4994

Abe J, Moriya Y, Saito M, Sugawara Y, Suda T, Nishii Y (1986) 1,25-Dihydroxycholecalciferol-induced differentiation of myelomonocytic leukemic cells unresponsive to colony stimulating factors and phorbol esters. J Cell Physiol 129:295–302

Adams JS, Clemens TL, Horiuchi N, Quaroni A, Holick MF (1982) Vitamin D resistant rickets with alopecia: cultured skin fibroblasts exhibit defective cytoplasmic receptors and unresponsiveness to 1,25(OH)$_2$D$_3$. J Clin Endocrinol Metab 55:1020–1022

Adams JS, Sharma OR, Gacad MA, Singer FR (1983) Metabolism of 25-hydroxyvitamin D_3 by cultured pulmonary alveolar macrophages in sarcoidosis. J Clin Invest. 78:1856–1860

Adams JS, Singer FR, Gacad MA, Sharma OP, Hayes MJ, Vouros P, Holick MF (1985) Isolation and structural identification of 1,25-dihydroxyvitamin D_3 produced by cultured alveolar macrophages in sarcoidosis. J Clin Endocrinol Metab 60:960–966

Arnaud SB, Goldsmith RS, Lambert PW, Go VLW (1975) 25-Hydroxyvitamin D_3: evidence of an enterohepatic circulation in man. Proc Soc Exp Biol Med 149:570–572

Arnaud SB, Matthausen M, Gilkinson JB, Goldsmith RS (1977) Components of 25-hydroxyvitamin D_3 in serum of young children in upper midwestern US. Am J Clin Nutr 30:1082–1086

Bachrach S, Fisher J, Parks JS (1979) An outbreak of vitamin D deficiency rickets in a susceptible population. Pediatrics 64:871–877

Baker AR, McDonnell DP, Hughes M, Crisp TM, Mangelsdorf DJ, Haussler MR, Pike JW, Shine J, O'Malley BW (1988) Cloning and expression of full-length cDNA encoding human vitamin D receptor. Proc Natl Acad Sci USA 85:3294–3298

Balsan S, Garabedian M, Larchet M, Gorski AM, Cournot G, Tau C, Bourdeau A, Silve C, Ricur C (1986) Long-term nocturnal calcium infusions can cure rickets and promote normal mineralization in hereditary resistance to 1,25-dihydroxyvitamin D. J Clin Invest 77:1661–1667

Barbour GL, Coburn JW, Slatopolsky E, Norman AW, Horst RL (1981) Hypercalcemia in an anephric patient with sarcoidosis: evidence for extrarenal generation of 1,25-dihydroxyvitamin D. N Engl J Med 305:440–443

Bar-Shavit Z, Noff D, Edelstein S, Meyer M, Shibolet S, Goldman R (1981) 1,25-Dihydroxyvitamin D_3 and the regulation of macrophage function. Calcif Tissue Int 33:673–676

Bar-Shavit Z, Teitelbaum SL, Reitsma P, Hall A, Pegg LE, Trial J, Kahn AJ (1983) Induction of monocyclic differentiation and bone resorption by 1,25-dihydroxyvitamin D_3. Proc Natl Acad Sci USA 80:5907–5911

Baxter LA, DeLuca HF (1976) Stimulation of 25-hydroxyvitamin D_3-la-hydroxylase by phosphate depletion. J Biol Chem 251:3158–3161

Bell NH, Greene A, Epstein S, Oesmann MJ, Shaw S, Shary J (1985a) Evidence for alteration of the vitamin D-endocrine system in blacks. J Clin Invest 76:470–473

Bell NH, Shary J, Shaw S, Turner RT (1985b) Hypercalcemia associated with increased circulating 1,25-dihydroxyvitamin D in a patient with pulmonary tuberculosis. Calcif Tissue Int 37:588–91

Bell NH, Stern PH, Pantzer E, Sinka TK, DeLuca HF (1979) Evidence that increased circulating 1-alpha dihydroxyvitamin D is the probable cause of abnormal calcium metabolism in sarcoidosis. J Clin Invest 64:218–225

Berdal A, Cuisinier GP, Balmain N, Thomasset M, Brehier A, Deffez JP, Mathieu H (1989) On the molecular mechanism of intestinal calcium transport. Adv Exp Med Biol 249:45–65

Beresford JN, Gallagher JA, Russell RGG (1986) 1,25-Dihydroxyvitamin D_3 and bone-derived cells in vitro: effects on alkaline phosphatase, type I collagen and proliferation. Endocrinology 119:1776–1785

Bhattacharyya MH, DeLuca HF (1973) The regulation of rat liver calciferol 25-hydroxylase. J Biol Chem 248:2969–2973

Bikle DD, Munson S (1985) 1,25-Dihydroxyvitamin D increases calmodulin binding to specific proteins in the chick duodenal brush border membrane. J Clin Invest 76:2312–2316

Bikle DD, Rasmussen H (1975) The ionic control of 1,25-dihydroxyvitamin D_3 production in isolated chick renal tubules. J Clin Invest 55:292–298

Bikle DD, Rasmussen H (1978) A biochemical model for the ionic control of 25-hydroxyvitamin D_3 la-hydroxylase. J Biol Chem 253:3042–3048

Bikle DD, Nemanic MK, Gee E, Elias P (1986a) 1,25-Dihydroxyvitamin D_3 production by human keratinocytes. Kinetics and Regulation. J Clin Invest 78:557–566

Bikle DD, Nemanic MK, Whitney JO, Elias PW (1986b) Neonatal human foreskin keratinocytes produce 1,25-dihydroxyvitamin D_3. Biochemistry 25:1545–1548

Bilezikian JP, Canfield RE, Jacobs TB, Polay JS, D'Adamo AP, Eisman JA, DeLuca HF (1978) Response of 1,25-dihydroxyvitamin D_3 to hypocalcaemia in human subjects. N Engl J Med 299:437–441

Bishop CE, Kendrick NC, Dame MC, DeLuca HF (1985) 1a,25-Dihydroxyvitamin D-induced modification of a cytosolic protein in embryonic chick intestine. J Biol Chem 260:5209–5212

Blunt JW, DeLuca HF, Schnoes HK (1968) 25-Hydroxycholecalciferol. A biologically active metabolite of vitamin D_3. Biochemistry 7:3317–3322

Boass A, Toverud SU, McCain TA, Pike JW, Haussler MR (1977) Elevated serum levels of 1a,25-dehydroxycholecalciferol in lactating rats. Nature 267:630–631

Boland R (1986) Role of vitamin D in skeletal muscle function. Endocr Rev 7:434–448

Bouillon R, VanBaelen H, Rombauts W, DeMoor P (1978) The isolation and characterization of the vitamin D-binding protein from rat serum J Biol Chem 253:4426–4431

Bouillon R, VanBaelen H, DeMoor P (1980) Comparative study of the affinity of the serum vitamin D-binding protein. J Steroid Biochem 13:1029–1034

Bouillon R, VanAssche FA, VanBaelen H, Heyns W, DeMoor P (1981) Influence of the vitamin D-binding protein on the serum concentration of 1,25-dihydroxyvitamin D_3: significance of the free 1,25-dihydroxyvitamin D_3 concentration. J Clin Invest 67:589–596

Boyle I, Gray RW, DeLuca HF (1971) Regulation by calcium of in vivo synthesis of 1,25-dihydroxycholecalciferol and 21,25-dihydroxycholecalciferol. Proc Natl Acad Sci USA 68:2131–2134

Boyle IT, Miravet L, Gray RW, Holick MF, DeLuca HF (1972) The response of intestinal calcium transport to 25-hydroxy and 1,25-dihydroxyvitamin D in nephrectomized rats. Endocrinology 90:605–608

Boyle IT, Omdahl JL, Gray RW, DeLuca HF (1973) The biological activity and metabolism of 24,25-dihydroxyvitamin D₃. J Biol Chem 248:4174–4180

Brasitus TA, Dudeja PK, Eby B, Lau K (1986) Correction by 1,25-dihydroxycholecalciferol of the abnormal fluidity and lipid composition of enterocyte brush border membranes in vitamin D-deprived rats. J Biol Chem 261:16404–16409

Brooks MM, Bell NM, Love L, Stern PH, Orfei E, Queener SF, Hamstra A, DeLuca HF (1978) Vitamin D dependent rickets type II. Resistance of target organs to 1,25-dihydroxyvitamin D. N Engl J Med 298:996–999

Brumbaugh PF, Haussler DH, Bressler R, Haussler MR (1974) Radioreceptor assay for 1a,25-dihydroxyvitamin D₃. Science 183:1089–1091

Burmester JK, Maeda N, DeLuca HF (1988) Isolation and expression of rat 1,25-dihydroxyvitamin D₃ receptor cDNA. Proc Natl Acad Sci USA 85:1005–1009

Cadranel J, Hance AJ, Milleron B, Paillard F, Akoun GM, Garabedian M (1988) Vitamin D metabolism in tuberculosis. Production of 1,25-(OH)₂D₃ by cells recovered by bronchoalveolar lavage and the role of this metabolite in calcium homeostasis. Am Rev Respir Dis 138:984–989

Carpenter TO (1989) Mineral regulation of vitamin D metabolism. Bone Miner 5:259–69

Castillo L, Tanaka Y, DeLuca HF, Sunde ML (1977) The stimulation of 25-hydroxyvitamin D3-1a-hydroxylase by estrogen. Arch Biochem Biophys 179:211–217

Castillo L, Tanaka Y, DeLuca HF, Ikekawa N (1978) On the physiological role of 1,24,25-trihydroxyvitain D₃. Miner Electrolyte Metab 1:198–207

Chesney RW, Kaplan BS, Phelps M, DeLuca HF (1984) Renal tubular acidosis does not alter circulating values of calcitriol. J Pediatr 104:51–55

Chesney RW, Moorthy AV, Eisman JA, Jax DK, Mazess RB, DeLuca HF (1978) Increased growth after long-term oral 1,25(OH)₂-vitamin D₃ in childhood renal osteodystrophy. N Engl J Med 298:238–244

Chesney RW, Mazess RB, Rose P, Hamstra AJ, DeLuca HF, Breed AL (1983) Long-term influence of calcitriol (1,25(OH)₂vitamin D) and supplemental phosphate in X-linked hypophosphatemic rickets. Pediatrics 71:559–567

Christakos S, Gabrielides C, Rhoten WB (1989) Vitamin D-dependent calcium binding proteins: chemistry, distribution, functional considerations and molecular biology. Endocr Rev 10:3–26

Christiansen C, Rodbro P, Tjellesen L (1983) Pathophysiology behind anticonvulsant osteomalacia. Acta Neurol Scand 94:21S–28S

Clemens TL, Adams JS, Henderson SL, Holick MF (1982) Increased skin pigment reduces the capacity of the skin to synthesize vitamin D. Lancet 1:74–76

Clemens TL, Adams JS, Horinchi N, Gilchrest BA, Cho H, Tsuchiya Y, Matsuo N, Suda T, Holick MF (1983) Interaction of 1,25-dihydroxyvitamin D₃ with keratinocytes and fibroblasts from skin of normal subjects and a subject with vitamin D-dependent rickets, type II: a model for study of the mode of action of 1,25-dihydroxyvitamin D₃. J Clin Endocrinol Metab 56:824–830

Clements MR, Davies M, Fraser DR, Lumb GA, Mawer B, Adams PH (1987a) Metabolic inactivation of vitamin D is enhanced in primary hyperparathyroidism. Clin Sci 73:659–664

Clements MR, Johnson L, Fraser DR (1987b) A new mechanism for induced vitamin D deficiency in calcium deprivation. Nature 324:62–65

Colston K, Colston MJ, Felman D (1981) 1,25-Dihydroxyvitamin D_3 and malignant melanoma: the presence of receptors and inhibition of cell growth in culture. Endocrinology 108:1083–1086

Corvol MT, Dumontier MF, Garabedian M, Rappaport R (1978) Vitamin D and cartilage: II. Biological activity of 25-hydroxycholecalciferol and 24,25- and 1,25-dihydroxycholecalciferols on cultured growth plate chondrocytes. Endocrinology 102:1269–1273

Coty WA (1980) A specific high affinity binding protein for 1,25-dihydroxyvitamin D in the chick oviduct shell gland. Biochem Biophys Res Commun 93:285–292

DeLuca HF (1975) The kidney as an endocrine organ involved in the function of vitamin D. Am J Med 58:39–47

DeLuca HF (1978a) Vitamin D and calcium transport. Ann NY Acad Sci 307:356–376

DeLuca HF (1978b) Vitamin D metabolism and function. Arch Intern Med 138:836–847

DeLuca HF (1979) Recent advances in our understanding of the vitamin D endocrine system. J Steroid Biochem 11:35–52

Delvin EE, Glorieux FH, Marie PJ, Pettifor JM (1981) Vitamin D dependency rickets: replacement therapy with calcitriol. J Pediat 99:26–34

Demay MB, Roth DA, Kronenberg HM (1989) Regions of the rat osteocalcin gene which mediate the effect of 1,25-dihydroxyvitamin D_3 on gene transcription. J Biol Chem 264:2279–2282

Demay MB, Gerardi JM, DeLuca HF, Kronenberg HM (1990) DNA sequences in the rat osteocalcin gene that bind the 1,25-dihydroxyvitamin D_3 receptor and confer responsiveness to 1,25-dihydroxyvitamin D_3. Proc Natl Acad Sci USA 87:369–373

Dent CE, Richens A, Rowe DJF, Stamp TCB (1970) Osteomalacia with long-term anticonvulsant therapy in epilepsy. Br Med J 4:69–72

Dodd RC, Cohen MS, Newman SL, Gray TK (1983) Vitamin D metabolites change phenotype of monoblastic U937 cells. Proc Natl Acad Sci USA 80:7538–7541

Drezner MK, Neelon FA, Lebovitz HE (1973) Pseudohypoparathyroidism type II. A possible defect in the reception of the cyclic AMP signal. N Engl J Med 289:1056–1060

Dusso AS, Finch J, Brown A, Ritter C, Delmez J, Schreiner G, Slatopolsky E (1991) Extrarenal production of calcitriol in normal and uremic humans. J Clin Endocrinol Metab 72:157–164

Eastwood JBN, deWardener ME (1979) Normal plasma 1,25($OH)_2$-vitamin D concentrations in nutritional osteomalacia. Lancet i:1377–1378

Eil C, Liberman UA, Rosen JF, Marx SJ (1981) A cellular defect in hereditary vitamin-D-dependent rickets type II: defective nuclear uptake of 1,25-dihydroxyvitamin D in cultured skin fibroplasts. N Engl J Med 304:1588–1591

Eisman JA (1983a) 1,25-Dihydroxyvitamin D3 receptor and role of 1,25-($OH)_2D_3$ in human cancer cells. In: Kumar R (ed) Vitamin D metabolism: basic and clinical aspects. Nijhoff, Boston, pp 365–382

Eisman JA (1983b) Stress testing of plasma 1,25-dihydroxyvitamin D in man. In: Kumar R (ed) Vitamin D metabolism: basic and clinical aspects. Nijhoff, Boston, pp 479–496

Eisman JA (1983c) The study of 1,25-dihydroxyvitamin D_3 receptor. In: Agarwal MR (ed) Principles of receptorology. deGruyter, Berlin, pp 465–544

Eisman JA (1988) Osteomalacia. Baillieres Clin Endocrinol Metab 2:125–155

Eisman JA, DeLuca HF (1977) Intestinal, 1,25-dihydroxyvitamin D_3 binding protein: specificity of binding protein. Steroids 30:245–257

Eisman JA, DeLuca HF (1978) Determination of vitamin D metabolites. In: Colowick SP, Kaplan NO (ed) Methods in enzymology, volume 25, part C. Academic, New York, pp 388–393

Eisman JA, Hamstra AJ, Kream BE, DeLuca HF (1976) 1,25-Dihydroxyvitamin D in biological fluids. Simplified and sensitive assay. Science 193:1021–1023

Eisman JA, Wark JD, Prince RL, Moseley JM (1979a) Modulation of plasma 1,25-dihydroxyvitamin D in man by stimulation and supression tests. Lancet ii:931–933

Eisman JA, Martin TJ, MacIntyre I, Moseley JM (1979b) 1,25-Dihydroxyvitamin D receptors in breast cancer cells. Lancet ii:1335–1336

Eisman JA, Martin TJ, MacIntyre I, Frampton RJ, Moseley JM, Whitehead R (1980) 1,25-Dihydroxyvitamin D_3-receptor in a cultured human breast cancer cell line (MCF-7). Biochem Biophys Res Commun 93:9–15

Eisman JA, Suva LJ, Sher E, Pearce PT, Funder JW, Martin TJ (1981) Frequency of 1,25-dihydroxyvitamin D_3 receptor in human breast cancer. Cancer Res 41:5121–5124

Eisman JA, Sher E, Suva LJ, Frampton RJ, McLean FL (1984) 1,25-Dihydroxyvitamin D_3 specifically induces its own metabolism in a cancer cell line. Endocrinology 114:1225–1231.

Eisman JA, Suva LJ, Martin TJ (1986a) Significance of 1,25-dihydroxyvitamin D3 receptor in primary breast cancers. Cancer Res 46:5406–5408

Eisman JA, Frampton RJ, McLean FJ (1986b) Biochemical significance of enhanced activity of fluorinated 1,25-dihydroxyvitamin D_3 in human cultured cell lines. Cell Biochem Funct 4:115–121

Eisman JA, Barkla DH, Tutton PJM (1987) 1,25-Dihydroxyvitamin D_3 suppresses the in vivo growth of human cancer solid tumor xenografts. Cancer Res 47:21–25

Eisman JA, Fragonas J-C, McMenemy LM (1988) Rapid turnover of the 1,25-dihydroxyvitamin D_3 receptor in human target cells. Endocrinology 122:1613–1621

Ellis GW, Cooke WT (1978) Serum concentrations of 25-hydroxyvitamin D in Europeans and Asians after oral vitamin D_3. Br Med J 1:685–686

Ellis G, Woodhead JS, Cooke WT (1977) Serum 25-hydroxyvitamin-D concentrations in adolescent boys. Lancet 1:825–828

Esvelt RP, DeLuca HF (1981) Calcitroic acid: biological activity and tissue distribution studies. Arch Biochem Biophys 206:403–413

Farach-Carson MC, Sergeev I, Norman AW (1991) Non-genomic actions of 1,25-dihydroxyvitamin D_3 in rat osteosarcoma cells: structure-function studies using ligand analogs. Endocrinology 129:1876–1882

Feldman D, Chen T, Cone C, Hirst M, Shani S, Benderli A, Hochenburg Z (1982) Vitamin-D resistant rickets with alopecia: cultured skin fibroplasts exhibit defective cytoplasmic receptors and unresponsiveness to 1,25-dihydroxyvitamin D_3. J Clin Endocrinol Metab 55:1020–1022

Fontaine O, Pavlovitch H, Balsan S (1978) 25-Hydroxycholecalciferol metabolism in hypophysectomized rats. Endocrinology 102:1822–1826

Frampton RJ, Suva LJ, Eisman JA, Findlay DM, Moore GE, Moseley JM, Martin TJ (1982) Presence of 1,25-dihydroxyvitamin D_3 in established human cancer cell lines in culture. Cancer Res 42:116–119

Frampton RJ, Omond SA, Eisman JA (1983) Inhibition of human cancer cell growth by 1,25-dihydroxyvitamin D_3 metabolites. Cancer Res 43:4443–4447

Francis RM, Peacock M, Storer JH, Davies AE, Brown WB, Nordin BE (1983) Calcium malabsorption in the elderly: the effect of treatment with oral 25-hydroxyvitamin D3. Eur J Clin Invest 13:391–6

Frankel TL, Mason RS, Hersey P, Murray E, Posen S (1983) The synthesis of vitamin D metabolites by human melanoma cells. J Clin Endocrinol Metab 57:627–631

Fraser DR, Kodicek E (1970) Unique biosynthesis by kidney of a biologically active vitamin D metabolite. Nature 228:764–766

Fraser DR, Kodicek E (1973) Regulation of 25-hydroxycholecalciferol-1-hydroxylase activity in kidney by parathyroid hormone. Nature 241:163–166

Fraser DR, Scriver CR (1976) Familial forms of vitamin D-resistant rickets revisited: X-linked hypophosphatemia and autosomal recessive vitamin D dependence. Am J Clin Nutr 29:1315–1329

Fraser DR, Kooh SW, Kind P, Holick M, Tanaka Y, DeLuca F (1973) Pathogenesis of hereditary vitamin D-dependent rickets. N Engl J Med 289:817–822

Carabedian M, Holick MF, DeLuca HF, Boyle IT (1972) Control of 25-hydroxycholecalciferol metabolism by parathyroid glands. Proc Natl Acad Sci USA 69:1673–1676

Ghazarian JG, DeLuca HF (1974) 25-Hydroxycholecalciferol-1-hydroxylase: a specific requirement for NADPH and a hemoprotein component in chick kidney mitochondria. Arch Biochem Biophys 160:63–72

Ghazarian JG, Schnoes HK, DeLuca HF (1973) Mechanism of 25-hydroxycholecalciferol 1a–hydroxylation. Incorporation of oxygen-18 into the 1a-position of 25-hydroxycholecalciferol. Biochemistry 12:2555–2558.

Ghazarian JG, Jefcoate CR, Knutson JC, Orme-Johnson WH, DeLuca HF (1974) Mitochondrial cytochrome P_{450}: a component of chick kidney 25-hydroxycholecalciferol-1a-hydroxylase. J Biol Chem 249:3026–3033

Geigy Scientific Tables (1981) Lentner Cornelius Lentner Charlotte, Wink A (eds). Ciba-Geigy, Basle, Switzerland. 1:242–260

Gkonos PJ, London R, Hendler ED (1984) Hypercalcemia and elevated 1,25-dihydroxyvitamin D levels in a patient with end stage renal disease and active tuberculosis. N Engl J Med 311:1683–1685

Gray RW, Boyle I, DeLuca HF (1971) Vitamin D metabolism: the role of kidney tissue. Science 172:1232–1234

Gray RW, Omdahl JL, Ghazarian JG, DeLuca HF (1972) 25-Hydroxycholecalciferol-1-hydroxylase: subcellular location and properties. J Biol Chem 247:7528–7532

Gray TK, Lester GE, Loreno RS (1979) Evidence for extra-renal 1-alpha hydroxylation of 25-hydroxyvitamin D_3 in pregnancy. Science 204:1311–1313

Haddad JG Jr, Hahn TJ (1973) Natural and synthetic sources of circulating 25-hydroxyvitamin D in man. Nature 244:515–517

Haddad JG, Jennings AJ, Aw TC (1988) Vitamin D uptake and metabolism by perfused rat liver: influences of carrier proteins. Endocrinology 123:498–505

Hahn TJ, Birge SJ, Scharp CR, Avioli LV (1972) Phenolbarbital-induced alterations in vitamin D metabolism. J Clin Invest. 51:741–748

Hahn TJ, Halstead LR, Haddad JG Jr (1977) Serum 25-hydroxyvitamin D concentrations in patients receiving chronic corticosteroid therapy. J Lab Clin Med 90:399–404

Harnden D, Kumar R, Holick MF, DeLuca HF (1976) Side chain metabolism of 25-hydroxy-[26,27-^{14}C] vitamin D_3 and 1,25-dihydroxy-[26,27-^{14}C] vitamin D_3 in vivo. Science 193:493–494

Harvey JA, Zerwekh JE, Sakhaee K, Pak CY (1989) Lack of effect of 24,25-dihydroxyvitamin D_3 administration on parameters of calcium metabolism. J Clin Endocrinol Metab 69:467–469

Haussler MR (1986) Vitamin D receptors; nature and function. Ann Rev Nutr 6:527–562

Haussler MR, Boyce DW, Littledike ET, Rasmussen H (1971) A rapidly acting metabolite of vitamin D_3. Proc Natl Acad Sci USA 68:177–181

Haussler MR, Mangelsdorf DJ, Komm BS, Terpening CM, Yamaoka K, Allegretto EA, Baker AR, Shine J, McDonnell DP, Hughes M, Weigel NL, O'Malley BW, Pikes JW (1988) Molecular biology of the vitamin D hormone. Recent Prog Horm Res 44:263–305

Henry HL, Norman AW (1975) Studies on the mechanism of action of calciferol: VII. Localization of 1,25-dihydroxyvitamin D_3 in chick parathyroid glands. Biochem Biophys Res Commun 62:781–788

Henry HL, Norman AW (1978) Vitamin D: two dihydroxylated metabolites are required for normal chicken egg hatchability. Science 201:835–837

Henry HL, Midgett RJ, Norman AW (1974) Regulation of 25-hydroxyvitamin D_3-1-hydroxylase in vivo. J Biol Chem 249:7584–7592

Hodgins MB, Murad S (1986) 1,25-Dihydroxycholecalciferol stimulates conversion of androstenedione into oestrone by human skin fibroplasts in culture. J Endocrinol 110:R1–R4

Holick MF (1988) Skin: site of the synthesis of vitamin D and a target tissue for the active form, 1,25-dihydroxyvitamin D_3. Ann NY Acad Sci 548:14–26

Holick MF, Schnoes HK, DeLuca HF (1971) Identification of 1,25-dihydroxycholecalciferol, a form of vitamin D_3 metabolically active in the intestine. Proc Natl Acad Sci USA 68:803–804

Holick MF, Schnoes HK, DeLuca HF, Gray RW, Boyle IT, Suda T (1972a) Isolation and identification of 24,25-dihydroxycholecalciferol: a metabolite of vitamin D_3 made in the kidney. Biochemistry 11:4251–4255

Holick MF, Garabedian M, DeLuca HF (1972b) 1,25-Dihydroxycholecalciferol: metabolite of vitamin D_3 active on bone in anephric rats. Science 176:1146–1148

Holick MF, Kleiner-Bossaller A, Schnoes HK, Kaiten PM, Boyle IT, DeLuca HF (1973) 1,24,25-Trihydroxyvitamin D_3. A metabolite of vitamin D_3 effective on intestine. J Biol Chem 248:6691–6696

Holick MF, MacLaughlin JA, Clark MB, Holick SA, Potts JT Jr, Anderson RR, Blank IH, Parrish JA, Elias P (1980) Photosynthesis of previtamin D_3 in human skin and the physiologic consequences. Science 210:203–205

Holick MF, MacLaughlin JA, Doppelt SH (1981) Regulation of cutaneous previtamin D_3 photosynthesis in man: skin pigment is not an essential regulator. Science 211:590–593

Holick MF, Smith E, Pincus S (1987) Skin as the site of vitamin D synthesis and target tissue for 1,25-dihydroxyvitamin D_3. Arch Dermatol 123:1677–1683

Hollis BW, Iskerky VN, Chang MK (1989) In vitro metabolism of 25-hydroxyvitamin D_3 by human trophoblastic homogenates, mitochondria and microsomes: lack of evidence for the presence of 25-hydroxyvitamin D_3-1a- and 24R-hydroxylases. Endocrinology 125:1224–1230

Holtrop ME, Raisz LG (1979) Comparison of the effects of 1,25-dihydroxycholecalciferol, prostaglandin E_2, and osteoclast-activating factor with parathyroid hormone on the ultrastructure of osteoclasts in cultured long bones of fetal rats. Calcif Tissue Int 29:201–205

Honma Y, Hozumi M, Abe E, Konno K, Fukushima M, Hata S, Nishii Y, DeLuca HF, Suda T (1983) 1a,25-Dihydroxyvitamin D_3 and 1a,25-hydroxyvitamin D_3 prolong survival time of mice inoculated with myeloid leukemia cells. Proc Natl Acad Sci USA 80:201–204

Horst RL (1979) 25-OHD-$_3$-26,23-Lactone: a metabolite of vitamin D_3 that is 5 times more potent than 25-OHD3 in the rat plasma competitive protein binding radioassay. Biochem Biophys Res Commun 89:286–293

Hosoi J, Abe E, Suda T, Kuroki T (1985) Isolation and structural identification of 1,25-dihydroxyvitamin D_3 produced by cultured alveolar macrophages in sarcoidosis. J Clin Endocrinol Metab 60:960–966

Hosomi J, Hosoi J, Abe E, Suda T, Kuroki T (1983) Regulation of terminal differentiation of cultured mouse epidermal cells by 1a,25-dihydroxyvitamin D_3. Endocrinology 113:1950–1957

Howard GA, Turner RT, Sherrard DJ, Baylink DJ (1981) Human bone cells in culture metabolize 25-hydroxyvitamin D_3 to 1,25-dihydroxyvitamin D_3 and 24,25-dihydroxyvitamin D_3. J Biol Chem 256:7738–7740

Hughes MR, Brumbauch PF, Haussler MR, Wergedal JE, Baylink DJ (1975) Regulation of serum 1a,25-dihydroxyvitamin D_3 by calcium and phosphate in the rat. Science 190:578–580

Huh N, Satoh M, Nose K, Abe E, Suda T, Rajewsky MF, Kuroki T (1987) Formation of multinucleated cells that respond to osteotropic hormones in long term human bone marrow cultures. Endocrinology 120/6:2326–2333

Hunziker W, Siebert PD, King MW, Stucki P, Dugaiczyk A, Norman AW (1983) Molecular cloning of a vitamin D-dependent calcium binding protein mRNA sequence from chick intestine. Proc Natl Acad Sci USA 80:4228-4232

Jones G, Baxter LA, DeLuca HF, Schnoes HK (1976) Biological activity of 1,25-dihydroxyvitamin D_2 in the chick. Biochemistry 15:713-716

Kanis JA, Cundy T, Bartlett M, Smith R, Heynen G, Warner GT, Russell RG (1978) Is 24,25-dihydroxycholecalciferol a calcium-regulating hormone in man? Br Med J 1:1382-1386

Kawashima H, Kurikawa K (1983) Unique hormonal regulation of vitamin D metabolism in the mammalian kidney. Miner Electrolyte Metab 9:227-235

Kawashima H, Torikai S, Kurokawa K (1981) Localization of 25-dihydroxyvitamin D_3 1a-hydroxylase and 24-hydroxylase along the rat nephron. Proc Natl Acad Sci USA 78:1199-1203

Kawashima H, Kraut JA, Kurokawa K (1982) Metabolic acidosis suppresses 25-hydroxyvitamin D_3-1a-hydroxylase in rat kidney: distinct site and mechanism of action. J Clin Invest 70:135-140

Kerner SA, Scott BA, Pike JW (1989) Sequence elements in the human osteocalcin gene confer basal activation and inducible response to hormonal vitamin D_3. Proc Natl Acad Sci USA 86:4455-4459

King WJ, Greene GL (1984) Monoclonal antibodies localize oestrogen receptor in the nuclei of target cells. Nature 307:745-747

Knutson JC, DeLuca HF (1974) 25-Hydroxyvitamin D_3-24-hydroxylase. Subcellular location and properties. Biochemistry 13:1543-1548

Koeffler HP, Amatruda T, Ickckawa N, Kobayashi Y, DeLuca HF (1984) Induction of macrophage differentiation of human normal and leukemic myeloid cells by 1,25-dihydroxyvitamin D_3 and its fluorinated analogues. Cancer Res. 44:5624-5628

Koeffler HP, Reichel H, Bishop JE, Norman AW (1985a) g-Interferon stimulates production of 1,25-dihydroxyvitamin D_3 by normal human macrophages. Biochem Biophys Res Commun 127:596-603

Koeffler HP, Hirji K, Itri L (1985b) 1,25-Dihydroxyvitamin D_3: in vivo and in vitro effects on human preleukemic and leukemic cells. Cancer Treat Rep 69:1399-1407

Koo WWK (1988) Calcium, phosphorus and vitamin D requirements of infants receiving parenteral nutrition. J Perinatol 8:263-268

Kretsinger RH, Mann JE, Simmonds JG (1982) Model of facilitated diffusion of calcium by the intestinal calcium binding protein. In: Norman AW, Schaefger K, von Herrath D, Grigolert H-G (eds) Vitamin D: chemical, biochemical and clinical endocrinology of calcium metabolism. de Gruyter, New York, pp 233-248

Kumar R, DeLuca F (1976) Side chain oxidation of 25-hydroxy-[26,27-^{14}C]-vitamin D_3 and 1,25-dihydroxy-[26,27-^{14}C]-vitamin D_3 in vivo by chickens. Biochem Biophys Res Commun 69:197-200

Kumar R, DeLuca HF (1977) Side-chain oxidation of 1,25-dihydroxyvitamin D_3 in the rat: effect of removal of the intestine. Biochem Biophys Res Commun 76:253-258

Kumar R, Harnden D, DeLuca HF (1976) Metablism of 1,25-dihydroxyvitamin D_3: evidence for side-chain oxidation. Biochemistry 15:2420-2423

Kumar R, Schnoes HK, DeLuca HF (1978) Rat intestinal 25-hydroxyvitamin D_3- and 1a,25-dihydroxyvitamin D_3-24-hydroxylase. J Biol Chem 253:3804-3809

Kumar R, Silva P, Epstein FH (1979) In vivo 24-hydroxylation of 25-hydroxyvitamin D_3 in enterocolectomized rats. Endocrinology 104:1794-1796.

Kumar R, Wiesner R, Scott M, Go VLM (1982) Physiology of 24,25-dihydroxyvitamin D_3 in normal human subjects. Am J Physiol 243:E370-E374

Kurihara N, Suda T, Miura Y, Nakauchi H, Kodama H, Hiura K, Hakeda Y, Kumegawa M (1989) Generation of osteoclasts from isolated hematopoietic progenitor cells. Blood 74:1295-1302

Kuroki T, Sasaki K, Chida K, Abe E, Suda T (1983) Regulation of *myc* gene expression in HL-60 leukaemia cells by a vitamin D metabolite. Nature 306:492–494

Laitinen K, Valimaki M, Lamberg-Allardt C, Kivisaari L, Lalla M, Karkkainen M, Ylikahri R (1990) Deranged vitamin D metabolism but normal bone mineral density in Finnish noncirrhotic male alcoholics. Alcohol Clin Exp Res 14:551–556

Lambert PW, Stern PH, Avioli RC, Brackett NC, Turner RT, Green A, Fu IY, Bell NH (1982) Evidence for extrarenal production of 1a-dihydroxyvitamin D in man. J Clin Invest 69:722–725

Larkins RG, MacAuley SJ, Colston KW, Evans IMA, Galante LS, MacIntrye I (1973) Regulation of vitamin D metabolism without parathyroid hormone. Lancet ii:289–291

Larkins RG, MacAuley SJ, MacIntyre I (1974a) Feedback control of vitamin D metabolism by nuclear action of 1,25-dihydroxyvitamin D_3 on the kidney. Nature 252:412–414

Larkins RG, MacAuley SJ, Rapoport A, Martin TJ, Tulloch BR, Byfield PGH, Matthews EW, MacIntrye I (1974b) Effects of nucleotides, hormones, ions and 1,25-dihydroxycholecalciferol on 1,25-dihydroxycholecalciferol production in isolated chick renal tubules. Clin Sci Mol Med 46:569–582

Lawson DEM, Fraser DR, Kodicek E, Morris HR, Williams DH (1971) Identification of 1,25-dihydroxycholecalciferol, a new kidney hormone controlling calcium metabolism. Nature 230:228–230

Lester E, Skinner RK, Wills MR (1977) Seasonal variation in serum 25-hydroxyvitamin D in the elderly in Britain. Lancet 1:979–980

Lian J, Stewart C, Puchacz E, Mackowiak S, Shalhoub V, Collart D, Zambetti G, Stein G (1989) Structure of the rat osteocalcin gene and regulation of vitamin D-dependent expression. Proc Natl Acad Sci USA 86:1143–1147

Liberman UA, Eil C, Marx SJ (1983) Resistance to 1,25-dihydroxyvitamin D. Association with heterogeneous defects in cultured skin fibroblasts. J Clin Invest 71:192–200

Lichtler A, Stover ML, Angilly J, Kream B, Bowe DW (1989) Isolation and characterization of the rat a1(I) collagen promoter. Regulation by 1,25-dihydroxyvitamin D. J Biol Chem 264:3072–3077

Litwiller RD, Vernon RM, Jardine I, Kumar R (1982) Evidence for a monoglucuronide of 1,25-dihydroxyvitamin D_3 in rat bile. J Biol Chem 257:7491–7494

Lund B, Sorensen OH, Hilden M, Lund B (1977) The hepatic conversion of vitamin D in alcoholics with varying degrees of liver affection. Acta Med Scand 202:221–224

Madhok TC, Schnoes HK, DeLuca HF (1977) Mechanism of 25-hydroxyvitamin D_3 24-hydroxylation: incorporation of oxygen-18 into the 24 position of 25-hydroxyvitamin D_3. Biochemistry 16:2142–2145

Malluche HH, Henry H, Meyer-Sabelleck W, Sherman D, Massry SG, Norman AW (1980) Effects and interactions of 24R,25-dihydroxyvitamin D_3 and 1,25-dihydroxyvitamin D_3 on bone. Am J Physiol 238:E494–E498

Mangelsdorf DJ, Koeffler HP, Donaldson CA, Pike JW, Haussler MR (1984) 1,25-Dihydroxyvitamin D_3-induced differentiation in a human promyelocytic leukaemia cell line (HL60): receptor-mediated maturation to macrophage-like cells. J Cell Biol 98:391–398

Mason RS, Frankel T, Chan Y-L, Lissner D, Posen S (1984) Vitamin D conversion by sarcoid lymph node homogenate. Ann Intern Med 100:59–61.

McCarthy DM, San Miguel JF, Freake HC, Green PM, Zola H, Catovsky D, Goldman JM (1983) 1,25-Dihydroxyvitamin D_3 inhibits proliferation of human promyelocytic leukaemia (HL60) cells and induces monocyte-macrophage differentiation in HL60 and normal human bone marrow cell. Leuk Res 7:51–55

McDonnell DP, Mangelsdorf DJ, Pike JW, Haussler MR, O'Malley BW (1987) Molecular cloning of complementary DNA encoding the avian receptor for vitamin D. Science 235:1214–1217

McLaughlin M, Raggatt PR, Fairney A, Brown DJ, Lester E, Wills MR (1974) Seasonal variations in serum 25-hydroxycholecalciferol in healthy people. Lancet 1:536–538

McSheehy PMJ, Chambers TJ (1987) 1,25-Dihydroxyvitamin D_3 stimulates rat osteoblastic cells to release a soluble factor that increases osteoblastic bone resorption. J Clin Invest 80:425–429

Minghetti PP, Cancela L, Fujisawa Y, Thoefan G, Norman AW (1988) Molecular structure of the chicken vitamin D-induced calbindin-D28K gene reveals eleven exons, six Ca^{2+} binding domains and numerous promoter regulatory elements. Mol Endocrinol 2:355–367

Miyaura C, Abe E, Suda T, Kuroki T (1985) Cooperative regulation of c-*myc* expression in differentiation of human promyelocytic leukemia induced by recombinant gamma-interferon and 1,25-dihydroxyvitamin D3. Cancer Res 45:4366–4371

Miyaura C, Jin CH, Yamaguchi Y, Tomida M, Hozumi M, Matsuda T, Hirano T, Kishimoto T, Suda T (1989) 1 Alpha,25-dihydroxyvitamin D_3 receptor distribution and effects in subpopulations of normal human T lymphocytes. J Clin Endocrinol Metab 68:774–779

Morrison NA, Shine J, Fragonas JC, Verkest V, McMenemy LM, Eisman JA (1989) 1,25-Dihydroxyvitamin D responsive element and glucocorticoid repression in the human osteocalcin gene. Science 246:1158–1161

Napoli JL, Pramanik BC, Partridge JJ, Ushkokovic MR, Horst RL (1982) 23S,25-Dihydroxyvitamin D_3 as a circulating metabolite of vitamin D_3. Its role in 25-hydroxyvitamin D_3-26,23-lactone biosynthesis. J Biol Chem 257:9634–9639

Nemere I, Szego CM (1981) Early actions of parathyroid hormone and 1,25-dihydroxycholecalciferol on isolated epithelial cells from rat intestine: I Limited lysosomal enzyme release and calcium uptake. Endocrinology 108:1450–1462

Nemere I, Yoshimoto Y, Norman AW (1984) Studies on the mode of action of calciferol. Calcium transport in perfused duodena from normal chicks: enhancement within 14 minutes of exposure to 1,25-dihydroxyvitamin D_3. Endocrinology 115:1476–1483

Norman AW (1990) Intestinal calcium absorption: a vitamin D-hormone-mediated adaptive response. Am J Clin Nutr. 51:290–300

Norman AW, Henry HL, Malluche HH (1980) 24R,25-Dihydroxyvitamin D_3 and 1a,25-dihydroxyvitamin D_3 are both indispensable for calcium and phosphorus homeostasis. Life Sci 27:229–237

Ohyama Y, Noshiro M, Okuda K (1991) Cloning and expression of cDNA encoding 25-hydroxyvitamin D3 24-hydroxylase. FEBS Lett 278:195–198

Omdahl JL, Gray RW, Boyle IT, Knutson J, DeLuca HF (1972) Regulation of metabolism of 25-hydroxycholecalciferol by kidney tissue in vitro by dietary calcium. Nature 237:63–64

Ornoy A, Goodwin D, Noff D, Edelstein S (1978) 24,25-Dihydroxyvitamin D is a metabolite of vitamin D essential for bone formation. Nature 276:517–519

Paaren HE, Schones HK, DeLuca HF (1977) Synthesis of 1b-hydroxyvitamin D_3 and 1b,25-dihydroxyvitamin D_3. J Chem Soc Chem Commun 23:890–892

Paulson SK, DeLuca HF (1985) Subcellular location and properties of rat renal 25-hydroxyvitamin D_3-1-a-hydroxylase. J Biol Chem 290:11488–11492

Pederson JI, Ghazarian JG, Orme-Johnson NR, DeLuca HF (1976) Isolation of chick renal mitochondrial ferredoxin active in the 25-hydroxyvitamin D_3-1a-hydroxylase system. J Biol Chem 251:3933–3941

Pettiror JM, Ross FP, Solomon L (1978) Seasonal variation in serum 25-hydroxycholecalciferol concentrations in elderly South African patients with fractures of femoral neck. Br Med J 6116:826–827

Pike JW, Dokoh S, Haussler MR, Liberman UA, Marx SJ, Eil C (1984) Vitamin D$_3$-resistant fibroblasts have immunoassayable 1,25-dihydroxyvitamin D3 receptors. Science 224:879–881

Pillai S, Bikle DD, Elias PM (1988a) 1,25-Dihydroxyvitamin D production and receptor binding in human keratinocytes varies with differentiation. J Biol Chem 263:5390–5395

Pillai S, Bikle DD, Elias PM (1988b) Vitamin D and epidermal differentiation: evidence for a role of endogenously produced vitamin D metabolites in keratinocyte differentiation. Skin Pharmacol 1:149–160

Ponchon G, Kennan AL, DeLuca HF (1969) "Activation" of vitamin D by the liver. J Clin Invest 48:2032–2037

Price PA, Baukol SA (1980) 1,25-Dihydroxyvitamin D$_3$ increases synthesis of the vitamin K-dependent bone protein by osteosarcoma cells. J Biol Chem 255:11660–11663

Prince RL, Wark JD, Omond S, Opie JM, Eagle R, Eisman JA (1983) A test of 1,25-dihydroxyvitamin D$_3$ secretory capacity in normal subjects for application in metabolic bone diseases. Clin Endocrinol 18:127–133

Puzas JE, Turner RT, Howard GA, Baylink DJ (1983) Cells isolated from embryonic intestine synthesize 1,25-dihydroxyvitamin D$_3$ and 24,25-dihydroxyvitamin D$_3$ in culture. Endocrinology 112:378–380

Raisz LG (1990) Recent advances in bone cell biology: interactions of vitamin D with other local and systemic factors. Bone Miner 9:191–197

Raisz LG, Trummel CL, Holick MF, DeLuca HF (1972) 1,25-Dihydroxycholecalciferol: a potent stimulator of bone resorption in tissue culture. Science 175:768–769

Raisz LG, Maina DM, Gworek SC, Dietrich JW, Canalis EM (1978) Hormonal control of bone collagen synthesis in vitro: inhibitory effect of 1-hydroxylated vitamin D metabolites. Endocrinology 102:731–735

Ransom M, Posen S, Mason RS (1988) Human melanocytes as a target tissue for hormones: in vitro studies with 1,25-dihydroxyvitamin D$_3$, a melanocyte stimulating hormone and beta-estradiol. J Invest Dermatol 91:593–598

Rasmussen H, Wong M, Bikle D, Goodman DBP (1972) Hormonal control of the renal conversion of 25-hydroxycholecalciferol to 1,25-dihydroxycholecalciferol. J Clin Invest 51:2502–2504

Reasner II CA, Dunn JF, Fetchick DA, Liel Y, Hollis BW, Epstein S, Shary J, Mundy GR, Bell NH (1990) Alteration of vitamin D metabolism in Mexican Americans. J Bone Miner Res 5:13–17

Regnier M, Darmon M (1991) 1,25-Dihydroxyvitamin D$_3$ stimulates specifically the last steps of epidermal differentiation of cultured human keratinocytes. Differentiation 47:173–188

Reichel H, Koeffler HP, Norman AW (1987) Synthesis in vitro of 1,25-dihydroxyvitamin D$_3$ and 24,25-dihydroxyvitamin D$_3$ by interferon-g-stimulated normal human bone marrow and alveolar macrophages. J Biol Chem 262:10931–10937

Reichel H, Koeffler HP, Norman AW (1989) The role of the vitamin D endocrine system in health and disease. N Engl J Med 320:980–989

Reitsma PH, Rothberg PG, Astrin SM, Trial J, Bar-Shavit Z, Hall A, Teitelbaum SL, Kahn AJ (1983) Regulation of *myc* gene expression in HL-60 cells by a vitamin D metabolite. Nature 306:492–494

Rhoten WB, Bruns ME, Christakos S (1985) Presence and localization of two vitamin D-dependent calcium binding proteins in kidneys of higher vertebrates. Endocrinology 117:674–683

Robertson I, Glekin BM, Henderson JB, McIntosh WB, Lakhani A, Dunnigan MG (1982) Nutritional deficiencies among ethnic minorities in the United Kingdom. Proc Nutr Soc 41:243–256

Rosen JF, Fleischman AR, Finberg L, Eisman JA, DeLuca HF (1977) 1,25-Dihydroxycholecalciferol: its use in the long-term management of idiopathic hypoparathyroidism in children. J Clin Endocrinol Metab 45:457–468

Rowe DW, Kream BE (1982) Regulation of collagen synthesis in fetal rat calvaria by 1,25-dihydroxyvitamin D_3. J Biol Chem 257:8009–8015

Russell J, Lettieri D, Sherwood LM (1986) Suppression by $1,25(OH)_2D_3$ of transcription of the pre-proparathyroid hormone gene. Endocrinology 119:2864–2866

Sato T, Hong MH, Jin CH, Ishimi Y, Udagawa N, Shinki T, Abe E, Suda T (1991) The specific production of the third component of complement by osteoblastic cells treated with 1a,25-dihydroxyvitamin D_3. FEBS Lett 285:21–24

Scriver CR, Reade TM, DeLuca HF, Hamstra AJ (1978) Serum 1,25-dihydroxy-vitamin D levels in normal subjects and in patients with hereditary rickets or bone disease. N Engl J Med 299:976–979

Shepard RM, DeLuca HF (1980) Plasma concentrations of vitamin D_3 and its metabolites in the rat as influenced by vitamin D_3 or 25-hydroxyvitamin D_3 intakes. Arch Biochem Biophys 202:43–53

Sher E, Eisman JA, Moseley JM, Martin TJ (1981) Whole cell uptake and nuclear localisation of 1,25-dihydroxyvitamin D3 by cancer cells (T47 D) in culture. Biochem J 200:315–320

Sher E, Martin TJ, Eisman JA (1985a) Hormone-dependent transformation and nuclear localisation of 1,25-dihydroxy-vitamin D_3 receptors from human breast cancer cell lines and chick duodenum. Horm Metab Res 17:147–152

Sher E, Frampton RJ, Eisman JA (1985b) Regulation of the 1,25-dihydroxy-vitamin D_3 receptor in intact human cancer cells. Endocrinology 116:971–979

Shinki T, Takahashi N, Kadofuku T, Sato T, Suda T (1985) Induction of spermidine N^1-acetyltransferase by 1a,25-dihydroxyvitamin D_3 as an early common event in the target tissues of vitamin D. J Biol Chem 260:2185–2190

Shinki T, Kadofuku T, Sato T, Suda T (1986) Spermidine N^1-acetyltransferase has a larger role than ornithine decarboxylase in 1a,25-dihydroxyvitamin D_3-induced putresine synthesis. J Biol Chem 261:11712–11716

Shinki T, Tanaka H, Kadofuku T, Sato T, Suda T (1989) Major pathway for putrescine synthesis induced by 1a,25-dihydroxyvitamin D_3 in chick duodenum. Gastroenterology 96:1494–1501

Silver J, Naveh-Many T, Mayer H, Schmelzer HJ, Popovtzer MM (1986) Regulation by vitamin D metabolites of parathyroid hormone gene transcription in vivo in the rat. J Clin Invest 78:1296–1301

Smith EL, Walworth NC, Holick MF (1986) Effect of 1,25-dihydroxyvitamin D_3 on the morphology and biochemical differentiation of cultured human keratinocytes grown in serum-free conditions. J Invest Dermatol 86:709–714

Sone T, Kerner S, Pike JW (1991) Vitamin D receptor interaction with specific DNA: association as a 1,25-dihydroxyvitamin D_3-modulated heterodimer. J Biol Chem 266:23296–23305

Sonnenberg J, Pansini AR, Christakos S (1984) Vitamin D-dependent rat renal calcium-binding protein: development of a radioimmunoassay, tissue distribution, and immunologic identification. Endocrinology 115:640–648

Spanos E, MacIntyre I (1977) Vitamin D and the pituitary. Lancet 1:840–841

Spanos E, Freake H, Macauley SJ, Macintyre I (1981) Regulation or vitamin D metabolism by calcium and phosphate ions in isolated renal tubes. Biochem J 196:187–193

Spielvogel AM, Farley RD, Norman AW (1972) Studies on the mechanism of action of calciferol: V. Turnover time of chick intestinal epithelial cells in relation to the intestinal action of vitamin D. Exp Cell Res 74:359–366

Stamp TC, Round JM, Rowe DJ, Haddad JG (1972) Plasma levels and therapeutic effect of 25-hydroxycholecalciferol in epileptic patients taking anticonvulsant drugs. Br Med J 4:9–12

Steeves RM, Lawson DEM (1985) Effect of 1,25-dihydroxyvitamin D on S-adenosylmethionine decarboxylase in chick intestine. Biochim Biophys Acta 841:292–298

Stryd RP, Gilbertson TJ, Brunden MN (1979) A seasonal variation study of 25-hydroxyvitamin D_3 serum levels in normal humans. J Clin Endocrinol Metab 48:771–775

Suda T (1989) The role of 1 alpha,25-dihydroxyvitamin D3 in the myeloid cell differentiation. Proc Soc Exp Biol Med 191:214–220

Suda T, Horiuchi N, Sasaki S (1973) Direct control by calcium of 25-hydroxycholecalciferol 1a-hydroxylase activity in chick kidney mitochondria. Biochem Biophys Res Commun 54:512–518

Suda T, Shinki T, Takahashi N (1990) The role of vitamin D in bone and intestinal cell differentiation. Ann Rev Nutr. 10:195–211

Sunde ML, Turk CM, DeLuca HF (1978) The essentiality of vitamin D metabolites for embryonic chick development. Science 200:1067–1069

Tanaka H, Abe E, Miyaura C, Kuribayashi T, Konno K, Nishii Y, Suda T (1982) 1,25-Dihydroxycholecalciferol and a human myeloid leukemia cell line (HL60): the presence of a cytosol receptor and induction of differentiation. Biochem J 204:713–719

Tanaka Y, DeLuca HF (1971) Bone mineral mobilizing activity of 1,25-dihydroxycholecalciferol, a metabolite of vitamin D. Arch Biochem Biophys 46:574–578

Tanaka Y, DeLuca HF (1974) Stimulation of 24,25-dihydroxyvitamin D_3 production by 1,25-dihydroxyvitamin D_3. Science 183:1198–1200

Tanaka Y, DeLuca HF (1984) Rat renal 25-hydroxyvitamin D_3 1- and 24-hydroxylases: their in vivo regulation. Am J Physiol 246:168–173

Tanaka Y, Lorenc RS, DeLuca HF (1975) The role of 1,25-dihydroxyvitamin D_3 and parathyroid hormone in the regulation of chick renal 25-hydroxyvitamin D_3-24-hydroxylase. Arch Biochem Biophys 171:521–526

Tanaka Y, DeLuca HF, Kobayashi Y, Taguchi T, Ikekawa N, Morisaki M (1979a) Biological activity of 24,24-diflouro-25-hydroxyvitamin D_3: effect of blocking of 24-hydroxylation on the functions of vitamin D. J Biol Chem 254:7163–7167

Tanaka Y, Halloran B, Schnoes HK, DeLuca HF (1979b) In vitro production of 1,25-dihydroxyvitamin D_3 by rat placental tissues. Proc Natl Acad Sci USA 76:5033–5035

Tanaka Y, DeLuca HF, Schnoes HK, Ikekawa N, Eguchi T (1981) 23,25-Dihydroxyvitamin D_3: a natural precursor in the biosynthesis of 25-hydroxyvitamin D_3-26,23-lactone. Proc Natl Acad Sci USA 78:4805–4808

Theofan G, Nyguyen AP, Norman AW (1986) Regulation of calbindin-D 28K gene expression by 1,25-dihydroxyvitamin D_3 is correlated to receptor occupancy. J Biol Chem 261:16943–16947

Trechsel U, Eisman JA, Fischer JA, Bonjour JP, Fleisch H (1980) Calcium-dependent parathyroid hormone-independent regulation of 1,25-dihydroxy-vitamin D. Am J Physiol 239:E119–E124

Tsai HC, Norman AW (1973) Studies on calciferol metabolism: VIII. Evidence for a cytoplasmic receptor for 1,25-dihydroxyvitamin D_3 in the intestinal mucosa. J Biol Chem 54:5967–5975

Tsai HC, Wong RG, Norman AW (1972) Studies on calciferol metabolism: IV. Subcellular localization of 1,25-dihydroxyvitamin D_3 in intestinal mucosa and correlation with increase calcium transport. J Biol Chem 248:5511–5519

Tsoukas CD, Provvedini DM, Manogalas SC (1984) 1,25-Dihydroxyvitamin D_3: a novel immunoregulatory hormone. Science 224:1438–1440

Tucker G III, Gagnon RE, Haussler MR (1973) Vitamin D_3-25 hydroxylase: tissue occurrence and apparent lack of regulation. Arch Biochem Biophys 155:47–57

Turner RT, Puzas JE, Forte M, Lester GE, Gray TK, Howard GA, Baylink DJ (1980) In vitro synthesis of 1-alpha 25-dihydroxycholecalciferol and 24,25-dihydroxycholecalciferol by isolated calvarial cells. Proc Natl Acad Sci USA. 77:5720–5724

Turner RT, Howard GA, Puzas JE, Baylink DJ, Knapp DR (1983) Calvarial cells synthesize 1a,25-dihydroxyvitamin D_3 from 25-hydroxyvitamin D_3. Biochemistry 22:1073–1076

Usui E, Noshiro M, Ohyama Y, Okuda K (1990) Unique property of liver mitochondrial P450 to catalyze the two physiologically important reactions involved in both cholesterol catabolism and vitamin D activation. FEBS Lett 274:175–177

Van Baelen H, Bouillon R, DeMoor P (1977) Binding of 25-hydroxycholecalciferol in tissues. J Biol Chem 252:2515–2518

Van Baelen H, Bouillon R, De Moor P (1980) Vitamin-D-binding protein (Gc-globulin) binds actin. J Biol Chem 255:2270–2272

Walters MR (1984) 1,25-Dihydroxyvitamin D3 receptors in the seminiferous tubules of the rat testis increase at puberty. Endocrinology 114:2167–2174

Walters MR (1985) Steroid hormone receptors and the nucleus. Endocr Rev 6:512–543

Walters MR, Hunziker W, Norman AW (1980) Unoccupied 1,25-dihydroxyvitamin D3 receptors. Nuclear/cytosol ratio depends on ionic strength. J Biol Chem 255:6799–6805

Walters MR, Hunziker W, Norman AW (1981) Apparent nuclear localisation of unoccupied receptors for 1,25-dihydroxyvitamin D_3. Biochem Biophys Res Commun 98:990–996

Walters MR, Wicker DC, Riggle PC (1986) 1,25-Dihydroxyvitamin D_3 receptor identified in the rat heart. J Mol Cell Cardiol 18:67–72

Wark JD, Tashjian AH Jr (1983) Regulation of prolactin mRNA by 1,25-dihydroxyvitamin D_3 in GH4C1 cells. J Biol Chem 258:12118–12121

Wark JD, Larkins RG, Perry-Keene D, Peter CT, Ross DL, Sloman JG (1979) Chronic diphenylhydantoin therapy does not reduce plasma 25-hydroxyvitamin D. Clin Endocrinol 11:267–274

Wasserman RH, Fullmer CS (1989) On the molecular mechanism of intestinal calcium transport. Adv Exp Med Biol 249:45–65

Wasserman RH, Brindak ME, Buddle MM, Cai Q, Davis FC, Fullmer CS, Gilmour RF Jr, Hu C, Mykkanen HM, Tapper DN (1990) Recent studies on the biological actions of vitamin D on intestinal transport and the electrophysiology of peripheral nerve and cardiac muscle. Prog Clin Biol Res 332:99–126

Weisman J, Harell A, Edelstein S, David M, Spirer Z, Golander A (1979) 1-Alpha,25-dihydroxyvitamin D_3 and 24,25-dihydroxyvitamin D_3 in vitro synthesis by human decidua and placenta. Nature 81:317–319

Wichmann JK, Paaren HE, Fivizzani MA, Schnoes HK, DeLuca HF (1980) Tetrahedron Lett 21:4667–4670

Wong GL, Luben RA, Cohn DV (1977) 1,25-Dihydroxycholecalciferol and parathormone: effects on isolated osteoclast-like and osteoblast-like cells. Science 197:663–665

Yoon K, Buenaga R, Rodan GA (1987) Tissue developmental expression of rat osteopontin. Biochem Biophys Res Commun 148:1129–1136

Yoon K, Rutledge SJC, Buenaga RF, Rodan GA (1988) Characterisation of the rat osteocalcin gene: stimulation of promoter activity by 1,25-dihydroxyvitamin D_3. Biochemistry 27:8521–8526

Zelikovic I, Chesney RW (1989) Vitamin D and mineral metabolism: the role of the kidney in health and disease. In: Bourne GH (ed) Impact of nutrition on health and disease. Basel, Karger, pp 156–216 (World review of nutrion and dietetics, vol 59)

CHAPTER 11

Bisphosphonates: Mechanisms of Action and Clinical Use

H. Fleisch

A. Introduction

The bisphosphonates are a new class of drugs which have been developed in the past 2 decades for use in various diseases of bone, tooth, and calcium metabolism. This chapter will cover the chemistry, the mechanisms of action, and the clinical applications of these compounds. Since a review was published on the same topic in this handbook in 1988 (FLEISCH 1988), some parts which were extensively discussed there will be kept short. Emphasis will be on newer developments and on clinical aspects. For complete information the reader should consult both articles.

B. Chemistry and General Characteristics

Bisphosphonates, previously erroneously called diphosphonates, are compounds characterized by two C-P bonds. If the two bonds are located on the same carbon atom, the compounds are called geminal bisphosphonates. Only these have an activity on the skeleton. They are therefore analogs of pyrophosphate, which contain an oxygen instead of a carbon atom. For the sake of simplicity, they will be called just bisphosphonates.

Geminal bisphosphonic acid   Pyrophosphoric acid

The P-C-P structure allows a great number of possible variations, either by changing the two lateral chains on the carbon atom or by esterifying the phosphate groups. The following bisphosphonates in order of their chronological description have been investigated in humans in bone disease, the first three being commercially available.

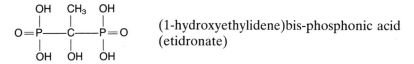

(1-hydroxyethylidene)bis-phosphonic acid (etidronate)

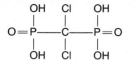

(dichloromethylene)bis-phosphonic acid
(clodronate)

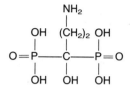

(3-amino-1-hydroxypropylidene)bis-phosphonic
acid (pamidronate)

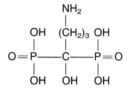

(4-amino-1-hydroxybutylidene)bis-phosphonic
acid (alendronate)

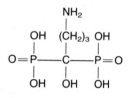

(6-amino-1-hydroxyhexylidene)bis-phosphonic
acid

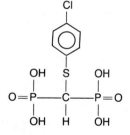

[[(4-chlorophenyl)thio]methylene]bis-phosphonic
acid (tiludronate)

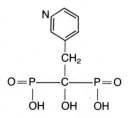

[1-hydroxy-2-(3-pyridinyl)ethylidene]bis-
phosphonic acid (risedronate)

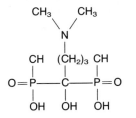

[3-(dimethylamino)-1-hydroxypropylidene]bis-phosphonic acid

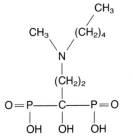

[1-hydroxy-3-(methylpentylamino)propylidene]bis-phosphonic acid (BM 210955)

Each bisphosphonate has its own physicochemical and biological characteristics, which is of great interest in the light of the future development of new compounds. This means, however, that it is not possible to extrapolate from the results of one compound to others.

The P-C-P bond of the bisphosphonates is stable to heat and most chemical reagents, and completely resistant to enzymatic hydrolysis. They have a strong affinity for metal ions. Some uncertainty still exists as to their state when in solution. Indeed, they are only partially ultrafiltrable in aqueous solutions as well as in plasma (WIEDMER et al. 1983), possibly because of the formation of complexes (LAMSON et al. 1984).

C. Synthesis

For a complete review of the synthesis of bisphosphates, see FLEISCH (1988).

D. Methods of Determination

Various methods are available to determine the structure, purity, and amount of bisphosphonates during synthesis. They include nuclear magnetic resonance, gel electrophoresis, gas chromatography (ISMAIL et al. 1987), and high-performance liquid chromatography (KWONG et al. 1990). The measurement in biologic fluids or in tissues is more difficult.

The first technique, which was however not sensitive, was described for etidronate (LIGGETT 1973). Later, methods which permit measurement of 1 nmol etidronate (BISAZ et al. 1975) and 7 nmol clodronate (CHESTER et al. 1981) were developed. More recently, high-performance liquid chromatography methods with a sensitivity of 20–50 nmol/l were developed for pamidronate (DALEY-YATES et al. 1989; FLESCH and HAUFFE 1989), alendronate (DE MARCO et al. 1989; KWONG et al. 1990; KLINE et al. 1990), and tiludronate (FELS et al. 1988). Clodronate can also be assessed by gas chromatography (AURIOLA et al. 1989).

E. History of the Development for Use in Bone Disease

Our knowledge of the biologic characteristics of bisphosphonates dates from the last 20 years only, the first report having appeared in 1968 (FLEISCH et al. 1968). The concept has been derived from our earlier studies on inorganic pyrophosphate. We had found that plasma and urine contained compounds inhibiting calcium phosphate precipitation, and that part of this inhibitory activity was due to inorganic pyrophosphate, a compound which had not been described previously in these media. Pyrophosphonate was then shown to impair in vitro the formation and dissolution of calcium phosphate crystals. Since pyrophosphate was able to inhibit ectopic calcification in vivo, it was suggested that it might be a physiological regulator of calcification and perhaps also of decalcification in vivo, its local concentration being determined by the activity of local pyrophosphatases (FLEISCH et al. 1966; for review see FLEISCH and RUSSELL 1970).

Because of its failure to act when given orally and its rapid hydrolysis when given parenterally, pyrophosphate found clinical use only in scintigraphy and against dental calculus, pyrophosphonate being now the main antitartar agent in toothpastes worldwide. This restricted use prompted us to search for analogs which would display similar physicochemical activity, but which would resist enzymatic hydrolysis and would therefore not be broken down metabolically. The bisphosphonates fulfilled these conditions.

F. Mode of Action

I. Physicochemical Effects

As was anticipated, the physicochemical effects of most of the bisphosphonates are very similar to those of pyrophosphate. Thus, most of them inhibit the formation of calcium phosphate crystals (FRANCIS 1969; FRANCIS et al. 1969; FLEISCH et al. 1970) and delay the aggregation of apatite crystals (HANSEN et al. 1976). They also slow down the dissolution of these crystals (FLEISCH et al. 1969; RUSSELL et al. 1970). All these effects appear to be related to the marked affinity of these compounds for solid phase calcium phosphate. Thus, they bind to the crystal surface by chemisorption onto calcium (JUNG et al. 1973), and then act as crystal poisons of both growth and dissolution. Bisphosphonates also inhibit the formation (FRASER et al. 1972) and the aggregation (ROBERTSON et al. 1973) of calcium oxalate crystals.

II. Effect on Calcification In Vivo

Like pyrophosphate, bisphosphonates inhibit calcification in vivo very efficiently. Thus, among others, they prevent experimentally induced calcification of many soft tissues such as arteries, kidneys, skin, and heart (FLEISCH et al. 1970; ROSENBLUM et al. 1977). In contrast to pyrophosphate, which acts only when given parenterally, they are also active when administered orally. In the arteries they decrease not only mineral deposition, but also the accumulation of cholesterol, elastin, and collagen (HOLLANDER et al. 1978; KRAMSCH and CHAN 1978).

Bisphosphonates can also inhibit the calcification of bioprosthetic heart valves. Thus, etidronate administered subcutaneously or locally inhibits the calcification of glutaraldehyde-treated porcine aortic valves implanted subcutaneously into rats (LEVY et al. 1985, 1987; GOLOMB et al. 1986, 1987) or sheep (JOHNSTON et al. 1989). It has also been tried with variable success to bind bisphosphonates covalently to the valve (WEBB et al. 1987; JONES et al. 1988).

Certain bisphosphonates also inhibit ectopic ossification when given systemically (PLASMANS et al. 1978) or locally (AHRENGART and LINDGREN 1986). Last, bisphosphonates also decrease the formation of experimental urinary stones (FRASER et al. 1972), and topical administration leads to a decreased formation of dental calculus (BRINER et al. 1971).

If administered in sufficient doses, bisphosphonates can also impair the mineralization of normal calcified tissues such as bone (JOWSEY et al. 1970; KING et al. 1971; SCHENK et al. 1973) and cartilage (SCHENK et al. 1973). The inhibition is eventually reversed after discontinuation of the drug (FLORA et al. 1980). The doses required to induce the block of mineralization vary according to the bisphosphonate used, the animal species, and the length of treatment.

The inhibition is not corrected by 1,25 $(OH)_2D_3$ or 24,25 $(OH)_2D_3$ (ATKIN et al. 1988) and can lead to an impairment of fracture healing (LENEHAN et al. 1985). Hypomineralization is also observed in dentine and in enamel (LARSSON 1974; OGAWA et al. 1989).

There is a close relationship between the ability of an individual bisphosphonate to inhibit the formation of calcium phosphate in vitro and its effectiveness on ectopic calcification in vivo (FLEISCH et al. 1970; SHINODA et al. 1983), suggesting that the latter can be explained in terms of a physicochemical mechanism. The mechanism of the inhibition of normal mineralization, although not completely clear yet, is likely to be also due, at least in part, to a physicochemical mechanism. However, an effect on matrix formation cannot be excluded. Indeed, when etidronate is given in doses which produce mineralization defects, changes in glycosaminoglycan synthesis are seen in teeth (Larsson 1976), articular cartilage (Palmoski and Brandt 1978), and growth plate cartilage (Howell et al. 1980). Furthermore, collagen synthesis seems to be also effected in dentine (Larsson 1974; Van Den Bos and Beertsen 1987; Ogawa et al. 1989) and heterotopic bone (Ostrowski et al. 1988).

III. Inhibition of Bone Resorption

1. Assessment of Activity

Bisphosphonates proved to be very powerful inhibitors of bone resorption when tested in a variety of conditions, both in vitro and in vivo.

a) In Vitro

Bisphosphonates block bone resorption induced by various means in organ culture (Fleisch et al. 1969; Reynolds et al. 1972; Boonekamp et al. 1986). They also impair dissolution of bone particles by macrophages (Chambers 1980; Reitsma et al. 1982).

b) Normal Animals

In growing rats, they block the degradation of both bone and cartilage and thus arrest the remodeling of the metaphysis which becomes club shaped and radiologically more dense than normal (Schenk et al. 1973; Reitsma et al. 1980). This effect is used as a model to study the potency of new compounds (Schenk et al. 1986). In the mouse, a similar effect has been found, leading to a picture like that seen in gray-lethal congenital osteope-trotic mice (Reynolds et al. 1973). The inhibition of endogenous bone resorption has also been documented by ^{45}Ca kinetic studies and by hydroxy-proline excretion (Gasser et al. 1972).

The decrease in resorption is accompanied by an increase in calcium balance and in the mineral content of bone (Gasser et al. 1972). However, this increase is in most cases smaller than predicted and, in addition, soon reaches a plateau (Reitsma et al. 1980). This is due to the fact that, after a certain time, bone formation decreases too (Gasser et al. 1972; Schenk et al. 1973; Reitsma et al. 1980; Wink and Hill 1988), possibly because of the so-called "coupling" between formation and resorption. The main effect of bisphosphonates is therefore a reduction of bone turnover. However, clodronate does not inhibit the anabolic effect of PTH in the rat (Hock et al. 1989), but tiludronate has an inhibitory effect in sheep when the effect is assessed by plasma osteocalcin (Delmas et al., personal communication).

c) Osteoporosis

Besides actually increasing bone mass in normal animals, the bisphosphonates are also effective in preventing bone loss in a number of experimental osteoporosis models. These include: sciatic nerve section (MÜHLBAUER et al. 1971; MICHAEL et al. 1971; SHIOTA 1985), spinal cord section (SCHOUTENS et al. 1988), hypokinesis, ovariectomy (SHIOTA 1985; WINK et al. 1985; WRONSKI et al. 1989; THOMPSON et al. 1992), heparin (HÄHNEL et al. 1973), lactation (BROMMAGE and BAXTER 1990), and corticosteroids (JEE et al. 1981). The effect on bone loss induced by a low Ca diet is ambiguous.

Only few studies address the question on the effect upon mechanical properties. Pamidronate shows a biphasic change, low doses improving elastic and ultimate strength in the rat, while higher doses have the opposite effect (GLATT et al. 1986; FERRETTI et al. 1990). Etidronate shows a positive effect in one study (SHIOTA 1985) and has no effect or a negative effect at higher doses in chicks (CHAN et al. 1977). The deleterious effect seems to be correlated to the inhibition of mineralization. An improvement of the mechanical properties was recently found with tiludronate (GENSENS et al. 1992).

d) Tumoral Bone Resorption

Bisphosphonates also inhibit tumoral bone resorption. In vitro, etidronate and clodronate inhibit the bone resorption induced by supernatants of tumor cultures (GALASKO et al. 1980; JUNG et al. 1981). In vivo various bisphosphonates partially correct the hypercalcemia induced in rats by subcutaneously implanted Walker 256 carcinomas (JOHNSON et al. 1982; GUAITANI et al. 1984; KOZAK et al. 1987) or Leydig tumors (MARTODAM et al. 1983). The effect is generally more pronounced on calciuria than on calcemia. This is explained by the fact that hypercalcemia is due to both bone resorption and increased tubular reabsorption of calcium (RIZZOLI et al. 1986), bisphosphonates acting only on the former.

Also bone resorption due to actual tumor invasion is slowed down, as shown in numerous models using different tumoral cells (JUNG et al. 1984; for later references see FLEISCH 1992). Practically all results indicate that the bisphosphonates do not inhibit the multiplication of tumor cells, and are therefore not active on the tumor itself, but exert their action by inhibiting the osteolytic process.

For a more detailed review see FLEISCH 1992.

e) Miscellaneous

Bisphosphonates also impair bone resorption induced by various agents such as parathyroid hormone (FLEISCH et al. 1969; RUSSELL et al. 1970) and retinoids (TRECHSEL et al. 1987). The latter effect has given a powerful screening assay for new compounds (MÜHLBAUER et al. 1991). They also slow down resorption of heterotopic experimentally induced bone (NILSSON et al. 1990), periodontal bone destruction, as well as the drift rate of teeth (HARDT 1988).

2. Activity of Various Bisphosphonates

The activity of bisphosphonates on bone resorption varies greatly from compound to compound (SHINODA et al. 1983). For etidronate, the dose inhibiting resorption is very near the one impairing normal mineralization. Therefore, one of the aims of bisphosphonate research has been to develop compounds with a more powerful antiresorptive activity, without a higher inhibition of mineralization. It was found that the dose inducing inhibition of mineralization is practically never below this level for etidronate. However, this is not the case for the dose inhibiting bone resorption. Already clodronate was more potent than etidronate (FLEISCH et al. 1969; RUSSELL et al. 1970) and was less active in inhibiting normal mineralization (SCHENK et al. 1973). Later, pamidronate was found to be still more active (REITSMA et al. 1980) and today compounds have been developed which are 10 000 times more powerful inhibitors than etidronate (MÜHLBAUER et al. 1991).

Up to now no clear-cut structure-activity relationship has been worked out. The length of the aliphatic carbon is important and adding a hydroxyl group to the carbon atom at position 1 increases potency (SHINODA et al. 1983). Derivatives with an amino group at the end of the side chain are very active. The first of these compounds to be described was pamidronate (BIJVOET et al. 1978; REITSMA et al. 1980). Again the length of the side chain is relevent, the highest activity being found with a backbone of four carbons (alendronate) (SCHENK et al. 1986). Alkylation of the amino group increases activity. Thus, if the amino group of pamidronate is dimethylated, the efficacy is enhanced (BOONEKAMP et al. 1987). Addition of larger alkyl groups added to the nitrogen results in even greater enhancement. Thus, [1-hydroxy-3-(methylpentylamino)propylidene]bis-phosphonate (BM 210955) is one of the most powerful bisphosphonates described up to now (MÜHLBAUER et al. 1991). Cyclic geminal bisphosphonates are also very active, especially those containing a nitrogen atom in the ring, such as risedronate. This effect of nitrogen is very intriguing and not yet explained. It appears that the activity sequence in increasing order is etidronate, tiludronate, clodronate, pamidronate, (6-amino-1-hydroxyhexylidene)bis-phosphonate, [3-(dimethylamino)-1-hydroxypropylidene]bis-phosphonate, alendronate, risedronate, and BM-210955.

Thus, while the P-C-P structure is a prerequisite for the activity, the intensity of the effect is exquisitely dependent upon the side chain.

3. Mechanisms of Action of Bone Resorption Inhibition

a) Effects on Osteoclasts

There is no doubt that the action in vivo is mediated through other mechanisms than the physicochemical inhibition of crystal dissolution initially postulated. The nature of these is, however, still unclear and it may well be that more than one mechanism is operating. The fact that the bisphosphonates alter the morphology of osteoclasts both in vitro and when administered in vivo (SCHENK et al. 1973; MILLER and JEE 1979) suggests an effect on the activity of these cells. This is supported by the finding that the addition of bisphosphonates to osteoclasts in vitro leads to an inhibition of their bone-resorbing activity and a retraction of lamellipodia (FLANAGAN and CHAMBERS 1989; SATO and GRASSER 1990). This activity is still present when the bone is exposed temporarily to the bisphosphonates before the osteoclasts are added, suggesting that the osteoclasts are inhibited when they come into contact with bisphosphonate-containing bone (FLANAGAN and CHAMBERS 1989). However, the finding that bisphosphonates with an up to 1000-fold different activity in the living animal show the same activity on the osteoclasts in vitro (SATO and GRASSER 1990) casts serious doubt on the conclusions drawn with this technique. Very recently, however, it was found that, when the osteoclasts were exposed to the bisphosphonates before being incubated with the hard tissues, the activity of various compounds correlated well with the activity in vivo (SAHNI et al., in press). Furthermore it was found that this effect was primarily not on the osteoclasts but on the accompanying osteoblasts, which produced less osteoclast stimulating activity (SAHNI et al., in press). This suggests that the bisphosphonates act on these cells before they adhere to the bone.

Another possibility is that the decrease in resorption is also due to a decrease in the number of osteoclasts, either because cells already present are destroyed or because recruitment of new cells is inhibited. Indeed in man, the number of osteoclasts is decreased after long-term treatment with various bisphosphonates. Furthermore, in culture systems where osteoclasts are already present such as new born calvaria, pamidronate is not more active than etidronate or clodronate (SHINODA et al. 1983; BOONEKAMP et al. 1986); however, this is not the case in systems where resorption depends upon formation of new osteoclasts (BOONEKAMP et al. 1986; LÖWIK et al. 1988). Moreover, the formation of multinuclear cells in long-term bone marrow culture is inhibited by bisphosphonates, the activity of various compounds being parallel to their potency in vivo (HUGHES et al. 1989). In contrast, however, recent studies in vivo fail to show any inhibition of osteoclast recruitment (CECCHINI et al. 1990). Moreover, in the rat, the number of osteoclasts is often increased, this in spite of the fact that bone resorption is blocked (SCHOUTENS et al. 1988; MÜHLBAUER et al. 1991).

b) Other Biochemical and Cellular Effects

A great number of different biochemical effects have been described. They are confusing and can sometimes even go in opposite directions with different compounds, or even with the same compound at different concentrations. Some may be relevant to bone resorption such as the reduction of lactic acid production (MORGAN et al. 1973; FAST et al. 1978) and of proton accumulation (CARANO et al. 1990), the inhibition of lysosomal enzymes in vitro (FELIX et al. 1976), in cultured calvaria (MORGAN et al. 1973; DELAISSE et al. 1985), and in vivo (ENDE 1979), the inhibition of pyrophosphatases (FELIX and FLEISCH 1975; SMIRNOVA et al. 1988), and the inhibition of prostaglandin synthesis (FELIX et al. 1981; OHYA et al. 1985).

It is also possible that the inhibitory effect is partly mediated through other cells. Macrophages are specially sensitive to bisphosphonates, which inhibit in vitro their activity (CHAMBERS 1980; STEVENSON and STEVENSON 1986) and their multiplication (CECCHINI et al. 1987). This effect appears to be specific for the mononuclear phagocyte lineage, since other marrow populations are not influenced (CECCHINI and FLEISCH 1990). Since macrophages produce a variety of bone-resorbing cytokines, and since the osteoclasts originate from the monocyte-phagocyte system, it is possible that the resorption inhibition is partly through an effect on macrophages.

Bisphosphonates have been used to selectively destroy macrophages in vivo. Thus, if they are administered encapsulated in liposomes, they are taken up by these cells mostly in the spleen and the liver and destroy them within 2 days (VAN ROOIJEN and VAN NIEUWMEGEN 1984). The activity is highest with clodronate, followed by pamidronate and then etidronate (VAN ROOIJEN and KORS 1989). This technique has been used to study repopulation kinetics of macrophages (VAN ROOIJEN et al. 1990) and the role of macrophages in the organism (THEPEN et al. 1989).

Numerous additional cellular actions have been described for individual bisphosphonates. These include: increase of fatty acid oxidation (FELIX and FLEISCH 1981) and amino acid oxidation (ENDE 1979); stimulation of the citric acid cycle (ENDE 1979); increase in cellular content of glycogen (FELIX et al. 1980); increase in production of alkaline phosphatase (FELIX and FLEISCH 1979); increase in the biosynthesis of bone and cartilage collagen (GUENTHER et al. 1981 a,b), possibly by impaired intracellular collagenolysis (GALLAGHER et al. 1982); impairment of dentin and cementum formation (BEERTSEN et al. 1985); increase in the synthesis of proteoglycans in vitro (GUENTHER et al. 1979), but decrease when administered in vivo (LARSSON 1976); inhibition of the $1,25(OH)_2D_3$-induced production of osteocalcin in vivo (STRONSKI et al. 1988); contradictory effects on cAMP production (PILCZYK et al. 1972; GEBAUER et al. 1976); decrease or increase in cellular multiplication (FAST et al. 1978; EVEQUOZ et al. 1985); inhibition of DNA polymerase (TALANIAN et al. 1989); inhibition of amebal phosphofructokinase (EUBANK and REEVES 1982) and inhibition of growth of the amebae of the slime mold *Dictostelyum discoideum* by means of the formation of nonhydrolyzable methylene analogues of ATP (KLEIN et al. 1988); inhibition of interleukin-1-induced enzyme release (EMONDS-ALT et al. 1985); and inhibition of the action of mitogens on mononuclear function and on the lymphoblastic response (DE VRIES et al. 1982). A few results point to an effect on the cellular calcium handling. These include: reduction in release of calcium from kidney mitochondria in vitro (GUILLAND et al. 1974) and increase in calcium of mitochondria in vivo (PLASMANS et al. 1980); inhibition in vitro of calcium-induced contraction of smooth muscle, possibly through inhibition of intracellular Ca mobilization and of influx of extra cellular Ca (PASPALIARIS and LEAVER 1990); and protection of the kidney from ischemia damage, possibly by preventing intracellular Ca accumulation (GREIF et al. 1990). Along this line it is interesting that nongeminal bisphosphonates act like Ca channel blockers (ROSSIER et al. 1989).

These findings suggest that bisphosphonates enter mammalian cells. This has been confirmed by studies in vitro, both for etidronate and clodronate (FAST et al. 1978). The cellular uptake is mostly in the cytosol and the concentration expressed in terms of cellular water can be severalfold higher than in the medium (FELIX et al. 1984). Cells with phagocytic properties display special avidity if the compounds are bound to apatite crystals (CHAMBERS 1980).

Unfortunately up to now no correlation between any of the biologic effects described and the inhibition of bone resorption in vivo could be found. Thus, none of the mechanisms discussed is likely to be the *only* explanation for the effect on bone resorption.

4. Other Effects In Vivo

Besides the effects on mineralized tissues, some other actions occur in vivo, often, however, after very large doses, so that the relevance to pharmacological doses is more than doubtful. They include (for references see FLEISCH 1988): decrease in the formation of antibody-secreting cells and impaired delayed and immediate hypersensitivity; atrophy of the thymus, disappearance of certain thymus-dependent macrophages, of natural killer cells, and diminution of the response of T lymphocytes to mitogens in newborn mice; increase in plasma high-density lipoproteins; and inhibition of passive cutaneous anaphylaxis. Of clinical interest is the inhibition of some of the changes seen in adjuvant-induced polyarthritis (FRANCIS et al. 1972, 1989; FLORA 1979; BARBIER et al. 1986), in some cases also of paw swelling (FRANCIS et al. 1989). However, collagen-induced arthritis is not influenced (MARKUSSE et al. 1990).

Some effects are secondary to the changes induced in bone like those on calcium absorption (GUILLAND et al. 1975; TRECHSEL et al. 1977), on $1,25(OH)_2D_3$ (HILL et al. 1973; BAXTER et al. 1974; GUILLAND et al. 1975), and on acid base metabolism (FREUDIGER and BONJOUR 1989).

G. Pharmacokinetics

Bisphosphonates are synthetic compounds which have not yet been found to occur naturally in animals or humans. No enzymes able to cleave the P-C-P bond have yet been described. The bisphosphonates investigated up to now, that is etidronate, clodronate and pamidronate, appear to be absorbed, stored, and excreted unaltered in the body. Thus, these bisphosphonates seem to be nonbiodegradable, both in animals and in solution (STEBER and

Wierich 1986). However, it cannot be excluded that other bisphosphonates may be altered in their side chain.

Relatively few pharmacokinetic studies are available up to now, partly because of the lack of sensitive chemical methods to measure the relevant compounds. Results with ^{99m}Tc compounds have to be interpreted with caution since they do not necessarily reflect the kinetics of the compound without technetium (Daley-Yates and Bennett 1988). Most of the data on bisphosphonates have been obtained with etidronate, clodronate, and pamidronate. The intestinal absorption lies between 1% or even less and 10% of an oral dose, is generally higher in the young, higher when ingestion increases, and shows a great inter- and intraspecies variation (Michael et al. 1972; Recker and Saville 1973; Gural 1975; Yakatan et al. 1982). In humans, absorption is 1%–9% for etidronate (Fogelman et al. 1986), and 1%–2% for clodronate (Yakatan et al. 1982). Absorption occurs, when assessed by experiments in situ, to some extent in the stomach and to a larger extent in the small intestine (Wasserman et al. 1973; Gural et al. 1985). It appears to occur by passive diffusion and is not mediated by the carrier mechanism responsible for phosphate absorption (Gural et al. 1985). It is diminished when the drug is given with meals and in the presence of calcium (Francis and Martodam 1983) and EDTA increases its absorption (Janner et al. 1992). Therefore, bisphosphonates always have to be given before meals and never together with milk products. The absorption is inversely related to the size of the compound. At least etidronate can be taken up by means of iontophoresis (Slough et al. 1988).

Between 20% and 50% of the absorbed etidronate is localized in bone, the remainder being rapidly excreted in the urine (Michael et al. 1972; Conrad and Lee 1981; Yakatan et al. 1982; Hanhijärvi et al. 1989). The retained part is somewhat smaller for Cl$_2$MBP (Conrad and Lee 1981).

Sometimes, bisphosphonates, especially pamidronate, can deposit in other organs such as the stomach (Larsson and Rohlin 1980), liver, and spleen (Wingen and Schmähl 1985; Mönkkönen et al. 1987, 1989a; Mönkkönen 1988). The deposition is percentually larger when large amounts of compounds are given (Wingen and Schmähl 1987; Mönkkönen et al. 1989a). Part of this extraosseous deposition appears to be due to the formation of complexes with iron liberated during the hemolysis induced by the infusion (Mönkkönen et al. 1989b; Mönkkönen and Ylitalo 1990). Furthermore, aggregates can be formed after too high or too rapid intravenous injection, which are then phagocytosed by the macrophages of the reticuloendothelial system. Thus, results obtained with large amounts of labeled compounds given rapidly intravenously have to be interpreted with caution.

The half-life of circulating bisphosphonates is short, in the rat only of the order of minutes (Bisaz et al. 1978). In man it is somewhat longer, about 2 h (Conrad and Lee 1981; Yakatan et al. 1982; Hanhijärvi et al. 1989). The rate of entry into bone is very fast, similar to that of calcium and phosphate. It has been calculated that the bone clearance is compatible with a complete extraction from the skeleton after the first passage, so that skeletal uptake might be determined above all by the vascularization of the bone (BISAZ et al. 1978) and its turnover. The areas of deposition are mostly those of bone formation. However, bisphosphonates are also enriched under the osteoclasts (SATO et al. 1991). Consequently, soft tissues are exposed to these compounds for only short periods, explaining that, despite the many cellular effects described in vitro, in vivo practically only bone is affected.

Once in the skeleton, the bisphosphonates are liberated again either in free or bound form only when the bone where they are deposited is destroyed. This may explain why one administration of bisphosphonates can be active for long periods, both in animals (STUTZER et al. 1988) and in humans (THIEBAUD et al. 1986a). Thus the half-life in the body depends upon the rate of bone turnover itself. As the bisphosphonates slow down the resorption of the bone where they are embedded, their half-life will even be longer than that of the rest of the skeleton, and it is not impossible that part of the administered bisphosphonates remain in the body in man for life. Half-life has been evaluated up to a year in mice or rats (WINGEN and SCHMÄHL 1987; MÖNKKÖNEN 1988; MÖNKKÖNEN et al. 1989a). Etidronate and pamidronate have a similar retention time, while clodronate is cleared somewhat more rapidly (MÖNKKÖNEN et al. 1989a).

The renal clearance of bisphosphonates is high, often around that of inulin (CONRAD and LEE 1981; HANHIJÄRVI et al. 1989) or even higher, suggesting the presence of a secretory pathway (TROEHLER et al. 1975; LIN et al. 1992).

H. Animal Toxicology

Published toxicologic animal studies reported to date are scanty and deal almost exclusively with etidronate and clodronate. Acute, subacute, and chronic administration in several animal species have revealed little toxicity. Teratogenic, mitogenic, and carcinogenic tests were negative (NOLEN and BUEHLER 1971; NIXON et al. 1972). The acute toxicity appears to be due to the formation of complexes with calcium, leading to hypocalcemia. When the compound is administered intravenously, toxicity varies with the speed of infusion (FRANCIS and SLOUGH 1984).

For etidronate the first chronic adverse event is the inhibition of bone calcification described above. Fractures can occur, but can in the long term be induced also when mineralization is not impaired, since a long-term decrease of bone turnover can lead itself to an increased fragility (FLORA et al. 1980). At higher doses, renal lesions appear with various bisphosphonates (HINTZE and D'AMATO 1980; ALDEN et al. 1989; CAL and DALEY-YATES 1990). Furthermore, inflammatory gastric lesions, noted even when the compounds are given parenterally, as well as pulmonary lesions have been reported. Clodronate is less toxic than etidronate (HINTZE and

D'Amato 1980). As mentioned above, atrophy of the thymus and some immunological alterations can occur after very high doses of clodronate in new-born animals (Milhaud et al. 1983; Labat et al. 1983, 1984). Six-month toxicology studies with clodronate have shown that a daily oral amount of 200 mg/kg and 40 mg/kg are the highest nontoxic dose in the rat and dog respectively (Boehringer Mannheim 1986).

Bisphosphonates cross the placenta and can affect the fetus. Thus large doses (200 mg/kg s.c.) of etidronate to pregnant rats given daily from day 7 to 11 of pregnancy lead to fetal abnormalities involving weight (Sakiyama et al. 1985), skeleton (Eguchi et al. 1982), and skin (Ikeo et al. 1987), and induce malformations and hemorrhages (Sakiyama et al. 1986).

It must be stressed that the results with one bisphosphonate cannot necessarily be extrapolated to other bisphosphonates. Indeed, toxicity, both in culture and in vivo, varies greatly from one compound to another, so that great caution has to be applied when using new compounds clinically.

I. Drug Interactions

No interactions have been described up to now. Large oral doses of bisphosphonates may enhance the absorption of other compounds, possibly by chelating calcium and changing the intestinal permeability, an example being the effect on cefoxitin in rats (Van Hoogdalem et al. 1989).

J. Clinical Use

Clinical applications in medicine have focused upon three main areas: (a) use as skeletal markers in the form of ^{99m}Tc derivatives for diagnostic purposes in nuclear medicine; (b) therapeutic use in patients with ectopic calcification and ossification; and (c) use in patients with increased bone destruction. Only the therapeutic aspects will be discussed here, scintigraphy being beyond the scope of this chapter. Until now, three bisphosphonates, namely etidronate, clodronate, and pamidronate, have been investigated on a larger scale in humans and are available commercially. Some clinical results are available also for a few others.

I. Ectopic Calcification and Ossification

Only etidronate has been investigated for these indications. The results are ambiguous in ectopic calcification, more encouraging in ectopic ossification.

1. Soft Tissue Calcification

Etidronate has been given in some cases of scleroderma, dermatomyositis, idiopathic infantile arterial calcification (Stuart et al. 1990), and calcinosis universalis. Efficacy is uncertain since these disorders often show spontaneous remissions (for other references see FLEISCH 1988).

2. Urolithiasis

The hope that the inhibitory effect on crystal growth and aggregation of both calcium phosphate and calcium oxalate would be useful for the prevention of urinary stones has not been fulfilled, at least with etidronate. Although pilot studies showed a certain effect in chronic stone formers (BAUMANN et al. 1978; BONE et al. 1979), the necessary dose to obtain inhibition of crystal growth in urine is high, about 1600 mg/day orally (OHATA and PAK 1974; BAUMANN et al. 1978), so that it will also induce skeletal effects. Furthermore, the clinical benefit is uncertain, large-scale studies having failed to show efficacy. Bisphosphonates cannot therefore be recommended for use in urolithiasis.

3. Dental Calculus

Many investigations have shown that topical application of etidronate diminishes the development of dental calculus. Azacycloheptylidene-2,2-bisphosphonate is added to a toothpaste which has been marketed in various countries. This topic will not be covered in this review.

4. Fibrodysplasia Ossificans Progressiva

Despite a series of investigations (BASSETT et al. 1969; GEHO and WHITESIDE 1973; REINER et al. 1980) and many case reports, it remains to be established whether this drug is active in decreasing ectopic bone formation in this disease. Some retardation in the evolution of the disease can occur, but a complete standstill is rarely obtained. Already formed lesions are not influenced. Despite this uncertainty, in view of the outcome of the disease and the lack of alternative treatment, the use of etidronate in an oral dosage of 20 mg kg/day seems advisable. Since effective doses also inhibit mineralization of normal bone and can lead to rickets in children (REINER et al. 1980), the drug should not be given for longer than 3 months, but better for shorter periods of a few weeks, and only when a new exacerbation occurs.

5. Other Heterotopic Ossifications

Results seem more encouraging with other types of heterotopic ossifications. Etidronate has been found to diminish the appearance of ossifications in patients with spinal cord injury (FINERMAN and STOVER 1981; FREED et al. 1982), after cranial trauma (SPIELMAN et al. 1983), and after total hip replacement (SLOOFF et al. 1974; FINERMAN and STOVER 1981). In the latter, although ectopic bone formation reappears at least partially after discontinuation of the drug, the mobility of the hip seems nevertheless to be improved in the etidronate-treated patients. These results have, however, been questioned by others (Garland et al. 1983; Thomas and Amstutz 1985).

Although its efficacy is not absolutely established, it seems nevertheless justifiable to administer etidronate preventively, especially to those patients who are particularly liable to develop ectopic ossifications, for example, patients who require a second operation after total hip replacement because of ossifications after the first intervention. The daily oral dosage lies between 800 and 1600 mg, given for 3 months and starting just before the operation. A longer treatment should not be given because of the inhibition of normal mineralization.

II. Diseases with Increased Bone Resorption

1. Paget's Disease

One of the main clinical uses of bisphosphonates today is in patients with Paget's disease. All bisphosphonates tested are active, although their potency varies, in decreasing bone turnover as assessed by urinary hydroxy-proline and calcium excretion, serum alkaline phosphatase as well as other means.

The largest number of investigations have been performed with etidro-nate. Both bone resorption and formation are decreased (Smith et al. 1971; Altman et al. 1973; Russell et al. 1974; De Vries and Bijvoet 1974). The effect on hydroxyproline usually precedes that on alkaline phosphatase, suggesting that the primary effect is on bone resorption, the effect on bone formation being secondary to the coupling between the two processes. The action on bone turnover is also illustrated by ^{45}Ca kinetic studies (Guncaga et al. 1974; De Vries and Bijvoet 1974) and by morphological studies (Russell et al. 1974; Guncaga et al. 1974; De Vries and Bijvoet 1974; Meunier et al. 1975; Siris et al. 1980a). The bone formed under treatment is lamellar, in contrast to the woven bone typical of this disease. However, etidronate does not affect the virus-induced measles nucleocapsid-like inclu-sions in the nuclei, nor the measles-type viral antigens in the osteoclasts (Basle et al. 1984). Other changes like elevated cardiac output (Henley et al. 1979), bone pain (Altman et al. 1973; Meunier et al. 1975), and the deformity of the face (Bickerstaff et al. 1990) are also improved. On the other hand, no improvement in the X-ray picture is obtained (De Vries and Bijvoet 1974; Canfield et al. 1977). In fact, in certain cases the drug induces the appearance of radiolucent areas (Nagant De Deuxchaisnes et al. 1979; Boyce et al. 1984) or increases the size of such lesions already present (Dodd et al. 1987). These effects are usually seen at oral doses of 10 and 20 mg/kg, but can occur at 7 mg or even lower (Nagant De Deuxchaisnes et al. 1981) and appear to be related to the appearance of bone pain (Fromm et al. 1979). They probably reflect a focal impaired mineralization and are specific for etidronate, since they are not seen with the other bisphosphonates.

The currently recommended dose of etidronate is 5 mg/kg orally up to 6 months. However, quite a few patients do not show optimal responses (GRAY et al. 1987). An alternative treatment is, accepting the mineralization defect, a dose of 20 mg/kg or 1600 mg/day orally for 1 month, since this is as effective as a treatment for 6 months with the same dose, and more effective than treatment for 6 months with 400 mg/day (PRESTON et al. 1986; GRAY et al. 1987). Another possibility is the intravenous administration of 300–600 mg daily for 5 days (KANIS et al. 1987). Therapy is resumed when the clinical or biochemical effect subsides.

The combination of etidronate and calcitonin has been reported to give better or faster results than each of these drugs administered alone (O'DONOGHUE and HOSKING 1987; THIEBAUD et al. 1990a).

Although clodronate is more active than etidronate in decreasing bone turnover in Paget's disease (GRAY et al. 1987), the clinical experience is much smaller than for etidronate. Oral daily doses between 400 and 1600 mg can normalize biochemical parameters (MEUNIER et al. 1979; DOUGLAS et al. 1980; DELMAS et al. 1982a), 800 mg being apparently sufficient for a maximal effect. Treatment for 1 month is as effective as treatment of 6 months (CHAPUY et al. 1983). This is also true for 5 days intravenous administration of 300 mg/day (YATES et al. 1985).

Pamidronate appears to be the most active of the three compounds. Successful regimens include 250 mg or more orally for 6 months, 50 mg being less effective (FRIJLINK et al. 1979; HEYNEN et al. 1982), 1500 mg orally for 5 days (THIEBAUD et al. 1987), 60 mg i.v. for 1 day (THIEBAUD et al. 1988), or 16 mg i.v. for 6 days (STONE et al. 1990).

Other bisphosphonates showing activity include (6-amino-1-hydroxy-lidene)bis-phosphonate given orally at 400 mg daily for 1–3 months or intravenously at 25–50 mg for 4 days (ATKINS et al. 1987; DELMAS et al. 1987); tiludronate orally for 6 months at 200 mg or 400 mg daily (REGINSTER et al. 1988; AUDRAN et al. 1989); alendronate intravenously for 4 days at 5 mg/kg daily (PEDRAZZONI et al. 1989; O'DOHERTY et al. 1990); [3-dimethyl-amino-1-hydroxypropylidene]bis-phosphonate intravenously at 2–8 mg or orally at 100–400 mg for 10 days (PAPAPOULOS et al. 1989).

In view of the many different doses given it is difficult to compare the activities of the various compounds. Furthermore, the doses which have to be given to normalize turnover vary from patient to patient. This is due not only to variable absorption but because the effective dose depends on the severity of the disease. Indeed, the bisphosphonates are deposited preferentially in locations of high bone turnover, so that, if these are more numerous, less compound will be available for each of them. It appears, however, that the sequence of activity is similar to that determined in animals.

All the bisphosphonates maintain their action for months or years after discontinuation of therapy, in contrast to calcitonin, which is active only as long as it is administered. Again, it is difficult to compare the various bisphosphonates in this respect, since the duration seems to depend upon the total dose administered (GRAY et al. 1987).

The effect of bisphosphonates in Paget's disease has been reviewed in two recent publications (HOSKING 1990; KANIS 1991).

2. Hypercalcemia of Malignancy and Tumoral Bone Destruction

Most studies have been performed with etidronate, clodronate, and pamidronate, and one or more of these three are now registered for therapeutic use in many countries. The effects assessed were mostly the lowering of blood calcium, calciuria and hydroxyproliuria, the action on pain, the occurrence of fractures, and the development of new osteolytic lesions. The effect on the biochemical parameters starts usually after 2 days, normalization occurring as quickly as 4 days, usually within 1 week. All three bisphosphonates are active, etidronate being the least, pamidronate the most potent.

It must be stressed that the correction of hypercalcemia is not always a good reflection of the antiosteolytic action of the compound, in contrast to the effect on calciuria or hydroxyprolinuria. This is due to the fact that hypercalcemia is induced not only be bone destruction, but also by an increase in tubular reabsorption of calcium (KANIS et al. 1980; BONJOUR et al. 1988). Since the bisphosphonates have no direct effect on the renal handling of calcium (BONJOUR et al. 1978; TROEHLER et al. 1982; RIZZOLI and BONJOUR 1989), they act only on that part of hypercalcemia induced by bone destruction. Thus, they are especially effective in tumors in which the increase in blood calcium is due principally to increased bone resorption, for example in myeloma. In contrast, the effect is less pronounced in tumors which induce an increase in renal reabsorption of calcium as seen in humoral hypercalcemia of malignancy (BONJOUR et al. 1988; THIEBAUD et al. 1990b).

Etidronate diminishes calcemia, calciuria, and hydroxyprolinuria when given intravenously (JUNG 1982; RYZEN et al. 1985; HASLING et al. 1986; JACOBS et al. 1987; KANIS et al. 1987; SINGER et al. 1991). The effect on pain is unclear (CAREY and LIPPERT 1988; SMITH 1989).

No data are available with respect to an effect on the appearance of new osteolytic lesions. The usual dose is 7.5 mg/kg i.v. for 3 days, the treatment being repeated when the effect subsides or is insufficient. It is not entirely clear to what extent oral treatment is efficacious. For more information see proceedings of a symposium held in 1987 (CANFIELD 1987).

Clodronate is very effective in diminishing or normalizing calcemia, calciuria, and hydroxyprolinuria (CHAPUY et al. 1980; DOUGLAS et al. 1980; SIRIS et al. 1980b; JACOBS et al. 1981; DELMAS et al. 1982a; JUNG 1982; PATERSON et al. 1983; ADAMI et al. 1987b; RASTAD et al. 1987; URWIN et al. 1987). It also decreases bone pain, leading sometimes to a marked improvement in the quality of life (JACOBS et al. 1981; DELMAS et al. 1982; ADAMI et al. 1985; ELOMAA et al. 1983; ASCARI et al. 1989), and decreases the occurrence of fractures (ELOMAA et al. 1983, 1987; ASCARI et al. 1989; McCLOSKEY et al. 1990). Furthermore it slows down the formation of new osteolytic lesions in bone, as well as the further growth of already existing ones, this in myeloma (DELMAS et al. 1982) as well as in metastases from solid tumors (ELOMAA et al. 1983, 1987; ASCARI et al. 1989), the effect being lost after discontinuation of the drug (ELOMAA et al. 1987). The development of metastases in soft tissues is not altered (ELOMAA et al. 1983).

Most of the studies used intravenous treatment. A 1-day infusion of 1500 mg is as efficient as 5 infusions of 300 mg (KANIS and McCLOSKEY 1990). Certain centers use 300 mg/day for 2–3 days or 600 mg for 1 day. If for some reason an oral medication is preferred, a dose of 3200 mg daily seems appropriate until calcemia normalizes (CHAPUY et al. 1980; DOUGLAS et al. 1980; SIRIS et al. 1980b). For long-term treatment the most practical procedure is to follow calcemia and resume treatment when blood calcium increases again. Another possibility is to give clodronate orally as maintenance therapy immediately after the intravenous regimen, starting with 800 mg daily and increasing up to 1600 mg or even 3200 mg if the desired effect is not obtained. However, this treatment is not efficacious in all patients.

Only very few data are available to determine the dose to give to nonhypercalcemic patients in order to slow down the development of new osteolytic lesions. The original study was done with 1600 mg daily (ELOMAA et al. 1983), the same dose being used in an ongoing multicenter study (McCLOSKEY et al. 1990).

The use of clodronate in tumor-induced osteolysis has been reviewed (BONJOUR and RIZZOLI 1990; KANIS and McCLOSKEY 1990) and discussed in a workshop (BRUNNER et al. 1989).

Also pamidronate decreases calcemia, calciuria, and hydroxyprolinuria most effectively (VAN BREUKELEN et al. 1979, 1982; SLEEBOOM et al. 1983; BODY et al. 1986; THIEBAUD et al. 1986a; HARINCK et al. 1987; RALSTON et al. 1988). Pamidronate also has a striking effect on bone pain (VAN HOLTEN-VERZANTVOORT et al. 1987; CLETON et al. 1989), myeloma responding particularly well (THIEBAUD et al. 1991), decreases fractures and prevents the development of new metastases (VAN HOLTEN-VERZANTVOORT et al. 1987; CLETON et al. 1989).

Most studies have been performed using intravenous infusions. Initially between 15 mg and 30 mg were infused daily until calcemia was normalized or reached a nadir (SLEEBOOM et al. 1983; BODY et al. 1986; HARINCK et al. 1987). When it was realized, however, that similar effects can be obtained when the same total dose is given once rather than on separate days (THIEBAUD et al. 1986a; YATES et al. 1987; MORTON et al. 1988; RALSTON et al. 1988; RODY et al. 1989), the protocol with a 1-day infusion gained popularity. The optimal dose is still a matter of debate. It lies between 30 mg and 80 mg and possibly has to be related to the preexistent calcemia

(Thiebaud et al. 1988a). The treatment is repeated if normocalcemia is not attained or when blood calcium rises again. At present the optimal chronic therapy to prevent the development of new osteolytic foci and fractures is still unknown.

Although it has been known for a long time that pamidronate is also active orally (Van Breukelen et al. 1979, 1982), intravenous application has been preferred by most investigators, mostly because of adverse gastrointestinal events. It seems that 1200 mg p.o. daily lies in the range of activity of 30 mg i.v. daily (Thiebaud et al. 1986b). To our knowledge, no oral formulation is yet commercially available.

The actions of pamidronate have recently been reviewed in a symposium (Burckhardt 1989) and an article (Fitton and McTavish 1991).

Data on other bisphosphonates are still scant. Alendronate is very active in lowering calcemia, a single infusion of 5 mg or six infusions of 2.5 mg being effective (Adami et al. 1987b). In a preliminary investigation, BM 210955 has proven active at a single dose below 1 mg i.v. (Wüster et al. 1990) and appears to be one of the most potent bisphosphonates available today also in man.

Finally some bisphosphonates have been used to target radioactive compounds onto bone. Among the compounds which have been tried are bisphosphonates made radioactive with ^{131}I (Eisenhut et al. 1986), ^{32}P (Potsaid et al. 1978), and ^{186}Re (Maxon et al. 1988).

For a more detailed review on the use of bisphosphonates in tumoral bone disease, see Fleisch (1992).

3. Hyperparathyroidism and Other Causes of Hypercalcemia

In primary hyperparathyroidism the oral administration of etidronate was ineffective (Kaplan et al. 1977). In contrast, 1200–3200 mg clodronate decrease hypercalcemia to some extent, serum alkaline phosphatase, calciuria, and hydroxypoliniuria (Douglas et al. 1980; Shane et al. 1981; Hamdy et al. 1987). Another study was, however, less positive (Adami et al. 1990). Pamidronate given at 30 mg/day intravenously is also active (Schmidli et al. 1990).

Bisphosphonates can also be effective in secondary and tertiary hyperparathyroidism (Hamdy et al. 1987). Clodronate 300–600 mg intravenously daily followed by 1600 mg orally daily completely corrected calcemia and hydroxyprolinuria in chronic renal failure, in some patients over months (Hamdy et al. 1990). In contrast 15 mg pamidronate intravenously three times a week, or 200 mg orally daily, had no effect (Hene et al. 1990), possibly because the PTH level of these patients was very high.

As is the case with tumoral hypercalcemia, the failure to normalize calcemia in all patients is explained by the fact that the hypercalcemia is due in part to increased renal reabsorption of calcium.

Hypercalcemia due to other causes also responds to bisphosphonates. This is the case in immobilization (YATES et al. 1984; GALLACHER et al. 1990), in thyrotoxicosis (TAN et al. 1988), and in sarcoidosis (GIBBS and PEACOCK 1986).

4. Osteoporosis

Until recently there have been only few studies using bisphosphonates in patients with osteoporosis. The first controlled study was performed with etidronate at a dose of 20 mg/kg daily p.o. for 6 months in senile osteoporosis (HEANEY and SAVILLE 1976). The results were not very encouraging since bone resorption and formation decreased approximately to the same extent, so that the effect on Ca balance was only small. Intestinal Ca absorption as well as urinary Ca was increased. However, at the above dose an inhibition of mineralization was likely to occur. Thus, a positive effect on bone balance, if present, would have been obscured. Later studies confirmed the increase in intestinal Ca absorption (NUTI et al. 1981), probably through an increase in $1,25(OH)_2D_3$.

Later, in bed rest studies, etidronate administered orally at 20 mg P/kg diminished the negative balance. However, calcaneal loss assessed by gamma absorptiometry was not altered (LOCKWOOD et al. 1975; SCHNEIDER and McDONALD 1984). A daily dose of 400 mg etidronate for 3 months reversed the increase in calcemia and urinary calcium occurring after surgical menopause (SMITH et al. 1989).

A series of studies used so-called coherence therapies, namely multiple cycles of short periods of etidronate with or without an activator of bone resorption (ANDERSON et al. 1984; HESCH et al. 1988; HODSMAN 1989; MALLETTE et al. 1989). Since they were not controlled, they are difficult to interpret, but with one exception (PACIFICI et al. 1988) seem to suggest an increase in vertebral mass. Recently, two controlled double-blind studies investigated the effect of discontinuous oral administration of 400 mg/day for 2 weeks every 16 weeks over a period of 3 years or more in postmenopausal women (STORM et al. 1990; WATTS et al. 1990). Both led to a small increase of vertebral bone mineral content instead of a loss or no change in the controls. Furthermore a small decrease in vertebral fractures was found. However, it is not yet clear whether this increase was significant. A small increase of the fracture rate in the third year found in one of the studies was apparently not significant and fortuitous.

Fewer studies have been carried out with clodronate. The first results were encouraging, since after 18 months the discontinuous oral administration of this compound led to an increase of about 6% in total body Ca measured by neutron activation as compared to a decrease of 2% in patients given placebo (CHESNUT 1988). Daily oral doses of 400 and 1600 mg given continuously prevent the bone loss occurring in paraplegia (Minaire et al. 1981).

Information is also available for pamidronate, which led to an increase of Ca balance still present after 1 year of treatment (Valkema et al. 1989). This finding was supported by bone mineral measurements in patients treated between 1 and 6 years, showing an annual increase of about 3% as compared to a nonsignificant change in nontreated patients. In steroid-induced osteoporosis pamidronate was found not only to prevent both metacarpal cortical loss and vertebral loss but actually to increase bone (Reid et al. 1988), the biochemical parameters indicating a decrease in bone turnover (Reid et al. 1990). Pamidronate also normalizes calcemia in acute spinal injury (Gallacher et al. 1990).

Tiludronate at an oral dose of 100 mg daily for 6 months also prevents the decrease in vertebral body mass over 1 year (Reginster et al. 1989).

Finally, alendronate given at one dose of 5 mg iv every 2 months also prevents vertebral bone loss (Passeri et al. 1991).

In summary it appears that bisphosphonates not only reverse a negative Ca balance but may transform it into a positive one, leading to an increase in bone mass.

III. Other Indications

In view of the effect of bisphosphonates on experimental Freund's adjuvant arthritis, various groups investigated the effect on rheumatoid arthritis in humans. While a preliminary study seemed to show positive effects of pamidronate in the disease (Bijvoet et al. 1980), this has not been sustained by later studies, which showed no effect on the clinical indices of arthritis using etidronate (Bird et al. 1988) or pamidronate (Ralston et al. 1989; Tan et al. 1989).

K. Adverse Events

As in animals, studies in humans have revealed only few important adverse events.

Caution must be taken with the intravenous administration of all bisphosphonates, since a rapid injection has led to renal failure (Bounameaux et al. 1983), possibly because of the precipitation of calcium bisphosphonate or the formation of calcium bisphosphonate aggregates in the blood. No further such events have been observed since care has been taken to administer all bisphosphonates given intravenously by slow infusion in a large volume of fluid.

With etidronate the first and major complication is the inhibition of normal skeletal mineralization. This effect appears at daily oral doses between 800 and 1600 mg (Jowsey et al. 1971; De Vries and Bijvoet 1974; Guncaga et al. 1974; Russell et al. 1974; Khairi et al. 1977; Mautalen et al. 1986) and has been well documented in Paget's disease (Meunier et al. 1979; Douglas et al. 1980). The inhibition regresses after discontinuation of therapy. As mentioned above, the inhibition of mineralization can induce focal osteomalacia at areas of high bone turnover, this at doses as low as 400 mg p.o. (Nagant De Deuxchaisnes et al. 1981; Boyce et al. 1984).

Fractures have occurred in children (Reiner et al. 1980) and possibly also in adults in Paget's disease when high doses are given over longer periods (Altman et al. 1973; Canfield et al. 1977; Khairi et al. 1977; Fromm et al. 1979; Johnston et al. 1983; Mautalen et al. 1986). However, fractures are also more frequent in untreated patients in this disease, so that the role of treatment is difficult to assess (Johnston et al. 1983). In children, long-term treatment at an oral dosage of 20 mg/kg may induce proximal muscular weakness leding to abnormal gait, similar to that seen in rickets (Reiner et al. 1980). Etidronate also causes a conspicuous rise in plasma phosphate, often to high levels, both in healthy persons and in patients. The change is associated with an increase in renal tubular reabsorption of phosphate (Recker et al. 1973; Walton et al. 1975). While it was first thought that this effect was specific for etidronate, it occurs also with other bisphosphonates, although to a much lower degree, and especially in hypoparathyroid patients (McCloskey et al. 1988). Lastly, some gastrointestinal disturbances can occur occasionally when the compound is given orally, which can, however, be overcome by dividing the dose (Russell et al. 1974; Canfield et al. 1977; Khairi et al. 1977). Intravenous infusions induce a transient loss or alteration of taste with a metallic flavor in some patients (Jones et al. 1987; Singer et al. 1991).

Except for a mild diarrhea when given orally, no proven side effects have been described as yet for clodronate. In contrast to etidronate, this compound does not inhibit mineralization of bone at the dosage used. In the course of the clinical evaluation of this compound, some of the treated patients have developed acute leukemia. However, an extremely careful further evaluation led an ad hoc panel of experts to the conclusion that causes other than the drug, especially preselection of patients, were at least as likely or more likely than clodronate as an explanation for the observed cases.

Also pamidronate does not inhibit bone mineralization at doses active on bone resorption. When given orally, pamidronate leads, especially at a dose of 600 mg or more daily, to gastrointestinal disturbances such as nausea, vomiting, pain, and diarrhea (van Breukelen et al. 1982; Harinck et al. 1987; Dodwell et al. 1990). The intensity of these reactions seem to depend upon the preparation used. At the beginning mucosal alterations were reported, which were eliminated by decreasing the dose and using enterocoated tablets.

Both the intravenous and the oral administration of pamidronate induce a transient pyrexia in up to 30% of the patients. This is the case also for other aminobisphosphonates, but contrasts with clodronate, which has no such effect. The pyrexia is maximal within 24–28 h and disappears after approximately 3 days, even when continuing treatment (VAN BREUKELEN et al. 1979; BIJVOET et al. 1980; ADAMI et al. 1987a). The effect is dose dependent and is only observed once, even if treatment is discontinued and restarted later. In the same time there is a decrease in peripheral lymphocytes, an increase in serum C-reactive protein, and a decrease in serum zinc (ADAMI et al. 1987a). The mechanism of these changes, which resemble an acute phase response, is still not understood, but could involve the stimulation of macrophages to release cytokines such as IL-1 and IL-6.

Other adverse effects include local thrombophlebitis at the infusion site (HARINCK et al. 1987), possibly because of an infusion fluid with too high a concentration of bisphosphonate.

No results are available for the other bisphosphonates.

L. Contraindications

Up to now no absolute contraindications have been described. The question is often raised of whether bisphosphonates can be administered in renal failure. Since these compounds are cleared from blood to a large extent by the skeleton, there is no theoretical reason to strictly avoid them in this condition. Actually, pamidronate has been successfully used for hypercalcemia in patients with renal failure (YAP et al. 1990). However, plasma levels are likely to be higher so that the dosage should be reduced. The amount of this reduction will only be known when plasma data becomes available.

Another open question is whether bisphosphonates should be given during fracture healing. Unfortunately only very few data are available on this question. It would appear that large doses of etidronate which are likely to inhibit mineralization should be avoided, while there is no evidence for harm from lower doses of this bisphosphonate or other bisphosphonates. Similar considerations can be made in patients with cementless implantation of porous devices which depend on osseous ingrowth for stabilization. Indeed etidronate administered at 2 mg/kg s.c. per day in dogs, a dose which inhibited mineralization, led to a decrease of bone implant interfacial shear strength (RIVERO et al. 1987).

M. Future Prospects

The bisphosphonates present a most interesting new development in the field of the treatment of bone diseases. It is probable that this is only the beginning of a new area of therapy. Indeed, since the effects vary greatly from one bisphosphonate to another, it is quite possible that new bisphosphonates may be synthesized which are superior to those known up to now. It might thus be possible in the future to find bisphosphonates which act more on ectopic calcification than on normal mineralization. Since the persistent presence of bisphosphonates in the body is a concern, it may be possible to find active analogues which do not show a P-C-P structure and are therefore biodegradable or eliminated faster. Finally, the possible use of bisphosphonates as carriers of drugs acting on the skeleton may be an interesting development.

References

Adami S, Salvagno G, Guarrera G, Bianchi G, Dorizzi R, Rosini S, Morbilio G, Lo Casco V (1985) Dichloromethylene-diphosphonate in patients with prostatic carcinoma metastatic to the skeleton. J Urol 134:1152–1154

Adami S, Bhalla AK, Dorizzi R, Montesanti F, Rosini S, Salvagno G, Lo Cascio V (1987a) The acute-phase response after bisphosphonate administration. Calcif Tissue Int 41:326–331

Adami S, Bolzicco GP, Rizzo A, Salvagno G, Bertoldo F, Rossini M, Suppi R, Lo Cacio V (1987b) The use of dichloromethylene bisphosphonate and aminobutane bisphosphonate in hypercalcemia of malignancy. Bone Miner 2:395–404

Adami S, Mian M, Bertoldo F, Rossini M, Jayawerra P, O'Riordan JLH, Lo Cascio V (1990) Regulation of calcium-parathyroid hormone feedback in primary hyperparathyroidism: effects of bisphosphonate treatment. Clin Endocrinol (Oxf) 33:391–397

Ahrengart L, Lindgren U (1986) Prevention of ectopic bone formation by local application of ethane-1-hydroxy-1,1-diphosphonate (EHDP): an experimental study in rabbits. J Orthop Res 4:18–26

Alden CL, Parker R, Eastman DF (1989) Development of an acute model for the study of chloromethanediphosphonate nephrotoxicity. Toxicol Pathol 17:27–32

Altman RD, Johnston CC, Khairi MRA, Wellman H, Serafini AN, Sankey RR (1973) Influence of disodium etidronate on clinical and laboratory manifestations of Paget's disease of bone (osteitis deformans). N Engl J Med 289:1379–1384

Anderson C, Cape RDT, Crilly RG, Hodsman AB, Wolfe BMJ (1984) Preliminary observations of a form of coherence therapy for osteoporosis. Calcif Tissue Int 36:341–343

Ascari E, Attardo-Parrinello G, Merlini G (1989) Treatment of painful bone lesions and hypercalcemia. Eur J Haematol 43(51):135–139

Atkin I, Ornoy A, Pita JC, Muniz OE, Agundez A, Castiglione G, Howell DS (1988)
EHDP-induced rachitic syndrome in rats is not reversed by vitamin D metabolites. Anat Rec 220:22–30

Atkins RM, Yates AJP, Gray RES, Urwin GH, Hamdy NAT, Beneton MNC, Rosini S, Kanis JA (1987) Aminohexane diphosphonate in the treatment of Paget's disease of bone. J Bone Miner Res 2(4):273–279

Audran M, Clochon P, Etghen D, Mazières B, Renier JC (1989) Treatment of Paget's disease of bone with (4-chloro-phenyl) thiomethylene bisphosphonate. Clin Rheumatol 8(1):71–79

Auriola S, Kostiainen R, Ylinen M, Mönkkönen J, Ylitalo P (1989) Analysis of (dichloromethylene)bisphosphonate in urine by capillary gas chromatography-mass spectrometry. J Pharm Biomed Anal 7:1623–1629

Barbier A, Brelière JC, Remandet B, Roncucci R (1986) Studies on the chronic phase of adjuvant arthritis: effect of SR 41319, a new diphosphonate. Ann Rheum Dis 45:67–74

Basle MF, Rebel A, Renier JC, Audran M, Filmon R, Malkani K (1984) Bone tissue in Paget's disease treated by ethane-1-hydroxy-1,1-diphosphonate (EHDP). Clin Orthop 184:281–288

Bassett CAL, Donath A, Macagno F, Preisig R, Fleisch H, Francis MD (1969) Diphosphonates in the treatment of myositis ossificans. Lancet 2:845

Baumann JM, Bisaz S, Fleisch H, Wacker M (1978) Biochemical and clinical effects of ethane-1-hydroxy-1,1-diphosphonate on calcium nephrolithiasis. Clin Sci Mol Med 54:509–516

Baxter LA, DeLuca HF, Bonjour JP, Fleisch H (1974) Inhibition of vitamin D metabolism by ethane-1-hydroxy-1,1-diphosphonate. Arch Biochem Biophys 164: 655–662

Beertsen W, Niehof A, Everts V (1985) Effects of 1-hydroxyethylidene-1,1-bisphosphonate (HEBP) on the formation of dentin and the periodontal attachment apparatus in the mouse. Am J Anat 174:83–103

Bickerstaff DR, Douglas DL, Burke PH, O'Doherty DP, Kanis JA (1990) Improvement in the deformity of the face in Paget's disease treated with disphosphonates. J Bone Joint Surg [Br] 72:132–136

Bijvoet OLM, Frijlink WB, Jie K, van der Linden H, Meijer CJLM, Mulder H, van Paassen HC, Reitsma PH, te Velde J, de Vries E, van der Wey JP (1980) APD in Paget's disease of bone. Role of the mononuclear phagocyte system? Arthritis Rheum 23:1193–1204

Bird HA, Hill J, Sitton NG, Dixon JS, Wright V (1988) A clinical and biochemical assessment of etidronate disodium in patients with active rheumatoid arthritis. Clin Rheumatol 7(1): 91–94

Bisaz S, Felix R, Fleisch H (1975) Quantitative determination of ethane-1-hydroxy-1,1-diphosphonate in urine and plasma. Clin Chim Acta 65:299–307

Bisaz S, Jung A, Fleisch H (1978) Uptake by bone of pyrophosphate, diphosphonates and their technetium derivatives. Clin Sci Mol Med 54:265–272

Body JJ, Borkowski A, Cleeren A, Bijvoet ALM (1986) Treatment of malignancy-associated hypercalcemia with intravenous aminohydroxypropylidene diphosphonate. J Clin Oncol 4:1177–1183

Body JJ, Magritte A, Seraj F, Sculier JP, Borkowski A (1989) Aminohydroxypropylidene bisphosphonate (APD) treatment for tumor-associated hypercalcemia: a randomized comparison between a 3-day treatment and single 24-hour infusions. J Bone Miner Res 4:923–928

Boehringer Mannheim (Schweiz) (1986) OSTAC pro infusione – zur symptomatischen Therapie der Tumor-Hyperkalzaemie – zur palliativen Therapie der Tumor-Osteolyse infolge Knochenmetastasen oder haemotologischer Neoplasien. Boehringer Mannheim (Schweiz), Rotkreuz

Bone HG, Zerwekh JE, Britton F, Pak CYC (1979) Treatment of calcium urolithiasis with diphosphonate: efficacy and hazards. J Urol 121:568–571

Bonjour JP, Rizzoli R (1990) Clodronate in hypercalcemia of malignancy. Calcif Tissue Int 46:20–25

Bonjour JP, Tröhler U, Preston C, Fleisch H (1978) Parathyroid hormone and renal handling of Pi: effect of dietary Pi and diphosphonates. Am J Physiol 234: F487–F505

Bonjour JP, Philippe J, Guelpa G, Bisetti A, Rizzoli R, Jung A, Rosini S, Kanis JA (1988) Bone and renal components in hypercalcemia of malignancy and responses to a single infusion of clodronate. Bone 9:123–130

Boonekamp PM, van der Wee-Pals LJA, van Wijk-Lennep MML, Thesing CW, Bijvoet OLM (1986) Two modes of action of bisphosphonates on osteoclastic resorption of mineralized matrix. Bone Miner 1:27–39

Boonekamp PM, Löwik CWGM, van der Wee-Pals LJA, van Wijk-van Lennep MLL, Bijvoet OLM (1987) Enhancement of the inhibitory action of APD on the transformation of osteoclast precursors into resorbing cells after dimethylation of the amino group. Bone Miner 2:29–42

Bounameaux HM, Schifferli J, Montani JP, Jung A, Chatelanat F (1983) Renal failure associated with intravenous diphosphonate. Lancet 1:471

Boyce BF, Fogelman I, Ralston S, Smith L, Johnston E, Boyle IT (1984) Focal osteomalacia due to low-dose diphosphonate therapy in Paget's disease. Lancet 1:821–824

Briner WW, Francis MD, Widder JS (1971) The control of dental calculus in experimental animals. Int Dent J 21:61–73

Brommage R, Baxter DC (1990) Inhibition of bone mineral loss during lactation by Cl$_2$MBP. Calcif Tissue Int 47:169–172

Brunner KW, Fleisch H, Senn HJ (eds) (1989) Bisphosphonates and tumor osteolysis. Recent Results Cancer Res 116

Burckhardt P (ed) (1989) Disodium pamidronate (APD) in the treatment of malignancy-related disorders. Huber, Bern

Cal JC, Daley-Yates PT (1990) Disposition and nephrotoxicity of 3-amino-1-hydroxypropylidene-1,1-bisphosphonate (APD), in rats and mice. Toxicology 65:179–197

Canfield RE (1987) Etidronate disodium: a new therapy for hypercalcemia of malignancy. Am J Med 82:1–78

Canfield RE, Rosner W, Skinner J, McWorther J, Resnick L, Feldman F, Kammerman S, Ryan K, Kunigonis M, Bohne W (1977) Diphosphonate therapy of Paget's disease of bone. J Clin Endocrinol Metab 44:96–106

Carano A, Teitelbaum SL, Konsek JD, Schlesinger PH, Blair HC (1990) Bisphosphonates directly inhibit the bone resorption activity of isolated avian osteoclasts in vitro. J Clin Invest 85:456–461

Carey PO, Lippert MC (1988) Treatment of painful prostatic bone metastases with oral etidronate disodium. Urology 32:403–407

Cecchini MG, Fleisch H (1990) Bisphosphonates in vitro specifically inhibit, among the hematopoietic series, the development of the mouse mononuclear phagocyte lineage. J Bone Min Res 5:1019–1027

Cecchini MG, Felix R, Cooper PH, Fleisch H (1987) Effect of bisphosphonates on proliferation and viability of mouse bone marrow-derived macrophages. J Bone Min Res 2:135–142

Cecchini MG, Castagna M, Schenk R, Fleisch H (1990) A new "in vivo" model for studying "de novo" osteoclastogenesis: the post-natal mouse caudal vertebrae. J Bone Min Res 5 Suppl 2:S223

Chambers TJ (1980) Diphosphonates inhibit bone resorption by macrophages in vitro. J Pathol 132:255–262

Chan MM, Riggins RS, Rucker RB (1977) Effect of ethane-1-hydroxy-1,1-diphosphonate (EHDP) and dietary fluoride on biomechanical and morphological changes in chick bone. J Nutr 107:1747–1754

Chapuy MC, Meunier PJ, Alexandre CM, Vignon EP (1980) Effects of disodium dichloromethylene diphosphonate on hypercalcemia produced by bone metastases. J Clin Invest 65:1243–1247

Chapuy MC, Charhon SA, Meunier PJ (1983) Sustained biochemical effects of short treatment of Paget's disease of bone with dichloromethylene diphosphonate. Metab Bone Dis Relat Res 4:325–328

Chesnut CH III (1988) Drug therapy: calcitonin, bisphosphonates, anabolic steroids, and hPTH (1–34). In: Riggs BL, Melton LJ (eds) Osteoporosis: etiology, diagnosis, and management. Raven, New York, pp 403–414

Chester TL, Lewis EC, Benedict JJ, Sunberg RJ, Tettenhorst WC (1981) Determination of (dichloromethylene)diphosphonate in physiological fluids by ion-exchange chromatography with phosphorus-selective detection. J Chromatogr Sci 225:17–25

Cleton FJ, van Holten-Verzantvoort AT, Zwinderman A, Kroon HM, Hermans J, Bijvoet OLM (1989) Long-term bisphosphonate treatment of bone metastases in breast cancer patients – effects on morbidity and quality of life. In: Burckhardt P (ed) Disodium pamidronate (APD) in the treatment of malignancy-related disorders. Huber, Bern, pp 113–119

Conrad KA, Lee SM (1981) Clodronate kinetics and dynamics. Clin Pharmacol Ther 30:114–120

Cram RL, Barmade R, Geho WB, Ray BD (1971) Diphosphonate treatment of calcinosis universalis. N Engl J Med 285:1012–1013

Daley-Yates PT, Bennett R (1988) A comparison of the pharmacokinetics of ^{14}C-labelled APD and [99]mTc-labelled APD in the mouse. Calcif Tissue Int 43:125–127

Daley-Yates P, Gifford LA, Hoggarth CR (1989) Assay of 1-hydroxy-3-amino-propylidene-1,1-bisphosphonate and related bisphosphonates in human urine and plasma by high-performance ion chromatography. J Chromatogr 490:329–338

Delaissé J-M, Eeckhout Y, Vaes G (1985) Bisphosphonates and bone resorption: effects on collagenase and lysosomal enzyme excretion. Life Sci 37:2291–2296

Delmas PD, Chapuy MC, Vignon E, Charhon S, Briançon D, Alexandre C, Edouard C, Meunier PJ (1982a) Long term effects of dichloromethylene diphosphonate in Paget's disease of bone. J Clin Endocrinol Metab 54(4):837–844

Delmas PD, Charhon S, Chapuy MC, Vignon E, Briançon D, Edouard C, Meunier PJ (1982b) Long-term effects of dichloromethylene diphosphonate (Cl_2MDP) on skeletal lesions in multiple myeloma. Metab Bone Dis Relat Res 4:163–168

Delmas PD, Chapuy MC, Edouard C, Meunier PJ (1987) Beneficial effects of aminohexane diphosphonate in patients with Paget's disease of bone resistant to sodium etidronate. Am J Med 83:276–282

De Marco JD, Biffar SE, Reed DG, Brooks MA (1989) The determination of 4-amino-1-hydroxybutane-1,1-diphosphonic acid monosodium salt trihydrate in pharmaceutical dosage forms by high-performance liquid chromatography. J Pharm Biomed Anal 7:1719–1727

De Vries E, van der Weij JP, van der Veen CJP, van Paassen HC, Jager MJ, Sleeboom HP, Bijvoet OLM, Cats A (1982) In vitro effect of (3-amino-1-hydroxypropylidene)-1,1-bisphosphonic acid (APD) on the function of mononuclear phagocytes in lymphocyte proliferation. Immunology 47:157–163

De Vries HR, Bijvoet OLM (1974) Results of prolonged treatment of Paget's disease of bone with disodium ethane-1-hydroxy-1,1-diphosphonate (EHDP). Neth J Med 17:281–298

Dodd GW, Ibbertson HK, Fraser TRC, Holdaway IM, Wattie D (1987) Radiological assessment of Paget's disease of bone after treatment with the bisphosphonates EHDP and APD. Br J Radiol 60:849–860

Dodwell DJ, Howell A, Ford J (1990) Reduction in calcium excretion in women with breast cancer and bone metastases using the oral bisphosphonate pamidronate. Br J Cancer 61:123–125

Douglas DL, Russell RGG, Preston CJ, Prenton MA, Duckworth T, Kanis JA, Preston FE, Woodhead JS (1980) Effect of dichloromethylene diphosphonate in Paget's disease of bone and in hypercalcaemia due to primary hyperparathyroidism or malignant disease. Lancet 1:1043–1047

Eguchi M, Yamaguchi T, Shiota E, Handa S (1982) Fault of ossification and calcification and angular deformities of long bones in the mouse fetuses caused by high doses of ethane-1-hydroxy-1,1-diphosphonate (EHDP) during pregnancy. Congenital Anom 22:47–52

Eisenhut M, Berbereich R, Kimmig B, Oberhausen E (1986) Iodine-131-labeled diphosphonates for palliative treatment of bone metastases. II. Preliminary clinical results with iodine-131 BDP3. J Nucl Med 27:1255–1261

Elomaa I, Blomqvist C, Gröhn P, Porkka L, Kairento AL, Selander K, Lamberg-Allardt C, Holmström T (1983) Long-term controlled trial with diphosphonate in patients with osteolytic bone metastases. Lancet 1:146–149

Elomaa I, Blomqvist C, Porkka L, Lamberg-Allardt C, Borgström GG (1987) Treatment of skeletal disease in breast cancer: a controlled clodronate trial. Bone 8(1):53–56

Emonds-Alt X, Brelière J-C, Roncucci R (1985) Effects of 1-hydroxyethylidene-1,1 bisphosphonate and (chloro-4 phenyl) thiomethylene bisphosphonic acid (SR 41319) on the mononuclear cell factor-mediated release of neutral proteinases by articular chondrocytes and synovial cells. Biochem Pharmacol 34:4043–4049

Ende JJ (1979) Effects of some diphosphonates on the metabolism of bone in vivo and in vitro. Thesis, University of Leiden

Eubank WB, Reeves RE (1982) Analog inhibitors for the pyrophosphate-dependent phosphofructokinase of *Entamoeba histolytica* and their effect of culture growth. J Parasitol 68:599–602

Evêquoz V, Trechsel U, Fleisch H (1985) Effect of bisphosphonates on production of interleukin 1-like activity by macrophages and its effect on rabbit chondrocytes. Bone 6:439–444

Fast DK, Felix R, Dowse C, Neumann WF, Fleisch H (1978) The effects of diphosphonates on the growth and glycolysis of connective-tissue cells in culture. Biochem J 172:97–107

Felix R, Fleisch H (1975) Properties of inorganic pyrophosphatase of pig scapula cartilage. Biochem J 147:111–118

Felix R, Fleisch H (1979) Increase in alkaline phosphatase activity in calvaria cells cultured with diphosphonates. Biochem J 183:73–81

Felix R, Fleisch H (1981) Increase in fatty acid oxidation in calvaria cells cultured with diphosphonates. Biochem J 196:237–245

Felix R, Russell RGG, Fleisch H (1976) The effect of several diphosphonates on acid phosphohydrolases and other lysosomal enzymes. Biochim Biophys Acta 429:429–438

Felix R, Fast DK, Sallis JD, Fleisch H (1980) Effect of diphosphonate on glycogen content of rabbit ear cartilage cells in culture. Calcif Tissue Int 30:163–166

Felix R, Bettex JD, Fleisch H (1981) Effect of diphosphonates on the synthesis of prostaglandins in cultured calvaria cells. Calcif Tissue Int 33:549–552

Felix R, Guenther HL, Fleisch H (1984) The subcellular distribution of ^{14}C dichloromethylenebisphosphonate and ^{14}C 1-hydroxyethylidene-1,1-bisphosphonate in cultured calvaria cells. Calcif Tissue Int 36:108–113

Fels JP, Guyonnet J, Berger Y, Cautreels W (1988) Determination of (4-chlorophenyl) thiomethylene bisphosphonic acid, a new bisphosphonate, in biological fluids by high-performance liquid chromatography. J Chromatogr 430:73–79

Ferretti JL, Cointry G, Capozza R, Montuori E, Roldán E, Pérez Lloret A (1990) Biomechanical effects of the full range of useful doses of (3-amino-1-hydroxy-propylidene)-1,1-bisphosphonate (APD) on femur diaphyses and cortical bone tissue in rats. Bone Miner 11:111–122

Finerman GAM, Stover SL (1981) Heterotopic ossification following hip replacement or spinal cord injury. Two clinical studies with EHDP. Metab Bone Dis Relat Res 4:337–342

Fitton A, McTavish D (1991) A review of its pharmacological properties and therapeutic efficacy in resorptive bone disease. Drugs 41:289–318

Flanagan AM, Chambers TJ (1989) Dichloromethylenebisphosphonate (Cl$_2$MBP) inhibits bone resorption through injury to osteoclasts that resorb Cl$_2$MBP-coated bone. Bone Miner 6:33–43

Fleisch H (1988) Bisphosphonates: a new class of drugs in diseases of bone and calcium metabolism. In: Baker PF (ed) Handbook of experimental pharmacology, vol 83. Springer, Berlin Heidelberg New York, pp 441–466

Fleisch H (1991) Bisphosphonates: pharmacology and use in the treatment of tumour-induced hypercalcaemic and metastatic bone disease. Drugs 42:913–944

Fleisch H, Russell RGG (1970) Pyrophosphate and polyphosphate. In: Rasmussen H (ed) Pharmacology of the endocrine system and related drugs. Pergamon, Oxford, pp 61–100, Encyclopaedia of pharmacology and therapeutics, sect 51

Fleisch H, Russell RGG, Straumann F (1966) Effect of pyrophosphate on hydroxy-apatite and its implications in calcium homeostasis. Nature 212:901–903

Fleisch H, Russell RGG, Bisaz S, Casey PA, Mühlbauer RC (1968) The influence of pyrophosphate analogues (diphosphonates) on the precipitation and dissolution of calcium phosphate in vitro and in vivo. Calcif Tissue Res 2 Suppl:10–10A

Fleisch H, Russell RGG, Francis MD (1969) Diphosphonates inhibit hydroxyapatite dissolution in vitro and bone resorption in tissue culture and in vivo. Science 165:1262–1264

Fleisch H, Russell RGG, Bisaz S, Mühlbauer RC, Williams DA (1970) The inhibitory effect of phosphonates on the formation of calcium phosphate crystals in vitro and on aortic and kidney calcification in vivo. Eur J Clin Invest 1:12–18

Flesch G, Hauffe SA (1989) Determination of the bisphosphonate pamidronate dis-odium in urine by pre-column derivatization with fluorescamine, high-performance liquid chromatography and fluorescence detection. J Chromatogr 489:446–451

Flora L (1979) Comparative antiinflammatory and bone protective effects of two diphosphonates in adjuvant arthritis. Arthritis Rheum 4:340–346

Flora L, Hassing GS, Parfitt AM, Villanueva AR (1980) Comparative skeletal effects of two diphosphonates in dogs. Metab Bone Dis Relat Res 2:389–407

Fogelman I, Smith L, Mazess R, Wilson MA, Bevan JA (1986) Absorption of oral diphosphonate in normal subjects. Clin Endocrinol (Oxf) 24:57–62

Francis MD (1969) The inhibition of calcium hydroxyapatite crystal growth by polyphosphates. Calcif Tissue Res 3:151–162

Francis MD, Martodam PR (1983) Chemical, biochemical, and medicinal properties of the diphosphonates. In: Hilderbrand RL (ed) The role of phosphonates in living systems. CRC, Boca Raton, p 55

Francis MD, Slough CL (1984) Acute intravenous infusion of disodium dihydrogen (1-hydroxyethylidene)diphosphonate: mechanism of toxicity. J Pharm Sci 73:1097–1100

Francis MD, Russell RGG, Fleisch H (1969) Diphosphonates inhibit formation of calcium phosphate crystals in vitro and pathological calcification in vivo. Science 165:1264–1266

Francis MD, Flora LF, King WF (1972) The effects of disodium ethanc-1-hydroxy-1,1-diphosphonate on adjuvant induced arthritis in rats. Calcif Tissue Res 9:109–121

Francis MD, Hovancik K, Boyce RW (1989) NE-58095: a diphosphonate which prevents bone erosion and preserves joint architecture in experimental arthritis. Int J Tissue React 11:239–252

Fraser D, Russell RGG, Pohler O, Robertson WG, Fleisch H (1972) The influence of disodium ethane-1-hydroxy-1,1-diphosphonate (EHDP) on the development of experimentally induced urinary stones in rats. Clin Sci 42:197–207

Freed JH, Hahn H, Menter R, Dillon T (1982) The use of three-phase bone scan in the early diagnosis of heterotopic ossification (HO) and in the evaluation of didronel therapy. Paraplegia 20:208–216

Freudiger H, Bonjour JP (1989) Bisphosphonates and extrarenal acid buffering capacity. Calcif Tissue Int 44:3–10

Frijlink WB, te Velde J, Bijvoet OLM, Heynen G (1979) Treatment of Paget's disease with (3-amino-1-hydroxypropylidene)-1,1-bisphosphonate (A.P.D.). Lancet 1:799

Fromm GA, Schajowicz F, Casco C, Ghiringhelli G, Mautalen C (1979) The treatment of Paget's bone disease with sodium ethidronate. Am J Med Sci 227:29–37

Galasko CSB, Samuel AW, Rushton S, Lacey E (1980) The effect of prostaglandin synthesis inhibitors and diphosphonates on tumour-mediated osteolysis. Br J Surg 67:493–496

Gallacher SJ, Ralston SH, Dryburgh FJ, Fraser CL, Allam BF, Boyce BF, Boyle IT (1990) Immobilization-related hypercalcaemia – a possible novel mechanism and response to pamidronate. Postgrad Med J 66:918–922

Gallagher JA, Guenther HL, Fleisch H (1982) Rapid intracellular degradation of newly synthesized collagen by bone cells. Effect of dichloromethylenebisphosphonate. Biochim Biophys Acta 719:349–355

Garland DE, Betzabe A, Venos KG, Vogt JC (1983) Diphosphonate treatment for heterotopic ossification in spinal cord injury patients. Clin Orthop 176:197–200

Gasser AB, Morgan DB, Fleisch HA, Richelle LJ (1972) The influence of two diphosphonates on calcium metabolism in the rat. Clin Sci 43:31–45

Gebauer U, Russell RGG, Touabi M, Fleisch H (1976) Effect of diphosphonates on adenosine 3′:5′ cyclic monophosphate in mouse calvaria after stimulation by parathyroid hormone in vitro. Clin Sci Mol Med 50:473–478

Geho WB, Whiteside JA (1973) Experience with disodium etidronate in diseases of ectopic calcification. In: Frame B, Parfitt AM, Duncan H (eds) Clinical aspects of metabolic bone disease. Excerpta Medica, Amsterdam, p 506

Geusens P, Nijs J, van der Perre G, van Audekercke R, Lowet G, Goovaerts S, Barbier A, Lacheretz F, Remandet B, Jiang Y, Dequeker J (1992) Longitudinal effect of tiludronate on bone mineral density, resonant frequency, and strength in monkeys. J Bone Min Res 7:599–609

Gibbs CJ, Peacock M (1986) Hypercalcaemia due to sarcoidosis corrects with bisphosphonate treatment. Postgrad Med J 61:937–938

Glatt M, Pataki A, Blättler A, Reife R (1986) APD longterm treatment increases bone mass and mechanical strength of femora of adult mice. Calcif Tissue Int 39:A72

Golomb G, Langer R, Schoen FJ, Smith MS, Choi YM, Levy RJ (1986) Controlled release of diphosphonate to inhibit bioprosthetic heart valve calcification: dose-response and mechanistic studies. J Contr Rel 4:181–194

Golomb G, Dixon M, Smith MS, Schoen FJ, Levy RJ (1987) Controlled-release drug delivery of diphosphonates to inhibit bioprosthetic heart valve calcification: release rate modulation with silicone matrices via drug solubility and membrane coating. J Pharm Sci 76:271–276

Gray RES, Yates AJP, Preston CJ, Smith R, Russell RGG, Kanis JA (1987) Duration of effect of oral diphosphonate therapy in Paget's disease of bone. Q J Med 245:755–767

Greif F, Anais D, Frei L, Arbeit L, Sorroff HS (1990) Blocking the calcium cascade in experimental acute renal failure. Isr J Med Sci 26:301–305

Guaitani A, Polentarutti N, Filippeschi S, Marmonti L, Corti F, Italia C, Coccioli G, Donelli MG, Mantovani A, Garattini S (1984) Effects of disodium etidronate in murine tumor models. Eur J Cancer Clin Oncol 20:685–693

Guaitani A, Sabatini M, Coccioli G, Cristina S, Garattini S, Bartosek I (1985) An experimental rat model of local bone cancer invasion and its responsiveness to ethane-1-hydroxy-1,1-bis(phosphonate). Cancer Res 45:2206–2209

Guenther HL, Guenther HE, Fleisch H (1979) Effects of 1-hydroxyethane-1,1-diphosphonate and dichloromethane on rabbit articular chondrocytes in culture. Biochem J 184:203–214

Guenther HL, Guenther HE, Fleisch H (1981a) The effects of 1-hydroxyethane-1,1-diphosphonate and dichloromethanedisphosphonate on collagen synthesis by rabbit articular chondrocytes and rat bone cells. Biochem J 196:293–301

Guenther HL, Guenther HE, Fleisch H (1981b) The influence of 1-hydroxyethane-1,1-diphosphonate and dichloromethanediphosphonate on lysine hydroxylation and cross-link formation in rat bone, cartilage and skin collagen. Biochem J 196:303–310

Guilland DF, Sallis JD, Fleisch H (1974) The effect of two diphosphonates on the handling of calcium by rat kidney mitochondria in vitro. Calcif Tissue Res 15:303–314

Guilland D, Trechsel U, Bonjour JP, Fleisch H (1975) Stimulation of calcium absorption and apparent increased intestinal, 1,25-dihydroxycholecalciferol in rats treated with low doses of ethane-1-hydroxy-1,1-diphosphonate. Clin Sci Mol Med 48:157–160

Guncaga J, Lauffenburger R, Lentner C, Dambacher MA, Haas HG, Fleisch H, Olah AJ (1974) Diphosphonate treatment of Paget's disease of bone. A correlated metabolic, calcium kinetic and morphometric study. Horm Metab Res 6:62–69

Gural RP (1975) Pharmacokinetics and gastrointestinal absorption behavior of etidronate. Dissertation, University of Kentucky

Gural RP, Chungi VS, Shrewsbury RP, Dittert LW (1985) Dose-dependent absorption of disodium etidronate. J Pharm Pharmacol 37:443–445

Hähnel H, Mühlbach R, Lindenhayn K, Schaetz P, Schmidt UJ (1973) Zum Einfluß von Diphosphonat auf die experimentelle Heparinosteopathie. Z Altersforsch 28:289–292

Hamdy NAT, Gray RES, McCloskey E, Galloway J, Rattenbury JM, Brown CB, Kanis JA (1987) Clodronate in the medical management of hyperparathyroidism. Bone 8(1):69–77

Hamdy NAT, McCloskey EV, Brown CB, Kanis JA (1990) Effects of clodronate in severe hyperparathyroid bone disease in chronic renal failure. Nephron 56:6–12

Hanhijärvi H, Elomaa I, Karlsson M, Lauren L (1989) Pharmacokinetics of disodium clodronate after daily intravenous infusions during five consecutive days. Int J Clin Pharmacol Ther Toxicol 27:602–606

Hansen NM Jr, Felix R, Bisaz S, Fleisch H (1976) Aggregation of hydroxyapatite crystals. Biochim Biophys Acta 451:549–559

Hardt AB (1988) Bisphosphonate effects on alveolar bone during rat molar drifting. J Dent Res 67:1430–1433

Harinck HIJ, Papapoulos SE, Blanksma HJ, Moolenaar AJ, Vermeij P, Bijvoet OLM (1987) Paget's disease of bone: early and late responses to three different modes of treatment with aminohydroxypropylidene bisphosphonate (APD). Br Med J 295:1301–1305

Hasling C, Charles P, Mosekilde L (1986) Etidronate disodium for treating hypercalcaemia of malignancy: a double blind, placebo-controlled study. Eur J Clin Invest 16:433–437

Heaney RP, Saville PD (1976) Etidronate disodium in postmenopausal osteoporosis. Cin Pharmacol Ther 20:593–604

Hené RJ, Visser WJ, Duursma SA, Raymakers JA, de Bos Kuil RJ, Dorhout Mees EJ (1990) No effect of APD (amino hydroxypropylidene bisphosphonate) on hypercalcemia in patients with renal osteodystrophy. Bone 11:15–20

Henley JW, Croxson RS, Ibbertson HK (1979) The cardiovascular system in Paget's disease of bone and the response to therapy with calcitonin and diphosphonate. Aust NZ J Med 9:390–397

Hesch RD, Heck J, Delling G, Keck E, Reeve J, Canzler H, Schober O, Harms H, Rittinghaus EF (1988) Results of a stimulatory therapy of low bone metabolism in osteoporosis with (1–38)hPTH and diphosphonate EHDP. Protocol of study I, osteoporosis trial Hannover. Klin Wochenschr 66:976–984

Heynen G, Delwaide P, Bijvoet OLM, Franchimont P (1982) Clinical and biological effects of low doses of (3 amino-1-hydroxypropylidene)-1,1-bisphosphonate (APD) in Paget's disease of bone. Eur J Clin Invest 11:29–35

Hill LF, Lumb GA, Mawer EB, Stanbury SW (1973) Indirect inhibition of the biosynthesis of 1,25-dihydroxycholecalciferol in rats treated with a diphosphonate. Clin Sci 44:335–347

Hintze KL, d'Amato RA (1980) Comparative toxicity of two diphosphonates. Toxicology 2:192

Hock JM, Hummert JR, Boyce R, Fonseca J, Raisz LG (1989) Resorption is not essential for the stimulation of bone growth by hPTH-(1-34) in rats in vivo. J Bone Miner Res 4:449–458

Hodsman AB (1989) Effects of cyclical therapy for osteoporosis using an oral regimen of inorganic phosphate and sodium etidronate: a clinical and bone histomorphometric study. Bone Miner 5:201–212

Hollander W, Prusty S, Nagraj S, Kirkpatrick B, Paddock J, Colombo M (1978) Comparative effects of cetaben (PHB) and dichloromethylene diphosphonate (Cl_2MBP) on the development of atherosclerosis in the cynomolgus monkey. Atherosclerosis 31:307–325

Hosking DJ (1990) Advances in the management of Paget's disease of bone. Drugs 40(6):829–840

Howell DS, Muniz OE, Blanco LN, Pita JC (1980) A micropuncture study of growth cartilage in phosphonate (EHDP) induced rickets. Calcif Tissue Int 30:35–42

Hughes DE, MacDonald BR, Russell RGG, Gowen M (1989) Inhibition of osteoclast-like cell formation by bisphosphonates in long-term cultures of human bone marrow. J Clin Invest 83:1930–1935

Ikeo T, Takaya T, Yamauchi K, Miwa M, Shioji I, Sakiyama Y (1987) Effect of ethane-1-hydroxy-1,1-diphosphonate (EHDP) on fetal mice during pregnancy: chemical changes in skin collagen. J Osaka Dent Univ 21:45–53

Ismail Z, Aldous S, Triggs EJ, Smithurst BA, Barry HD (1987) Gas chromatographic analysis of didronel tablets. J Chromatogr 404:372–377

Jacobs TP, Siris ES, Bilezikian JP, Baquiran DC, Shane E, Canfield RE (1981) Hypercalcemia of malignancy: treatment with intravenous dichloromethylene diphosphonate. Ann Intern Med 94:312–316

Jacobs TP, Gordon AC, Silverberg SJ, Shane E, Reich L, Clemens TL, Gundberg CH (1987) Neoplastic hypercalcemia: physiologic response to intravenous etidronate disodium. Am J Med 82(2a):42–50

Janner M, Mühlbauer RC, Fleisch H (1991) Sodium EDTA enhances intestinal absorption of two bisphosphonates. Calcif Tissue Int 49:280–283

Jee WSS, Black HE, Gotcher JE (1981) Effect of dichloromethane disphosphonate on cortisol-induced bone loss in young adult rabbits. Clin Orthop 156:39–51

Johnson KY, Wesseler MA, Olson IIM, Martodam RR, Poser JW (1982) The effects of diphosphonates on tumor-induced hypercalcemia and osteolysis in Walker carcinosarcoma 256 (W-256) of rats. In: Donath A, Courvoisier B (eds) Diphosphonates and bone. Médecine et Hygiène, Genéva, pp 386–389

Johnston CC Jr, Altman RD, Canfield RE, Finerman GAM, Taulbee JD, Ebert ML (1983) Review of fracture experience during treatment of Paget's disease of bone with etidronate disodium (EHDP). Clin Orthop 172:186–194

Jones M, Eidbo EE, Hilbert SL, Ferrans VJ, Clark RE (1988) The effects of anticalcification treatments on bioprosthetic heart valves implanted in sheep. Trans Am Soc Artif Intern Organs 34:1027–1031

Jones RG, McLasky EVM, Kanis JA (1987) Transient taste-loss during treatment with etidronate. Lancet 2:637

Jowsey J, Holley KE, Linman JW (1970) Effect of sodium etidronate in adult cats. J Lab Clin Med 76:126–133

Jowsey J, Riggs BL, Kelly PJ, Hoffman DL, Bordier P (1971) The treatment of osteoporosis with disodium ethane-1-hydroxy-1,1-diphosphonate. J Lab Clin Med 78:574–584

Jung A (1982) Comparison of two parenteral diphosphonates in hypercalcemia of malignancy. Am J Med 72:221–226

Jung A, Bisaz S, Fleisch H (1973) The binding of pyrophosphate and two diphosphonates on hydroxyapatite crystals. Calcif Tissue Res 11:269–280

Jung A, Mermillod B, Barras C, Baud M, Courvoisier B (1981) Inhibition by two diphosphonates of bone lysis in tumor conditioned media. Cancer Res 41:3233–3237

Jung A, Bornand J, Mermillod B, Edouard C, Meunier PJ (1984) Inhibition by diphosphonates of bone resorption induced by the Walker tumor of the rat. Cancer Res 44:3007–3011

Kanis JA (1991) Pathophysiology and treatment of Paget's disease of bone. In: Kanis JA (ed) Pathophysiology and treatment of Paget's disease. Dunitz, London

Kanis JA, McCloskey EV (1990) The use of clodronate in disorders of calcium and skeletal metabolism. In: Kanis JA (ed) Calcium metabolism. Karger, Basel, pp 89–136

Kanis JA, Cundy T, Heynen G, Russell RGG (1980) The pathophysiology of hypercalcaemia. Metab Bone Dis Relat Res 2:151–159

Kanis JA, Urwin GH, Gray Res, Beneton MNC, McCloskey EV, Hamdy NAT, Murray SA (1987) Effects of intravenous etidronate disodium on skeletal and calcium metabolism. Am J Med 82(2A):55–70

Kaplan RA, Geho WB, Pointdexter C, Haussler M, Dietz GW, Pak CYC (1977) Metabolic effects of diphosphonate in primary hyperparathyroidism. J Clin Pharmacol 17:410–419

Khairi MRA, Altman RD, DeRosa GP, Zimmermann J, Schenk RK, Johnston CC (1977) Sodium etidronate in the treatment of Paget's disease of bone. Ann Intern Med 87:656–663

King WR, Francis MD, Michael WR (1971) Effect of disodium ethane-1-hydroxy-1,1-diphosphonate on bone formation. Clin Orthop 78:251–270

Klein G, Martin JB, Satre M (1988) Methylenediphosphonate, a metabolic poison in Dictyostelium discoideum. ^{31}P NMR evidence for accumulation of adenosine $5'$-(β,τ-methylenetriphosphate) and diadenosine $5',5'''$-P^1,P^4-(P^2,P^3-methylenetetraphosphate). Biochemistry 27:1897–1901

Kline WF, Matuszewski BK, Bayne WF (1990) Determination of 4-amino-1-hydroxy-butane-1,1-bisphosphonic acid in urine by automated precolumn derivatization with 2,3-naphthalene dicarboxyaldehyde and high-performance liquid chromatography with fluorescence detection. J Chromatogr 534:139–149

Kozak ST, Rizzoli R, Trechsel U, Fleisch H (1987) Effect of a single injection of two new bisphosphonates on the hypercalcemia and hypercalciuria induced by Walker carcinosarcoma 256/B in thyroparathyroidectomized rats. Cancer Res 47:6193–6197

Kramsch DM, Chan CT (1978) The effect of agents interfering with soft tissue calcification and cell proliferation on calcific fibrous fatty plaques in rabbits. Circ Res 42:562–571

Kwong E, Chiu AMY, McClintock SA, Cotton ML (1990) HPLC analysis of an amino bisphosphonate in pharmaceutical formulations using postcolumn derivatization and fluorescence detection. J Chromatogr Sci 28:563–566

Labat ML, Tzehoval E, Moricard Y, Feldmann M, Milhaud G (1983) Lack of a T-cell dependent subpopulation of macrophages in (dichloromethylene) diphosphonate-treated mice. Biomed Pharmacother 37:270–276

Labat ML, Florentin I, Davigny M, Moricard Y, Milhaud G (1984) Dichloromethylene diphosphonate (Cl_2MDP) reduces natural killer (NK) cell activity in mice. Metab Bone Dis Relat Res 5:281–287

Lamson ML, Fox JL, Huguchi WI (1984) Calcium and 1-hydroxyethylidene-1,1-bisphosphonic acid: polynuclear complex formation in the physiological range of pH. Int J Pharm 21:143–154

Larsson A (1974) The short-term effects of high doses of ethylene-1-hydroxy-1,1-diphosphonates upon early dentine formation. Calcif Tissue Res 16:109–127

Larsson SE (1976) The metabolic heterogeneity of glycosaminoglycans of the different zones of the epiphyseal growth plate and the effect of ethane-1-hydroxy-1,1-diphosphonate (EHDP) upon glycosaminoglycan synthesis in vivo. Calcif Tissue Res 21:67–82

Larsson A, Rohlin M (1980) In vivo distribution of ^{14}C-labeled ethylene-1-hydroxy-1,1-diphosphonate in normal and treated young rats. An autoradiographic and ultrastructural study. Toxicol Appl Pharmacol 52:391–399

Lenehan TM, Balligand M, Nunamaker DM, Wood FE Jr (1985) Effect of EHDP on fracture healing in dogs. J Orthop Res 3:499–507

Levy RJ, Wolfrum J, Schoen FJ, Hawley MA, Lund SA (1985) Inhibition of calcification of bioprosthetic heart valves by local controlled release diphosphonate. Science 228:190–192

Levy RJ, Schoen FJ, Lund SA, Smith MS (1987) Prevention of leaflet calcification of bioprosthetic heart valves with diphosphonate injection therapy. J Thorac Cardiovasc Surg 94:551–557

Liggett SJ (1973) Determination of ethane-1-hydroxy-1,1-diphosphonic acid (EHDP) in human feces and urine. Biochem Med 7:68–77

Lin JH, Chen IW, Deluna FA, Hichens M (1992) Renal handling of alendronate in rats. An uncharacterized renal transport system. Drug Metab Dispos 20:608–613

Lockwood DR, Vogel JM, Schneider VS, Hulley SB (1975) Effect of the diphosphonate EHDP on bone mineral metabolism during prolonged bed rest. J Clin Endocrinol Metab 41:533–541

Löwik CWGM, van der Pluijm G, van der Wee-Pals LJA, van Bloys Treslong-de Groot H, Bijvoet OLM (1988) Migration and phenotypic transformation of osteoclast precursors into mature osteoclasts: the effect of a bisphosphonate. J Bone Miner Res 3:185–191

Mallette LE, LeBlanc AD, Pool JL, Mechanick JI (1989) Cyclic therapy of osteoporosis with neutral phosphate and brief, high-dose pulses of etidronate. J Bone Miner Res 4(2):143–148

Markusse HM, Lafeber GJM, Breedveld FC (1990) Bisphosphonates in collagen arthritis. Rheumatol Int 9:281–283

Martodam RR, Thornton KS, Sica DA, Souza SM, Flora L, Mundy GR (1983) The effects of dichloromethylene diphosphonate on hypercalcemia and other parameters of the humoral hypercalcemia of malignancy in the rat Leydig cell tumor. Calcif Tissue Int 35:512–519

Mautalen C, Gonzalez D, Blumenfeld EL, Santini Araujo E, Schajowicz F (1986) Spontaneous fractures of uninvolved bones in patients with Paget's disease during unduly prolonged treatment with disodium etidronate (EHDP). Clin Orthop 207:150–155

Maxon HR, Deutsch EA, Thomas SR, Libson K, Lukes SJ, Williams CC, Ali S (1988) Re-186(Sn) HEDP for treatment of multiple metastatic foci in bone: human biodistribution and dosimetric studies. Radiology 166:501–507

McCloskey EV, Yates AJP, Gray RES, Hamdy NAT, Galloway J, Kanis JA (1988) Diphosphonates and phosphate homocostasis in man. Clin Sci 74:607–612

McCloskey EV, Paterson AHG, Powles T, Kanis JA (1990) Clodronate decreases the incidence of hypercalcaemia and major vertebral fractures in metastatic breast cancer. J Bone Miner Res 5(2):241

Meunier P, Chapuy MC, Courpron P, Vignon E, Edouard C, Bernard J (1975) Effects cliniques, biologiques et histologiques de l'éthane-1-hydroxy-1,1-diphosphonate (EHDP) dans la maladie de Paget. Rev Rhum Mal Osteoartic 42:699–705

Meunier PJ, Alexandre C, Edouard C, Mathieu L, Chapuy MC, Bressot C, Vignon E, Trechsel U (1979) Effects of disodium dichloromethylenediphosphonate on Paget's disease of bone. Lancet 2:489–492

Michael WR, King WR, Francis MD (1971) Effectiveness of diphosphonates in preventing "osteoporosis" of disuse in the rat. Clin Orthop 78:271–276

Michael WR, King WR, Wakim JM (1972) Metabolism of disodium ethane-1-hydroxy-1,1-diphosphonate (disodium etidronate) in the rat, rabbit, dog and monkey. Toxicol Appl Pharmacol 21:503–515

Milhaud G, Labat ML, Moricard Y (1983) (Dichloromethylene) diphosphonate-induced impairment of T-lymphocyte function. Proc Natl Acad Sci USA 80:4469–4473

Miller SC, Jee WSS (1979) The effect of dichloromethylene-diphosphonate, a pyrophosphate analog, on bone and bone cell structure in the growing rat. Anat Rec 193:439–462

Minaire P, Bérard E, Meunier PJ, Edouard C, Goedert G, Pilonchéry G (1981) Effects of disodium dichloromethylene diphosphonate on bone loss in paraplegic patients. J Clin Invest 68:1086–1092

Mönkkönen J (1988) A one year follow-up study of the distribution of ^{14}C-clodronate in mice and rats. Pharmacol Toxicol 62:51–53

Mönkkönen J, Ylitalo P (1990) The tissue distribution of clodronate (dichloromethylene bisphosphonate) in mice. The effects of vehicle and the route of administration. Eur J Drug Metab Pharmacokinet 15:239–294

Mönkkönen J, Ylitalo P, Elo HA, Airaksinen MM (1987) Distribution of ^{14}C-clodronate (dichloromethylene bisphosphonate) disodium in mice. Toxicol Appl Pharmacol 89:287–292

Mönkkönen J, Koponen HM, Ylitalo P (1989a) Comparison of the distribution of three bisphosphonates in mice. Pharmacol Toxicol 65:294–298

Mönkkönen J, Urtti A, Paronen P, Elo HA, Ylitalo P (1989b) The uptake of clodronate (dichloromethylene bisphosphonate) by macrophages in vivo and in vitro. Drug Metab Dispas 17:690–693

Morgan DB, Monod A, Russell RGG, Fleisch H (1973) Influence of dichloromethylene diphosphonate (Cl_2MDP) and calcitonin on bone resorption, lactate production and phosphatase and pyrophosphatase content of mouse calvaria treated with parathyroid hormone in vitro. Calcif Tissue Res 13:287–294

Morton AR, Cantrill JA, Craig AE, Howell A, Davies M, Anderson DC (1988) Single dose versus daily intravenous aminohydroxypropylidene bisphosphonate (APD) for the hypercalcaemia of malignancy. Br Med J 296:811–814

Mühlbauer RC, Russell RGG, Williams DA, Fleisch H (1971) The effects of diphosphonates, polyphosphonates, and calcitonin on immobilisation osteoporosis in rats. Eur J Clin Invest 1:336–344

Mühlbauer RC, Bauss F, Schenk R, Janner M, Bosies E, Strein K, Fleisch H (1991) BM 21.0955 A potent new bisphosphonate to inhibit bone resorption. J Bone Miner Res 6:1003–1011

Mühlemann HR, Bowles D, Schatt A, Bernimoulin JP (1970) Effect of diphosphonate on human supragingival calculus. Helv Odontol Acta 14:31–33

Nagant de Deuxchaisnes C, Rombouts-Lindemans C, Huaux JP, Malghem J, Madlague B (1979) Roentgenologic evaluation of the action of the diphosphonate EHDP and of combined therapy (EHDP and calcitonin) in Paget's disease of bone. Mol Endocrinol 1:405–433

Nagant de Deuxchaisnes C, Rombouts-Lindemans C, Huaux JP, Devogelaer JP, Malghem J, Madague B, Withofs H, Meersseman F (1981) Paget's disease of bone. Br Med J 283:1054–1055

Nemoto R, Uchida K, Tsutsumi M, Koiso K, Satou S, Satou T (1987) A model of localized osteolysis induced by the MBT-2 tumor in mice and its responsiveness to etidronate disodium. J Cancer Res Clin Oncol 113:539–543

Nilsson OS, Bauer HCF, Brosjö O, Törnkvist H (1990) Bone resorption in orthotopic and heterotopic bone of dichloromethylene bisphosphonate-treated rats. J Orthop Res 8:213–219

Nixon GA, Buehler EV, Newmann EA (1972) Preliminary safety assessment of disodium etidronate as an additive to experimental oral hygiene products. Toxicol Appl Pharmacol 22:661–671

Nolen GA, Buehler EV (1971) The effects of disodium etidronate on the reproductive functions and embryogeny of albino rats and New Zealand rabbits. Toxicol Appl Pharmacol 18:548–561

Nuti R, Righi G, Turchetti V, Vattimo A (1981) Etidronato sodico (EHDP) ed osteoporosi. Clin Ter 99:33–42

O'Doherty DP, Bickerstaff DR, McCloskey EV, Hamdy NAT, Beneton MNC, Harris S, Mian M, Kanis JA (1990) Treatment of Paget's disease of bone with aminohydroxybutylidene bisphosphonate. J Bone Miner Res 5(5):483–491

O'Donoghue DJ, Hosking DJ (1987) Biochemical response to combination of disodium etidronate with calcitonin in Paget's disease. Bone 8:219–225

Ogawa Y, Adachi Y, Hong S, Yagi T (1989) 1-Hydroxyethylidene-1,1-bisphosphonate (HEPB) simultaneously induces two distinct types of hypomineralization in the rat incisor dentine. Calcif Tissue Int 44:46–60

Ohata M, Pak CY (1974) Preliminary study of the treatment of nephrolithiasis (calcium stones) with diphosphonate. Metabolism 23:1167–1173

Ohya K, Yamada S, Felix R, Fleisch H (1985) Effect of bisphosphonates on prostaglandin synthesis by rat bone cells and mouse calvaria in culture. Clin Sci 69:403–411

Ostrowski K, Wojtowicz A, Dziedzic-Goclawska A, Rozycka M (1988) Effect of 1-hydroxyethylidene-1,1-bisphosphonate (HEBP) and dichloromethylidene-bisphosphonate (Cl_2MBP) on the structure of the organic matrix of heterotopically induced bone tissue. Histochemistry 88:207–212

Pacifici R, McMurtry C, Vered I, Rupich R, Avioli LV (1988) Coherence therapy does not prevent axial bone loss in osteoporotic women: a preliminary comparative study. J Clin Endocrinol Metab 88:747–753

Palmoski M, Brandt K (1978) Effects of diphosphonates on glycosaminoglycan synthesis and proteoglycan aggregation in normal adult articular cartilage. Arthritis Rheum 21:942–949

Papapoulos SE, Hoekman K, Löwik CWGM, Vermeij P, Bijvoet OLM (1989) Application of an in vitro model and a clinical protocol in the assessment of the potency of a new bisphosphonate. J Bone Miner Res 4(5):775–781

Paspaliaris V, Leaver DD (1990) The bisphosphonate, clodronate, inhibits calcium-induced contraction in vascular smooth muscle. Eur J Pharmacol 183:1257

Passeri M, Baroni MC, Pedrazzoni M, Pioli G, Barbagallo M, Costi D, Biondi M, Girasole G, Arlunnoo B, Palummeri E (1991) Intermittent treatment with intravenous 4-amino-1-hydroxybutylidene-1,1-bisphosphonate (AHBuBP) in the therapy of postmenopausal osteoporosis. Bone Min 15:237–248

Paterson AD, Kanis JSA, Cameron EC, Douglas DL, Beard DJ, Preston FE, Russell RGG (1983) The use of dichloromethylene diphosphonate for the management of hypercalcaemia in multiple myeloma. Br J Haematol 54:121–131

Pedrazzoni M, Palummeri E, Ciotti G, Davoli L, Pioli G, Girasole G, Passeri M (1989) Short-term effects on bone and mineral metabolism of 4-amino-1-hydroxybutylidene-1,1-diphosphonate (ABDP) in Paget's disease of bone. Bone Miner 7:301–307

Pilzyk R, Sutcliffe H, Martin TJ (1972) Effect of bisphosphonates on prostaglandin synthesis by rat bone cells and mouse calvaria in culture. Clin Sci 69:403–411

Plasmans CMT, Kuypers W, Slooff TJJH (1978) The effect of ethane-1-hydroxy-1,1-diphosphonic acid (EHDP) on matrix induced ectopic bone formation. Clin Orthop 132:233–243

Plasmans CMT, Jap PHK, Kujipers W, Slooff TJJH (1980) Influence of diphosphonate on the cellular aspect of young bone tissue. Calcif Tissue Int 32:247–256

Potsaid MS, Irwin RJ, Castronovo FP, Prout GR Jr, Harvey WJ, Francis MD, Tofe AJ, Zamenhof RG (1978) (^{32}P)Diphosphonate dose determination in patients with bone metastases from prostatic carcinoma. J Nucl Med 19:98–104

Preston CJ, Yates AJP, Beneton MNC, Russell RGG, Gray RES, Smith R, Kanis JA (1986) Effective short term treatment of Paget's disease with oral etidronate. Br Med J 292:79–80

Ralston SH, Alzaid AA, Gallacher SJ, Gardner MD, Cowan RA, Boyle IT (1988) Clinical experience with aminohydroxypropylidene bisphosphonate (APD) in the management of cancer-associated hypercalcaemia. Q J Med 81:258–266

Ralston SH, Hacking L, Willocks L, Bruce F, Pitkeathly DA (1989) Clinical, biochemical, and radiographic effects of aminohydroxypropylidene bisphosphonate treatment in rheumatoid arthritis. Ann Rheum Dis 48:396–399

Rastad J, Benson L, Johansson H, Knuutila M, Pettersson B, Wallfelt C, Akerstrom G, Ljunghall S (1987) Clodronate treatment in patients with malignancy-associated hypercalcemia. Acta Med Scand 221:489–494

Recker RR, Saville PD (1973) Intestinal absorption of disodium ethane-1-hydroxy-1,1-diphosphonate (disodium etidronate) using a deconvolution technique. Toxicol Appl Pharmacol 24:580–589

Recker RR, Hassing GS, Lau JR, Saville PD (1973) The hyperphosphatemic effect of disodium ethane-1-hydroxy-1,1-diphosphonates (EHDP™): renal handling of phosphorus and the renal response to parathyroid hormone. J Lab Clin Med 81:258–266

Reginster JY, Jeugmans-Huynen AM, Albert A, Denis D, Deroisy R, Lecart MP, Fontaine MA, Collette J, Franchimont P (1988) Biological and clinical assessment of a new bisphosphonate, (chloro-4 phenyl) thiomethylene bisphosphonate, in the treatment of Paget's disease of bone. Bone 9:349–354

Reginster JY, Lecart MP, Deroisy D, Sarlet N, Denis D, Collette J, Ethgen D, Franchimont P (1989) Prevention of postmenopausal bone loss by tiludronate. Lancet 2:1469–1471

Reid IR, Alexander CJ, King AR, Ibbertson HK (1988) Prevention of steroid-induced osteoporosis with (3-amino-1-hydroxypropylidene)-1,1-bisphosphonate (APD). Lancet 1:143–146

Reid IR, Schooler BA, Stewart AW (1990) Prevention of glucocorticoid-induced osteoporosis. J Bone Miner Res 5(6):619–623

Reiner M, Sautter V, Olah A, Bossi A, Largiadèr U, Fleisch H (1980) Diphosphonate treatment in myositis ossificans progressiva. In: Caniggia A (ed) Etidronate. Istituto Gentili, Pisa, p 237

Reitsma PH, Bijvoet OLM, Verlinden-Ooms H, van der Wee-Pals LJA (1980) Kinetic studies of bone and mineral metabolism during treatment with (3-amino-1-hydroxy-propylidene)-1,1-bisphosphonate (ADP) in rats. Calcif Tissue Int 32:145–147

Reitsma PH, Teitelbaum SL, Bijvoet OLM, Kahn AJ (1982) Differential action of the bisphosphonates (3-amino-1-hydroxypropylidene)-1,1-bisphosphonate (ADP) and disodium dichloromethylidene bisphosphonate (Cl_2MDP) on rat macrophage-mediated bone resorption in vitro. J Clin Invest 70:927–933

Reynolds JJ, Minkin C, Morgan DB, Spycher D, Fleisch H (1972) The effect of two diphosphonates on the resorption of mouse calvaria in vitro. Calcif Tissue Res 10:302–313

Reynolds JJ, Murphy H, Mühlbauer RC, Morgan DB, Fleisch H (1973) Inhibition by diphosphonates of bone resorption in mice and comparison with grey lethal osteopetrosis. Calcif Tissue Res 12:59–71

Rivero DP, Skipor AK, Singh M, Urban RM, Galante JO (1987) Effect of disodium etidronate (EHDP) on bone ingrowth in a porous material. Clin Orthop 215:279–286

Rizzoli R, Bonjour JP (1989) High extracellular calcium increases the production of a parathyroid hormone-like activity by cultured Leydig tumor cells associated with humoral hypercalcemia. J Bone Miner Res 4:839–844

Rizzoli R, Caverzasio J, Fleisch H, Bonjour JP (1986) Parathyroid hormone-like changes of renal calcium and phosphate reabsorption induced by Leydig cell tumor in thyroparathyroid-ectomized rats. Endocrinology 119:1004–1009

Robertson WG, Peacock M, Nordin BEC (1973) Inhibitors of the growth and aggregation of calcium oxalate crystals in vitro. Clin Chim Acta 43:31–37

Rosenblum IY, Black HE, Ferrell JF (1977) The effects of various diphosphonates on a rat model of cardiac calciphylaxis. Calcif Tissue Res 23:151–159

Rossier JR, Cox JA, Niesor EJ, Bentzen CL (1989) A new class of calcium entry blockers defined by 1,3-diphosphonates. J Biol Chem 264:16598–16607

Russell RGG, Mühlbauer RC, Bisaz S, Williams DA, Fleisch H (1970) The influence of pyrophosphate, condensed phosphates, phosphonates and other phosphate compounds on the dissolution of hydroxyapatite in vitro and on bone resorption induced by parathyroid hormone in tissue culture and in thyroparathyroidec-tomised rats. Calcif Tissue Res 6:183–196

Russell RGG, Preston C, Smith R, Walton RJ, Woods CG (1974) Diphosphonates in Paget's disease. Lancet 1:894–898

Ryzen E, Martodam RR, Troxell M, Benson A, Paterson A, Shepard K, Hicks R (1985) Intravenous etidronate in the management of malignant hypercalcemia. Arch Intern Med 145:449–452

Sahni M, Guenther HL, Collin P, Martin TJ, Fleisch H (1993) Bisphosphonates act on rat bone resorption through the mediation of osteoblasts. J Clin Invest (in press)

Sakiyama Y, Tada I, Yamamoto H, Nakanishi T, Yasuda Y, Soeda Y, Oda M (1985) The effect of ethane-1-hydroxy-1,1-diphosphonate (EHDP) on fetal mice during pregnancy: with emphasis on implantation and fetal weight. J Osaka Dent Univ 19:87–90

Sakiyama Y, Yamamoto H, Soeda Y, Tada I, Oda M, Nagasawa S, Ikeo T (1986) The effect of ethane-1-hydroxy-1,1-diphosphonate (EHDP) on fetal mice during pregnancy. II. Anomalies. J Osaka Dent Univ 20:91–100

Sato M, Grasser W (1990) Effects of bisphosphonates on isolated rat osteoclasts as examined by reflected light microscopy. J Bone Miner Res 5:31–40

Sato M, Grasser W, Endo N, Akins R, Simmons H, Thompson DD, Golub E, Rodan GA (1991) Bisphosphonate action. Alendronate localization in rat bone and effects of osteoclast ultrastructure. J Clin Invest 88:2095–2105

Schenk R, Merz WA, Mühlbauer R, Russell RGG, Fleisch H (1973) Effect of ethane-1-hydroxy-1,1-diphosphonate (EHDP) and dichloromethylene diphosphonate (Cl_2MDP) on the calcification and resorption of cartilage and bone in the tibial epiphysis and metaphysis of rats. Calcif Tissue Res 11:196–214

Schenk R, Eggli P, Felix R, Fleisch H, Rosini S (1986) Quantitative morphometric evaluation of the inhibitory activity of new aminobisphosphonates on bone resorption in the rat. Calcif Tissue Int 38:342–349

Schmidli RS, Wilson I, Espiner EA, Richards AM, Donald RA (1990) Aminopropylidene diphosphonate (APD) in mild primary hyperparathyroidism: effect on clinical status. Clin Endocrinol (Oxf) 32:293–300

Schneider VS, McDonald J (1984) Skeletal calcium homeostasis and countermeasures to prevent disuse osteoporosis. Calcif Tissue Int 36(1):151–154

Schoutens A, Verhas M, Dourov N, Bergmann P, Caulin F, Verschaeren A, Mone M, Heilporn A (1988) Bone loss and bone blood flow in paraplegic rats treated with calcitonin, diphosphonate, and indomethacin. Calcif Tissue Int 42:136–143

Shane E, Baquiran DC, Bilezikian JP (1981) Effect of dichloromethylene diphosphonate on serum and urinary calcium in primary hyperparathyroidism. Ann Intern Med 95:23–27

Shinoda H, Adamek G, Felix R, Fleisch H, Schenk R, Hagan P (1983) Structure-activity relationship of various bisphosphonates. Calcif Tissue Int 35:87–99

Shiota E (1985) Effects of diphosphonate on osteoporosis induced in rats. Roentgeneological, histological and biomechanical studies. Fukuoka Acta Med 76(6): 317–342

Singer FR, Ritch PS, Lad TE, Ringenberg QS, Schiller JH, Recker RR, Ryzen E (1991) Treatment of hypercalcemia of malignancy with intravenous etidronate. Arch Intern Med 151:471–476

Siris ES, Canfield RE, Jacobs TP, Baquiran DC (1980a) Long-term therapy of Paget's disease of bone with EHDP. Arthritis Rheum 23:1177–1183

Siris ES, Sherman WH, Baquiran DC, Schlatterer JP, Osserman EF, Canfield RE (1980b) Effects of dichloromethylene diphosphonate on skeletal mobilization of calcium in multiple myeloma. N Engl J Med 302:310–315

Sleeboom HP, Bijvoet OLM, van Oosterom AT, Gleed JH, O'Riordan JLH (1983) Comparison of intravenous (3-amino-1-hydroxypropylidene)-1,1-bisphosphonate and volume repletion in tumor-induced hypercalcemia. Lancet 2:239–243

Slooff TJJH, Feith R, Bijvoet OLM, Nollen AJG (1974) The use of a disphosphonate in para-articular ossification after total hip replacement. A clinical study. Acta Orthop Belg 40:820–828

Slough CL, Spinelli MJ, Kasting GB (1988) Transdermal delivery of etidronate (EHDP) in the pig via iontophoresis. J Membr Sci 35:161–165

Smith JA (1989) Pallation of painful bone metastases from prostate cancer using sodium etidronate: results of a randomized, prospective double-blind, placebo-controlled study. J Urol 141:85–87

Smith ML, Fogelman I, Hart DM, Scott E, Bevan J, Leggate I (1989) Effect of etidronate disodium on bone turnover following surgical menopause. Calcif Tissue Int 44:74–79

Smith R, Russell RGG, Bishop M (1971) Diphosphonates and Paget's disease of bone. Lancet 1:945–947

Smirnova IN, Kudryavtseva NA, Komissarenko SV, Tarusova NB, Baykov AA (1988) Diphosphonates are potent inhibitors of mammalian inorganic pyrophosphatase. Arch Biochem Biophys 267:280–284

Spielman G, Gennarelli TA, Rogers CR (1983) Disodium etidronate: its role in preventing heterotopic ossification in severe head injury. Arch Phys Med Rehabil 64:539–542

Steber J, Wierich P (1986) Properties of hydroxyethane disphosphonates affecting its environmental fate: degradability, sludge adsorption, mobility in soils, and bioconcentration. Chemosphere 15:929–945

Stevenson PH, Stevenson JR (1986) Cytotoxic and migration inhibitory effects of bisphosphonates on macrophages. Calcif Tissue Int 38:227–233

Stone MD, Hawthorne AB, Kerr D, Webster G, Hosking DJ (1990) Treatment of Paget's disease with intermittent low-dose infusions of disodium pamidronate (APD). J Bone Miner Res 5(12):1231–1235

Storm T, Thamsborg G, Steiniche T, Genant HK, Soerensen OH (1990) Effect of intermittent cyclical etidronate therapy on bone mass and fracture rate in women with postmenopausal osteoporosis. N Engl J Med 322(18):1265–1271

Stronski S, Bettschen-Camin L, Wetterwald A, Felix R, Trechsel U, Fleisch H (1988) Bisphosphonates inhibit 1,25-dihydroxyvitamin D3-induced increase of osteocalcin in plasma of rats in vivo and in culture medium of rat calvaria in vitro. Calcif Tissue Int 42:248–254

Stuart G, Wren C, Bain H (1990) Idiopathic infantile arterial calcification in two siblings: failure of treatment with diphosphonate. Br Heart J 64:156–159

Stutzer A, Fleisch H, Trechsel U (1988) Short- and long-term effects of a single dose of bisphosphonates on retinoid-induced bone resorption in thyroparathyroidectomized rats. Calcif Tissue Int 43:294–299

Talanian RV, Brown NC, McKenna CE, Ye TG, Levy JN, Wright GE (1989) Carbonyldiphosphonate, a selective inhibitor of mammalian DNA polymerase. Biochemistry 28:8270–8274

Tan PLJ, Ames R, Yeoman S, Ibbertson HK, Caughey DE (1989) Effects of aminobisphosphonate infusion on biochemical indices of bone metabolism in rheumatoid arthritis. Br J Rheum 28:325–328

Tan TT, Alzaid AA, Sutcliffe N, Gardner MD, Thomson JA, Boyle IT (1988) Treatment of hypercalcaemia in thyrotoxicosis with aminohydroxypropylidene diphosphonate. Postgrad Med J 64:224–227

Thepen T, van Rooijen N, Kraal G (1989) Alveolar macrophage elimination in vivo is associated with an increase in pulmonary immune response in mice. J Exp Med 170:499–509

Thiébaud D, Jaeger P, Jacquet AF, Burckhardt P (1986a) A single-day treatment of tumor-induced hypercalcemia by intravenous amino-hydroxypropylidene bisphosphonate. J Bone Miner Res 1:555–562

Thiébaud D, Portmann L, Jaeger PH, Jacquet AF, Burckhaardt P (1986b) Oral versus intravenous AHPrBP (APD) in the treatment of hypercalcemia of malignancy. Bone 7:247–253

Thiébaud D, Jaeger P, Burckhardt P (1987) Paget's disease of bone treated in five days with AHPrBP (APD) per os. J Bone Miner Res 2(1):45–52

Thiébaud D, Jaeger P, Jacquet AF, Burckhardt P (1988a) Dose-response in the treatment of hypercalcemia of malignancy by a single infusion of the bisphosphonate AHPrBP. J Clin Oncol 6:762–768

Thiébaud D, Jaeger P, Gobelet C, Jacquet AF, Burckhardt P (1988b) A single infusion of the bisphosphonate AHPrBP (APD) as treatment of Paget's disease of bone. Am J Med 85:207–212

Thiébaud D, Jacquet AF, Burckhard P (1990a) Fast and effective treatment of malignant hypercalcemia: combination of suppositories of calcitonin and a single infusion of 3-amino 1-hydroxypropylidene-1-bisphosphonate. Arch Intern Med 150:2125–2128

Thiébaud D, Jaeger P, Burckhardt P (1990b) Response to retreatment of malignant hypercalcemia with the bisphosphonate AHPrBP (ABD): respective role of kidney and bone. J Bone Miner Res 5:221–226

Thiébaud D, Leyvraz S, von Fliedner V, Perey L, Cornu P, Thiébaud S, Burckhardt P (1991) Treatment of bone metastases from breast cancer and myeloma with pamidronate. Eur J Cancer 27:37–41

Thomas BJ, Amstutz HC (1985) Results of the administration of diphosphonate for the prevention of heterotopic ossification after total hip arthroplasty. J Bone Joint Surg [Am] 67:400–403

Thompson DD, Seedor JG, Quartuccio H, Solomon H, Fioravanti C, Davidson J, Klein H, Jackson R, Clair J, Frankenfield D, Brown E, Simmons HA, Rodan GA (1992) The bisphosphonate, alendronate, prevents bone loss in ovariectomized baboons. J Bone Min Res 7:951–960

Trechsel U, Schenk R, Bonjour JP, Russell RGG, Fleisch H (1977) Relation between bone mineralization. Ca absorption, and plasma Ca in phosphonate-treated rats. Am J Physiol 232:E298–E305

Trechsel U, Stutzer A, Fleisch H (1987) Hypercalcemia induced with an arotinoid in thyroparathyroidectomized rats. A new model to study bone resorption in vivo. J Clin Invest 80:1679–1686

Troehler U, Bonjour JP, Fleisch H (1975) Renal secretion of diphosphonates in rats. Kidney Int 8:6–13

Troehler U, Bonjour JP, Fleisch H (1982) Interference of dichloromethylene diphosphonate with parathyroid hormone effects at the bone but not at the kidney level. Miner Electrolyte Metab 7:122–126

Urwin GH, Yates AJP, Gray Res, Hamdy NAT, McCloskey EV, Preston FE, Greaves M, Neil FE, Kanis JA (1987) Treatment of the hypercalcaemia of malignancy with intravenous clodronate. Bone 8(1):43–51

Valkema R, Vismans F-JFE, Papapoulos SE, Pauwels EKJ, Bijvoet OLM (1989) Maintained improvement in calcium balance and bone mineral content in patients with osteoporosis treated with the bisphosphonate APD. Bone Miner 5:183–192

Van Breukelen FJM, Bijvoet OLM, von Oosterom AT (1979) Inhibition of osteolytic bone lesions by (3-amino-1-hydroxypropylidene)-1,1-bisphosphonate (A.P.D.). Lancet 1:803–805

Van Breukelen FJM, Bijvoet OLM, Frijlink WB, Sleebloom HP, Mulder H, von Oosterom AT (1982) Efficacy of amino-hydroxypropylidene bisphosphonate in hypercalcemia: observations on regulation of serum calcium. Calcif Tissue Int 34:321–327

Van den Bos T, Beertsen W (1987) Effects of 1-hydroxyethylidene-1,1-bisphosphonate (HEBP) on the synthesis of dentine matrix proteins in the mouse. Coll Relat Res 7:135–147

Van Holten-Verzantvoort AT, Bijvoet OLM, Cleton FJ, Hermans J, Kroon DM, Harinck HIJ, Vermey P, Elte JWF, Neijt JP, Beex LVAM, Blijham G (1987) Reduced morbidity from skeletal metastases in breast cancer patients during long-term bisphosphonate (APD) treatment. Lancet 2:983–985

Van Hoogdalem EJ, Wackwitz ATE, de Boer AG, Breimer DD (1989) 3-Amino-1-hydroxypropylidene-1,1-diphosphonate (APD): a novel enhancer of rectal cefoxitin absorption in rats. J Pharm Pharmacol 41:339–341

Van Rooijen N, Kors N (1989) Effects of intracellular diphosphonates on cells of the mononuclear phagocyte system: in vivo effects of liposome-encapsulated diphosphonates on different macrophage subpopulations in the spleen. Calcif Tissue Int 45:153–156

Van Rooijen N, van Nieuwmegen R (1984) Elimination of phagocytic cells in the spleen after intravenous injection of liposome-encapsulated dichloromethylene diphosphonate: an enzyme-histochemical study. Cell Tissue Res 238:355–358

Van Rooijen N, Kors N, van den Ende M, Dijkstra CD (1990) Depletion and repopulation of macrophages in spleen and liver of rat after intravenous treatment with liposome-encapsulated dichloromethylene diphosphonate. Cell Tissue Res 260:215–222

Walton RJ, Russell RGG, Smith R (1975) Changes in the renal and extrarenal handling of phosphate induced by disodium etidronate (EHDP) in man. J Clin Sci Mol Med 49:45–56

Wasserman RH, Bonjour JP, Fleisch H (1973) Ileal absorption of disodium ethane-1-hydroxy-1,1-diphosphonate (EHDP) and disodium dichloromethylene diphosphonate (Cl$_2$MDP) in the chick. Experientia 29:1110–1111

Watts NB, Harris ST, Genant HK, Wasnick RD, Miller PD, Jackson RD, Licata AA, Ross P, Woodson G, Yanover MJ, Mysiw WJ, Kohse L, Rao MB, Steiger P, Richmond B, Chesnut CH (1990) Intermittent cyclical etidronate treatment of postmenopausal osteoporosis. N Engl J Med 323(2):73–79

Webb CL, Benedict JJ, Schoen FJ, Linden JA, Levy RJ (1987) Inhibition of bioprosthetic heart valve calcification with covalently bound aminopropanehydroxy-diphosphonate. Trans Am Soc Artif Intern Organs 33:592–595

Wiedmer WH, Zbinden AM, Trechsel U, Fleisch H (1983) Ultrafiltrability and chromatographic properties of pyrophosphate, 1-hydroxyethylidene-1,1-bisphosphonate, and dichloromethylenebisphosphonate in aqueous buffers and in human plasma. Calcif Tissue Int 35:397–400

Wingen F, Schmähl D (1985) Distribution of 3-amino-1-hydroxypropane-1,1-diphosphonic acid in rats and effects on rat osteosarcoma. Arzneimittelforsching 35:1565–1571

Wingen F, Eichmann T, Manegold C, Krempien B (1986) Effects of new bisphosphonic acids on tumor-induced bone destruction in the rat. J Cancer REs Clin Oncol 111:35–41

Wink CS, Hill EM (1988) Dichloromethylene bisphosphonate retards femoral expansion in normal and castrated adult male rats. Acta Anat (Basel) 132:321–323

Wink CS, Onge MS, Parker B (1985) The effects of dichloromethylene bisphosphonate on osteoporotic femora of adult castrate male rats. Acta Anat 124:117–121

Wronski TJ, Dann LM, Scott KS, Crooke LR (1989) Endocrine and pharmacological suppressors of bone turnover protect against osteopenia in ovariectomized rats. Endocrinology 125:810–816

Wüster C, Scharla SH, Schmidt J, Ziegler R (1990) Efficacy and safety of BM 21.0955, a new bisphosphonate in patients with humoral hypercalcemia of malignancy. J Bone Miner Res 5(2):102

Yakatan GJ, Poynor WJ, Talbert RL, Floyd BF, Slough CL, Ampulski RS, Benedict JJ (1982) Clodronate kinetics and bioavailability. Clin Pharmacol Ther 31:402–410

Yap AS, Hockings GI, Fleming SJ, Khafagi FA (1990) Use of aminohydroxy-propylidene bisphosphonate (AHPrBP, "APD") for the treatment of hypercalcemia in patients with renal impairment. Clin Nephrol 34:225–229

Yates AJP, Jones TJ, Mundy KI, Hague RV, Brown CB, Guilland-Cumming D, Kanis JA (1984) Immobilisation hypercalcaemia in adults and treatment with clodronate. Br Med J 289:1111–1112

Yates AJP, Percival RC, Gray RES, Urwin GH, Hamdy NAT, Preston CJ, Beneton MNC, Russell RGG, Kanis JA (1985) Intravenous clodronate in the treatment and retreatment of Paget's disease of bone. Lancet 1:1474–1477

Yates AJP, Murray RML, Jerums GJ, Martin TJ (1987) A comparison of single and multiple intravenous infusions of 3-amino-1-hydroxypropylidene-1,1-bisphosphonate (APD) in the treatment of hypercalcemia of malignancy. Aust N Z J Med 17:387–391

CHAPTER 12

Paget's Disease

D.C. ANDERSON

A. Introduction

Paget's disease is a chronic focal slowly progressive bone disease of unknown aetiology. The first clear description of the disorder was made in 1877 by the London surgeon Sir James PAGET (1877), who coined the name "osteitis deformans", although others had described the condition earlier (WILKS 1860; CZERNY 1873). PAGET of course described what we would now recognise as very extensive and long-standing disease (Fig. 1); and circumstantial evidence suggests that cases such as his index case with gross bony deformities and skull expansion exhibit the end result of 50 or more years of disease. Since the cause of the disease is still not established, it is possible that some of the clinical variability is due to host response to the aetiological agent(s), and some is due to involvement of more than one (closely related) agent; it is to be hoped that the next few years will, with the application of powerful molecular biology techniques, see the resolution of these issues.

Fortunately for patients, in recent years there have been major advances in the treatment, first with the advent of calcitonin and more recently with the development of a range of drugs of the bisphosphonate class. It is highly likely that a substantial fraction of patients can be cured if the latter drugs are used in the optimal way.

B. Nature of the Underlying Disease Process

There is a great deal of circumstantial evidence to indicate that the primary abnormality in Paget's disease lies in the structure and function of the osteoclast. First, both the number and size of osteoclasts in affected bones are greatly increased in affected but not in unaffected bones of the same patient. Their morphology is abnormal also by virtue of their containing inclusion bodies visible on electron microscopy, which consist of arrays of fibrils suggestive of viral nucleocapsids (REBEL et al. 1987; MILLS and SINGER 1976) (Fig. 2). This led to the suggestion that the disease might be caused by a persistent infection of the osteoclast by a paramyxovirus. A third strand of evidence is that not infrequently the progression of the disease can be observed through a bone – and it consists of a lytic leading edge visible radiologically and marked histologically by an advancing front of bone-

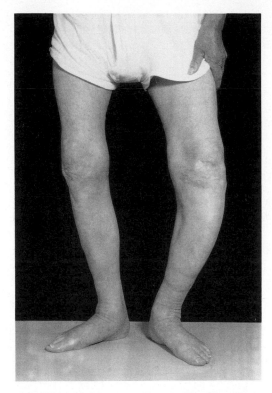

Fig. 1. A patient with advanced Paget's disease affecting the left femur and tibia, with gross bowing and expansion

resorbing osteoclasts with the typical abnormal morphology. Typically, this moves at a rate of about 1 cm/year. Behind this advancing front of osteoclasts, bone becomes progressively remodelled over time, with osteoblastic activity locally accelerated to keep pace with that of the abnormal osteoclasts. Our most effective agents against the disease appear to attack osteoclasts or at least to inhibit bone resorption, and once this is suppressed bone formation appears to return to normal progressively over a few months.

C. Epidemiology

Epidemiological studies have pointed to wide disparities in the incidence of Paget's disease in different parts of the world. Some of this variation may be racial or genetic, but family and other studies suggest that the major explanation is environmental. Across western Europe, despite relative genetic homogeneity of the population the incidence of the disease varies at least 20-fold. The best evidence comes from studies of BARKER and colleagues (BARKER et al. 1980; DETHERIDGE et al. 1982), and was based on studies of

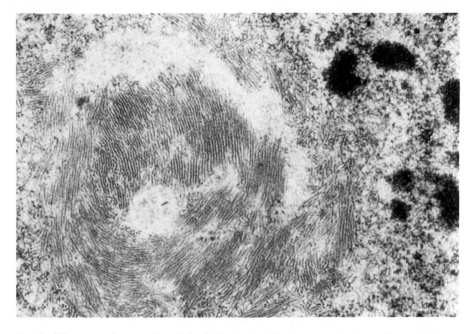

Fig. 2. Electron micrographs of the inclusion bodies in a pagetic osteoclast; evidence to suggest the involvement of a paramyxovirus. (Courtesy of Barbara Mills)

plain X-rays of the abdomen and pelvis taken from X-ray archives (plain X-rays associated with barium studies and intravenous pyelograms). These studies reveal that the highest incidence is in parts of the Northwest of Britain, where in some towns as much as 8%–10% of the elderly population (aged over 55 years) have Paget's disease. There is a fourfold variation in incidence in Britain, with levels varying even more widely across Europe and being as low as 0.5% or less in Sweden and Greece (Figs. 3, 4). Elsewhere in the world, moderately high levels are seen in Australia, New Zealand, and the northern United States. There is a focus of high disease incidence in Argentina in the plain around Buenos Aires, and mainly in whites of European extraction. In the United States, the incidence in whites and blacks appears to be similar. The disease is virtually unheard of in Japan, and infrequent in China.

Family studies indicate that someone with a first-degree relative with Paget's disease has about a five times greater than average chance of having Paget's disease themselves – the disease does not, however, follow Mendelian laws of inheritance, and the pattern within families is felt to be compatible with common exposure to a causative agent.

An exception to this generalisation may be the form of Paget's disease seen in Avellino in Italy and in emigrés from there; in contrast to "normal" Paget's disease, the affected individuals have a high incidence of osteo-

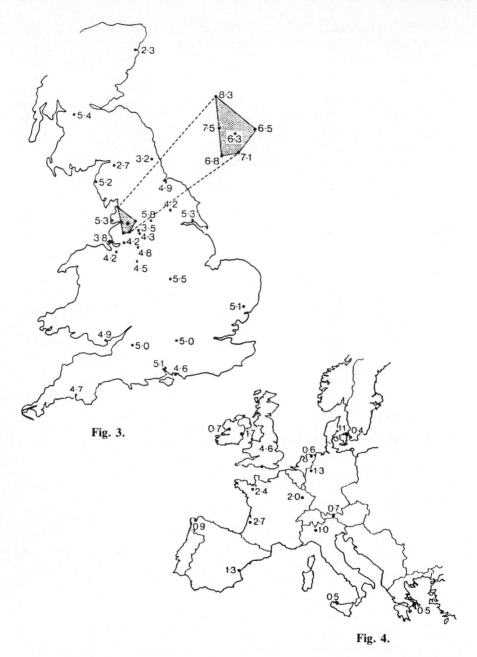

Fig. 3.

Fig. 4.

Fig. 3. Percentages of patients aged 55 years or more with radiological Paget's disease on an X-ray of pelvis, lumbosacral spine and femoral heads, in 31 British towns. (BARKER et al. 1980)

Fig. 4. Percentages of patients aged 55 years or more with Paget's disease in different parts of Europe. (DETHERIDGE et al. 1982)

clastomas, which are generally rare tumours to complicate Paget's disease (JACOBS et al. 1979). In Northern Ireland, there is an extensive family with an osteolytic bone condition termed familial expansile osteolysis (FEO), which appears to be inherited as an autosomal dominant condition. This is associated with generalised osteolysis of long bones, and finally the development of focal painful lesions which resemble those of Paget's (OSTERBERG et al. 1988). The inclusion bodies typical of Paget's disease have been described in the osteoclasts of such lesions.

D. Direct Studies on the Etiology of Paget's Disease

Several studies have examined for viral antigens using poly- or monoclonal antibodies directed against a number of paramyxoviruses – measles, respiratory syncytial virus, simian virus 5, and parainfluenza virus 3 have all been reported as positive (REBEL et al. 1980; MILLS et al. 1984). In retrospect, these studies are of uncertain significance – immunocytochemistry on bone is difficult to conduct and the potential for false positives (and negatives) is considerable. One study using DNA probes to the nucleocapsid protein of measles labelled by nick-translation showed positive in situ hybridisation (BASLÉ et al. 1986); however, our group was unable to confirm this in 25 cases of Paget's disease using a (much more specific) RNA probe (GORDON et al. 1991); we likewise found no evidence for respiratory syncytial virus or simian virus 5 in smaller numbers of cases using specific RNA probes.

E. Possible Role of Canine Distemper Virus

Our own group has obtained evidence in two case control studies (O'DRISCOLL and ANDERSON 1985; O'DRISCOLL et al. 1990) to suggest that in the northwest of England patients with Paget's disease have a significantly higher rate of recalled domestic exposure to dogs than do age- and sex-matched control subjects. These differences are most marked for decades from 30–60 years before present. These findings, which have been essentially confirmed in one study from New Zealand (HOLDAWAY et al. 1990) (but not others), suggested to us that the disease might be caused by a canine virus, and canine distemper seemed the most obvious candidate in view of its close relationship to measles.

We have so far examined biopsied bone from 42 cases of Paget's disease and find evidence by in situ hybridisation for CDV viral sequences in about half the cases studied (Figs. 5, 6). Several findings suggest that this is of relevance and not due to artefacts.

1. The antisense probes (which hybridise with messenger RNA) used are of high specificity, and associated with appropriate positive and negative controls. Sense probes, in contrast, have been consistently negative.

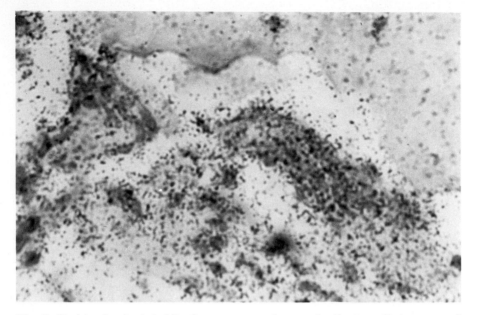

Fig. 5. Positive in situ hybridisation over osteoclasts and adjacent cells in a case of Paget's disease, using an ^{35}S-labelled probe to canine distemper virus messenger RNA. (GORDON et al. 1991)

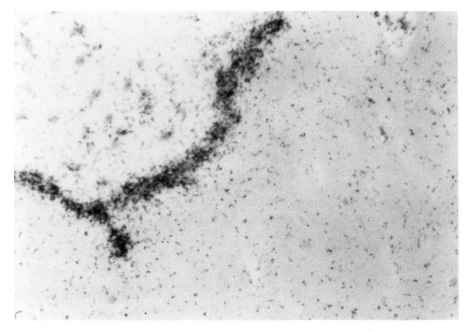

Fig. 6. As for Fig. 4, showing strong hybridisation in a line of osteoblasts. (GORDON et al. 1991)

2. Measles is consistently negative with both sense and antisense probes to nucleocapsid mRNA.
3. There is internal consistency observed when probes to three different genes were examined – the same individuals positive with a probe to nucleocapsid mRNA were positive to the fusion protein mRNA. In a subgroup there was likewise consistency between those positive for nucleocapsid and p-protein genes (unpublished).

Interestingly, our group has recently found convincing evidence that the virus message is present in abundance in osteoclasts of dogs with active CDV infection (MEE et al. 1992); however, here there is evidence for similar amounts of signal to genomic and messenger RNA. In Paget's bone, only messenger RNA (with antisense probe) was detected, pointing to much greater abundance of messenger than genomic RNA.

Finally, we have recently been successful in detecting CDV RNA in bone by the polymerase chain reaction (PCR) technique. Clearly the role of paramyxoviruses is still subjudice, and indeed it is quite possible that more than one virus is involved – perhaps two paramyxoviruses are required; of which one may be CDV.

F. Properties of the Osteoclast That Might Make It Particularly Susceptible to Persistent Infection with an RNA Virus

As discussed elsewhere (Chap. 3), the osteoclast is a highly specialised multinuclear cell formed by fusion of precursor cells of haemopoietic origin. It possesses a sealing ring (the clear zone), enclosing the so-called ruffled border through which protons and enzymes are extruded. Bone is attacked therefore by acid (pH 4) to dissolve the hydroxyapatite mineral phase, and by proteolytic enzymes to dissolve the collagenous matrix. Osteoclasts normally "hunt in packs" and once bone resorption has started in one area of bone there is evidence to suggest that there is a feed-ahead process. In cortical bone a tunnel is cut out by an advancing phalanx of osteoclasts, followed by osteoblast precursors which proliferate and differentiate into osteoblasts which eventually fill in the space to form an haversian system. It appears highly likely that osteoclastic bone resorption leads to local recruitment and/or replication of the osteoclast precursor. The bone-resorbing osteoclast may produce growth factors which promote local replication of both osteoclast and osteoblast precursors.

If paramyxoviruses are involved, the most obvious relevant new property that they might confer on the cells they infect is that they make them fuse, since they each code for a fusion protein which is incorporated in the cell membrane. Our simplest hypothetical model is illustrated in Fig. 7. The suggestion is that the fusion protein, expressed in the osteoclast, would alter

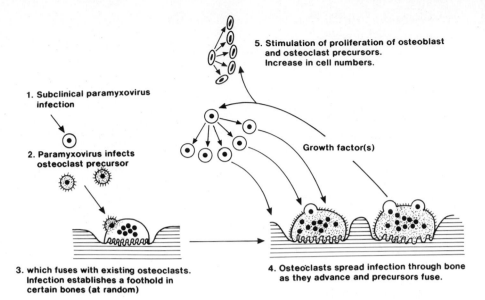

1. Subclinical paramyxovirus infection

2. Paramyxovirus infects osteoclast precursor

3. which fuses with existing osteoclasts. Infection establishes a foothold in certain bones (at random)

4. Osteoclasts spread infection through bone as they advance and precursors fuse.

5. Stimulation of proliferation of osteoblast and osteoclast precursors. Increase in cell numbers.

Growth factor(s)

Fig. 7. Hypothetical model of how a persistent paramyxovirus infection might lead to Paget's disease; the "spikes" on the cell surface depict the viral fusion protein which we postulate to enhance fusion, and alter the properties of the osteoclasts; increased production of a growth factor(s) would enhance proliferation of both osteoclast and osteoblast precursors

its properties in such a way as to promote replication, recruitment and fusion of its own precursors. Once established in a given area of bone the disease might be expected to spread outwards radially, as the osteoclasts resorb bone. All osteoclasts behind the leading edge of disease would be affected, and would transmit the virus to the cytoplasm of precursors as these fused with them. The process would spread provided that large osteoclasts can separate again into smaller units.

One of the surprising findings in our study is that canine distemper virus probes hybridise with osteoblasts and osteocytes as well as osteoclasts in pagetic bone; this suggests that although they appear to behave normally these cells may also be involved in persistence of the virus in infected bone. In their natural hosts, it is evident that CDV and measles virus replicate best in rapidly dividing cells, and as close contact occurs between osteoclasts and stromal cells it seems possible that the virus is transmitted from one cell type to another.

It seems likely that the next few years will see further advances in understanding of the role of CDV and/or other paramyxoviruses in Paget's disease, and that such studies will also throw more light on the nature of cell-cell communication between osteoclasts and bone-forming cells.

G. Clinical Features

Nothing is known of the initial onset of Paget's disease – whether for example it is associated with a flu-like or gastrointestinal illness. This situation will remain until the causative agent is discovered.

It is evident from the extent of bony involvement at presentation and from observations of the rate of spread of the disease through bone (about 1 cm/year) that there is in most cases a very long silent interval before the patient presents with the disease. Indeed the vast majority of affected individuals never present, and may have no symptoms of the disease. When symptoms do develop, they vary enormously in nature and severity, depending presumably upon the extent and duration of disease, the host response to it, and its precise location. Contrary to dogma, we have seen evidence on bone scan of new lesions appearing in patients with advanced disease, though this appears to be relatively uncommon.

I. Bones Affected and Extent

Any bone in the body may be involved in Paget's disease, although it is seldom seen in very small bones such as the phalanges and the carpal bones. This can be explained if the disease starts as single foci in one or more bones at one point in time. The chances of the disease taking hold may be a function of the initial infective dose of virus, the number of active osteoclasts in a given bone at the time of infection (a property determined partly by the total mass of the individual bone) and by the extent of bone resorption within it. The disease appears to be distributed at random in any individual case. Bones that are commonly affected are the pelvis, skull and vertebrae and the large long bones of the lower and upper limbs, notably femora, tibiae, humerus and radius. Less commonly involved are the ulna, fibula, clavicles, ribs, mandible, patella, facial bones, and bones of the hands and feet. If one bone is shown to be affected, there is a two in three chance of a second also being affected; and so on up to six or seven bones (Harinck et al. 1986); this probably does not hold for more extensive disease.

The disease appears to start at one or other end of a long bone, and seldom in the middle; presumably it starts at the epiphyseal plate where osteoclasts are most active; it is clearly the case that in canine distemper in the dog the virus replicates most actively at the epiphyseal plate (MEE et al. 1992).

The disease does not appear to "leap across" cartilaginous joints, and may be arrested at fibrous joints – as for example the sacroiliac joints and occasionally the sutures of the skull. In the skull it will usually spread also to the bones of the upper face; and sometimes it is evident that it is most severe in the maxilla or zygoma, and appears to have started there.

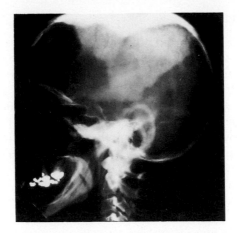

Fig. 8. Osteoporosis circumscripta of the skull

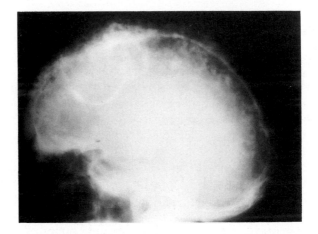

Fig. 9. Paget's disease of the skull with massive new bone proliferation

II. Symptoms and Signs

These, as expected, vary enormously. The process is initially one of bone resorption, followed by secondary bone formation. This seems to vary markedly in extent between cases. Thus one occasionally sees a patient with osteoporosis circumscripta of the skull, and little if any sign of new bone formation (Fig. 8). In other cases, in all bones affected it is evident that there is an enormous amount of new bone formed (Fig. 9), and the predominant impression is of severe osteosclerosis, and massive bone proliferation.

1. Features Due to Long-standing Excessive Bony Remodeling

Turnover in affected bones is increased 20-fold or more. Bone that is replaced becomes progressively more abnormal in macroscopic and micro-scopic form. The histopathology is discussed below. Over many years the macroscopic form of the bone changes, depending among other things on the stresses to which it is subjected. The tibia becomes particularly obviously deformed, with expansion and forward bowing (Fig. 1), which is most marked at the end where the disease has clearly been longest active (i.e. away from the leading edge). When this process is advanced, incremental fractures may develop, located characteristically on the inner aspect of the outermost cortex of the bone. These are virtually only seen in the tibia and the femur (Fig. 10), and normally more than one is "stacked up" in an array along the bone, and at right angles to the cortex.

There are some other bones that are subject to characteristic deformities when the disease is extensive. These include the skull, which becomes expanded, sometimes generally and sometimes focally giving rise to a "bumpy skull" (Fig. 9). Increase in hat size was one of the complaints of Sir James Paget's index case. It is also subject to characteristic deformity, the

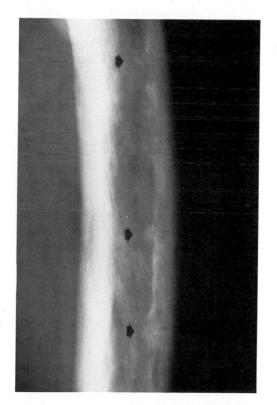

Fig. 10. Paget's disease of femur with typical incremental fractures (*arrows*)

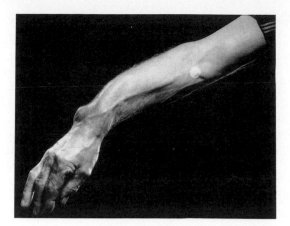

Fig. 11. Paget's disease of the radius showing typical expansion and deformity

base collapsing progressively onto the vertebral column, giving an appearance of "platybasia" and basilar invagination.

The radius when affected becomes expanded and bent, rotational forces presumably leading to remodelling such that it eventually becomes fixed in pronation (Fig. 11). Not infrequently, other bones become obviously expanded in patients in whom the disease is associated with production of a lot of new bone. In the vertebral column, there is often a combination of expansion and compression of a (sclerotic) bone. In the pelvis, long-standing disease may be associated with inward bulging of the acetabulum.

2. Features Due to Secondary Arthritis

Where Paget's disease affects a bone adjacent to a joint this is commonly associated with secondary osteoarthritis. Doubtless this is in part due to the adverse effects of increased vascularity on articular cartilage. Vascularity makes joint replacements bloody and hazardous procedures in the face of active disease.

3. Features Due to Pressure on Surrounding Structures

The principal structures involved are nerves, nerve roots and the drainage system of cerebrospinal fluid. Root pain is common with vertebral involvement. Deafness is particularly common with involvement of the skull, and is in part due to damage to the VIIIth nerve, and in part to damage to the ossicles. Pressure on the optic nerves is, fortunately, less common. Severe platybasia may lead to obstruction at the level of the fourth ventricle, with internal hydrocephalus, which may be the cause of severe headache. Fortunately this is an uncommon complication, even when the skull is extensively involved.

Pressure on the spinal cord is occasionally seen, with involvement of one or more vertebral bodies; since this may respond to effective treatment it seems probable that some of the damage results from soft tissue swelling due to increased vascularity of the bone surrounding the spinal cord, and some probably from diversion of blood supply from the cord.

4. Neoplasia

Paget's disease is associated with an increased incidence of osteogenic sarcoma, and a number of other sarcomas such as fibrosarcoma and malignant histiocytic fibrosarcoma. These are presumably the consequence of dramatically increased cell division in the stromal cell lines in active disease, since increased cell division and turnover in general predisposes to mutations and translocations necessary for malignant transformation. Nevertheless, less than 1% of cases develop tumours. Osteoclastomas are also increased in incidence (though they are thought not to be tumours of the osteoclasts, but rather stromal cell tumours invaded by normal (or at least non-neoplastic) osteoclasts).

H. Histopathology (Figs. 12, 13)

Most information results from examination of transiliac bone biopsies. The bone cells show evidence of greatly excessive number and activity, with osteoclasts much larger than normal, more numerous (by a factor of 200 or more) and apparently engaged in totally uncontrolled resorption of bone and sometimes even unmineralised bone matrix. There are also greatly increased numbers of active osteoblasts, covering 20%–40% of bone surfaces, and marrow fibrosis which seems to accompany any cause of increased osteoclasis. The bone matrix itself consists of a mosaic of connected "islands", each the residue of a wave of bone formation and subsequent bone resorption. These islands are demarcated by cement lines marking the reversal phase; the bone itself consists of some true woven bone with rounded osteocytes in the lacunae, and some lamellar bone. The osteoblasts appear to commence by filling in holes with woven bone, and finish the process with layers of lamellar bone; with effective bisphosphonate treatment they make apparently completely normal lamellar bone. The iliac bone, as with other bones affected, may become greatly expanded, a process which involves formation of increasing amounts of periosteal new bone – primary lamellar bone laid down by periosteal osteoblasts; not infrequently islands of such bone are found "buried" deep in the biopsy (RICHARDSON et al. 1990).

I. Clinical Assessment and Investigation

Clinical examination can only generally reveal the presence of advanced disease. *Bone scans*, conducted by gamma camera imaging of the skeleton

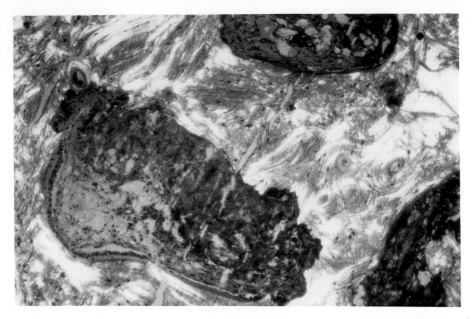

Fig. 12. Bone biopsy, stained with haematoxylin and eosin, and viewed under polarised light. Note typical mixture of mosaics containing woven and chopped up lamellar bone, irregular resorption surfaces containing osteoclasts, and other surfaces with active osteoblasts laying down bone (*bottom left*)

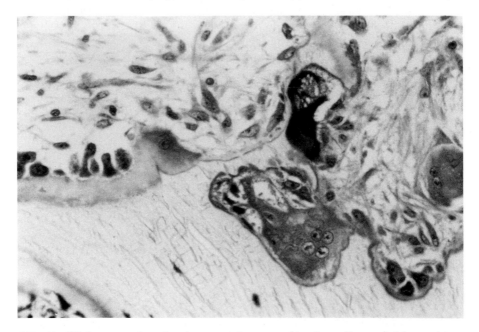

Fig. 13. High-power view showing osteoclasts resorbing bone (*lower right*) osteoblasts (*middle left*) and marrow fibrosis

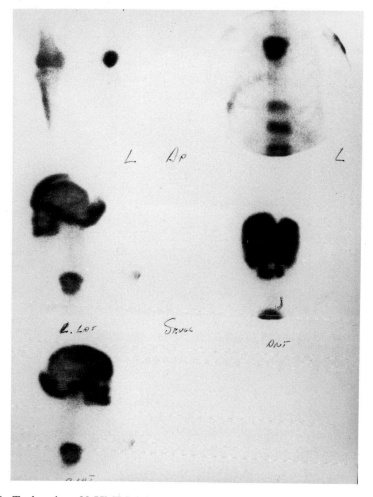

Fig. 14. Technetium-99 HMDP labelled bone scan images of patient showing Paget's disease (osteoporosis circumscripta) of skull, and disease also in right femur and tibia, left patella, manubrium sterni, a rib and several vertebrae

after injection of ^{99}Tc-labelled bisphosphonates, are generally highly reliable in revealing the extent and location of bone involvement (Fig. 14); although occasionally on bone scan Paget's disease may be confused with other bone diseases, the focal nature, combined with relatively uniform uptake of radioisotope through much or all of the bone (depending upon the duration of disease at the time of presentation), is generally diagnostic.

Radiology of bones demonstrated to be involved on bone scan is helpful; early in the disease, and at the leading edge of advance of the disease, there is generally a lytic "front" (Fig. 15), behind which there is increasing thickening of the bone, distortion, and loss of normal architecture. In the

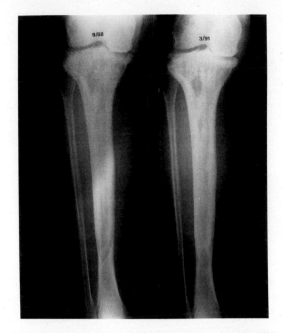

Fig. 15. V-shaped lytic front of advancing Paget's disease in the tibia; during the 2½ years between the two X-rays one course of etidronate had been given which may have showed the advance of the disease. Lytic clefts are seen over the proximal tibia

skull there are sometimes extensive areas of radiolucency – so-called osteoporosis circumscripta (Fig. 8). In other bones, a radiolucent appearance is generally confined either to the advancing edge of disease, or to focal areas generally within the cortex – the so-called lytic clefts. These lytic areas, which are associated with greatly increased uptake on bone scan, are particularly informative markers of the response to treatment with osteoclast-inhibiting agents (see below). A further important radiological feature which is seen in weight-bearing long bones are "incremental fractures", discussed above. They are presumably caused by stress caused by tension transmitted along their cortex of the bone, coupled with the disturbed microarchitecture (see below).

Finally, a fortunately infrequent development is of malignant transformation in pagetic bone. Tumours are usually sarcomas, and may be osteogenic, or non-osteogenic (see above under "neoplasia".)

Biochemistry: The mainstay of biochemical assessment of disease activity is the serum alkaline phosphatase, a crude marker of osteoblastic function. Broadly, this correlates with a product of disease extent and activity. As expected, it varies in its value as a marker of activity of Paget's disease, being highly informative in extensive disease ("mega-Paget's") and uninformative when, for example, only a single vertebra is involved. It is likely that the osteoblasts function normally although with greatly increased activity, so this is an indirect marker of the primary abnormality (in the osteoclasts).

A more direct marker of bone resorption is the urinary hydroxyproline, a measure of the breakdown of collagen; this is best measured on a fasting morning sample expressed as a ratio to creatinine; this is practical and also minimises the effect of variations in dietary intake of collagen or gelatin. More specific markers of type I collagen breakdown are now being used – these depend upon the fact that collagen fibres become covalently linked, forming pyridinium cross-links; when collagen is degraded, hydroxypyridinium compounds are released which are excreted in urine.

J. Treatment of Paget's Disease

(CANTRILL and ANDERSON 1990; SINGER and WALLACH 1991; KANIS 1991)

Until about 20 years ago there was no specific treatment for Paget's disease. In the severe symptomatic case only palliative measures (pain killers) were available. The first major advance came with the introduction of calcitonin.

Although the physiological role of calcitonin is still not fully understood, one of its major actions is to bind to and act upon the mature osteoclast. It acts via surface receptors in part at least by activating adenylate cyclase, and via released cyclic AMP acutely inhibits osteoclastic bone resorption. Clinically, calcitonin exerts a significant beneficial effect on bone pain and leads to a reduction in all indices of bone activity – with for example a 50% reduction in serum alkaline phosphatase being seen over a period of months. Unfortunately it does not appear to exert any major lasting effect on the course or extent of disease. The major form of (synthetic) calcitonin used is salmon calcitonin, which has a very long half-life, and is much more potent than human or porcine calcitonin. Unfortunately it has to be given by subcutaneous injection at least three times a week and up to daily, and is associated with troublesome flushing and headaches. Because of these problems, the much greater efficacy of bisphosphonates, and the frequent development of refractoriness to non-human calcitonin (due to antibody formation), I believe that calcitonin will eventually be of purely historical interest in Paget's disease.

I. Bisphosphonates (Diphosphonates)

The generic structure of the bisphosphonates is illustrated in Fig. 16. These compounds are analogues of pyrophosphate, and bind to hydroxyapatite. They have two separate effects on bone – (1) they inhibit nucleation of hydroxyapatite crystals and so lead to impaired mineralisation and (2) they inhibit osteoclastic bone resorption. The first effect is undesirable, especially in Paget's disease, where bone structure is already weakened. Different bisphosphonates vary considerably in the absolute potency and in the relative

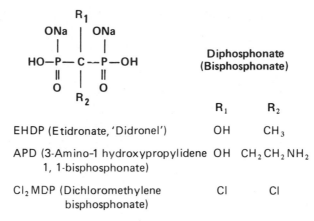

Fig. 16. Generic structure of the bisphosphonates, and the structure of the three most readily available. In pyrophosphate, of which they are analogues, the phosphates are joined by oxygen

ratios of the two effects. Etidronate, the first bisphosphonate to be marketed, has a narrow therapeutic margin, and is in any case relatively ineffective in Paget's disease. Much better are the second (clodronate and pamidronate) and third generation bisphosphonates (e.g. alendronate).

A further major problem with these drugs is their poor absorption from the GI tract. In fact in Paget's disease this is not a major disadvantage, because once in bone the drug has a very long half-life of 1 year or more and a long-term beneficial effect on disease activity. This makes a short course of intravenous infusions a practical possibility, which is not the case with other situations such as prevention of bone resorption by metastases or treatment of osteoporosis.

Over the past 6 years we have developed the use of *intravenous pamidronate* for the primary treatment of Paget's disease, and have treated nearly 400 cases (CANTRILL et al. 1986; RICHARDSON et al. 1990; CANTRILL and ANDERSON 1990). We now adopt the following strategy (which is still not fully optimised). Patients receive a "test" dose of 30 mg pamidronate i.v., given in saline over 2 h; 1 week later they have the first of a series of infusions of 60 mg pamidronate given in 500 ml isotonic saline by drip over 4 h. We give either three infusions of 60 mg (total dose, 210 mg) or six infusions of 60 mg (total dose, 390 mg), depending upon the initial level of serum alkaline phosphatase (the cutoff point being 500 IU/l (normal 30–130 IU/l)). The result is monitored by serum and urine biochemistry, with a bone scan repeated 6 months after the last infusion. Retreatment is given for the following indications: (a) incomplete biochemical remission or residual "hot" bone scan and (b) evidence of relapse, either on biochemical or bone scan criteria.

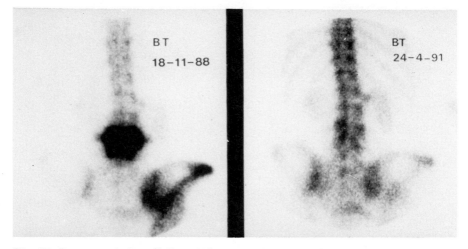

Fig. 17. Bone scan before (*left*) and 2½ years after a single course of i.v. pamidronate (total dose 180 mg) in a woman whose serum alkaline phosphatase fell from 330 to 75 IU/l and has remained suppressed. Such cases give strong encouragement that bisphosphonates may at least sometimes cure the disease

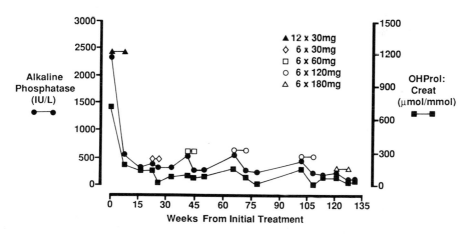

Fig. 18. Serum alkaline phosphatase and urinary hydroxyproline response to six courses of i.v. pamidronate, with increasing doses, in one woman with extensive Paget's disease. Total dose over 2½ years = 3.42 g

For relatively refractory cases we have found that retreatment can be given repeatedly – with increasing individual doses of up to 180 mg given at 2 weekly intervals on six occasions in some cases. Figure 17 shows the bone scan in a woman whose serum alkaline phosphatase has fallen to low normal and remained so over 3 years, after a single course of low-dose i.v. pamidronate. Figure 18 shows the biochemical response to repeated courses

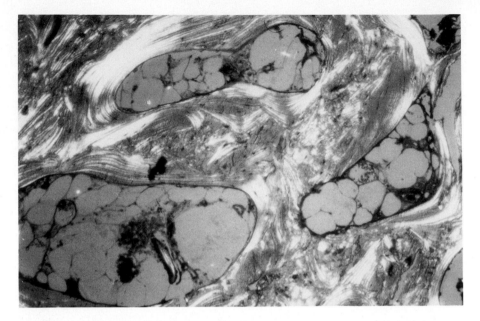

Fig. 19. Histological appearance of bone in pamidronate-treated Paget's disease: note original bone is now overlaid with nearly inactive bone cells overlying surface lamellar bone; as in normal bone, osteoclasts are now scanty

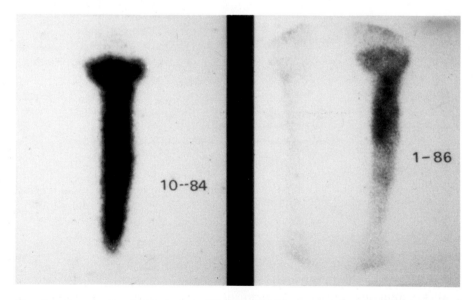

Fig. 20. Bone scan of tibia before (10–84) and 12 months after (1–86) a course of i.v. pamidronate (180 mg); note continuing patchy increased uptake, indicating continuing active disease, despite now-normal biochemistry. This was associated with progressive biochemical evidence of relapse

of infusions in a woman with extensive Paget's disease who was very resistant, but showed an excellent response to higher doses.

Histologically, pamidronate is associated with a marked reduction in bone turnover and a reduction in size and number of osteoclasts. There remains evidence of old disordered bone turnover, but the surface is now covered with lamellar bone (Fig. 19). In partially treated cases there remain residual foci of active pagetic osteoclasts.

At present, in about 10% of cases all evidence (biochemistry and bone scans, supported by bone biopsy in some cases) points to cure of the disease. For example, even grossly abnormal bone scans can return to normal (Fig. 17), and remain normal for years. At the other extreme, a further 10% are relatively resistant, while the remainder show excellent responses, but with continuing activity (Fig. 20).

In conclusion, therefore, the omens are extremely good for cure of a substantial fraction of patients, especially if the third-generation bisphophonates prove to be even more effective than pamidronate.

II. Probable Mode of Action of Bisphosphonates in Paget's Disease

Recent studies by SATO et al. (1991) indicate that alendronate, which is related in structure to pamidronate, is concentrated beneath the bone-resorbing osteoclast (SATO et al. 1990). There is dispute as to whether the major effect is on recruitment or activity of the mature osteoclast; the abrupt reduction in urinary hydroxyproline excretion suggests that the latter is the major effect. We suspect that once bone resorption is inhibited a vicious cycle is broken and the osteoclast no longer stimulates recruitment and/or proliferation of its own precursors; furthermore, the precursors no longer fuse with pagetic osteoclasts, so infecting themselves. We believe that if this cycle is interrupted for long enough then all infected pagetic osteoclasts may die out, leaving a bone which is cured of active disease.

III. Future Work

Clearly the major need is to discover more of the cause(s) and pathophysiology of this intriguing disease, so that effective prevention can be implemented. Meanwhile, much work is going on to refine the treatment of the established case. This seems to be best achieved with short courses of intravenous bisphosphonates: more work is needed to establish which is the best. At present, pamidronate seems to be the front runner!

Acknowledgements. I gratefully acknowledge the help and support of my former patients and colleagues at Hope Hospital, Salford, UK. Notable among the latter are Judy Cantrill, John Denton, Margaret Gordon, John O'Driscoll, Tony Freemont, Peter Richardson, Paul Sharpe, Sylvia Mercer, and the staff of the Medical Illustration Unit. The study was supported by the Sir Jules Thorn Trust, the Wellcome Trust, Salford Paget's Disease Appeal and the National Association for the Relief of Paget's Disease.

References

Barker DJP, Chamberlain AT, Guyer PB, Gardner MJ (1980) Paget's disease of bone: the Lancashire focus. Br Med J 280:1105–1107

Baslé MF, Fournier JG, Rozenblatt S, Rebel A, Bouteille M (1986) Measles virus RNA detected in Paget's disease bone tissue by in situ hybridization. J Gen Virol 67:907–913

Cantrill JA, Anderson DC (1990) Treatment of Paget's disease of bone. Clin Endocrinol (Oxf) 32:507–518

Cantrill JA, Buckler HM, Anderson DC (1986) Low dose intravenous 3-aminohydroxypropylidine 1-1 bisphosphonate (APD) for the treatment of Paget's disease of bone. Ann Rheum Dis 45:1012–1018

Czerny V (1873) Eine lokale Malacie des Unterschenkels. Wien Med Wochenschr 1:1–3

Detheridge FM, Gryer PB, Barker DJP (1982) European distribution of Paget's disease of bone. Br Med J 285:1005–1008

Gordon M, Anderson DC, Sharpe PT (1991) Canine distemper virus localised in bone cells of patients with Paget's disease. Bone 12:195–201

Harinck HIJ, Bijvoet OLM, Vellenga CJRL, Blacksma HJ, Frijlink WB (1986) Relation between signs and symptoms in Paget's disease of bone. QJ Med 58:133–151

Holdaway IM, Ibbertson HK, Wattie D, Scragg R, Graham P (1990) Previous dog ownership in Paget's disease. Bone Miner 8:53–58

Jacobs TP, Michelsen J, Polay JS, D'Adanio AC, Canfield RE (1979) Giant cell tumor in Paget's disease of bone. Familial and geographical clustering. Cancer 44:742–747

Kanis JA (1991) Pathophysiology and treatment of Paget's disease of bone. Dunitz, London

Mee AP, Webber DM, May C, Bennett D, Sharpe PT, Anderson DC (1992) Detection of canine distemper virus in bone cells in the metaphysis of distemper-infected dogs. J Bone Miner Res 7:829–834

Mills BG, Singer FR (1976) Nuclear inclusions in Paget's disease of bone. Science 194:201–206

Mills BG, Singer FR, Weiner LP, Suffin SC, Stabile E, Holt P (1984) Evidence for both respiratory syncytial virus and measles virus antigens in osteoclasts of patients with Paget's disease of bone. Clin Orthop 184:303–311

O'Driscoll JB, Anderson DC (1985) Past pets and Paget's disease. Lancet 2:919–921

O'Driscoll JB, Buckler HM, Jeacock J, Anderson DC (1990) Dogs, distemper and osteitis deformans: a further epidemiological study. Bone Miner 11:209–216

Osterberg PH, Wallace RGH, Adams DA, Crone RS, Dickson GR, Kanis JA, Mollen RA, Neven NC, Sloan J, Toner PG (1988) Familial expansile osteolysis – a new dysplasia. J Bone Joint Surg [Br] 70:255–260

Paget J (1877) On a form of chronic inflammation of bones (osteitis deformans). Med Chir Trans Lond 60:37–63

Rebel A, Baslé MF, Pouplard A, Filmon R, Kouyoumdjiam S, Lepatezour A (1980) Viral antigens in osteoclasts from Paget's disease of bone. Lancet 2:344–346

Rebel A, Malkani K, Basle M et al. (1987) Osteoclast ultrastructure in Paget's disease of bone. Clin Orthop 217:4–8

Richardson PC, Anderson DC, Denton J, Freemont AJ (1990) Changes in bone morphology following treatment of Paget's disease of bone with APD. In: Takahashi HE (ed) Bone morphometry, 1990. Nishimura/Smith-Gordon, Niigata, pp 235–238

Sato M, Grasser W, Endo N, Akine R, Simmons H, Thompson DD, Golub E, Rodan GA (1991) Biophosphonate action. Alendronate localization in rat bone and effects on osteoclast ultrastructure J Clin Invest 88:2095–2105

Singer FR, Wallach S (eds) (1991) Paget's disease of bone: clinical assessment, present and future therapy. Elsevier, Amsterdam

Wilks S (1860) Case of osteoporosis or spongy hypertrophy of the bones (calvaria clavicle os femoris and rib exhibited at the Society). Trans Pathol Soc Lond 20:273–277

CHAPTER 13
Hyperparathyroid and Hypoparathyroid Bone Disease

M. Peacock

A. Introduction

Hyperparathyroid and hypoparathyroid diseases provide unique insights into the action of parathyroid hormone (PTH) on bone. Diseases of excess PTH arise either as a primary abnormality in hormone secretion, or as a compensatory response to a disorder of serum calcium homeostasis. Hypoparathyroidism usually arises from surgical removal of the parathyroids, although it may arise as an idiopathic disease. Uncommonly, the parathyroid receptor is defective, giving rise to increased PTH secretion but with failure of biological action.

By their nature, hyperparathyroidism and hypoparathyroidism are chronic diseases of variable severity that evolve with time. As such, the information they provide on the physiological action of PTH on bone is indirect. Furthermore, each parathyroid disease, and each patient, carries biochemical and environmental factors that modify and modulate the effect of PTH on bone. Nevertheless, since the original clinical descriptions of hyperparathyroidism by Mandl (1926) and by Hannon et al. (1930) and of hypoparathyroidism by Albright and Reifenstein (1948), studies of skeletal changes in diseases of over- or undersecretion of PTH have greatly advanced the understanding of the action of the hormone on bone.

B. Parathyroid Hormone Function: Calcium Homeostasis

The main function of PTH, reviewed in detail in this volume in Chapters 4, 15 and 18, is to regulate plasma ionized calcium concentration. Central to this regulation, is the inversely sigmoidal relationship between plasma calcium and parathyroid secretion and gland mass, (Fig. 1) and the action of PTH on calcium transport directly in kidney and bone and indirectly in gut (Peacock 1980), (Fig. 2). In humans, the effects of over- or under secretion of PTH on the kidney (Figs. 3, 4), bone (Fig. 5), and gut (Fig. 6) account for many of the biochemical and skeletal abnormalities found in diseases of the parathyroids.

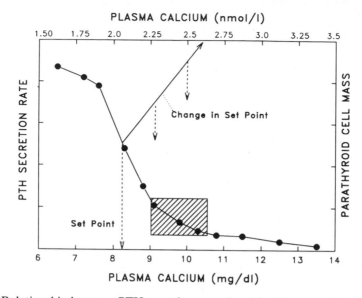

Fig. 1. Relationship between PTH secretion, parathyroid cell mass, and total plasma calcium concentration. The shape of the secretion curve (●–●) in relation to acute changes in serum calcium is inversely sigmoidal (MAYER and HURST 1978). The shape of the cell mass curve may be similar but has not been established. In the normal range for plasma calcium (9–10.5 mg/dl, 2.25–2.63 nmol/l), the normal mass of parathyroid tissue is about 160 mg (AKERSTROM et al. 1984) and the normal secretion rate about 400 ng/min (MAYER and HURST 1978). The serum calcium concentration at which PTH secretion is 50% inhibited ("set point") is shown (---) but is displaced to the right (→) as cell mass increases and in pathological states of the parathyroid gland

C. Classification of Parathyroid Disease

Diseases of chronic over- and under secretion of PTH encompass a variety of pathologies (Table 1). Increased parathyroid cell mass with oversecretion of PTH may be classified into primary and secondary hyperparathyroidism. In primary disease a defect within the cell results in enlargement of the gland and oversecretion of PTH. In secondary hyperparathyroidism, secretion and mass are also excessive, but are a response to disease disturbing calcium homeostasis. Chronic renal failure and vitamin D deficient osteomalacia are the commonest causes of secondary hyperparathyroidism. However, it is being increasingly recognized that secondary hyperparathyroidism occurs with aging. Although a less severe form of secondary hyperparathyroidism than that occurring with vitamin D deficiency and chronic renal failure, it has important implications because of its effects on skeletal strength and on fracture incidence in the elderly. In some subjects who have had secondary hyperparathyroidism for many years, the parathyroid gland may transform from a state of hypertrophy to one of autonomy. When this

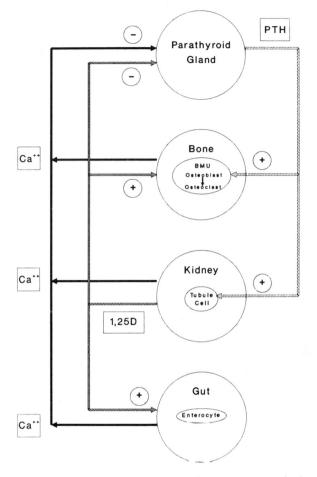

Fig. 2. Diagrammatic representation of the regulatory organs and stimuli involved in blood calcium homeostasis. PTH increases blood-ionized calcium (Ca) level directly by increasing both tubular calcium reabsorption in kidney and BMU activation frequency in bone; and indirectly by increasing calcium absorption efficiency in gut via increased renal 1,25(OH)$_2$ vitamin D (1,25D) secretion. The resultant increase in Ca^{2+} level, together with the raised 1,25D secretion, suppresses PTH secretion by the parathyroid gland. $-$, inhibition; $+$ stimulation

occurs, PTH secretion is no longer under calcium regulation, hypercalcemia ultimately develops, and the disease is known as tertiary hyperparathyroidism.

Hypoparathyroidism is most commonly due to removal of the parathyroid glands at surgery for diseases of the neck affecting the anatomic distribution of the parathyroid glands. It also occurs, however, as an idiopathic disease. Pseudohypoparathyroidism is a disease characterized by a lack of responsiveness in the parathyroid receptors and parathyroid secretion is generally considered to be normally regulated.

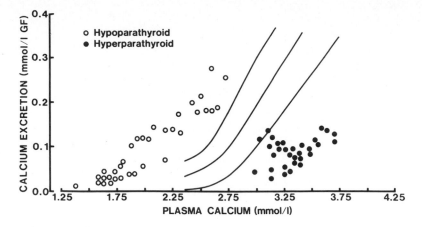

Fig. 3. Relationship between urine calcium excretion (expressed per liter glomerular filtrate) and filtered calcium (expressed per liter plasma) established in patients with acquired hypoparathyroidism (○) and primary hyperparathyroidism (●) and in healthy subjects with normal parathyroid function (mean and range). At the same urinary calcium excretion, and thus calcium input into blood, PTH is able to set plasma calcium concentration within a 2.5-mmol/l (6-mg/dl) range. (PEACOCK et al. 1969)

D. Primary Hyperparathyroidism

I. Incidence

A number of studies suggest that the incidence of primary hyperparathyroidism is about 25/100000 per year (STEINSTROM and HERDMAN 1974; HEATH et al. 1980; MUNDY et al. 1980) with a prevalence of 1 to 4 per 1000 in the general population (CHRISTENSSON et al. 1976; DENT et al. 1987; PALMER et al. 1988). Because asymptomatic patients outnumber those with symptoms, the incidence of primary hyperparathyroidism varies with the availability and length of use of biochemical screening for serum calcium concentration (MELTON 1991). All age groups are affected, but the incidence increases with age and there is a marked increase in women after the menopause (HEATH et al. 1980; PEACOCK 1978; MUNDY et al. 1980). The disease is two to five times more common in women than men. The higher incidence of hyperparathyroidism in women is unexplained, but the increase following menopause may be due to unmasking of mild hypercalcemia by estrogen deficiency (SELBY and PEACOCK 1986).

II. Diagnosis

The diagnosis of primary hyperparathyroidism is established biochemically. Serum calcium concentration must be persistently increased above the normal

Table 1. Classification of hyperparathyroid and hypoparathyroid disease. Major biochemical changes and modifiers of PTH response on bone

	Serum						CaAbs	Other modifiers
	PTH	Ca	P	pH	1,25D	25D		
Hyperparathyroidism								
Primary	↑	↑	↓	↓	↑	N	↑	
Secondary								
Renal failure	↑	↓	↑	↓	↓	N	↓	PO$_4$ depletion, Al retention, dialysis
Vitamin D deficient osteomalacia	↑	↓	↓	N	↓	↓	↓	General malabsorption
Ageing	↑	N	N	N	↓	↓	↓	Drugs, ill health
Others								
Oral phosphate	↑	↓	↑	N	↓	N	↓	
Calcium "leak"	↑	↓	↓	N	↑	N	↑	
Tertiary hyperparathyroidism								
Hypoparathyroidism								
Surgical and idiopathic	↓	↓	↑	N	↓	N	↓	Vitamin D treatment, thyroxine treatment
Pseudo-hypoparathyroidism	↑	↓	↑	N	↓	N	↓	Vitamin D treatment

range in the presence of an increased serum concentration of PTH. However, in milder cases, serum PTH concentration is often within the upper half of the normal range. Assays for intact PTH have increased the reliability of biochemical diagnosis of primary hyperparathyroidism from normal subjects and from patients with nonparathyroid hypercalcemia, with few false-positive and false-negative diagnoses (NUSSBAUM and POTTS 1991). Because the disease is defined by the upper limit of normal serum calcium concentration, usually the mean + 2 SD, there are subjects with the disease whose serum calcium and PTH concentrations lie within the normal range, and there are normal subjects whose serum calcium concentration is higher than the 2 SD range. In these problematic cases, decreased serum phosphate and tubular reabsorption of phosphate, and increased serum $1,25(OH)_2$ vitamin D may help in corroborating the diagnosis of primary hyperparathyroidism. The relationship between PTH, $1,25(OH)_2$ vitamin D, and calcium absorption from the gut is depicted in Figs. 4 and 6. In such subjects, thiazide treatment readily causes hypercalcemia and may also be helpful in diagnosis (CHRISTENSSON et al. 1977). However, the distinction between patients with mild primary hyperparathyroidism who have renal stones and patients with

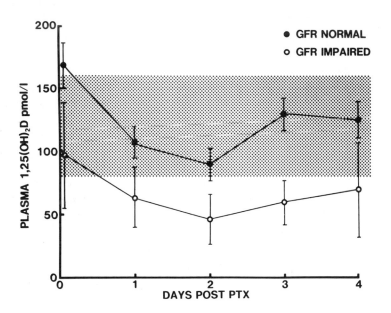

Fig. 4. Relationship between plasma $1,25(OH)_2$ vitamin D and time after parathyroidectomy (*PTX*) in primary hyperparathyroid patients with (○) and without (●) impaired glomerular filtration rate (GFR). The normal range is shown as a *stippled bar*. Immediately after PTX the increased levels of $1,25(OH)_2$ vitamin D decrease into the low normal range in patients with normal GFR. A similar response is present in patients with impaired GFR although the values for $1,25(OH)_2$ vitamin D are lower

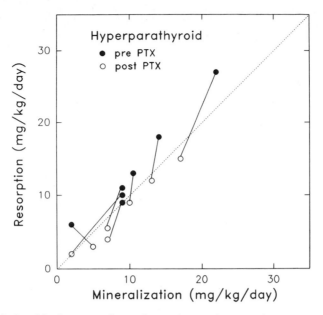

Fig. 5. Relationship between bone formation and resorption rates measured by calcium isotope kinetics and balance in patients with primary hyperparathyroidism before (●) and after (○) parathyroidectomy (*PTX*). The line of equality is shown. Before operation most patients have higher resorption than formation rates and after surgery higher formation than resorption, but both before and after PTX formation and resorption remain coupled

idiopathic urinary stone formation, particularly those with hypophosphatemia and hyperabsorption of calcium, remains a challenging diagnostic problem (PEACOCK and ROBERTSON 1989; PAK 1990).

It is important to distinguish subjects with familial hypocalciuric hypercalcemia from patients with primary hyperparathyroidism. The former is a benign condition that does not respond to parathyroidectomy (LAW and HEATH 1985). In familial hypocalciuric hyperparathyroidism, the hypercalcemia is probably due to an abnormality in renal reabsorption of calcium (ATTIE et al. 1983), although it has been argued that there is also an abnormality in parathyroid gland (MARX 1991; LAW et al. 1984). Patients with both primary hyperparathyroidism and any disease causing disturbances in calcium metabolism, such as sarcoidosis (PEACOCK and KRADIN 1981b), may also give rise to diagnostic difficulties requiring extensive biochemical investigation (LAFFERTY 1991).

III. Pathogenesis

Primary hyperparathyroidism is a disease of oversecretion of PTH due to a neoplastic increase in the mass of the parathyroid glands. In 90% of patients it is due to a single adenoma. More than one gland is affected in less than

10% of cases and classifiable as hyperplasia, although the histological diagnosis of multiple adenomas from hyperplasia is not absolute (ROTH 1971; THOMPSON et al. 1982; GHANDUR-MNAYMNEH and KIMURA 1984; AKERSTROM et al. 1986). A small percentage of patients have cancer of the gland that spreads locally or metastasizes (SCHANTZ and CASTLEMAN 1973). The increase in PTH secretion in the absence of renal failure and vitamin D deficiency generally remains proportional to the increase in parathyroid mass (MURRAY et al. 1972).

The pathogenesis is generally considered to be due to the clonal growth of a single cell, transformed by a neoplastic event (ARNOLD et al. 1988; FRIEDMAN et al. 1989). The latter has been related to several genetic abnormalities (MARX 1991). In a minority of adenomas, one copy of chromosome 11, containing the PTH gene, has undergone reciprocal conservative recombination between two loci on either side of the centromere (ARNOLD et al. 1988, 1989). In others, somatic inactivation of the MEN1 gene on chromosome 11, probably a normal growth suppressor gene, may be involved in up to 25% of sporadic parathyroid adenomas (FRIEDMAN et al. 1989; BISHOP 1991). In patients with familial multiple endocrine neoplasia type I (FMEN1), this abnormality may be present in about 60% of cases (FRIEDMAN et al. 1989; THAKKER et al. 1989).

In familial hyperparathyroidism the genetic abnormality is inherited. In the more common sporadic form, the genetic abnormality is presumably due to somatic mutation. In some cases this can be related to radiation to the neck in childhood (COHEN et al. 1990). Very rarely, the disease is due to PTH secretion from a cancer not derived from parathyroid tissue, so-called ectopic primary hyperparathyroidism (NUSSBAUM et al. 1990).

IV. Nonskeletal Signs

A wide spectrum of symptoms and signs can be elicited in patients with primary hyperparathyroidism (CLARK et al. 1991; HEATH 1991; HABENER and POTTS 1990). Some, such as polyuria, polydipsia, urinary stone formation, renal failure, pancreatitis, pyrophosphate arthritis, frank myopathy, and peptic ulcer (PIPELEERS-MARICHAL et al. 1990), can be attributed directly to the effects of PTH or $1,25(OH)_2$ vitamin D on calcium metabolism. Others, such as hypertension, muscle fatigue, and neuropsychiatric symptoms, are more difficult to relate to the parathyroid disease, but are considered by some workers to be common and due to oversecretion of PTH (JOBORN et al. 1989; LJUNGHALL et al. 1991).

V. Skeletal Signs

The prevalence of bone disease in primary hyperparathyroidism varies with both referral bias in the population examined and criteria used for diagnosis. Radiological changes are the least sensitive and diagnose only the most

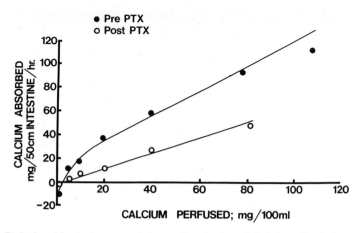

Fig. 6. Relationship between calcium absorbed and calcium load (measured by direct perfusion of calcium through the small intestine) in a patient with primary hyperparathyroidism before (○) and after (●) parathyroidectomy. Parathyroidectomy decreases the absorptive component responsible for active calcium transport at low calcium loads. (PEACOCK 1976)

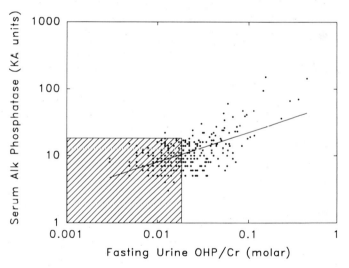

Fig. 7. Relationship between bone formation (serum alkaline phosphate) and bone resorption (fasting urine hydroxyproline) in patients with primary hyperparathyroidism. The normal ranges are shown (▨)

severely affected patients. Histomorphometry on biopsied bone is more sensitive, and biochemical markers of bone turnover are the most sensitive. Using biomarkers as the criteria of bone involvement, only about half of the patients have increased bone turnover (Fig. 7).

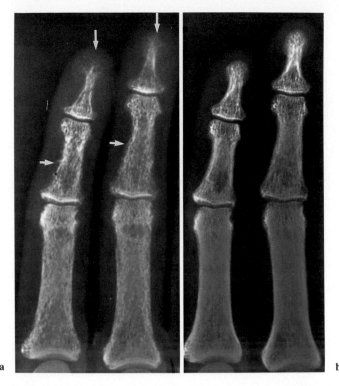

a   b

Fig. 8a,b. Radiographs of index and middle finger of a patient with primary hyperparathyroidism. **a** Before parathyroidectomy, subperiosteal erosions (→) are marked
on the radial aspect of the middle phalanges giving rise to the characteristic lacework
pattern. Resorption of the ungual tufts (↓) is prominent and tunneling of the
cortices has resulted in extensive loss of cortical bone. **b** One year after parathyroidectomy the bone pattern has returned to normal, although cortical thickness
remains reduced

1. Radiology

The effects of PTH on the skeleton in severely affected patients are well
recognized (GREENFIELD 1990a). The bone disease is referred to as osteitis
fibrosa cystica or generalisata. The term is inappropriate because, although
there may be cystic changes and fibrosis, there is no inflammation. More
importantly, it does not describe the diagnostic feature of primary hyperparathyroidism on the skeleton, which is subcortical erosions (PUGH 1951;
RICHARDSON et al. 1986; GENANT et al. 1973; WEISS 1974; GREENFIELD
1990a) (Fig. 8a,b). Radiologically, these first appear subperiostially, but
later occur at endosteal surfaces resulting in loss of cortical diameter. Within
cortical bone, marked tunneling occurs producing linear striations on
radiographs (Fig. 8a). The latter, however, are not unique to primary
hyperparathyroidism and may be seen where there is rapid loss in cortical

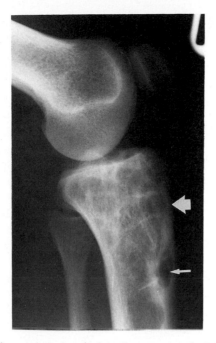

Fig. 9. Radiograph of a cystic lesion (⬅) in the upper end of the tibia in an 18-year-old women with primary hyperparathyroidism. Biopsy of the lesion (⬅) showed a brown tumor (see Fig. 11)

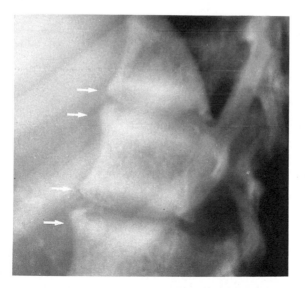

Fig. 10. Radiograph of the lateral lumbar vertebrae in the patient shown in Fig. 8. Sclerosis of the end plates (→) contrasts with the osteopenia of the center giving an appearance of alternating bands (rugger jersey)

bone secondary to conditions such as disuse osteoporosis. Subperiosteal erosions are best seen, and diagnosed at an earlier stage of the disease, if fine detail film is used for radiography (Weiss 1974; Genant et al. 1973). Any cortical surface of the skeleton may be affected (Greenfield 1990a) but the best diagnostic site is the radial aspects of the middle phalanges. Hand radiographs may also show characteristic resorption of the terminal phalanges (Fig. 8a). Other common sites for visualizing cortical erosions are the peripheral ends of the clavicles and their lower borders, the margins of the symphysis pubis and the sacroiliac joints, the medial aspects of the femoral neck, and the cranium. Cystic lesions within bone may appear at any skeletal site and may be multiple or solitary (Huvos 1991; Mirra 1989) (Fig. 9).

Patchy osteosclerosis is not common in primary hyperparathyroidism (Greenfield 1990a). When it occurs, it usually affects the vertebrae, causing increased bone density of the end plates and giving rise to a banded appearance in the spine, referred to radiologically as "rugger jersey" (Fig. 10). The metaphysis of long bones, the skull, the pelvis, and the rib cage may also be affected.

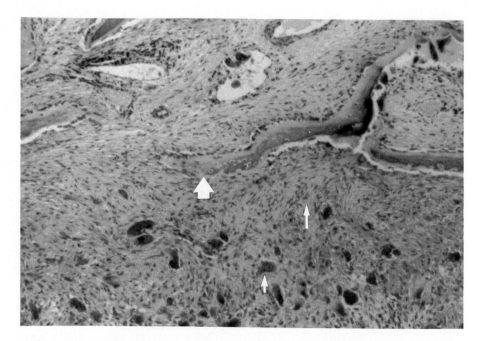

Fig. 11. Histology of the brown tumor removed from the cystic lesion shown in Fig. 9. Spindle-shaped mesenchymal cells (↑) with scattered osteoclasts (↑) occupy the center of the cyst. At the periphery trabeculae are being completely removed by osteoclastic resorption (⬆)

2. Histology

The histological basis of subperiosteal erosion, cortical tunneling, and trabecular perforation is osteoclastic bone resorption. In cancellous bone there is proliferation of mesenchymal cells and fibrosis. Woven bone is produced but fails to be remodeled into lamellar bone and radiologically appears as sclerosis. Cystic lesions contain a population of spindle-shaped mesenchymal cells with scattered osteoclasts and hemorrhagic tissue giving them the macroscopic appearance of brown tumors (HUVOS 1991; MIRRA 1989) (Fig. 11). Distant from the periphery of the cyst, where osteoclastic bone resorption is occurring, the tissue is unrecognizable histologically from a giant cell tumor of bone (HUVOS 1991; MIRRA 1989). Within the cyst there is clear evidence that it develops by complete perforation and removal of trabeculae and that bone formation, although it may not be uncoupled from resorption, is ineffective, producing only fibrosis and woven bone.

In milder cases the main abnormality is an increase in the numbers of active BMUs (DELMAS et al. 1986; CHARLES et al. 1987). The increased rate of activation results in an increase in the number of osteoclasts and in the number of trabecular surfaces covered in osteoid. Osteoid thickness, however, remains normal unless osteomalacia develops, in which case the osteoid seam width thickens and osteoid volume greatly expand (PARFITT 1990; PEACOCK 1984).

3. Bone Mass and Fracture

In severe primary hyperparathyroidism both localized and generalized osteopenia are marked and can be readily diagnosed from radiographs indicating that over 30% of the bone mass has been lost (RICHARDSON et al. 1986). The commonest clinical manifestation is fracture occurring through localized bone loss produced by cysts or cortical erosions. Parathyroidectomy is absolutely indicated in such patients. On the other hand, in mild asymptomatic primary hyperparathyroidism, surgical treatment may cause complications (LAFFERTY and HUBAY 1989; MALMAEUS et al. 1988; CLARK et al. 1991) and, because many do not show an increase in parathyroid activity with time (RAO et al. 1988), there is a trend to manage these patients by regular follow-up only (POTTS 1990; NCH Consensus Development Conferences 1991). Such an approach raises the question of whether untreated subjects develop parathyroid-dependent osteopenia, leading in later life to an increase in age-related fractures (PEACOCK 1991).

The prevalence of fractures in mild or asymptomatic hyperparathyroidism is not agreed. Some studies indicate that the number of fractures is no greater than expected (WILSON et al. 1988a), whereas others show an increased incidence in both vertebral and peripheral fracture (PEACOCK et al. 1984; DAUPHINE et al. 1975; KOCHERSBERGER et al. 1987; LARSSON et al. 1989) (Fig. 12). Most studies show a decrease in cortical bone mass (PEACOCK et al. 1984; WILSON et al. 1988b; SILVERBERG et al. 1989; LARSSON

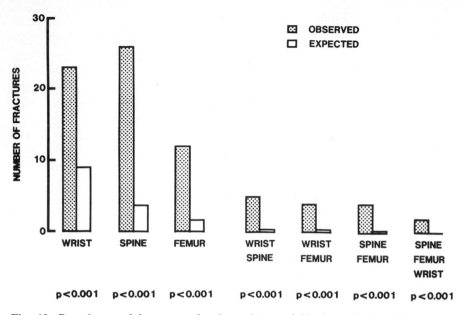

Fig. 12. Prevalence of fractures of wrist, spine, and hip in patients with primary hyperparathyroidism (▦ n = 174) as compared to age and sex-matched normals (□). (Peacock et al. 1984)

et al. 1989; Leppla et al. 1982), which is not totally replaced after parathyroidectomy (Mautalen et al. 1986; Martin et al. 1990; Leppla et al. 1982). Cancellous bone, however, is less affected, with some studies showing preservation of density at the spine (Silverberg et al. 1989) and bone volume in the iliac crest (Parisien et al. 1990). In asymptomatic patients who choose not to have surgery, bone density needs to be assessed at skeletal sites with a high content of cortical bone (mid-radius) and at sites with a high content of cancellous bone (spine) (Richardson et al. 1986).

Bone density predicts the risk of future fracture in age-related bone loss (Wasnich et al. 1985; Gardsell et al. 1989; Hui et al. 1989; Cummings et al. 1990) and can probably be used to identify those patients needing surgical treatment because of low bone density from those with normal density who may be managed by medical follow-up.

VI. Human Parathyroid Hormone

Animals injected daily with PTH increase their cancellous bone mass without developing cortical bone loss (Liu and Kalu 1990; Hori et al. 1988; Tada et al. 1990; Hock et al. 1989; Liu et al. 1991). Several pilot studies in humans with osteoporosis have been carried out using a similar regimen with amino-terminal hPTH given as a dose that increases serum calcium but does not produce hypercalcemia. Using hPTH alone, an increase in cancellous bone volume is observed in osteoporotic women (REEVE et al. 1980). However, this is accompanied by no change in calcium retention or absorption and by a decrease in cortical bone mass (HESP et al. 1981), suggesting that the increase in cancellous bone occurs at the expense of cortical bone. When hPTH is given along with oral 1,25(OH)$_2$ vitamin D, calcium absorption increases but the gain in cancellous bone is still accompanied by cortical bone loss (SLOVIK et al. 1986; NEER et al. 1990). A striking feature of these studies is the unexplained wide variability in the bone responses. The variability may relate to confounding factors (Table 1) such as the level of serum phosphate, acidosis, and calcium absorption. The biological basis for the anabolic response in cancellous bone and catabolic response in cortical bone remains unexplained but clearly highlights basic differences in the behavior of bone at different sites in the skeleton and differences in response to changes in PTH levels as compared to steady state levels.

E. Secondary Hyperparathyroidism

Secondary hyperparathyroidism is common and caused by a variety of disease that stress the calcium homeostatic mechanisms (Table 1). Unlike primary hyperparathyroidism, symptoms attributable to PTH oversecretion are not clinically evident.

I. Renal Failure

1. Diagnosis

Chronic renal disease is common and affects all age groups and both sexes. Secondary hyperparathyroidism in chronic renal failure is established by measuring increased serum PTH concentration. Because the carboxy-terminal fragment of PTH is cleared from blood by the kidney, assays measuring only intact hormone should be used to avoid overestimating the degree of hyperparathyroidism (SEGRE and POTTS 1989). Serum calcium concentrations and 1,25(OH)$_2$ vitamin D are either low or subnormal (HAUSSLER and MCCAIN 1977) and serum phosphate is increased (Table 1). The decreased serum 1,25(OH)$_2$ vitamin D levels may be associated with low 25OH vitamin D levels in serum because of reduced sunlight exposure due to chronic ill health (PEACOCK et al. 1977; EASTWOOD et al. 1979).

A number of factors may alter these diagnostic biochemistries. Treatment with dietary phosphate-binding agents and with dialysis tend to normalize serum calcium and phosphate concentrations. On the other hand, hyper-calcemia may develop because of either hypophosphatemia from excessive use of phosphate-binding agents (PIERIDES 1977) or excessive use of calcium carbonate as a phosphate-binding agent (HERCZ et al. 1986; SLATOPOLSKY et al. 1986). Hypercalcemia may also arise from vitamin D metabolites causing increased calcium absorption efficiency relative to decreased glomerular filtration rate (PEACOCK et al. 1977a) or from the onset of tertiary hyperparathyroidism (CASTLEMAN and KIBBLE 1963). The use of oral aluminum hydroxide as a phosphate-binding agent, and dialysis fluids containing aluminum, may lead to toxic levels of aluminum in bone and low bone turnover osteomalacia with fractures (HODSMAN et al. 1982; PARKINSON et al. 1979; GOODMAN et al. 1984; DRUEKE 1980). A feature of this condition is hypercalcemia produced by small doses of $1,25(OH)_2$ vitamin D that do not heal the osteomalacia (PIERIDES et al. 1976).

2. Pathogenesis

Secondary hyperparathyroidism (REISS et al. 1968; ARNAUD 1973) with a high incidence of bone disease (STANBURY and LUMB 1966; SLATOPOLSKY and COBURN 1990) is an inevitable outcome of the hypocalcemia caused by any chronic reduction in glomerular filtration rate. A number of factors contribute to the decrease in serum calcium including phosphate retention and calcium malabsorption from reduced $1,25(OH)_2$ vitamin D secretion.

a) Phosphate Retention

Phosphate retention leads to hyperphosphatemia (KLEEMAN et al. 1969), which produces hypocalcemia by least two mechanisms. The most immediate is a physicochemical reduction in serum-ionized concentration (HERBERT et al. 1966; REISS et al. 1970), driving calcium from the extracellular fluid compartment to the tissues as insoluble calcium phosphate deposits. Hyperphosphatemia also reduces $1,25(OH)_2$ vitamin D secretion (GRAY et al. 1977; PORTALE et al. 1986), which, in turn, reduces calcium absorption efficiency, and probably promotes or facilitates parathyroid gland growth and PTH secretion. The central role of chronic phosphate retention in the pathogenesis of secondary hyperparathyroidism of renal failure is illustrated by studies on the time course of biochemical changes in chronic renal failure in animals induced by partial nephrectomy (SLATOPOLSKY et al. 1972; RUTHERFORD et al. 1977). When phosphate retention is prevented by reducing dietary phosphate intake in proportion to the decreasing glomerular filtration rate, hyperparathyroidism is greatly attenuated as compared to animals allowed to become hyperphosphatemic. When both normophosphatemia and normal calcium absorption, achieved with vitamin D supplementation, are maintained, hyperparathyroidism does not develop (RUTHERFORD et al. 1977). Clinically, the maintenance of normophosphatemia by diet and oral phosphate-binding agents is universally accepted as a major therapeutic goal in the management of patients with chronic renal failure (SLATOPOLSKY and COBURN 1990).

b) Deficiency of $1,25(OH)_2$ Vitamin D

The secretion of $1,25(OH)_2$ vitamin D is decreased in chronic renal failure by reduced renal cell mass, independent of the effect of hyperphosphatemia

(HAUSSLER and McCAIN 1977), although it remains under PTH control (Fig. 4). The reduction in 1,25(OH)$_2$ vitamin D results in severe calcium malabsorption (PEACOCK et al. 1977, 1980; COBURN et al. 1973). Perhaps the most persuasive evidence that 1,25(OH)$_2$ vitamin D may also play a direct role in the development of hyperparathyroidism is that 1,25(OH)$_2$ vitamin D given intravenously, thus avoiding hypercalcemia by bypassing an action on calcium absorption, substantially decreases PTH secretion independent of an increase in serum calcium concentration (SLATOPOLSKY et al. 1984; DELMEZ et al. 1989). There is substantial evidence that 1,25(OH)$_2$ vitamin D, acting indirectly through absorption and probably also by direct action on PTH secretion, when taken daily by patients with chronic renal failure, decreases the severity of secondary hyperparathyroidism (MEMMOS et al. 1982; BAKER et al. 1986; NORDAL and DAHL 1988; ANDRESS et al. 1989). Moreover, patients with early chronic renal failure given replacement doses of 1,25(OH)$_2$ vitamin D orally develop much milder secondary hyperparathyroidism than those taking a placebo (BAKER et al. 1989). Resistance of the skeleton to the action of PTH, in chronic renal failure, if it exists, probably relates to the levels of 1,25(OH)$_2$ vitamin D present (MASSRY et al. 1975) and to the levels of phosphate in serum (SOMERVILLE and KAYE 1982).

3. Skeletal Signs

a) Radiology and Histology

The effect of PTH on the skeleton in chronic renal failure is indistinguishable from that in primary hyperparathyroidism both radiologically (JENSEN and KLIGER 1977; GREENFIELD 1990b) and histologically (DEBNAM et al. 1977; ELLIS et al. 1977; PEACOCK et al. 1977). Subperiosteal erosions are extensive, but, in relation to the degree of hyperparathyroidism present, cystic changes are less common and sclerosis more common than in primary disease (GREENFIELD 1990b).

Pure parathyroid bone disease only occurs as one extreme of a spectrum of changes in the skeleton known collectively as renal osteodystrophy. At the other extreme, osteomalacia and rickets predominate (STANBURY 1972; ELLIS et al. 1977; SHERRARD 1986). Furthermore, the osteomalacic component has multiple pathogenesis. The calcification defect may be induced by vitamin D deficiency, giving rise to high turnover osteomalacia, or by phosphate depletion or aluminum accumulation, giving rise to low turnover osteomalacia (PEACOCK 1984; PARFITT 1990). In children, renal rickets is accompanied by sevvere growth failure which, in part, is due to vitamin D deficiency (PEACOCK 1984). Biomarkers of bone turnover are generally increased, reflecting high bone turnover, and, as in primary hyperparathyroidism, remain coupled. In the presence of aluminum or phosphate-induced bone disease biomarkers may decrease into the normal range in severely affected subjects.

b) Bone Mass and Fracture

Bone density and fracture prevalence in chronic renal failure have not been extensively or systematically studied. Most studies have examined the effect of dialysis on bone mass on subjects on multiple treatments. From studies that have been reported it appears, as would be predicted, that cortical bone is lost from the peripheral skeleton in excess of cancellous bone loss at the spine, and dialysis appears to slow the rate of loss (Piraino et al. 1988; Eeckhout et al. 1989; Overton et al. 1976; Rickers et al. 1983; Lindergard 1981). In 74 patients the annual rate of bone loss at cortical bone was about 5% before dialysis treatment, which fell to about 1% on dialysis (Lindergard 1981). The incidence of fractures in chronic renal failure is equally difficult to interpret. Fractures are common, sometimes referred to as fracturing renal osteodystrophy, but are related much more to low bone turnover caused by aluminum, phosphate depletion, and vitamin D deficiency osteomalacia (Cochran et al. 1981) than to osteopenic bone loss. Many of these are pseudofractures, occurring at skeletal sites subjected to greatest mechanical stress such as the ribs, metatarsals and metacarpals, and upper end of the femora and the pelvis. If parathyroid-induced bone loss is involved, it does so by reducing bone mass at a stage before the calcification defect develops.

II. Vitamin D Deficient Osteomalacia/Rickets

1. Pathogenesis and Diagnosis

Secondary hyperparathyroidism is an inevitable outcome of the failure of vitamin D to express its biological action on gut and bone. This may be due to a deficiency in vitamin D, an abnormality in its metabolism, or a defect in its receptor in target tissues (Table 2). The diagnosis is established by increased serum concentrations of PTH in the face of hypocalcemia, and a deficit either in the concentration of serum $1,25(OH)_2$ vitamin D and 25OH vitamin D, or in the biological action of $1,25(OH)_2$ vitamin D.

The major regulator of calcium absorption efficiency in humans is vitamin D, and as serum vitamin D levels fall calcium absorption efficiency decreases (Haussler and McCain 1977; Reichel et al. 1989). The initial hypocalcemic stress is caused by calcium malabsorption. As vitamin D level decreases further, there is failure to express its biological action on the calcification mechanism in bone and, in association with the secondary hyperparathyroidism, produces high bone turnover osteomalacia. In this state, bone has an increased avidity for calcium and over 90% of the calcium delivered intravenously is swept into bone, producing only a marginal increase in serum calcium (Peacock 1980). This skeletal avidity for calcium helps sustain the chronic hypocalcemia. PTH resistance in bone may also develop and, although difficult to corroborate experimentally, clinically the skeletal

Table 2. Biochemisty of hyperparathyroidism secondary to the vitamin D osteomalacias

	Vitamin D			
	Vitamin D deficiency	Renal failure	VDDR type I	VDDR type II VDR-gene defect
Se vitamin D	↓	N	N	N
Vitamin D 25OHase	N	N	N	N
Se 25OH vitamin D	↓	N	N	N
25OH vitamin D 1αOHase	N	↓	↓	N
Se 1,25 vitamin D	↓	↓	↓	↑
Calcium absorption	↓	↓	↓	↓
Vitamin D receptor (VDR)	N	N	N	↓
Se PTH	↑	↑	↑	↑
Se calcium	↓	↓	↓	↓
Ur calcium/creatinine	↓	↓	↓	↓
Calcium tubular reabsorption	↑	N	↑	↑
Se Phosphate	↓	↑	↓	↓
Phosphate tubular reabsorption	↓	↓	↓	↓
Creatinine clearance	N	↓	N	N
Bone turnover biomarkers	↑	↑	↑	↑

Se, serum; Ur, urine; ↓, decreased; ↑, increased; N, normal

signs of hyperparathyroidism secondary to vitamin D abnormalities are different from those present in primary disease.

Vitamin D osteomalacia and rickets are caused by several defects, resulting in a failure of vitamin D to express its biological action (Table 2). Globally, the most common cause of vitamin D-related osteomalacia/rickets is vitamin D deficiency (PEACOCK 1984). Vitamin D has limited natural distribution in foods and dietary vitamin D accounts for only about half, particularly in the elderly (OMDAHL et al. 1982), of the recommended allowance of $50 \mu g$/day (1989). The major fraction of the vitamin D requirement is produced by the action of UV radiation from sunlight on the skin (LAWSON et al. 1979; ADAMS et al. 1982). Because sunlight exposure plays such a major role in meeting daily requirements, certain populations are at risk of developing vitamin D deficient osteomalacia/rickets. Immigrants, particularly those with deeply pigmented skin, from subtropical regions, moving to countries of higher latitude are at particular risk because of inappropriate clothing, habits and skin pigmentation (STAMP et al. 1980; PEACOCK et al. 1979). Vitamin D deficient rickets, however, may occur in tropical countries where environmental factors reduce sunlight exposure (VAISHNAVA 1975; CHAPMAN 1971). Becoming housebound also increases the risk of developing vitamin D deficiency osteomalacia (Hodkinson et al. 1973; Aaron et al. 1974; Hordon and Peacock 1990; Johnston et al. 1987). The population at greatest risk are the infirm elderly, but any chronic illness that reduces outdoor activity promotes vitamin D deficiency. Vitamin D deficient osteomalacia is common in malabsorptive bowel disease (Morgan et al. 1970; Meredith and Rosenberg 1980; Rao 1985; Driscoll et al. 1977; Compston et al. 1978a,b; Peacock et al. 1981; Parfitt et al. 1978). It can be cured by ultraviolet radiation, indicating that lack of sunlight exposure is a major risk factor (Jung et al. 1978; Adams et al. 1982). However, loss of vitamin D metabolites from disruption of the intrahepatic circulation and reduced absorption of vitamin D, a fat-soluble vitamin, may also be involved (Wiesner et al. 1980; Kumar 1984). In vitamin D resistant rickets type I, there is a hereditary absence of the 1-α hydroxylase enzyme (Labuda et al. 1990) in the kidney and, despite adequate serum concentrations of 25OH vitamin D, serum $1,25(OH)_2$ vitamin D is low and leads to hyperparathyroidism and rickets (Fraser et al. 1973). In vitamin D resistant rickets type II, there is a hereditary defect in the vitamin D receptor (Hughes et al. 1991; Pike 1991), resulting in the inability of vitamin D to express its biological action (Brooks et al. 1978; Rosen et al. 1979; Liberman et al. 1980). In these children the hyperparathyroidism develops in the presence of increased concentrations of serum of $1,25(OH)_2$ vitamin D.

2. Skeletal Signs

a) Radiology, Histology, and Biochemistry

Subperiosteal erosions do not occur in vitamin D deficient osteomalacia/ rickets, despite PTH serum concentrations as high as those found in primary hyperparathyroidism with radiological changes (Greenfield 1990c). This difference supports the concept that PTH requires vitamin D to express its full activity. On the other hand, there is loss of cortical bone (Peacock et al. 1984; Matloff et al. 1982; Deller and Begley 1983; Parfitt et al. 1985). Radiologically, the pathogenomonic feature of vitamin D deficient osteomalacia is the pseudofracture. In vitamin D deficient rickets it is the failure of mineralization of the growth plate.

A prolongation of the mineralization lag time and an increase in osteoid seam thickness due to reduction in the rate of mineralization are the diagnostic histological features (Parfitt 1990). These abnormalities result in an increase in osteoid volume that manifests by softening of bone, loss of rigidity, and skeletal deformity. The secondary hyperparathyroidism increases the frequency of BMU activation, resulting in a high-bone turnover osteomalacia and rickets (Parfitt 1990). The effect of hyperparathyroidism on bone, a preosteomalacic state (Parfitt 1990; Nordin et al. 1980), precedes the calcification defect, increasing the number of surfaces covered by osteoid. The latter must be distinguished from osteoid accumulating due to reduction in the mineralization rate.

Biomarkers of bone formation and resorption are increases. Moreover, they remain coupled, as they do in primary hyperparathyroidism, indicating that the level of formation markers reflects osteoblast activity and not its ability to lay down the mineral component of the calcification front. Both resorption markers and/or formation markers can, therefore, be used to assess the severity of the disease and its response to treatment.

b) Bone Density and Fracture

Like other hyperparathyroid states, increased activation frequency causes negative skeletal balance which reverses with the normalization of the activation frequency. However, in vitamin D osteomalacia and rickets, particularly that occurring in small bowel disease, malabsorption of calcium and phosphorus is marked and the bone deficit, particularly in cortical bone, may be severe (PARFITT et al. 1985; PEACOCK 1984). Even with appropriate vitamin D treatment and calcium supplementation, the cortical bone deficit may persist. Furthermore, the response by bone to vitamin D treatment may be attenuated if calcium and phosphate are not supplied in adequate amounts.

The fracture of vitamin D osteomalacia is the pseudofracture occurring at sites of mechanical stress. They are common in the pubic rami, the metatarsals, the metacarpals, the upper end of the femur, and the outer margins of the scapulae (GREENFIELD 1990c).

III. Ageing

1. Diagnosis and Pathogenesis

Serum PTH concentrations increase with ageing (GALLAGHER et al. 1980b; CHAPUY et al. 1983; DANDONA et al. 1986; PEACOCK and HORDON 1989;

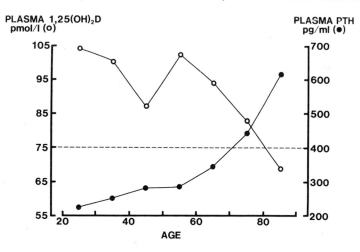

Fig. 13. Relationship between mean plasma 1,25(OH)₂ vitamin D (○) and mean plasma PTH (●) and age in normal women. (PEACOCK and HORDON 1989)

Wiske et al. 1979; Orwoll and Meier 1986) (Fig. 13). The increase has been found using assays directed at both intact PTH and its fragments (Young et al. 1987). It is increasingly accepted that secondary hyperparathyroidism in the elderly has important biological implications for bone in the pathogenesis of age-related fractures (Johnston et al. 1985; Riggs and Melton 1986, 1990; Orwoll and Meier 1986). The hyperparathyroidism occurs with a low normal or subnormal serum calcium concentration and a normal or increased serum phosphate concentration. Four main etiological factors have been identified: vitamin D status, glomerular filtration rate, calcium absorption efficiency, and dietary calcium intake.

a) Vitamin D

Serum 25OH D concentrations decrease with age (Baker et al. 1980; Chapuy et al. 1983; Peacock and Hordon 1989a; McKenna et al. 1985; Tsai et al. 1984). The decrease appears in the 5 decade and continues into the 9th and 10th decades. By the 8th decade mean serum 25OH vitamin D concentration has fallen by about two-thirds of the young normal and about 50% of the elderly population have a serum 25OH vitamin D less than 10 nmol/l (Fig. 14). In the institutionalized elderly (Corless et al. 1975; Lips et al. 1988) and in patients hospitalized because of femoral fracture (Baker et al. 1979; Lips et al. 1982), serum 25 vitamin D levels are particularly low. In the elderly, serum 25OH vitamin D and PTH are inversely related (Francis et al. 1983; Hordon and Peacock 1987). Despite reduced levels, seasonal variation in serum 25OH vitamin D concentration occurs, resulting in levels being highest in late summer and lowest in early spring (Bouillon et al. 1987; Webb et al. 1988). Accompanying this seasonal variation in serum 25OH vitamin D, there is reciprocal variation in scrum PTH (Bouillon et al. 1987; Krall et al. 1989), strongly suggesting that it is the decrease in serum 25OH vitamin D levels that stresses the calcium homeostatic mechanisms. Low serum 25OH vitamin D concentrations in the elderly are due to reduction in sunlight exposure and are most marked in those subjects who are housebound from chronic ill health (Webb et al. 1990). The reduced ability of skin to produce vitamin D with ultraviolet radiation exposure with age may be a contributing factor (Holick et al. 1989; MacLaughlin and Holick 1985). As 25OH vitamin D in serum falls below a concentration of about 60 nmol/l, the production of $1,25(OH)_2$ vitamin D becomes increasingly substrate dependent (Peacock et al. 1985; Bouillon et al. 1987; Peacock and Hordon 1989). The biological effect of this relationship is seen in calcium absorption efficiency, which decreases as serum 25OH vitamin D decreases (Peacock and Hordon 1989). The range of serum 25OH vitamin D from 60 to 10 nmol/l represents vitamin D insufficiency and less than 10 nmol/l, in which the response in $1,25(OH)_2$ vitamin D to changes in substrate is supranormal, represents vitamin D deficiency. It is not known whether serum levels of 25OH vitamin D between 60 and 10 nmol/l have adverse direct effects on bone in addition to that produced by reduced calcium efficiency. They probably do, since $1,25(OH)_2$ vitamin D appears to be an important regulator of osteoblast activity within the normal range (DUDA et al. 1987).

b) Glomerular Filtration

With age glomerular filtration rate decreases (SHOCK 1987; ANDERSON et al. 1987; EPSTEIN et al. 1986; BUCHANAN et al. 1988; YENDT et al. 1991; KOKOWICZ et al. 1990), starting in the 4th decade and continuing into the 10th decade (Fig. 14). Because lean body mass also decreases with age, age-related changes in glomerular filtration are not accurately reflected by serum creatinine concentration. Disturbances in calcium homeostasis caused by decreased glomerular filtration are subtle and fall far short of the changes present in chronic renal failure. They probably account in part for the decrease in $1,25(OH)_2$ vitamin D concentration that occurs with ageing (EPSTEIN et al. 1986; SOWERS et al. 1990; TSAI et al. 1984) (Fig. 13), although the decrease is not a universal finding (CLEMENS et al. 1986; SHERMAN et al. 1990).

c) Calcium Absorption

Calcium absorption efficiency falls with age (NORDIN et al. 1976; IRELAND and FORDTRAN 1973; GALLAGHER et al. 1979). The decrease appears in the 6th decade and continues through to the 9th and 10th decades (Fig. 14).

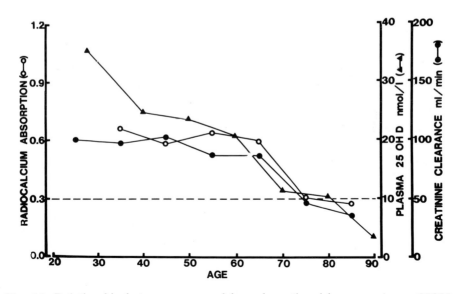

Fig. 14. Relationship between mean calcium absorption (○), mean plasma 25OH vitamin D (▲), and mean creatinine clearance (●) and age in normal women. (PEACOCK and HORDON 1989)

However, calcium absorption in the elderly remains responsive to standard amounts of oral 1,25(OH)$_2$ vitamin D (Francis and Peacock 1987) and only in a small number of subjects does the malabsorption represent a resistance to the action of 1,25(OH)$_2$ vitamin D (Francis et al. 1984). The decrease in absorption is probably multifactorial, with the combined effects of decreased glomerular filtration and serum 25(OH) vitamin D being major factors.

d) Dietary Calcium

Calcium intake in the diet in the elderly is low (Block et al. 1985), and in many subjects is well below the RDA of 1 g calcium/day (Recommended Dietary Allowances 1989). Calcium supplementation of elderly subjects taking less than 500 mg calcium/day results in a reduction in serum PTH and bone turnover and an increase in bone mass (Dawson-Hughes et al. 1987, 1990). Thus, in those subjects, low calcium intake is a factor in the secondary hyperparathyroidism which, in turn, adversely affects bone mass. Calcium supplementation in postmenopausal women and subjects with osteoporosis increases bone mass, particularly in cortical bone (Nordin and Heaney 1990; Dawson-Hughes 1991), supporting the idea that suppression of secondary hyperparathyroidism has a beneficial effect on cortical bone mass.

The prevalence of secondary hyperparathyroidism in the elderly may be estimated from the number of subjects having a serum PTH concentration above the young normal range. Criteria, however, for the diagnosis have not been agreed upon. In general, the mean serum PTH concentration doubles between the age of 20 to 40 years and age 70 years and older (Epstein et al. 1986; Kokowicz et al. 1990) (Fig. 13).

e) Bone Mass and Fracture

The main significance of hyperparathyroidism with ageing is the effect it has on bone mass and fracture incidence. With ageing there is a universal decrease in bone mass over the age of 50 years, and an increase in the incidence of all fractures (Newton-John and Morgan 1970; Smith et al. 1975; Johnston et al. 1989). The rise is marked in fractures of the wrist, spine, and particularly the upper femur (Gallagher et al. 1980a; Horsman et al. 1985). For every standard deviation decrease in bone mass, the relative risk of fractures approximately doubles (Ross et al. 1990; Hui et al. 1989; Gardsell et al. 1989; Cummings et al. 1990). The bone loss attributable to secondary hyperparathyroidism is unknown but the contribution to cortical bone loss is probably greater than to trabecular bone loss and, thus, has a relatively greater impact on hip fractures than vertebral fractures. The increase in serum PTH and the relative incidence of spine and hip fractures has suggested that age-related osteoporosis is two overlapping conditions, type I and II (Riggs and Melton 1986). In type II, the fracture patients are older, the PTH serum concentrations are higher, and hip fractures are commoner than vertebral fractures (Riggs and Melton 1990). Evidence is accumulating that treatment with supplements of calcium (DAWSON-HUGHES et al. 1990; DAWSON-HUGHES 1991; KOCHERSBERGER et al. 1991; CHAPUY et al. 1987) or vitamin D (NORDIN et al. 1985; LIPS et al. 1988; CHAPUY et al. 1987) increases bone mass and may reduce fracture incidence. Bone histomorphometry in subjects over the age of 65 years has been largely directed at patients who have sustained a femoral fracture rather than subjects with evidence of secondary hyperparathyroidism. In femoral fracture patients, the incidence of low bone mass and abnormal histology are high, but only a proportion show increased bone turnover typical of hyperparathyroidism (HORDON and PEACOCK 1990; LIPS et al. 1982; AARON et al. 1974; WILTON et al. 1987). On the other hand, frank osteomalacia (LIPS et al. 1982; HORDON and PEACOCK 1990; AARON et al. 1974) and primary hyperparathyroidism (CHALMERS and IRVINE 1988) are not uncommon.

IV. Others

Secondary hyperparathyroidism may occur in a number of less common conditions. Dietary phosphate supplements, if taken chronically in large amounts, lead to secondary hyperparathyroidism. In the management of the hypophosphatemic osteomalacias (PEACOCK 1984; PARFITT 1990), phosphate supplements are standard treatment and lead to hyperparathyroidism (GLORIEUX et al. 1980; RASMUSSEN et al. 1981) and parathyroid bone disease. Other conditions treated with phosphate supplements, having the same potential for causing secondary hyperparathyroidism, are idiopathic renal stone disease (PEACOCK and ROBERTSON 1989) and osteoporosis treated with an "ADFR" regimen (RASSMUSSEN et al. 1980; HODSMAN 1989).

A "renal leak" of calcium leading to secondary hyperparathyroidism has been reported to be relatively common, although this is disputed (PEACOCK and ROBERTSON 1989), in urinary store disease (PAK and GALOSY 1979; SHAKHALL et al. 1985; PAK 1990) and leads to decreased bone mass (LAWOYIN et al. 1979).

F. Tertiary Hyperparathyroidism

The term "tertiary hyperparathyroidism" describes a state of autonomous secretion of the parathyroid that develops in the course of a disease causing prolonged chronic secondary hyperparathyroidism such as vitamin D deficient osteomalacia (DAVIES et al. 1956) and chronic renal failure (CASTLEMAN and KIBBLE 1963). Since these earliest descriptions, tertiary hyperparathyroidism has been shown to develop in vitamin D deficiency osteomalacia secondary to various malabsorption states (DAVIES et al. 1968) in chronic renal failure (DAVIES et al. 1968), following renal transplant (DOMINQUEZ et al. 1970) in patients with various forms of hypophosphatemic osteomalacia on treatment with high doses of phosphate (FIRTH et al. 1985), and in vitamin D deficient osteomalacia (PEACOCK 1984).

The effects of tertiary hyperparathyroidism on the skeleton does not differ from that of primary or secondary hyperparathyroidism. Where it arises secondary to chronic renal failure, it has to be distinguished from aluminum bone disease incorrectly treated with $1,25(OH)_2$ vitamin D_3. It must also be distinguished from hypercalcemia produced by $1,25(OH)_2$ vitamin D or calcium carbonate used as a phosphate binding agent.

With better understanding of the factors involved in secondary hyperparathyroidism and the therapeutic use of vitamin D and its metabolites, tertiary hyperparathyroidism is a preventable disease and its incidence should be decreasing.

G. Hypoparathyroidism

I. Diagnosis and Pathogenesis

Hypoparathyroidism is usually caused by the absence of PTH and diagnosed by unmeasurable serum PTH concentrations in the face of chronic hypocalcemia. The hypocalcemia is a direct consequence of the absence of PTH action on kidney and to a lesser extent on bone. Tubular reabsorption of calcium, serum $1,25(OH)_2$ vitamin D, calcium absorption efficiency, bone turnover, and biomarkers of bone turnover are reduced. Hyperphosphatemia is present as a direct consequence of increased renal phosphate reabsorption.

Most cases of hypoparathyroidism result from damage to the parathyroid glands. Surgery to the neck, particularly to the thyroid gland, is the commonest cause (surgical hypoparathyroidism) but damage from radioiodine treatment of thyrotoxicosis (BURCH and POSILLICO 1983), and from iron (BREZIS et al. 1982), copper (CARPENTER et al. 1983), and aluminum (CANN et al. 1979) accumulation, and destruction by infiltrating diseases are also causes. Less commonly, hypoparathyroidism may appear as a sporadic disease (idiopathic hypoparathyroidism) affecting both sexes and all ages. In the adult the disease may develop at any age, even in the elderly (GRAHAM et al. 1979). In children hypoparathyroidism may be due to hereditary aplasia (WHYTE et al. 1986; AHN et al. 1986) and as part of the DiGeorge's syndrome (MILLER et al. 1983) or in older children as a component of the autoimmune polyglandular syndrome (AHONEN 1985). In familial isolated hypoparathyroidism a point mutation in the signal peptide-encoding region of the preproparathyroid hormone gene has been shown to be the underlying defect (ARNOLD et al. 1990).

Chronic hypoparathyroidism may occasionally be due to an abnormality in the PTH receptor (LEVINE and AURBACH 1989; SPIEGEL 1989). In these patients the hypocalcemia occurs in the presence of increased serum concentrations of PTH and represents a state of PTH resistance. A deficiency of a guanine nucleotide-binding protein, Gs, in the PTH receptor complex is a primary abnormality accounting for the resistance, but the disease can be

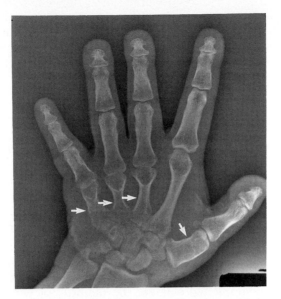

Fig. 15. Radiograph of the hand in a 31-year-old woman with hypocalcemia due to pseudohypoparathyroidism. Bradydactyly (➤) is present in the first, third, fourth, and fifth metacarpal and there is generalized reduction in skeletal size. Cortical thickness is reduced, suggesting that bone is responding to PTH despite resistance to PTH action by the kidney

further classified into type Ia, if there is a universal lack of Gs, and type Ib and II depending on biochemical differences in the receptor response to PTH (LEVINE and AURBACH 1989; SPIEGEL 1989).

Albright's hereditary osteodystrophy (ALBRIGHT et al. 1952) with short stature and bradydactyly (Fig. 15) in which pseudohypoparathyroidism may, or may not, occur (pseudo-pseudohypoparathyroidism) is a closely related hereditary condition.

1. Nonskeletal Signs

The signs and symptoms in hypoparathyroidism are dominated by the effect of hypocalcemia on the neuromuscular system and include tetany, convulsions, and paresthesia. Ectopic calcification in the basal ganglia, early onset lenticular cataract, and enamel hypoplasia, in children, may also relate to hypocalcemia and hyperphosphatemia.

2. Skeletal Signs

a) Radiology, Histology, and Biochemistry

Hypoparathyroidism gives rise to no diagnostic radiographic features. Transverse calcification in the vertebrae are reported (ROSEN and DESHMUKH

1985), but probably represent periods of growth failure, related more to treatment than to specific effects of PTH on the skeleton. There are little histomorphometric data on bone in hypoparathyroidism, but biomarkers of bone turnover are low, reflecting the greatly reduced activation frequency of the BMU.

b) Bone Mass and Fracture

Bone mass measurements in hypoparathyroidism are few but they suggest that there is either no change in bone mass (Breslau et al. 1983; Parfitt 1977) or that it may be increased (Seeman et al. 1982; Shukla et al. 1990; Hossain et al. 1970; Orr-Walker et al. 1990). Interpretation of the significance of these changes in relation to the absence of PTH is confounded by preexisting diseases affecting bone mass and by treatment of hypoparathyroidism with vitamin D and calcium supplements. In a case of postsurgical hypoparathyroidism untreated for 42 years, there was a substantial increase in bone density of both the spine and wrist (Orr-Walker et al. 1990). In 24 hypoparathyroid women, the majority of whom had surgical hypoparathyroidism, cortical to total area of the metacarpal was only slightly greater than control subjects, but was greater than in subjects with primary hyperparathyroidism, particularly in menopausal women (Hossain et al. 1970). In a study of 20 patients with postsurgical hypoparathyroidism, bone mineral density at the lumbar spine, mid radius, and distal radius was increased above normal (Seeman et al. 1982). Increased bone density in the spine and normal cortical bone in the metacarpals in seven women with long-standing hypoparathyroidism has also been reported (Shukla et al. 1990). On the other hand, in 61 subjects with hypoparathyroidism the metacarpal bone mass was decreased as compared to expected values, although greater than in patients with primary hyperparathyroidism (Parfitt 1977). The fracture incidence in hypoparathyroidism has not been established, but fracture is not a recognized clinical feature of the disease. Whether hypoparathyroidism protects the skeleton from fracture has not been established.

In pseudohypoparathyroidism developmental abnormalities in the skeleton may be present, particularly bradydactyly and short stature (Albright et al. 1952). Cortical bone mass as compared to that in surgical hypoparathyroidism is reduced by about 15% (Breslau et al. 1983) (Fig. 15). The decrease in bone mass can probably be ascribed to the effect of PTH, since the patients with pseudohypoparathyroidism had a normal response in bone biomarkers to PTH injections (Breslau et al. 1983), indicating that the PTH receptors in bone may often be normal in this disease. Indeed, some patients with pseudohypoparathyroidism not only have normal bone turnover but may develop secondary hyperparathyroid bone disease (Drezner and Nelson 1983) and even high-turnover osteomalacia (Wilson and Hadden 1980).

References

(1989) Recommended dietary allowances, 10th edn. National Academy Press, Washington

(1991) Proceedings of the NIH Consensus Development Conference on diagnosis and management of asymptomatic primary hyperparathyroidism. Liebert, New York

Aaron JE, Gallagher JC, Anderson J, Stasiak L, Longton EB, Nordin BEC, Nicholson M (1974) Frequency of osteomalacia and osteoporosis in fractures of the proximal femur. Lancet 1:229–233

Adams JS, Clemens TL, Parrish JA, Holick MF (1982) Vitamin D synthesis and metabolism after ultraviolet radiation of normal and vitamin D-deficient subjects. N Engl J Med 306:722–725

Ahn TG, Antonarakis SE, Kronenberg HM et al. (1986) Familial isolated hypoparathyroidism: a molecular genetic analysis of 8 families with 23 affected persons. Medicine (Baltimore) 65:73–81

Ahonen P (1985) Autoimmune polyendocrinopathy – candidiasis – ectodermal dystrophy (APECED): autosomal recessive inheritance. Clin Genet 27:535–542

Akerstrom G, Malmaeus J, Bergstrom R (1984) Surgical anatomy of human parathyroid glands. Surgery 95:14–21

Akerstrom G, Rudberg C, Cyrimelius L et al. (1986) Histologic parathyroid adenoma and chief cell hyperphasia. Hum Pathol 17:520–527

Albright F, Reifenstein EC (1948) The parathyroid glands and metabolic bone disease. Williams and Wilkins, Baltimore

Albright F, Forbes AP, Henneman PH (1952) Pseudopseudohypoparathyroidism. Trans Assoc Am Physicians 65:337

Anderson S, Meyer TW, Brenner BM (1987) Mechanisms of age-associated glomerular sclerosis. In: Cameron JS, Nunez JFM (eds) Renal function and disease in the elderly. Butterworth, London, pp 49–66

Andress DL, Norris KC, Coburn JW, Slatopolsky EA, Sherrard DJ (1989) Intravenous calcitriol in the treatment of refactory osteitis fibrosa cystica of chronic renal failure. N Engl J Med 274–279

Arnaud CD (1973) Hyperparathyroidism and renal failure. Kidney Int 4:89–95

Arnold A, Staunton CE, Kim HG, Gaz RD, Kronenberg HM (1988) Monoclonality and abnormal parathyroid hormone genes in parathyroid adenoma. N Engl J Med 318:658–662

Arnold A, Kim HG, Gaz RD, Eddy RL, Fukushima R, Byers MG, Shous TB, Kronenberg HM (1989) Molecular cloning and chromosomal mapping of DNA rearranged with the parathyroid hormone gene in a parathyroid adenoma. J Clin Invest 83:2034–2040

Arnold A, Horst SA, Gardella TJ, Baba H, Levine MA, Kronenberg HM (1990) Mutation of the signal peptide-encoding region of the preproparathyroid hormone gene in familial isolated hypoparathyroidism. J Clin Invest 86: 1084–1087

Attie MF, Gill JR Jr, Stock JL et al. (1983) Urinary calcium excretion in familial hypocalciuric hypercalcemia: persistence of relative hypocalcuria after induction of hypoparathyroidism. J Clin Invest 72:667–676

Baker LRI, Muir JW, Sharman VL, Abrams SML, Greenwood RN, Cattell WR, Goodwin FJ, Marsh FP, Adami S, Hately W, Hattersley LA, Morgan AG, Papapoulos SE, Revell PA, Tucker AK, Chaput de Saintonge DM, O'Riordan JLH (1986) Controlled trial of calcitriol in hemodialysis patients. Clin Nephrol 26(4):185–191

Baker LRI, Abrams SML, Roe CJ, Faugere M-C, Fanti P, Subayti Y, Malluche HH (1989) 1,25(OH)2D3 administration in moderate renal failure: a prospective double-blind trial. Kidney Int 35:661–669

Baker MR, McDonnell H, Peacock M, Nordin BEC (1979) Plasma 25-hydroxy vitamin D concentrations in patients with femoral fracture. Br Med J 1:589–591

Baker MR, Peacock M, Nordin BEC (1980) The decline of vitamin D status with age. Age Ageing 9:249–252

Bishop JM (1991) Molecular themes in oncogenesis. Cell 64:235–248

Block G, Dresser CM, Hartman AM, Carroll MD (1985) Nutrient sources in the American diet: quantitative data from the Hanes II survey. Am J Epidemiol 122:13–26

Bouillon RA, Auwerx JH, Lissens WD, Pelemans WK (1987) Vitamin D status in the elderly: seasonal substrate deficiency causes 1,25-dihydroxycholecalciferol deficiency. Am J Clin Nutr 45:755–763

Breslau NA, Moses AM, Pak CY (1983) Evidence for bone remodeling but lack of calcium mobilization response to parathyroid hormone in pseudohypoparathyroidism. J Clin Endocrinol Metab 57:638–644

Brezis M, Shaler O, Leibel B et al. (1982) The spectrum of parathyroid function in thalassaemia subjects with transfusional iron overload. Miner Electrolyte Metab 8:307

Brooks MH, Bell NH, Love L, Stern PH, Orfei E, Queener SF, Hamstra AJ, DeLuca HF (1978) Vitamin D-dependent rickets, type II resistance of target organs to 1,25-dihydroxy vitamin D. N Engl J Med 298:996–999

Buchanan JR, Myers CA, Greer RB (1988) Effect of declining renal function on bone density in aging women. Calcif Tissue Int 43:1–6

Burch WM, Posillico JT (1983) Hypoparathyroidism after I-131 therapy with subsequent return of parathyroid function. J Clin Endocrinol Metab 57:398

Cann CE, Prussia SG, Gordon GS (1979) Aluminum uptake by the parathyroid glands. J Clin Endocrinol Metab 49:543–545

Carpenter TO, Carnes DL, Anast CS (1983) Hypoparathyroidism in Wilson's disease. N Engl J Med 309:873

Castleman B, Kibble B (1963) Case records of the Massachusetts General Hospital. Case 29. N Engl J Med 268:943–953

Chalmers J, Irvine GB (1988) Fractures of the femoral neck in elderly patients with hyperparathyroidism. Clin Orthop 125–130

Chapman K (1971) Osteomalacia in Iran. J Obstet Gynaecol Br Commonw 78: 851–860

Chapuy MC, Durr F, Chapuy P (1983) Age-related changes in parathyroid hormone and 25 hydroxycholecalciferol levels. J Gerontol 38:19–22

Chapuy MC, Chapuy P, Meunier PJ (1987) Calcium and vitamin D supplements: effects on calcium metabolism in elderly people. Am J Clin Nutr 46:324 328

Charles P, Eriksen EF, Mosekilde L, Melsen F, Jensen FT (1987) Bone turnover and balance evaluated by a combined calcium balance and 47calcium kinetic study and dynamic histomorphometry. Metabolism 36:1118–1124

Christensson T, Hellstrom K, Wengle B, Alveryd A, Wiland B (1976) Prevalence of hypercalcemia in a health screening in Stockholm. Acta Med Scand 200:131–137

Christensson T, Hellstrom K, Wengle B (1977) Hypercalcemia and primary hyperparathyroidism. Arch Intern Med 137:1138–1142

Clark OH, Wilkes W, Siperstein AE, Duh Q-Y (1991) Diagnosis and management of asymptomatic hyperparathyroidism: safety, efficacy, and deficiencies in our knowledge. J Bone Miner Res 6 Suppl 2:S135–S142

Clemens T, Zhou X, Myles M, Endres D, Lindsay R (1986) Serum vitamin D_2 and vitamin D_3 metabolite concentrations and absorption of vitamin D_2 in elderly subjects. J Clin Endocrinol Metab 63(3):656–660

Coburn JW, Hartenbower DL, Massry SG (1973) Intestinal absorption of calcium and the effect of renal insufficiency. Kidney Int 4:96–104

Cochran M, Platts MM, Moorhead PJ, Buxton H (1981) Spontaneous hypercalcaemia in maintenance dialysis patients: an association with a typical osteomalacia and fracture. Miner Electrolyte Metab 5:280–286

Cohen J, Gierlowski TC, Schneider AB (1990) A prospective study of hyperparathyroidism in individuals exposed to radiation in childhood. JAMA 264:581–584

Compston JE, Ayers AB, Horon LWL, Tighe JR, Creamer B (1978a) Osteomalacia after small bowel resection. Lancet 1:9–12

Compston JE, Laker MF, Woodhead JS (1978b) Bone disease after jejuno-ileal bypass for obesity. Lancet 2:1–4

Corless D, Beer M, Boucher BJ, Gupta SP, Cohen RD (1975) Vitamin D status in long-stay geriatric patients. Lancet 1:1404–1406

Cummings SR, Black DM, Nevitt MC, Browner WS, Cauley JA, Genant HK, Mascioli SR, Scott JC, Seeley DG, Steiger P, Vogt TM (1990) Appendicular bone density and age predict hip fracture in women. JAMA 263:665–668

Dandona P, Menon RK, Shenoy R, Houlder S, Thomas M, Mallinson WJW (1986) Low 1,25-dihydroxyvitamin D, secondary hyperparathyroidism, and normal osteocalcin in elderly subjects. J Clin Endocrinol Metab 63(2):459–462

Dauphine RT, Riggs BL, Scholz DA (1975) Back pain and vertebral crush fractures: an unemphasized mode of presentation for primary hyperparathyroidism. Ann Intern Med 83:365–367

Davies DR, Dent CE, Willcox A (1956) Hyperparathyroidism and steatorthsea. Br Med J 2:1133–1137

Davies DR, Dent CE, Watson L (1968) Tertiary hyperparathyroidism. Br Med J 2:395–399

Dawson-Hughes B (1991) Calcium supplementation and bone loss: a review of controlled clinical trials. Am J Clin Nutr 54 Suppl:274S–280S

Dawson-Hughes B, Jacques P, Shipp C (1987) Dietary calcium intake and bone loss from the spine in healthy postmenopausal women. Am J Clin Nutr 46:685–687

Dawson-Hughes B, Dallal GE, Krall EA, Sadowski L, Sahyoun N, Tannenbaum S (1990) A controlled trial of the effect of calcium supplementation on bone density in postmenopausal women. N Engl J Med 323:878–883

Debnam JW, Bates ML, Kopelman RC, Teitelbaum SL (1977) Radiological/pathological correlations in uremic bone disease. Diagn Radiol 125:653–658

Deller DJ, Begley MD (1983) Calcium metabolism and the bones after partial gastrectomy. I. Clinical features and radiology of the bones. Australas Ann Med 12:282–294

Delmas PD, Demlaux B, Malaval L et al. (1986) Serum bone gamma carboxy-lutamic acid containing protein in primary hyperparathyroidism and maligant hypercalcemia. Comparison with bone histomorphometry. J Clin Invest 77:985

Delmez JA, Tindira C, Grooms P, Dusso A, Windus DW, Slatopolsky E (1989) Parathyroid hormone suppression by intravenous 1,25dihydroxyvitamin D. J Clin Invest 83:1349–1355

Dent DM, Miller JL, Klatt L, Barron J (1987) The incidence and causes of hypercalcemia. Postgrad Med J 63:745–750

Dominquez JM, Mautalln CA, Rodo JE, Barcat JA, Molins ME (1970) Tertiary hyperparathyroidism diagnosed after renal homotransplantation. Am J Med 49:423–428

Drezner MK, Nelson FA (1983) Pseudohypoparathyroidism. In: Stanbury JB (ed) The metabolic basis of inherited disease. McGraw-Hill, New York, p 1508

Driscoll RH, Meredith SC, Wagonfeld JW, Rosenberg IH (1977) Bone histology and vitamin D status in Crohn's disease. Assessment of vitamin D therapy. Gastroenterology 72:1051

Drueke T (1980) Dialysis osteomalacia and aluminium intoxication. Nephron 26:207–210

Duda RJ Jr, Kumar R, Nelson K, Zinsmeister AR, Mann KG, Riggs BL (1987) 1,25-Dihydroxyvitamin D stimulation test for osteoblast function in normal and osteoporotic postmenopausal women. J Clin Invest 79:1249–1253

Eastwood JB, Daly A, Carter GD, Alaghband-Zahek, DeWardener HE (1979) Plasma 25-hydroxy vitamin D in normal subjects and patients with terminal renal failure, on maintenance haemodialysis and after transplantation. Clin Sci 57:473

Eeckhout E, Verbeelen D, Sennesael J, Kaufman I, Jonckheer MH (1989) Monitoring of bone mineral content in patients on regular hemodialysis. Nephron 52:158–161

Ellis HA, Pierides AM, Feest TG, Ward MK, Kerr DNS (1977) Histopathology of renal osteodystrophy with particular reference to the effects of 1-hydroxy vitamin D3 in patients treated by long-term dialysis. Clin Endocrinol (Oxf) 7:31S–38S

Epstein S, Bryce G, Hinman JW, Miller ON, Riggs BL, Hui SL, Johnston CC Jr (1986) The influence of age on bone mineral regulating hormones. Bone 7:421–425

Firth RG, Grant CS, Riggs BL (1985) Development of hypercalcemic hyperparathyroidism after long-term phosphate supplementation in hypophosphatemic osteomalacia. Am J Med 78:669–673

Francis RM, Peacock M (1987) Local action of oral 1,25-dihydroxycholecalciferol on calcium absorption in osteoporosis. Am J Clin Nutr 46:315–318

Francis RM, Peacock M, Storer JH, Davies AEJ, Brown WB, Nordin BEC (1983) Calcium malabsorption in the elderly: the effect of treatment with oral 25 hydroxyvitamin D3. Eur J Clin Invest 13:391–396

Francis RM, Peacock M, Taylor GA, Storer JH, Nordin BEC (1984) Calcium malabsorption in elderly women with vertebral fractures: evidence for resistance to the action of vitamin D metabolites on the bowel. Clin Sci 66:103–107

Fraser DR, Kooh SW, Kind HP, Holick MF, Tanaka Y, DeLuca HF (1973) Pathogenesis of hereditary vitamin D dependent rickets. An inborn error of vitamin D metabolism involving defective conversion of 25-hydroxyvitamin D to 1,25 dihydroxyvitamin D. N Engl J Med 289:817–822

Friedman E, Sakaguchhi K, Bale AE, Falchetti A, Streeten E, Zimering MB, Weinstein LS, McBride WD, Nakamura Y, Brandi M-L, Norton JA, Aurbach GD, Spiegel AM, Marx SJ (1989) Clonality of parathyroid tumors in familial multiple endocrine neoplasia type 1. N Engl J Med 321:213–218

Gallagher JC, Riggs BL, Eisman J, Hamstra A, Arnaud SB, DeLuca HF (1979) Intestinal calcium absorption and serum vitamin D. J Clin Invest 64:729–736

Gallagher JC, Melton LJ, Riggs BL, Bergstrath E, DeLuca HF (1980a) Epidemiology of fractures of the proximal femur in Rochester, Minnesota. Clin Orthop 150:163–171

Gallagher JC, Riggs BL, Jerpbak CM, Arnaud CD (1980b) The effect of age on serum immunoreactive parathyroid hormone in normal and osteoporotic women. J Lab Clin Med 95(3):373–385

Gardsell P, Johnell O, Nilsson BE (1989) Predicting fracture in women by using forearm bone densitometry. Calcif Tissue Int 44:235–242

Genant HK, Heck LL, Lanzl LH, Rossman K, VanderHorst J, Paloyan E (1973) Primary hyperparathyroidism. Diagn Radiol 109:513–524

Ghandur-Mnaymneh L, Kimura N (1984) The parathyroid adenoma: a histopathological definition with a study of 172 cases of primary hyperparathyroidism. Am J Pathol 115:70–83

Glorieux FH, Marie PJ, Pettifor JM, Delvin EE (1980) Bone response to phosphate salts, ergocalciferol and calcitriol in hypophosphatemic vitamin D-resistant rickets. N Engl J Med 303:1023–1031

Goodman WG, Henry DA, Horst R et al. (1984) Parenteral aluminium administration in the dog: induction of osteomalacia and effect on vitamin D metabolism. Kidney Int 25:370–375

Graham K, Williams BO, Rowe MJ (1979) Idiopathic hypoparathyroidism: a cause of fits in the elderly. Br Med J 1:1460–1461

Gray RW, Wilz DR, Caldas AE, Lemann J (1977) The importance of phosphate in regulating plasma 1,25(OH)2 vitamin D levels in humans: studies in healthy subjects in calcium stone formers and patients with primary hyperparathyroidism. J Clin Endocrinol Metab 45:299–306

Greenfield BG (1990a) Hyperparathyroidism. In: Greenfield GB (ed) Radiology of bone diseases, 5th edn. Lippincott, Philadelphia, pp 43–61

Greenfield GB (1990b) Renal osteodystrophy. In: Greenfield GB (ed) Radiology of bone diseases, 5th edn. Lippincott, Philadelphia, pp 62–73

Greenfield GB (ed) (1990c) Radiology of bone diseases, 5th edn. Lippincott, Philadelphia

Habener JF, Potts JT Jr (1990) Primary hyperparathyroidism. In: Avioli LV, Krane SM (eds) Metabolic bone disease. Saunders, Philadelphia, pp 475–545

Hannon RR, Shorr E, McClellan WS, Dubois EF (1930) A case of osteites fibrosa cystica (osteomalacia?) with evidence of hyperactivity of the parathyroid bodies, metabolic study I. J Clin Invest 8:215–277

Haussler MR, McCain TA (1977) Vitamin D metabolism and action. N Engl J Med 297:974–983, 1041–1050

Heath H III (1991) Clinical spectrum of primary hyperparathyroidism: evolution with changes in medical practice and technology. J Bone Miner Res 6 Suppl 2:S63–S70

Heath H III, Hodgson SF, Kennedy MA (1980) Primary hyperparathyroidism: incidence, morbidity, and potential economic impact in a community. N Engl J Med 302(4):189–193

Herbert LA, Lemann J, Petersen JR, Lennon EJ (1966) Studies of the mechanism by which phosphate infusion lowers serum calcium concentration. J Clin Invest 45:1886–1894

Hercz G, Kraut JA, Andress DA et al. (1986) Use of calcium carbonate as a phosphate binder in dialysis patients. Mineral Electrolyte Metab 12:314–319

Hesp R, Hulme P, Williams D, Reeve J (1981) The relationship between changes in femoral bone density and calcium balance in patients with involutional osteoporosis treated with human parathyroid hormone fragment (hPTH 1 34). Metab Bone Dis Relat Res 2:331–334

Hock JM, Hummert JR, Boyce R, Fonseca J, Raisz LG (1989) Resorption is not essential for the stimulation of bone growth by hPTH-(1–34) in rats in vivo. J Bone Miner Res 4:449–458

Hodkinson HM, Round P, Stanton BR, Morgan C (1973) Sunlight, vitamin D and osteomalacia in the elderly. Lancet 1:910–912

Hodsman AB (1989) Effects of cyclical therapy of osteoporosis using an oral regimen of inorganic phosphate and sodium etidronate: a clinical and bone histomorphometric study. Bone Miner 5:201–212

Hodsman AB, Sherrard DJ, Alfrey AC et al. (1982) Bone aluminium and histomorphometric features of renal osteodystrophy. J Clin Endocrinol Metab 54:539–546

Holick MF, Matsuoka LY, Wortsman J (1989) Age, vitamin D, and solar ultraviolet. Lancet 11:

Hordon LD, Peacock M (1987) Vitamin D metabolism in women with femoral neck fracture. Bone Miner 2:413–426

Hordon LD, Peacock M (1990) Osteomalacia and osteoporosis in femoral neck fracture. Bone Miner 11:247–259

Hori M, Uzawa T, Morita K, Noda T, Takahashi H, Inoue J (1988) Effect of human parathyroid hormone (PTH(1–34)) on experimental osteopenia of rats induced by ovariectomy. Bone Miner 3:193–199

Horsman A, Marshall DH, Peacock M (1985) A stochastic model of age-related bone loss and fractures. Clin Orthop 195:207–215

Hossain M, Smith DA, Nordin BEC (1970) Parathyroid activity and postmenopausal osteoporosis. Lancet 1:809–811

Hughes MR, Malloy PJ, O'Malley BW, Pike JW, Feldman D (1991) Genetic defects of the 1,25-dihydroxyvitamin D_3 receptor. J Recept Res 11:699–716

Hui SL, Slemenda CW, Johnston CC Jr (1989) Baseline measurement of bone mass predicts fracture in white women. Ann Intern Med 111:355–361

Huvos AG (1991) Giant-cell tumor of bone. In: Huvos AG (ed) Bone tumors. Saunders, Philadelphia, pp 429–467

Ireland P, Fordtran JS (1973) Effect of dietary calcium and age on jejunal calcium absorption in humans studied by intestinal perfusion. J Clin Invest 52:2672–2681

Jensen PS, Kliger AS (1977) Early radiographic manifestations by secondary hyperparathyroidism associated with chronic renal disease. Diagn Radiol 125:645–652

Joborn C, Rastad J, Stalberg E, Akerström G, Ljunghall S (1989) Muscle function in patients with primary hyperparathyroidism. Muscle Nerve 12:87–94

Johnston CC, Norton J, Khairi MR, Kernek C, Edouard C, Arlot M, Meunier PJ (1985) Heterogeneity of fracture syndromes in postmenopausal women. J Clin Endocrinol Metab 61:551–556

Johnston CC, Peacock M, Meunier P (1987) Osteomalacia as a risk factor for hip fractures in the U.S.A. In: Christiansen C, Johansen JS, Riis BJ (eds) Osteoporosis 1987. Norhaven, Viborg, pp 317–320

Johnston CC, Melton LJ III, Lindsay R, Eddy DM (1989) Clinical indications for bone mass measurements. J Bone Miner Res 4:1–27

Jung RT, Davie M, Hunter S, Chalmers TM (1978) Ultraviolet light: an effective treatment of osteomalacia in malabsorption. Br Med J 1:1668–1669

Kleeman CR, Massry SG, Coburn JW, Popovtzer MM (1969) Renal osteodystrophy, soft tissue calcification and disturbed divalent ion metabolism in chronic renal failure. Arch Intern Med 124:262

Kochersberger G, Buckley NJ, Leight GS, Martinez S, Studenski S, Volger J, Lyles KW (1987) What is the clinical significance of bone loss in primary hyperparathyroidism? Arch Intern Med 147:1951–1953

Kochersberger G, Westlund R, Lyles KW (1991) The metabolic effects of calcium supplementation in the elderly. J Am Geriatr Soc 39:192–196

Kokowicz MA, Melton J III, Cedel SL, O'Fallon WM, Riggs BL (1990) Effect of age on variables relating to calcium and phosphorus metabolism in women. J Bone Miner Res 5:345–352

Krall EA, Sahyoun N, Tannenbaum S, Dallal GE, Dawson-Hughes B (1989) Effect of vitamin D intake on seasonal variations in parathyroid hormone secretion in postmenopausal women. N Engl J Med 321:1777–1783

Kumar R (1984) Metabolism of 1,25-dihydroxy-vitamin D3. Physiol Rev 64:478–504

Labuda M, Morgan K, Glorieux FH (1990) Mapping autosomal recessive vitamin D dependency type I to chromosome 12q14 by linkage analysis. Am J Hum Genet 47:28–36

Lafferty FW (1991) Differential diagnosis of hypercalcemia. J Bone Miner Res 6 Suppl 2:S51–S59

Lafferty FW, Hubay CA (1989) Primary hyperparathyroidism. A review of the long-term surgical and nonsurgical morbidities as a basis for a rational approach to treatment. Arch Intern Med 149:789–796

Larsson K, Lindh E, Lind L, Persson I, Ljunghall S (1989) Increased fracture risk in hypercalcemia. Bone mineral content measured in hyperparathyroidism. Acta Orthop Scand 60:268–270

Law WM Jr, Heath H (1985) Familial benign hypercalcemia (hypocalciuric hypercalcemia). Clinical and pathogenetic studies in 21 families. Ann Intern Med 102:511–519

Law WM Jr, Carney JA, Health H III (1984) Parathyroid glands in familial benign hypercalcemia (hypocalciuric hypercalcemia). Am J Med 76:1021–1026

Lawoyin S, Sismilich S, Browne R, Pak CYC (1979) Bone mineral content in patients with calcium urolithiasis. Metabolism 28:1250–1254

Lawson DEM, Paul AA, Black AE, Cole TJ, Mandel AR, Davie M (1979) Relative contributions of diet and sunlight to vitamin D state in the elderly. Br Med J 1:303–305

Leppla DC, Snyder W, Pak CY (1982) Sequential changes in bone density before and after parathyroidectomy in primary hyperparathyroidism. Invest Radiol 17:604–606

Levine MA, Aurbach GD (1989) Pseudohypoparathyroidism. In: DeGroot LJ (ed) Endocrinology. Saunders, Philadelphia, pp 1065–1079

Liberman UA, Samuel R, Halabe A et al. (1980) End-organ resistance to 1,25 dihydroxycholecalciferol. Lancet 1:504–506

Lindergard B (1981) Changes in bone mineral content evaluated by photon absorptiometry before the start of active uremia treatment. Clin Nephrol 16:126–130

Lips P, Netelenbos JC, Jongen M, van Ginkel FC, Althuis AL, van Schaik CL, van der Vijgh WJF, Vermeider JPW, van der Meer C (1982) Histomorphometric profile and vitamin D status in patients with femoral neck fracture. Metab Bone Dis Relat Res 4(2):85–93

Lips P, Wiersinga A, van Ginkel FC, Jongen MJM, Netelenbos JC, Hackeng WHL, Delmas PD, van der Vighn WJF (1988) The effect of vitamin D supplementation on vitamin D status and parathyroid function in elderly subjects. J Clin Endocrinol Metab 67:644–650

Liu CC, Kalu DN (1990) Human parathyroid hormone-(1–34) prevents bone loss and augments bone formation in sexually mature ovariectomized rats. J Bone Miner Res 5:973–982

Liu CC, Kalu DN, Salerno E, Echon R, Hollis BW, Ray M (1991) Preexisting bone loss associated with ovariectomy in rats is reversed by parathyroid hormone. J Bone Miner Res 6:1071–1080

Ljunghall S, Jakobsson S, Joborn C, Palmér M, Rastad J, Åkerström G (1991) Longitudinal studies of mild primary hyperparathyroidism. J Bone Miner Res 6 Suppl 2:S111–S116

MacLaughlin J, Holick MF (1985) Aging decreases the capacity of human skin to produce vitamin D3. J Clin Invest 76:1536–1538

Malmaeus J, Granberg P-O, Halvosen J, Akerstrom G, Johannson H (1988) Parathyroid surgery in Scandinavia. Acta Chir Scand 154:409–413

Mandl F (1926) Klinisches und Experimentelles zur Frage der lokalisierten Ostitis fibrosa. B. Die generaliserte Form der Ostitis fibrosia. Arch Klin Chir 143:245

Martin P, Bergmann P, Gillet C, Fuss M, Corvilain J, van Geertruyden J (1990) Long-term irreversibility of bone loss after surgery for primary hyperparathyroidism. Arch Intern Med 150:1495–1497

Marx SJ (1991) Etiologies of parathyroid gland dysfunction in primary hyperparathyroidism. J Bone Miner Res 6 Suppl 2:S19–S24

Massry SG, Stein R, Garty J et al. (1975) Skeletal resistance to the calcemic action of parathyroid hormone in uremia. Role of 1,25(OH)2D3 (Abstr). Kidney Int 1:467–474

Matloff DS, Kaplan MM, Neer RM et al. (1982) Osteoporosis in primary biliary cirrhosis: effects of 25-hydroxyvitamin D3 treatment. Gastroenterology 83:97–102

Mautalen C, Reyes HR, Ghiringhelli G, Fromm G (1986) Cortical mineral content in primary hyperparathyroidism. Changes after parathyroidectomy. Acta Endocrinol (Copenh) 111:494–497

Mayer GP, Hurst JG (1878) Sigmoidal relationship between parathyroid hormone secretion rates and plasma calcium concentration in calves. Endocrinology 102: 1803–1807

McKenna MJ, Freany R, Meade A, Muldowney FP (1985) Hypovitamin D and elevated serum alkaline phosphatase in elderly Irish people. Am J Clin Nutr 41:101

Melton LJ III (1991) Epidemiology of primary hyperparathyroidism. J Bone Miner Res 6 Suppl 2:S25–S30

Memmos DE, Eastwood JB, Tarner B et al. (1982) Double-blind trial of oral 1,25-dihydroxy vitamin D3 versus placebo in asymptomatic hyperparathyroidism in patients receiving maintenance haemodialysis. Br Med J 282:1919–1924

Meredith SC, Rosenberg IH (1980) Gastrointestinal hepatic disorders and osteomalacia. Clin Endocrinol Metab 9:131–150

Miller JD, Bowker BM, Cole DEC et al. (1983) DeGeorge's syndrome in monozygotic twins. Am J Dis Child 137:438–440

Mirra JM (1989) Brown tumor of hyperparathyroidism. In: Mirra JM (ed) Bone tumors. Lea and Febiger, Philadelphia, pp 1785–1799

Morgan DB, Hunt G, Pasterson CR (1970) The osteomalacia syndrome after stomach operations. Q J Med 34:394–410

Mundy GR, Core DH, Fisken R (1980) Primary hyperparathyroidism: changes in the pattern of clinical presentation. Lancet 1:1317–1321

Murray TM, Peacock M, Powell D, Manchik JM, Potts JT (1972) Non-autonomy of hormone secretion in primary hyperparathyroidism. Clin Endocrinol (Oxf) 1:235–246

Neer RM, Slovik DM, Daly M, Lo C, Potts JT, Jr, Nussbaum SR (1990) Treatment of postmenopausal osteoporosis with daily parathyroid hormone plus calcitriol. In: Christiansen C, Overgaard K (eds) Osteoporosis 1990. Proceedings of the Third International Symposium on Osteoporosis. Osteopress, Copenhagen, pp 1314–1317

Newton-John H, Morgan B (1970) The loss of bone with age: osteoporosis and fractures. Clin Orthop71:229–252

Nordal KP, Dahl E (1988) Low dose calcitriol versus placebo in patients with predialysis chronic renal failure. J Clin Endocrinol Metab 67:929–936

Nordin BEC, Heaney RP (1990) Calcium supplementation of the diet: justified by present evidence. Br Med J 300:1056–1060

Nordin BEC, Wilkinson R, Marshall DH, Gallagher JC, Williams A, Peacock M (1976) Calcium absorption in the elderly. Calc Tiss Res 21:442–451

Nordin BEC, Peacock M, Aaron J, Crilly RG, Heyburn PJ, Horsman A, Marshall DH (1980) Osteoporosis and osteomalacia. Clin Endocrinol Metab 9:177–205

Nordin BEC, Baker MR, Horsman A, Peacock M (1985) A prospective trial of the effect of vitamin D supplementation on metacarpal bone loss in elderly women. Am J Clin Nutr 42:470–474

Nussbaum SR, Potts JT Jr (1991) Immunoassays for parathyroid hormone 1–84 in the diagnosis of hyperparathyroidism. J Bone Miner Res 6 Suppl 2:S43–S50

Nussbaum SR, Gaz RD, Arnold A (1990) Hypercalcemia and ectopic excretion of parathyroid hormone by an ovarian carcinoma with rearrangement of the gene for parathyroid hormone. N Engl J Med 323:1324–1328

Omdahl JL, Garry PJ, Hunsaker LA, Hunt WC, Goodwin JS (1982) Nutritional status in a healthy elderly population: vitamin D. Am J Clin Nutr 36:1225–1233

Orr-Walker B, Harris R, Holdaway IM, Foote G, Reid IR (1990) High peripheral and axial bone densities in a postmenopausal woman with untreated hypoparathyroidism. Postgrad Med J 66:1061–1063

Orwoll ES, Meier DE (1986) Alterations in calcium, vitamin D, and parathyroid hormone physiology in normal men with aging: relationship to the development of senile osteopenia. J Clin Endocrinol Metab 63:1262–1269

Overton TR, Silverberg DS, Grace M et al. (1976) Bone demineralization in renal failure: a longitudinal study of the distal femur using photon absorptiometry. Br J Radiol 49:921–925

Pak CYC (1990) Kidney stones: pathogenesis, diagnosis and therapy. In: Avioli LV, Krane SM (eds) Metabolic bone disease. Saunders, Philadelphia, pp 823–849

Pak CYC, Galosy RA (1979) Fasting urinary calcium and adenosive 3, 5 monophosphate: a discriminant analysis for the identification of renal absorptive hypercalcuria. J Clin Endocrinol Metab 48:260–265

Palmer M, Jakobsson G, Akerstrom G, Ljunghall S (1988) Prevalence of hypercalcemia in a health survey: a 14-year-fellowship study of serum calcium values. Eur J Clin Invest 18:39–46

Parfitt AM (1977) Metacarpal cortical dimensions in hypoparathyroidism, primary hyperparathyroidism and chronic renal failure. Calcif Tissue Res Suppl:S329–S331

Parfitt AM (1990) Osteomalacia and related disorders. In: Avioli LV, Krane SM (eds) Metabolic bone disease. Saunders, Jovanovich, Philadelphia, pp 329–396

Parfitt AM, Miller MJ, Frame B, Villanueva AR, Rao DS, Oliver I, Thompson DL (1978) Metabolic bone disease after intestinal bypass for treatment of obesity. Ann Intern Med 89:193–199

Parfitt AM, Rao D, Stanciu J, Villanueva A, Kleerekoper M, Frame B (1985) Irreversible bone loss in osteomalacia. J Clin Invest 76:2403–2412

Parisien M, Silverberg SJ, Shane E, de La Cruz L, Lindsay R, Bilezikian JP, Dempster DW (1990) The histomorphometry of bone in primary hyperparathyroidism: preservation of cancellous bone structure. J Clin Endocrinol Metab 70:930–938

Parkinson IS, Ward MK, Feest TG et al. (1979) Fracturing dialysis osteodystrophy and dialysis encephalopathy: an epidemiological survey. Lancet 1:406–409

Peacock M, Robertson WG, Nordin BEC (1969) Relation between serum and urinary calcium with particular reference to parathyroid activity. Lancet 384–386

Peacock M (1976) Parathyroid hormone and calcitonin. In: Nordin BEC (ed) Calcium, phosphate and magnesium metabolism. Churchill Livingstone, Edinburgh, pp 405–443

Peacock M (1978) The endocrine control of calcium and phosphorus metabolism. Medicine (Baltimore) 9:407–417

Peacock M (1980) Hypercalcaemia and calcium homeostasis. Metab Bone Dis Rel Res 2:143–150

Peacock M (1984) Osteomalacia and rickets. In: Nordin BEC (ed) Metabolic bone and stone disease. Churchill Livingstone, Edinburgh, pp 71–111

Peacock M (1991) Interpretation of bone mass determinations as they relate to fracture: implications for asymptomatic primary hyperparathyroidism. J Bone Miner Res 6 Suppl 2.S77–S82

Peacock M, Hordon L (1989) Femoral fracture: the role of vitamin D. In: Kleerekoper M, Krane SM (eds) Clinical disorders of bone and mineral metabolism. Liebert, New York, pp 265–271

Peacock M, Kradin RL (1981) A 76 year old women with intermittent hypercalcemia. Case records of the Massachusetts General Hospital. N Engl J Med 305: 1457–1464

Peacock M, Robertson WG (1989) Urinary calcium stone disease. In: DeGroot LJ et al. (eds) Endocrinology. Saunders, Philadelphia, pp 1111–1132

Peacock M, Aaron JE, Walker GS, Davison AM (1977a) Bone disease and hyperparathyroidsm in chronic renal failure: the effect of 1 alpha hydroxyvitamin D3. Clin Endocrinol (Oxf) 7:73S–81S

Peacock M, Heyburn PJ, Aaron JE et al. (1979) Osteomalacia: treated with 1-hydroxy or 1,25 dihydroxy vitamin D. In: Norman AW et al. (eds) Vitamin D, basic research and its clinical application. deGruyter, Berlin, pp 1177–1183

Peacock M, Taylor GA, Brown W (1980) Plasma 1,25(OH)2 D measured by radioimmunoassay and cytosol radioreceptor assay in normal subjects and patients with primary hyperparathyroidism and renal failure. Clin Chim Acta 101:93–101

Peacock M, Bambach CP, Robertson WG, Aaron JE, Hill GL (1981) Urinary stone formation in bowel disease. In: Smith LH, Robertson WG, Finlayson B (eds) Urolithiasis: clinical and basic research. Plenum, New York, pp 159–168

Peacock M, Horsman A, Aaron JE, Marshall DH, Selby PL, Simpson M (1984) The role of parathyroid hormone in bone loss. In: Christiansen et al. (ed) Osteoporosis. Aalborg Stifsbogtrykkeri, Aalborg, pp 463–468

Peacock M, Selby PL, Francis RM, Brown WB, Hordon L (1985) Vitamin D deficiency, insufficiency, sufficiency and intoxication. What do they mean? In: Normal AW, Schaefer K, Grigoleit H-G, Herrath Dv (eds) Sixth workshop on vitamin D. de Gruyter, Berlin pp 569–570

Pierides AM (1977) The role of phosphate in renal bone disease. Clin Endocrinol (Oxf) 7:101S–107S

Pierides AM, Ellis HA, Simpson W et al. (1976) Variable response to long term 1-hydroxycholecalciferol in haemodialysis osteodystrophy. Lancet 1:1903-1095

Pike JW (1991) Vitamin D_3 receptors: structure and function in transcription. Annu Rev Nutr 11:189–216

Pipeleers-Marichal M, Somers G, Williams G et al. (1990) Gastrinomas in the duodenum of patients with multiple endocrine neoplasia type I and the Zollinger-Ellison syndrome. N Engl J Med 322:723–727

Piraino B, Chen T, Cooperstein L, Segre G, Puschett J (1988) Fractures and vertebral bone mineral density in patients with renal osteodystrophy. Clin Nephrol 30:57–62

Portale AA, Halloran BP, Murphy MM, Morris RC Jr (1986) Oral intake of phosphorus can determine the serum concentration of 1,25-dihydroxy vitamin D by determining its production rate in humans. J Clin Invest 77:7–12

Potts JT (1990) Management of asymptomatic hyperparathyroidism. J Clin Endocrinol Metab 70:1489–1493

Pugh DG (1951) Subperiosteal resorption of bone. A roentgenologic manifestation of primary hyperparathyroidism and renal osteodystrophy. AJR 66(4):577–586

Rao DS (1985) Bone and mineral metabolism. In: Berk JE (ed) Bockus gastroenterology. Saunders, Philadelphia, pp 4629–4638

Rao DS, Wilson RJ, Kleerekoper M, Parfitt AM (1988) Lack of biochemical progression or continuation of accelerated bone loss in mild asymptomatic primary hyperparathyroidism: evidence for biphasic disease course. J Clin Endocrinol Metab 67:1294–1298

Rasmussen H, Pechet M, Anast C, Mazur A, Gertner J, Broadus AE (1981) Long term treatment of familial hypophosphatemic rickets with oral phosphate and 1 alpha-hydroxy vitamin D3. J Pediatr 99:16–25

Rassmussen H, Bordier P, Marie P, Auquier L, Eisinger JB, Kuntz D et al. (1980) Effect of combined therapy with phosphate and calcitonin on bone volume in osteoporosis. Metab Bone Dis Relat Res 2:107–111

Reeve J, Meunier PJ, Parsons JA, Bernat M, Bijvoet OLM, Courpron P, Edouard C, Klenerman L, Neer RM, Renier JC, Slovik D, Vismans FJFE, Potts JT Jr (1980) The anabolic effect of human parathyroid hormone fragment (hPTH 1-34) therapy on trabecular bone in involutional osteoporosis: report of a multicenter trial. Br Med J 280:1340–1344

Reichel H, Koeffler HP, Norman AW (1989) The role of the vitamin D endocrine system in health and disease. N Engl J Med 320(15):980–991

Reiss E, Canterbury J, Egdahl RH (1968) Experience with a radioimmunoassay of parathyroid hormone in human sera. Trans Assoc Am Physiol 81:104–115

Reiss E, Canterberry JM, Bercovile MA, Kaplan EL (1970) The role of phosphate in the secretion of parathyroid hormone in man. J Clin Invest 49:2146–2149

Richardson ML, Pozzi-Mucelli RS, Kanter AS, Kolb FO, Ettinger B, Genant HK (1986) Bone mineral changes in primary hyperparathyroidism. Skeletal Radiol 15:85–95

Rickers H, Christensen M, Rodbro P (1983) Bone mineral content in patients on prolonged maintenance hemodialysis: a three year follow-up study. Clin Nephrol 20:302–307

Riggs BL, Melton LJ (1986) Involutional osteoporosis. N Engl J Med 314:1676–1686

Riggs BL, Melton LJ III (1990) Clinical heterogeneity of involutional osteoporosis: implications for preventive therapy. J Clin Endocrinol Metab 70:1229–1232

Rosen JF, Fleischman AR, Fineberg L, Hamstra A, DeLuca HF (1979) Rickets with alopecia, an inborn error of vitamin D metabolism, J Pediatr 94:729–735

Rosen RA, Deshmukh SM (1985) Growth arrest recovery lines in hypoparathyroidism. Radiology 155:61–62

Ross PD, Davis JW, Vogel JM, Wasnich RD (1990) A critical review of bone mass and the risk of fractures in osteoporosis. Calcif Tissue Int 46:149–161

Roth SI (1971) Recent advances in parathyroid gland pathology. Am J Med 50: 612–622

Rutherford WE, Bordier P, Marie P, Hruska K, Harter H, Greenwalt A, Blondin J, Haddad J, Bricker N, Slatopolsky E (1977) Phosphate control and 25-hydroxycholecalciferol administration in preventing experimental renal osteodystrophy in the dog. J Clin Invest 60:332–341

Schantz A, Castleman B (1973) Parathyroid carcinoma: a study of 70 cases. Cancer 31:600–605

Seeman E, Wahner HW, Offord KP, Kumar R, Johnson WJ, Riggs BL (1982) Differential effects of endocrine dysfunction on the axial and the appendicular skeleton. J Clin Invest 69:1302–1309

Segre GV, Potts JT (1989) Differential diagnosis of hypercalcemia: methods and clinical applications of parathyroid assays. In: DeGroot LJ et al. (eds) Endocrinology. Saunders, Philadelphia, pp 984–1001

Selby PL, Peacock M (1986) Ethinyl estradiol and norethindrone in the treatment of primary hyperparathyroidism in postmenopausal women. N Engl J Med 314: 1481–1485

Shakhall K, Nicar MJ, Brater DC et al. (1985) Exaggerated natriuretic and calciuric response to hydrochlorothiazide in renal hypercalcuria but not in absorptive hypercalcuria. J Clin Endocrinol Metab 61:825–829

Sherman SS, Hollis BW, Tobin JD (1990) Vitamin D status and related parameters in a healthy population: the effects of age, sex and season. J Clin Endocrinol Metab 71:405–413

Sherrard DJ (1986) Renal osteodystrophy. Semin Nephrol 6:56–67

Shock NW (1987) The kidney: a model for the study of aging in a physiological system. In: Cameron JS, Nunez JFM (eds) Renal function and disease in the elderly. Butterworth, London, pp 1–2

Shukla S, Gillespy T, Thomas WC Jr (1990) The effect of hypoparathyroidism on the aging skeleton. J Am Geriatr Soc 38:884–888

Silverberg SJ, Shane E, de La Cruz L, Dempster DW, Feldman F, Seldin D, Jacobs TP, Siris ES, Cafferty M, Parisien MV, Lindsay R, Clemens TL, Bilezikian JP (1989) Skeletal disease in primary hyperparathyroidism. J Bone Miner Res 4:283–291

Slatopolsky E, Coburn JW (1990) Renal osteodystrophy. In: Avioli LV, Krane SM (eds) Metabolic bone disease. Saunders, Philadelphia, pp 452–474

Slatopolsky E, Caglar S, Gradowska L, Centerbury J, Reiss E, Bricker NS (1972) On the prevention of secondary hyperparathyroidism in experimental chronic renal disease using "proportional reduction" of dietary phosphorus intake. Kidney Int 2:147–151

Slatopolsky E, Weerts C, Thielan J, Horst R, Harter H, Martin KJ (1984) Marked suppression of secondary hyperparathyroidism. J Clin Invest 74:2136–2143

Slatopolsky E, Weerts C, Lopex-Hilkir S et al. (1986) Calcium carbonate as a phosphate binder in patients with chronic renal failure undergoing dialysis. N Engl J Med 315:157–161

Slovik DM, Rosenthal DI, Doppelt SH, Potts JT Jr, Daly MA, Campbell JA, Neer RM (1986) Restoration of spinal bone in osteoporotic men by treatment with human parathyroid hormone (1–34) and 1,25-dihydroxyvitamin D. J Bone Miner Res 1:377–381

Smith DM, Khairi MRA, Johnston CC Jr (1975) The loss of bone mineral with ageing and its relationship to the risk of fracture. J Clin Invest 56:311–318

Somerville PJ, Kaye M (1982) Action of phosphorus on calcium release in isolated perfused rat tails. Kidney Int 22:348–354

Sowers MR, Wallace RB, Hollis BW (1990) The relationship of 1,25-dihydroxyvitamin D and radial bone mass. Bone Miner 10:139–148

Spiegel AM (1989) Pseudohypoparathyroidism. In: Scriver CR et al. (eds) The metabolic basic of inherited disease. McGraw-Hill, New York, pp 2013–2027

Stamp TCB, Walker PG, Perry W, Jenkins MV (1980) Nutrition osteomalacia and late rickets in Greater London 1974–1979. Clinical and metabolic studies in 45 patients. Clin Endocrinol Metab 9:81–105

Stanbury SW (1972) Azotaemic renal osteodystrophy. Clin Endocrinol 1:267–304

Stanbury SW, Lumb GA (1966) Parathyroid function in chronic renal failure. Q J Med 35:1–23

Steinstrom G, Herdman PA (1974) Clinical findins in patients with hypercalcemia. Acta Med Scand 195:473–477

Tada K, Yamamuro T, Okumura H, Kasai R, Takahashi H (1990) Restoration of axial and appendicular bone volumes by h-PTH(1-34) in parathyroidectomized and osteopenic rats. Bone 11:163–169

Thakker RV, Bouloux P, Wooding C, Chotai K, Broad PM, Spurr NK, Besser GM, O'Riordan JLH (1989) Association of parathyroid tumors in multiple endocrine neoplasia type 1 with loss of alleles on chromosome 11. N Engl J Med 321:218–224

Thompson NW, Eckhauser FE, Harness JK (1982) The anatomy of primary hyperparathyroidism. Surgery 92:814–824

Tsai KS, Health H, Kumar R, Riggs BL (1984) Impaired vitamin D metabolism with aging in women. Possible role in pathogenesis of senile osteoporosis. J Clin Invest 73:1668–1672

Vaishnava HP (1975) Vitamin D deficiency osteomalacia in Northern India. J Assoc Physicians India 23:477–484

Wasnich RD, Ross PD, Heilbrun LK, Vogel JM (1985) Prediction of postmenopausal fracture risk with use of bone mineral measurements. Am J Obstet Gynecol 153:745–751

Webb AR, Kline L, Holick MF (1988) Influence of season and latitude on the cutaneous synthesis of vitamin D3. J Clin Endocrinol Metab 67:373–378

Webb AR, Pilbeam C, Hanafin N, Holick MF (1990) An evaluation of the relative contributions of exposure to sunlight and of diet to the circulating concentrations of 25-hydroxyvitamin D in an elderly nursing home population in Boston. Am J Clin Nutr 51:1075–1081

Weiss A (1974) Incidence of subperiosteal resorption in hyperparathyroidism studied by fine detail bone radiography. Clin Radiol 25:273–276

Whyte MP, Kim GS, Kosanovich M (1986) Absence of parathyroid tissue in sex-linked recessive hypoparathyroidism. J Pediatr 109:915

Wiesner RH, Kumar R, Seeman E, Go VLH (1980) Enterohepatic physiology of 1,25 dihydroxy vitamin D metabolites in normal man. J Lab Clin Med 96:1094–1100

Wilson JD, Hadden DR (1980) Pseudohypoparathyroidism presenting with rickets. J Clin Endocrinol Metab 51:1184–1189

Wilson RJ, Rao S, Ellis B, Kleerekoper M, Parfitt AM (1988b) Mild asymptomatic primary hyperparathyroidism is not a risk factor for vertebral fractures. Ann Intern Med 109:959–962

Wilton TJ, Hosking DJ, Pawley E, Stevens A, Harvey L (1987) Osteomalacia and femoral neck fractures in the elderly patient. J Bone Joint Surg [Br] 69(3):388–390

Wiske PS, Epstein S, Bell NH, Queener SF, Edmondson J, Johnston CC Jr (1979) Increases in immunoreactive parathyroid hormone with age. N Engl J Med 300:1419–1421

Yendt ER, Cohanim M, Jarzylo S, Jones G, Rosenberg G (1991) Bone mass is related to creatinine clearance in normal elderly women. J Bone Miner Res 6:1043–1050

Young G, Marcus R, Minkogg JR, Kim LY, Segre GV (1987) Age-related rise in parathyroid hormone in man: the use of intact and midmolecule antisera to distinguish hormone secretion from retention. J Bone Miner Res 2:367–374

CHAPTER 14

Skeletal Responses to Physical Loading

L.E. LANYON

A. Introduction

The principal functions of most bones are to provide shape and withstand repetitive load-bearing. The function of bone tissue is to provide both a load-bearing material and an available repository for mineral. The functional responsibilities of bone and bones can only be discharged through the agency of populations of cells whose activity must be regulated, coordinated, and controlled accordingly.

Studies on the control of bone cell function have traditionally concentrated on the effects of systemic hormones, and more recently the influence of local growth factors, cytokines, and changes in cellular ion concentration. These are reviewed elsewhere in this book. Studies which relate the biochemical function of bone cells to changes in their biochemical milieu are ideally suited to investigating the metabolic role of bone tissue. Unfortunately they leave practically unexamined the functions of bones as structures, and bone tissue as a load-bearing constituent of these structures. This is a substantial deficiency since one of the most obvious, and arguably the most important, features of bones is their ability to adapt their shape, their mass, and the organisation of their tissue so that they may withstand without damage the loads they customarily experience.

The reasons for neglecting the mechanisms of functionally adaptive architecture are not hard to find. Those interested in cell regulation are accustomed to investigations based on biochemical manipulation and biochemical assessment of cell function. Those interested in functional adaptability to load-bearing tend to be better suited for mathematical stress analysis, the conclusions of which are not yet generally helpful in relation to cellular metabolism. What is most urgently required are investigations at the interface of organ and tissue level biology, cell biology, and biomechanics.

This chapter will focus on this interface by considering the significance, and possible mechanisms, of loading-related control of bone architecture. It will concentrate on those bones whose primary role is functional load-bearing.

B. Influences on Bone Form

Many skeletal features such as the overall shape of each bone, the location of joint surfaces and muscle attachments, the presence of medullary cavities, and even the gross distribution of cortical and cancellous regions are genetically determined and will develop in the absence of functional load-bearing.

However, despite the inherent structural suitability of the genetically determined arrangement, bones whose primary role is load-bearing (such as the long bones, and the vertebrae) if they have developed in the absence of load-bearing would fail if immediately subjected to normal functional loads. This is because the specific features upon which load-bearing competence depends, girth, cortical thickness, medullary cavity diameter, cross-sectional shape, the orientation connectivity and spatial arrangement of trabeculae, all develop "normally", and are maintained "normal" only in the presence of "normal" functional load-bearing (JAWORSKI and UHTHOFF 1986).

For any bone to grow, develop, and maintain its structural competence it must undergo the continuous processes of modelling and remodelling. These processes are performed by populations of osteoblasts and osteoclasts. The same processes are involved in functionally deprived bones as in those subjected to normal load-bearing. They are also the processes by which mineral is cycled into and out of bone tissue. Modelling and remodelling are therefore common pathways for separate mechanisms designed to meet different needs.

Control of growth will not be considered here although it naturally has a considerable influence on bone architecture. Each individual's genetic inheritance determines the form of the template on which functional and metabolic influences act, and the sensitivity of this template's responsiveness to these influences. In some bones nearly all the information necessary to produce the "normal" adult structure is determined genetically or relies only upon normal physical relationships with other structures (for instance the bones of the vault of the skull). In other bones (for instance antlers in male deer) genetic information needs a suitable hormonal environment for full adult expression (LINCOLN 1975). However, in bones with a primary load-bearing responsibility it is evident that there is no genetic regulation of the specific architectural features on which their structural competence depends, or the remodelling activity within them necessary to maintain serum calcium. Both these parameters vary throughout an individual's life according to their particular circumstances and so require control mechanisms which depend on continuous functional feedback.

The controlling inputs for modelling and remodelling include: (a) the stimuli associated with growth itself, (b) influences associated with inherent coupling of formation and resorption, (c) the influence of the calcium-regulating hormones, (d) the influence of functional load-bearing, and (e) the influence of microdamage. Healing of frank fractures while not unimportant cannot be regarded as a normal functional influence, or a consequence of normal functional activity.

The control mechanism for maintaining serum calcium depends substantially upon calcium-regulating hormones. These hormones are capable of adjusting serum calcium because they have profound and well-documented concentration-dependent effects on bone remodelling, intestinal absorption, and renal excretion of calcium. Their own secretion into the bloodstream is regulated by serum calcium concentration. This constitutes a classic feedback loop.

Production and maintenance of structurally appropriate architecture requires a similarly relevant feedback for the control of bone form and bone mass. The purpose of this control is presumably to influence modelling and remodelling behaviour to ensure that at each location there is sufficient bone tissue, with appropriate material properties, advantageously placed to withstand, with only an easily reparable level of microdamage, the functional load-bearing prevailing at that location. In order to be able to maintain this satisfactory relationship between customary load-bearing and the load-bearing capacity of the existing architecture throughout the skeleton it is necessary for the cells responsible for controlling bone architecture to have relevant feedback on the appropriateness of the relationship between the existing architecture and the prevailing loads at each skeletal location. The feedback for this mechanically related control of modelling/remodelling is more complex than that for calcium regulation and since it is related to the local situation at a number of skeletal sites it cannot be orchestrated systemically.

For us to appreciate the nature of this loading-related feedback, we must define those aspect(s) of mechanical load-bearing which provide a controlling influence on bone cell behaviour. To appreciate the significance of this control process as a determinant of bone architecture we need to know how loading-derived stimuli interact with the other influences on bone cell behaviour, notably the effect of calcium-regulating hormones. This knowledge should allow the rational development of therapeutic strategies for maintaining or enhancing bone mass.

C. Hierarchy of Functional Control

Growth itself provides a programme of development which is influenced by a number of factors. Once growth has ceased the primary functional influences on remodelling within the skeleton are those related to control of serum calcium and continued provision of a structurally appropriate architecture. As well as these two functionally-adaptive influences, there is the influence of function-related microdamage, which is essentially repair, and influences of non-skeletal origin such as changes in hormonal and nutritional status, age, and drug therapy or abuse.

Demands for skeletal calcium require bone resorption and are thus in direct competition with mechanically based requirements to preserve bone mass for load-bearing. Hormonal demands for resorption are, however, synergistic with those demands for resorption necessary to repair microdamage which is itself mechanically engendered. These competing and complementary mechanically and hormonally derived influences on remodelling are presumably resolved at each location within the bone as a result of the combination of cellular responses, cytokines, and local growth factors which they separately produce. Thus at different levels of both load-bearing and hormonal activity there may be either synergy or competition for any particular local modelling or remodelling behaviour (LANYON 1984, 1986). Since calcium-regulating hormones are primarily concerned with resorption to provide serum calcium, and since their demands usually have priority, their potential for structurally deleterious modelling/remodelling is profound. In contrast their potential for controlling, rather than enabling, structurally appropriate remodelling is negligible since they have no relevant functional control input. In normal individuals peak bone mass, and mass (and architecture) at any time, are therefore primarily determined by the individual's genetic inheritance, and their bones' strain history acting through mechanisms whose responsiveness is also part of their genetic makeup. Bone architecture will only be affected by the level of nutrition, hormonal, and metabolic balance etc., if these influences enhance distort or limit this mechanically derived response.

For tissue loading to influence modelling or remodelling it must elicit some chemical response within a sensitive cell population. We have documented some instances of this response which may be parts of the early stages in a cascade of reactions in this and other populations of cells involved in the control of modelling/remodelling. Our data suggest an immediate response in osteocytes which is related to the magnitude of the dynamic strain change in their vicinity (SKERRY et al. 1989). Because of their location, osteocytes do not themselves participate in the modelling or remodelling response. This suggests that these cells have a primary strain-sensitive role. They are certainly well placed to function in this way. Not only are they distributed throughout the bone matrix, but they communicate with each other and with the cells on the bone surface, through gap junction connections (DOTY 1981; MENTON et al. 1984). Such connections are specifically designed for the passage of information from one cell to another. In the experiments referred to here we have attempted (a) to define those aspects of a bone's strain regime that influence its modelling and remodelling behaviour and (b) to investigate in vivo and in vitro the sequence of events in the resident bone cells which follow exposure to a potentially osteogenic strain-related stimulus.

These investigations are at a potentially interesting stage since by identifying the early strain-generated biochemical events we will be well placed to understand the relationships of these events with the other, intrinsically biochemically-based stimuli, to which bone modelling and remodelling are subjected.

Although many of the active agents involved in metabolic control of modelling/remodelling have been identified, it has been a source of frustration for many workers that none of them has proved capable of providing a sustained net osteogenic effect with accompanying improvement in structural properties. The reason for this is not hard to find. None of the known agents responsible for metabolically related remodelling has any "interest" in bone mass or in bone architecture. Bone mass is always sufficient for immediate calcium requirements, and a trabecula oriented in one direction is as available and useful a source of mineral as one oriented in another.

Not only does the calcium-regulating process have no interest in bone mass or architecture, it has no means by which to derive feedback from these variables in order to control them. Any expectation that there should be an "osteogenic hormone" is therefore doomed. Regulating bone mass is the responsibility of a system whose feedback is derived from the only functional variable to which bone mass at each location is of interest, namely load-bearing. Total skeletal mass (and architecture), and the structural competence it implies, is the cumulative effect of these local loading-related stimuli.

Although the agents of calcium-regulation cannot themselves contribute a functional stimulus to the synthesis or placement of tissue to produce a mechanically suitable architecture, it is evident that, without the mechanisms of calcium metabolism, structurally appropriate anatomical features, if produced, could not be mineralized, and the processes of modelling and remodelling could not be completed. However, in this respect calcium itself, and the calcium-regulating hormones, are enabling, rather than controlling, the achievement and maintenance of bone architecture. It is clear also that changes in an individual's nutritional and hormonal circumstances can disable the capacity of any loading-related functionally adaptive process either to establish or maintain a structurally competent skeleton. Specific insufficiencies such as a low-calcium diet or vitamin deficiences are obvious examples, but hormonal imbalance, the effect of age per se, and the effect of drugs can all prevent the attainment and maintenance of the architecture necessary for structural competence.

In a perfect situation with no nutritional, metabolic, or hormonal impediment there would be full expression of the bone mass and architecture which the load-bearing stimulus requires. It is logical therefore that the flow path of the various influences on bone mass should involve a primary functional stimulus derived from some measure of the appropriateness of current bone architecture in relation to current load-bearing, and that this pathway should be modified by non-mechanically derived influences downstream. Rectifying deficiencies in these modifying influences can only allow full expression of the mechanical stimulus, it cannot produce a bone mass which is greater, or a bone architecture which is more appropriate, than that which is required mechanically.

In practice it is evident that inadequate bone architecture may result from age-related, hormonally-related, and nutritionally-related constraints on the consequences of the mechanically related stimulus; or inadequacies and/or inappropriateness of the stimulus itself.

D. Nature of the Loading-Related Stimulus

The structural variables controlled by the bone cell population are the mass, material properties, and spatial organization of the bone tissue present. The product of these variables and the structure's applied load are the strains[1] which the load engenders. Since the objective of the bone cell population is presumably to ensure that the variables over which they have control are appropriate in relation to the applied load, it is logical to propose that their mechanically-related feedback should be the strain which such loading engenders within the bone matrix.

Not only is load-induced strain a functional variable which contains all the information necessary for the control of bone architecture in relation to bone loading, it can also affect cells directly, or indirectly through one of its derivatives such as intralacunar pressure, fluid flow, or charged fluid flow.

The proposal that dynamic strain change in the matrix is a functional input capable of influencing bone cell behaviour is supported by a number of experimental findings. These show both in vivo and in vitro that there are relevant functional relationships between the components of the strain environment, and both short-term bone cell behaviour and longer-term bone modelling and remodelling.

E. Experimental Studies: In Vivo

One of the most productive models for studying the effects of load-bearing on bone architecture has been the functionally isolated, externally loadable avian ulna preparation. This preparation allows quantified loads to be repetitively applied in vivo over a period of weeks to large segments of bone in adult animals (Lanyon and Rubin 1984). Using this prepa ation we have been able to establish:

1. That in the situation of surgically induced disuse daily exposure to extremely short periods of dynamic loads not only prevents the resorption which normally accompanies reduced loading, but also results in an increase in bone formation proportional to the peak strain magnitude (Figs. 1, 2)

---

[1] It is not uncommon for stress and strain to be used interchangeably. This is incorrect. When a load is applied to a structure it deforms until the intermolecular forces within the structure prevent further deformation. These intermolecular forces are the stresses, and in a simple situation equate to the applied load distributed across the load-carrying area (hence stress = force per unit area). The deformation produced by the applied load (and resisted by the stresses) can be resolved into strains which are defined as the ratio of change in any dimension to the original dimension. A strain of 1 (sometimes expressed as a percentage, 1 = 100%) represents a doubling of a particular dimension. Functional strains in bone tissue are normally less than 0.003 (also sometimes referred to as 0.3% or 3000 microstrain). In contrast to strains which can easily be measured stresses can only be calculated. There is no way in which stresses can be either measured or sensed directly.

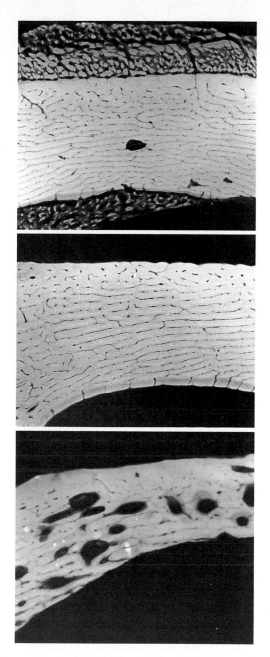

Fig. 1. Microradiographs of cortical bone from adult turkey ulnas (*middle*) under normal circumstances showing little or no modelling or remodelling activity (*bottom*) from a similar bone deprived of functional loading for 8 weeks. The situation has been transformed into one of intense activity. The endosteal surface has been eroded with resulting thinning of the cortex and there is substantial intracortical activity characterised by incompletely infilled haversian remodelling. This section shows the classic features of the active phase of disuse osteopenia. *Top*, a section from a bone in which the disuse was interrupted by a short daily period of intermittent loading. This not only prevents the resorption seen in disuse alone but is associated with new bone formation on both periosteal and endosteal surfaces. The changes in bone cross-sectional area under these different loading circumstances are illustrated in Fig. 2. (From RUBIN and LANYON 1985)

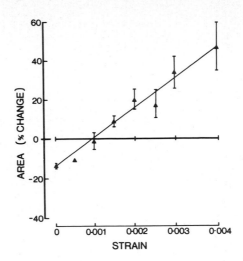

Fig. 2. Dose : response relationship between peak strain magnitude and change in bone cross-sectional area in disuse preparations of turkey ulnas subjected to intermittent compressive loads producing peak strains of different magnitudes in the experiment in Fig. 1. Disuse and peak strains of less than 0.001 were associated with bone loss whereas strains above this level were associated with a proportional increase in bone cross-sectional area. (After RUBIN and LANYON 1985)

(RUBIN and LANYON 1985). This response which occurs on both periosteal and endosteal surfaces is initially diffuse woven bone, but if daily loading is maintained for 16 weeks this consolidates and undergoes haversian remodelling as it becomes a structurally integral part of the expanded cortex (RUBIN, personal communication). Static load applied continuously produces no different effect from disuse (LANYON and RUBIN 1984).

2. The osteogenic response to a single period of daily dynamic loading saturates after as few as 36 consecutive 1-Hz loading cycles/day occupying only 72 s. Further loading cycles up to 1800 produce no significant additional osteogenic response. As few as four loading cycles/day of a potentially osteogenic stimulus are sufficient to prevent resorption while being insufficient to stimulate formation (RUBIN and LANYON 1984).

3. Different strain distributions produce different dose : response relationships between peak strain magnitude and change in bone cross-sectional area. In the avian ulna peak principal strain levels presented in the distribution produced by loading in torsion appear less osteogenic than the same levels presented in the distribution produced by loading in longitudinal compression (PEAD and LANYON 1990).

4. The strain-related, potentially osteogenic, response to intermittent loading can act in direct competition with hormonally derived stimuli for resorption during calcium insufficiency.

This is evident from the finding that bone loss due to disuse is additional to that due to calcium insufficiency, and can be modulated by external

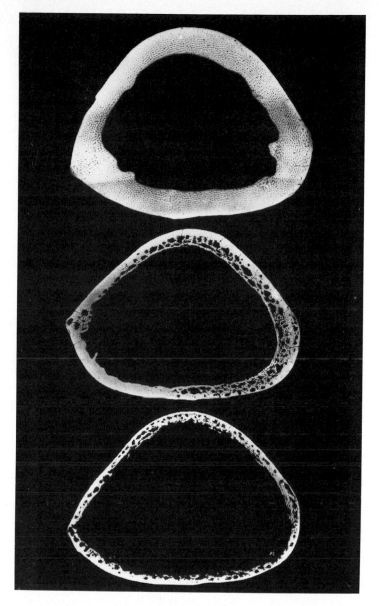

Fig. 3. Microradiographs of sections taken from the midshaft of turkey ulnas to show the interactions between hormonally-derived and mechanically-derived stimuli. The upper two bones are from animals of similar size and age, and share a similar loading environment, being in normal, intact, functional wings. The differences in cross-sectional area between these bones can be attributed to their different hormonal environment. The top bone was from an animal on a calcium-sufficient diet, the middle bone from an animal after 6 weeks of calcium insufficiency. The lower two bones are the left and right ulnas from the same animal and thus share a common hormonal environment. However, the bottom bone has experienced no functional load-bearing over the period of calcium insufficiency. The bone loss due to calcium insufficiency and that due to disuse are additive. This suggested that even during severe calcium insufficiency mechanical loading provides a conservative effect on bone remodelling. This was confirmed by modulating the degree of bone loss by a short period of applied external loading. (After LANYON et al. 1986)

loading (Lanyon et al. 1986) (Fig. 3). In this experiment a strain regime which was osteogenic in male animals on a calcium-sufficient diet served only to modulate resorption in calcium-insufficient females.

5. A single period of loading on a single day can stimulate transformation of a quiescent periosteum into one actively forming new bone 6 days later (Pead et al. 1988a). The magnitude of this osteogenic response is modulated by a single large dose of indomethacin at the time of loading (Pead and Lanyon 1989).

6. Twenty-four hours after a single period of loading there is a sixfold increase in the number of osteocytes incorporating [^{3}H]uridine (Pead et al. 1988b). This is consistent with increased synthetic activity in these cells.

7. Five minutes after a single period of loading there is a local strain magnitude-related increase in the number of osteocytes showing G6PD (glucose 6 phosphate dehydrogenase) activity, and in the level of G6PD activity of periosteal cells (Skerry et al. 1989). This response is unaccompanied by any increase in the activity of aldolase or GA3PD. G6PD activity is the rate-limiting step of the pentose monophosphate shunt. An increase in G6PD activity is consistent with the production of RNA and increased synthetic activity.

8. Immediately after a single period of loading there is an increased orientation in the proteoglycan molecules within the cortical bone which, in the absence of further loading, persists for over 24 h (Skerry et al. 1988, 1990). Long-term disuse (Dodds et al. 1990) and human clinical osteoporosis (Ferris et al. 1987) are both associated with decreased proteoglycan orientation in bone tissue.

F. Experimental Studies: In Vitro

In vitro we have investigated bone cell responses to mechanical loading in cancellous bone core biopsy explants which were loaded while being perfused, and in 17-day embryonic chick tibias which were loaded in culture.

These studies allowed us to demonstrate the following:

9. Five minutes after loading in both cancellous cores and embryonic tibias there is a loading-related increase in G6PD activity similar to that seen in vivo in resident bone cells. In bone cores this increase in G6PD activity is inhibited by indomethacin (Dallas et al. 1993).

10. Six hours after loading in bone cores there is a similar loading-related increase in [^{3}H]uridine uptake in osteocytes and surface bone cells to that seen in vivo (Dallas et al. 1993).

11. Six hours after loading in both cores and embryonic tibias there is a loading-related increase in the specific activity of [^{3}H]uridine in the RNA extracted from bone cores. In cores this loading-related response is also substantially modified by indomethacin (El Haj et al. 1988a,b, 1990; Minter 1991; Dallas et al. 1993).

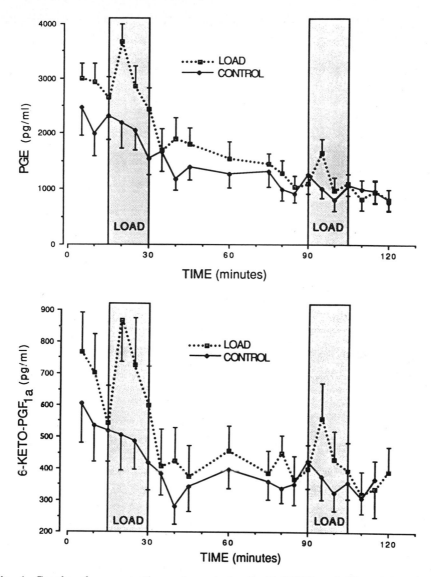

Fig. 4. Graphs of concentrations of prostaglandin E (PGE) and 6-keto-PGF$_1$ (the metabolite of prostacyclin) released into the perfusing medium from cores of adult canine cancellous bone subjected to two 15-min periods of intermittent loading 1 h apart. Both loading periods show elevated levels in the 0 to 5 min and the 5 to 10 min samples for both compounds but these had fallen to preload levels by the 10 to 15 min sample (from Rawlinson et al. 1991b)

12. Within 5 min of the beginning of loading in bone cores there is a transient increase in 6 Keto PGF$_1$ (the stable metabolite of prostacyclin) and prostaglandin E in the perfusate (Fig. 4). There is also immunocytochemical evidence of the presence of PGE in surface cells and PGI$_2$ in both surface cells and osteocytes (Rawlinson et al. 1991a,b).

13. Both prostacyclin and prostaglandin E_2 added to the perfusate of bone cores produces within 8 min an increased activation of G6PD in ostisocytes and lining cells (RAWLINSON et al. 1991b). However, the increase in specific activity of [^{3}H]uridine in extracted RNA is stimulated by prostacyclin and not PGE_2 (RAWLINSON et al. in preparation). Autoradiography confirms the site of this PGI_2-induced incorporation of [^{3}H]uridine to be osteocytes and lining cells.

G. Loading of Bone Cell Cultures

In primary bone cell cultures and in cell lines we have not yet been able to demonstrate the same range of mechanically-related changes in bone cell behaviour seen in organ culture or in vivo. To be able to do so would provide substantial experimental advantage.

H. Implications of Experiments In Vivo

The in vivo results from the avian wing preparation (1–7) all support the concept of a bone cell population swiftly responsive to changes in mechanical events in its tissue. The two effects of mechanical loading on bone modelling/remodelling, which appear in a strain magnitude related fashion, are inhibition of resorption and increase in formation.

It seems that functional levels of bone mass are only maintained in the presence of intermittent loading, and that this loading has to occur at roughly daily intervals but need only occupy a brief period each day. Failure to maintain exposure to functional loading results in disuse osteopenia. BURKHART and JOWSEY's (1967) experiments showing that disuse osteopenia occurs only in the presence of intact parathyroids suggests that the stimulus for bone loss arises from the (resorptive) effect of the hormonal environment unopposed by the (conservational and potentially osteogenic) effects of mechanical loading. The calcium deficiency experiment (4) is consistent with the hypothesis of opposing mechanically-derived and hormonally-derived stimuli. This experiment also shows the overwhelming effect that calcium-regulating hormones can have over mechanically-derived, potentially osteogenic responses.

The lack of any inflexion in the strain response curve (1) (Fig. 2) suggests that stimulation of new bone formation, and inhibition of bone resorption, may be dose-related aspects of the same mechanism, with the potentially osteogenic response to load-bearing being antagonistic to the potentially resorptive influence of calcium-regulating hormones.

The osteogenic response to a single period of loading (5) demonstrates that in a disuse situation at least only a single short exposure to an osteogenic strain regime is necessary to engender the full cascade of events which culminate in new bone formation. Presumably the long-term modelling/

remodelling response to repeated exposure to such stimuli (1–4) is the cumulative effect of each individual daily cascade.

The finding that exposure to short periods of artificial loading can produce substantial new bone formation, despite peak physiological strain levels never being exceeded, supports the idea [originally proposed in relation to much longer duration adaptive experiments in sheep (LANYON et al. 1982)] that the origin of the adaptive stimulus may be responsive to differences in strain distribution rather than changes in local strain magnitudes. Thus for each strain distribution there may be a different slope to the dose:response curve, but in each case the slope is peak dynamic strain magnitude-dependent. This hypothesis is supported by the different dose: response relationship between torsion and compression (3). Together with (2) and (5), these results are consistent with adaptive modelling/remodelling being dominated by the effects of short-duration signals with unusual strain distributions rather than many repetitions of strain cycles with a normal strain distribution. In effect this would mean that mechanically adaptive modelling/remodelling is error-driven and thus not necessarily related to the predominant load-bearing activity.

Finding 8 is consistent with this hypothesis since it provides a mechanism by which intermittent strain experienced in "real time" induces more persistent but recoverable strain-related changes in the bone matrix which could subsequently influence bone cell behaviour. This could be interpreted as a "strain memory". There would be no need for such a memory (or a swift cellular response to strain change) if adaptive bone cell responses were driven by many repetitions of a uniform pattern of loading. Although there is as yet no positive evidence that strain-related proteoglycan orientation has any functional consequences, it is of interest that the degree of orientation of proteoglycans in the matrix appears to be deficient in bone specimens from human clinical osteoporotics (FERRIS et al. 1987).

In vivo modulation of the osteogenic response to loading by large concentrations of indomethacin is consistent with a prostanoid-dependent step early in the cascade of events between strain transduction and subsequent osteogenesis. However, since the high concentration of indomethacin could have inhibited recruitment of preosteoblasts, the prostanoid-dependent step could be part of the osteogenic response to the mechanically-derived stimulus, rather than the early transduction and formulation of the stimulus into biochemical terms. These two effects could not easily be disentangled in vivo but were resolved in vitro.

I. Implications of Experiments In Vitro

I. Organ Culture

The in vitro findings expand our knowledge from that available from the in vivo experiments and allow us to identify a number of the steps in the putative cascade of events between a period of loading capable of engendering an osteogenic response and the osteogenic response itself. It is of course impossible at this early stage to say whether these are really part of a sequence or not.

The local strain magnitude-related increase in the number of osteocytes showing G6PD activity in vivo; the finding that indomethacin blocks this strain-related response both in vivo and in vitro; the immediately increased levels of prostaglandin and the metabolite of prostacyclin in the perfusate of loaded cancellous bone cores in vitro; the finding that PGE_2 and PGI_2 both stimulate G6PD activity; and that exogenous prostacyclin added to the medium in this preparation imitates (quantitatively) the RNA production stimulated by loading: all imply that G6PD activation is an intermediate step between strain-related prostacyclin production and stimulation of RNA. Increased G6PD activity is not a specific response but merely reflects a strain magnitude-related increase in synthetic activity possibly to produce RNA. This RNA could, but need not be, coded for the production of a specific growth factor or cytokine.

One significant feature of the adaptive response to increased strain is that the maximum amount of new bone formation does not seem to occur at the site of the greatest local overstrain (LANYON et al. 1982; RUBIN and LANYON 1985). This is presumably because strategic placement of new bone, and removal of redundant tissue, requires an appreciation of the mismatch between the actual and the desirable strain distribution for each location, rather than just the differences in local peak strain magnitude. The need for this assessment of strain distribution has led us to propose that following the "capture" and transduction of strain information into biochemical information there is an integrative phase during which the strain magnitude-dependent consequences of strain in the locality of each cell are modulated in relation to the strain distribution prevailing throughout a wider volume of tissue. The location of the new bone formation (and resorption) of the adaptive response is presumably related to this modulated information.

The nature of this "strain distribution-modifying" step is practically unstudied. Indeed it is largely unappreciated probably because it is disguised by the equation of the local strain magnitude-related increase in the number of osteocytes showing G6PD activity in short-term experiments, and the global strain distribution mismatch-dependent, but peak strain magnitude-related, overall increases in bone mass in long-term experiments.

Assuming that such as assessment of strain distribution does exist, the bone cells' response to strain involves at least three phases: (a) immediate transduction of mechanical strain into biochemical information followed by a series of biochemical reactions including prostanoid production all of which (from the G6PD evidence) are related directly to the initiating local peak strain magnitude, (b) a "strain environment-modifying phase" when local strain magnitude-related biochemical events are modified in relation to other features of the strain environment (including distribution) throughout a wider volume of bone tissue, and (c) an adaptive response when both resorption and formation are influenced by the stimulus, modified as in (b), opposed, enabled, or enhanced according to the local biochemical environment including the hormonal milieu.

As yet we have accumulated some information as to how the strain-generated biochemical "signal" is generated. It appears that PGE_2 and PGI_2 stimulate increased G6PD activity in a local strain magnitude-dependent fashion and that the increased prostacyclin production is followed by increased RNA synthesis. Although the evidence is not good, it appears that the RNA response in osteocytes more closely parallels the disposition of subsequent new bone formation than the local strain magnitude related G6PD activity. If this is the case then some account of strain distribution will have occurred between these two phases. Although we have no information as to what form the "signal processing" might take, any appreciation of strain distribution requires communication between strain-sensitive cells. Such communication is a feature of osteocytes.

It is attractive to presume that the strain distribution-modulated RNA response involves the production of some cytokine or growth factor which then interrelates with all the other local and systemic influences on bone cell populations responsible for the control of modelling and remodelling. Since osteocytes do not produce matrix, it is logical to suppose that what they do provide in response to strain is designed to influence the modelling/remodelling process indirectly.

J. Discussion

Mechanically-related control of bone architecture is of clinical importance in relation to occupational or athletic adaptation of bone structure, long-term functional compatibility of skeletal implants particularly prostheses, and postmenopausal osteoporosis. In vivo studies of the relationship between bone mass and physical activity in humans have been largely confined to attempts to relate levels of physical activity, or changes in the level of activity, with noninvasive assessments of bone mass (i.e., CHOW et al. 1987; KANDERS et al. 1988; SIMKIN et al. 1987; SMITH et al. 1989; review by SMITH and GILLIGAN 1987; GUTIN and QASPER 1992). Assessments of the suitability, or load-bearing capacity, of bone architecture are rarely made since the criteria are not defined. Few of the studies on bone mass are longitudinal, and only recently have studies been published which relate loading at a particular bone site with change in the architecture of that site. Since strain-related remodelling is essentially a local response to loading, this is of course essential. Relating bone mass at a site chosen for its convenience, and relating it to some measure of cardiovascular performance is as clearly unacceptable as it would be to assess cardiac performance, by measuring bone density. Nevertheless, despite the inappropriateness of many of the measurements frequently used, and the poor definition of the loading regimes actually employed, the consensus of exercise-related studies is unmistakable. Increased functional loading is associated with a location-specific increase in bone mass, and decreased functional loading with bone loss (LEICHTER et al. 1989; JACOBSON et al. 1984; KIRK et al. 1989; POCOCK et al. 1989; COLLETTI et al. 1989; KANDERS et al. 1988). This carries with it the strong implication that normal loading activity at each location is an important, if not the most important, functional determinant for normal bone mass.

Since it is evident that most people do not radically change their exercise habits at the time of menopause, when rapid bone loss occurs, it is legitimate to ask the question "what is the failure of the mechanism which ensures structural competence premenopausally and yet allows the structural incompetence characteristic of senile and postmenopausal osteoporosis?" (LANYON 1984, 1986). Among the answers are effects downstream from the functional response to load-bearing which modify or inhibit this response. These effects include those due to age per se, dietary and absorptive insufficiencies which increase the pressure for bone resorption, kidney failure which has a similar effect, hormonal imbalances, and treatment with anti-inflammatory drugs. The association between bone loss and estrogen levels is so obvious that it cannot be ignored.

It is evident that the functionally adaptive response in bone tissue evolved to produce an appropriate bone mass and architecture in the situation of a complete repertoire of hormones. Estrogen appears to act on the same side of the balance of influences as physical load-bearing to provide at least a conservational effect on bone mass by reducing the activation frequency of remodelling units (STEINICHE et al. 1989). It may also enhance the osteogenic components of the remodelling cycle and may be specifically synergistic to the strain-related stimulus to modelling/remodelling activity. When estrogen is removed and the remodelling frequency increased, if the hormonal: mechanical equilibrium is also reset to a position where resorptive influences have a greater advantage, then there will be a rapid movement towards a lower bone mass. Such a movement is a feature of the postmenopausal period.

For a loading-related conservational and potentially osteogenic stimulus to compensate for the loss of the synergistic effects of estrogen, it would have to be increased beyond the level operating before the menopause. In fact the opposite is usually the case because the functionally-adaptive process also evolved to produce a bone architecture appropriate to the spectrum of physical activity characteristic of young adults in societies accustomed to an active life. This spectrum involves a wide range of loading situations some with quite high strains and high strain rates. [The osteogenic potential of a strain regime appears to be related to the maximum strain rate as well as the peak strain magnitude (O'CONNOR et al. 1982)]. One feature of increasing age particularly in "advanced" societies is the reduction in both the vigour and diversity of physical activity. Activity with normal, or even higher than normal, peak strain magnitudes but low strain rates or error-free strain distributions will be perceived by the bone cells as relative disuse, and lead quite appropriately (as far as the mechanism is concerned) to bone loss. Indeed if our suggestion is correct and normal bone mass is maintained primarily by the constant stimulus from everyday error signals, the less vigorous, stereotyped activity of the aged (and some middle aged) would be interpreted as error-free, and thus osteogenic stimulus-free. Coincidence of a reduced loading-related stimulus per se and the removal of estrogen, will produce an additional tendency to bone loss.

Consideration of these points raises a number of practical questions:

1. "To what extent can appropriate exercise provide a conservational or osteogenic stimulus adequate to prevent sufficient bone loss to remove a significant proportion of the population from being "at risk" from osteoporotic fractures?" Evidence such as that presented by CHOW et al. (1987), JACOBSON et al. (1984), SMITH et al. (1989), SIMKIN et al. (1987), COOPER et al. (1988), WICKHAM et al. (1989), and reviewed by SMITH and GILLIGAN (1987) suggests that the use of exercise in this fashion is feasible. The efficacy of various specific exercise regimens has been reviewed by GUTIN and KASPER (1992). Most of the studies referred to show exercise-related increases in bone mass, or reduction of bone loss in post-menopausal women.

2. "What constitutes appropriate exercise in relation to preserving or increasing bone mass?" Our experimental evidence suggests that bone modelling and remodelling are profoundly affected by short periods of dynamic strain change, the most osteogenic response being produced by high strains, high strain rates, and unusual strain distributions. We consider that these are more likely to be generated by sporadic error signals than repetitive coordinated functional loading. From our data we predict that short periods of diverse weight-bearing exercise will be far more effective therefore than long periods of running, bicycling, or swimming. These predictions have been supported by GUTIN and KASPER (1992) who conclude "appropriate exercise can contribute to bone density and play a role in the prevention of osteoporosis. To be most effective a combination of relatively vigorous aerobic and strength training seems sensible". NOTELOVITZ et al. (1990) have demonstrated the potential of combined therapy. They used variable resistance weight training combined with estrogen replacement in women following surgical menopause and demonstrated not only prevention of bone loss but quite dramatic increases in bone mass.

3. "To what extent can we get the benefits of exercise without the exercise?" This is the key question for those interested in the pharmacology of bone. With the possible exception of fluoride treatment (the structural consequences of which are open to doubt), there are few, if any, therapeutic agents which are inherently osteogenic in that they produce a sustained increase in bone mass. In the absence of such substances, treatment is

essentially supportive. Therapy with hormones, vitamins, and/or calcium will at best make possible full expression of the bone architecture demanded by the mechanically-related stimulus. If this stimulus is lacking, then maintenance of a robust bone structure cannot be expected. Devising a means for therapeutic intervention to achieve exercise-related benefits without exercise depends upon either (a) imitating the osteoregulatory effect of load-bearing by other means, and thus essentially deceiving the homeostatic mechanism that there is less bone, or more load-bearing, than actually exists or (b) making possible full expression of the bone mass and architecture that the homeostatic mechanism demands but which for various reasons it is prevented from obtaining. To successfully achieve either of these objectives requires an understanding of the normal mechanisms of mechanically-related control of bone architecture and the normal inter-relationships of these pathways with those other influences on bone modelling and remodelling.

K. Summary

The continuing ability of the skeleton to resist fracture depends upon maintaining at each location sufficient bone tissue with adequate material properties, appropriately placed to withstand applied loads. At each location the product of bone mass, architecture, material properties, and applied load is the dynamic strain situation within the tissue. Functional strains therefore carry the information necessary for the feedback control of bone architecture in relation to load-bearing requirement. Such information cannot be provided by systemic influences.

The importance of local functional strains in the control of bone architecture is supported by the findings of immediate strain-related changes in the activity of resident bone cells, and long-term strain-related changes in modelling and remodelling behaviour. We propose that the modelling and remodelling which actually determines bone architecture, and thus fracture resistance, at each location, is primarily the result of the balance of potentially competing and complementary influences derived from local strain-related factors, and the local effects of systemic hormones. The change in this equilibrium of influences postmenopausally is in favour of increased, negatively balanced remodelling and so in the absence of an enhanced mechanically-derived stimulus bone loss will result.

Since loading-related functional adaptation in bone is a local response to local loading, it follows that any exercise regime intended to increase or maintain bone mass must be designed to produce a conservational or "osteogenic" strain regime at each location concerned. Current evidence strongly suggests that appropriate exercise can modulate or even reverse postmenopausal bone loss. Appropriately controlled studies in humans using properly characterized loading regimes to determine the most effective loading regime for each location remain to be performed. At present animal data suggest that short periods of diverse weight-bearing activity will be far more effective than long periods of repetitive loading, which involve lower peak loads applied in habitual loading situations. This prediction is supported by some human studies.

Sensible therapeutic interference with the processes of bone modelling/remodelling to maintain or enhance the skeleton's structural competence requires further knowledge of the normal mechanisms whereby structure is related to function. Our current work is directed towards determining the sequence of events between a period of loading with osteoregulatory potential and the modelling/remodelling changes themselves. This work is at present only rudimentary; however, we have identified certain events in vivo and in vitro which are consistent with an almost immediate prostaglandin response in osteocytes and lining cells followed by an increase in G6PD activity in bone cells and an increase in their RNA production. Although the earliest biochemical responses appear to be related to local peak strain magnitude, the sites of adaptive new bone formation are not necessarily similarly distributed. The modification of the potentially osteogenic stimulus in the light of strain distribution is a significant step in the cascade of modelling/remodelling which is as yet practically unstudied.

We hypothesize, as yet with no verification, that the RNA produced by osteocytes in response to dynamic strain in their matrix is coded for some cytokine or growth factor which then interacts with the other factors influencing bone modelling and remodelling. If this is so there is significant potential to influence this stage therapeutically by enhancing the effect of the conservational or potentially osteogenic, mechanically-derived stimulus at the expense of the resorptive stimulus derived from calcium-regulating hormones.

Acknowledgements. Over the years the work reported here has been supported by the MRC (UK), the Wellcome Trust, the Wolfson Foundation, SERC, NASA, and the USDA.

References

Burkhart JM, Jowsey J (1967) Parathyroid and thyroid hormone in the development of immobilisation osteoporosis. Endocrinology 81:1053–1062

Chow R, Harrison JE, Notarius C (1987) Effect of two randomised exercise programmes on bone mass of healthy postmenopausal women. Br Med J 295: 1441–1444

Colletti LA, Edwards J, Gordon L, Shary J, Bell NH (1989) The effects of muscle building exercise on bone mineral density in the radius, spine, and hip, in young men. Calcif Tissue Int 45:12–14

Cooper C, Barker DJP, Wickham CAC (1988) Physical activity muscle strength and calcium intake in fracture of the proximal femur in Britain. Br Med J 297: 1443–1446

Dallas SC, Zaman G, Pead MJ, Lanyon LE (1993) Early strain-related changes in cultured embryonic chick tibiotarsi parallel those associated with adaptive modeling in vivo J Bone Miner Res 8:251–259

Dodds R, Skerry TM, Pead MJ, Lanyon LE (1990) Proteoglycan orientation in bone; its relationship to loading, disuse and clinical osteoporosis. Orthop Trans 14:511

Doty SB (1981) Morphological evidence of gap junctions between bone cells. Calcif Tissue Int 33:509–512

El Haj AJ, Minter S, Lanyon LE (1988a) Pathways of activation in adult adaptive bone remodelling. Calcif Tissue Int 42:A30

El Haj AJ, Minter S, Pead MJ, Skerry TM, Lanyon LE (1988b) Cellular response to mechanical loading in explants of adult cancellous bone. J Bone Miner Res 3:S200

El Haj AJ, Minter L, Rawlinson SCF, Suswillo R, Lanyon LE (1990) Cellular responses to mechanical loading in vitro. J Bone Miner Res 5:923–932

Ferris B, Klenerman L, Dodds RA, Bitensky L, Chayen J (1987) Altered organisation of non collagenous bone matrix in osteoporosis. Bone 8:285–288

Gustin B, Kasper MJ (1992) Can vigorous exercise play a role in osteoporosis? A review. Osteoporosis Int 2:55–59

Jacobson PC, Beaver W, Grubb SA, Taft TN, Talmage RV (1984) Bone density in women: college athletes and older athletic women. J Orthop Res 2:328–332

Jaworski ZG, Uhthoff HK (1986) Reversibility of non traumatic disuse osteoporosis during its active phase. Bone 7:431–439

Kanders B, Dempster DW, Lindsay R (1988) Interaction of calcium nutrition and physical activity on bone mass in young women. J Bone Miner Res 3:145–149

Kirk S, Sharp CF, Elbaum N, Endres DB, Simon SM, Mohler JG, Rude RK (1989) Effect of long distance running on bone mass in women. J Bone Miner Res 4:515–522

Lanyon LE (1984) Functional strain as a determinant of bone remodelling. Calcif Tissue Int 36:S56–S61

Lanyon LE (1986) Biomechanical factors in adaptation of bone structure to function. In: Uhthoff HK, Jaworski ZFG (eds) Current concepts of bone fragility. Springer, Berlin Heidelberg New York, pp 19–33

Lanyon LE, Rubin CT (1984) Static versus dynamic loads as an influence on bone remodelling. J Biomech 17:892–905

Lanyon LE, Goodship AE, Pye CJ, MacFie H (1982) Mechanically adaptive bone remodelling. A quantitative study on functional adaptation in the radius following ulna osteotomy in sheep. J Biomech 15:767–781

Lanyon LE, Rubin CT, Baust G (1986) Modulation of bone loss during calcium insufficiency by controlled dynamic loading. Calcif Tissue Int 38:209–216

Leichter I, Simkin A, Margulies JY, Bivas A, Steinberg R, Giladi M, Milgrom C (1989) Gain in mass density of bone following strenuous physical activity. J Orthop Res 7:86–90

Lincoln A (1975) An effect of the epididymis on the growth of antlers of castrated red deer. J Reprod Fertil 42:159–161

Menton DN, Simmons DJ, Chang A-L, Orr Y (1984) From lining cell to osteocyte – an SEM study. Anat Rec 209:29–39

Minter SC (1991) Use of in vitro techniques to investigate cellular responses to mechanical load in bone. PhD thesis, University of London

Notelovitz M, Martin D, Tesar R, Khan Y, Probart C, Fields C, McKenzie L (1990) Estrogen therapy and variable-resistance weight training increase bone mineral in surgically menopausal women. J Bone Miner Res 6:583–590

O'Connor JA, Lanyon LE, MacFie H (1982) The influence of strain rate on adaptive bone remodelling. J Biomech 15:767–781

Pead MJ, Lanyon LE (1989) Indomethacin modulation of load-related stimulation of new bone formation in vivo. Calcif Tissue Int 45:34–40

Pead MJ, Lanyon LE (1990) Adaptive remodelling in bone: torsion versus compression. Proc Orthop Trans 14:340

Pead MJ, Skerry TM, Lanyon LE (1988a) Direct transformation from quiescence to formation in the adult periosteum following a single brief period of loading. J Bone Miner Res 3:647–656

Pead MJ, Suswillo R, Skerry TM, Vedi S, Lanyon LE (1988b) Increased 3H uridine levels in osteocytes following a single short period of dynamic loading in vivo. Calcif Tissue Int 43:92–97

Pocock N, Eisman J, Gwinn T, Sambrook P, Kelly P, Freund J, Yeates M (1989) Muscle strength, physical fitness and weight but not age predict femoral neck bone mass. J Bone Miner Res 4:441–448

Rawlinson SCF, El-Haj AJ, Minter SC, Tavares IA, Bennet A, Lanyon LE (1991a) Prostacyclin production in osteocytes may be an early strain-related step in mechanically adaptive bone remodelling. J Anat 179:218

Rawlinson SCF, El-Haj AJ, Minter SC, Bennett A, Tavares IA, Lanyon LE (1991b) Load-related release of prostaglandins in cores of cancellous bones in culture – A role for prostacyclin in adaptive remodelling? J Bone Miner Res 6:1345–1351

Rubin CT, Lanyon LE (1984) Regulation of bone formation by applied dynamic loads. J Bone Joint Surg [Am] 66:397–402

Rubin CT, Lanyon LE (1985) Regulation of bone mass by mechanical strain magnitude. Calcif Tissue Int 37:411–417

Simkin A, Ayalon, Leichter I (1987) Increased trabecular bone density due to bone loading exercise in post-menopausal osteoporotic women. Calcif Tissue Int 40: 59–63

Skerry TM, Bitensky L, Chayen J, Lanyon LE (1988) Loading-related reorientation of bone proteoglycans. A strain memory in bone tissue? J Orthop Res 6:547–552

Skerry TM, Bitensky L, Chayen J, Lanyon LE (1989) Early strain-related changes in enzyme activity in osteocytes following bone loading in vivo. J Bone Miner Res 4:783–788

Skerry TM, Suswillo R, El Haj AJ, Ali NN, Dodds RA, Lanyon LE (1990) Load-induced proteoglycan orientation in bone tissue vivo and in vitro. Calcif Tissue Int 46:318–326

Smith EL, Gilligan C (1987) Effects of inactivity and exercise on bone. Physician Sports Med 15:91–100

Smith EL, Gilligan C, McAdam M, Ensign CP, Smith P (1989) Deterring bone loss by exercise intervention in premenopausal and postmenopausal women. Calcif Tissue Int 44:312–321

Steiniche T, Hasling C, Charles E, Eriksen EF, Mosekilde L, Melsen F (1989) A randomised study on the effects of estrogen/gestagen or high dose oral calcium on trabecular bone remodelling in post menopausal osteoporosis. Bone 10: 313–320

Wickham CAC, Walsh K, Cooper C, Barker DJP, Margetts BM, Morris J, Bruce SA (1989) Dietary calcium, physical activity and risk of hip fracture: A prospective study. Br Med J 299:889–892

CHAPTER 15
Parathyroid Hormone: Biosynthesis, Secretion, Chemistry, and Action

H.M. Kronenberg, F.R. Bringhurst, S. Nussbaum, H. Jüppner, A.-B. Abou-Samra, G. Segre, and J.T. Potts, Jr.

The parathyroid hormone (PTH) story was once fairly simple. PTH raises blood calcium by resorbing bone, conserving urinary calcium, and activating vitamin D in order to increase intestinal calcium absorption. Blood calcium, in turn, decreases PTH secretion. The PTH-calcium homeostatic loop acts to maintain a constant level of blood calcium in the face of varying dietary and skeletal demands. This physiologically appealing story remains a powerful organizing principle for understanding parathyroid function, but has been modified by important observations in the last few years.

   1. The characterization of parathyroid hormone-related protein (PTHrP) has introduced important new ideas: this predominantly paracrine factor shares receptors with PTH; the structure and sequence of PTHrP is only beginning to lead to greater understanding of PTH structure.
   2. The parathyroid cell is regulated not only by calcium but also by $1,25(OH)_2D_3$.
   3. The PTH receptor shares striking homology with receptors for calcitonin and secretin; together these receptors begin to define a new subfamily of G protein-linked receptors.
   4. Parathyroid hormone not only activates adenylate cyclase in cells, but also activates phospholipase C. The precise roles of these and other candidate pathways of PTH action remain unclear.
   5. In bone, PTH can stimulate trabecular bone formation at the same time that it stimulates cortical bone resorption.

   These new observations are all still imperfectly understood but suggest complicated levels of regulation and roles for PTH that substantially expand the classical model. In this chapter, the actions of PTH at the tissue level will first be summarized. Then, the biosynthesis and secretion of PTH by the parathyroid cell will be discussed. An analysis of PTH chemistry and structure will then be followed by new information about PTH receptors and the second messengers responsible for initiating the cell's responses to PTH.

A. Physiologic Actions

Recognition of the physiologic effects of PTH originally derived from observations in humans and animals with hypoparathyroidism and in patients with severe primary hyperparathyroidism. In hyperparathyroidism, in particular, progressive osteopenia, hypercalcemia, hypophosphatemia, hypercalciuria, and kidney stones had implicated bone, kidney, and possibly intestine as the major putative target tissues of the hormone. The roles of these tissues as mediators of PTH action were subsequently borne out by an enormous volume of scientific investigation. Thus, although stimulation of intestinal calcium absorption is now thought to occur mainly indirectly, via enhanced renal synthesis of $1,25(OH)_2D_3$, alterations in cellular activities of bone and kidney are now understood to be the principal mechanisms whereby PTH maintains mineral-ion and skeletal hemeostasis.

Extensive investigations over the past 50 years have greatly refined understanding of the specific PTH-responsive cell types within these tissues, as well as the critical biochemical events that underlie the homeostatic effects of the hormone. More recently, actions of PTH have been reported in a wide variety of "nonclassical" target tissues, including cartilage, vascular and other smooth muscle, placenta, liver, pancreatic islets, brain, dermal fibroblasts, and lymphocytes. These findings have been further supported by very recent initial observations of the widespread tissue expression of mRNA encoding a cloned PTH receptor. The physiologic significance of these "nonclassical" actions of PTH remains unclear, however, particularly in view of the possibility that some or all of these effects may reflect physiologic actions of PTHrP rather than of PTH per se.

I. Actions in Bone

Numerous studies in vivo and in vitro have confirmed that sustained exposure to PTH, particularly at high concentrations, leads to activation and recruitment of osteoclasts, accelerated bone resorption, and subsequent net bone loss. These changes are accompanied by activation of osteoclastic membrane proton pumps, local release of acid hydrolases, release of calcium, phosphate, and degraded matrix components into blood, and a variety of other responses that are not specific to PTH but rather constitute the generic response of osteoclasts to a variety of different bone-resorbing agents. Other, more rapid responses to PTH precede evidence of osteoclastic bone resorption and may be of particular importance for the minute-to-minute regulation of blood calcium. Thus, administration of PTH is followed within minutes by a transient decrease in blood calcium, due at least in part to uptake by bone cells (PARSONS and ROBINSON 1971). This is succeeded by an increased mobilization of calcium from bone. This calcium may be derived from a pool distinct from the mineralized matrix phase; release may be mediated by (nonosteoclastic) osteocytes distributed along the endosteum of bone

(TALMAGE et al. 1976). The specific cellular or anatomic basis of these early responses remains unsettled, but the low abundance of osteoclasts in normal bone is also consistent with the hypothesis that the involvement of bone in short-term calcium homeostasis is mediated by mechanisms other than osteoclastic bone resorption per se.

1. Effects upon Osteoclasts

It is now generally accepted that mature osteoclasts do not possess receptors for PTH (RODAN and MARTIN 1981). This conclusion is based upon findings that isolated osteoclasts fail to respond directly to added PTH in vitro (CHAMBERS et al. 1985; NICHOLSON et al. 1986), as well as upon failure to demonstrate binding of radioiodinated PTH to osteoclasts auto-radiographically in vivo (ROULEAU et al. 1988) or in vitro (SILVE et al. 1982). Although direct effects of PTH on osteoclasts in vitro have been reported (MEARS 1971; FERRIER et al. 1986), contamination by nonosteoclastic bone cells may well explain these observations. More recently, TETI et al. (1991) described specific binding of $[^{125}I]bPTH(1-84)$ to individual avian osteoclasts visualized by autoradiography, although the binding was of relatively low affinity. Also, HAKEDA et al. (1989) reported high-affinity binding of $[^{125}I]bPTH(1-34)$ to murine hematopoietic blast cells, which were then stimulated by PTH to differentiate into multinucleated osteoclast-like cells that no longer bound the hormone. These findings raise the interesting possibility that PTH may act directly upon early marrow osteoclast precursors to promote recruitment of new osteoclasts but that the activity of mature osteoclasts is controlled indirectly via other PTH target cells in bone. It is likely that more direct information about the possible existence of PTH-responsive cells within the osteoclast lineage will derive from use of in situ hybridization or immunohistochemical approaches made possible by the recent cloning of the PTH receptor.

If mature osteoclasts lack PTH receptors, what are the signals that activate them in response to PTH (FELDMAN et al. 1980)? It is clear from coculture or conditioned-medium experiments that PTH-stimulated osteoblasts release one or more paracrine factors that recruit new osteoclasts and/or activate mature osteoclasts (CHAMBERS et al. 1984; WONG 1984; PERRY et al. 1989; McSHEEHY and CHAMBERS 1986). Such a paracrine mechanism is thought to underlie, at least in part, the apparent coupling between bone resorption and formation observed across a wide range of cellular activity in bone (RODAN and MARTIN 1981; HOWARD et al. 1981). Candidate molecules identified to date include interleukin-6, GM-CSF, and a partially characterized 9-kDa peptide, all of which have been shown to be secreted from osteoblasts or other osteogenic cells (LOWIK et al. 1989; PALIWAL and INSOGNA 1991; FELIX et al. 1989). Other work suggests a PTH-responsive mechanism that requires direct contact between osteoblastic cells and osteoclastic precursors (YAMASHITA et al. 1990). It seems likely that the local, indirect regulation of osteoclastic bone resorption by PTH will prove to be quite complex and will involve multiple secreted factors or cellular mechanisms specific for different phases of osteoclastic differentiation and activation.

2. Effects upon Osteoblasts

Osteoblasts appear to be the major direct cellular target of PTH action in bone. Osteoblasts, as well as various osteoblast-like transformed cell lines widely used for in vitro studies of osteoblastic function, possess high-affinity surface receptors for PTH and generate a variety of intracellular signals in response to the hormone, including changes in cAMP, IP_3, DAG, Ca^{2+}, membrane potential, and pH (reviewed below). High concentrations of PTH lead acutely to inhibition of many osteoblastic functions, both in vivo and in vitro, although a delayed increase in osteoblast number, seen both in vivo and in bone organ cultures, is associated with an overall increase in osteoblastic activity that ultimately may or may not approach the accelerated rate of osteoclastic bone resorption. In any event, the net result is an increase in activity of both populations of bone cells and a corresponding increase in overall rates of bone turnover (BINGHAM et al. 1969; FELDMAN et al. 1980; HOWARD et al. 1981; RODAN and MARTIN 1981; WONG 1984). PTH regulates a vast array of osteoblastic activities (Table 1), including many aspects of cellular carbohydrate, lipid, protein, and nucleotide metabolism; rates of membrane transport of Ca^{2+}, H^+, Na^+, K^+, and PO_4 ions and of nutrients such as glucose and amino acids; cytoskeletal assembly and cell shape; synthesis and secretion of type-1 collagen, osteonectin, osteopontin, and other components of bone matrix; activity of critical enzymes such as alkaline phosphatase, collagenase, and plasminogen activator; and secretion of putative autocrine or paracrine growth factors and cytokines such as IGFs I and II, various IGF-binding proteins (IGFBPs), TGF-β, M-CSF, IL-6, PGE_2, and partially characterized "coupling factors" (vide supra). Cellular responsiveness to other hormones and growth factors, as well as to PTH itself, is also modulated via mechanisms that include receptor regulation, desensitization, and, in the case of IGFs, altered secretion of specific IGFBPs that either potentiate or inhibit IGF effects (TORRING et al. 1991). In many cases, the details of these regulatory phenomena vary dramatically among different experimental systems. These differences probably reflect the importance of the PTH concentration per se, the duration and pattern of exposure to the hormone, and, in vitro, important biological differences of the "osteoblast(s)" under study. This diversity is perhaps not surprising, in light of the abundant evidence of heterogeneity among osteoblastic cells, even within a particular tissue such as a rat calvarium (GUENTHER et al. 1989; RODAN et al. 1988; YOON et al. 1987; CIVITELLI et al. 1989). Indeed, recent in vivo autoradiographic data indicate that the bone cell to which intravenously administered [^{125}I]PTH(1–34) binds most intensely in young

Table 1. Osteoblast functions regulated by parathyroid hormone

Proliferation	Matrix protein synthesis and secretion
	Collagen
Cellular metabolism	Osteocalcin
Glucose and amino acid transport	Osteonectin
Citrate, ornithine decarboxylation	Osteopontin
Glycogen synthesis, glucose	
oxidation	Enzyme synthesis and secretion
Synthesis of RNA, protein, lipids	Alkaline phosphatase
Ion Transport	Collagenase
Ca^{2+}, PO_4, H^+	Plasminogen activator/inhibitor
Na^+/K^+ ATPase	Metalloproteinase inhibitor
Cytoskeletal and membrane structure	
Cytokines and other factors	Release of paracrine growth factors
Actin, vimentin, tubulin, and	IGF-1, IGF-2, IGF-binding
actinin synthesis	proteins, TGFβ
Phosphatidylethanolamine synthesis	M-CSF
Hormonal responsiveness	Interleukin-6
PTH receptor expression	Prostaglandin E_2, others
EGF receptor expression	Unidentified "coupling factors"
1,25-Dihydroxyvitamin D	
receptor expression	

rat long bones is not the mature osteoblast but a morphologically distinct cell possessed of elongated cytoplasmic extensions interpositioned between blood vessels and the trabecular bone surface (ROULEAU et al. 1988). The possibility that such cells might mediate the rapid alterations in bone-blood calcium flux following PTH administration, noted above, must be addressed further.

One topic of obvious interest is the effect of PTH on osteoblast proliferation and differentiation and the associated issue of the net effect of PTH on bone mass. The variety of experimental approaches that have been applied to this question highlights the complexity of PTH action in bone. As noted above, continuous exposure to high circulating concentrations of PTH in vivo clearly leads to progressive bone loss and osteopenia, although osteoblasts do increase in number (reviewed in HABENER and POTTS 1978). The response to PTH differs among various anatomic regions of bone: patients with mild hyperparathyroidism exhibit loss of cortical but not cancellous (trabecular) bone (SILVERBERG et al. 1989). In contrast, intermittent (daily) injection of low doses of PTH increases bone mass in normal, parathyroidectomized, or ovariectomized rats (KALU et al. 1970; TAM et al. 1982; GUNNESS-HEY and HOCK 1984; HOCK et al. 1988) and in osteoporotic humans (SLOVIK et al. 1986). In vitro, PTH inhibits the differentiation of fetal rat calvarial preosteoblastic cells required for bone-nodule formation, if the hormone is administered continuously, but not if it is given intermittently (BELLOWS et al. 1990). In intact cultured fetal rodent calvaria, continuous exposure to PTH selectively inhibits collagen synthesis (BRINGHURST and POTTS 1981; CANALIS et al. 1989), despite enhanced total DNA synthesis. In contrast, limited (24 h) exposure to PTH is followed by an increase in collagen synthesis over several days. This effect is blocked by neutralizing antibodies to IGF-I and is thus presumably due to local release of IGF-I stimulated by PTH (Canalis et al. 1989; McCarthy et al. 1989). The delayed stimulation of proliferation induced by PTH in these cultures is not mediated by IGF, however (Canalis et al. 1989). Direct experiments in vitro with isolated osteoblasts from adult human or embryonic rat or chick bone demonstrate stimulation of DNA synthesis by PTH (Somjen et al. 1987; Van der Plas et al. 1985; Macdonald et al. 1986), whereas PTH inhibits growth of UMR 106-01 and dexamethasone-treated ROS 17/2.8 rat osteosarcoma cells (Partridge et al. 1985). These differences in PTH action thus appear to relate mainly to the concentration and temporal pattern of exposure to the hormone, although certain effects may predominate in unusual cellular contexts (i.e., UMR cells) or following exposure to other hormones or growth factors. As discussed below, it seems likely that these differences may result from modulation of the activation of different osteoblastic second messenger signals, due either to differential susceptibility of individual signaling pathways to homologous desensitization (Bidwell et al. 1991) or to intrinsic differences in sensitivity to hormone/receptor activation. Such an explanation of varying responses to PTH is supported by studies showing differences in the relative efficacy of various PTH fragments in stimulation of cAMP, Ca^{2+}, and growth in cultured chondrocytes (Schlüter et al. 1989).

II. Actions in Kidney

Parathyroid hormone exerts a variety of actions on the kidney, including decreased reabsorption of phosphate and bicarbonate, increased reabsorption of calcium and magnesium, and enhanced synthesis of $1,25(OH)_2D$. Most of these effects have been recognized for many years, although understanding of the specific cellular subtypes and mechanisms that mediate them has unfolded only gradually. Early in vivo micropuncture analysis progressed to in vitro studies with microdissected nephron segments, isolated perfused tubules, intact cells, membrane fractions, and, most recently, use of cultured cells derived from specific regions of the nephron or cell lines that model particular aspects of renal epithelial function. Analysis of the renal actions of PTH has been complicated by the wide diversity and topographical heterogeneity of cellular functions that exist within the kidney. The variety of distinct transport mechanisms arrayed in close succession along the nephron, functional differences between otherwise similar cortical vs. medullary nephrons, and the relative lack of well-characterized cell lines suitable for studying renal epithelial functions specific for different nephron segments have challenged the ingenuity of investigators. Despite these difficulties, substantial progress has been made in defining critical aspects of PTH control of renal function.

1. Calcium Reabsorption

Calcium reabsorption occurs throughout the nephron, but the mechanisms involved differ strikingly from one location to the next (SUKI 1979). In the proximal tubule, which reabsorbs over half of total filtered Ca^{2+}, Ca^{2+} reabsorption is closely linked to that of Na^+ (although these can be dissociated) and is likely due entirely to passive, isosmotic transport down the ambient electrochemical gradient (DUARTE and WATSON 1967; MURAYAMA et al. 1972; NG et al. 1984). Proximal tubular cells express abundant functional PTH receptors on their basolateral membranes (TORIKAL et al. 1981; MOREL et al. 1981), but micropuncture studies have shown that regulation of Ca^{2+} reabsorption by PTH is essentially restricted to the distal nephron (GREGER et al. 1978; AGUS et al. 1973; IMAI 1981; SHAREGHI and STONER 1978). Within the distal nephron, several contiguous segments – the cortical thick ascending loop of Henle (cTAL), the distal convoluted tubule (DCT), and the connecting tubule (CNT) – exhibit PTH-stimulated Ca^{2+} transport, although the mechanisms involved appear to differ.

In the cTAL, basal Ca^{2+} transport occurs passively along paracellular pathways in response to the (lumen-positive) transepithelial electrochemical gradient (BOURDEAU and BURG 1980). In this segment, PTH increases the transepithelial voltage gradient further and thereby supports additional Ca^{2+} transport (WITTNER and DISTEFANO 1990). In more distal segments (DCT and CNT), by contrast, Ca^{2+} reabsorption occurs via active transport against a steep electrochemical gradient and is dissociated from lumenal Na transport (COSTANZO and WINDHAGER 1980). The CNT, in particular, appears to be the major site at which PTH regulates active transport of Ca^{2+} (IMAI 1981; SHAREGHI and STONER 1978). Several recent observations have helped to clarify some details of the mechanisms involved.

Active transport of Ca^{2+} ultimately depends upon extrusion of Ca^{2+} against the steep chemical gradient that exists at the basolateral surface of the polarized renal epithelial cell. This active transport may be mediated by either (a) a primary "Ca^{2+} pump" (Ca^{2+}/Mg ATPase) or (b) a Na^+/Ca^{2+} exchanger driven, in turn, by the Na^+/K^+ ATPase(s) that maintains the transmembrane Na^+ gradient. In membrane vesicles from rabbit distal tubules, BOUHTIAUY et al. (1991) found that PTH nearly doubles the maximal rate of Na^+/Ca^{2+} exchange across the basolateral membrane (BLM) but does not increase the activity of the primary Ca^{2+}/Mg ATPase "Ca^{2+} pump." Interestingly, expression of the Na^+/Ca^{2+} exchanger, like PTH-stimulated active transport of Ca^{2+}, is apparently limited to the distal nephron, whereas the Ca^{2+}/Mg ATPase is present in both proximal and distal nephron segments (RAMACHANDRAN and BRUNETTE 1989). In intact isolated rabbit CNTs, BOURDEAU and LAU (1989) found that PTH increased cytosolic Ca^{2+} slowly (over several minutes) by promoting entry of extracellular Ca^{2+}, while SHIMIZU et al. (1990) observed a delayed (20–30 min) depolarization of the membrane potential at the apical pole of the CNT cells (but not cTAL or DCT cells). These rather leisurely changes in cytosolic Ca^{2+} and membrane potential are unlike the more rapid transients typical of receptor-dependent signaling events (see below) and more likely reflect downstream alterations in the activities of membrane channels or transporters for Ca^{2+} and Na^+, respectively. Finally, in single distal tubular epithelial cells derived from cTAL and DCT, BACSKAI and FRIEDMAN (1990) reported that PTH induces the appearance of functional dihydropyridine-sensitive Ca^{2+} channels and an associated rise in cytosolic Ca^{2+} over 30 min (at 25°C), both of which were blocked when microtubular assembly was inhibited with colchicine.

Overall, these observations suggest that, in response to PTH, pre-formed Ca^{2+} channels, sequestered within distal tubular cells, are rapidly translocated to the surface to mediate enhanced apical (luminal) Ca^{2+} entry (Fig. 1). Such channels could require further activation, i.e., via phosphorylation association with specific G proteins, or other modifications, to become fully functional. At the same time, PTH enhances the activity of Na^+/Ca^{2+} exchangers in the basolateral (antiluminal) membrane. Driven by the underlying transmembrane Na^+ gradient, these exchangers mediate active basolateral extrusion of the increased flow of Ca^{2+} ions arriving through the apical surface (SHIMIZU et al. 1990). The availability of appropriate cell models, such as the MDCK cells recently reported to exhibit PTH-stimulated transcellular Ca^{2+} transport as well as other distal tubular characteristics (KENNEDY et al. 1989), should provide convenient approaches to further elucidating the cellular mechanisms whereby PTH controls Ca^{2+} reabsorption in the distal nephron. The involvement of specific intracellular second messenger responses to PTH in the genesis of these changes in distal renal epithelial function will be reviewed below.

2. Phosphate Reabsorption

Parathyroid hormone is the major hormonal factor that controls proximal renal tubular phosphate reabsorption and, hence, the serum phosphate concentration (reviewed in BRINGHURST 1989; GMAJ and MURER 1986). The inhibition of phosphate reabsorption by PTH is most evident in the early proximal tubule, although effects of the hormone have also been described in more distal regions of the nephron. Proximal tubular phosphate transport proceeds mainly via a Na^+-P cotransport mechanism at the luminal (apical) surface of the epithelial cells which, like distal Ca reabsorption, is ultimately driven by the transmembrane Na^+ gradient generated by the Na^+, K^+ ATPase. PTH rapidly inhibits the V_{max} of this Na^+-P cotransporter by a mechanism that does not require new protein synthesis (GMAJ and MURER 1986). Recent data suggest that endocytosis and sequestration of apical membranes containing the transporters may be involved, as the PTH effect is blocked by colchicine and other maneuvers that inhibit endocytosis (KEMPSON et al. 1990). Functional PTH receptors linked to adenylate cyclase have been localized exclusively to the basolateral membranes of isolated proximal tubular cells (SHLATZ et al. 1975). Thus, inhibition of phosphate

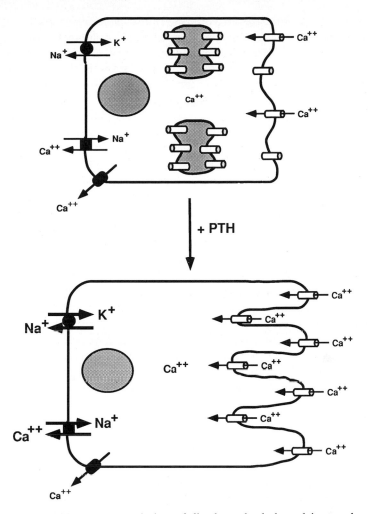

Fig. 1. Parathyroid hormone regulation of distal renal tubular calcium reabsorption. PTH triggers the translocation of preformed voltage-dependent calcium channels from sites of intracellular sequestration to the apical membrane, which also undergoes rapid morphological changes that greatly increase its surface area. Intracellular free calcium rises significantly, and increased net transepithelial calcium transport occurs, mainly via enhanced Na/Ca exchange at the basolateral membrane, supported in turn by the Na/K ATPase. Activity of the basolateral Mg-ATP-dependent calcium pump is not increased. Analogous events underlie PTH regulation of proximal tubular phosphate transport

transport is presumably mediated by a soluble messenger generated on the cytoplasmic surface of the basolateral membrane and not by direct coupling between the cotransporter and apical PTH receptors. On the other hand, studies with the opossum kidney ("OK") cell line, a proximal tubule-like epithelial cell line which has been used extensively to study PTH-dependent inhibition of phosphate transport, suggest that PTH receptors may be present on both the apical and basolateral surfaces of the cell (HELMLE-KOLB et al. 1990a; RESHKIN et al. 1990). It is not yet clear whether the lack of polarization of functional PTH receptors in OK cells is due to the artificial in vitro environment, the transformed phenotype of the cells, or their nonidentity with bona fide proximal tubular epithelial cells. Direct immunofluorescence analysis using antibodies directed against cloned PTH receptors will perhaps soon enable more definitive analysis of this issue to be made.

Some evidence has emerged recently for multiple PTH-responsive Na^+-P cotransporters in the proximal tubule with different kinetic properties, as well as for a distinct, Na^+-independent mechanism driven by a (lumenacidic) transmembrane pH gradient (QUAMME 1990). The precise anatomical location(s) and molecular characteristics of these various transporters have not yet been defined, but it appears that multiple tubular mechanisms of phosphate transport may be regulated by PTH, as well as by other factors such as phosphate deprivation (QUAMME et al. 1989a; QUAMME 1990). In any event, the major mechanism whereby PTH inhibits renal phosphate reabsorption appears to be the rapid removal, via membrane internalization, of functional Na^+-P cotransporters from the luminal cell surface of early proximal tubular cells. The possibilities of additional actions, such as reduced transcription, altered mRNA stability, or covalent modification of the Na^+-P cotransporters, remain largely unexplored. Pursuit of these questions will likely require isolation or molecular cloning of the Na^+-P cotransporter molecule(s).

3. Other Renal Effects

Apart from regulation of calcium and phosphate reabsorption, PTH is known to exert a variety of other effects on the kidney. These include inhibition of sodium, water, and bicarbonate reabsorption (WEN 1974; IINO and BURG 1979; ALPERN 1990), metabolic effects such as increased gluconeogenesis (NAGATA and RASMUSSEN 1970), increased 1-α-hydroxylation of 25OH-vitamin D, and regulation of the vitamin D receptor and the 24-hydroxylase enzyme that metabolizes $1,25(OH)_2$-vitamin D (REINHARDT and HORST 1990). Most of these actions have been localized to the proximal tubule. Regulation of bicarbonate reabsorption by PTH occurs mainly in the late, straight segment of the proximal tubule (IINO and BURG 1979) but otherwise shares many features in common with the control of phosphate reabsorption that occurs mainly in the early, convoluted portion. In the case of bicarbonate reabsorption, the transporter involved is the apical Na^+/H^+ antiporter, which also is driven by the transmembrane sodium gradient and which is rapidly removed by internalization in response to PTH (HENSLEY et al. 1989; HELMLE-KOLB et al. 1990a,b).

Thus, with respect to the regulation of renal epithelial function, a general theme of PTH action has emerged in which acute changes in ion transport are mediated by the rapid translocation of membranes containing active transporters either to or from the cell surface. Direct evidence of such rapid morphological changes in renal epithelial cells after PTH exposure has already been obtained (GOLIGORSKY et al. 1986a). The precise biochemical events triggered by PTH that mediate these movements have not yet been elucidated, although some progress has been made toward understanding the molecular basis of analogous changes in cell shape and microtubular assembly in osteoblasts (LOMRI and MARIE 1990; EGAN et al. 1991). It seems clear that PTH also engenders additional, more sustained changes in the levels or intrinsic activities of specific transporters or enzymes via alterations in rates of transcription or steady-state mRNA levels (WATFORD and MAPES 1990; REINHARDT and HORST 1990), or through posttranslational modifications such as phosphorylation by cyclic AMP-dependent protein kinase (WEINMAN et al. 1987) or protein kinase C, but these possibilities will remain incompletely explored until more specific probes (cDNA, antibodies, etc.) are available for the various transporters and enzymes involved.

B. Biosynthesis and Secretion of PTH

The ability of PTH to rapidly change the blood level of calcium mandates that the synthesis and secretion of PTH be carefully regulated. The parathyroid chief cell is characterized by three properties needed for its physiologic function: it is designed to produce large amounts of PTH in a regulated manner, to secrete stored hormone in response to decreases in blood calcium, and to replicate when chronically stimulated. A series of investigations over the last decade have begun to clarify the interacting mechanisms responsible for chief cell function.

I. Parathyroid Hormone Biosynthesis

Parathyroid hormone is synthesized as a larger precursor, preproparathyroid hormone (preproPTH). Figure 2 illustrates the known preproPTH sequences. These preproPTH sequences (human: HENDY et al. 1981; bovine: KRONENBERG et al. 1979; rat: HEINRICH et al. 1984; pig: SCHMELZER et al. 1987; chicken: KHOSLA et al. 1988; RUSSELL and SHERWOOD 1989) share a 25-residue "pre" or signal sequence and a 6-residue "pro" sequence. The signal sequence, helped by the short "pro" sequence, functions to direct the hormone into the secretory pathway. The hydrophobic signal sequence resembles similar sequences at the amino termini of most proteins destined for secretion. As the nascent signal sequence emerges from the ribosome during protein synthesis, it binds to a signal recognition particle. This recognition particle then binds to a receptor on the rough endoplasmic reticulum (ER), thereby selecting which polysomes bind to the rough ER. In a still poorly understood fashion, the signal sequence then directs the preproPTH across the membrane

```
         -31                                    -6        +1
human    M I PAK DMAKVMI VMLAI CFLTKSDG  KSVKKR  SVSE I QL MHNLGKHL
bovine   MMSA KDMVKVMI VMLAI CFLARSDG  KSVKKR  AVSE I Q FMHNLGKHL
porcine  MMSA KDTVKVMVVMLAI CFLARSDG  KP I KKR  SVSEI Q LMHNL GKHL
rat      MMSASTMAKVMI L MLAVCLLTQADG  KPV KKR  AVSEI Q LMHNL GKHL
chicken  M TSTKNLAKA I VI L YAI CFFTNSDG  RPMMKR  SVSEMQLMHNL GEHR


human    NSMERV EWLRKKL QDVHNFVALGAPL  APRDAGSQRPRKKEDNVLVE
bovine   SSMERV EWL RKKLQDV HNFVALGASI  AYRDGSSQRPRKKEDNVLVE
porcine  SS LERV EWL RKKLQDV HNFVALGASI  VHR DGGSQRPRKKEDNVLVE
rat      ASVERMQWL RKKLQDV HNFVSLGVQMAAR EGSYQRPTKKEENVLVD
chicken  HTVERQ DWLQMKLQDVH     SAL E          DARTQRPRNKEDI VLGE


human       S HEKSLGEA           DKADVNVLTKAKSQ
bovine      SHQKSLGEA            DKADVDVLI KAKPQ
porcine     SHQKSLGEA            DKAAVDVLI KAKPQ
rat         GNSKSLGEG            DKADVDVLVKAKSQ
chicken  IRNR RLLPEHLRAAVQKKSIDLDKAYMNVLFKTKP
```

Fig. 2. Sequences of preproparathyroid hormones from human (Hᴇɴᴅʏ et al. 1981), bovine (Kʀᴏɴᴇɴʙᴇʀɢ et al. 1979), porcine (Sᴄʜᴍᴇʟᴢᴇʀ et al. 1987), rat (Hᴇɪɴʀɪᴄʜ et al. 1984), and chicken (Kʜᴏsʟᴀ et al. 1988). Residues -31 to -7 represent the "pre" sequences; residues -6 to -1 the "pro" sequences. The sequences are aligned to maximize similarities. Sequences is expressed in single-letter code: ala, A; arg; R; asn, N; asp, D; cys, C; gln, Q; glu, E; gly, G; his, H; ile, I; leu, L; lys, K; met, M; phe, F; pro, P; ser, S; thr, T; trp, W; tyr, Y; val, V

into the cisternae of the rough ER. As the protein is transported across the membrane, the signal sequence is cleaved by an endopeptidase and rapidly degraded. Since the cleavage occurs before the full length of preproPTH has been synthesized, only trace amounts of intact preproPTH are found in the cell.

The importance of the signal sequence for normal secretion is illustrated by the finding of inherited hypoparathyroidism in a family carrying a preproPTH gene with a mutant signal sequence (Aʀɴᴏʟᴅ et al. 1990). A point mutation at residue 18 changes the cysteine to arginine and thereby inserts a charged residue into the hydrophobic core of the signal sequence. When this mutant preproPTH is expressed in cell-free extracts or in cultured cells, a dramatic deficiency in translocation across the endoplasmic reticulum, in signal sequence cleavage, and in subsequent secretion is apparent.

The role of the "pro" sequence is not completely understood. ProPTH is cleaved to PTH when the precursor reaches the end of the Golgi apparatus and is packed into secretory granules (Hᴀʙᴇɴᴇʀ et al. 1975). No proPTH is secreted from the chief cell; thus, the "pro" sequence must have an intra-cellular function. One role of the "pro" sequence is to help the signal sequence work efficiently in guiding the precursor across the endoplasmic reticulum (Wɪʀᴇɴ et al. 1988). If a mutant preproPTH gene, missing precisely the codons encoding the pro-specific sequence, is expressed in cultured cells, the precursor is inefficiently cleaved, and both the normal and an abnormal signal cleavage site are used. Presumably, some property of the amino-terminal portion of mature PTH is incompatible with efficient signal function, if the mature PTH sequence is placed next to the signal sequence. The "pro" sequence thus acts as a spacer to keep the signal sequence and the amino-terminal portion of PTH apart.

Portions of the mature PTH molecule have an intracellular function, as well (LIM et al. 1991b). When the human prepro PTH DNA was engineered to encode preproPTH (1–40) (where the numbers refer to the mature PTH sequence) and was expressed in cultured cells, the signal sequence functioned and proPTH (1–40) was produced. The proPTH (1–40) was not further processed, however, and no PTH peptides were secreted from cells. A similar though less dramatic defect in secretion was exhibited by preproPTH (1–52). These short precursors are long enough to get across the endoplasmic reticulum, but are not able to traverse the complete secretory pathway. These results may partly explain the continuing enigma of the function of the carboxy-terminal portion of the PTH molecule. The amino-terminal fragment PTH (1–34) exhibits most of the known biologic functions of PTH (1–84), and yet nature has chosen to conserve much of the sequence of the longer molecule. Perhaps one function of the longer molecule is an intra-cellular function; that is, the longer peptide is required for efficient transport through the secretory apparatus. Since all secreted peptides, even short ones, are synthesized as rather large precursors, this intracellular function of large precursors may be a general one.

Mature PTH is stored in secretory granules, but is not completely stable. Carboxy-terminal fragments of PTH are secreted from parathyroid glands in vivo, and can represent a substantial fraction of secreted hormone when secretion is suppressed by hypercalcemia (MAYER et al. 1979). When newly synthesized PTH molecules were pulse-labeled in parathyroid cells in vitro, analogous intracellular degradation of PTH was noted (HABENER et al. 1975; CHU et al. 1973). In these studies, when PTH secretion was stimulated by lowering the level of calcium in the medium, less PTH was degraded. Thus, calcium influences the amount of available intact PTH by causing intracellular degradation of the hormone. This regulation at the post-translational level allows the cell to provide more biologically active hormone in response to hypocalcemia. This effect could be caused by activation by calcium of a PTH-degrading pathway. Alternatively, the intracellular degradation rate may be constant; the decrease in total degradation of PTH caused by low calcium may simply result from rapid secretion of PTH and the consequent decreased intracellular exposure of PTH to the degradation mechanism.

Phorbol ester treatment of parathyroid cells has also been shown to increase the fraction of PTH secreted as fragments, both at high and low calcium levels (TANGUAY et al. 1991). Phorbols, presumably by activating protein kinase C, may be activating a proteolytic mechanism or may be selectively stimulating the secretion from granules containing mostly degraded PTH. The physiologic correlate of the action of phorbol esters needs further exploration.

II. Parathyroid Hormone Gene

Genomic DNA encoding preproPTH has been isolated from the human (VASICEK et al. 1983; REIS et al. 1990), bovine (WEAVER et al. 1984), and rat (HEINRICH et al. 1984) genomes. These three mammalian genes share a common, simple structure consisting of three exons and two introns. The first exon encodes the messenger RNA's 5'-noncoding region; the second exon encodes the signal sequence and the first four residues of the "pro" sequence; and the third exon encodes the mature PTH sequence and the mRNA's 3'-noncoding region.

Though a small amount of PTH mRNA is synthesized in the hypothalamus (FRASER et al. 1990), transcription of the PTH gene otherwise occurs exclusively in the parathyroid gland. The DNA sequences responsible for this striking tissue specificity have not been well defined. An 'experiment of nature" suggests, however, that such sequences probably are located upstream of the first intron. In a subset of parathyroid adenomas, the sequences upstream from the PTH gene and the first, noncoding exon are separated from the rest of the PTH gene and positioned adjacent to the PRAD1 gene on the long arm of chromosome 11 (ROSENBERG et al. 1991; MOTOKURA et al. 1991). As a consequence of this gene rearrangement, the PRAD1 gene is dramatically overexpressed. This overexpression may well favor growth of the adenomas. The overexpression of PRAD1 in this subset of tumors strongly suggests that the rearranged upstream PTH gene DNA sequences direct vigorous gene transcription and presumably drive the expression of the PTH gene when they are in their normal location.

The major regulators of PTH gene transcription are 1,25 dihydroxyvitamin D ($1,25(OH)_2D_3$) and calcium. Both high and low levels of $1,25(OH)_2D_3$ alter PTH gene expression. $1,25(OH)_2D_3$ inhibits PTH gene transcription, when primary, dispersed bovine parathyroid cells are exposed to high levels of the sterol (SILVER et al. 1985; RUSSELL et al. 1986a). Further, in intact rats, intraperitoneal injections of $1,25(OH)_2D_3$ rapidly lead to a dramatic fall in PTH gene transcription and mRNA levels (SILVER et al. 1986). The precise blood levels of $1,25(OH)_2D_3$ required to suppress PTH gene transcription in vivo have not been established. The effects of low levels of $1,25(OH)_2D_3$ have not been studied extensively in vivo. Such studies are difficult to perform because of confounding effects of vitamin D deficiency on blood calcium and parathyroid cell number. Weanling rats fed a vitamin D-deficient diet for 3 weeks had a modest increase in their PTH mRNA levels (NAVEH-MANY and SILVER 1990). This increase occurred with no apparent change in blood calcium and with only a slight, statistically nonsignificant fall in blood levels of $1,25(OH)_2D_3$.

Calcium is also an important regulator of *PTH* gene transcription. In dispersed primary cultures of bovine parathyroid cells, PTH mRNA levels and *PTH* gene transcription rate fall, in response to elevation of calcium in the medium (RUSSELL et al. 1983, 1986b). Two groups have studied the acute effects of calcium on PTH mRNA levels in vivo. Both agree that acute lowering of blood calcium (with phosphate, calcitonin, or EDTA) leads to a prompt increase in PTH mRNA levels (NAVEH-MANY et al. 1989; YAMAMOTO et al. 1989). Elevations in blood calcium, in contrast, led to no change in PTH mRNA after 6 h (NAVEH-MANY et al. 1989) and to a modest decrease in PTH mRNA levels after 48 h (YAMAMOTO et al. 1989). The parathyroid gland is apparently more prepared to increase PTH mRNA levels in response to hypocalcemia than to decrease PTH mRNA in response to hypercalcemia. This pattern resembles the pattern of PTH secretion in response to calcium. In each case, the gland responds dramatically to hypocalcemia, but decreases its activity incompletely in response to hypercalcemia.

In vivo, of course, changes in calcium or $1,25(OH)_2D_3$ seldom occur in isolation. The interactions between calcium and $1,25(OH)_2D_3$ are, therefore, important, but have not been exhaustively analyzed. When rats were made acutely hypocalcemic with phosphate and were at the same time given $1,25(OH)_2D_3$ intraperitoneally, the suppressive effect of $1,25(OH)_2D_3$ dominated over that of hypocalcemia, and PTH mRNA levels fell (NAVEH-MANY et al. 1989). In contrast, when rats were fed a low-calcium diet for 3 weeks, blood calcium fell and $1,25(OH)_2D_3$ increased dramatically. In this case, PTH mRNA levels increased severalfold. While cell number was not measured, other experiments done by the same investigators (NAVEH-MANY and SILVER 1990) suggest that this combination of low calcium and high $1,25(OH)_2D_3$ lead to an increase in PTH mRNA/cell. The differing results of the acute and chronic studies suggest that the net effects of changes in calcium and $1,25(OH)_2D_3$ will depend on the chronicity and degree of the changes in each variable.

Glucocorticoids may be another regulator of PTH gene transcription, though the effects of glucocorticoids have not been extensively evaluated. In in vitro studies, dexamethasone increased PTH mRNA in dispersed, hyperplastic human parathyroid cells (PERALDI et al. 1990), and cortisol abolished the decrease in PTH mRNA in response to $1,25(OH)_2D_3$ in dispersed bovine parathyroid cells (KARMALI et al. 1989).

Not much is yet known about specific DNA sequences that mediate the effects of calcium and $1,25(OH)_2D_3$ on *PTH* gene transcription. Lack of well-differentiated, established cell line secreting PTH has made transfection studies cumbersome or difficult to interpret. Consequently, the picture is still quite incomplete. Nevertheless, a broad outline is fairly clear. When a fusion gene containing 684 bp DNA upstream of the human *PTH* gene was introduced into rat pituitary GH_4 cells, expression of the gene was specifically suppressed by $1,25(OH)_2D_3$ (OKAZAKI et al. 1988). Two groups have identified DNA sequences upstream of the *PTH* gene that bind to $1,25(OH)_2D_3$

receptors in vitro. Filter binding assays showed that $1,25(OH)_2D_3$ receptors can bind to bovine *PTH* gene sequences between -485 and -100 base pairs upstream from the start site of transcription (FARROW et al. 1990). Subsequently, gel mobility shift assays were used to identify a specific 26-bp sequence, located 125 bp upstream from the human *PTH* gene, which binds vitamin D receptors (DEMAY et al. 1991). When a somewhat larger oligonucleotide containing this sequence was linked to a reporter gene and expressed in GH4 cells, $1,25(OH)_2D_3$ decreased expression of the reporter gene. Thus, this sequence is a negative response element that responds to $1,25(OH)_2D_3$.

DNA sequences responsible for calcium regulation of the *PTH* gene have been sought by the use of similar strategies. A DNA sequence far upstream of the human *PTH* gene regulates gene transcription in response to changes in extracellular calcium, after transfection of this sequence into fibroblasts (OKAZAKI et al. 1990). This sequence can also act as a silencer of gene transcription (OKAZAKI et al. 1991). Further work is needed to establish how this sequence senses changes in calcium and whether this sequence regulates transcription in normal parathyroid cells.

III. Parathyroid Hormone Secretion

1. Physiology

Extracellular calcium (more precisely, ionized calcium) is the major regulator of PTH secretion (reviewed in BROWN 1991; POCOTTE et al. 1991). Extensive studies, both in vitro and in vivo, document that the dose-response curve for PTH secretion in response to extracellular calcium levels is sigmoidal. PTH secretion is maximal at low calcium concentrations, falls steeply as the physiologic level of calcium is reached, and plateaus, with incomplete suppression when calcium is further elevated. Since normal blood calciums are near the bottom of the curve, the system is designed to respond more dramatically to falls in blood calcium than to increases in blood calcium. The chief cell responds not only to the absolute level of calcium; it also responds to the rate of change in calcium (BRENT et al. 1988; GRANT et al. 1990). Sudden drops in calcium, in particular, stimulate PTH secretion more than would be predicted by the level of calcium alone. This rate dependence of secretion is probably teleologically useful; it may partly explain the pulsatile nature of PTH secretion, as well. From the perspective of the investigator, the rate dependence mandates great attention to detail when characterizing the changes of PTH secretion in response to changes in calcium in vivo.

Magnesium's effect on PTH secretion is similar to that of calcium. Unlike calcium, though, magnesium's effect is quantitatively modest within the relevant physiologic range. Catecholamines stimulate PTH secretion through a cyclic AMP-mediated mechanism. The physiologic importance of this effect, which can easily be demonstrated in vivo and in vitro, remains to be established, however. A large and somewhat contradictory literature documents the effects of metabolites of vitamin D on PTH secretion. The evidence that $1,25(OH)_2D_3$ dramatically suppresses PTH synthesis, summarized earlier, reconciles much of the data. Thus, $1,25(OH)_2D_3$ probably has little direct effect on the secretory process itself. The suppression of PTH secretion seen in response to $1,25(OH)_2D_3$ results from suppression of synthesis and from indirect effects of $1,25(OH)_2D_3$ that are mediated by increases in blood calcium.

2. Cellular Mechanisms

The parathyroid chief cell's ability to sense modest changes in blood calcium and increase PTH secretion when calcium falls remains unexplained. In the last few years, however, a series of important observations have filled in portions of the still incomplete picture. Calcium sensors, G proteins, and, possibly, intracellular second messengers, may be linked together in a pathway that leads from a fall in extracellular calcium to stimulation of PTH secretion.

A series of indirect arguments suggest that an extracellular receptor for calcium may initiate the pathway. Extracellular calcium, along with a series of other divalent cations (Mg^{2+}, Sr^{2+}, Ba^{2+}), induces transient elevation of intracellular calcium that can be detected using intracellular fluorescent indicators, such as fura-2 (NEMETH and SCARPA 1987; BROWN et al. 1990; FITZPATRICK 1990). This transient increase in response to extracellular divalent cations occurs even in the absence of extracellular calcium and is accompanied by an increase in cytosolic inositol 1,4,5-triphosphate (IP_3) levels (BROWN et al. 1987; SHOBACK et al. 1988). Since many extracellular ligands bind to specific membrane receptors and stimulate IP_3 synthesis and subsequent increases in intracellular calcium, the existence of a receptor for divalent cations on parathyroid chief cells is suggested. The ability of these same divalent cations to inhibit PTH secretion, along with other correlations, suggests that this (or these) receptor mediates the effect of calcium on PTH secretion. While these physiologic arguments are suggestive, substantial work remains to be done before the relevance of an extracellular receptor for calcium is established.

An independent body of data suggests that calcium channels in the plasma membrane mediate or at least affect calcium's action. Antibodies to the α-subunit of the skeletal muscle calcium channel blocked the secretion of PTH in response to low calcium levels (FITZPATRICK et al. 1988). Calcium channel agonists inhibit PTH secretion and calcium channel antagonists stimulate PTH secretion (FITZPATRICK et al. 1986a, 1989), though not in every investigator's experience (MUFF et al. 1988). Studies using the diltiazem analog TA-3090 suggest that calcium channels may participate in transmembrane signaling. This analog acts as a calcium channel agonist in parathyroid cells and inhibits PTH secretion. In a calcium-dependent fashion, the analog also blocked the rise in intracellular cAMP caused by dopamine. This effect could be blocked by pertussis toxin (CHEN and BROWN 1990). Thus, a channel activator participates in an activity that is probably mediated by an extracellular receptor.

A third candidate for a calcium-sensing molecule (not necessarily distinct from a receptor or a channel) has been defined by a monoclonal antibody to a protein found only on parathyroid, renal, and placental cells (JUHLIN et al. 1987, 1990). This monoclonal antibody blocks secretion of PTH in response to low calcium. The protein recognized by the antibody is decreased in amount on parathyroid adenomas (JUHLIN et al. 1989). Further evidence will be needed to establish the physiologic role of this intriguing protein, however. Thus, at the moment, the biochemical nature and the physiologic character of the initial sensor of extracellular calcium remains uncertain.

Evidence from several experimental approaches suggests that G proteins may mediate the response to extracellular calcium in the parathyroid cell. Pertussis toxin, which inactivates several G proteins, blocks the inhibition of PTH secretion caused by calcium (FITZPATRICK et al. 1986b). Pertussis toxin also blocks the decrease in cAMP (elevated by dopamine) caused by extracellular calcium (CHEN et al. 1989). Further, the GTP analog, GppNHp, stimulates PTH secretion from permeabilized parathyroid cells (OETTING et al. 1986). This effect might be mediated by known second messengers, though it is also possible that a G protein directly stimulates the PTH secretory apparatus.

Several second messenger systems function in parathyroid cells and can be affected by changes in extracellular calcium. In no case, however, has the role for any second messenger in calcium-directed inhibition of PTH secretion of PTH been established. Calcium modestly lowers cellular cAMP levels (BROWN et al. 1978) and blocks the rise of cyclic AMP stimulated by catecholamines and dopamine (BROWN and THATCHER 1982). This blockage cannot quantitatively explain the effect of calcium on secretion, however. Calcium also stimulates production of diacyl glycerol and IP_3 in parathyroid cells (BROWN et al. 1987; SHOBACK et al. 1988). IP_3 releases calcium from vesicular stores into the intracytosolic space. If this calcium then inhibited PTH secretion, the pathway from extracellular calcium to inhibition of secretion would be complete. However, when the effect of intracellular calcium on PTH secretion was tested directly in electropermeabilized parathyroid chief cells, no such role for intracellular calcium could be established. Instead, increased levels of intracellular calcium stimulated hormone secretion (OETTING et al. 1986). Either intracellular calcium (and therefore IP_3) does not suppress PTH secretion normally, or, perhaps the mediator of calcium's effect is destroyed or diluted by permeabilization of parathyroid cells.

Protein kinase C might play a role in calcium signaling. Phorbol esters stimulate PTH secretion, when extracellular calcium is elevated (MORRISSEY 1988; BROWN et al. 1984; MEMBRENO et al. 1989). Furthermore, membrane-bound (and presumably active) protein kinase C increases when extracellular calcium is lowered (KOBAYASHI et al. 1988). Nevertheless, the role of protein kinase C is not straightforward. At low levels of calcium, phorbol esters do not stimulate PTH secretion. Further, elevations of extracellular calcium lead to increases of parathyroid cell diacylglycerol (BROWN et al. 1987; SHOBACK et al. 1988). This increase would be expected to activate protein kinase C. This expected activation must be reconciled with the observed increase in membrane-bound, presumably active, protein kinase C, when calcium is lowered. A role for protein kinase C in calcium signaling thus remains possible, but the relevant regulators of protein kinase C need to be established and a role in mediating the effects of low calcium remains to be clarified.

A novel autocrine system may interact with the calcium-sensing mechanism in unanticipated ways. Chromogranin-A is a major secretory product of parathyroid and many other secretory cells (KEMPER et al. 1974; COHN et al. 1982). Within the chromogranin A sequence is the sequence of pancreastatin, a potent inhibitor of glucose-stimulated insulin release. Interestingly, pancreastatin also inhibits PTH secretion stimulated by either low calcium or phorbol ester (FASCIOTTO et al. 1989). Furthermore, antibodies to chromogranin A potentiate secretion from cultured parathyroid cells (FASCIOTTO et al. 1990). The inhibitory effects of chromogranin A itself are considerably weaker than those of pancreastatin, however. Further, it is not clear what fragments of chromogranin A, if any, are found in or near the parathyroid cell in vivo. Nevertheless, the idea that chromogranin A and/or its fragments may be involved in the autoregulation of PTH secretion is an attractive hypothesis. This mechanism might control the pulsatility of PTH secretion, for example. Further physiologic studies in a variety of in vivo and in vitro models are needed to clarify chromogranin A's role.

To summarize, several types of data suggest that calcium binds to a parathyroid plasma membrane calcium sensor. This binding is associated with activation of G proteins. Increases in extracellular calcium lead to stimulation of IP_3 synthesis, an increase in intracellular ionized calcium, and a blunting of agonist-induced cAMP production. Decreases in extracellular calcium lead to membrane binding of protein kinase C. These changes occur at physiologically relevant concentrations of extracellular calcium. A complete pathway linking extracellular calcium to changes in PTH secretion remains to be established, however.

C. Structural Basis of PTH Function

Although parathyroid hormone is secreted as an 84 amino acid peptide, all of the hormone's known physiological effects on mineral ion homeostasis can be produced by the amino-terminal peptide PTH 1–34 (TREGEAR et al. 1973; POTTS et al. 1971). This fundamental insight has made possible an extensive structure-function analysis of short PTH peptides synthesized using automated, solid phase techniques (see ROSENBLATT 1982, 1984; POTTS et al. 1982 for a review of the earlier literature). Recent advances have made it possible to study full-length analogs of PTH 1–84; fragment condensation peptide synthesis and production by recombinant DNA methods have been used (RABBANI et al. 1990; BORN et al. 1988; ZAMAN et al. 1991; GARDELLA et al. 1991). Studies using circular dichroism and two-dimensional nuclear magnetic resonance have begun to define aspects of PTH's secondary and tertiary structure (ZULL et al. 1987; BARDEN and KEMP 1989; CODDINGTON and BARLING 1989; LEE and RUSSELL 1989; KLAUS et al. 1991). The activities of the PTH-related protein have clarified the roles of analogous sequences in the PTH molecule (CAULFIELD et al. 1990; ABOU-SAMRA et al. 1989a; NISSENSON et al. 1988). The cloning of the PTH receptor (JÜPPNER et al. 1991) and the consequent ability to alter the structure of the receptor as well as the hormone should provide a new approach to defining the interactions of PTH residues with the receptor. In the following section, four areas of current interest will be reviewed: the importance of the amino-terminal portion of PTH for bioactivity; current concepts of PTH conformation and secondary structure; the impact of the study of PTHrP, which is structurally related to PTH; and possible bioactivity determined by carboxy-terminal sequences.

I. Parathyroid Hormone Binding and Activation Domains

Advances in protein isolation and sequencing and the development of the Merrifield solid-phase method for protein synthesis were the stimuli for the earliest understanding of structure-activity relationships for PTH. The isolation and complete amino acid sequence of bovine PTH 2 decades ago (NIALL et al. 1970) was followed by a series of syntheses which defined the 1–34 region of the molecule as essential and sufficient for full biological activity in multiple bioassay systems (TREGEAR et al. 1973; POTTS et al. 1971). The initial effort to confirm the structure deduced for bovine PTH led to the synthesis of a biologically active amino-terminal fragment, PTH 1–34. Selection of chain length to synthesize was somewhat arbitrary: The selection of the phenylalanine residue found at position 34 as the point to initiate synthesis was based on the knowledge that it was midway between the first two aspartic acid residues found at the amino terminus. It was known that dilute acid hydrolysis, which favors cleavage at aspartic acid residues, led to production of a biologically active fragment. Many years later investigation of the peripheral metabolism of PTH revealed the endogenous production of fragments such as PTH 1–33.

Many fragments and analogues of the PTH sequence from several mammalian species have been made and tested in a variety of biological response systems. In vitro assays featuring the stimulation of cyclic AMP production in membranes and whole cells, as well as in vivo bioassays based on stimulation of calcium mobilization from bone, have been used for several decades. A considerable breakthrough occurred when techniques were developed that permitted the radioiodination of a PTH fragment that retained biological activity and bound to receptors (SEGRE et al. 1979).

Modification of the PTH molecule with an isosteric substitution of norleucine for methionine at positions 8 and 18 and the substitution of tyrosine for phenylalanine at position 34 permitted the development of a radioreceptor binding assay based on the biologically active iodinated peptide [Nle^{8,18},Tyr^{34}] bPTH(1–34) amide and purified canine renal membranes (ROSENBLATT et al. 1976, 1980; NUSSBAUM et al. 1980; SEGRE et al. 1979). The radioreceptor binding assay, with modifications over the past 10 years involving its performance using bone and kidney-derived cell lines rather than renal membranes, has allowed fine discrimination of the specific effects of modifications to the PTH structure on alteration of binding affinity (COLE et al. 1989; GOLDMAN et al. 1988; COHEN et al. 1991; GARDELLA et al. 1991). A large series of PTH analogs, truncated at either their amino-terminal or their carboxy-terminal ends, have been tested for receptor binding and for the ability to stimulate synthesis of adenylate cyclase (NUSSBAUM et al. 1980; ROSENBLATT et al. 1980; McKEE et al. 1988; NG et al. 1984). Three major conclusions can be drawn from these studies (see Fig. 3). First, the peptide PTH 25–34 can bind specifically to PTH receptors (NUSSBAUM et al. 1980; ROSENBLATT et al. 1980). The relatively high affinity of this peptide for the receptor led to its designation as the hormone's principal binding domain. Second, the amino-terminal fragment PTH 1–27 can stimulate adenylate cyclase. Thus, this sequence, which contains only two residues of the PTH 25–34 peptide, can bind to the receptor without the need for the carboxy-terminal sequence (NUSSBAUM et al. 1980). In fact, PTH 10–27 can bind weakly to receptors (NUSSBAUM et al. 1980). Thus, at least two separate regions, PTH 10–27 and PTH 25–34, can bind PTH receptors. Third, amino-terminal residues are crucial for activation of adenylate cyclase.

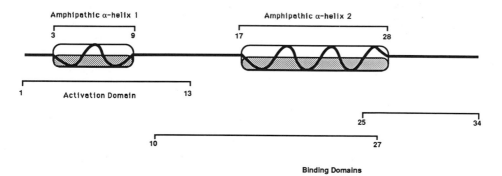

Fig. 3. Composite topologic map of PTH 1–34. Included are PTH sequences identified as binding domains, 10–27, 25–34; and activation domain 1–13. NMR analysis suggests that sequences 3–9 and 17–28 are *a*-helical in 10.7% trifluoreothanol

Modification of the amino-terminal residue by, for example, acetylation, or addition of tyrosine at position-1 caused marked loss of activity (TREGEAR et al. 1973). The deletion of the amino-terminal residue from chemically synthesized peptides based on the bovine or human sequences resulted in peptides with dramatic loss of activity. The additional removal of position 2 valine resulted in peptides with very low adenylate cyclase-stimulating activity. PTH 3–34 binds well to PTH receptors (K_D = 1.0–2.0 × $10^{-9} M$, depending on the binding assay employed), but activates adenylate cyclase poorly. PTH 7–34 binds to receptors poorly (ROSENBLATT et al. 1980; KUBOTA et al. 1986), but has no or very little ability to stimulate adenylate cyclase. PTH 7–34 has been shown to function as an antagonist of PTH action on kidney (HORIUCHI et al. 1983) and bone in vivo (DOPPELT et al. 1986). PTH 3–34 was shown to be a partial agonist in parathyroidectomized dogs (SEGRE et al. 1985). Thus, PTH must contact the receptor at multiple sites; contacts through the amino terminus of the hormone are crucial for transmembrane signaling.

The advent of molecular biology as a powerful and practical tool in the production and chemical characterization of polypeptides has been very helpful in further defining structure-activity relationships for PTH. In order to analyze a large series of specific amino acid substitutions in the amino-terminal region of PTH, a strategy using recombinant DNA was devised. Partially degenerate oligonucleotides were used to introduce random mutations in the 1–4 region of human PTH 1–84 (GARDELLA et al. 1991). These PTH mutants were expressed in a mammalian cell line, the COS-7 cell, after transfection of the mutant PTH DNA. The receptor-binding and cAMP-stimulating activities of each mutant were assessed by directly applying the supernatant media from transfected cells into radioreceptor and cell-based cAMP-stimulating assays using ROS 17/2.8 cells. Serine 1 and serine 3 could be substituted with several amino acids without severe decreases in receptor binding or cyclase activity. In marked contrast, mutations involving valine 2 reduced bioactivity to less than 2% of the native hormone. What was unusual about the valine 2 substitutions was that some of the mutants displayed substantial binding affinity. This was a different pattern than that observed for mutations of glutamic acid 4, which were associated with parallel declines in both receptor-binding affinity and bioactivity. These data suggested that valine 2 was an important determinant for receptor activation, whereas glutamic acid 4 was an important determinant for receptor binding (GARDELLA et al. 1991).

Furthermore, the exploration of the role of position 2 by site-directed mutagenesis led to GARDELLA's finding that substitution of valine at position 2 by arginine resulted in a unique peptide analog. The [Arg2] PTH 1–34 synthetic peptide showed marked disparity in receptor activation and binding in osteosarcoma cells, ROS 17/2.8 cells. In contrast, this disparity was only modest, when the analog was tested in an opossum kidney cell line, the OK cell. This species difference in the activity of [Arg 2] PTH 1–34 was also seen when the Arg 2 PTH analog was bound to COS 7 cells expressing either the cloned rat bone or opossum kidney PTH receptors (see below). In an attempt to define the structural basis for the effect of the arginine 2 substitution on receptor activation, PTH analogs containing citrulline or lysine at position 2 were synthesized and studied. Results of analysis of these analogs indicated that position 2 amino acids that are polar or occupy a large volume cannot activate the ROS cell PTH receptor.

Studies of analogs designed to probe the similarities and differences in the PTH and PTHrP sequences have suggested that amino-terminal residues of PTH extending as far as residues 10 and 11 can influence the activation of adenylate cyclase (NUTT et al. 1990) (see Sect. IV, below). Thus, the activation domain of PTH extends through most of the sequence shared by PTH and PTHrP.

II. Evolutionary Lessons: Rat and Chicken PTH

Systematic comparisons of a polypeptide's varying sequences across a wide range of species can provide insight into structure/function relationships and a better understanding of the diversity of the peptide's functions. So far, PTH's structural analysis has been confined to mammalian species (human, cow, pig, rat) and to one species of bird, the chicken. Efforts are now underway to determine the structure of PTH in fish (ROSENBERG et al. 1991). Although earlier work suggested that only amphibians and their descendents have parathyroid glands, DNA encoding a PTH-like molecule has been identified in trout.

Functional implications of evolutionary diversity have been studied in both the rat and chicken models. Synthetic replicates of the 1–34 sequences of rat (KEUTMANN et al. 1985) and chicken PTH (CAULFIELD et al. 1988) have been synthesized and analyzed. Furthermore, chicken PTH 1–88 has been produced by recombinant techniques, and the full-length hormone has been evaluated for bioactivity (LIM et al. 1991a).

There are five sequence differences between rat and human PTH 1–34 (HEINRICH et al. 1984). Like bovine PTH, rat PTH has the activity-enhancing alanine for serine substitution at position 1. The four other amino acid changes occur in residues 16, 18, 21, and 22. The region PTH 25–34, representing the principal binding region, is conserved in rat PTH, as it is in all other sequences (bovine, human, porcine) with the exception of chicken PTH. The potency of rat PTH in the canine renal adenylate cyclase system is eight- to tenfold higher than the potency of human PTH and two- to fourfold higher than that of bovine PTH.

Chicken PTH has marked differences from all other PTH sequences. A portion of the 25–34 region, absolutely conserved in all of the known mammalian PTHs, has been deleted, and there is an absence of the tribasic region extending from residues 25–27. More dramatic differences, again resulting from deletion and substitution, are present in the remainder of the full-length molecule. Early reports using chicken PTH partially purified from chicken parathyroids suggested unusual potency for the chicken hormone (Rosenberg et al. 1987, 1988). Additionally, chicken PTH was reported to stimulate adrenal steroidogenesis (Rosenberg et al. 1987). Subsequent studies of synthetic chicken PTH 1–34, however, showed that this peptide has only 10% of the bioactivity of human PTH 1–34 in multiple in vitro assay systems (Caulfield et al. 1988; Lim et al. 1991a). Furthermore, using chicken PTH 1–88 produced using a recombinant DNA strategy, the full-length chicken hormone was found to be devoid of steroidogenic potency and was comparable in activity to the synthetic chicken PTH 1–34 peptide (Lim et al. 1991a).

III. Three-Dimensional Structure of PTH

As noted above, analysis of PTH analogs has suggested that two different regions of PTH 1–34 can bind independently to the receptor and that the amino-terminal sequence is needed for transmembrane signaling. Evolutionary comparisons and analysis of additional analogs suggest that a somewhat loosely conserved region from residues 16–22 joins two highly conserved regions containing residues 1–15 and 23–34. The constraints on specific residues may arise either from requirements for direct contact of these residues with PTH receptors or from requirements for maintenance of secondary and tertiary structure of the hormone. Because no definitive structure for PTH has been established through two-dimensional NMR analysis, and the molecule has not yet been crystallized for X-ray analysis, only an outline of PTH structure can be suggested, by combining the results of a series of spectroscopic studies with modeling based on secondary structure predictions. Uncertainty about the appropriate solvents to use for analysis of secondary or tertiary structure has limited the ability to design experimental conditions that resemble the environment of the hormone when it interacts with the PTH receptor. Recent cocrystallization and analyses of epidermal growth factor (Günther et al. 1990) and growth hormone (Cunningham et al. 1991) with extracellular fragments of their respective receptors provide instructive models for the future.

The earliest spectroscopic studies of PTH conformation indicated that there was a pH-dependent increase in helical structure. The gel filtration pattern of bovine PTH 1–84 suggested that the molecule was asymmetric and became more compact at alkaline pH. Further analysis of PTH 1–34 and PTH 53–84 and comparison of the Stokes' radii of these two synthetic peptides with globular peptides of similar molecular weight suggested that the 1–34 fragment was more compact than the carboxyl-terminal fragment. Further credence to these ideas followed the demonstration, by dark-field electron microscopy, that there were two connected domains of unequal mass (Fiskin et al. 1977).

Several groups have analyzed the secondary structure of PTH 1–34 and relevant analogs using circular dichroism (ZULL et al. 1990; NUSSBAUM et al. 1985). Such analyses show little α-helical content in aqueous solution. When CD spectra were analyzed for PTH 1–34 in increasing concentrations of trifluoroethanol, increasing α-helix was predicted. Comparisons of the helical content of amino-terminal truncated molecules suggested that both amino-terminal and carboxy-terminal regions contributed to the α-helical structure. Analysis of PTH 1–34 structure by two-dimensional NMR has importantly extended the CD data (FRELINGER and ZULL 1986; ZULL et al. 1987; CODDINGTON and BARLING 1989; LEE and RUSSELL 1989; KLAUS et al. 1991). No well-defined tertiary structure could be discerned for PTH 1–34 in aqueous solution. In 10.7% trifluoroethanol, however, two α-helices were identified, containing PTH 3–9 and 17–28 (KLAUS et al. 1991). The region between the helices was without secondary structure. The entire molecule was extremely flexible; no long-range interactions between the two helices could be identified.

Several groups have used programs that predict secondary structure from primary sequence data to predict possible secondary structures for PTH 1–34. These studies have disagreed in minor details, but generally identify potential α-helices that roughly coincide with those found by two-dimensional NMR in the presence of trifluorethanol (NUSSBAUM et al. 1985; FRELINGER and ZULL 1986; COHEN et al. 1991). Edmonson wheel analysis predicts that the putative carboxy-terminal helix would be an amphipathic helix, with polar and charged residues on one side of the helix and a hydrophobic face on the other side. Such amphipathic helices have been found in other hormonal systems, in which they may play a functional role. A predicted amphipathic α-helix in a functionally vital region of the calcitonin molecule, for example, could be replaced with a second amphipathic α-helix of different primary structure, with retention of biologic activity (MOE and KAISER 1985).

While the physical studies and structural modeling provide useful perspectives and potentially testable hypotheses, they all have uncertain relevance to the structure of PTH when the hormone interacts with the receptor. Trifluorethanol may mimic the environment of the hormone when it interacts with the hydrophobic environment of the plasma membrane or perhaps with a hydrophobic surface of the receptor itself. Since the receptor contains a large extracellular domain, (JÜPPNER et al. 1991), however, the hormone may well make few contacts with the plasma membrane and may function in a largely aqueous environment. The flexibility of the hormone in aqueous solution suggests that convincing three-dimensional structural information about the physiologically relevant conformations of PTH will be difficult to establish. Nevertheless, even the imprecise predictions currently possible provide a framework for designing PTH analogs. The activities of these analogs can be used to support or reject the structural predictions. For example, a generic amphipathic *a*-helix was substituted at positions 25–34; the resultant peptide was inactive (Zwerling and Nussbaum, preliminary data). Thus, more than simply an amphipathic helix is needed for receptor binding. Multiple individual substitutions designed to disrupt the predicted amphipathic helix also resulted in peptides that failed to bind receptors (Gardella and Nussbaum, unpublished). Studies such as these will incrementally make clearer the structural determinants of PTH action.

IV. Lessons from the Structure and Activity of PTHrP

The discovery of PTHrP, the peptide responsible for humoral hypercalcemia associated with malignancy, and the identification of a common receptor for PTH and PTHrP on osteoblast- and kidney-derived target tissue, has permitted a more complete understanding of how the structural attributes of these two peptides can lead to similarities and differences in their actions. As discussed elsewhere in this volume by Martin and his colleagues, PTHrP may exist in three related forms with different carboxyl termini, as a result of alternative exon splicing: PTHrP 1–139, PTHrP 1–141, and PTHrP 1–173. The circulating form(s) of the hormone have not yet been defined.

Most importantly, PTH and PTHrP have extraordinary sequence homology in their amino-terminal 13 amino acids. In addition, there is preservation of two to three conserved residues in the remainder of the 1–34 sequences of the molecules (see Fig. 4). Thus, the major region of sequence identity between the two hormones resides in the portion of the hormone important for trans-membrane signaling. Nevertheless, PTH 1–34 and PTHrP 1–34 compete for identical binding sites in radioreceptor assays with virtually identical affinities (Nissenson et al. 1988).

The vital importance of the amino termini of both PTH and PTHrP is supported by the loss of bioactivity and the impressive decline in binding

```
                 5          10         15         20         25        30
bPTH     A V S E I Q F M H N L G K H L S S M E R V E W L R K K L Q D V H N F
hPTH     S V S E I Q L M H N L G K H L N S M E R V E W L R K K L Q D V H N F
rPTH     A V S E I Q L M H N L G K H L N S V E R M Q W L R K K L Q D V H N F
cPTH     S V S E M Q L M H N L G E H R H T V E R Q D W L Q M K L Q D V H S A
pPTH     S V S E I Q L M H N L G K H L S S L E R V E W L R K K L Q D V H N F
hPTH rP  A V S E H Q L L H D K G K S I Q D L R R R F F L H H L I A E I H T A
rPTH rP  A V S E H Q L L H D K G K S I Q D L R R R F F L H H L I A E I H T A
cPTH rP  A V S E H Q L L H D K G K S I Q D L R R R F F L Q N L I E G V N T A
```

Fig. 4. Sequence homologies within the known PTH and PTHrP sequences. *Boxed* amino acids are identical. Note the sequence identities within the amino-terminal 13 residues of PTH and PTHrP. Single-letter amino acid codes are represented in Fig. 2

affinity with the deletion of the first five to seven amino acids. Although there are sequence similarities within the 15–34 sequences of both peptides, they are quite modest. Nevertheless, the binding data suggest that the 15–34 regions of both peptides must have important structural similarities (CAULFFILD et al. 1990; ABOU-SAMRA et al. 1989a). The hypothesis that peptides containing the distinct 14–34 sequences of either PTH or PTHrP contain sufficient structural information for binding to the PTH receptor has been tested by two groups (CAULFIELD et al. 1990; ABOU-SAMRA et al. 1989a). Through the use of [Nle^{8,18},Tyr^{34}] bPTH 1–34 amide and [Tyr^{36}] PTHrP 1–36 amide iodinated radioligands and synthetic PTH and PTHrP peptides encompassing the sequences 14–34, these carboxyl-terminal fragments were shown to compete for a common PTH/PTHrP receptor. [Tyr^{36},Cys^{38}] PTHrP 14–38 and [Tyr^{34}] bPTH 14–34 amide competed with an iodinated PTH analog for binding sites on ROS cells with apparent K_ds of 10 and 50 μM respectively and with an iodinated PTHrP analog with apparent K_ds of 30 and 10 μM respectively. These studies indicated that although PTH and PTHrP 14–34 share very limited amino acid homology, their secondary structures may be sufficiently similar to permit binding to a common PTH/PTHrP receptor.

The properties of PTHrP analogs have revealed interesting features of the activation domains of PTHrP and PTH. [Tyr^{34}] PTHrP 7–34 amide is eightfold more potent than [Tyr^{34}] PTH 7–34 amide in inhibiting PTH-stimulated cAMP production in ROS 17/2.8 cells (McKEE et al. 1988). In addition, [Tyr^{34}] PTHrP 7–34 amide is a weak partial agonist in many systems, whereas the corresponding PTH 7–34 peptide has not displayed any agonism in multiple in vitro and in vivo bioassay systems for cAMP generation, phosphate transport, or hypercalcemia.

The basis for differences in PTH and PTHrP 7–34 agonist actions has been investigated. Substitution of Asn 10 and Leu 11 from PTH in the place of Asp 10 and Lys 11 of PTHrP resulted in a peptide devoid of bioactivity (NUTT et al. 1990). No agonist action was observed in an assay system based on highly responsive ROS 17/2.8 cells pretreated with dexamethasone and pertussis toxin. Even more interestingly, the reciprocal peptide, in which Asn 10 and Lys 11 from PTHrP were placed in the PTH 7–34 backbone, gained agonist activity. These data establish that the activation domain of PTH and PTHrP extends to residue 11 and is virtually coextensive with the highly conserved region of the peptides. One can speculate that these sequences may interact with a discrete domain of the PTH receptor that is distinct from regions of the receptor that bind to the carboxy-terminal portions of the peptide.

Two-dimensional NMR analysis of PTHrP 1–34 differed strikingly from the two-dimensional NMR analysis of PTH 1–34 (BARDEN and KEMP 1989; KLAUS et al. 1991). Most importantly, in aqueous solution, structural regularities in the PTHrP structure could be discerned. Too few proton interactions were defined to allow determination of a complete structure, but sufficient data were collected to argue for the presence of α-helix at residues 4–9, β-turns at residues 10–13 and 16–19, and multiple interactions between the amino-terminal and carboxy-terminal portions of the molecule. The resulting model predicts a compact structure maintained by multiple interactions between the amino-terminal helix and carboxy-terminal coil. In aqueous solution, PTH does not exhibit analogous interactions (KLAUS et al. 1991). Nevertheless, since both peptides bind to the same receptor with comparable affinities, the structural outline of PTHrP is likely to be relevant to the active conformation of PTH.

V. Structure-Activity Relationships for Middle and Carboxyl Regions of PTH

Considerable information is accumulating that indicates that distal regions of PTH 1–84 may be responsible for novel biologic actions. An area of intense investigation has focussed on the role of PTH on chondrocyte proliferation (SCHLÜTER et al. 1989; SILBERMANN et al. 1991; KOIKE et al. 1990). PTH 1–34 induced a 12- to 15-fold increase in the efficiency of colony formation in soft agar by embryonic chondrocytes. The fragment PTH 28–48, which does not stimulate cAMP production, had activity comparable to that of PTH 1–84 or PTH 1–34 in stimulating DNA synthesis in chicken chondrocytes (SCHLÜTER et al. 1989). A series of synthetic peptides, each containing the residues PTH 30–34, delineated this chondrocyte mitogenic domain (SCHLÜTER et al. 1989). Other regions of PTH may alter chondrocyte response to PTH-1–34. When PTH 53–84 was added to neonatal chondrocytes along with PTH 1–34 and PTH 28–48, the mitogenic effects of PTH were completely abolished and normal structural features throughout the mineralized hypertrophic cartilage were disrupted (SILBERMANN et al. 1991). In vivo studies will be required to establish the physiologic relevance of these effects of distal PTH fragments on chondrocytes.

Several studies suggest biologically important interactions of the carboxy-terminal portion (MURRAY et al. 1989, 1991) of PTH with cells. Discrete binding sites for carboxyl-terminal PTH 53–84 exist in both renal and skeletal tissues. PTH 53–84 can stimulate alkaline phosphatase activity in dexamethasone-treated ROS 17/2.8 cells. Cytochemical bioassays for PTH are sensitive to the presence of carboxy-terminal determinants. The substitution of Asp for Asn at position 76 of human PTH results in a peptide that can inhibit PTH 1–84's action in a renal cytobiochemical assay. In contrast, in cAMP-based assays that respond to PTH 1–34, Asp 76 hPTH 1–84 and Asn 76 hPTH 1–84 behaved identically (ZAMAN et al. 1991). Contributions of the carboxyl terminus of PTH to inhibitory potency in cytobiochemical assays were also demonstrated by the greater inhibitory potency of PTH 3–84 than that of PTH 3–34 (BORN et al. 1988).

All of these studies suggest that PTH has biologic actions through receptors other than the one that recognizes PTH 1–34. The physiologic importance and even the existence of these actions in the intact organism need to be established.

D. Parathyroid Hormone Receptors

Like other peptide hormones, PTH initiates its cellular actions by binding with high affinity and specificity to receptor proteins located on the plasma membranes of target cells. The study of these receptors has been pursued using three kinds of experimental approaches. First, receptors were defined as sites on cells or membranes that bound PTH or PTH analogs with high affinity and specificity. Large numbers of studies (reviewed in ORLOFF et al. 1989b), typically using biologically active, radiolabeled, amino-terminal PTH analogs, demonstrated that classical PTH target cells possess receptors and that nonclassical target cells, such as fibroblasts, contained similar receptors, generally fewer in number. These studies showed that PTH receptors bind PTH with an apparent affinity $[K_d]$ of less than $5\,nM$ (NISSENSON et al. 1986). In isolated renal membranes, GTP analogs reduced the affinity of receptors for PTH; this property is typical of G protein-coupled receptors (GILMAN 1987). Further, as discussed in the previous section, PTHrP and its amino-terminal fragments bind to these receptors on bone- and kidney-derived tissues with identical affinity and specificity (NISSENSON et al. 1988; ORLOFF et al. 1989a; JÜPPNER et al. 1988; SHIGENO et al. 1988c; HORIUCHI et al. 1987; KEMP et al. 1987). Thus, radioligand assays have provided important information linking binding proteins to signaling by PTH and PTHrP. Analogous assays have also been used to define bone- and kidney-binding sites for full-length PTH (1–84) that recognize the carboxy-terminal portion of the peptide (McKEE and MURRAY 1985; RAO and MURRAY 1985; DEMAY et al. 1985). However, these receptors for carboxy-terminal PTH need further analysis before their possible biological roles can be defined.

The second approach used to characterize PTH receptors involved cross-linking strategies to identify proteins from classical and nonclassical target tissues that bind PTH and its analogs. Such approaches allowed, for the first time, more detailed biochemical characterization of receptor proteins. Recently, the use of recombinant DNA technology has allowed the cloning of cDNA-encoding PTH receptors, and thus provided precise molecular definition of receptors. This methodology provides new probes for assessing receptor expression and for deliberately manipulating receptor structure. Both the cross-linking studies and recombinant DNA studies have allowed the beginning of a structural understanding of receptor function.

The structural properties of the PTH receptor were first evaluated (COLTERA et al. 1981; DRAPER et al. 1982) using ^{125}I-labeled, photoreactive analogs of [Nle^{8,18},Tyr^{34}]bPTH(1–34)amide. Both groups identified PTH-binding proteins in canine renal membranes with an M_r of 60–70 kDa. These proteins were similar to those subsequently identified in human cells of skeletal and dermal origin (GOLDRING et al. 1984; PUN et al. 1988). More recently, chemically defined photoderivatives of NlePTH (SHIGENO et al. 1989) and PTHrP (JÜPPNER et al. 1990) were synthesized. Both peptides were first reacted with 4-fluoro-3 nitrophenylazide (FNPA); the mixture of FNPA-derivatized peptide analogs was then resolved by HPLC and the various peptides were purified to homogeneity. The derivatized residue was subsequently identified by amino acid and sequence analysis. Derivatization of Lys^{13} resulted in an NlePTH analog with only slightly impaired affinity for the receptor, while derivatization of positions Lys^{26,27} or the amino-terminal α-amino function revealed a more significant reduction of affinity (SHIGENO et al. 1989). FNPA derivatization of [Tyr^{36}]PTHrP(1–36)amide led to the synthesis of three well-defined analogs. The peptide modified on Lys^{13} showed impaired affinity for the receptor, while modification of Lys^{11} did not change affinity or biological activity. Derivatization of the amino-terminal residue revealed only a minor decrease in ligand affinity for the receptor, yet a largely improved cross-linking efficiency, and a dramatically impaired efficacy in stimulating cAMP production (JÜPPNER et al. 1988). These chemically defined, high-affinity FNPA derivatives of NlePTH and PTHrP proved invaluable in characterizing their common receptor on ROS 17/2.8 cells. The PTH receptor in these osteoblast-like cells was shown to be a glycoprotein with an apparent molecular size of ~80 kDa. Comparative studies using radiolabeled, photoderivatized analogues of both PTH and PTHrP revealed that both peptides bind equivalently to the same receptor protein and that both radioligands are displaced by either PTH and PTHrP with equivalent affinity and efficacy (JÜPPNER et al. 1988).

Using a different approach, NISSENSON et al. (1987), first demonstrated high-affinity, Gpp(NH)p-sensitive, specific cross-linking of ^{125}I-labeled bPTH(1–34) to several proteins from canine renal membranes. After radioligand binding, the heterobifunctional cross-linker N-hydroxysuccinimidyl-4-azido-benzoate (HSAB) was used to covalently attach the ligand to the receptor; SDS-PAGE revealed a major receptor-ligand band with a size of 85 kDa, a size confirmed in subsequent observations (SHIGENO et al. 1988a,b; JÜPPNER et al. 1988). Not only did these investigations provide the first compelling evidence for the specificity of the receptor affinity labeling techniques, they also indicated that the PTH receptor, at least in plasma membrane preparations, is very sensitive to enzymatic degradation. Various enzyme inhibitors successfully diminished the conversion of the major 85-kDa receptor protein into smaller fragments: a fully functional, G protein-sensitive 70-kDa degradation product and a 55-kDa fragment (NISSENSON et al. 1987; KARPF et al. 1988). This finding was later also confirmed for receptors which were affinity-labeled with radioiodinated, amino-terminal PTHrP (ORLOFF et al. 1989a; KARPF et al. 1991). PTH/PTHrP receptors in renal plasma membranes (KARPF et al. 1987) and bone-derived ROS 17/2.8 cells (SHIGENO et al. 1988b) are glycoproteins with asparagine-linked oligosaccharides. The two functionally intact receptor proteins, the 55-kDa receptor fragment, and the 50-kDa fragment derived from elastase, chymotrypsin, or *Staphylococcus aureus* V8 protease treatment were quantitatively retained on wheat germ lectin affinity columns (KARPF et al. 1987; SHIGENO et al. 1988a). This result confirms that the receptor is a glycoprotein and implies that the PTH-binding region is located within a 50-kDa receptor fragment (KARPF et al. 1991). After enzymatic removal of the asparagine-linked oligosaccharides, the size of the protein backbone was predicted to be ~59 kDa (SHIGENO et al. 1988a,b).

Treatment of renal plasma membranes with disulfide bond-reducing agents completely abolished ligand binding to the PTH/PTHrP receptor. This result indicates that disulfide bonds stabilize a secondary structure of the receptor protein essential for ligand binding. Further, treatment of the partially purified covalent ligand-receptor complex with DTT and proteolytic enzymes released a presumably nonglycosylated ≤14-kDa extramembranous fragment that is thought to contain a principle ligand-binding domain (KARPF et al. 1991).

Further structural analysis of the PTH/PTHrP receptor has required the isolation of cDNA encoding the receptors. Using an expression-cloning strategy, cDNA clones that encode common PTH/PTHrP receptors from opossum kidney (OK) and rat osteosarcoma (ROS 17/2.8 cells) were purified (JÜPPNER et al. 1991; ABOU-SAMRA et al. 1992). The sequences of these receptors contain identical residues at 78% of their corresponding positions and thus demonstrate a remarkable degree of phylogenetic conservation. These PTH receptors share common structural features with other G protein-linked receptors; these are predicted to include an extracellular, amino-terminal portion, seven membrane-spanning domains, three extra-cellular loops, and three intracellular loops, and an intracellular, carboxy-terminal tail (Fig. 5). The amino terminus contains a hydrophobic segment, which is thought to represent a signal peptide. If the signal sequence is cleaved off the amino terminal, the extracellular domain contains approximately 155 amino acids. Both PTH/PTHrP receptors contain eight conserved extracellular cysteine residues, four potential N-linked glycosylation sites, and multiple potential phosphorylation sites in the third intracellular loop and the carboxy-terminal, intracellular region. Despite the predicted structual similarity, the PTH/PTHrP receptor has virtually no sequence homology with other G protein-linked receptors, except for striking homology for the calcitonin and secretin receptors (LIN et al. 1991; ISHIKARA et al. 1991). The overall amino acid identity with the calcitonin receptor, for example, is 32%, with an overall similarity of 56% and with multiple regions of complete identity. Comparison with the secretin receptor revealed an even higher degree of conservation with both PTH/PTHrP receptors. Also, all of the eight extracellular cysteines residues are conserved, as are two of the four potential, N-linked glycosylation sites and multiple proline residues. Northern blot analysis of total A^+-selected RNA from ROS 17/2.8 cells, rat bone, and kidney revealed one prominent, approximately 3-kb hybridizing species. An

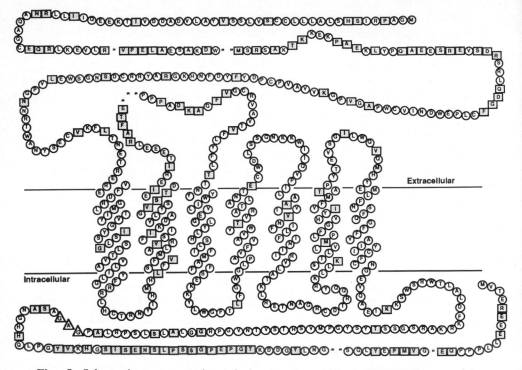

Fig. 5. Schematic representation of the opossum kidney PTH/PTHrP receptor (Jüppner et al. 1991). Comparison with the rat bone PTH/PTHrP receptor (Abou-samra et al. 1992). Residues that are identical in each receptor are *circled*; residues that differ in sequence between the two receptors are *enclosed by shaded squares*; residues present only in the opossum kidney receptor are *enclosed by triangles*; residues present only in the rat bone receptor are *shown by asterisks*

identical, although dramatically less abundant, hybridizing RNA species was also observed in a variety of other rat organs (unpublished data). The presence of this receptor RNA in "nonclassical" target tissues and in F9 embryonic carcinoma cells, a model for early embryonic cells, suggests that the same, or very closely related receptors are found both in classic PTH endocrine target tissues and in targets of the paracrine/autocrine factor PTHrP.

The biological properties of the cDNA clones encoding the PTH/PTHrP receptors were first evaluated in transiently transfected COS cells (Jüppner et al. 1991; Abou-Samra et al. 1992). Both expressed receptors bind PTH(1–34) and PTHrP(1–36) equivalently, yet with about tenfold lower affinity than is displayed by native receptors in the parent cell lines. The apparent K_d of either peptide is about $0.5\,nM$ for native OK cells and $0.9\,nM$ for native ROS 17/2.8 cells. The cloned OK and ROS cell receptors expressed in COS cells exhibited affinities of $4\,nM$ and $10\,nM$, respectively. This discrepancy between the native receptors and the cloned receptors expressed in COS cells may result from limited availability of G proteins, and, thus, inadequate coupling of G proteins to the abundantly expressed receptor protein ($>1 000 000$ receptor copies/cell). This explanation is supported by findings in AtT-20 and LLC-PK$_1$ cells that are stably transfected with the receptor clones. At a receptor copy number of $10 000–100 000$/cell, which is approximately that of the OK and ROS 17/2.8 cell lines, the apparent K_d of both receptors was about $0.5 nM$ (BRINGHURST et al. 1991; ABOU-SAMRA et al. 1991b). PTH(3–34) and (7–34) bind with progressively lower affinity to COS cells transiently transfected with either cloned receptor, a finding which is similar to that observed in native OK and ROS 17/2.9 cells. As in the native cell lines, PTH(7–34) binds with more than tenfold higher affinity to the expressed opossum kidney receptor than to the rat bone receptor. This discrepancy in binding, probably reflecting species differences, has proven useful for defining ligand-binding sites within the receptor protein. Indeed, preliminary studies using hybrid receptor clones revealed that the improved affinity of the OK cell receptor for PTH(7–34) can be mapped to the amino-terminal, extracellular domain and the first extracellular loop of the OK clone. Analogous studies that exploit the differing interactions of the two receptors with the human PTH analog, [Arg-2] PTH(1–34) (GARDELLA et al. 1991), have shown that an area between the third and the seventh transmembrane domain of the receptor recognizes the alteration of residue 2 of PTH. These studies suggest that PTH interacts with multiple regions of the receptor over much of its length.

Parathyroid hormone (1–34) and PTHrP(1–36) both stimulate cAMP accumulation in transfected COS cells equivalently. The ED$_{50}$s are similar to those obtained with both ligands in native OK and ROS 17/2.8 cells ($0.4–1 nM$). This high potency supports the hypothesis that insufficient G protein coupling causes the decrease in apparent K_ds of the transiently expressed receptors. That is, receptors coupled to G proteins, as reflected in cAMP accumulation, respond to low concentrations of PTH. Interestingly, a mutant cDNA clone, OK-H, with a 69 amino acid deletion from the carboxy-terminal tail, was fully functional in radioreceptor assays and revealed no impairment of cAMP accumulation when stimulated with PTH or PTHrP. This indicates that the terminal portion of the carboxy-terminal tail of the PTH/PTHrP receptor is not required for expression, ligand binding, or Gs coupling (JÜPPNER et al. 1991).

In addition to stimulating cAMP production, the expressed PTH/PTHrP receptors have the capacity to increase intracellular free calcium when exposed to either PTH(1–34) or PTHrP(1–36). Similarly, [^{3}H]myoinositol-loaded COS cells that were transfected with either cloned receptor showed an increase of IP$_2$ and IP$_3$ when treated with PTH(1–34) or PTHrP(1–36). Intracellular free calcium revealed only a small increase, when the studies were performed with COS cells transfected with OK-H, and there was no detectable increase in IP$_2$ and IP$_3$ generation after treatment with PTH(1–34) or PTHrP(1–36) (ABOU-SAMRA et al. 1992). These data strongly argue that the carboxyl-terminal, intracellular PTH/PTHrP receptor region is necessary for coupling to phospholipase C but not to adenylate cyclase.

Thus, the cloning of PTH receptors has clarified a series of issues. These receptors are part of a new subfamily of G protein-linked receptors. The similarities of the structures of receptors for PTH/PTHrP, calcitonin, and secretin suggest that shared functional patterns will be found, as well. For example, the amino-terminal regions of both PTH and secretin are important for transmembrane signaling. The striking similarities of the rat bone and opossum kidney receptors suggest that one identical receptor is found in both bone and kidney. Determination of sequences from both targets in one species will be needed to address this question. The cloned receptors bind amino-terminal fragments of PTH and PTHrP and may well represent mediators of the physiologic actions of both peptides. The cloned receptors both couple to adenylate cyclase and to phospholipase C signaling pathways. However, a systematic search is now needed to explore the possible existence of additional receptors, for amino-terminal fragments of PTH and PTHrP, for other fragments, and for the full-length peptides.

Hormonal responsiveness to PTH is not only dependent upon the levels of circulating hormone but also is determined by the sensitivity of target tissues to the hormone; the latter is influenced by the number of functional PTH receptors in these tissues. The number and the function of receptors in the target tissues are tightly regulated by the hormonal milieu. Glucocorticoids, for example, upregulate the number of PTH receptors in some bone-derived cells (YAMAMOTO et al. 1988b). Also, glucocorticoids enhance both the coupling of the PTH receptor to the adenylate cyclase apparatus (RODAN et al. 1984) and the activation of the cAMP-dependent protein kinase by cAMP (ZAJAC et al. 1986). These two effects of glucocorticoids on adenylate cyclase and on the cAMP-dependent protein kinase are independent from their effect on PTH receptor number (RODAN et al. 1984; ZAJAC et al. 1986). $1,25(OH)_2$ vitamin D and retinoic acid can also modulate the number and the functions of the PTH receptors in osteoblastic osteosarcoma cells (Ros 17/2.8). In these cells, $1,25(OH)_2$ vitamin D dramatically downregulates the PTH receptor for a prolonged time (TITUS et al. 1991). Conversely, downregulation of the PTH receptor by retinoic acids is reversed after removing retinoic acid from the medium (GU and SEGRE, unpublished). A discussion of how cells use different pathways to modulate the number and function of PTH receptors in response to various stimuli can be found in the next section of this chapter.

E. Second Messengers in PTH Action

I. Cyclic AMP

Rapid activation of adenylate cyclase by PTH was first described 25 years ago (CHASE and AURBACH 1967), and many of the effects of PTH on bone and kidney are reproduced by cyclic AMP analogs or phosphodiesterase inhibitors (RASMUSSEN et al. 1968; WELLS and LLOYD 1969; AGUS et al. 1971; BOURDEAU and BURG 1980; McKINNEY and MYERS 1980). In vivo, administration of cAMP analogs elevates serum calcium and enhances urinary phosphate excretion (WELLS and LLOYD 1969; AGUS et al. 1971), whereas PTH infusion rapidly increases cAMP production by bone and kidney (CHASE and AURBACH 1967; BROADUS 1979; SUGIMOTO et al. 1985). Similarly, in vitro, PTH increases cAMP formation in primary cell or organ cultures of bone and kidney and in hormonally responsive transformed cell lines with renal epithelial or osteoblastic characteristics (NISSENSON and ARNAUD 1979; MAJESKA et al. 1980; PARTRIDGE et al. 1981; HERRMANN-ERLEE et al. 1983; RODAN and RODAN 1974; AUSIELLO et al. 1980; LIVESEY et al. 1982). Many of the cellular biologic responses to PTH in these systems can be reproduced by pharmacologic activation of PK-A. In renal cells, these include inhibition of phosphate and bicarbonate transport, increased calcium transport, cytosolic acidification, and stimulated phosphoenolpyruvate carboxykinase gene transcription (CAVERZASIO et al. 1986; HANAI et al. 1986; GOOD 1990; POLLOCK et al. 1986), and, in bone cells, regulation of alkaline phosphatase, citrate decarboxylase, ornithine decarboxylase, and glucose-6-phosphate dehydrogenase activities; DNA, collagen, matrix protein, and phospholipid synthesis; collagenase and plasminogen activator secretion; calcium and phosphate uptake; cytoskeletal structure; and others (MAJESKA and RODAN 1982; WONG et al. 1979; LOWIK et al. 1986; SAKAGUCHI et al. 1987; REID et al. 1988; DIETRICH et al. 1976; ALLAN et al. 1986; MATSUMOTO et al. 1986; NODA et al. 1988; CIVITELLI et al. 1989; FUKAYAMA and TASHJIAN 1990; SELZ et al. 1989; LOMRI and MARIE 1990; TORRING et al. 1991) It thus is considered likely that cAMP, via activation of PK-A and subsequent phosphorylation of various enzymes, ion channels, transcription factors, and other proteins, mediates many of the actions of PTH in target tissues. More direct evidence for the role of PK-A in PTH action has been obtained recently by stable transfection into PTH-responsive cell lines of DNA-encoding mutant, cAMP-resistant regulatory subunits of PK-A (BRINGHURST et al. 1989; FUKAYAMA et al. 1991; SEGAL and POLLOCK 1990). When overexpressed in such cells, these mutant proteins combine with the catalytic subunits of PK-A and prevent subsequent dissociation (activation) of active catalytic subunits by endogenous cAMP generated in response to the hormone. The resulting dominant-negative mutation of PK-A has been employed in both osteoblastic and renal cells to demonstrate directly that specific biologic responses to PTH, such as regulation of alkaline phosphatase, membrane phospholipid synthesis, inorganic phosphate transport, and cell proliferation, require PK-A activation.

II. Other Second Messengers

Recently, however, it has become clear that PTH elicits a number of rapid signaling events within target cells apart from adenylate cyclase activation alone. Thus, PTH activates PLC and subsequent generation of DAG and inositol polyphosphates (IP_3, IP_4, etc.) within seconds of addition to kidney or bone cells (Bidot-Lopez et al. 1981; Meltzer et al. 1982; Rappaport and Stern 1986; Quamme et al. 1989b,c; Coleman and Bilezikian 1990; Civitelli et al. 1988; Farndale 1988; Suzuki et al. 1989; Babich et al. 1989; Cosman et al. 1989). Concomitant increases in intracellular free Ca^{2+} or Ca^{2+} uptake also are observed in a variety of experimental systems, including normal primary kidney and bone cells as well as transformed opossum kidney and rat osteosarcoma cells (Dziak and Stern 1975; Marcus and Orner 1980; Yamaguchi et al. 1987; Civitelli et al. 1988; Reid et al. 1987; Lowik et al. 1985; Donahue et al. 1988; Hruska et al. 1986; Filburn and Harrison 1990; Lieberherr 1987). These rapid increases in cytosolic Ca^{2+}, which are not due to cAMP or PK-A activation, result mainly from release of Ca^{2+} from intracellular stores, although influx of Ca^{2+} from the extra-cellular compartment also occurs in some cells. In some cases, a secondary, more gradual rise in intracellular Ca^{2+} occurs which is dependent upon influx of extracellular Ca^{2+} and may be mimicked by cyclic AMP analogs (Yamaguchi et al. 1987). In this regard, a variety of Ca^{2+} channels have been reported in the plasma membranes of osteoblastic cells, including typical L- and T-type dihydropyridine-sensitive channels as well as others (Chesnoy-Marchais and Fritsch 1988; Guggino et al. 1989; Karpinski et al. 1989; Duncan and Misler 1989). Because all of the PTH receptors cloned to date exhibit both coupling (through Gs) to adenylate cyclase and a 7-transmembrane-domain structure typical of other G-protein-linked receptors, it is presumed that coupling of occupied PTH receptors to PLC, ion channels, and other effectors occurs via specific G-proteins (Gq, etc.), although this has not yet been demonstrated directly. It is also possible, however, that PTH receptors may bind directly to and activate Ca^{2+} and other ion channels within the plasma membrane, without intervention of a specific G-protein. In both renal and osseous systems, generation of DAG, IP_3, and Ca^{2+} signals by PTH is associated with activation of PKC, which then phosphorylates specific protein substrates, at least some of which are distinct from those phosphorylated by PKA (Abou-Samra et al. 1989b; Iida-Klein et al. 1989; Chakravarthy et al. 1990; Nemani et al. 1991).

Studies in several systems involving synthetic PTH analogs with truncated amino termini have suggested that activation of adenylate cyclase by PTH may be dissociated from stimulation of Ca^{2+} transients and PKC. Thus, $[Nle^{8,18},Tyr^{34}]bPTH(3-34)$ and $[Tyr^{34}]bPTH(7-34)$ increased cytosolic Ca^{2+} in perifused aequorin-loaded ROS 17/2.8 cells without augmenting medium cAMP (Donahue et al. 1988). Single-cell recordings of fura-2-loaded UMR 106-01 cells showed stimulation of cytosolic Ca^{2+} by bPTH(3-34) and propionyl-bPTH(2-34) at concentrations of these peptides that did not augment cAMP, even in the presence of phosphodiesterase inhibitors (Lowik et al. 1986; Fujimori et al. 1991). In ROS 17/2 cells, bPTH(3-34), like bPTH(1-34), strongly induced membrane-associated PKC activity without concomitant activation of adenylate cyclase (CHAKRAVARTY et al. 1990). An earlier study with isolated rat T cells had also shown that bPTH(3–34) was equipotent with bPTH(1–34) in stimulating mitosis and intracellular Ca^{2+} transients (ATKINSON et al. 1987). As reviewed earlier, these truncated PTH analogs were designed originally as PTH antagonists, as they lack intrinsic adenylate cyclase activation but inhibit receptor binding of PTH(1–34). The unanticipated finding, though still controversial (REID et al. 1987; TAMURA et al. 1989; FILBURN and HARRISON 1990), that these antagonists of PTH adenylate cyclase activation may actually induce, at least partially, alternate second messengers, suggests spatial separation within the PTH(1–34) molecule of structural determinants critical for activation of different signal-transduction pathways. Indeed, such observations, together with other demonstrations of unique biologic effects (independent of cAMP) of even more severely truncated fragments such as PTH(13–34) (reviewed earlier and below), have been taken as evidence of the existence of separate classes of PTH receptors in these cells. While this possibility remains, recent studies with cloned PTH receptors do indicate that a single PTH receptor can activate both adenylate cyclase and PLC in the same cell.

Other early signals generated by PTH have also been described, including changes in membrane potential (EDELMAN et al. 1986; FERRIER and WARD 1986), cytosolic acidification (via inhibition of Na^+-H^+ antiport) (POLLOCK et al. 1986), increased Cl^- conductance (CHESNOY-MARCHAIS and FRITSCH 1989) and stimulation of PLA2 with generation of prostaglandins such as PGE2 (MACDONALD et al. 1984; FEYEN et al. 1984). Whether these events reflect additional, parallel pathways of receptor-dependent signaling or, perhaps more likely, secondary responses to the primary messages cAMP, DAG, IP_3, and Ca^{2+}, remains to be established.

III. Physiologic Roles of Different Second Messengers in PTH Action

The potential physiologic importance of alternate signaling pathways, such as those involving Ca^{2+} and PKC, is underscored by the fact that numerous biological responses to PTH in target cells cannot be explained readily by activation of adenylate cyclase alone and that pharmacologic activation of these alternate pathways may reproduce some of the effects of the hormone, independent of cAMP. Thus, for example, rapid uptake of radioactive Ca^{2+} into osteoblasts appears not to be mediated by cAMP (DZIAK and STERN 1975; FUKAYAMA and TASHJIAN 1989). This effect could involve a cAMP-independent messenger system or receptor-operated Ca^{2+} channels, as discussed above. Collagenase production stimulated by PTH in UMR 106-01 cells in only partly mimicked by cAMP analogs, whereas combinations of cAMP, phorbol ester, and a Ca^{2+} ionophore more fully reproduce the strong hormonal effect (CIVITELLI et al. 1988). Similarly, homologous downregulation of PTH receptors in UMR 106-01 or ROS 17/2.8 cells has been found to be partly or entirely independent of cAMP, respectively

(Abou-Samra et al. 1989c, 1991a); receptor downregulation in ROS cells, moreover, is mimicked completely by phorbol esters (Abou-Samra et al. 1989c). In proximal renal tubular cells, increased gluconeogenesis and rapid morphological changes (microvillar shortening) induced by PTH are dependent upon Ca^{2+} and are not reproduced by cAMP (Goligorsky et al. 1986a,b).

As noted earlier, in studies with synthetic peptide fragments, the proliferative effects of PTH on osteoblasts and chondrocytes have been mapped to sequences of the hormone [PTH(13–34), PTH(28–48), etc.] that are fully active yet clearly do not stimulate adenylate cyclase (Schlüter et al. 1989; Somjen et al. 1990). In the case of osteoblasts, proliferation stimulated by these fragments is strikingly dependent upon availability of extracellular Ca^{2+} (Somjen et al. 1990). In guinea pig distal tubular cells, measurements of G6PD activation in a sensitive cytochemical bioassay showed that synthetic PTH analogs such as $[Tyr^{34}]hPTH(7–34)NH_2$ and $[Tyr^{34}]hPTH(13–34)NH_2$, which do not elicit detectable cAMP production in other systems, were equipotent with bPTH(1–84) (Sakaguchi et al. 1987). Although the G6PD response is also stimulated by cAMP analogs in these cells, the disparity between the cAMP and G6PD responses to these analogs strongly suggests a cAMP-independent pathway for generation of the G6PD effect.

Finally, several investigators have shown that the resorptive response to PTH in cultured rodent calvaria can be dissociated somewhat from cAMP generation and that inhibitors of adenylate cyclase fail to alter the resorptive response to the hormone (Lerner et al. 1989; Reid et al. 1990). Attempts to inhibit PTH-dependent bone resorption in vitro with specific antagonist analogs such as bPTH(3–34) have succeeded in some hands (Rosol and Capen 1988) but not in others (Herrmann-Erlee et al. 1983; Klein et al. 1987). In fact, analogs such as bPTH(2–34) and bPTH(3–34) have been shown to mimick effects of PTH(1–34), albeit with reduced efficacy, in organ cultures of bone (Herrmann-Erlee et al. 1983; Bringhurst and Potts 1981). Although this too has been cited as evidence that bone resorption caused by PTH may be mediated by cAMP-independent mechanisms, the intact bones used in these assays are composed of heterogeneous cell populations, including osteoclasts sensitive to cAMP-dependent inhibition by calcitonin. Clearly, attempts to determine mechanisms of PTH effects in such complex systems are fraught with great difficulty.

IV. Second Messengers in PTH Regulation of Renal Phosphate Transport

Efforts to clarify the roles of specific second messengers in PTH regulation of renal epithelial phosphate transport have been particularly illustrative with respect to the strategies employed and, as well, the difficulties inherent in approaching these issues. As discussed earlier, renal tubular phosphate reabsorption is inhibited by PTH in vivo by a mechanism that involves rapid endocytosis of functional transporters from the apical membranes of proximal renal tubular cells (KEMPSON et al. 1990). This effect is mimicked in vivo by administration of active cAMP analogs (AGUS et al. 1971) and is inhibited by coinfusion of $[Tyr^{34}]bPTH(7-34)$ amide, which also antagonizes the adenylate cyclase response to $PTH(1-34)$ in vitro (HORIUCHI et al. 1983). In OK opossum kidney cells, the V_{max} of the Na^+/phosphate cotransporter is inhibited by $PTH(1-34)$, as well as by cAMP analogs, cholera toxin, and forskolin. These results accord with observations in vivo and support a role for PKA in this effect of the hormone (CAVERZASIO et al. 1986; COLE et al. 1988; QUAMME et al. 1989a,b; NAKAI et al. 1990).

Interest in the possible role of cAMP-independent signals, however, derived from observations that inhibition of phosphate transport occurs at concentrations of PTH $(1-34)$ 10- to 100-fold lower than those required for adenylate cyclase activation (COLE et al. 1987, 1988). Also, PTH analogs, such as $[Nle^{8,18},Tyr^{34}]bPTH(3-34)NH_2$ and others truncated or modified at the N-terminus to minimize or eliminate adenylate cyclase activation, were noted nevertheless to inhibit OK-cell phosphate transport directly, even in the absence of detectable generation of cAMP (COLE et al. 1987, 1988). Moreover, in coincubations, marked inhibition of the cAMP response to $PTH(1-34)$ by such analogs was not accompanied by concurrent inhibition of the phosphate effect (COLE et al 1989; PIZURKI et al. 1990; MUFF et al. 1990). Similar results were obtained using pharmacologic inhibitors of adenylate cyclase such as $2',5'$-dideoxyadenosine (COLE et al. 1988). Subsequently, it was shown that IP_3 and DAG production are stimulated in OK cells by $PTH(1-34)$ at concentrations $(0.001-0.01 nM)$ that are comparable to those that block phosphate transport but much lower than those needed to activate adenylate cyclase in these cells (QUAMME et al. 1989b,c), and that phorbol esters are potent inhibitors of phosphate transport in these cells (COLE et al. 1987; NAKAI et al. 1989; MALSTROM et al. 1988). Other studies served to discount a role for Ca^{2+} per se, as ionophores and EGTA did not alter phosphate transport, either directly or in response to PTH (QUAMME et al. 1989c; HELMLE-KOLB et al. 1990b), and other agents that elevate Ca^{2+} in these cells, such as thrombin, failed to reproduce the phosphate regulation seen with PTH (MALSTROM et al. 1988). The possible importance of PKC activation in the PTH effect was supported also by findings that downregulation or inhibition of PKC by prolonged exposure to phorbols or staurosporine, respectively, did block regulation of phosphate transport by PTH and, interestingly, by forskolin also (MALSTROM et al. 1988).

Thus, the cumulative data indicate that regulation of phosphate transport by PTH in OK cells can be mimicked by pharmacologic activation of either PKA or PKC. Whether or not PKC is the principal mediator of the PTH effect, it appears that active PKC enzyme is at least necessary, even when the primary signal is cAMP (as with forskolin stimulation). The significance of the apparent dissociation between cAMP and phosphate regulation highlighted by the work with PTH analogs has been discounted by several subsequent observations. First, MARTIN et al. (1989) showed that, despite the absence of a measurable cAMP response, the synthetic analog [Nle^{8,18},Tyr^{34}]bPTH(3–34)NH$_2$ does activate PKA in OK cells, as does PTH(1–34) at concentrations well below the K_m for cAMP accumulation. Second, reexamination of the activities of PTH "antagonists" in dexamethasone- and pertussis toxin-pretreated ROS 17/2.8 cells has revealed significant agonism for adenylate cyclase activation in the case of both [Nle^{8,18},Tyr^{34}]bPTH(3–34)NH$_2$ and [Tyr^{34}]bPTH(7–34)NH$_2$ (MCKEE et al. 1990). Finally, studies with cAMP-resistant OK cells stably transfected with a dominant-negative mutation of PKA have shown that active PKA is required for regulation of phosphate transport by PTH (SEGAL and POLLOCK 1990). Recent evidence that dexamethasone treatment blocks the effect of PTH and forskolin on phosphate transport, but not that of phorbol esters (KAUFMANN et al. 1991) also supports a major role for PKA in mediating this biologic effect of the hormone, although, as with most of the evidence available, several interpretations are still possible. The precise mechanism(s) whereby PTH regulates phosphate transport thus remains unsettled. The available data are most consistent with parallel activation of kinases A and C and a necessary role for at least basal levels of both enzymes for effective transmission of the hormonal signal. The full extent to which such dual signaling may be important for this or other effects of the hormone in kidney and bone cells has yet to be determined.

V. Modulation of PTH Signal Transduction

While it is clear that PTH activates multiple messengers within target cells and that such plurality in signaling is probably needed to adequately explain the various actions of the hormone, relatively little is known about the possible modulation of the pattern of second messenger responses generated by the hormone within target cells under different physiologic circumstances. Numerous possibilities, most already demonstrated in various other G protein-linked receptor systems, exist for such regulation, including *differential surface expression of functionally distinct PTH receptor subtypes* via changes in synthesis, inactivation, or clearance of specific receptor species; *altered coupling of a single receptor to one or more G proteins* via chemical modification of the receptor or the G protein(s), changes in the proportions of different G proteins available within the cell, or control of critical cofactors necessary for receptor/G protein interaction; *modifications of effector kinases or ion channels* (PKA, PKC(s), etc.) via analagous transcriptional controls, posttranslational modifications or allosteric interactions; and *altered stability of the second messenger molecules per se*, such as the induction of cAMP phosphodiesterase, DAG kinase, IP phosphatase or

Ca^{2+}-ATPase activities that rapidly terminate these signals. These regulatory effects could be produced in response to initial PTH exposure, to the actions of other hormones, or to local ionic or other environmental factors, such as mechanical stress.

Such opportunities for alteration of the pattern of the multiple signals generated by the hormone clearly provide a basis for enormous diversity in cellular responsiveness to PTH, including modulated feedback or "cross-talk" between different signaling pathways and differential regulation of critical enzyme systems and transcription factors that mediate more distal actions of the hormone. Moreover, the possibility that more than one active chemical form of the hormone might exist in the circulation cannot yet be definitively excluded, even without considering the possibility of functional receptors for circulating carboxy-terminal fragments of PTH, and work with N-truncated PTH analogs has already shown that ligand structure is a critical determinant of the pattern of intracellular messengers generated by the PTH receptor(s). Thus, the diversity already apparent in this system predicts that further understanding of the structural basis of PTH receptor signaling and of postreceptor regulatory phenomena will provide important opportunities for pharmacologic control of cellular activity in bone and kidney.

At present, efforts to approach these issues have merely scratched the surface of the problem. It is clear from studies both in vivo and in vitro that chronic (hours–days) exposure to high concentrations of PTH rather routinely induces homologous downregulation of surface PTH receptors as well as desensitization of the subsequent adenylate cyclase response to receptor activation. Such homologous desensitization has been described in several in vitro systems, including UMR 106, ROS 17/2.8, and SaOS-2 osteosarcoma cells and OK kidney cells, although the mechanisms involved appear to differ. In UMR 106 cells, for example, desensitization of adenylate cyclase by PTH occurs within 30–60 min, does not involve a pertussis toxin-sensitive G protein, and is mimicked by phorbol esters or calcium ionophores (MITCHELL and GOLTZMAN 1990; PUN et al. 1990; IKEDA et al. 1991a,b). The role of cAMP in this process is controversial, as is the role of alterations in Gs. By contrast, in another rat osteoblast-like osteosarcoma cell line, ROS 17/2.8, preincubation with phorbol esters or high extracellular calcium actually increases PTH-activated adenylate cyclase, whereas cAMP has no effect (PINES et al. 1986; YAMAMOTO et al. 1988a; ABOU-SAMRA et al. 1989c; RAO and MURRAY 1989). Notably, in ROS cells prior exposure to PTH also desensitizes the subsequent PKC response to the hormone, whereas the intracellular Ca^{2+} transient is well preserved – an example of differential desensitization of messenger responses (ABOU-SAMRA et al. 1989b; BIDWELL et al. 1991). Dissociation of second messenger responses to PTH has also been observed in response to pertussis toxin or following preincubation with insulin or different concentrations of extracellular phosphate (CIVITELLI et al. 1988; IIDA-KLEIN and HAHN 1991; GREEN et al. 1991).

Mechanisms of PTH receptor downregulation also appear to differ among these cell lines. In UMR cells, receptor downregulation is mimicked by cAMP analogs, whereas cAMP appears not to be involved in ROS cells, despite a comparable magnitude and time course (16–72 h). In ROS cells but not in UMR cells, homologous downregulation is partly dependent upon a pertussis toxin-sensitive G protein (Abou-Samra et al. 1989c; Ikeda et al. 1991a). Studies with mutant UMR cells that express a regulated cAMP-resistant phenotype have shown that PTH receptor downregulation is partly mimicked by [Nle^{8,18},Tyr^{34}]bPTH(3–34) amide and that this effect of the analog does not require PKA, whereas downregulation caused by PTH(1–34) involves both cAMP-dependent and -independent mechanisms (Abou-Samra et al. 1991a). Similar recent experiments with OK kidney cells indicate that homologous desensitization of adenylate cyclase by PTH in these cells may be mediated by PKC but that receptor downregulation may involve other, as yet unidentified, mechanisms (Pernalete et al. 1990). Thus, the details of intracellular regulation of hormonal responsiveness following prior exposure to PTH appear to vary strikingly among different target cell systems, possibly due to differences in populations of expressed G proteins, regulation and coupling of specific effector kinases, aspects of the trans-formed phenotype of these cells, or other poorly understood factors.

Finally, it is quite clear that cellular responsiveness to PTH may be modulated substantially by a variety of exogenous influences, such as other hormones, growth factors, extracellular ion concentrations, and other factors. Most of the available data concern the adenylate cyclase response to PTH, and many such interactions have been described, including effects of cortisol, estrogens, androgens, 1,25-dihydroxyvitamin D, insulin, EGF, phosphate and calcium ions, and prostaglandins, among others (Hahn et al. 1984; Rizzoli and Fleisch 1986; Ikeda et al. 1991b; Fukayama and Tashjian 1989; Iida-Klein and Hahn 1991; Guiterrez et al. 1987; Rao and Murray 1989; Green et al. 1991). The putative locus of these interactions is typically unclear, although direct modulation of PTH receptor/Gs coupling is a common theme, as assessed by comparing responsiveness to PTH vs. forskolin in whole cells or vs. guanine nucleotides or fluoride in isolated membranes. These heterologous effects add yet another layer of complexity to the regulation of cellular responsiveness to PTH.

It is obvious that transduction of the signal(s) generated by interaction of PTH with surface receptors on target cells involves an exceeding complex pattern of parallel and intersecting pathways that are modulated in response to a host of environmental determinants, the most important of which may be prior exposure to the hormone itself. These intracellular signals ultimately become integrated and converge upon individual distal cellular regulatory proteins, thereby altering critical aspects of metabolic activity, cytoskeletal structure, ion transport, gene transcription, and other cellular functions which together define specific physiologic actions of the hormone. The potential importance of differential desensitization of specific second messenger signals in response to the temporal pattern and level of prior exposure to PTH is highlighted by observations, reviewed earlier, that intermittent administration of PTH may lead to anabolic effects on bone mass that are quite distinct from the catabolic effects observed during continuous exposure to high hormone concentrations. Additional specificity for particular messenger pathways may be resident in separate structural domains of the PTH molecule, as revealed by studies with N-truncated and other hormone analogs. Alternatively, specificity may be dictated by the number and type(s) of PTH receptors on the cell surface, concurrent hormonal stimuli, local environmental factors, the state of cellular differentiation, the stage of the cell cycle, or any of a variety of other possible variables mentioned earlier. Understanding the mechanisms and interactions of even a handful of the most critical of these factors will provide a major challenge for PTH research in the next decade.

F. Conclusion

A number of important questions have been raised by new information about parathyroid hormone. What are the biochemical mechanisms governing PTH secretion and how are these related to the regulation of PTH synthesis and parathyroid cell proliferation? How does PTH stimulate both bone formation and bone resorption? Do different PTH analogs, PTH receptors, or second messenger pathways favor one physiologic action or another? How does the organism use one receptor to mediate both the homeostatic actions of PTH and some paracrine effects of PTHrP without undesirable cross-talk? How many receptors are needed to mediate all the actions of these peptides?

Each of these questions suggests opportunities for improving the diagnosis and therapeutics of diseases of mineral metabolism. Vitamin D analogs that specifically decrease PTH biosynthesis may find use in disorders of PTH excess. PTH analogs may be found that favor one or another action of PTH, particularly the anabolic action on bone. Antibodies to the PTH receptor may be powerful and specific antagonists of PTH/PTHrP action in the setting of life-threatening hypercalcemia. As is often the case, these clinical interventions are, in turn, likely to yield new basic insights into PTH physiology.

References

Abou-Samra A-B, Uneno S, Jüppner H, Keutmann H, Potts JT Jr, Segre GV, Nussbaum SR (1989a) Non-homologous sequences of parathyroid hormone and the parathyroid hormone related peptide bind to a common receptor on ROS 17/2.8 cells. Endocrinology 125:2215–2217

Abou-Samra A-B, Jüppner H, Westerberg D, Potts JT Jr, Segre GV (1989b) Parathyroid hormone causes translocation of protein kinase-C from cytosol to membranes in rat osteosarcoma cells. Endocrinology 124:1107–1113

Abou-Samra A-B, Jüppner H, Potts JT Jr, Segre GV (1989c) Inactivation of pertussis-toxin-sensitive guanyl nucleotide-binding proteins increases parathyroid hormone receptors and reverses agonist-induced receptor down-regulation in ROS 17/2.8 cells. Endocrinology 125:2594–2599

Abou-Samra A-B, Zajac JD, Schiffer-Alberts D, Skurat R, Kearns A, Segre GV, Bringhurst FR (1991a) Cyclic adenosine 3′,5′-monophosphate (cAMP)-dependent and cAMP-independent regulation of parathyroid hormone receptors in UMR 106-01 osteoblastic osteosarcoma cells. Endocrinology 129:2547–2554

Abou-Samra A-B, Jüppner H, Alberts D, Kong F, Segre G (1991b) Activation of PTH/PTHrP receptors stably expressed in the mouse corticotroph tumor ATT-20 cells stimulates ACTH secretion. J Bone Miner Res 6 Suppl 1:S111

Abou-Samra A-B, Jüppner H, Force T, Freeman M, Kong XF, Schipani E, Urena P, Richards J, Bonventre JV, Potts JT Jr, Kronenberg HM, Segre GV (1992) A single PTH/PTHrP receptor activates both adenylate cyclase and phospholipase C. Proc Natl Acad Sci USA 89:2132–2736

Agus ZS, Puschett JB, Senesky D, Goldberg M (1971) Mode of action of parathyroid hormone and adenosine 3′,5′-cyclic monophosphate on renal tubular phosphate reabsorption in the dog. J Clin Invest 50:617–626

Agus ZS, Gardner LB, Beck LH, Goldber M (1973) Effects of parathyroid hormone on renal tubular reabsorption of calcium, sodium and phosphate. Am J Physiol 224:1143–1148

Allan EH, Hamilton JA, Medcalf RL, Kubota M, Martin TJ (1986) Cyclic AMP-dependent and -independent effects on tissue-type plasminogen activator activity in osteogenic sarcoma cells: evidence from phosphodiesterase inhibition and parathyroid hormone antagonists. Biochim Biophys Acta 888:199–207

Alpern RJ (1990) Cell mechanisms of proximal tubule acidification. Physiol Rev 70:79–114

Arnold A, Horst SA, Gardella RJ, Baba H, Levine MA, Kronenberg HM (1990) Mutation of the signal peptide-encoding region of the preproparathyroid hormone gene in familial isolated hypoparathyroidism. J Clin Invest 86:1084–1087

Atkinson M, Hesch R-D, Cade C, Wadwah M, Perris AD (1987) Parathyroid hormone stimulation of mitosis in rat thymic lymphocytes in independent of cyclic AMP. J Bone Miner Res 2:303–309

Ausiello DA, Rosenblatt M, Dayer JR (1980) Parathyroid hormone modulates protein kinase in giant cell tumors of human bone. Am J Physiol 239:E144–E149

Babich M, King KL, Nissenson RA (1989) G protein-dependent activation of a phosphoinositide-specific phospholipase C in UMR-106 osteosarcoma cell membranes. J Bone Miner Res 4:549–556

Bacskai BJ, Friedman PA (1990) Activation of latent Ca^{2+} channels in renal epithelial cells by parathyroid hormone. Nature 347:388–391

Barden JA, Kemp BE (1989) NMR study of a 34-residue N-terminal fragment of the parathyroid-hormone-related protein secreted during humoral hypercalcemia of malignancy. Eur J Biochem 184:379–394

Bellows CG, Ishida H, Aubin JE, Heersche JNM (1990) Parathyroid hormone reversibly suppresses the differentiation of osteoprogenitor cells into functional osteoblasts. Endocrinology 127:3111–3116

Bidot-Lopez P, Farese RV, Sabir MA (1981) Parathyroid hormone and adenosine-3′,5′-monophosphate activity increase phospholipids in the phosphadidate-polyphosphoinositol pathway in rabbit kidney cortex tubules in vitro by a cyclohexamide-sensitive process. Endocrinology 108:2078–2081

Bidwell JP, Fryer MJ, Firek AF, Donahue JH, Heath H III (1991) Desensitization of rat osteoblast-like cells (ROS 17/2.8) by parathyroid hormone uncouples the adenosine 3′,5′-monophosphate and cytosolic ionized calcium response limbs. Endocrinology 128:1021–1028

Bingham PJ, Brazell IA, Owen M (1969) The effect of parathyroid extract on cellular activity and plasma calcium levels in vivo. J Endocrinol 45:387–400

Born W, Loveridge N, Petermann JB, Kronenberg HM, Potts JT Jr, Fischer JA (1988) Inhibition of parathyroid hormone bioactivity by human parathyroid hormone (PTH)-(3–84) and PTH-(8–84) synthesized in Escherichia coli. Endocrinology 123:1848–1853

Bouhtiauy I, LaJeunesse D, Brunette MG (1991) The mechanism of parathyroid hormone action on calcium reabsorption by the distal tubule. Endocrinology 128:251–258

Bourdeau JE, Burg MB (1980) Effect of PTH on calcium transport across the cortical thick ascending limb of Henle's loop. Am J Physiol 239:F121–F126

Bourdeau JE, Lau K (1989) Effects of parathyroid hormone on cytosolic free calcium concentration in individual rabbit connecting tubules. J Clin Invest 83:373–379

Brent GA, LeBoff MS, Seely EW, Conlin PR, Brown EM (1988) Relationship between the concentration and rate of change of calcium and serum intact parathyroid hormone levels in normal humans. J Clin Endocrinol Metab 67:944–950

Bringhurst FR (1989) Calcium and phosphate distribution, turnover, and metabolic actions. In: DeGroot LJ (ed) Endocrinology, vol 2, 2nd edn. Saunders, Philadelphia, pp 805–843

Bringhurst FR, Potts JT Jr (1981) Bone collagen synthesis in vitro. Structure-activity relations among parathyroid hormone fragments and analogs. Endocrinology 108:103–108

Bringhurst FR, Zajac JD, Daggett AS, Skurat RN, Kronenberg HM (1989) Inhibition of parathyroid hormone responsiveness in clonal osteoblastic cells expressing a mutant form of 3′,5′-cyclic adenosine monophosphate-dependent protein kinase. Mol Endocrinol 3:60–67

Bringhurst FR, Jüppner H, Kronenberg HM, Abou-Samra AB, Segre GV (1991) Stable expression of functional PTH receptors in LLC-PK1 porcine renal epithelial cells. J Bone Miner Res 6 Suppl 1:S134

Broadus AE (1979) Nephrogenous cyclic AMP as a parathyroid function test. Nephron 23:136–141

Brown EM (1991) Extracellular Ca^{2+} sensing, regulation of parathyroid cell function, and role of Ca^{2+} and other ions as extracellular (first) messengers. Physiol Rev 71:371–411

Brown EM, Thatcher JG (1982) Adenosine 3′,5′-monophosphate (cAMP)-dependent protein kinase and the regulation of parathyroid hormone release by divalent cations and agents elevating cellular cAMP in dispersed bovine parathyroid cells. Endocrinology 110:1374–1380

Brown EM, Gardner DG, Windeck RA, Aurbach GD (1978) Relationship of intracellular 3′,5′-adenosine monophosphate accumulation to parathyroid hormone release from dispersed bovine parathyroid cells. Endocrinology 103: 2323–2333

Brown EM, Redgrave J, Thatcher J (1984) Effect of the phorbol ester TPA on PTH secretion: evidence for a role for protein kinase C in the control of PTH release. FEBS Lett 175:72–75

Brown EM, Enyedi P, LeBoff M, Rotberg J, Preston J, Chen C (1987) High extracellular Ca^{2+} and Mg^{2+} stimulate accumulation of inositol phosphates in bovine parathyroid cells. FEBS Lett 218:113–118

Brown EM, Fuleihan GE-H, Chen CJ, Kifor O (1990) A comparison of the effects of divalent and trivalent cations on parathyroid hormone release, 3′,5′-cyclic-adenosine monophosphate accumulation, and the levels of inositol phosphates in bovine parathyroid cells. Endocrinology 127:1064–1072

Canalis E, Centrella M, Burch W, McCarthy TL (1989) Insulin-like growth factor I mediates selective anabolic effects of parathyroid hormone in bone cultures. J Clin Invest 83:60–65

Caulfield MP, Levy JJ, McKee RL, Goldman ME, DeHaven PA, Reagan JE, Heaney L, Nutt RF, Winquist RJ, Russell J, Sherwood LM, Rosenblatt M

(1988) Avian (chicken) parathyroid hormone: synthesis and comparative biological evaluation of the 1–34 fragment. Endocrinology 123:2949–2951

Caulfield MP, McKee RL, Goldman ME, Duong LT, Fisher JE, Gay CT, DeHaven PA, Levy JJ, Roubini E, Nutt RF, Chorev M, Rosenblatt M (1990) The bovine renal parathyroid hormone (PTH) receptor has equal affinity for two different amino acid sequences: the receptor binding domains of PTH and PTH-related protein are located within the 14–34 region. Endocrinology 127:83–87

Caverzasio J, Rizzoli R, Bonjour JV (1986) Sodium-dependent phosphate transport inhibited by parathyroid hormone and cyclic AMP stimulation in an opossum kidney cell line. J Biol Chem 261:3233–3237

Chakravarthy BR, Durkin JP, Rixon RH, Whitfield JF (1990) Parathyroid hormone fragment [3–34] stimulates protein kinase-C (PKC) activity in rat osteosarcoma and murine T-lymphoma cells. Biochem Biophys Res Commun 171:1105–1110

Chambers TJ, Athanasou NA, Fuller K (1984) Effect of parathyroid hormone and calcitonin on the cytoplasmic spreading of isolated osteoclasts. J Endocrinol 102:281–286

Chambers TJ, McSheehy PM, Thomson BM, Fuller K (1985) The effect of calcium-regulating hormones and prostaglandins on bone resorption by osteoclasts disaggregated from neonatal rabbit bones. Endocrinology 116:234–239

Chase LR, Aurbach GD (1967) Parathyroid function and the renal secretion of 3',5'-adenylic acid. Proc Natl Acad Sci USA 58:518–525

Chen CJ, Brown EM (1990) The diltiazem analog TA-3090 mimics the actions of high extracellular Ca^{2+} on parathyroid function in dispersed bovine parathyroid cells. J Bone Miner Res 5:581–587

Chen CJ, Barnett JV, Congo DA, Brown EM (1989) Divalent cations suppress 3',5'-adenosine monophosphate accumulation by stimulating a pertussis toxin-sensitive guanine nucleotide-binding protein in cultured bovine parathyroid cells. Endocrinology 124:233–240

Chesnoy-Marchais D, Fritsch J (1988) Voltage-gated sodium and calcium currents in rat osteoblasts. J Physiol (Lond) 398:291–311

Chesnoy-Marchais D, Fritsch J (1989) Chloride current activated by cyclic AMP and parathyroid hormone in rat osteoblasts. Pflugers Arch 415:104–114

Chu LLH, MacGregor RR, Anast CS, Hamilton JW, Cohn DV (1973) Studies on the biosynthesis of rat parathyroid hormone and proparathyroid hormone: adaptation of the parathyroid gland to dietary restriction of calcium. Endocrinology 93:915–924

Civitelli R, Reid IR, Westbrook S, Avioli LV, Hruska KA (1988) PTH elevates inositol polyphosphates and diacylglycerol in a rat osteoblast-like cell line. Am J Physiol 255:E660–E667

Civitelli R, Hruska KA, Jeffrey JJ, Kahn AJ, Avioli LV, Partridge NC (1989) Second messenger signaling in the regulation of collagenase production by osteogenic osteosarcoma cells. Endocrinology 124:2928–2934

Coddington JM, Barling PM (1989) Proton nuclear magnetic resonance studies of intact native bovine parathyroid hormone. Mol Endocrinol 3:749–753

Cohen FE, Strewler GJ, Bradley MS, Carlquist M, Nilsson M, Ericsson M, Ciardelli TL, Nissenson RA (1991) Analogues of parathyroid hormone modified at positions 3 and 6: effects on receptor binding and activation of adenylyl cyclase in kidney and bone. J Biol Chem 266:1997–2004

Cohn DV, Zangerle R, Fischer-Colbrie R, Chu LLH, Elting JJ, Hamilton JW, Winkler H (1982) Similarity of secretory protein-I from parathyroid gland to chromagranin A from adrenal medulla. Proc Natl Acad Sci USA 79:6056–6059

Cole JA, Eber SL, Peolling RE, Thorne PK, Forte LR (1987) A dual mechanism for regulation of kidney phosphate transport by parathyroid hormone. Am J Physiol 253:E221–E227

Cole JA, Forte LR, Eber S, Thorne PK, Poelling RE (1988) Regulation of sodium-dependent phosphate transport by parathyroid hormone in opossum kidney cells: adenosine 3′,5′-monophosphate-dependent and -independent mechanisms. Endocrinology 122:2981–2989

Cole JA, Carnes DL, Forte LR, Eber S, Poelling RE, Thorne PK (1989) Structure-activity relationships of parathyroid hormone analogs in the opossum kidney cell line. J Bone Miner Res 4:723–730

Coleman DT, Bilezikian JP (1990) Parathyroid hormone stimulates formation of inositol phosphates in a membrane preparation of canine renal cortical tubular cells. J Bone Miner Res 5:299–306

Coltera MD, Potts JT Jr, Rosenblatt M (1981) Identification of a renal receptor for parathyroid hormone by photoaffinity radiolabeling using a synthetic analogue. J Biol Chem 256:10555–10559

Cosman F, Morrow BS, Kopal MA, Bilezikian JP (1989) Stimulation of inositol phosphate formation in ROS 17/2.8 cell membranes by guanine nucleotide, calcium and parathyroid hormone. J Bone Miner Res 4:413–420

Costanzo LS, Windhager EE (1980) Effect of PTH, ADH and cAMP on distal tubular Ca and Na reabsorption. Am J Physiol 239:F478–F485

Cunningham BC, Ultsch M, deVos AM, Mulkerrin MG, Clauser KR, Wells JA (1991) Dimerization of the extracellular domain of the human growth hormone receptor by a single hormone molecule. Science 254:821–825

Demay M, Mitchell J, Goltzman D (1985) Comparison of renal and osseous binding of parathyroid hormone and hormonal fragments. Am J Phyisol 249:E437–E446

Demay M, DeLuca H, Kronenberg HM (1991) Identification of sequences in the human parathyroid hormone gene that binds the 1,25-dihydroxyvitamin D_3 receptor. J Bone Miner Res 5 Suppl 2:616

Dietrich JW, Canalis EM, Maina DM, Raisz LG (1976) Hormonal control of bone collagen synthesis in vitro: effects of parathyroid hormone and calcitonin. Endocrinology 98:943–949

Donahue HJ, Fryer MJ, Eriksen EF, Heath H III (1988) Differential effects of parathyroid hormone and its analogues on cytosolic calcium ion and cAMP levels in cultured rat osteoblast-like cells. J Biol Chem 263:13522–13527

Doppelt SH, Neer RM, Nussbaum SR, Federico P, Potts JT Jr, Rosenblatt M (1986) Inhibition of the in vivo parathyroid hormone-mediated calcemic response in rats by a synthetic hormone antagonist. Proc Natl Acad Sci USA 83:7557–7560

Draper MW, Nissenson RA, Winer J, Ramachandran J, Arnaud CD (1982) Photo-affinity labeling of the canine renal receptor for parathyroid hormone. J Biol Chem 257:3714–3718

Duarte CG, Watson JF (1967) Calcium reabsorption in proximal tubule of the dog nephron. Am J Physiol 212:1355–1360

Duncan R, Misler S (1989) Voltage-activated and stretch-activated Ba^{2+} conducting channels in an osteoblast-like cell line (UMR 106). FEBS Lett 251:17–21

Dziak R, Stern PH (1975) Calcium transport in isolated bone cells. III. Effects of parathyroid hormone and cyclic 3′,5′-AMP. Endocrinology 104:493–499

Edelman A, Fritsch J, Balsan S (1986) Short-term effects of PTH on cultured rat osteoblasts: changes in membrane potential. Am J Physiol 251:C483–C490

Egan JJ, Gronowicz G, Rodan GA (1991) Parathyroid hormone promotes the disassembly of cytoskeletal actin and myosin in cultured osteoblastic cells: mediation by cyclic AMP. J Cell Biochem 45:101–111

Farndale RW, Sandy JR, Atkinson SJ, Pennington SR, Meghji S, Meikle MC (1988) Parathyroid hormone and prostaglandin E_2 stimulate both inositol phosphate and cyclic AMP accumulation in mouse osteoblast cultures. Biochem J 252:263–268

Farrow SM, Hawa NS, Karmali R, Hewison M, Walters JC, O'Riordan JLH (1990) Binding of the receptor for 1,25-dihydroxyvitamin D_3 to the 5′-flanking region of the bovine parathyroid hormone gene. J Endocrinol 126:355–359

Fasciotto BH, Gorr S-U, DeFranco DJ, Levine MA, Cohn DV (1989) Pancreastatin, a presumed product of chromogranin-A (secretory protein-I) processing, inhibits secretion from porcine parathyroid cells in culture. Endocrinology 125:1617–1622

Fasciotto BH, Gorr S-U, Bourdeau AM, Cohn DV (1990) Autocrine regulation of parathyroid secretion: inhibition of secretion by chromogranin-A (secretory protein-I) and potentiation of secretion by chromogranin-A and pancreastatin antibodies. Endocrinology 127:1329–1335

Feldman RS, Krieger NS, Tashjian AH Jr (1980) Effects of parathyroid hormone and calcitonin on osteoclast formation in vitro. Endocrinology 107:1137–1143

Felix R, Fleisch H, Elford PR (1989) Bone-resorbing cytokines enhance release of macrophage colony-stimulating activity by the osteoblastic cell MC3T3-E1. Calcif Tissue Int 44:356–360

Ferrier J, Ward A (1986) Electrophysiological differences between bone cell clones: membrane potential responses to parathyroid hormone and correlation with cAMP response. J Cell Physiol 126:237–242

Ferrier J, Ward A, Kanehisa J, Heersche JN (1986) Electrophysiological responses of osteoclasts to hormones. J Cell Physiol 128:23–26

Feyen JHM, van der Wilt G, Moonen P, DiBon A, Nijweide PJ (1984) Stimulation of arachidonic acid metabolism in primary cultures of osteoblast-like cells by hormones and drugs. Prostaglandins 28:769–781

Filburn CR, Harrison S (1990) Parathyroid hormone regulation of cytosolic Ca^{2+} in rat proximal tubules. Am J Physiol 258:F545–F552

Fiskin AM, Cohn DV, Peterson GS (1977) A model for the structure of bovine parathormone derived by dark field electron microscopy. J Biol Chem 252:8261–8268

Fitzpatrick LA (1990) Differences in the actions of calcium versus lanthanum to influence parathyroid hormone release. Endocrinology 127:711–715

Fitzpatrick LA, Brandi ML, Aurbach GD (1986a) Control of PTH secretion is mediated through calcium channels and is blocked by pertussis toxin treatment of parathyroid cells. Biochem Biophys Res Commun 138:960–965

Fitzpatrick LA, Brandi ML, Aurbach GD (1986b) Calcium-controlled secretion is effected through a guanine nucleotide regulatory protein in parathyroid cells. Endocrinology 119:2700–2703

Fitzpatrick LA, Chin H, Nirenberg M, Aurbach GD (1988) Antibodies to an alpha subunit of skeletal muscle calcium channels regulate parathyroid cell secretion. Proc Natl Acad Sci USA 85:2115–2119

Fitzpatrick LA, Yasumoto T, Aurbach GD (1989) Inhibition of parathyroid hormone release by maitotoxin, a calcium channel activator. Endocrinology 124:97–103

Fraser RA, Kronenberg HM, Pang PK, Harvey S (1990) Parathyroid hormone messenger ribonucleic acid in the rat hypothalamus. Endocrinology 127:2517–2522

Frelinger AL III, Zull JE (1986) The role of the methionine residues in the structure and function of parathyroid hormone. Arch Biochem Biophys 244:641–649

Fujimori A, Cheng S-L, Avioli LV, Civitelli R (1991) Dissociation of second messenger activation by parathyroid hormone fragments in osteosarcoma cells. Endocrinology 128:3032–3039

Fukayama S, Tashjian AH Jr (1989) Direct modulation by androgens of the response of human bone cells (SaOS-2) to human parathyroid hormone (PTH) and PTH-related protein. Endocrinology 125:1789–1794

Fukayama S, Tashjian AH Jr (1990) Stimulation by parathyroid hormone of $^{45}Ca^{2+}$ uptake in osteoblast-like cells: possible involvement of alkaline phosphatase. Endocrinology 126:1941–1949

Fukayama S, Kearns AK, Skurat RN, Tashjian AH Jr, Bringhurst FR (1991) Protein kinase-A-dependent inhibition of alkaline phosphatase release by SaOS-2 human osteoblastic cells: studies in new mutant cell lines that express a cyclic AMP-resistant phenotype. Cell Regul 2:889–896

Gardella TJ, Axelrod D, Rubin D, Keutmann HT, Potts JT Jr, Kronenberg HM, Nussbaum SR (1991) Mutational analysis of the receptor-activating region of human parathyroid hormone. J Biol Chem 266:13141–13146

Gilman AG (1987) G proteins: transducers of receptor-generated signals. Annu Rev Biochem 56:615–649

Gmaj P, Murer H (1986) Cellular mechanisms of inorganic phosphate transport in kidney. Physiol Rev 66:36–70

Goldman ME, Chorev M, Reagan JE, Nutt RF, Levy JJ, Rosenblatt M (1988) Evaluation of novel parathyroid hormone analogs using a bovine renal membrane receptor binding assay. Endocrinology 123:1468–1475

Goldring SR, Tyler GA, Krane SM, Potts JT Jr, Rosenblatt M (1984) Photoaffinity labeling of parathyroid hormone receptors: comparison of receptors across species and target tissues and after densensitization to hormone. Biochemistry 23:498–502

Goligorsky MS, Menton DN, Hruska KA (1986a) Parathyroid hormone-induced changes of the brush border membrane topography and cytosketelon in cultured renal proximal tubular cells. J Membr Biol 92:151–162

Goligorsky MS, Loftus DJ, Hruska KA (1986b) Cytoplasmic calcium in individual proximal tubular cells in culture. Am J Physiol 251:F938–F944

Good DW (1990) Inhibition of bicarbonate absorption by peptide hormones and cyclic adenosine monophosphate in rat medullary thick ascending loop. J Clin Invest 85:1006–1013

Grant FD, Conlin PR, Brown EM (1990) Rate and concentration dependence of parathyroid hormone dynamics during stepwise changes in serum ionized calcium in normal humans. J Clin Endocrinol Metab 71:370–378

Green J, Kleeman CR, Schotland S, Chaimovitz C (1991) Acute phosphate depletion dissociates hormonal stimulated second messengers in osteoblast-like cells. Endocrinology 129:848–858

Greger R, Lang F, Oberleithner H (1978) Distal site of calcium reabsorption in the rat nephron. Pflugers Arch 374:153–157

Guenther HL, Hofstetter W, Stutzer A, Muhlbauer R, Fleisch H (1989) Evidence for heterogeneity of the osteoblastic phenotype determined with clonal rat bone cells established from transforming growth factor-B-induced cell colonies grown anchorage independently in semisolid medium. Endocrinology 125:2092–2102

Guggino SE, Lajeunesse D, Wagner JA, Synder SH (1989) Bone remodeling signaled by a dihydrophyridine- and phenylalkylamine-sensitive calcium channel. Proc Natl Acad Sci USA 86:2957–2960

Guitierrez GE, Mundy GR, Derynck R, Hewlett EL, Katz MS (1987) Inhibition of parathyroid hormone-responsive adenylate cyclase in clonal osteoblast-like cells by transforming growth factor α and epidermal growth factor. J Biol Chem 262:15845–15850

Gunness-Hey M, Hock JM (1984) Increased trabecular bone mass in rats treated with human synthetic parathyroid hormone. Metab Bone Dis Relat Res 5:177–181

Günther N, Betzel C, Weber W (1990) The secreted form of the epidermal growth factor receptor: characterization and crystallization of the receptor-ligand complex. J Biol Chem 265:22082–22085

Habener JF, Potts JT Jr (1978) Parathyroid physiology and primary hyperparathyroidism. In: Avioli LV, Krane SM E (eds) Metabolic bone disease. vol 2. Academic, New York, pp 1–147

Habener JF, Kemper B, Potts JT Jr (1975) Calcium-dependent intracellular degradation of parathyroid hormone: a possible mechanism for the regulation of hormone stores. Endocrinology 97:431–441

Hahn TJ, Westbrook SL, Halstead LR (1984) Cortisol modulation of osteoblast metabolic activity in cultured neonatal rat bone. Endocrinology 114:1864–1870

Hakeda Y, Hiura K, Sato T, Okazaki R, Matsumoto T, Ogata E, Ishitani R, Humegawa M (1989) Existence of parathyroid hormone binding sites on murine hemopoietic blast cells. Biochem Biophys Res Commun 163:1481–1486

Hanai H, Ishida M, Liang CT, Sacktor B (1986) Parathyroid hormone increases sodium/calcium exchange activity in renal cells and the blunting of the response in ageing. J Biol Chem 261:5419–5425

Heinrich G, Kronenberg HM, Potts JT Jr, Habener JF (1984) Gene encoding parathyroid hormone: nucleotide sequence of the rat gene and deduced amino acid sequence of rat preproparathyroid hormone. J Biol Chem 259:3320–3329

Helmle-Kolb C, Montrose MH, Murer H (1990a) Parathyroid hormone regulation of Na^+/H^+ exchange in opossum kidney cells: polarity and mechanisms. Pflugers Arch 416:615–623

Helmle-Kolb C, Montrose MH, Stange G, Murer H (1990b) Regulation of Na^+/H^+ exchange in opossum kidney cells by parathyroid hormone, cyclic AMP and phorbol esters. Pflugers Arch 415:461–470

Hendy GN, Kronenberg HM, Potts JT Jr, Rich A (1981) Nucleotide sequence of cloned cDNAs encoding human preproparathyroid hormone. Proc Natl Acad Sci USA 78:7365–7369

Hensley CB, Bradley ME, Mircheff AK (1989) Parathyroid hormone-induced translocation of Na-H antiporters in rat proximal tubules. Am J Physiol 257:C637–C645

Herrman-Erlee MPM, Nijweide PJ, van der Meer JM, Ooms MAC (1983) Action of bPTH and bPTH fragments on embryonic bone in vitro: dissociation of cyclic AMP and bone resorbing response. Calcif Tissue Int 35:70–77

Hock JM, Gera I, Fonseca J, Raisz LG (1988) Human parathyroid hormone (1–34) increases bone mass in ovariectomized and orchidectomized rats. Endocrinology 122:2899–2904

Horiuchi N, Holick MF, Potts JT Jr, Rosenblatt M (1983) A parathyroid hormone inhibitor in vivo: design and biologic evaluation of a hormone analog. Science 220:1053–1055

Horiuchi N, Caulfield MP, Fisher JE, Goldman ME, McKee RL, Reagan JE, Levy JJ, Nutt RF, Rodan SB, Schofield TL, Clemens TL, Rosenblatt M (1987) Similarity of synthetic peptide from human tumour to parathyroid hormone in vivo and in vitro. Science 238:1566–1568

Howard GA, Bottemiller BL, Turner RT, Rader JT, Baylink DL (1981) Parathyroid hormone stimulates bone formation and resorption in organ culture: evidence for a coupling mechanism. Proc Natl Acad Sci USA 78:3208

Hruska KA, Goligorsky M, Scoble J, Tsutsumi M, Westbrook S, Moskowitz D (1986) Effects of parathyroid hormone on cytosolic calcium in renal proximal tubular primary cultures. Am J Physiol 251:F188–F198

Iida-Klein A, Hahn TJ (1991) Insulin acutely suppresses parathyroid hormone second messenger generation in UMR-106-01 osteoblast-like cells: differential effects on phospholipase C and adenylate cyclase activation. Endocrinology 129:1016–1024

Iida-Klein A, Varlotta V, Hahn TJ (1989) Protein kinase C activity in UMR 106-01 cells: effects of parathyroid hormone and insulin. J Bone Miner Res 4:767–774

Iino Y, Burg MB (1979) Effect of parathyroid hormone on bicarbonate absorption by proximal tubules in vitro. Am J Physiol 236:F387–F391

Ikeda K, Imai Y, Fukase M, Fujita T (1990) The effect of 1,25 dihydroxyvitamin D_3 on human osteoblast-like osteosarcoma cell: modification of response to PTH. Biochem Biophys Res Commun 168:889–897

Ikeda K, Sugimoto T, Fukase M, Fujita T (1991a) Protein kinase C is involved in PTH-induced homologous desensitization by directly affecting PTH receptors in the osteoblastic osteosarcoma cells. Endocrinology 128:2901–2906

Ikeda K, Sugimoto T, Fukase M, Fujita T (1991b) Role of increase in intracellular calcium in PTH-induced homologous desensitization in UMR 106-01 cells. Biochem Biophys Res Commun 176:1033–1036

Imai M (1981) Effects of parathyroid hormone and N6,O2-dibutyryl cyclic AMP on Ca^{2+} transport across the rabbit distal nephron segments perfused in vitro. Pflugers Arch 390:145–151

Ishikara T, Nakamura S, Kaziro Y, Takahashi T, Takahashi K, Nagata S (1991) Molecular cloning and expression of a cDNA encoding the secretin receptor. EMBO J 10:1635–1641

Juhlin CR, Holmdahl R, Johannsson H, Rastad J, Akerstrom G, Klareskog G (1987) Monoclonal antibodies with exclusive reactivity against parathyroid cells and tubule cells of the kidneys. Proc Natl Acad Sci USA 84:2990–2994

Juhlin C, Rastad J, Klareskog L, Grimelius L, Akerstrom G (1989) Parathyroid histology and cytology with monoclonal antibodies recognizing a calcium sensor of parathyroid cells. Am J Pathol 135:321–328

Juhlin C, Lundgren S, Johannsson H, Lorentzen J, Rask L, Larsson E, Rastad J, Akerstrom G, Klareskog L (1990) 500 kilodalton calcium sensor regulating cytoplasmic Ca^{2+} in cytotrophoblast cells of human placenta. J Biol Chem 265:8275–8280

Jüppner H, Abou-Samra AB, Uneno S, Gu WX, Potts JT Jr, Segre GV (1988) The parathyroid hormone-like peptide associated with humoral hypercalcemia of malignancy and parathyroid hormone bind to the same receptor on the plasma membrane of ROS 17/2.8 cells. J Biol Chem 263:8557–8560

Jüppner H, Abou-Samra AB, Uneno S, Keutmann HT, Potts JT Jr, Segre GV (1990) Preparation and characterization of N^{α}-(4-azido-2-nitrophenyl) [Ala^1, Tyr^{36}]-parathyroid hormone related peptide (1–36) amide: a high-affinity, partial agonist having high cross-linking efficiency with its receptor on ROS 17/2.8 cells. Biochemistry 29:6941–6946

Jüppner H, Abou-Samra A-B, Freeman M, Kong X-F, Schipani E, Richards J, Kolakowski LF Jr, Hock J, Potts JT Jr, Kronenberg HM, Segre GV (1991) A G protein-linked receptor for parathyroid hormone and parathyroid hormone-related peptide. Science 254:1024–1026

Kalu DN, Ennock JP, Doyle FH, Foster GV (1970) Parathyroid hormone and experimental osteosclerosis. Lancet 1:1363–1366

Karmali R, Farrow S, Hewison M, Barker S, O'Riordan JLH (1989) Effects of 1,25-dihydroxyvitamin D_3 and cortisol on bovine and human parathyroid cells. J Endocrinol 123:137–142

Karpf DB, Arnaud CD, King K, Bambino T, Winer J, Nyiredy K, Nissenson RA (1987) The canine renal parathyroid hormone receptor is a glycoprotein: characterization and partial purification. Biochemistry 26:7825–7833

Karpf DB, Arnaud CD, Bambino T, Duffy JD, King KL, Winer J, Nissenson RA (1988) Structural properties of the renal parathyroid hormone receptor: hydrodynamic analysis and protease sensitivity. Endocrinology 123:2611–2620

Karpf DB, Bambino T, Alford G, Nissenson RA (1991) Features of the renal parathyroid hormone-parathyroid hormone-related protein receptor derived from structural studies of receptor fragments. J Bone Miner Res 6:173–182

Karpinski E, Wu L, Civitelli R, Avioli LV, Hruska KA, Pang PKT (1989) A dihydropyridine-sensitive calcium channel in rodent osteoblastic cells. Calcif Tissue Int 45:54–57

Kaufmann M, Muff R, Fischer JA (1991) Effects of dexamethasone on parathyroid hormone (PTH) and PTH-related protein regulated phosphate uptake in opossum kidney cells. Endocrinology 128:1819–1824

Kemp BE, Mosely JM, Rodda CP, Ebeling PR, Wettenhall REH, Stapleton D, Diefenbach-Jagger H, Ure F, Michelangali VP, Simmons HA, Raisz LG, Martin TJ (1987) Parathyroid hormone-related protein of malignancy: active synthetic fragments. Science 238:1568–1570

Kemper B, Habener JF, Rich A, Potts JT Jr (1974) Parathyroid hormone secretion: discovery of a major calcium-dependent protein. Science 184:167–169

Kempson SA, Helmle C, Abraham MI, Murer H (1990) Parathyroid hormone action on phosphate transport is inhibited by high osmolality. Am J Physiol 258: F1336–F1344

Kennedy SM, Flanagan JL, Mills JW, Friedman PA (1989) Stimulation by parathyroid hormone of calcium absorption in confluent Madin-Darby canine kidney cells. J Cell Physiol 139:83–92

Keutmann HT, Griscom AW, Nussbaum SR, Reiner BF, Goud AN, Potts JT Jr, Rosenblatt M (1985) Rat parathyroid hormone-(1–34) fragment: renal adenylate cyclase activity and receptor binding properties in vitro. Endocrinology 117:1230–1234

Khosla S, Demay M, Pines M, Hurwitz S, Potts JT Jr, Kronenberg HM (1988) Nucleotide sequence of cloned cDNAs encoding chicken preproparathyroid hormone. J Bone Miner Res 3:689–698

Klaus W, Dieckmann T, Wray V, Schomburg D, Wingender E, Mayer H (1991) Investigation of the solution structure of the human parathyroid hormone fragment (1–34) by ^{1}H NMR spectroscopy, distance geometry, and molecular dynamics calculations. Biochemistry 30:6936–6942

Klein RF, Strewler GJ, Leung SC, Nissenson RA (1987) Parathyroid hormone-like adenylate cyclase-stimulating activity from a human carcinoma is associated with bone-resorbing activity. Endocrinology 120:504–511

Kobayashi N, Russell J, Lettieri D, Sherwood LM (1988) Regulation of protein kinase C by extracellular calcium in bovine parathyroid cells. Proc Natl Acad Sci USA 85:4857–4860

Koike T, Iwamoto M, Shimazu A, Nakashima K, Suzuki F, Kato Y (1990) Potent mitogenic effects of parathyroid hormone (PTH) on embryonic chick and rabbit chondrocytes: differential effects of age on growth, proteoglycan, and cyclic AMP responses of chondrocytes to PTH. J Clin Invest 85:626–631

Kronenberg HM, McDevitt BE, Majzoub JA, Nathans J, Sharp PA, Potts JT Jr, Rich A (1979) Cloning and nucleotide sequence of DNA coding for bovine preproparathyroid hormone. Proc Natl Acad Sci USA 76:4981–4985

Kubota M, Ng KW, Murase J, Noda T, Moseley JM, Martin TJ (1986) Efficacy and specificity of human parathyroid hormone analogues as antagonists in intact clonal osteogenic sarcoma cells. J Endocrinol 108:261–265

Lee SC, Russell AF (1989) Two-dimensional ^{1}H-NMR study of the 1–34 fragment of human parathyroid hormone. Biopolymers 28:1115–1127

Lerner UH, Ransjo M, Sahlberg K, Ljunggren O, Fredholm BB (1989) Forskolin sensitizes parathyroid hormone-induced cyclic AMP response, but not the bone resorptive effect, in mouse calvarial bones. Bone Miner 5:169–181

Lieberherr M (1987) The effects of vitamin D_3 metabolites on cytosolic free calcium in confluent mouse osteoblasts. J Biol Chem 262:13168–13173

Lim S-K, Gardella T, Thompson A, Rosenberg J, Keutmann H, Potts JT Jr, Kronenberg H, Nussbaum S (1991a) Full length chicken parathyroid hormone: biosynthesis in E. coli and analysis of biologic activity. J Biol Chem 266:3709–3714

Lim SK, Gardella TJ, Baba H, Nussbaum SR, Kronenberg HM (1992) The carboxy-terminus of PTH is essential for hormone processing and secretion. Endocrinol 131:2325–2330

Lin HY, Harris TL, Flannery MS, Aruffo A, Kaji EH, Gorn A, Kolakowski LF Jr, Lodish HF, Goldring SR (1991) Expression cloning of an adenylate cyclase-coupled calcitonin receptor. Science 254:1022–1024

Livesey SA, Kemp BE, Re CA, Partridge NC, Martin TJ (1982) Selective hormonal activation of cyclic AMP-dependent protein kinase isoenzymes in normal and malignant osteoblasts. J Biol Chem 257:14983–14987

Lomri A, Marie PJ (1990) Distinct effects of calcium- and cyclic AMP-enhancing factors on cytoskeletal synthesis and assembly in mouse osteoblastic cells. Biochim Biophys Acta 1052:179–186

Lowik CWGM, van Leeuwen JPTM, van der Meer JM, van Zeeland JK, Scheven BAA, Herrmann-Erlee MPM (1985) A two-receptor model for the action of parathyroid hormone on osteoblasts: a role for intracellular free calcium and cAMP. Cell Calcium 6:311–326

Lowik CWGM, van Zeeland JK, Herrmann-Erlee MPM (1986) An in situ assay system to measure ornithine decarboxylase activity in primary cultures of chicken osteoblasts: effects of bone-seeking hormones. Calcif Tissue Int 38:21–26

Lowik CWGM, van der Pluijm G, Bloys H, Hoekman K, Bijvoet OLM, Aarden LA, Papapoulos SE (1989) Parathyroid hormone (PTH) and PTH-like protein (PLP) stimulate interleukin-6 production by osteogenic cells: a possible role of interleukin-6 in osteoclastogenesis. Biochem Biophys Res Commun 162: 1546–1552

MacDonald BR, Gallagher JA, Ahnfelt-Ronne I, Beresford JN, Gowen M, Russell RGG (1984) Effects of bovine parathyroid hormone and 1,25-dihydroxyvitamin D on the production of prostaglandins by cells derived from human bone. FEBS Lett 169:49–52

MacDonald BR, Gallagher JA, Russell RGG (1986) Parathyroid hormone stimulates the proliferation of cells derived from human bone. Endocrinology 118: 2445–2449

Majeska RJ, Rodan GA (1982) Alkaline phosphatase inhibition by parathyroid hormone and isoproterenol in a clonal rat osteosarcoma cell line: possible modulation by cyclic AMP. Calcif Tissue Int 34:59–66

Majeska RJ, Rodan SB, Rodan GA (1980) Parathyroid hormone-responsive clonal cell lines from rat osteosarcoma. Endocrinology 107:1494–1503

Malstrom K, Stange G, Murer H (1988) Intracellular cascades in the parathyroid-hormone dependent regulation of Na^+/phosphate cotransport in OK cells. Biochem J 251:207–213

Marcus R, Orner FB (1980) Parathyroid hormone as a calcium ionophore in bone cells: tests of specificity. Calcif Tissue Int 32:1207–1211

Martin KJ, McConkey CL, Garcia JC, Montani D, Betts CR (1989) Protein kinase A and the effects of parathyroid hormone on phosphate uptake in opossum kidney cells. Endocrinology 125:295–301

Matsumoto T, Morita K, Kawanobe Y, Ogata E (1986) Effects of parathyroid hormone on phospholipid metabolism in osteoblast-like rat osteogenic sarcoma cells. Biochem J 236:605–608

Mayer GP, Keaton JA, Hurst JG, Habener JF (1979) Effects of plasma calcium concentration on the relative proportion of hormone and carboxyl fragments in parathyroid venous blood. Endocrinology 104:1778–1784

McCarthy TL, Centrella M, Canalis E (1989) Parathyroid hormone enhances the transcript and polypeptide levels of insulin-like growth factor I in osteoblast-enriched cultures from fetal rat bone. Endocrinology 124:1247–1253

McKee MD, Murray TM (1985) Binding of intact parathyroid hormone to chicken renal membranes: evidence for a second binding site with carboxyl-terminal specificity. Endocrinology 117:1930–1939

McKee RL, Goldman ME, Caulfield MP, DeHaven PA, Levy JJ, Nutt RF, Rosenblatt M (1988) The 7–34 fragment of human hypercalcemia factor is a partial agonist/antagonist for parathyroid hormone-stimulated cAMP production. Endocrinology 122:3008–3010

McKee RL, Caulfield MP, Rosenblatt M (1990) Treatment of bone-derived ROS 17/2.8 cells with dexamethasone and pertussis toxin enables detection of partial agonist activity for parathyroid hormone antagonists. Endocrinology 127:76–82

McKinney TD, Myers P (1980) PTH inhibition of bicarbonate transport by proximal convoluted tubules. Am J Physiol 1980:F127–F134

McSheehy PMGJ, Chambers TJ (1986) Osteoblastic cells mediate osteoclastic responsiveness to parathyroid hormone. Endocrinology 118:824–828

Mears DC (1971) Effects of parathyroid hormone and thyrocalcitonin on the membrane potential of osteoclasts. Endocrinology 88:1021–1028

Meltzer V, Weinreb S, Bellorin-Font E, Hruska KA (1982) Parathyroid hormone stimulation of renal phosphoinositol metabolism is a cyclic nucleotide-independent effect. Biochim Biophys Acta 712:258–267

Membreno L, Chen T-H, Woodley S, Gagucas R, Shoback D (1989) The effects of protein kinase-C agonists on parathyroid hormone release and intracellular free Ca^{2+} in bovine parathyroid cells. Endocrinology 124:789–797

Mitchell J, Goltzman D (1990) Mechanisms of homologous and heterologous regulation of parathyroid hormone receptors in the rat osteosarcoma cell line UMR 106. Endocrinology 126:2650–2660

Moe GR, Kaiser ET (1985) Design, synthesis and characterzation of a model peptide having potent calcitonin-like biological activity. Implications for calcitonin structure/activity. Biochemistry 24:1971–1976

Morel F, Imbert-Teboul M, Charbardes D (1981) Distribution of hormone-dependent adenylate cyclase in the nephron and its physiological significance. Annu Rev Physiol 43:569–581

Morrissey JJ (1988) Effect of phorbol myristate acetate on secretion of parathyroid hormone. Am J Physiol 254:63–70

Motokura T, Bloom T, Kim HG, Jüppner H, Ruderman JV, Kronenberg HM, Arnold A (1991) A BCL1-linked candidate oncogene which is rearranged in parathyroid tumors encodes a novel cyclin. Nature 350:512–515

Muff R, Nemeth EF, Haller-Brem S, Fischer JA (1988) Regulation of hormone secretion and cytosolic Ca^{2+} by extracellular Ca^{2+} in parathyroid cells and C-cells: role of voltage-sensitive Ca^{2+} channels. Arch Biochem Biophys 265:128–135

Muff R, Caulfield MP, Fischer JA (1990) Dissociation of cAMP accumulation and phosphate uptake in opossum kidney (OK) cells with parathyroid hormone (PTH) and parathyroid hormone related protein (PTHrp). Peptides 11:945–949

Murayama Y, Morel F, LeGrimellec C (1972) Phosphate, Ca^{++} and Mg^{++} transfers in proximal tubules and loops of Henle, as measured by single nephron microperfusion experiments in the rat. Pflugers Arch 333:1–6

Murray TM, Rao LG, Muzaffar SA, Ly H (1989) Human parathyroid hormone carboxyterminal peptide (53–84) stimulates alkaline phosphatase activity in dexamethasone-treated rat osteosarcoma cells in vitro. Endocrinology 124:1097–1099

Murray TM, Rao LG, Muzaffar SA (1991) Dexamethasone-treated ROS 17/2.8 rat osteosarcoma cells are responsive to human carboxylterminal parathyroid hormone peptide hPTH (53–84): stimulation of alkaline phosphatase. Calcif Tissue Int 49:120–123

Nagata N, Rasmussen H (1970) Parathyroid hormone, 3′,5′-AMP, Ca^{++} and gluconeogenesis. Proc Natl Acad Sci USA 64:368–374

Nakai M, Kinoshita Y, Fukase M, Fujita T (1989) Phorbol esters inhibit phosphate uptake in opossum kidney cells: a model of proximal renal tubular cells. Biochem Biophys Res Commun 145:303–308

Nakai M, Fukase M, Yamaguchi T, Tsukamoto T, Fujii N, Fujita T (1990) Human PTH-(3–34) inhibited the effects of human parathyroid hormone-related protein on phosphate uptake in a cultured renal cell line (OK cells). J Bone Miner Res 5:995–1002

Naveh-Many T, Silver J (1990) Regulation of parathyroid hormone gene expression by hypocalcemia, hypercalcemia, and vitamin D in the rat. J Clin Invest 86:1313–1319

Naveh-Many T, Friedlaender MM, Mayer H, Silver J (1989) Calcium regulates parathyroid hormone messenger ribonucleic acid (mRNA), but not calcitonin mRNA in vivo in the rat. Dominant role of 1,25-dihydroxyvitamin D. Endocrinology 125:275–280

Nemani R, Wongsurawat N, Armbrecht HJ (1991) Effect of parathyroid hormone on rat renal cAMP-dependent protein kinase and protein kinase C activity measured using synthetic peptide substrates. Arch Biochem Biophys 285:153–157

Nemeth EF, Scarpa A (1987) Rapid mobilization of cellular Ca^{2+} in bovine parathyroid cells evoked by extracellular divalent cations: evidence for a cell surface calcium receptor. J Biol Chem 262:5188–5196

Ng RCK, Rouse D, Suki WN (1984) Calcium transport in the rabbit superficial proximal convoluted tubule. J Clin Invest 74:832–842

Niall HD, Keutmann HT, Sauer RT, Hogan ML, Dawson BF, Aurbach GD, Potts JT Jr (1970) The amino-acid sequence of bovine parathyroid hormone I. Hoppe Seylers Z Physiol Chem 351:1586–1588

Nicholson GC, Livesey SA, Moseley JM, Martin TJ (1986) Actions of calcitonin, parathyroid hormone, and prostaglandin E2 on cyclic AMP formation in chicken and rat osteoclasts. J Cell Biochem 31:229–241

Nickols GA, Nickols MA, Helwig J-J (1990) Binding of parathyroid hormone and parathyroid hormone-related protein to vascular smooth muscle of rabbit renal microvessels. Endocrinology 126:721–727

Nissenson RA, Arnaud CD (1979) Properties of the parathyroid hormone receptor-adenylate cyclase system in chicken renal plasma membranes. J Biol Chem 254:1469–1475

Nissenson RA, Mann E, Winer J, Teitelbaum AP, Arnaud CD (1986) Solubilization of a guanine nucleotide-sensitive parathyroid hormone-receptor complex from canine renal cortex. Endocrinology 118:932–939

Nissenson RA, Karpf D, Bambino T, Winer J, Canga M, Nyiredy K, Arnaud CD (1987) Covalent labeling of a high-affinity, guanyl nucleotide sensitive parathyroid hormone receptor in canine renal cortex. Biochemistry 26:1874–1878

Nissenson RA, Diep D, Strewler GJ (1988) Synthetic peptides comprising the amino-terminal sequence of a parathyroid hormone-like protein from human malignancies: binding to parathyroid hormone receptors and activation of adenylate cyclase in bone cells and kidney. J Biol Chem 263:12866–12871

Noda M, Yoon K, Rodan GA (1988) Cyclic AMP-mediated stabilization of osteocalcin mRNA in rat osteoblast-like cells treated with parathyroid hormone. J Biol Chem 263:18574–18577

Nussbaum SR, Rosenblatt M, Potts JT Jr (1980) Parathyroid hormone/renal receptor interactions: demonstration of two receptor-binding domains. J Biol Chem 255:10183–10187

Nussbaum SR, Beaudette NV, Fasman GD, Potts JT Jr, Rosenblatt M (1985) Design of analogues of parathyroid hormone: a conformational approach. J Protein Chem 4:391–406

Nutt RF, Caulfield MP, Levy JJ, Gibbons SW, Rosenblatt M, McKee RL (1990) Removal of partial agonism from parathyroid hormone (PTH)-related protein-(7–34)NH$_2$ by substitution of PTH amino acids at positions 10 and 11. Endocrinology 127:491–493

Oetting M, LeBoff MS, Swiston L, Preston J, Brown E (1986) Guanine nucleotides are potent secretagogues in permeabilized parathyroid cells. FEBS Lett 208:99–104

Okazaki T, Igarashi T, Kronenberg HM (1988) 5′-Flanking region of the parathyroid hormone gene mediates negative regulation by 1,25(OH)$_2$ vitamin D$_3$. J Biol Chem 263:2203–2208

Okazaki T, Igarashi T, Ogata E (1990) Calcium-responsive DNA element in the human parathyroid hormone gene. J Bone Miner Res 5 Suppl 2:268

Okazaki T, Zajac JD, Igarashi T, Ogata E, Kronenberg HM (1991) Negative regulatory elements in the human parathyroid hormone gene. J Biol Chem 266:21903–21910

Orloff JJ, Wu TL, Heath HW, Brady TG, Brines ML, Stewart AF (1989a) Characterization of canine renal receptors for the parathyroid hormone-like protein associated with humoral hypercalcemia of malignancy. J Biol Chem 264:6097–6103

Orloff JJ, Wu TL, Stewart AF (1989b) Parathyroid hormone-like proteins: biochemical responses and receptor interactions. Endocr Rev 10:476–495

Paliwal I, Insogna K (1991) Partial purification and characterization of the 9000-dalton bone-resorbing activity from parathyroid hormone-related protein-treated SaOS2 cells (Abstr 245). J Bone Miner Res 6 Suppl 1:S144

Parsons JA, Robinson CJ (1971) Calcium shift into bone causing transient hypocalcaemia after injection of parathyroid hormone. Nature 230:581–582

Partridge NC, Kemp BE, Veroni MC, Martin TJ (1981) Activation of 3',5'-monophosphate-dependent protein kinase in normal and malignant bone cells by parathyroid hormone, prostaglandin E_2 and prostacyclin. Endocrinology 108:220–225

Partridge NC, Opie AL, Opie RT, Martin TJ (1985) Inhibitory effects of parathyroid hormone on growth of osteogenic sarcoma cells. Calcif Tissue Int 37:519–525

Peraldi M-N, Rondeau E, Jousset V, El M'Selmi A, LaCave R, DeLarue F, Garel J-M, Sraer J-D (1990) Dexamethasone increases preproparathyroid hormone messenger RNA in human hyperplastic parathyroid cells in vitro. Eur J Clin Invest 20:392–397

Pernalete N, Garcia JC, Betts CR, Martin KJ (1990) Inhibitors of protein kinase-C modulate desensitization of the parathyroid hormone receptor-adenylate cyclase system in opossum kidney cells. Endocrinology 126:407–413

Perry HM III, Skogen W, Chappel J, Kahn AJ, Wilner G, Teitelbaum SL (1989) Partial characterization of a parathyroid hormone-stimulated resorption factor(s) from osteoblast-like cells. Endocrinology 125:2075–2082

Pines M, Santora A, Spiegal A (1986) Effects of phorbol esters and pertussis toxin on agonist-stimulated cyclic AMP production in rat osteosarcoma cells. Biochem Pharmacol 35:3639–3641

Pizurki L, Rizzoli R, Bonjour J-P (1990) Inhibition by (D-Trp^{12},Tyr^{34})bPTH (7–34) amide of PTH and PTHrp effects on Pi transport in renal cells. Am J Physiol 259:F389–F392

Pocotte SL, Ehrenstein G, Fitzpatrick LA (1991) Regulation of parathyroid hormone secretion. Endocr Rev 12:291–301

Pollock AS, Warnock DG, Strewler GJ (1986) Parathyroid hormone inhibition of Na^+-H^+ antiporter activity in a cultured renal cell line. Am J Physiol 250:F217–F225

Potts JT Jr, Tregear GW, Keutmann HT, Niall HD, Sauer R, Deftos LJ, Dawson BF, Hogan ML, Aurbach GD (1971) Synthesis of a biologically active N-terminal tetratriacontapeptide of parathyroid hormone. Proc Natl Acad Sci USA 68:63–67

Potts JT Jr, Kronenberg HM, Rosenblatt M (1982) Parathyroid hormone: chemistry, biosynthesis and mode of action. Adv Protein Chem 35:323–396

Pun KK, Arnaud CD, Nissenson RA (1988) Parathyroid hormone receptors in human dermal fibroblasts: structural and functional characterization. J Bone Miner Res 3:453–460

Pun K-K, Ho PWM, Nissenson RA, Arnaud CD (1990) Desensitization of parathyroid hormone receptors on cultured bone cells. J Bone Miner Res 5:1193–1200

Quamme GA (1990) Effect of parathyroid hormone and dietary phosphate on phosphate transport in renal outer cortical and outer medullary brush-border membrane vesicles. Biochim Biophys Acta 1024:122–130

Quamme G, Biber J, Murer H (1989a) Sodium-phosphate co-transport in OK cells: inhibition by PTH and "adaptation" to low phosphate. Am J Physiol 257:F967–F973

Quamme G, Pfeilschifter J, Murer H (1989b) Parathyroid hormone inhibition of Na^+/phosphate cotransport in OK cells: generation of second messengers in the regulatory cascade. Biochem Biophys Res Commun 158:951–957

Quamme G, Pfeilschifter J, Murer H (1989c) Parathyroid hormone inhibition of Na^+/phosphate cotransport in OK cells: requirement of protein kinase C-dependent pathway. Biochim Biophys Acta 1013:159–165

Rabbani SA, Kaiser SM, Henderson JE, Bernier SM, Mouland AJ, Roy DR, Zahab DM, Sung WL, Goltzman D, Hendy GN (1990) Synthesis and characterization of extended and deleted recombinant analogues of parathyroid hormone-(1–84): correlation of peptide structure with function. Biochemistry 29:10080–10089

Ramachandran C, Brunette MG (1989) The renal Na^+/Ca^{++} exchange system is located exclusively in the distal tubule. Biochem J 257:259–264

Rao LG, Murray TM (1985) Binding of intact parathyroid hormone to rat osteosarcoma cells: major contribution of binding sites for the carboxyl-terminal region of the hormone. Endocrinology 117:1632–1638

Rao LG, Murray TM (1989) Calcium and protein kinase C enhance parathyroid hormone- and forskolin-stimulated adenylate cyclase in ROS 17/2.8 cells. Calcif Tissue Int 45:354–359

Rappaport MS, Stern PH (1986) Parathyroid hormone and calcitonin modify inositol phospholipid metabolism in fetal rat limb bones. J Bone Miner Res 1:173–179

Rasmussen H, Pechet M, Fast D (1968) Effect of dibutyryl cyclic adenosine 3',5'-monophosphate, theophylline, and other nucleotides upon calcium and phosphate metabolism. J Clin Invest 47:1843–1850

Reid IR, Civitelli R, Halstead LR, Avioli LV, Hruska KA (1987) Parathyroid hormone acutely elevates intracellular calcium in osteoblast-like cells. Am J Physiol 253:E45–E51

Reid IR, Civitelli R, Avioli LV, Hruska KA (1988) Parathyroid hormone depresses cytosolic pH and DNA synthesis in osteoblast-like cells. Am J Physiol Physiol 255:E9–E15

Reid IR, Lowe C, Cornish J, Gray DH, Skinner SJM (1990) Adenylate cyclase blockers dissociate PTH-stimulated bone resorption from cAMP production. Am J Physiol 258:E708–E714

Reinhardt TA, Horst RL (1990) Parathyroid hormone down-regulates 1,25-dihydroxy-vitamin D receptors (VDR) and VDR messenger ribonucleic acid in vitro and blocks homologous up-regulation of VDR in vivo. Endocrinology 127:942–948

Reis A, Hecht W, Groger R, Bolim I, Cooper DN, Lindenmaier W, Mayer H, Schmidtke J (1990) Cloning and sequence analysis of the human parathyroid hormone gene region. Hum Genet 84:119–124

Reshkin SJ, Forgo J, Murer H (1990) Functional asymmetry in phosphate transport and its regulation in opossum kidney cells: parathyroid hormone inhibition. Pflugers Arch 416:624–631

Rizzoli R, Fleisch H (1986) Heterologous desensitization by 1,25-dihydroxyvitamin D-3 of cyclic AMP response to parathyroid hormone in osteoblast-like cells and the role of the stimulatory guanine nucleotide regulating protein. Biochim Biophys Acta 887:214–221

Rodan GA, Martin TJ (1981) Role of osteoblasts in hormonal control of bone resorption – a hypothesis. Calcif Tissue Int 33:349–351

Rodan GA, Heath JK, Yoon K, Noda M, Rodan SB (1988) Diversity of the osteoblastic phenotype. Ciba Found Symp 136:78

Rodan SB, Rodan GA (1974) The effects of parathyroid hormone and thyrocalcitonin on the accumulation of cyclic adenosine 3',5'-monophosphate in freshly isolated bone cells. J Biol Chem 249:3068–3074

Rodan SB, Fischer MK, Egan JJ, Epstein PM, Rodan GA (1984) The effect of dexamethasone on parathyroid hormone stimulation of adenylate cyclase in ROS 17/2.8 cells. Endocrinology 115:951–957

Rosenberg J, Pines M, Hurwitz S (1987) Response of adrenal cells to parathyroid hormone stimulation. J Endocrinol 112:431–437

Rosenberg J, Pines M, Hurwitz S (1988) Stimulation of chick adrenal steroidogenesis by avian parathyroid hormone. J Endocrinol 116:91–95

Rosenberg CL, Kim HG, Shows TB, Kronenberg HM, Arnold A (1991) Rearrangement and overexpresion of D115287E, a candidate oncogene on chromosome 11q13 in benign parathyroid tumors. Oncogene 6:449–454

Rosenblatt M (1982) Structure-activity relations in the calcium-regulating peptide hormones. In: Parsons JA (ed) Endocrinology of calcium metabolism. Raven, New York, pp 103–142 (Comprehensive endocrinology)

Rosenblatt M (1984) Parathyroid hormone: intracellular transport, secretion, and receptor interaction. Pept Protein Rev 2:209–296

Rosenblatt M, Goltzman D, Keutmann HT, Tregear GW, Potts JT Jr (1976) Chemical and biological properties of synthetic, sulfur-free analogues of parathyroid hormone. J Biol Chem 251:159–164

Rosenblatt M, Segre GV, Tyler GA, Shepard GL, Nussbaum SR, Potts JT Jr (1980) Identification of a receptor-binding region in parathyroid hormone. Endocrinology 107:545–550

Rosol TJ, Capen CC (1988) Inhibition of in vitro bone resorption by a parathyroid hormone receptor antagonist in the canine adenocarcinoma model of humoral hypercalcemia of malignancy. Endocrinology 122:2098–2102

Rouleau MF, Mitchell L, Goltzman D (1988) In vivo distribution of parathyroid hormone receptors in bone: evidence that a predominant osseous target cell is not the mature osteoblast. Endocrinology 123:187–191

Russell J, Sherwood LM (1989) Nucleotide sequence of the DNA complementary to avian (chicken) preproparathyroid hormone mRNA and the deduced sequence of the hormone precursor. Mol Endocrinol 3:325–331

Russell J, Lettieri D, Sherwood LM (1983) Direct regulation by calcium of cytoplasmic messenger ribonucleic acid coding for pre-proparathyroid hormone in isolated bovine parathyroid cells. J Clin Invest 72:1851–1855

Russell J, Lettieri D, Sherwood LM (1986a) Suppression by $1,25(OH)_2D_3$ of transcription of the pre-proparathyroid hormone gene. Endocrinology 119:2864–2866

Russell J, Lettieri D, Sherwood LM (1986b) Direct suppression by calcium of transcription of the parathyroid hormone gene. 68th Annual Meeting of the Endocrine Society, Anaheim

Sakaguchi K, Fukase M, Kobayashi I, Kimura T, Sakakibara S, Katsuragi S, Morita K, Noda T, Fujita T (1987) Synthetic parathyroid hormone fragments shortened at the amino terminus stimulate glucose-6-phosphate dehydrogenase activity in the distal renal tubule. J Bone Miner Res 2:83–90

Schlüter K-D, Hellstern H, Wingender E, Mayer H (1989) The central part of parathyroid hormone stimulates thyrmidine incorporation of chondrocytes. J Biol Chem 264:11087–11092

Schmelzer H-J, Gross G, Widera G, Mayer H (1987) Nucleotide sequence of a full-length cDNA clone encoding preproparathyroid hormone from pig and rat. Nucleic Acids Res 15:6740

Segal JH, Pollock AS (1990) Transfection-mediated expression of a dominant cAMP-resistant phenotype in the opossum-kidney (OK) cell line prevents parathyroid hormone-induced inhibition of Na-phosphate cotransport. J Clin Invest 86:1442–1450

Segre GV, Rosenblatt M, Reiner BL, Mahaffey JE, Potts JT Jr (1979) Characterization of parathyroid hormone receptors in canine renal cortical plasma membranes using a radioiodinated sulfur-free hormone analogue: correlation of binding with adenylate cyclase activity. J Biol Chem 254:6980–6986

Segre GV, Rosenblatt M, Tully GL III, Laugharn J, Reit B, Potts JT Jr (1985) Evaluation of an in vitro parathyroid hormone antagonist in vivo in dogs. Endocrinology 116:1024–1029

Selz T, Caverzasio J, Bonjour JP (1989) Regulation of Na-dependent Pi transport by parathyroid hormone in osteoblast-like cells. Am J Physiol 256:E93–E100

Shareghi GR, Stoner LC (1978) Calcium transport across segments of the rabbit distal nephron in vitro. Am J Physiol 235:F367–F375

Shigeno C, Hiraki Y, Westerberg DP, Potts JT Jr, Segre GV (1988a) Photoaffinity labelling of parathyroid hormone receptors in clonal rat osteosarcoma cells. J Biol Chem 263:3864–3871

Shigeno C, Hiraki Y, Westerberg DP, Potts JT Jr, Segre GV (1988b) Parathyroid hormone receptors are plasma membrane glycoproteins with asparagine-linked oligosaccharides. J Biol Chem 263:3872–3878

Shigeno C, Yamamoto I, Kitamura N, Noda T, Lee K, Sone T, Shiomi K, Ohtaka A, Fujii N, Yajima H, Konish J (1988c) Interaction of human parathyroid hormone-related peptide with parathyroid hormone receptors in clonal rat osteosarcoma cells. J Biol Chem 34:18369–18377

Shigeno C, Hiraki Y, Keutmann HT, Stern AM, Potts JT Jr, Segre GV (1989) Preparation of a photoreactive analog of parathyroid hormone [Nle[8],Lys(N-ε-4-azido-2-nitrophenyl)[13],Nle[18],Tyr[34]]bovine parathyroid hormone (1–34)NH$_2$, a selective, high-affinity ligand for characterization of parathyroid hormone receptors. J Anal Biochem 179:268–273

Shimizu T, Yoshitomi K, Nakamura M, Imai M (1990) Effect of parathyroid hormone on the connecting tubule from the rabbit kidney: biphasic response of transmural voltage. Pflugers Arch 416:254–261

Shlatz IJ, Schwartz IL, Kinne-Safran E, Kinne R (1975) Distribution of PTH-stimulated adenylate cyclase in plasma membranes of cells of the kidney cortex. J Membr Biol 24:131–144

Shoback DM, Membreno LA, McGhee JG (1988) High calcium and other divalent cations increase inositol trisphosphate in bovine parathyroid cells. Endocrinology 123:382–389

Silbermann M, Shurtz-Swirski R, Lewinson D, Shenzer P, Mayer H (1991) In vitro response of neonatal condylar cartilage to simultaneous exposure to the parathyroid hormone fragments 1–34, 28–48, and 53–84 hPTH. Calcif Tissue Int 48:260–266

Silve CM, Hradek GT, Jones AL, Arnaud CD (1982) Parathyroid hormone receptor in intact embryonic chicken bone: characterization and cellular localization. J Cell Biol 94:379–386

Silver J, Russell J, Sherwood LM (1985) Regulation by vitamin D metabolites of messenger ribonucleic acid for preproparathyroid hormone in isolated bovine parathyroid cells. Proc Natl Acad Sci USA 82:4270–4273

Silver J, Naveh-Many T, Mayer H, Schmelzer HJ, Popovtzer MM (1986) Regulation by vitamin D metabolites of parathyroid hormone gene transcription in vivo in the rat. J Clin Invest 78:1296–1301

Silverberg SJ, Shane E, Cruz Ldl, Dempster DW, Feldman F, Seldin D, Jacobs TP, Siris ES, Cafferty M, Parisien MV, Lindsay R, Clemens TL, Bilezikian JP (1989) Skeletal disease in primary hyperparathyroidism. J Bone Miner Res 4:283–291

Slovik DM, Rosenthal DI, Doppelt SH, Potts JT Jr, Dalt MA, Campbell JA, Neer RM (1986) Restoration of spinal bone in osteoporotic men by treatment with human parathyroid hormone (1–34) and 1,25-dihydroxyvitamin D. J Bone Miner Res 1:377–381

Somjen D, Zor U, Kaye AM, Harell A, Binderman I (1987) Parathyroid hormone induction of creatine kinase activity and DNA synthesis is mimicked by phospholipase C, diacylglycerol and phorbol ester. Biochim Biophys Acta 931:215–23

Somjen D, Binderman I, Schluter K, Wingender E, Mayer H, Kaye AM (1990) Stimulation by defined parathyroid hormone fragments of cell proliferation in skeletal-derived cell cultures. Biochem J 272:781–785

Sugimoto T, Fukase M, Tsutsumi M, Imai Y, Hishikawa R, Yoshimoto Y, Fujita T (1985) Additive effects of parathyroid hormone and calcitonin on adenosine 3′,5′-monophosphate release in newly established perfusion system of rat femur. Endocrinology 117:1901–1905

Suki WN (1979) Calcium transport in the nephron. Am J Physiol 237:F1–F6

Suzuki Y, Hruska KA, Reid I, Alvarez UM, Avioli LV (1989) Characterization of phospholipase C activity of the plasma membrane and cytosol of an osteoblast-like cell line. Am J Med Sci 297:135–144

Talmage RV, Doppelt SH, Fondren FB (1976) An interpretation of acute changes in plasma [45]Ca following parathyroid hormone administration to thyroparathyroidectomized rats. Calcif Tissue Res 22:117–28

Tam CS, Heersche JNM, Murray TM, Parsons JA (1982) Parathyroid hormone stimulates the bone apposition rate independently of its resorptive action: differential effects of intermittent and continuous administration. Endocrinology 110:506–512

Tamura T, Sakamoto H, Filburn CR (1989) Parathyroid hormone 1–34, but not 3–34 or 7–34, transiently translocates protein kinase C in cultured renal (OK) cells. Biochem Biophys Res Commun 159:1352–1358

Tanguay KE, Mortimer ST, Wood PH, Hanley DA (1991) The effects of phorbol myristate acetate on the intracellular degradation of bovine parathyroid hormone. Endocrinology 128:1863–1868

Teti A, Rizzoli R, Zallone AZ (1991) Parathyroid hormone binding to cultured avian osteoclasts. Biochem Biophys Res Commun 174:1217–1222

Titus L, Jackson E, Nanes MS, Rubin JE, Catherwood BD (1991) 1,25-Dihydroxy-vitamin D reduces parathyroid hormone receptor number in ROS 17/2.8 cells and prevents the glucocorticoid-induced increase in these receptors: relationship to adenylate cyclase activation. J Bone Miner Res 6:631–637

Torikai S, Wang M-S, Klein KL, Kurokawa K (1981) Adenylate cyclase and cell cyclic AMP of rat cortical thick ascending limb of Henle. Kidney Int 20:649–654

Torring O, Firek AF, Heath H III, Conover CA (1991) Parathyroid hormone and parathyroid hormone-related peptide stimulate insulin-like growth factor binding protein secretion by rat osteoblast-like cells through an adenosine $3',5'$-monophosphate-dependent mechanism. Endocrinology 128:1006–1014

Tregear GW, van Rietschoten J, Greene E, Keutmann HT, Niall HD, Reit B, Parsons JA, Potts JT Jr (1973) Bovine parathyroid hormone: minimum chain length of synthetic peptide required for biological activity. Endocrinology 93:1349–1353

Van der Plas A, Feyen JHM, Nijweide PJ (1985) Direct effect of parathyroid hormone on the proliferation of osteoblast-like cells; a possible involvement of cyclic AMP. Biochem Biophys Res Commun 129:918–925

Vasicek T, McDevitt BE, Freeman MW, Potts JT Jr, Rich A, Kronenberg HM (1983) Nucleotide sequence of genomic DNA encoding human parathyroid hormone. Proc Natl Acad Sci USA 80:2127–2131

Watford M, Mapes RE (1990) Hormonal and acid-base regulation of phospho-enolpyruvate carboxykinase mRNA levels in rat kidney. Arch Biochem Biophys 282:399–403

Weaver CA, Gordon DF, Kissil MS, Mead DA, Kemper B (1984) Isolation and complete nucleotide sequence of the gene for bovine parathyroid hormone. Gene 28:319–329

Weinman EJ, Shenolikar S, Kahn AM (1987) cAMP-associated inhibition of Na^+-H^+ exchanger in rabbit kidney brush-border membranes. Am J Physiol 252: F19–F25

Wells H, Lloyd W (1969) Hypercalcemic and hypophosphatemic effects of dibutyryl cyclic AMP in rats after parathyroidectomy. Endocrinology 84:861–867

Wen SF (1974) Micropuncture studies of phosphate transport in the proximal tubule of the dog: the relationship to sodium reabsorption. J Clin Invest 53:143–153

Wiren KM, Potts JT Jr, Kronenberg HM (1988) Importance of the propeptide sequence of human preproparthyroid hormone for signal sequence function. J Biol Chem 263:19771–19777

Wittner M, DiStefano A (1990) Effects of antidiuretic hormone, parathyroid hormone and glucagon on transepithelial voltage and resistance of the cortical and medullary thick ascending limb of Henle's loop of the mouse nephron. Pflugers Arch 415:707–712

Wong GL (1984) Paracrine interactions in bone-secreted products of osteoblasts permit osteoclasts to respond to parathyroid hormone. J Biol Chem 259: 4019–4022

Wong GL, Kent GN, Ku KY, Cohn DV (1979) The interaction of parathormone and calcium on the hormone-regulated synthesis of hyaluronic acid and citrate decarboxylation in isolated bone cells. Endocrinology 103:2274–2282

Yamaguchi DT, Hahn TJ, Iida-Klein A, Kleeman CR, Muallem S (1987) Parathyroid hormone-activated calcium channels in an osteoblast-like clonal osteosarcoma cell line. J Biol Chem 262:7711–7718

Yamamoto I, Shigeno C, Potts JT Jr, Segre GV (1988a) Characterization and agonist-induced down-regulation of parathyroid hormone receptors in clonal rat osteosarcoma cells. Endocrinology 122:1208–1217

Yamamoto I, Potts JT Jr, Segre GV (1988b) Glucocorticoids increase parathyroid hormone receptors in osteoblastic osteosarcoma cells (ROS 17/2). J Bone Miner Res 3:707–712

Yamamoto M, Igarashi T, Muramatsu M, Fukagawa M, Motokura T, Ogata E (1989) Hypocalcemia increases and hypercalcemia decreases the steady state level of parathyroid hormone messenger ribonucleic acid in the rat. J Clin Invest 83:1053–1058

Yamashita T, Asano K, Takahashi N, Akatsu T, Udagawa N, Sasaki T, Martin TJ, Suda T (1990) Cloning of an osteoblastic cell line involved in the formation of osteoclast-like cells. J Cell Physiol 145:587–595

Yoon K, Buenaga R, Rodan GA (1987) Tissue specificity and developmental expression of rat osteopontin. Biochem Biophys Res Commun 148:1129–1136

Zajac JD, Livesey SA, Michelangeli VP, Rodan SB, Rodan GA, Martin TJ (1986) Glucocorticoid treatment facilitates cyclic adenosine 3',5'-monophosphate-dependent protein kinase response in parathyroid hormone-responsive osteogenic sarcoma cells. Endocrinology 118:2059

Zaman G, Saphier PW, Loveridge N, Kimura T, Sakakibara S, Bernier SM, Hendy GN (1991) Biological properties of synthetic human parathyroid hormone: effect of deamidation at position 76 on agonist and antagonist activity. Endocrinology 128:2583 2590

Zull JE, Smith LM, Chuang J, Jentoft J (1987) Deletion of lysine 13 alters the structure and function of parathyroid hormone. Mol Cell Endocrinol 51:267–271

Zull JE, Smith SK, Wiltshire R (1990) Effect of methionine oxidation and deletion of amino-terminal residues on the conformation of parathyroid hormone: circular dichroism studies. J Biol Chem 265:5671–5676

CHAPTER 16
Calcitonin Gene Products: Molecular Biology, Chemistry, and Actions*

W. Born and J.A. Fischer

A. Introduction

Calcitonin was discovered by Copp et al. (1961) as a hypocalcemic hormone and the neuropeptide calcitonin gene-related peptide (CGRP) recognized through analysis of the calcitonin gene structure (Amara et al. 1982).

Calcitonin/CGRP genes I (or α) (*CALC I*) and second closely related genes (*CALC II* (or β)) have been identified in man and rat (Steenbergh et al. 1986; Amara et al. 1985). Two distinct messenger RNA (mRNA) species are individually formed through splicing of initial *CALC I* gene transcripts along two alternative RNA-processing pathways (Rosenfeld et al. 1983). Thyroid C cells in mammals and ultimobranchial bodies in fish and chicken predominantly produce mRNA encoding a calcitonin precursor protein that consists of calcitonin and amino (N)- and carboxyl(C)-terminal flanking peptides. Messenger RNA encoding CGRP and an N-terminal flanking peptide is the major mature transcription product in neuronal tissues. A region within the human *CALC II* gene with homology to the calcitonin-encoding sequence in the *CALC I* gene contains translation stop codons in front of an open reading frame for a second calcitonin-like peptide, and is therefore not expressed. Besides the *CALC I* and *II* genes, molecular cloning identified a homologous nonexpressed *CALC III* pseudogene (Höppener et al. 1988), and distantly related islet amyloid polypeptide (*IAPP*) genes in man (Mosselman et al. 1988) and rat (Van Mansfeld et al. 1990). IAPP has about 50% structural homology with CGRP (Westermark et al. 1986) and is principally synthesized in the pancreas.

All known calcitonins are single-chain polypeptides with 32 and all CGRP with 37 amino acid residues. They have N-terminal ring structures in common, linked by disulfide bridges of cysteines, and amidated C-termini. Limited structural homology between calcitonin and CGRP peptides suggests that they may have arisen through duplication of ancestral calcitonin/CGRP genes. As a result, calcitonin and CGRP share some biological targets. Calcitonin inhibits bone resorption in low and CGRP in high amounts. The effects are probably mediated by the same calcitonin receptors on osteoclasts

* Supported in part by the Swiss National Science Foundation (Grant No. 32-28297.90) and the Kanton of Zurich.

(Roos et al. 1986; Goltzman and Mitchell 1985). Both peptides cause vasodilatation of skin blood vessels presumably through interaction with CGRP receptors (Brain et al. 1985; Gennari and Fischer 1985).

In the present review the biosynthesis, structure, and receptors and biological targets of calcitonin/CGRP gene products are compared and functional and clinical implications discussed.

B. Calcitonin/CGRP Genes

Analyses of cloned rat and human calcitonin gene structures have identified coding sequences within a single transcription unit for individual calcitonin and CGRP precursor proteins which include N- and C-terminal flanking peptides of up to now unknown physiological function. Related genes encoding the structurally similar IAPP have also been recognized. DNA sequence analysis of complementary DNA (cDNA) encoding calcitonin peptides of mammals, birds, and fish has elucidated the evolution of the calcitonin genes. Expression of *CALC I* genes is independently regulated at the level of transcription and in a tissue-specific manner at the level of primary transcript processing.

I. Structure of DNA

Structurally similar single-copy genes for calcitonin, referred to as *CALC I* genes (Fig. 1), have been identified in man (Steenbergh et al. 1984, 1985a; Jonas et al. 1985), rat (Amara et al. 1984), and chicken (Minvielle et al. 1987). Detailed restriction endonuclease mapping and DNA sequence analysis revealed complex transcription units of 6.2 kilobases in man and 8.2 kilobases in the rat, both consisting of six exons. Alignment and sequence comparison with cloned mRNA from rat and human medullary thyroid carcinoma (MTC) cell lines encoding calcitonin and CGRP precursor proteins (Amara et al. 1982; Nelkin et al. 1984) revealed that calcitonin mRNA contained the exons 1, 2, and 3 combined with exon 4, and that CGRP mRNA corresponded precisely in sequence to the exons 1, 2, and 3 linked to the exons 5 and 6 (Fig. 1). Equivalent transcription rates through all six exons of the rat gene observed in MTC tissue (Amara et al. 1984) and the identification by Northern blot analysis of poly(A)-tailed primary *CALC I* gene transcripts containing all six exons in human MTC tissue (Bovenberg et al. 1986) indicated that calcitonin and CGRP mRNA are formed through selection of alternative splice sites defining the 3'-ends of intron 3 and intron 4, respectively. Sequences involved in the alternative splicing events are conserved between the human and rat genes (Steenbergh et al. 1984). Detailed sequence analysis of the six exons indicated that they encode functionally distinct regions (Fig. 1). Exons 1, 2, and 3 code for 5'-non-translated sequences (exon 1), the secretion signal peptides (exon 2), and

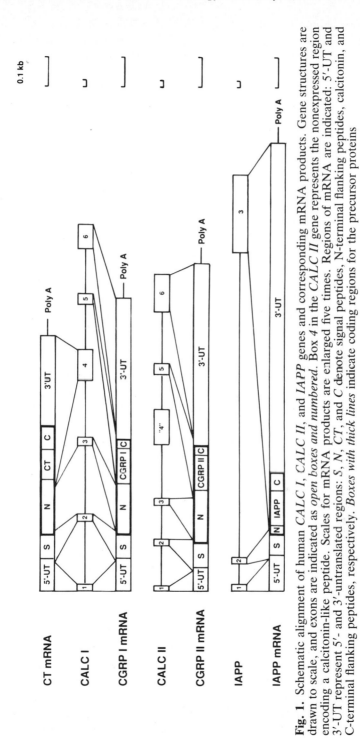

Fig. 1. Schematic alignment of human *CALC I*, *CALC II*, and *IAPP* genes and corresponding mRNA products. Gene structures are drawn to scale, and exons are indicated as *open boxes and numbered*. Box 4 in the *CALC II* gene represents the nonexpressed region encoding a calcitonin-like peptide. Scales for mRNA products are enlarged five times. Regions of mRNA are indicated: 5'-UT and 3'-UT represent 5'- and 3'-untranslated regions: *S*, *N*, *CT*, and *C* denote signal peptides, N-terminal flanking peptides, calcitonin, and C-terminal flanking peptides, respectively. *Boxes with thick lines* indicate coding regions for the precursor proteins

common N-terminal regions of the calcitonin and CGRP precursor proteins (exon 3). The fourth exon contains the entire coding sequence for calcitonin and its C-terminal flanking peptide together with 3'-noncoding sequences. Exon 5 encodes CGRP and exon 6 contains CGRP mRNA 3'-nontranslated sequences.

Complementary DNA to mRNA encoding precursor proteins of CGRP II in man and rat have been cloned from MTC tissue. They were detected with hybridization probes derived from exon 5 sequences of the *CALC I* genes that recognized corresponding regions of over 90% sequence homology (Amara et al. 1985; Steenbergh et al. 1985b). Southern blot analysis of total human and rat DNA confirmed the existence of *CALC II* genes in both species. The cloned human *CALC II* gene exhibits a striking resemblance in overall structure to the *CALC I* gene (Fig. 1) (Steenbergh et al. 1986). Detailed sequence analysis revealed regions with 90% homology to exons 2, 3, and 5 of the *CALC I* gene. The noncoding exon 6 of the human *CALC I* gene exhibits only 65% sequence homology to the corresponding sequence of the *CALC II* gene. Located between exons 3 and 5 is a region with about 50% homology to exon 4 of the *CALC I* gene (Fig. 1). The presence of stop codons in all three reading frames within the exon 4-like sequence of the *CALC II* gene, however, suggests that the *CALC II* gene is a pseudogene for a second human calcitonin. Besides, Northern blot analysis of RNA from several tissues and tumor cell lines failed to detect mature mRNA species containing "exon 4" sequences of *CALC II* (Steenberg et al. 1986; Alevizaki et al. 1986).

Sequence comparison of the calcitonin and CGRP exons of the *CALC I* gene suggests that they both arose from a common primordial sequence and that rearrangement events were responsible for the generation of the transcription units (Jonas et al. 1985). The human *CALC I* and *CALC II* genes, and a third human genomic locus, *CALC III*, containing nucleotide sequences highly homologous to both exon 2 and exon 3 of the *CALC I* and *CALC II* gene, but no calcitonin- or CGRP-encoding regions, are located on chromosome 11 (Höppener et al. 1984, 1985, 1988). This and the identification of a *CALC II* gene in the rat suggests that the so far identified members of the *CALC* gene family arose through local duplication of a common ancestral gene prior to the rodent-primate split.

Based on structural similarity to human and rat *CALC* genes, the recently cloned islet amyloid polypeptide (*IAPP*) genes in man (Mosselman et al. 1988; Nishi et al. 1989) and rat (Van Mansfeld et al. 1990) have also been considered to be members of this neuroendocrine peptide gene family. The human *IAPP* gene is a single-copy gene, similar in size and exon-intron organization to the rat gene, and localized on the short arm of chromosome 12 rather than on chromosome 11 with the *CALC I*, *II*, and *III* genes. As a result, the exon 2- and 3-like sequences of *CALC III* are not directly related to the *IAPP* gene. The structural organization of the *IAPP* genes with only three exons is simpler than that of the *CALC* genes (Fig. 1). Exons 2 and 3, including positions and type of splice junctions, are closely related to exons 2 and 5 of the *CALC I* and *II* genes and encode an *IAPP* precursor protein. Like *CGRP, IAPP* consists of 37 amino acids with an N-terminal ring structure and an amidated C-terminus. The sequence homology between human *IAPP* and *CGRP II* is 46%. Predicted N- and C-terminal flanking peptides are different from the corresponding peptides of the calcitonin and CGRP precursor proteins. Analysis of the nucleotide and predicted amino acid sequence of the relatively long intron 2 (4.9 kilobases) of the human *IAPP* gene revealed no homology to either exon 3 or exon 4 of the *CALC I* and *II* genes. This indicates that the human *IAPP* gene is only distantly related to the *CALC I* and *II* genes, and encodes a single-protein product.

Molecular cloning of calcitonin-encoding cDNA of rabbit (MARTIAL et al. 1990) and salmon (PÖSCHL et al. 1987) revealed structures similar to those of man, rat, and chicken. The overall homology of mRNA sequences encoding calcitonin precursor proteins is rather low whereas the regions encoding calcitonin alone are more closely related. Salmon calcitonin genes have so far not been cloned. It would be interesting to know whether CGRP-like peptides are present in the calcitonin genes. Besides, three different, but closely homologous salmon calcitonin isohormones have been identified (DEFTOS and ROOS 1989).

Sequences of DNA flanking the *CALC I* transcription unit have been analyzed in the human genome with respect to methylation patterns of upstream regulatory regions and to restriction fragment length polymorphism (RFLP). Restriction sites involved in RFLP are a *Taq*I site 2.4 kilobases 3' to exon 6 giving rise to alleles of 7.0 and 9.0 kilobases (HÖPPENER et al. 1984) and a *Pvu*II site 13 kilobases downstream of the 3'-end of the gene generating alleles of 8.5 and 9.5 kilobases (BROAD et al. 1989). Two regions within the *CALC I* gene with the potential to be involved in the regulation of *CALC I* gene expression mediated by alterations in methylation are located at the 5'-end of the gene, spanning a sequence from the center of intron 1 up to 1.8 kilobases of upstream sequence, and within intron 2. The region at the 5'-end of the *CALC I* gene is nonmethylated in normal and MTC tissues (BROAD et al. 1989). But the same region becomes frequently methylated in small-cell lung carcinoma cell lines expressing the *CALC I* gene (BAYLIN et al. 1986). Demethylation of the intron 2 region correlates with the activation and maintenance of *CALC I* gene expression in tumor tissue.

Transient expression of reporter genes under the control of the *CALC I* gene promoter region in different tumor cell lines, including those of MTC or neuronal origin, identified regulatory elements within 1.3 kilobases of DNA upstream of the *CALC I* gene transcription start site. Complex tissue-specific enhancers were located in regions spanning 1362 to 827 base pairs upstream from the start of transcription in the rat gene (STOLARSKY-FREDMAN et al. 1990), and 1060 to 905 base pairs 5' to the transcription start site in the human gene (PELEG et al. 1990). The human enhancer contains E-box-like elements. Enhanced expression mediated by these elements integrated in homologous or heterologous promotors was only observed in neuronal or MTC-derived cell lines. A cyclic AMP-responsive element active in a human MTC cell line (TT line) but inactive in a small-cell lung carcinoma (DMS53 line) is located between 252 and 132 base pairs upstream from the transcription start site of the human *CALC I* gene (DE BUSTROS et al. 1990).

II. Regulation of Transcription

The primordial cellular mediator of the calcium-evoked secretion of calcitonin from thyroid C cells is a transient rise of the intracellular free calcium concentration (HALLER-BREM et al. 1988). Messenger RNA synthesis is only minimally if at all affected by changes of the free cytosolic calcium levels, but stimulated by the phorbol ester 12-*O*-tetradecanoyl phorbol 13-acetate (TPA) and by cyclic AMP analogues (DE BUSTROS et al. 1985, 1986). Activation of protein kinase C and A pathways also enhances cell differentiation, and suppresses proliferation and c-*myc* gene mRNA levels.

Calcitonin gene transcription is regulated by vitamin D and glucocorticoids as shown in vivo in the rat, and in vitro in human and rat MTC cell lines. Conflicting results have been obtained with respect to the action of 1,25-dihydroxyvitamin D on the thyroid calcitonin mRNA content in the rat. A twofold increase of calcitonin mRNA was observed in female rats 1 and 2 h after subcutaneous administration of 500 pmol 1,25-dihydroxyvitamin D_3 (SEGOND et al. 1985), whereas almost total suppression and parallel inhibition of the *CALC I* gene transcription rate has been reported in normal male rats at 6 and 24 h after intraperitoneal injections of 100 pmol 1,25-dihydroxyvitamin D_3 (NAVEH-MANY and SILVER 1988). The later findings correspond to a time- and dose-dependent lowering of calcitonin and CGRP mRNA levels by 1,25-dihydroxyvitamin D_3 in a human MTC (TT) cell line (COTE et al. 1987b).

In the same human MTC (TT) cell line, the synthetic glucocorticoid dexamethasone, on the other hand, stimulates the levels of calcitonin gene transcripts in a dose- and time-dependent manner. The levels of total *CALC I* gene transcripts and the ratio between calcitonin and CGRP mRNA are raised, but cell growth is concomitantly suppressed (COTE and GAGEL 1986). The demonstration of lowered calcitonin to CGRP mRNA ratio in fast-growing TT cells as compared to resting TT cells (NELKIN et al. 1989) suggests that in this particular cell line dexamethasone indirectly regulates alternative splicing through inhibition of cell growth and presumably enhanced cell differentiation. In rat MTC cells dexamethasone selectively stimulates the *CALC I* gene transcription rate, but does not affect *CALC II* gene activity (RUSSO et al. 1988). In female adrenalectomized rats in vivo thyroid calcitonin mRNA levels are reduced to 40% of the levels observed in control animals. They can be restored to 70% by dexamethasone treatment and by calcium supplementation, and the two effects are additive (BESNARD et al. 1989).

Little is known of the regulation of the *CALC I* and *II* genes in neuronal tissues expressing CGRP. Peripheral axotomy selectively raised CGRP I mRNA and CGRP immunoreactivity in motoneurons of rat spinal cord, but CGRP II mRNA remained unaffected (NOGUCHI et al. 1990a). Axotomy of the rat facial nerve led to a transient induction of CGRP gene expression in motoneurons of the facial nucleus (HAAS et al. 1990). Studies in adult rat dorsal root ganglion neurons in primary culture demonstrated that a continuous supply of nerve growth factor is required to maintain steady state levels of substance P and CGRP I and the corresponding mRNA (LINDSAY and HARMAR 1989). In situ hybridization histochemistry and immunohistochemistry in the spinal cord of castrated rats revealed suppression of CGRP I mRNA levels and CGRP immunoreactivity in the androgen-sensitive motoneurons of the spinal nucleus of the bulbocavernosus by testosterone (POPPER and MICEVYCH 1990).

III. Tissue-Specific Expression of Messenger RNA

Tissue-specific selection of alternative splice sites in initial *CALC I* gene transcripts results in the production of calcitonin predominantly in thyroid C cells and of CGRP in neuronal tissue (AMARA et al. 1982; ROSENFELD et al. 1983).

Differential regulation of tissue-specific processing of *CALC I* gene transcripts in vivo has been investigated in normal and tumor tissues and in tumor cell lines by in situ hybridization, Northern blot analysis and S_1 nuclease mapping of mRNA, and immunological characterization of peptide products. Calcitonin and CGRP mRNA are present in the rat thyroid at a ratio of 95:1 (SABATE et al. 1985), and calcitonin and CGRP are synthesized in the same thyroid C cells in similar proportion. Coproduction of calcitonin and CGRP has also been described in human and monkey pituitary glands, but the levels of CGRP mRNA were only 2%–4% of the small amounts present in the rat thyroid gland (JONAS et al. 1985). In human MTC tissue the amounts of calcitonin mRNA exceed those of CGRP mRNA. In individual tumor cells of familiar or sporadic MTC, calcitonin mRNA levels were at least five times higher than those of CGRP mRNA (HÖPPENER et al. 1986; NOEL et al. 1990). Growth-related changes in the ratio of calcitonin to CGRP mRNA, and highest relative amounts of CGRP mRNA during rapid growth, have been observed in a human MTC (TT) cell line (NELKIN et al. 1989), suggesting that alternative RNA processing in this cell line depends on growth conditions and differentiation.

CALC I gene expression is also observed in lung carcinoma and pheochromocytoma, and the calcitonin mRNA was indistinguishable from that of MTC tissue (HÖPPENER et al. 1986). Lung tumor tissue, in contrast to lung tumor cell lines, contained no detectable CGRP mRNA (EDBROOKE et al. 1985; HÖPPENER et al. 1986; NELKIN et al. 1984; RILEY et al. 1986; SCHIFTER et al. 1989). Studies in normal rats suggest that CGRP expression in the lung is developmentally regulated. CGRP mRNA appeared on the 18th day of gestation in endocrine cells of the lung, and the levels were highest on the 20th day of gestation, and then decreased postnatally (WADA et al. 1988).

The splicing choice of a variety of tissues that normally do not express the *CALC I* gene has been studied in transgenic mice transfected with the rat *CALC I* transcription unit under the control of the mouse metallothionein-I promoter (CRENSHAW et al. 1987). Over 90% of the fusion gene transcripts identified on Northern blots of mRNA from liver, kidney, skeletal muscle, spleen, gut, and lung corresponded to calcitonin mRNA. The heart was the only non-neuronal tissue that expressed over 10% CGRP mRNA. The brain contained 58% CGRP mRNA and 42% calcitonin mRNA. But in situ hybridization localized calcitonin mRNA predominantly in nonneuronal cells of the brain, such as the choroid plexus, ependyma, and pia mater. Among neurons, only the Purkinje cell layer of the cerebellum and the inferior colliculus contained predominantly calcitonin mRNA. The results suggest that the splice machinery dictating CGRP expression is widely distributed in transgenic mice, but to a large extent restricted to neuronal tissue.

Analysis of splicing patterns obtained with wild-type and different mutant calcitonin/CGRP transcription units in human epithelial (HeLa) and mouse teratocarcinoma (F9) cell lines demonstrated that nucleotide sequences near the calcitonin-specific splice acceptor site inhibit the production of calcitonin mRNA in the cell line of neuronal origin (F9) (EMESON et al. 1989). The analysis of intermediate splicing products produced by the HeLa cell nuclear extracts from in vitro primary transcripts containing the exon 3 to exon 5 region of the human *CALC I* gene identified an unusual uridine branch acceptor upstream of the calcitonin splice acceptor site (ADEMA et al. 1988). Mutation of this uridine residue into an adenosine residue results in a markedly raised calcitonin-splicing efficiency in pheochromocytoma cells (PC12) of neuronal origin as well as in a human embryonic kidney cell line (ADEMA et al. 1990). The results imply that unusual branch acceptors such as cytidine in the rat and uridine in man function as *cis*-active elements which inhibit the formation of calcitonin mRNA in CGRP-producing cells.

Messenger RNA-encoding CGRP II precursor proteins have been cloned from rat and human MTC tissue, indicating that *CALC I* and *II* genes are both active in some MTC (STEENBERGH et al. 1958b; AMARA et al. 1985). In the rat, CGRP I and II mRNA have been identified in the trigeminal ganglia, lateral medulla, hypothalamus, and midbrain, but in each region the level of expression of CGRP II mRNA was lower than 20% of that of CGRP I mRNA (AMARA et al. 1985). CGRP I and II mRNA have also been colocalized in small and medium-sized neurons of the rat dorsal root ganglion. CGRP I mRNA was predominantly found in large neurons, but CGRP II mRNA alone was identified in enteric neurons of the intestine (MULDERRY et al. 1988; NOGUCHI et al. 1990a). Selective expression of the *CALC II* gene has also been observed in cell lines from several Ewing sarcomas, a malignant neoplasm of bone (HÖPPENER et al. 1987).

C. Calcitonin Gene Products

Calcitonin and CGRP are synthesized as parts of larger precursor proteins. Calcitonin and its N- and C-terminal flanking peptides are predominantly produced in thyroid C cells and the stimulation of their secretion by raised extracellular calcium is well established. CGRP was mainly found in the central and peripheral nervous system in capsaicin-sensitive sensory nerve fibers and in motoneurons. CGRP overflow from nerve fibers is obtained through calcium-dependent depolarization by potassium and acute administration of capsaicin.

I. Biosynthesis

Analysis of cloned calcitonin gene structures of man, rat, rabbit, chicken, and fish revealed conservation of the structural organization of calcitonin and CGRP precursor proteins throughout evolution. In the initial translation products calcitonin and CGRP are flanked by N- and C-terminal cryptic peptides (Fig. 1). Conserved sequences of basic amino acid residues flanking calcitonin and CGRP are recognition sites for proteolytic processing enzymes. Glycine residues next to the c-terminal amino acids of calcitonin and CGRP are required for C-terminal amidation. Comparison between known coding sequences for calcitonin precursor proteins revealed different divergence rates for calcitonin, and the N- and C-terminal flanking peptides (LASMOLES et al. 1985). Sequence variability is highest in coding regions for N-terminal flanking peptides, intermediate in those for C-terminal peptides, and lowest for those of calcitonin. The intact human calcitonin and CGRP precursor proteins have been identified in tissue culture medium of a human MTC (TT) cell line and microsequencing revealed identical N-termini. This indicates that the same site of cotranslational cleavage of the signal sequence from the prohormone is used (GKONOS et al. 1986). Corresponding components have been recognized in plasma of MTC patients and in tissue culture medium of a small cell lung tumor cell line (TSCHOPP et al. 1982). In a rat MTC cell line processing of the calcitonin precursor protein occurs first, proteolytically, at the dibasic site preceding the calcitonin sequence, and subsequently at the cleavage and amidation site between calcitonin and the C-terminal flanking peptide (BIRNBAUM et al. 1986).

II. Structure and Tissue Distribution

Calcitonin and CGRP are single-chain polypeptides of 32 and 37 amino acid residues, respectively. Common structural features include N-terminal ring structures and amidated C-termini. The structure of CGRP in contrast to that of calcitonin and the N- and C-terminal flanking peptides has been highly conserved throughout evolution.

Presently known structures of 11 different calcitonin peptides include those of man, cow, sheep, pig, rat, rabbit, chicken, and eel and of 3 distinct peptides in salmon (Deftos and Roos 1989; Martial et al. 1990). In all known calcitonin peptides eight amino acids are in invariant positions. They include five of seven amino acid residues of the N-terminal ring structure linked by a disulfide bridge of cysteines in positions 1 and 7, a leucine in position 9, a glycine in position 28, and the C-terminal prolineamide. Human, rat, and rabbit calcitonin are closely related (94% homology). The fish and chicken calcitonins are 81% homologous, and the bovine, porcine, and ovine calcitonins exhibit 91% homology. Between themselves the three groups of calcitonins diverge considerably.

Calcitonin is predominantly produced in the C cells of the thyroid gland of mammals and in ultimobranchial glands of fish (Copp et al. 1967) and chicken (Homma et al. 1986). But calcitonin has also been identified in the hypothalamus, the pituitary gland, lung tumor tissue and cell lines, and pheochromocytoma (Bone et al. 1983; Catherwood et al. 1987; Fischer et al. 1981b; Gropp et al. 1985; Voelkel et al. 1973). Plasma levels of calcitonin in normal human subjects range from 5 to 40 pg Eq/ml (Body and Heath 1983), and major components include intact calcitonin(1–32) and its methionine-sulfoxide form, and the calcitonin precursor protein (Tobler et al. 1984; Born et al. 1991). Evidence for additional calcitonin peptides with human- or salmon-like structures has been obtained in fish, amphibians, birds, and mammals including man (Perez-Cano et al. 1982a,b; Fischer et al. 1983; Gropp et al. 1985; Lasmoles et al. 1985).

Amino acid sequences of human and rat CGRP I and II (Steenbergh et al. 1986; Amara et al. 1985) and porcine (Kimura et al. 1987) and chicken CGRP (Minvielle et al. 1986) are over 80% homologous. Human CGRP I and II share greater structural homolgy with salmon (24% and 27%) than with human calcitonin (16% and 19%). Human and rat CGRP I and II differ in only three and one amino acids, respectively. All CGRPs have in common an N-terminal ring structure linked by a disulfide bridge of cysteines in positions 2 and 7 and a C-terminal phenylalanineamide. The N-terminal amino acid sequence 1–13 is invariant except for alterations in positions 1 and 3. In human CGRP I and II the extreme N-terminus and the N-terminal ring structure appear unimportant for receptor binding, because the affinity and the molecular weights of binding proteins were indistinguishable from human CGRP (1–37) I and II, and human CGRP I (8–37) (Stangl et al. 1991). Furthermore, photoaffinity labeling of Asp in position 3 of human

CGRP I and the naturally occurring substitution of Asp by Asn in human CGRP II were without consequence for receptor binding. Amino acid substitutions in the middle and C-terminal regions (amino acids 14–37) of all known CGRPs are restricted to positions 14, 15, 22, 23, 25, 31, and 35. Ligand displacement in radioreceptor studies of human CGRP with the C-terminal fragments 15–37, 21–37, and 28–37 of human CGRP I suggests that the invariant amino acid residues between positions 8 and 13 include important binding epitopes. They form part of a proposed amphiphilic α-helix between position 8 and 18 of rat CGRP I (LYNCH and KAISER 1988). This is consistent with results of circular dichroism measurements of human CGRP I in aqueous solution at 4°C that revealed α-helical structure involving eight to ten amino acid residues (MANNING 1989).

Immunoreactive CGRP is mainly found in capsaicin-sensitive nerve fibers supplying the cardiovascular system, the respiratory and gastrointestinal tract, and the skin and bone. It is synthesized in primary afferent nerve cell bodies of dorsal root and vagal and trigeminal ganglia. CGRP frequently coexists with substance P and to a lesser extent with other neuropeptides in the same neuron (CADIEUX et al. 1986; DALSGAARD et al. 1989; EDVINSSON et al. 1987; FRANCO-CERECEDA et al. 1987b; GEPPETTI et al. 1989; GIBBINS et al. 1987; GIBSON et al. 1984; HILL and ELDE 1988; HUA et al. 1987; JU et al. 1987; KRUGER et al. 1989; MULDERRY et al. 1985; NILSSON et al. 1990; REINECKE and FORSSMANN 1988; SKOFITSCH and JACOBOWITZ 1985; SU et al. 1987). Ultrastructural immunohistochemistry colocalized CGRP and substance P in single secretory granules (GULBENKIAN et al. 1986; MERIGHI et al. 1988) and biochemical analyses demonstrated that both peptides are costored in synaptosomal vesicles (FRIED et al. 1989). CGRP has also been found in spinal cord motoneurons (FONTAINE et al. 1986; VILLAR et al. 1989), at the human neuromuscular junction (MORA et al. 1989), in the brain (KAWAI et al. 1985), and in the thyroid (TSCHOPP et al. 1984; ARIAS et al. 1989). Evidence for CGRP biosynthesis in sensory and motoneurons (ARVIDSSON et al. 1990; CORTÉS et al. 1990; GIBSON et al. 1988; RÉTHELYI et al. 1989) and in thyroid parafollicular C cells (ZABEL and SCHÄFER 1988) has been obtained by in situ hybridization histochemistry. CGRP I and II have been isolated from the human spinal cord (MORRIS et al. 1984; PETERMANN et al. 1987; WIMALAWANSA et al. 1990). CGRP I and II mRNA are coexpressed in rat dorsal root ganglion cells (NOGUCHI et al. 1990b). Axonal transport of CGRP and substance P has been described in dorsal roots (GIBBINS et al. 1985) and in sensory and motor fibers of the sciatic nerve (KASHIHARA et al. 1989).

A parallel, rapid, and transient overflow of CGRP and neurokinin A in response to the acute administration of capsaicin suggests that circulating CGRP originates at least in part from sensory nerve endings. To this end, chronic treatment with capsaicin and blockage of axonal transport with colchicine lowers plasma levels of CGRP (DIEZ-GUERRA et al. 1988; ZAIDI et al. 1985). Major circulating CGRP components include mature

CGRP(1–37) and a CGRP precursor protein (Born et al. 1991). CGRP I and II are found in similar amounts in the circulation (Wimalawansa et al. 1989). CGRP-like material has also been detected immunohistochemically with antibodies recognizing mammalian CGRP in neuronal tissue and ultimobranchial glands of amphibians and fish (Batten and Cambre 1989; Kline et al. 1988; Murphy et al. 1990; Ohtani et al. 1989; Venesio et al. 1987), and interestingly in nervous tissue of invertebrates such as the earthworm and the sea squirt (Sasayama et al. 1989). This provides additional evidence for high structural conservation of CGRP-like peptides during evolution.

Structures of N- and C-terminal flanking peptides of calcitonin and CGRP have been predicted from cloned sequences of *CALC I* (human, rat, and chicken) and *CALC II* genes (human and rat) and from calcitonin-encoding cDNA of rabbit and salmon (Amara et al. 1984; Jonas et al. 1985; Steenbergh et al. 1985; Minvielle et al. 1987; Martial et al. 1990; Pöschl et al. 1987). The amino acid sequence of the human N-terminal flanking peptide of calcitonin isolated from MTC tissue confirmed the DNA-predicted structure (Conlon et al. 1988a). The corresponding peptides have also been identified in the circulation of normal human subjects and of MTC patients (Born et al. 1991) and in rat MTC tissue (Burns et al. 1989a). Predicted N-terminal flanking peptides vary in length between 52 (N-terminal flanking peptide of CGRP in chicken) and 60 amino acids (N-terminal flanking peptide of CGRP II in the rat). N-terminal flanking peptides of calcitonin and CGRP I have the amino acid residues 1–50 in common that are encoded by the same exon 3. Sequence homology between the N-terminal flanking peptides of calcitonin and CGRP in man, rat, and rabbit, and between those of chicken and salmon, respectively, exceeds 60%.

The structure of the C-terminal flanking peptides of calcitonin and CGRP are variable. Those of calcitonin vary in length between 16 amino acids in the rat and 21 amino acids in man, rabbit, and chicken. Highest sequence homology (48%) exists between man and rabbit. The human peptide, PDN-21, has been isolated from MTC tissue (Conlon et al. 1988b), and it coexists with calcitonin in thyroid C cells (Ali-Rachedi et al. 1983) and in the brain (Fischer et al. 1983), as well as in the circulation of normal subjects and MTC patients (Ittner et al. 1985). DNA-predicted C-terminal flanking peptides of all known CGRPs have four amino acids. Those of human CGRP I and II and of rat CGRP I have the sequence Asp-Leu-Gln-Ala in common, but their expression at the level of peptides has not been verified so far.

III. Regulation of Release

Calcitonin and its N- and C-terminal flanking peptides are cosecreted from thyroid C cells in normal human subjects and in MTC patients in calcium-responsive manner (Born et al. 1991; Ittner et al. 1985). An acute increase of serum calcium levels stimulated translatable calcitonin mRNA levels in rat thyroid glands within 2 min; it was inhibited by actinomycin D (SEGOND et al. 1989). Similarly, serum levels of calcitonin and its N- and C-terminal flanking peptides increased within minutes after intravenous calcium administration in man (BORN et al. 1991; ITTNER et al. 1985). In patients with chronic hypercalcemia, however, e.g., with primary hyperparathyroidism, serum levels of calcitonin and of its C-terminal flanking peptide are within the normal range. Calcitonin appears unlikely to be important as a homeostatic regulator of the extracellular calcium concentration (ITTNER et al. 1985). The physiological relevance of other stimulators of calcitonin secretion such as pentagastrin, glucagon, catecholamines, and potassium remains to be delineated (AVIOLI et al. 1971; Cooper et al. 1971; McLEAN et al. 1984; VORA et al. 1978).

Circulating levels of CGRP are not affected by acute or chronic changes of the serum calcium concentration in normal human subjects (BORN et al. 1991), but elevated CGRP concentrations seen in some MTC patients were raised further in response to calcium and pentagastrin administration (MASON et al. 1986; KIM et al. 1989). A calcium-dependent parallel increase of calcitonin and CGRP was also observed in perfused dog thyroid glands (AHRÉN et al. 1989). In a human MTC (TT) cell line and in rat MTC cell lines the stimulation of secretion of calcitonin and CGRP is mediated by raised intracellular free calcium concentrations and protein kinase C and A activation (COTE et al. 1987a; HALLER-BREM et al. 1988; SEITZ and COOPER 1989). A slowly inactivating calcium current, defective in the human TT-cell line not responding to changes of the extracellular calcium concentration, has been proposed to function as a sensor in calcium-responsive rat MTC cells (SCHERÜBL et al. 1990).

Depletion by capsaicin from neuronal tissue localized CGRP in afferent nerve fibers. The release of intact CGRP from rat spinal cord slices and rat trigeminal ganglion cells was stimulated, in calcium-dependent manner, by capsaicin and 60 mM potassium presumably through voltage-dependent calcium channels (MASON et al. 1984; SARIA et al. 1986). The proposed role for CGRP as an extracellular neuromodulator in the sensory nervous system is consistent with the observed inhibition of the veratridine-stimulated release of CGRP from dispersed rat trigeminal ganglion cells by tetrodotoxin and local anesthetics which block sodium channels (PETERFREUND and VALE 1986). Differential regulation of CGRP and substance P content was observed in primary cultures of neonatal rat vagal sensory neurons (MACLEAN et al. 1989). Forskolin increased the levels of both peptides, but CGRP was selectively raised by TPA. Nerve growth factor predominantly raised the substance P content and corticosterone selectively suppressed substance P levels. In the perfused guinea pig heart, calcium-dependent stimulation of the release of intact CGRP from capsaicin-sensitive cardiac afferents by total ischemia and by bradykinin, ouabain, and nicotine has been observed (FRANCO-CERECEDA et al. 1989). Simultaneous release of substance P by bradykinin was also seen (Geppetti et al. 1988). Inhibition of the bradykinin-stimulated release of CGRP by indomethacin suggested this effect to be mediated by prostaglandins. The mode of sensory nerve activation seemed to be different here from that produced by capsaicin or electric field stimulation (Geppetti et al. 1990). Noxious thermal or mechanical cutaneous stimuli and electrical stimulation of unmyelinated primary afferents stimulated the release of both substance P and CGRP from the substantia gelatinosa region in the lower lumbar spinal cord, but the role of CGRP in primary afferent transmission of nociceptive information remains to be established (Morton and Hutchison 1989). The CGRP content in lumbar motoneurons was decreased after spinal cord transection, and it appears that alterations in the balance of inputs by signal substances received by motoneurons and/or changes of their mobility may modify intracellular CGRP levels (Arvidsson et al. 1989; Marlier et al. 1990). Electrical or high potassium stimulation of the motor nerve in phrenic nerve-diaphragm preparations caused release of CGRP from the neuromuscular junction and increased the cyclic AMP content of skeletal muscle, and potentiated twitch contraction (Uchida et al. 1990).

IV. Metabolism

In man the kidney removes two-thirds of the intravenously administered calcitonin (Ardaillou et al. 1973). Additional sites for the extraction of human, porcine, and salmon calcitonin in dogs and rats include the liver and possibly bone and muscle (Clark et al. 1974; Singer et al. 1972a). In the isolated perfused rat kidney removal of calcitonin proceeds through filtration and filtration-independent pathways. Calcitonin-degrading enzymatic activity was located in brush border membranes (Simmons et al. 1988). The urinary clearance of calcitonin(1–32) in man was less than 1% of the metabolic clearance rate, which amounted to 8 ml/kg per minute, and degradation of calcitonin by plasma proteins was negligible (Huwyler et al. 1979). Less is known about the metabolism of CGRP. The metabolic clearance rates of human CGRP I and II and of rat CGRP I were similar to those of calcitonin (Beglinger et al. 1988; Kraenzlin et al. 1985).

D. Biological Action

Calcitonin and CGRP present discrete structural homology, limited cross-reactivity of receptors, and overlapping biological effects in several target tissues which include the skeleton, the kidney, and the cardiovascular system (Table 1).

Table 1. Biological effects of calcitonin and CGRP

	Route of administration	Calcitonin	CGRP
Bone resorption	s/in vitro	↓↓	↓
Pain perception	icv/s	↓	?
Gastrointestinal			
Acid output	icv/s/in vitro	↓	↓
Food intake	icv/s	↓	↓
Cardiovascular			
Hypertension	icv	↑↑	↑↑
Tachycardia	icv	↑↑	↑↑
Vasodilatation	s/in vitro	↑	↑↑
Hypotension	s	0	↑↑
Tachycardia	s/in vitro	0	↑↑
Contractility heart	s/in vitro	0	↑
Renal			
Blood flow	s	0	↑ [a]
Glomerular filtration rate	s	0	↑ [a]
Renin secretion	s/in vitro	↑	↑↑
Urinary flow	s	↑↑ [a]	↑
Fractional excretion			
Na, Cl	s	↑↑	↑
Ca, PO$_4$	s	↑↑	0

s, systemic; icv, intracerebroventricular.
[a] Arterial pressure maintained.

I. Calcitonin Receptor and Targets

1. Receptors

Calcitonin receptors linked to adenylate cyclase activation have been recognized in bone and kidney, which are known target organs of the hormone (MARX et al. 1972). There, they are localized in osteoclasts, and in the medullary and cortical portions of the thick ascending limb and in the distal convoluted kidney tubules (NICHOLSON et al. 1986; SEXTON et al. 1987; MOREL 1983). Binding of radioactive salmon [^{125}I]calcitonin has also been observed in the central nervous system. There specific binding is highest in the midbrain and brainstem, and low in the neocortex, cerebellum, and spinal cord (Figs. 2, 3) (FISCHER et al. 1981b; OLGIATI et al. 1983; HENKE et al. 1983). A bronchial carcinoma cell line (BEN) produces calcitonin (predominantly precursor forms) and possesses calcitonin receptors and hormone-responsive adenylate cyclase (HAM et al. 1980; MOSELEY et al. 1986). The osteogenic UMR 106-01 CGRP receptor positive cells, on the other hand, release a CGRP-like peptide (MICHELANGELI et al. 1986; ZAIDI et al. 1989). The biological relevance of the autocrine pathways remains to be elucidated.

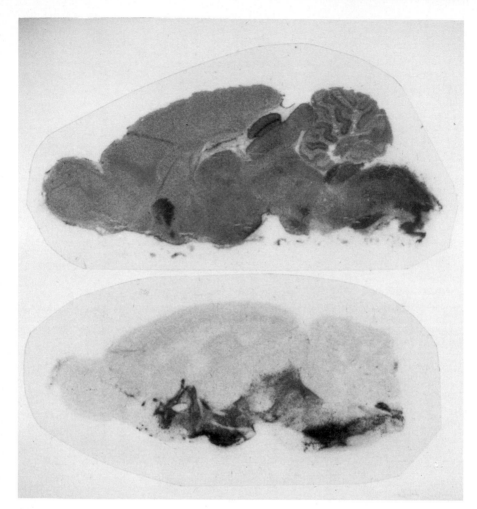

Fig. 2. Receptor autoradiography of [^{125}I]rat CGRP I (*top panel*) and [^{125}I]salmon calcitonin (*bottom panel*) of the rat brain

Covalent cross-linking techniques have revealed proteins binding [^{125}I]calcitonin specifically in rat osteoclasts, human breast cancer cells, and placental membranes (M_r, 85 000) (Nicholson et al. 1986, 1988; Moseley et al. 1986), and in the rat kidney (M_r, 70 000, 40 000, 33 000) (Bouizar et al. 1986). Expression cloning of a complementary DNA from a porcine kidney epithelial cell line (LLC-PK$_1$) revealed the structure of a 482-amino acid receptor protein with high affinity for salmon calcitonin (Lin et al. 1991). This calcitonin receptor is a member of a new family of G-protein-coupled receptors including the rat secretin receptor (Ishihara et al. 1991) and common receptors for parathyroid hormone and parathyroid hormone-

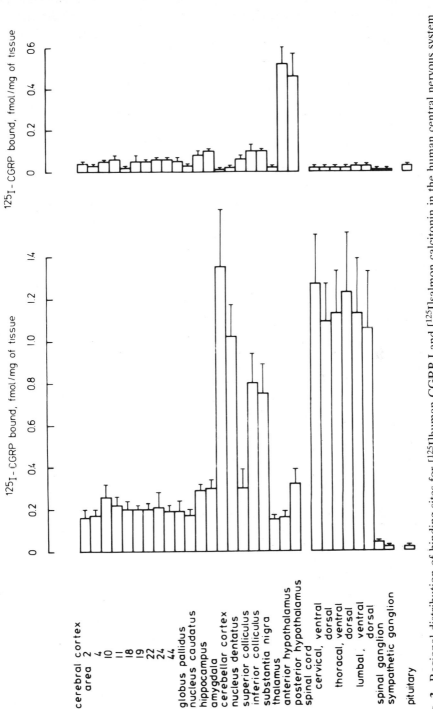
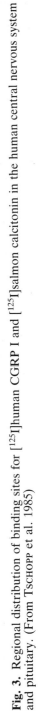

Fig. 3. Regional distribution of binding sites for [125I]human CGRP I and [125I]salmon calcitonin in the human central nervous system and pituitary. (From Tschopp et al. 1985)

related peptide cloned from Oppossum kidney and rat bone cell lines (Jüppner et al. 1991; Abou-Samra et al. 1992). Transient expression of the cloned porcine calcitonin receptor activated both the adenylate cyclase and phospholipase C pathways by CT in a human kidney cell line (HEK-293) (Chabre et al. 1992).

Specific [125I]salmon calcitonin binding is largely irreversible and associated with persistent activation of adenylate cyclase activity (Fischer et al. 1981a; Nicholson et al. 1987). This unique phenomenon makes the study of receptor downregulation using [125I]calcitonin binding and conventional washing of cells and particulate fractions questionable. Independently, phorbol ester evoked reduction of receptor binding and adenylate cyclase activation by calcitonin in breast and bronchial carcinoma cell lines suggest that protein kinase C is involved in the densitization of calcitonin receptors (Findlay et al. 1989). Prolonged infusions of salmon calcitonin in vivo reduced the number of rat kidney calcitonin binding sites as evidenced by autoradiography, and suppressed the hypocalcemic response (Bouizar et al. 1987).

Besides stimulation of cyclic AMP formation, free cytosolic calcium was also raised in osteoclasts (Malgaroli et al. 1989; Zaidi et al. 1990). The effects were mimicked by 8-bromocyclic AMP, suggesting that the cytosolic calcium response is distal to cyclic AMP formation. Inhibition of lipogenesis by calcitonin is a calcium calmodulin-dependent pathway in the rat liver also distal to cyclic AMP accumulation (Nishizawa et al. 1988). In rabbit medullary thick ascending limb tubules cytosolic free calcium was raised independent of changes of cyclic AMP concentrations (Murphy et al. 1986).

The weak hypocalcemic action of CGRP in relation to that of calcitonin and cross-tachyphylaxis on the inhibition of ^{45}calcium release from prelabeled bone explants suggests that CGRP interacts with calcitonin receptors on osteoclasts (Roos et al. 1986). Similarly, in kidney membranes and cultured kidney cells, CGRP inhibits [125I]salmon calcitonin binding and enhances adenylate cyclase activity, and plasminogen activator production, albeit at 500- to 1000-fold higher concentrations than salmon calcitonin (Goltzman and Mitchell 1985; Wohlwend et al. 1985). The stimulation in both osteoclasts and kidney tubules is probably mediated by calcitonin receptors, revealing cross-reactivity to CGRP.

2. Biological Targets

Calcitonin is known to lower serum calcium levels through inhibition of bone resorption and stimulation of the urinary calcium excretion. The antiresorptive effect is shared by CGRP albeit in higher amounts than calcitonin probably through interaction with calcitonin receptors (Roos et al. 1986).

Inhibition of bone resorption by calcitonin is obtained through suppression of osteoclastic activity. To this end, cell motility is arrested and retraction of osteoclastic spreading has been recognized on time-lapse video recording (CHAMBERS et al. 1986). This is associated with an inhibition of the secretion of lysosomal enzymes at the apical pole of the osteoclasts facing the bone compartment (BARON et al. 1990). The enzymes are rerouted to intracellular vacuoles, and eventually their synthesis is also arrested.

In the kidney, calcitonin stimulates the excretion of calcium, phosphate, sodium, and chloride and enhances 1,25-dihydroxyvitamin D production (GNAEDINGER et al. 1989; BIJVOET et al. 1971; HAAS et al. 1971; HORIUCHI et al. 1979; JAEGER et al. 1986). Inhibition of Na^+-dependent phosphate transport occurs primarily in proximal kidney tubules where cyclic AMP simulation has not been observed (YUSUFI et al. 1987; MOREL 1983).

Intracerebroventricular administration of calcitonin and perfusion of jejunum, ileum, and colon with calcitonin or CGRP revealed chloride secretion and inhibition of active sodium absorption (PRIMI and BUENO 1986; GRAY et al. 1976; McCULLOCH and COOKE 1989). The effects were only obtained with pharmacological amounts of calcitonin, but may explain the diarrhea seen in some patients with MTC with excessive secretion of calcitonin.

In view of the presence of calcitonin and of its receptors in the circumventricular region of the brain (FISCHER et al. 1981a,b), it would seem that some central actions of the peptide are physiologically relevant. The earliest discovered neural action of calcitonin represents inhibition of pain perception, also used therapeutically in man (PECILE et al. 1975). The effect was not suppressed by the opiate antagonist naloxone, and may involve serotonergic and adrenergic pathways (BRAGA et al. 1978; CLEMENTI et al. 1985; GUIDOBONO et al. 1986). Similarly, CGRP also has antinociceptive properties (PECILE et al. 1987).

Intracerebroventricular administration of calcitonin inhibits gastric secretion in far lower amounts than systemic injections (MORLEY et al. 1981). The effect may therefore be centrally mediated. After intracerebroventricular injections of calcitonin, specific effects brought about through interaction with receptors in the periventricular region of the brain need to be interpreted with caution since intact calcitonin-(1–32) reaches the general circulation within minutes (MORIMOTO et al. 1985; SABBATINI et al. 1985). Calcitonin, moreover, stimulates the release of somatostatin from the isolated stomach and may therefore suppress gastric acid secretion indirectly (CHIBA et al. 1980; WOLOSZCZUK et al. 1986). Central and peripheral administration of calcitonin also inhibits food intake (FREED et al. 1979; DE BEAUREPAIRE and SUAUDEAU 1988; SHIMIZU and OOMURA 1986). The central anoretic and gastrointestinal motor effects of calcitonin appear to be mediated in part by prostaglandins (FARGEAS et al. 1984).

Stimulation of prolactin secretion through centrally administered calcitonin (IWASAKI et al. 1979; CHIHARA et al. 1982) is opposite to the inhibition recognized in cultured pituitary cells (SHAH et al. 1990). Inhibition of prolactin secretion also observed after central administration of calcitonin

(CLEMENTI et al. 1983) and inhibition of growth hormone and prolactin release by intracerebroventricular CGRP (TANNENBAUM and GOLTZMAN 1985; FAHIM et al. 1990) may be caused by overflow of the peptides into the peripheral circulation (see above), and direct interaction with the pituitary gland. There calcitonin inhibits thyroliberin-stimulated prolactin release through suppression of increased cytosolic free calcium concentrations (SHAH et al. 1990). In vivo both calcitonin and CGRP suppress prolactin secretion (ISAAC et al. 1980; ELIE et al. 1990). Calcitonin, moreover, inhibits the pulsatile growth hormone secretion after both central and peripheral administration (LENGYEL and TANNENBAUM 1987; LOOIJ et al. 1988). Besides, peripheral administration of calcitonin suppresses the secretion of thyoliberin, and the hypothalamus appears to be involved (MITSUMA et al. 1984).

With regard to behavioral effects, calcitonin promotes haloperidol-induced catalepsy, and inhibits amphetamine-induced locomotor activity and avoidance behavior (NICOLETTI et al. 1982; TWERY et al. 1986; CLEMENTI et al. 1984).

II. Calcitonin Gene-Related Peptide Receptors and Targets

Calcitonin gene-related peptide is principally a neuropeptide acting locally through interaction with receptors at its target organs.

1. Receptors

Membrane homogenates and receptor autoradiography have revealed an extensive distribution of CGRP-specific binding sites throughout the nervous system, and among peripheral organs the heart, spleen, blood vessels, lung, kidney, and in T lymphocytes (TSCHOPP et al. 1985; GOLTZMAN and MITCHELL 1985; SEIFERT et al. 1985; SKOFITSCH and JACOBOWITZ 1985; INAGAKI et al. 1986; SEXTON et al. 1986; McCORMACK et al. 1989; UMEDA and ARISAWA 1989). High density of specific binding sites has been recognized in the cerebellum and spinal cord (Fig. 3). The cerebellum is a rich source of solubilized binding proteins for receptor identification and purification. Both in membrane homogenates and in CHAPS-solubilized human cerebellum specific binding proteins with apparent molecular weights of 95 000, 60 000, 54 000, and 17 000 have been identified through cross-linking of [125I]human CRGP I and II, but also with the CGRP antagonist [125I]human CRGP-I(8–37) (DOTTI-SIGRIST et al. 1988; STANGL et al. 1991). Along the same lines, human CGRP(8–37) potently inhibited binding of [125I]human CGRP(1–37) to guinea pig atrial and ileal preparations (DENNIS et al. 1990). Related results have been obtained using a photoreactive analog interacting with the aspartate residue in position 3 within the N-terminal ring structure of CGRP I (STANGL et al. 1991). The binding data indicate that the N-terminal ring structure of CGRP is not essential for the interaction with its receptor. The 60 000 and 54 000 molecular weight components are N-glycosylated. Even though biochemical cross-linking has not revealed differences in the molecular weights of the CGRP-binding proteins using [^{125}I]human CGRP I and II, subtle differences in the regional distribution of [^{125}I]human CGRP I and II binding have been found using receptor auto-radiography, e.g., in the ventromedial hypothalamus (HENKE et al. 1987).

A CGRP-specific binding protein (M_r, 60000) was recognized in cultured rat vascular smooth muscle cells and in bovine endothelial cells (HIRATA et al. 1988). CGRP-specific binding proteins (M_r, 120000, 90000, 70000) have also been identified in porcine coronary arteries, and in the heart atrium and ventricular muscles, and in the spinal cord (MIYAUCHI et al. 1988; SANO et al. 1989).

In the rat atrium and spleen as well as in the rat and human brain, salmon and human calcitonin inhibit [^{125}I]CGRP binding in high concentrations in parallel fashion to CGRP, indicating receptor cross-reactivity (SIGRIST et al. 1986; SEIFERT et al. 1985; MATON et al. 1990; HENKE et al. 1985). Receptor-binding studies revealing superimposable inhibition curves with CGRP and salmon calcitonin, and autoradiographic examination of the nucleus accumbens in the rat brain, are consistent with a unique CGRP/calcitonin-binding protein (SEXTON et al. 1988). On biological grounds, DENNIS et al. (1990) have also presented evidence for CGRP receptor heterogeneity (see below).

In arterial blood vessels, the heart, myotubes, spleen, kidney, liver and in osteoblast-enriched bone cells the CGRP receptors are linked to cyclic AMP accumulation (KUBOTA et al. 1985; EDVINSSON et al. 1985; SIGRIST et al. 1986; JENNINGS and MUDGE 1989; KURTZ et al. 1988; CHIBA et al. 1989; MICHELANGELI et al. 1989). In the liver, spleen, heart, atrium, and vas deferens the human CGRP I antagonist-(8–37) was shown to inhibit receptor binding and cyclic AMP formation (CHIBA et al. 1989; DENNIS et al. 1990). As a result of cyclic AMP formation, the calcium conductance is prolonged with CGRP in cat parasympathetic ganglia and in guinea pig atria (ONO et al. 1989; OHMURA et al. 1990). Likewise, CGRP produced hyperpolarization of the smooth musculature of cerebral arteries and vasodilatation independent of endothelial cells (SAITO et al. 1989). In cultured rat neurons reduction of calcium and potassium currents by CGRP was associated with increased cellular cyclic AMP concentrations; the effects were also obtained with forskolin (ZONA et al. 1991).

2. Biological Targets

Calcitonin gene-related peptide is a neuropeptide acting locally at its target sites in paracrine fashion. Predominant effects are on the cardiovascular system and include vasodilatation, and positive chronotropic and inotropic effects in the heart (BRAIN et al. 1985; FISHER et al. 1983; FRANCO-CERECEDA et al. 1987a). In addition to the vasodilatory effects CGRP inhibits contractile responses in other smooth muscles such as of the intestine, anus, uterus, ureter, bladder, vas deferens, and spleen (Holzer et al. 1989; Pennefather et al. 1990; Samuelson et al. 1985; Hua et al. 1987; Stief et al. 1990; Goto et al. 1987; Sigrist et al. 1986). The cardiovascular effects of CGRP are only shared to a limited extent by calcitonin, whereas the opposite is true concerning the inhibition of bone resorption by calcitonin (Roos et al. 1986). The different potencies are explained by receptor cross-reactivity of calcitonin and CGRP due to their limited structural homology (see above).

The N-terminal fragments human CGRP I(1–12), -(1–15), and -(1–22) lowered arterial pressure in rats albeit at doses higher than that of the intact peptide (Maggi et al. 1990). The C-terminal fragments, human CGRP I(8–37) and -(12–37), in contrast, caused vasoconstriction and antagonized vasodilatory effects and the stimulation of the heart rate by the intact CGRP(1–37) (Dennis et al. 1989, 1990; Han et al. 1990; Gardiner et al. 1990). Similarly, rat [Tyr^0]CGRP(28–37) antagonized the relaxation of the anal smooth musculature and stimulation of amylase secretion (Chakder and Rattan 1990; Maton et al. 1990). Human CGRP(8–37) was a potent antagonist of the stimulation of the heart rate, but the antagonistic potency was much weaker in the rat vas deferens (Dennis et al. 1990). The results suggest the existence of more than one CGRP receptor type, tentatively termed by Dennis et al. (1990) CGRP$_1$ and CGRP$_2$. Along similar lines, the linear analog, [acetamidomethyl-Cys^{2,7}]CGRP retained high potency in the relaxation of the rat vas deferens but did not stimulate the heart rate (Dennis et al. 1989). Thus it appears that the N-terminal amino acid ring structure of CGRP is essential for the cardiovascular effects of CGRP which are antagonized by the C-terminal fragments-(8–37) and -(12–37).

The most remarkable effect of CGRP at least in humans is potent vasodilatation of skin blood vessels visible as flushing of the face and chest (Gennari and Fischer 1985). More intensive facial flushing was noted with CGRP than with calcitonin. Vasodilatation of skin blood vessels was also recognized following the intradermal administration of CGRP (Brain et al. 1985). Infusions of low doses of CGRP enhanced blood flow in the skin and in the common carotid artery without concomitant changes of the heart rate and the arterial pressure (Gardiner et al. 1989; Jäger et al. 1990). Since the arterial pressure and heart rate remained largely unchanged, a redistribution of blood flow as a compensatory mechanism is implied. In fact, blood flow to the superior mesenteric artery was decreased (Jäger et al. 1990). In another study carotid blood flow was also raised in normal human subjects by a dose which increased the heart rate but left the arterial pressure unchanged (Macdonald et al. 1989). Stimulation of coronary blood flow is a sensitive response of CGRP (Holman et al. 1986; Greenberg et al. 1987). It is even recognizable when the arterial pressure is lowered with CGRP and the renal blood flow is concomitantly reduced (Dipette et al. 1989).

On a molar basis, CGRP is a very potent vasodilator (Franco-Cereceda et al. 1987a). To this end, human CGRP relaxed small arteries from human skeletal muscle precontracted with norepinephrine with an EC$_{50}$ of 0.5 nM.

Stimulation of cyclic AMP formation and activation of an ATP-sensitive potassium channel are involved in the vasodilatory responses of CGRP (KUBOTA et al. 1985; NELSON et al. 1990). Unlike relaxation in the aorta of the rat, which required the presence of the endothelium, relaxation persisted in the absence of the endothelium in cerebral arteries of the cat (KUBOTA et al. 1985; EDVINSSON et al. 1985). Activation of adenylate cyclase in bovine aortic endothelial cells by CGRP by itself does not prove that the endothelium is required for the relaxation of blood vessels (CROSSMAN et al. 1990).

The potent cardiovascular action of CGRP was discovered in rat and man using higher amounts than those enhancing blood flow alone, and hypotension as well as positive chronotropic and inotropic effects were predominant features (FISHER et al. 1983; GENNARI and FISCHER 1985; STRUTHERS et al. 1986; FRANCO-CERECEDA et al. 1987a). It appears possible that the hypotension is secondary to generalized vasodilatation. CGRP exerts direct and indirect positive chronotropic and inotropic effects, and also stimulates the release of atrial natriuretic peptide through a cyclic AMP-dependent mechanism (SIGRIST et al. 1986; YAMAMOTO et al. 1988; SCHIEBINGER and SANTORA 1989). The increase of rate and tension of the isolated rat atrium in response to CGRP is still obtained in the presence of adrenergic and histaminergic antagonists and of indomethacin blocking prostaglandin synthesis (SIGRIST et al. 1986). Consistent rises of circulating levels of norepinephrine and epinephrine indicate reflex activation of sympathetic tone. But adrenergic blocking agents did not affect positive chronotropic and inotropic effects of CGRP on isolated atria of rat and guinea pig in vitro. Moreover, the positive chronotropic and hypotensive effects and skin vasodilatation (facial flushing) of CGRP were left unchanged during the administration of the combined α- and β-adrenergic blocking agent labetalol in vivo in man, but the ventricular inotropic effect of CGRP was prevented (GENNARI and FISCHER 1985). The ventricular inotropic response of CGRP, which is negligible in the rat, therefore probably depends on sympathetic activation and catecholamine release due to the concomitant fall in arterial pressure (FISHER et al. 1983; GENNARI and FISCHER 1985; STRUTHERS et al. 1986). The negligible direct effects of CGRP on the heart ventricle are also consistent with lower endogenous CGRP levels as well as receptor density compared to the atrium (SIGRIST et al. 1986).

Intracerebroventricular administration of CGRP, on the other hand, evoked elevations of the arterial pressure and heart rate concomitant with enhanced sympathetic outflow (FISHER et al. 1983). The detailed pathways remain to be delineated.

In the kidney, CGRP-containing nerve fibers have been localized in the proximity of arteries and arterioles (including the juxtaglomerular apparatus) (KURTZ et al. 1988; REINECKE and FORSSMANN 1988). The smooth musculature of the renal pelvis and the ureter are, moreover, densely innervated with CGRP-immunoreactive nerve fibers (HUA et al. 1987; MAGGI et al. 1987b; KURTZ et al. 1988). The localization of immunoreactive nerve fibers together with CGRP receptors on autoradiographic examination is indicative that CGRP is probably locally released. The physiological relevance of the renal effects of CGRP remains to be elucidated. Acute treatment with capsaicin enhances the release of neuropeptides such as CGRP from afferent nerve fibers (see above). Raised tension is a well-established stimulator of afferent nerve fibers. To this end, increased intrapelvic volume and pressure enhance the tension of the smooth musculature of the pelvis and thus activate afferent nerve fibers. This presumably brings about the release of CGRP in antidromic fashion, which in turn reduces the spontaneous activity of the renal pelvis and ureter.

Calcitonin gene-related peptide enhances renal blood flow concomitant with a dose-dependent fall of the renal vascular resistance (Villarreal et al. 1988). As a result, the glomerular filtration, filtration fraction, and urinary flow are increased (Villarreal et al. 1988; Kurtz et al. 1989). In vitro CGRP blunts the contraction of mesangial cells obtained with angiotensin II. Relaxation of mesangial cells by CGRP is presumably responsible for the increased filtration fraction seen in vivo and in vitro. There CGRP stimulates cyclic AMP formation which mediates the dilatory effect of CGRP much like in other smooth muscle cells (Kubota et al. 1985; Edvinsson et al. 1985; Kurtz et al. 1989), but CGRP does not interfere with the rise of free cytosolic calcium obtained with angiotensin II (Kurtz et al. 1989). Similarly, CGRP, unlike calcitonin, stimulates cyclic AMP formation in isolated glomeruli (Edwards and Trizna 1990). Taken together the results reveal that CGRP causes relaxation of renal mesangial cells and vasodilatation, and as a result presumably increases glomerular filtration. In the absence of calcitonin receptors in renal glomeruli and mesangial cells, direct effects of CGRP seem probable (Kurtz et al. 1989; Morel 1983; Sexton et al. 1987).

Besides its vasodilatory effects CGRP enhances the renin-angiotensin-aldosterone system as counterregulatory action to the vasodilatation and hypotension (Kurtz et al. 1988). CGRP also stimulates renin activity directly in isolated juxtaglomerular cells through a cyclic AMP-dependent pathway. The contribution of sympathetic reflex activation as recognized by raised plasma levels of norepinephrine and epinephrine cannot be differentiated in vivo from the direct stimulation of renin secretion. Stimulation of renin activity in isolated renal juxtaglomerular cells is shared with calcitonin in high concentrations presumably because of cross-reactivity of receptors (Kurtz et al. 1988).

Renal tubular effects such as stimulation of the urinary fractional excretion of sodium, chloride, potassium, calcium, and phosphate are predominantly obtained with calcitonin (Bijvoet et al. 1971; Haas et al. 1971; Gnaedinger et al. 1989; Morel 1983) (see above). With CGRP, the fractional excretion of sodium and chloride is also raised, but the effect is less pronounced than that of equimolar amounts of calcitonin (Gnaedinger et al. 1989). Lowered excretion of sodium and potassium and reduction of urinary flow was also found with CGRP concomitant with reduction of arterial pressure (VILLARREAL et al. 1988). Interference of hypotension with tubular function due to excessive amounts of CGRP appears probable. In the isolated rat kidney, on the other hand, perfused at constant pressure, stimulation of sodium excretion by CGRP and urinary flow has been observed (KURTZ et al. 1989). Renal tubular effects are presumably brought about through interaction with calcitonin receptors (WOHLWEND et al. 1985; GOLTZMAN and MITCHELL 1985). Nonetheless, localized release of CGRP from nerve fibers may be physiologically as relevant as the hormonal effect of calcitonin.

The role(s) of the lung as a target for CGRP is controversial. While vasodilatation is a recognized effect of CGRP, epithelium-dependent contraction of tracheal strips in the guinea pig, absent effect in vivo in rats, and inhibition of constriction of airway smooth muscle cells of the rat have been reported (PALMER et al. 1987; TSCHIRHART et al. 1990; LUNDBERG et al. 1985; CADIEUX et al. 1990).

In contrast to the relaxation of the smooth musculature, CGRP stimulates the contraction of the striated skeletal musculature (TAKAMORI and YOSHIKAWA 1989). To this end, CGRP is present in motoneurons of the ventral spinal cord and in muscular end plates, where the peptide enhances neuromuscular transmission, and bungaratoxin binding, and stimulates acetylcholine receptor synthesis (FONTAINE et al. 1987; NEW and MUDGE 1986). Cyclic AMP formation and phosphorylation of the acetylcholine receptor, and phosphosoinositide turnover by CGRP may be involved in the trophic actions of the neuropeptide (MILES et al. 1989; LAUFER and CHANGEUX 1989). Colocalization and release of the classical neurotransmitter acetylcholine with the neuropeptide CGRP would therefore have a defined purpose, with acetylcholine being responsible for fast and transient contraction of the skeletal musculature, and the neuropeptide CGRP for longer-lasting synthesis of the acetylcholine receptor. In a similar way CGRP is involved in the differentation of dopaminergic neurons in the olfactory bulb, and this effect is blocked by CGRP antibodies (DENIS-DONINI 1989).

Intracerebroventricular and systemic injections of CGRP, but also of calcitonin, inhibit gastric acid secretion (HUGHES et al. 1984; LENZ et al. 1984, 1985; KRAENZLIN et al. 1985; PAPPAS et al. 1986; UMEDA and OKADA 1987; MORLEY et al. 1981). Intravenous injection of antibodies to CGRP prevented the systemic, but not the central, inhibition of gastric acid secretion by CGRP (LENZ et al. 1984). Inhibition of gastric secretion in rats was recognized with unchanged mucosal blood flow (LEUNG et al. 1987). Human CGRP II, unlike CGRP I, and calcitonin inhibit gastric acid secretion in humans (BEGLINGER et al. 1988). Pentagastrin-stimulated acid secretion was also suppressed by human CGRP II, unlike human CGRP I, in rabbits where the stimulation of blood flow to the stomach was indistinguishable (BAUERFEIND et al. 1989). The results point to differentiated regulatory functions of the two closely related CGRPs on gastric blood flow and gastric acid secretion. CGRP and calcitonin inhibit the secretion of gastrointestinal hormones such as somatostatin, gastrin, and pancreatic glucagon in man (Koop et al. 1987; Kraenzlin et al. 1985; Stevenson et al. 1985; Yamatani et al. 1986; Dunning and Taborsky 1987; Scott Helton et al. 1990; Chiba et al. 1980). Relaxation of gastric smooth muscle by CGRP was linked to calcium channels and may be mediated by prostaglandins (Katsoulis and Conlon 1989). Subcutaneous injections of CGRP prevented ulcers in rats (Maggi et al. 1987a).

Both central and peripheral administration of CGRP and calcitonin suppress pancreatic exocrine function, esophageal contraction, food intake, intestinal motility, and gastrointestinal transit (Rattan et al. 1988; Lenz and Brown 1990; Nealon et al. 1989; Krahn et al. 1984; Freed et al. 1979; Bueno et al. 1986; Lenz 1988). Incubation of pancreatic acini with CGRP, on the other hand, stimulated amylase secretion by a cyclic AMP-dependent mechanism (Zhou et al. 1986). Intravenous administration of human calcitonin also enhanced salivary amylase output (Drack et al. 1976). Differential responses of the two peptides administered centrally, systemi-cally, and locally, and CGRP and/or calcitonin receptor interaction, and detailed dose-response relationships remain to be carried out in the gastro-intestinal system.

Hypocalcemic action of CGRP obtained in high amounts in relation to those of calcitonin is presumably mediated through calcitonin receptors on osteoclasts, exhibiting cross-reaction and cross-tachyphylaxis between the two peptides (Roos et al. 1986; D'Souza et al. 1986) (see above).

The CGRP potentiation of irritant actions and plasma protein extravasation brought about by substance P may be related to the presence of the two peptides in the same spinal neurons (Wiesenfeld-Hallin et al. 1984; Gamse and Saria 1985). To this end, CGRP was found to inhibit a substance P endopeptidase, and this may represent a rationale for the colocalization and cosecretion of the two peptides (Le Greves et al. 1985; Saria et al. 1986). Besides, CGRP was shown to stimulate the release of acetylcholine from myenteric plexus neurons (Mulholland and Jaffer 1990).

III. Other Gene Products

The N- and C-terminal peptides flanking calcitonin within the procalcitonin sequence are released in normal human subjects in response to intravenous calcium (Born et al. 1991) (see above). Consistent biological effects remain to be elucidated. According to Burns et al. (1989b), the N-terminal flanking peptide PAS-57 is a growth factor with mitogenic activity in normal and neoplastic human osteoblasts. The originally described hypocalcemic action of the C-terminal flanking peptide PDN-21, or katacalcin, was subsequently not confirmed (Macintyre et al. 1984; Roos et al. 1986). These peptides, although released from thyroid C cells in a calcium-dependent manner, are in search of a defined biological function.

Islet amyloid polypeptide (IAPP) or amylin has about 50% structural homology with CGRP (WESTERMARK et al. 1986; NISHI et al. 1989). IAPP is principally synthesized and located in the pancreas. In response to glucose, IAPP is cosecreted with insulin (KANATSUKA et al. 1989; KAHN et al. 1990). Inhibition of insulin secretion by IAPP and CGRP is questionable (OHSAWA et al. 1989; O'BRIEN et al. 1990; PETTERSSON and AHRÉN 1988), but both IAPP and CGRP suppress glycogen synthesis in the skeletal musculature (LEIGHTON and COOPER 1988; KREUTTER et al. 1989). As a result, during hyper-insulinemic glucose-clamp studies in rats both IAPP and CGRP suppress glucose disposal and cause insulin resistance (MOLINA et al. 1990). The effects have evoked a potential role of IAPP in the pathogenesis of non-insulin-dependent diabetes mellitus (COOPER et al. 1989). Much like CGRP, IAPP inhibits bone resorption at concentrations very much higher than those of calcitonin (DATTA et al. 1989). The differential role(s) of IAPP and of CGRP have so far not been defined.

E. Clinical Implications

I. Calcitonin

Calcitonin together with the N-terminal and C-terminal flanking peptides PAS-57 and PDN-21 of procalcitonin are the predominant calcitonin gene products useful as tumor markers in C-cell hyperplasia and MTC (ITTNER et al. 1985; BORN et al. 1991). Both inhibition of bone resorption and stimulation of the urinary calcium excretion by calcitonin lower serum calcium levels. However, calcitonin only minimally contributes to the homeostatic regulation of serum calcium concentrations in man, which are unaltered in thyroidectomized patients with low circulating levels of calcitonin as well as in MTC patients with excessive secretion.

Nonetheless, calcitonin is useful as an antiresorptive agent in the treatment of patients with high bone turnover, and increased bone breakdown, e.g., in postmenopausal osteoporosis and in Paget's disease (GRUBER et al. 1984; ALOIA et al. 1985; MAZZUOLI et al. 1990; SINGER and MILLS 1984). Some patients are responsive to salmon calcitonin for only limited periods. Salmon calcitonin, differing from human calcitonin in 16 of the 32 amino acids, has been used widely in therapy, and antibody production is recognized in up to 78% of treated patients (SINGER et al. 1972b; HADDAD and CALDWELL 1972). As a result, clinical resistance due to neutralizing antibodies has been observed in up to 50% of the patients treated (LEVY et al. 1988; MUFF et al. 1991). The experience with the use of human calcitonin is more limited. Nonetheless, human calcitonin effectively lowered bone turnover in patients previously resistant to salmon calcitonin because of neutralizing antibodies (MUFF et al. 1990). The contribution of receptor downregulation and the sensitivity of osteoclasts to the prolonged administration of human calcitonin remain to be delineated (Tashjian et al. 1978; Bouizar et al. 1987). Potent analgesic properties of calcitonin in the absence of relevant side effects enhance the importance of the peptide as a useful therapeutic agent of raised bone breakdown (Pecile et al. 1975; Pontiroli 1985). Recently developed nasal formulations of both salmon and human calcitonin are more practical than the earlier used parenteral administration (Reginster et al. 1987; Muff et al. 1990).

II. Calcitonin Gene-Related Peptide

Calcitonin gene-related peptide is a neuropeptide released at target tissues locally. Nonetheless, intravenous administration of CGRP elicits biological effects such as arterial vasodilatation at rates lower than most hormones which reach their targets through the circulation in classical endocrine fashion. As a result, CGRP is probably the most potent vasodilator in normal human subjects. Tissue selectivity such as stimulation of the blood flow in the skin and the common carotid artery at the expense of the superior mesenteric artery are noteworthy actions (Jäger et al. 1990). As a consequence possibly of enhanced blood flow to the brain, CGRP corrected neurological deficits following surgery of intracranial aneurysms causing subarachnoid hemorrhage (Johnston et al. 1990).

In recent studies, CGRP improved myocardial contractility in patients with congestive heart failure refractory to digoxin (Gennari et al. 1990). As a result cardiac output was increased and the systemic and pulmonary vascular resistance were reduced (Anand et al. 1991).

F. Conclusions

Synthesis of calcitonin and CGRP I is directed by the same gene (*CALC I*), and distinct splice acceptor sites 5′ to calcitonin- and CGRP I-encoding exons are proposed to function as *cis*-regulatory elements for the predominant production of calcitonin mRNA in thyroid C cells and of CGRP mRNA in neuronal tissues (Emeson et al. 1989; Adema et al. 1990). Structural similarities between calcitonin and CGRP-coding sequences suggest that they are derived from a common primordial sequence (Jonas et al. 1985). Proposed local replications of a common ancestral gene are consistent with the observed colocalization on chromosome 11 in man of the three structurally closely related *CALC I*, *CALC II*, and *CALC III* genomic loci (Höppener et al. 1984, 1985, 1988). The minimal structural differences among all known CGRPs suggest strong evolutionary constraints and more vitally important functions of CGRP as compared to those of calcitonin.

Calcitonin and CGRP exert a wide spectrum of biological properties, but physiological functions, if any, of N- and C-terminal flanking peptides within the calcitonin and CGRP precursor proteins remain to be elucidated. Calcitonin is produced in the thyroid C cells, and main targets are the kidney and bone. However, calcitonin is also found in the hypothalamus and the pituitary gland, and high-affinity binding sites for salmon [^{125}I]calcitonin have been observed in the midbrain and brainstem (CATHERWOOD et al. 1987; FISCHER et al. 1981a,b). Suppression of osteoclastic bone resorption and stimulation of the urinary excretion of calcium, phosphate, sodium, and chloride, and of 1,25-dihydroxyvitamin D production in the kidney are brought about through interaction of calcitonin with specific receptors linked to adenylate cyclase activation and raised free cytosolic calcium concentrations (MARX et al. 1972; MALGAROLI et al. 1989). An important central effect of calcitonin is the inhibition of pain perception (PECILE et al. 1975).

Limited structural homology between calcitonin and CGRP probably accounts for a weak hypocalcemic effect by 500 to 1000 times higher amounts of CGRP as compared to calcitonin. Overlapping biological properties of calcitonin and CGRP are prominent in the gastrointestinal system. The most sensitive effect of CGRP shared by calcitonin in high amounts is the vasodilatation recognized as facial flushing, and stimulation of blood flow through the carotid and coronary arteries (BRAIN et al. 1985). With higher amounts of CGRP generalized suppression of vascular resistance causes a lowering especially of the diastolic arterial pressure, and directly and indirectly a stimulation of the heart rate (JÄGER et al. 1990). Relaxation of the smooth muscle tone is not restricted to the vascular system, but is also observed in the gastrointestinal tract, uterus, and kidney. In the latter, prominent effects include relaxation of renal mesangial cells and vasodilatation (VILLARREAL et al. 1988; KURTZ et al. 1989), but CGRP also enhances the renin-angiotensin-aldosterone system, through stimulation of renin activity in renal juxtaglomerular cells directly, and indirectly as a consequence of vasodilatation and hypotension (KURTZ et al. 1988). At the skeletal musculature end plates CGRP, which is colocalized with acetylcholine, stimulates acetylcholine receptor synthesis. Together with the rapid and short-acting acetylcholine, CGRP serves as a long-term activator of the motoneuron-muscular junction (FONTAINE et al. 1987; NEW and MUDGE 1986; MILES et al. 1989; LAUFER and CHANGEUX 1989). Most actions of CGRP are associated with stimulation of cyclic AMP production in target organs. The potentiation of biological effects of substance P (WIESENFELD-HALLIN et al. 1984; GAMSE and SARIA 1985) through inhibition of its proteolytic degradation (LE GREVES et al. 1985) by CGRP also confers physiological relevance to the observed coexistence of both peptides in the same nerve fiber.

The N-terminal amino acid ring structure of CGRP is essential for the cardiovascular effects of CGRP, whereas the C-terminal human CGRP I (8–37) and (12–37) fragments exert potent antagonistic properties (DENNIS et al. 1989, 1990; HAN et al. 1990; GARDINER et al. 1990). Receptor heterogeneity is suggested by the weaker antagonistic effects of CGRP-(8–37) on the relaxation of the rat vas deferens by intact CGRP (1–37) in relation to the suppression of the contractility of guinea pig atrial preparations (DENNIS et al. 1990). Distinct binding proteins for the highly homologous CGRP I and II have so far not been identified, but subtle differences in the regional distribution of [^{125}I]human CGRP I and II binding sites in the hypothalamus (Henke et al. 1987) and in the biological properties of the two peptides have been recognized. To this end, CGRP II, unlike CGRP I, inhibits gastric acid secretion in man (Beglinger et al. 1988). The structural analysis and expression of calcitonin and CGRP receptors, site-directed mutations, and generation of specific receptor antibodies are required to further elucidate distinct actions of calcitonin and of CGRP I and II.

References

Abou-Samra A-B, Jüppner H, Force T, Freeman MW, Kong X-F, Schipani E, Urena P, Richards J, Bonventre JV, Potts JT Jr, Kronenberg HM, Segre GV (1992) Expression cloning of a common receptor for parathyroid hormone and parathyroid hormone-related peptide from rat osteoblast-like cells: a single receptor stimulates intracellular accumulation of both cAMP and inositol trisphosphates and increases intracellular free calcium. Proc Natl Acad Sci 89:2732–2736

Adema GJ, Bovenberg RAL, Jansz HS, Baas PD (1988) Unusual branch point selection involved in splicing of the alternatively processed calcitonin/CGRP-I pre-mRNA. Nucleic Acids Res 16:9513–9526

Adema GJ, van Hulst KL, Baas PD (1990) Uridine branch acceptor is a *cis*-acting element involved in regulation of the alternative processing of calcitonin/CGRP-I pre-mRNA. Nucleic Acids Res 18:5365–5373

Ahrén B, Ekman R, Laurberg P (1989) Calcium stimulates the release of calcitonin gene-related peptide from the canine thyroid. Am J Physiol 256:E597–E599

Alevizaki M, Shiraishi A, Rassool FV, Ferrier GJM, MacIntyre I, Legon S (1986) The calcitonin-like sequence of the β CGRP gene. FEBS Lett 206:47–52

Ali-Rachedi A, Varndell IM, Facer P, Hillyard CJ, Craig RK, MacIntyre I, Polak JM (1983) Immunocytochemical localisation of katacalcin, a calcium-lowering hormone cleaved from the human calcitonin precursor. J Clin Endocrinol Metab 57:680–682

Aloia JF, Vaswani A, Kapoor A, Yeh JK, Cohn SH (1985) Treatment of osteoporosis with calcitonin, with and without growth hormone. Metabolism 34:124–129

Amara SG, Jonas V, Rosenfeld MG, Ong ES, Evans RM (1982) Alternative RNA processing in calcitonin gene expression generates mRNAs encoding different polypeptide products. Nature 298:240–244

Amara SG, Evans RM, Rosenfeld MG (1984) Calcitonin/calcitonin gene-related peptide transcription unit: tissue-specific expression involves selective use of alternative polyadenylation sites. Mol Cell Biol 4:2151–2160

Amara SG, Arriza JL, Leff SE, Swanson LW, Evans RM, Rosenfeld MG (1985) Expression in brain of a messenger RNA encoding a novel neuropeptide homologous to calcitonin gene-related peptide. Science 229:1094–1097

Anand IS, Gurden J, Wander GS, O'Gara P, Harding SE, Ferrari R, Cornacchiari A, Panzali A, Wahi PL, Poole-Wilson PA (1991) Cardiovascular and hormonal effects of calcitonin gene-related peptide in congestive heart failure. J Am Coll Cardiol 17:208–217

Ardaillou R, Paillard F, Scraer J, Vallee G (1973) Compared kinetics of salmon and human radioiodinated calcitonin in man. Horm Metab Res 5:232–233

Arias J, Scopsi L, Fischer JA, Larsson LI (1989) Light- and electron-microscopic localization of calcitonin, calcitonin gene-related peptide, somatostatin and C-terminal gastrin/cholecystokinin immunoreactivities in rat thyroid. Histochemistry 91:265–272

Arvidsson U, Cullheim S, Ulfhake B, Hökfelt T, Terenius L (1989) Altered levels of calcitonin gene-related peptide (CGRP)-like immunoreactivity of cat lumbar motoneurons after chronic spinal cord transection. Brain Res 489:387–391

Arvidsson U, Schalling M, Cullheim S, Ulfhake B, Terenius L, Verhofstad A, Hökfelt T (1990) Evidence for coexistence between calcitonin gene-related peptide and serotonin in the bulbospinal pathway in the monkey. Brain Res 532:47–57

Avioli LV, Shieber W, Kipnis DM (1971) Role of glucagon and adrenergic receptors in thyrocalcitonin release in the dog. Endocrinology 88:1337–1340

Baron R, Neff L, Brown W, Louvard D, Courtoy PJ (1990) Selective internalization of the apical plasma membrane and rapid redistribution of lysosomal enzymes and mannose 6-phosphate receptors during osteoclast inactivation by calcitonin. J Cell Sci 97:439–447

Batten TFC, Cambre ML (1989) Calcitonin gene-related peptide-like immunoreactive fibres innervating the hypothalamic inferior lobes of teleost fishes. Neurosci Lett 98:1–7

Bauerfeind P, Hof R, Hof A, Cucala M, Siegrist S, von Ritter C, Fischer JA, Blum AL (1989) Effects of hCGRP I and II on gastric blood flow and acid secretion in anesthetized rabbits. Am J Physiol 256:G145–G149

Baylin SB, Höppener JWM, de Bustros A, Steenbergh PH, Lips CJM, Nelkin BD (1986) DNA methylation patterns of the calcitonin gene in human lung cancers and lymphomas. Cancer Res 46:2917–2922

Beglinger C, Born W, Hildebrand P, Ensinck JW, Burkhardt F, Fischer JA, Gyr K (1988) Calcitonin gene-related peptides I and II and calcitonin: distinct effects on gastric acid secretion in humans. Gastroenterology 95:958–965

Besnard P, Jousset V, Garel J-M (1989) Additive effects of dexamethasone and calcium on the calcitonin mRNA level in adrenalectomized rats. FEBS Lett 258:293–296

Bijvoet OLM, van der Sluys Veer J, de Vries HR, van Koppen ATJ (1971) Natriuretic effect of calcitonin in man. N Engl J Med 284:681–688

Birnbaum RS, Mahoney WC, Roos BA (1986) Biosynthesis of calcitonin by a rat medullary thyroid carcinoma cell line. J Biol Chem 261:699–703

Body J-J, Heath H III (1983) Estimates of circulating monomeric calcitonin: physiological studies in normal and thyroidectomized man. J Clin Endocrinol Metab 57:897–903

Bone HG III, Catherwood BD, Deftos LJ (1983) Extraction of a substance with calcitonin-like immunoreactivity from pituitary glands of intact and thyroidectomized rats. Calcified Tissue Int 35:620–623

Born W, Beglinger C, Fischer JA (1991) Diagnostic relevance of the amino-terminal cleavage peptide of procalcitonin (PAS-57), calcitonin and calcitonin gene-related peptide in medullary thyroid carcinoma patients. Regul Pept 32:311–319

Bouizar Z, Fouchereau-Peron M, Taboulet J, Moukhtar MS, Milhaud G (1986) Purification and characterization of calcitonin receptors in rat kidney membranes by covalent cross-linking techniques. Eur J Biochem 155:141–147

Bouizar Z, Rostène WH, Milhaud G (1987) Down-regulation of rat kidney calcitonin receptors by salmon calcitonin infusion evidenced by autoradiography. Proc Natl Acad Sci USA 84:5125–5128

Bovenberg RAL, van de Meerendonk WPM, Baas PD, Steenbergh PH, Lips CJM, Jansz HS (1986) Model for alternative RNA processing in human calcitonin gene expression. Nucleic Acids Res 14:8785–8803

Braga P, Ferri S, Santagostino A, Olgiati VR, Pecile A (1978) Lack of opiate receptor involvement in centrally induced calcitonin analgesia. Life Sci 22:971–978

Brain SD, Williams TJ, Tippins JR, Morris HR, MacIntyre I (1985) Calcitonin gene-related peptide is a potent vasodilator. Nature 313:54–56

Broad PM, Symes AJ, Thakker RV, Craig RK (1989) Structure and methylation of the human calcitonin/α-CGRP gene. Nucleic Acids Res 17:6999–7011

Bueno L, Fargeas MJ, Julie P (1986) Effects of calcitonin and CGRP alone or in combination on food intake and forestomach (reticulum) motility in sheep. Physiol Behav 36:907–911

Burns DM, Birnbaum RS, Roos BA (1989a) A neuroendocrine peptide derived from the amino-terminal half of rat procalcitonin. Mol Endocrinol 3:140–147

Burns DM, Forstrom JM, Friday KE, Howard GA, Roos BA (1989b) Procalcitonin's amino-terminal cleavage peptide is a bone-cell mitogen. Proc Natl Acad Sci USA 86:9519–9523

Cadieux A, Springall DR, Mulderry PK, Rodrigo J, Ghatei MA, Terenghi G, Bloom SR, Polak JM (1986) Occurrence, distribution and ontogeny of CGRP immunoreactivity in the rat lower respiratory tract: effect of capsaicin treatment and surgical denervations. Neuroscience 19:605–627

Cadieux A, Lanoue C, Sirois P, Barabé J (1990) Carbamylcholine- and 5-hydroxy-tryptamine-induced contraction in rat isolated airways: inhibition by calcitonin gene-related peptide. Br J Pharmacol 101:193–199

Catherwood BD, Deftos LJ, Spiess J (1987) Complete sequence analysis of calcitonin extracted from porcine pituitary. In: Cohn DV, Martin TJ, Meunier PJ (eds) Calcium regulation and bone metabolism. Basic and clinical aspects, vol 9. Excerpta Medica, Amsterdam, pp 82–87 (Proceedings of the 9th International Conference on Calcium Regulating Hormones and Bone Metabolism, 25 Oct–1 Nov, Nice 1986)

Chabre O, Conklin BR, Lin HY, Lodish HF, Wilson E, Ives HE, Catanzariti L, Hemmings BA, Bourne HR (1992) A recombinant calcitonin receptor independently stimulates 3',5'-cyclic adenosine monophosphate and Ca^{2+}/insitol phosphate signaling pathways. Mol Endocrinol 6:551–556

Chakder S, Rattan S (1990) [Tyr^0]-Calcitonin gene-related peptide 28–37 (rat) as a putative antagonist of calcitonin gene-related peptide responses on opossum internal anal sphincter smooth muscle. J Pharmacol Exp Ther 253:200–206

Chambers TJ, Chambers JC, Symonds J, Darby JA (1986) The effect of human calcitonin on the cytoplasmic spreading of rat osteoclasts. J Clin Endocrinol Metab 63:1080–1085

Chiba T, Taminato T, Kadowaki S, Goto Y, Mori K, Seino Y, Abe H, Chihara K, Matsukura S, Fujita T, Kondo T (1980) Effects of [$Asu^{1,7}$]-eel calcitonin on gastric somatostatin and gastrin release. Gut 21:94–97

Chiba T, Yamaguchi A, Yamatani T, Nakamura A, Morishita T, Inui T, Fukase M, Noda T, Fujita T (1989) Calcitonin gene-related peptide receptor antagonist human CGRP-(8–37). Am J Physiol 256:E331–E335

Chihara K, Iwasaki J, Iwasaki Y, Minamitani N, Kaji H, Fujita T (1982) Central nervous system effect of calcitonin: stimulation of prolactin release in rats. Brain Res 248:331–339

Clark MB, Williams CC, Nathanson BM, Horton RE, Glass HI, Foster GV (1974) Metabolic fate of human calcitonin in the dog. J Endocrinol 61:199–210

Clementi G, Nicoletti F, Patacchioli F, Prato A, Patti F, Fiore CE, Matera M, Scapagnini U (1983) Hypoprolactinemic action of calcitonin and the tuberoinfundibular dopaminergic system. J Neurochem 40:885–886

Clementi G, Drago F, Prato A, Cavaliere S, di Benedetto A, Leone F, Scapagnini U, Rodolico G (1984) Effects of calcitonin, parathyroid hormone and its related fragments on acquisition of active avoidance behavior. Physiol Behav 33:913–916

Clementi G, Amico-Roxas M, Rapisarda E, Caruso A, Prato A, Trombadore S, Priolo G, Scapagnini U (1985) The analgesic activity of calcitonin and the central serotonergic system. Eur J Pharmacol 108:71–75

Conlon JM, Grimelius L, Thim L (1988a) Structural characterization of a high-molecular-mass form of calcitonin [procalcitonin-(60–116)-peptide] and its corresponding N-terminal flanking peptide [procalcitonin-(1–57)-peptide] in a human medullary thyroid carcinoma. Biochem J 256:245–250

Conlon JM, McGregor GP, Wallin G, Grimelius L, Thim L (1988b) Molecular forms of katacalcin, calcitonin gene-related peptide and gastrin-releasing peptide, in a human medullary thyroid carcinoma. Cancer Res 48:2412–2416

Cooper CW, Schwesinger WH, Mahgoub AM, Ontjes DA (1971) Thyrocalcitonin: stimulation of secretion by pentagastrin. Science 172:1238–1240

Cooper GJS, Day AJ, Willis AC, Roberts AN, Reid KBM, Leighton B (1989) Amylin and the amylin gene: structure, function and relationship to islet amyloid and to diabetes mellitus. Biochim Biophys Acta 1014:247–258

Copp DH, Davidson AGF, Cheney B (1961) Evidence for a new parathyroid hormone which lowers blood calcium. Can Fed Biol Soc 4:17

Copp DH, Cockroft DW, Kueh Y (1967) Calcitonin from ultimobranchial glands of dogfish and chickens. Science 158:924–925

Cortés R, Arvidsson U, Schalling M, Ceccatelli S, Hökfelt T (1990) In situ hybridization studies on mRNAs for cholecystokinin, calcitonin gene-related peptide and choline acetyltransferase in the lower brain stem, spinal cord and dorsal root ganglia of rat and guinea pig with special reference to motoneurons. J Chem Neuroanat 3:467–485

Cote GJ, Gagel RF (1986) Dexamethasone differentially affects the levels of calcitonin and calcitonin gene-related peptide mRNAs expressed in a human medullary thyroid carcinoma cell line. J Biol Chem 261:15524–15528

Cote GJ, Gould JA, Huang S-CE, Gagel RF (1987a) Studies of short-term secretion of peptides produced by alternative RNA processing. Mol Cell Endocrinol 53:211–219

Cote GJ, Rogers DG, Huang ESC, Gagel RF (1987b) The effect of 1,25-dihydroxy-vitamin D3 treatment on calcitonin and calcitonin gene-related peptide mRNA levels in cultured human thyroid C-cells. Biochem Biophys Res Commun 149: 239–243

Crenshaw EB III, Russo AF, Swanson LW, Rosenfeld MG (1987) Neuron-specific alternative RNA processing in transgenic mice expressing a metallothioncin-calcitonin fusion gene. Cell 49:389–398

Crossman DC, Dashwood MR, Brain SD, McEwan J, Pearson JD (1990) Action of calcitonin gene-related peptide upon bovine vascular endothelial and smooth muscle cells grown in isolation and co-culture. Br J Pharmacol 99:71–76

Dalsgaard C-J, Jernbeck J, Stains W, Kjartansson J, Hægerstrand A, Hökfelt T, Brodin E, Cuello AC, Brown JC (1989) Calcitonin gene-related peptide-like immunoreactivity in nerve fibers in the human skin. Histochemistry 91:35–38

Datta HK, Zaidi M, Wimalawansa SJ, Ghatei MA, Beacham JL, Bloom SR, MacIntyre I (1989) In vivo and in vitro effects of amylin and amylin-amide on calcium metabolism in the rat and rabbit. Biochem Biophys Res Commun 162:876–881

De Beaurepaire R, Suaudeau C (1988) Anorectic effect of calcitonin, neurotensin and bombesin infused in the area of the rostral part of the nucleus of the tractus solitarius in the rat. Peptides 9:729–733

De Bustros A, Baylin SB, Berger CL, Roos BA, Leong SS, Nelkin BD (1985) Phorbol esters increase calcitonin gene transcription and decrease c-myc mRNA levels in cultured human medullary thyroid carcinoma. J Biol Chem 260:98–104

De Bustros A, Baylin SB, Levine MA, Nelkin BD (1986) Cyclic AMP and phorbol esters separately induce growth inhibition, calcitonin secretion, and calcitonin gene transcription in cultured human medullary thyroid carcinoma. J Biol Chem 261:8036–8041

De Bustros A, Lee RY, Compton D, Tsong TY, Baylin SB, Nelkin BD (1990) Differential utilization of calcitonin gene regulatory DNA sequences in cultured lines of medullary thyroid carcinoma and small-cell lung carcinoma. Mol Cell Biol 10:1773–1778

Deftos LJ, Roos BA (1989) Medullary thyroid carcinoma and calcitonin gene expression. Bone Miner Res 6:267–316

Denis-Donini S (1989) Expression of dopaminergic phenotypes in the mouse olfactory bulb induced by the calcitonin gene-related peptide. Nature 339:701–703

Dennis T, Fournier A, St Pierre S, Quirion R (1989) Structure-activity profile of calcitonin gene-related peptide in peripheral and brain tissues. Evidence for receptor multiplicity. J Pharmacol Exp Ther 251:718–725

Dennis T, Fournier A, Cadieux A, Pomerleau F, Jolicoeur FB, St Pierre S, Quirion R (1990) hCGRP$_{8-37}$, a calcitonin gene-related peptide antagonist revealing calcitonin gene-related peptide receptor heterogeneity in brain and periphery. J Pharmacol Exp Ther 254:123–128

Diez-Guerra FJ, Zaidi M, Bevis P, MacIntyre I, Emson PC (1988) Evidence for release of calcitonin gene-related peptide and neurokinin A from sensory nerve endings in vivo. Neuroscience 25:839–846

Dipette DJ, Schwarzenberger K, Kerr N, Holland OB (1989) Dose-dependent systemic and regional hemodynamic effects of calcitonin gene-related peptide. Am J Med Sci 297:65–70

Dotti-Sigrist S, Born W, Fischer JA (1988) Identification of a receptor for calcitonin gene-related peptides I and II in human cerebellum. Biochem Biophys Res Commun 151:1081–1087

Drack GT, Koelz HR, Blum AL (1976) Human calcitonin stimulates salivary amylase output in man. Gut 17:620–623

D'Souza SM, MacIntyre I, Girgis SI, Mundy GR (1986) Human synthetic calcitonin gene-related peptide inhibits bone resorption in vitro. Endocrinology 119:58–61

Dunning BE, Taborsky GJ Jr (1987) Calcitonin gene-related peptide: a potent and selective stimulator of gastrointestinal somatostatin secretion. Endocrinology 120:1774–1781

Edbrooke MR, Parker D, McVey JH, Riley JH, Sorenson GD, Pettengill OS, Craig RK (1985) Expression of the human calcitonin/CGRP gene in lung and thyroid carcinoma. EMBO J 4:715–724

Edvinsson L, Fredholm BB, Hamel E, Jansen I, Verrecchia C (1985) Perivascular peptides relax cerebral arteries concomitant with stimulation of cyclic adenosine monophosphate accumulation or release of an endothelium-derived relaxing factor in the cat. Neurosci Lett 58:213–217

Edvinsson L, Ekman R, Jansen I, McCulloch J, Uddman R (1987) Calcitonin gene-related peptide and cerebral blood vessels: distribution and vasomotor effects. J Cereb Blood Flow Metab 7:720–728

Edwards RM, Trizna W (1990) Calcitonin gene-related peptide: effects on renal arteriolar tone and tubular cAMP levels. Am J Physiol 258:F121–F125

Elie C, Moukhtar MS, Milhaud G, Cressent M (1990) Hypoprolactinemic effect of calcitonin gene-related peptide in the rat. Neuropeptides 16:109–113

Emeson RB, Hedjran F, Yeakley JM, Guise JW, Rosenfeld MG (1989) Alternative production of calcitonin and CGRP mRNA is regulated at the calcitonin-specific splice acceptor. Nature 341:76–80

Fahim A, Rettori V, McCann SM (1990) The role of calcitonin gene-related peptide in the control of growth hormone and prolactin release. Neuroendocrinology 51:688–693

Fargeas MJ, Fioramonti J, Buéno L (1984) Prostaglandin E$_2$: a neuromodulator in the central control of gastrointestinal motility and feeding behavior by calcitonin. Science 225:1050–1052

Findlay DM, Michelangeli VP, Robinson PJ (1989) Protein kinase-C-induced down-regulation of calcitonin receptors and calcitonin-activated adenylate cyclase in T47D and BEN cells. Endocrinology 125:2656–2663

Fischer JA, Sagar SM, Martin JB (1981a) Characterization and regional distribution of calcitonin binding sites in the rat brain. Life Sci 29:663–671

Fischer JA, Tobler PH, Kaufmann M, Born W, Henke H, Cooper PE, Sagar SM, Martin JB (1981b) Calcitonin: regional distribution of the hormone and its binding sites in the human brain and pituitary. Proc Natl Acad Sci USA 78:7801–7805

Fischer JA, Tobler PH, Henke H, Tschopp FA (1983) Salmon and human calcitonin-like peptides coexist in the human thyroid and brain. J Clin Endocrinol Metab 57:1314–1316

Fisher LA, Kikkawa DO, Rivier JE, Amara SG, Evans RM, Rosenfeld MG, Vale WW, Brown MR (1983) Stimulation of noradrenergic sympathetic outflow by calcitonin gene-related peptide. Nature 305:534–536

Fontaine B, Klarsfeld A, Hökfelt T, Changeux JP (1986) Calcitonin gene-related peptide, a peptide present in spinal cord motoneurons, increases the number of acetylcholine receptors in primary cultures of chick embryo myotubes. Neurosci Lett 71:59–65

Fontaine B, Klarsfeld A, Changeux JP (1987) Calcitonin gene-related peptide and muscle activity regulate acetylcholine receptor α-subunit mRNA levels by distinct intracellular pathways. J Cell Biol 105:1337–1342

Franco-Cereceda A, Gennari C, Nami R, Agnusdei D, Pernow J, Lundberg JM, Fischer JA (1987a) Cardiovascular effects of calcitonin gene-related peptides I and II in man. Circ Res 60:393–397

Franco-Cereceda A, Henke H, Lundberg JM, Petermann JB, Hökfelt T, Fischer JA (1987b) Calcitonin gene-related peptide (CGRP) in capsaicin-sensitive substance P-immunoreactive sensory neurons in animals and man: distribution and release by capsaicin. Peptides 8:399–410

Franco-Cereceda A, Saria A, Lundberg JM (1989) Differential release of calcitonin gene-related peptide and neuropeptide Y from the isolated heart by capsaicin, ischaemia, nicotine, bradykinin and ouabain. Acta Physiol Scand 135:173–187

Freed WJ, Perlow MJ, Wyatt RJ (1979) Calcitonin: inhibitory effect on eating in rats. Science 206:850–852

Fried G, Franck J, Brodin E, Born W, Fischer JA, Hiort W, Hökfelt T (1989) Evidence for differential storage of calcitonin gene-related peptide, substance P and serotonin in synaptosomal vesicles of rat spinal cord. Brain Res 499:315–324

Gamse R, Saria A (1985) Potentiation of tachykinin-induced plasma protein extravasation by calcitonin gene-related peptide. Eur J Pharmacol 114:61–66

Gardiner SM, Compton AM, Bennett T (1989) Regional hemodynamic effects of calcitonin gene-related peptide. Am J Physiol 256:R332–R338

Gardiner SM, Compton AM, Kemp PA, Bennett T, Bose C, Foulkes R, Hughes B (1990) Antagonistic effect of human α-CGRP [8–37] on the in vivo regional haemodynamic actions of human α-CGRP. Biochem Biophys Res Commun 171:938–943

Gennari C, Fischer JA (1985) Cardiovascular action of calcitonin gene-related peptide in humans. Calcif Tissue Int 37:581–584

Gennari C, Nami R, Agnusdei D, Fischer JA (1990) Improved cardiac performance with human calcitonin gene-related peptide in patients with congestive heart failure. Cardiovasc Res 24:239–241

Geppetti P, Maggi CA, Perretti F, Frilli S, Manzini S (1988) Simultaneous release by bradykinin of substance P- and calcitonin gene-related peptide immunoreactivities from capsaicin-sensitive structures in guinea-pig heart. Br J Pharmacol 94:288–290

Geppetti P, Baldi E, Castellucci A, del Bianco E, Santicioli P, Maggi CA, Lippe IT, Amann R, Skofitsch G, Theodorsson E, Manzini S (1989) Calcitonin gene-related peptide in the rat kidney: occurrence, sensitivity to capsaicin, and stimulation of adenylate cyclase. Neuroscience 30:503–513

Geppetti P, Tramontana M, Santicioli P, del Bianco E, Giuliani S, Maggi CA (1990) Bradykinin-induced release of calcitonin gene-related peptide from capsaicin-sensitive nerves in guinea-pig atria: mechanism of action and calcium requirements. Neuroscience 38:687–692

Gibbins IL, Furness JB, Costa M, MacIntyre I, Hillyard CJ, Girgis S (1985) Co-localization of calcitonin gene-related peptide-like immunoreactivity with substance P in cutaneous, vascular and visceral sensory neurons of guinea pigs. Neurosci Lett 57:125–130

Gibbins IL, Furness JB, Costa M (1987) Pathway-specific patterns of the co-existence of substance P, calcitonin gene-related peptide, cholecystokinin and dynorphin in neurons of the dorsal root ganglia of the guinea-pig. Cell Tissue Res 248:417–437

Gibson SJ, Polak JM, Bloom SR, Sabate IM, Mulderry PM, Ghatei MA, McGregor GP, Morrison JFB, Kelly JS, Evans RM, Rosenfeld MG (1984) Calcitonin gene-related peptide immunoreactivity in the spinal cord of man and of eight other species. J Neurosci 4:3101–3111

Gibson SJ, Polak JM, Giaid A, Hamid QA, Kar S, Jones PM, Denny P, Legon S, Amara SG, Craig RK, Bloom SR, Penketh RJA, Rodek C, Ibrahim NBN, Dawson A (1988) Calcitonin gene-related peptide messenger RNA is expressed in sensory neurones of the dorsal root ganglia and also in spinal motoneurones in man and rat. Neurosci Lett 91:283–288

Gkonos PJ, Born W, Jones BN, Petermann JB, Keutmann HT, Birnbaum RS, Fischer JA, Roos BA (1986) Biosynthesis of calcitonin gene-related peptide and calcitonin by a human medullary thyroid carcinoma cell line. J Biol Chem 261:14386–14391

Gnaedinger MP, Uehlinger DE, Weidmann P, Sha SG, Muff R, Born W, Rascher W, Fischer JA (1989) Distinct hemodynamic and renal effects of calcitonin gene-related peptide and calcitonin in men. Am J Physiol 257:E848–E854

Goltzman D, Mitchell J (1985) Interaction of calcitonin and calcitonin gene-related peptide at receptor sites in target tissues. Science 227:1343–1345

Goto K, Kimura S, Saito A (1987) Inhibitory effect of calcitonin gene-related peptide on excitation and contraction of smooth muscles of the rat vas deferens. J Pharmacol Exp Ther 241:635–641

Gray TK, Brannan P, Juan D, Morawski SG, Fordtran JS (1976) Ion transport changes during calcitonin-induced intestinal secretion in man. Gastroenterology 71:392–398

Greenberg B, Rhoden K, Barnes P (1987) Calcitonin gene-related peptide (CGRP) is a potent non-endothelium-dependent inhibitor of coronary vasomotor tone. Br J Pharmacol 92:789–794

Gropp C, Luster W, Havemann K (1985) Salmon and human calcitonin like material in lung cancer. Br J Cancer 51:897–901

Gruber HE, Ivey JL, Baylink DJ, Matthews M, Nelp WB, Sisom K, Chestnut CH III (1984) Long-term calcitonin therapy in postmenopausal osteoporosis. Metabolism 33:295–303

Guidobono F, Netti C, Pagani F, Sibilia V, Pecile A, Candeletti S, Ferri S (1986) Relationship of analgesia induced by centrally injected calcitonin to the CNS serotonergic system. Neuropeptides 8:259–271

Gulbenkian S, Merighi A, Wharton J, Varndell IM, Polak JM (1986) Ultrastructural evidence for the coexistence of calcitonin gene-related peptide and substance P in secretory vesicles of peripheral nerves in the guinea pig. J Neurocytol 15:535–542

Haas CA, Streit WJ, Kreutzberg GW (1990) Rat facial motoneurons express increased levels of calcitonin gene-related peptide mRNA in response to axotomy. J Neurosci Res 27:270–275

Haas HG, Dambacher MA, Guncaga J, Lauffenburger T (1971) Renal effects of calcitonin and parathyroid extract in man. J Clin Invest 50:2689–2702

Haddad JG, Caldwell JG (1972) Calcitonin resistance: clinical and immunologic studies in subjects with Paget's disease of bone treated with porcine and salmon calcitonins. J Clin Invest 51:3133–3141

Haller-Brem S, Muff R, Fischer JA (1988) Calcitonin gene-related peptide and calcitonin secretion from a human medullary thyroid carcinoma cell line: effects of ionomycin, phorbol ester and forskolin. J Endocrinol 119:147–152

Ham J, Ellison ML, Lumsden J (1980) Tumour calcitonin. Interaction with specific calcitonin receptors. Biochem J 190:545–550

Han S-P, Naes L, Westfall TC (1990) Inhibition of periarterial nerve stimulation-induced vasodilation of the mesenteric arterial bed by CGRP (8–37) and CGRP receptor desensitization. Biochem Biophys Res Commun 168:786–791

Henke H, Tobler PH, Fischer JA (1983) Localization of salmon calcitonin binding sites in rat brain by autoradiography. Brain Res 272:373–377

Henke H, Tschopp FA, Fischer JA (1985) Distinct binding sites for calcitonin gene-related peptide and salmon calcitonin in rat central nervous system. Brain Res 360:165–171

Henke H, Sigrist S, Lang W, Schneider J, Fischer JA (1987) Comparison of binding sites for the calcitonin gene-related peptides I and II in man. Brain Res 410: 404–408

Hill EL, Elde R (1988) Calcitonin gene-related peptide-immunoreactive nerve fibers in mandibular periosteum of rat: evidence for primary afferent origin. Neurosci Lett 85:172–178

Hirata Y, Takagi Y, Takata S, Fukuda Y, Yoshimi H, Fujita T (1988) Calcitonin gene-related peptide receptor in cultured vascular smooth muscle and endothelial cells. Biochem Biophys Res Commun 151:1113–1121

Holman JJ, Craig RK, Marshall I (1986) Human α- and β-CGRP and rat α-CGRP are coronary vasodilators in the rat. Peptides 7:231–235

Holzer P, Barthó L, Matusák O, Bauer V (1989) Calcitonin gene-related peptide action on intestinal circular muscle. Am J Physiol 256:G546–G552

Homma T, Watanabe M, Hirose S, Kanai A, Kangawa K, Matsuo H (1986) Isolation and determination of the amino acid sequence of chicken calcitonin I from chicken ultimobranchial glands. J Biochem 100:459–467

Höppener JWM, Steenbergh PH, Zandberg J, Bakker E, Pearson PL, Geurts van Kessel AHM, Jansz HS, Lips CJM (1984) Localization of the polymorphic human calcitonin gene on chromosome 11. Hum Genet 66:309–312

Höppener JWM, Steenbergh PH, Zandberg J, Geurts van Kessel AHM, Baylin SB, Nelkin BD, Jansz HS, Lips CJM (1985) The second human calcitonin/CGRP gene is located on chromosome 11. Hum Genet 70:259–263

Höppener JWM, Steenbergh PH, Moonen PJJ, Wagenaar SS, Jansz HS, Lips CJM (1986) Detection of mRNA encoding calcitonin, calcitonin gene-related peptide and proopiomelanocortin in human tumors. Mol Cell Endocrinol 47:125–130

Höppener JWM, Steenbergh PH, Slebos RJC, Visser A, Lips CJM, Jansz HS, Bechet JM, Lenoir GM, Born W, Haller-Brem S, Petermann JB, Fischer JA (1987) Expression of the second calcitonin/calcitonin gene-related peptide gene in Ewing sarcoma cell lines. J Clin Endocrinol Metab 64:809–817

Höppener JWM, Steenbergh PH, Zandberg J, Adema GJ, Geurts van Kessel AHM, Lips CJM, Jansz HS (1988) A third human CALC (pseudo)gene on chromosome 11. FEBS Lett 233:57–63

Horiuchi N, Takahashi H, Matsumoto T, Takahashi N, Shimazawa E, Suda T, Ogata E (1979) Salmon calcitonin-induced stimulation of $1\alpha,25$-Dihydroxychol-ecalciferol synthesis in rats involving a mechanism independent of adenosine $3':5'$-cyclic monophosphate. Biochem J 184:269–275

Hua XY, Theodorsson-Norheim E, Lundberg JM, Kinn A-C, Hökfelt T, Cuello AC (1987) Co-localization of tachykinins and calcitonin gene-related peptide in capsaicin-sensitive afferents in relation to motility effects on the human ureter in vitro. Neuroscience 23:693–703

Hughes JJ, Levine AS, Morley JE, Gosnell BA, Silvis SE (1984) Intraventricular calcitonin gene-related peptide inhibits gastric acid secretion. Peptides 5:665–667

Huwyler R, Born W, Ohnhaus EE, Fischer JA (1979) Plasma kinetics and urinary excretion of exogenous human and salmon calcitonin in man. Am J Physiol 236:E15–E19

Inagaki S, Kito S, Kubota Y, Girgis S, Hillyard CJ, MacIntyre I (1986) Autoradio-graphic localization of calcitonin gene-related peptide binding sites in human and rat brains. Brain Res 374:287–298

Isaac R, Merceron R, Caillens G, Raymond J-P, Ardaillou R (1980) Effects of calcitonin on basal and thyrotropin-releasing hormone-stimulated prolactin secretion in man. J Clin Endocrinol Metab 50:1011–1015

Ishihara T, Nakamura S, Kaziro Y, Takahashi T, Takahashi K, Nagata S (1991) Molecular cloning and expression of a cDNA encoding the secretin receptor. EMBO J 10:1635–1641

Ittner J, Dambacher MA, Born W, Ketelslegers JM, Buysschaert M, Albert PM, Lambert AE, Fischer JA (1985) Diagnostic evaluation of measurements of carboxyl-terminal flanking peptide (PDN-21) of the human calcitonin gene in human serum. J Clin Endocrinol Metab 61:1133–1137

Iwasaki Y, Chihara K, Iwasaki HA, Abe H, Fujita T (1979) Effect of calcitonin on prolactin release in rats. Life Sci 25:1243–1248

Jaeger P, Jones W, Clemens TL, Hayslett JP (1986) Evidence that calcitonin stimulates 1,25-dihydroxyvitamin D production and intestinal absorption of calcium in vivo. J Clin Invest 78:456–461

Jäger K, Muench R, Seifert H, Beglinger C, Bollinger A, Fischer JA (1990) Calcitonin gene-related peptide (CGRP) causes redistribution of blood flow in humans. Eur J Clin Pharmacol 39:491–494

Jennings CGB, Mudge AW (1989) Chick myotubes in culture express high-affinity receptors for calcitonin gene-related peptide. Brain Res 504:199–205

Johnston FG, Bell BA, Robertson IJA, Miller JD, Haliburn C, O'Shaughnessy D, Riddell AJ, O'Laoire SA (1990) Effect of calcitonin gene-related peptide on postoperative neurological deficits after subarachnoid haemorrhage. Lancet 335: 869–872

Jonas V, Lin CR, Kawashima E, Semon D, Swanson LW, Mermod J-J, Evans RM, Rosenfeld MG (1985) Alternative RNA processing events in human calcitonin/calcitonin gene-related peptide gene expression. Proc Natl Acad Sci USA 82: 1994–1998

Ju G, Hökfelt T, Brodin E, Fahrenkrug J, Fischer JA, Frey P, Elde RP, Brown JC (1987) Primary sensory neurons of the rat showing calcitonin gene-related peptide immunoreactivity and their relation to substance P-, somatostatin-, galanin-, vasoactive intestinal polypeptide- and cholecystokinin-immunoreactive ganglion cells. Cell Tissue Res 247:417–431

Jüppner H, Abou-Samra A-B, Freeman M, Kong XF, Schipani E, Richards J, Kolakowski LF Jr, Hock J, Potts JT Jr, Kronenberg HM, Segre GV (1991) A G protein-linked receptor for parathyroid hormone and parathyroid hormone-related peptide. Science 254:1024–1026

Kahn SE, d'Alessio DA, Schwartz MW, Fujimoto WY, Ensinck JW, Taborsky GJ Jr, Porte D Jr (1990) Evidence of cosecretion of islet amyloid polypeptide and insulin by β-cells. Diabetes 39:634–638

Kanatsuka A, Makino H, Ohsawa H, Tokuyama Y, Yamaguchi T, Yoshida S, Adachi M (1989) Secretion of islet amyloid polypeptide in response to glucose. FEBS Lett 259:199–201

Kashihara Y, Sakaguchi M, Kuno M (1989) Axonal transport and distribution of endogenous calcitonin gene-related peptide in rat peripheral nerve. J Neurosci 9:3796–3802

Katsoulis S, Conlon JM (1989) Calcitonin gene-related peptides relax guinea pig and rat gastric smooth muscle. Eur J Pharmacol 161:129–134

Kawai Y, Takami K, Shiosaka S, Emson PC, Hillyard CJ, Girgis S, MacIntyre I, Tohyama M (1985) Topographic localization of calcitonin gene-related peptide in the rat brain: an immunohistochemical analysis. Neuroscience 15:747–763

Kim S, Morimoto S, Kawai Y, Koh E, Onishi T, Ogihara T (1989) Circulating levels of calcitonin gene-related peptide in patients with medullary thyroid carcinoma. J Clin Chem Clin Biochem 27:423–427

Kimura S, Sugita Y, Kanazawa I, Saito A, Goto K (1987) Isolation and amino acid sequence of calcitonin gene-related peptide from porcine spinal cord. Neuropeptides 9:75–82

Kline LW, Kaneko T, Chiu K-W, Harvey S, Pang PKT (1988) Calcitonin gene-related peptide in the bullfrog, Rana catesbeiana: localization and vascular actions. Gen Comp Endocrinol 72:123–129

Koop H, Eissele R, Kühlkamp V, Bothe E, Dionysius J, Arnold R (1987) Calcitonin gene-related peptide stimulates rat gastric somatostatin release in vitro. Life Sci 40:541–546

Kraenzlin ME, Ch'ng JLC, Mulderry PK, Ghatei MA, Bloom SR (1985) Infusion of a novel peptide, calcitonin gene-related peptide (CGRP) in man. Pharmacokinetics and effects on gastric acid secretion and on gastrointestinal hormones. Regul Pept 10:189–197

Krahn DD, Gosnell BA, Levine AS, Morley JE (1984) Effects of calcitonin gene-related peptide on food intake. Peptides 5:861–864

Kreutter D, Orena SJ, Andrews KM (1989) Suppression of insulin-stimulated glucose transport in L6 myocytes by calcitonin gene-related peptide. Biochem Biophys Res Commun 164:461–467

Kruger L, Silverman JD, Mantyh PW, Sternini C, Brecha NC (1989) Peripheral patterns of calcitonin gene-related peptide general somatic sensory innervation: cutaneous and deep terminations. J Comp Neurol 280:291–302

Kubota M, Moseley JM, Butera L, Dusting GJ, MacDonald PS, Martin TJ (1985) Calcitonin gene-related peptide stimulates cyclic AMP formation in rat aortic smooth muscle cells. Biochem Biophys Res Commun 132:88–94

Kurtz A, Muff R, Born W, Lundberg JM, Millberg B-I, Gnädinger MP, Uehlinger DE, Weidmann P, Hökfelt T, Fischer JA (1988) Calcitonin gene-related peptide is a stimulator of renin secretion. J Clin Invest 82:538–543

Kurtz A, Schurek H-J, Jelkmann W, Muff R, Lipp H-P, Heckmann U, Eckardt K-U, Scholz H, Fischer JA, Bauer C (1989) Renal mesangium is a target for calcitonin gene-related peptide. Kidney Int 36:222–227

Lasmoles F, Jullienne A, Day F, Minvielle S, Milhaud G, Moukhtar MS (1985) Elucidation of the nucleotide sequence of chicken calcitonin mRNA: direct evidence for the expression of a lower vertebrate calcitonin-like gene in man and rat. EMBO J 4:2603–2607

Laufer R, Changeux J-P (1989) Calcitonin gene-related peptide and cyclic AMP stimulate phosphoinositide turnover in skeletal muscle cells. J Biol Chem 264:2683–2689

Le Greves P, Nyberg F, Terenius L, Hökfelt T (1985) Calcitonin gene-related peptide is a potent inhibitor of substance P degradation. Eur J Pharmacol 115:309–311

Leighton B, Cooper GJS (1988) Pancreatic amylin and calcitonin gene-related peptide cause resistance to insulin in skeletal muscle in vitro. Nature 335:632–635

Lengyel A-MJ, Tannenbaum GS (1987) Mechanisms of calcitonin-induced growth hormone (GH) suppression: roles of somatostatin and GH-releasing factor. Endocrinology 120:1377–1383

Lenz HJ (1988) Calcitonin and CGRP inhibit gastrointestinal transit via distinct neuronal pathways. Am J Physiol 254:G920–G924

Lenz HJ, Brown MR (1990) Cerebroventricular calcitonin gene-related peptide inhibits rat duodenal bicarbonate secretion by release of norepinephrine and vasopressin. J Clin Invest 85:25–32

Lenz HJ, Mortrud MT, Rivier JE, Brown MR (1985) Calcitonin gene-related peptide inhibits basal, pentagastrin, histamine, and bethanecol stimulated gastric acid secretion. Gut 26:550–555

Lenz HJ, Mortrud MT, Vale WW, Rivier E, Brown MR (1984) Calcitonin gene-related peptide acts within the central nervous system to inhibit gastric acid secretion. Regul Pept 9:271–277

Leung FW, Tallos EG, Taché YF, Guth PH (1987) Calcitonin gene-related peptide inhibits acid secretion without modifying blood flow. Am J Physiol 252:G215–G218

Levy F, Muff R, Dotti-Sigrist S, Dambacher MA, Fischer JA (1988) Formation of neutralizing antibodies during intranasal synthetic salmon calcitonin treatment of Paget's disease. J Clin Endocrinol Metab 67:541–545

Lindsay RM, Harmar AJ (1989) Nerve growth factor regulates expression of neuropeptide genes in adult sensory neurons. Nature 337:362–364

Looij BJ Jr, Roelfsema F, van der Heide D, Frölich M, Souverijn JHM, Nieuwenhuizen Kruseman AC (1988) The effect of calcitonin on growth hormone secretion in man. Clin Endocrinol (Oxf) 29:517–527

Lundberg JM, Franco-Cereceda A, Hua X, Hökfelt T, Fischer JA (1985) Co-existence of substance P and calcitonin gene-related peptide-like immuno-reactivities in sensory nerves in relation to cardiovascular and bronchoconstrictor effects of capsaicin. Eur J Pharmacol 108:315–319

Lynch B, Kaiser ET (1988) Biological properties of two models of calcitonin gene-related peptide with idealized amphiphilic α-helices of different lengths. Biochemistry 27:7600–7607

Macdonald NJ, Butters L, O'Shaughnessy DJ, Riddell AJ, Rubin PC (1989) A comparison of the effects of human alpha calcitonin gene-related peptide and glyceryl trinitrate on regional blood velocity in man. Br J Clin Pharmacol 28:257–261

MacIntyre I, Hillyard CJ, Reynolds JJ, Gaines Das RE, Craig RK (1984) A second plasma calcium-lowering peptide from the human calcitonin precursor – a re-evaluation. Nature 308:84

MacLean DB, Bennett B, Morris M, Wheeler FB (1989) Differential regulation of calcitonin gene-related peptide and substance P in cultured neonatal rat vagal sensory neurons. Brain Res 478:349–355

Maggi CA, Evangelista S, Giuliani S, Meli A (1987a) Anti-ulcer activity of calcitonin gene-related peptide in rats. Gen Pharmacol 18:33–34

Maggi CA, Giuliani S, Santicioli P, Abelli L, Meli A (1987b) Visceromotor responses to calcitonin gene-related peptide (CGRP) in the rat lower urinary tract: evidence for a transmitter role in the capsaicin-sensitive nerves of the ureter. Eur J Pharmacol 143:73–82

Maggi CA, Rovero P, Giuliani S, Evangelista S, Regoli D, Meli A (1990) Biological activity of N-terminal fragments of calcitonin gene-related peptide. Eur J Pharmacol 179:217–219

Malgaroli A, Meldolesi J, Zallone AZ, Teti A (1989) Control of cytosolic free calcium in rat and chicken osteoclasts. The role of extracellular calcium and calcitonin. J Biol Chem 264:14342–14347

Manning MC (1989) Conformation of the alpha form of human calcitonin gene-related peptide (CGRP) in aqueous solution as determined by circular dichroism spectroscopy. Biochem Biophys Res Commun 160:388–392

Marlier L, Rajaofetra N, Peretti-Renucci R, Kachidian P, Poulat P, Feuerstein C, Privat A (1990) Calcitonin gene-related peptide staining intensity is reduced in rat lumbar motoneurons after spinal cord transection: a quantitative immunocytochemical study. Exp Brain Res 82:40–47

Martial K, Minvielle S, Jullienne A, Segond N, Milhaud G, Lasmoles F (1990) Predicted structure of rabbit N-terminal, calcitonin and katacalcin peptides. Biochem Biophys Res Commun 171:1111–1114

Marx SJ, Woodard CJ, Aurbach GD (1972) Calcitonin receptors of kidney and bone. Science 178:999–1001

Mason RT, Peterfreund RA, Sawchenko PE, Corrigan AZ, Rivier JE, Vale WW (1984) Release of predicted calcitonin gene-related peptide from cultured rat trigeminal ganglion cells. Nature 308:653–655

Mason RT, Shulkes A, Zajac JD, Fletcher AE, Hardy KJ, Martin TJ (1986) Basal and stimulated release of calcitonin gene-related peptide (CGRP) in patients with medullary thyroid carcinoma. Clin Endocrinol (Oxf) 25:675–685

Maton PN, Pradhan T, Zhou Z-C, Gardner JD, Jensen RT (1990) Activities of calcitonin gene-related peptide (CGRP) and related peptides at the CGRP receptor. Peptides 11:485–489

Mazzuoli GF, Tabolli S, Bigi F, Valtorta C, Minisola S, Diacinti D, Scarnecchia L, Bianchi G, Piolini M, dell'Acqua S (1990) Effects of salmon calcitonin on the bone loss induced by ovariectomy. Calcif Tissue Int 47:209–214

McCormack DG, Mak JCW, Coupe MO, Barnes PJ (1989) Calcitonin gene-related peptide vasodilation of human pulmonary vessels. J Appl Physiol 67:1265–1270

McCulloch CR, Cooke HJ (1989) Human α-calcitonin gene-related peptide influences colonic secretion by acting on myenteric neurons. Regul Pept 24:87–96

McLean GW, Rabin D, Moore L, Deftos LJ, Lorber D, McKenna TJ (1984) Evaluation of provocative tests in suspected medullary carcinoma of the thyroid: heterogeneity of calcitonin responses to calcium and pentagastrin. Metabolism 33:790–796

Merighi A, Polak JM, Gibson SJ, Gulbenkian S, Valentino KL, Peirone SM (1988) Ultrastructural studies on calcitonin gene-related peptide-, tachykinins- and somatostatin-immunoreactive neurones in rat dorsal root ganglia: evidence for the colocalization of different peptides in single secretory granules. Cell Tissue Res 254:101–109

Michelangeli VP, Findlay DM, Fletcher A, Martin TJ (1986) Calcitonin gene-related peptide (CGRP) acts independently of calcitonin on cyclic AMP formation in clonal osteogenic sarcoma cells (UMR 106-01). Calcif Tissue Int 39:44–48

Michelangeli VP, Fletcher AE, Allan EH, Nicholson GC, Martin TJ (1989) Effects of calcitonin gene-related peptide on cyclic AMP formation in chicken, rat, and mouse bone cells. J Bone Miner Res 4:269–272

Miles K, Greengard P, Huganir RL (1989) Calcitonin gene-related peptide regulates phosphorylation of the nicotinic acetylcholine receptor in rat myotubes. Neuron 2:1517–1524

Minvielle S, Cressent M, Lasmoles F, Jullienne A, Milhaud G, Moukhtar MS (1986) Isolation and partial characterization of the calcitonin gene in a lower vertebrate. FEBS Lett 203:7–10

Minvielle S, Cressent M, Delehaye MC, Segond N, Milhaud G, Jullienne A, Moukhtar MS, Lasmoles F (1987) Sequence and expression of the chicken calcitonin gene. FEBS Lett 223:63–68

Mitsuma T, Nogimori T, Chaya M (1984) Peripheral administration of eel calcitonin inhibits thyrotropin secretion in rats. Eur J Pharmacol 102:123–128

Miyauchi T, Sano Y, Hiroshima O, Yuzuriha T, Sugishita Y, Ishikawa T, Saito A, Goto K (1988) Positive inotropic effects and receptors of calcitonin gene-related peptide (CGRP) in porcine ventricular muscles. Biochem Biophys Res Commun 155:289–294

Molina JM, Cooper GJS, Leighton B, Olefsky JM (1990) Induction of insulin resistance in vivo by amylin and calcitonin gene-related peptide. Diabetes 39:260–265

Mora M, Marchi M, Polak JM, Gibson SJ, Cornelio F (1989) Calcitonin gene-related peptide immunoreactivity at the human neuromuscular junction. Brain Res 492:404–407

Morel F (1983) Regulation of kidney functions by hormones: a new approach. Recent Prog Horm Res 39:271–304

Morimoto T, Okamoto M, Koida M, Nakamuta H, Stahl GL, Orlowski RC (1985) Intracerebroventricular injection of ^{125}I-salmon calcitonin in rats: fate, anorexia and hypocalcemia. Jpn J Pharmacol 37:21–29

Morley JE, Levine AS, Silvis SE (1981) Intraventricular calcitonin inhibits gastric acid secretion. Science 214:671–673

Morris HR, Panico M, Etienne T, Tippins J, Girgis SI, MacIntyre I (1984) Isolation and characterization of human calcitonin gene-related peptide. Nature 308:746–748

Morton CR, Hutchison WD (1989) Release of sensory neuropeptides in the spinal cord: studies with calcitonin gene-related peptide and galanin. Neuroscience 31:807–815

Moseley JM, Smith P, Martin TJ (1986) Identification of the calcitonin receptor by chemical cross-linking and photoaffinity labeling in human cancer cell lines. J Bone Miner Res 1:293–297

Mosselman S, Höppener JWM, Zandberg J, van Mansfeld ADM, Geurts van Kessel AHM, Lips CJM, Jansz HS (1988) Islet amyloid polypeptide: identification and chromosomal localization of the human gene. FEBS Lett 239:227–232

Muff R, Dambacher MA, Perrenoud A, Simon C, Fischer JA (1990) Efficacy of intranasal human calcitonin in patients with Paget's disease refractory to salmon calcitonin. Am J Med 89:181–184

Muff R, Dambacher MA, Fischer JA (1991) Formation of neutralizing antibodies during intranasal synthetic salmon calcitonin treatment of postmenopausal osteoporosis. Osteoporosis Int 1:72–75

Mulderry PK, Ghatei MA, Rodrigo J, Allen JM, Rosenfeld MG, Polak JM, Bloom SR (1985) Calcitonin gene-related peptide in cardiovascular tissues of the rat. Neuroscience 14:947–954

Mulderry PK, Ghatei MA, Spokes RA, Jones PM, Pierson AM, Hamid QA, Kanse S, Amara SG, Burrin JM, Legon S, Polak JM, Bloom SR (1988) Differential expression of α-CGRP and β-CGRP by primary sensory neurons and enteric autonomic neurons of the rat. Neuroscience 25:195–205

Mulholland MW, Jaffer S (1990) Stimulation of acetylcholine release in myenteric plexus by calcitonin gene-related peptide. Am J Physiol 259:G934–G939

Murphy E, Chamberlin ME, Mandel LJ (1986) Effects of calcitonin on cytosolic Ca in a suspension of rabbit medullary thick ascending limb tubules. Am J Physiol 251:C491–C495

Murphy S, Osborne PB, Adamson S, Campbell G (1990) Co-localization of calcitonin gene-related peptide- and substance P-like immunoreactivity in mucosal intra-epithelial nerves in the toad colon. Neurosci Lett 116:7–11

Naveh-Many T, Silver J (1988) Regulation of calcitonin gene transcription by vitamin D metabolites in vivo in the rat. J Clin Invest 81:270–273

Nealon WH, Beauchamp RD, Townsend CM, Thompson JC (1990) Additive interactions of calcitonin gene-related peptide and calcitonin on pancreatic exocrine function in conscious dogs. Surgery 107:434–441

Nelkin BD, Rosenfeld KI, de Bustros A, Leong SS, Roos BA, Baylin SB (1984) Structure and expression of a gene encoding human calcitonin and calcitonin gene-related peptide. Biochem Biophys Res Commun 123:648–655

Nelkin BD, Chen KY, de Bustros A, Roos BA, Baylin SB (1989) Changes in calcitonin gene RNA processing during growth of a human medullary thyroid carcinoma cell line. Cancer Res 49:6949–6952

Nelson MT, Huang Y, Brayden JE, Hescheler J, Standen NB (1990) Arterial dilations in response to calcitonin gene-related peptide involve activation of K^+ channels. Nature 344:770–773

New HV, Mudge AW (1986) Calcitonin gene-related peptide regulates muscle acetylcholine receptor synthesis. Nature 323:809–811

Nicholson GC, Moseley JM, Sexton PM, Mendelsohn FAO, Martin TJ (1986) Abundant calcitonin receptors in isolated rat osteoclasts. J Clin Invest 78:355–360

Nicholson GC, Moseley JM, Yates AJP, Martin TJ (1987) Control of cyclic adenosine 3',5'-monophosphate production in osteoclasts: calcitonin-induced persistent activation and homologous desensitization of adenylate cyclase. Endocrinology 120:1902–1908

Nicholson GC, D'Santos CS, Evans T, Moseley JM, Kemp BE, Michelangeli VP, Martin TJ (1988) Human placental calcitonin receptors. Biochem J 250:877–882

Nicoletti F, Clementi G, Patti F, Canonico PL, di Giorgio RM, Matera M, Pennisi G, Angelucci L, Scapagnini U (1982) Effects of calcitonin on rat extrapyramidal motor system: behavioral and biochemical data. Brain Res 250:381–385

Nilsson G, Alving K, Ahlstedt S, Hökfelt T, Lundberg JM (1990) Peptidergic innervation of rat lymphoid tissue and lung: relation to mast cells and sensitivity to capsaicin and immunization. Cell Tissue Res 262:125–133

Nishi M, Sanke T, Seino S, Eddy RL, Fan Y-S, Byers MG, Shows TB, Bell GI, Steiner DF (1989) Human islet amyloid polypeptide gene: complete nucleotide sequence, chromosomal localization, and evolutionary history. Mol Endocrinol 3:1775–1781

Nishizawa Y, Okui Y, Inaba M, Okuno S, Yukioka K, Miki T, Watanabe Y, Morii H (1988) Calcium/calmodulin-mediated action of calcitonin on lipid metabolism in rats. J Clin Invest 82:1165–1172

Noel M, Gavoille A, Lasmoles F, Kahn E, Caillou B, Gardet P, Fragu P (1990) Quantification of intracellular calcitonin gene transcripts in human medullary thyroid carcinoma (MTC) by in situ hybridization. J Endocrinol Invest 13:567–573

Noguchi K, Senba E, Morita Y, Sato M, Tohyama M (1990a) α-CGRP and β-CGRP mRNAs are differentially regulated in the rat spinal cord and dorsal root ganglion. Mol Brain Res 7:299–304

Noguchi K, Senba E, Morita Y, Sato M, Tohyama M (1990b) Co-expression of α-CGRP and β-CGRP mRNAs in the rat dorsal root ganglion cells. Neurosci Lett 108:1–5

O'Brien TD, Westermark P, Johnson KH (1990) Islet amyloid polypeptide (IAPP) does not inhibit glucose-stimulated insulin secretion from isolated perfused rat pancreas. Biochem Biophys Res Commun 170:1223–1228

Ohhashi T, Jacobowitz DM (1988) Effects of calcitonin gene-related peptide on neuromuscular transmission in the isolated rat diaphragm. Peptides 9:613–617

Ohmura T, Nishio M, Kigoshi S, Muramatsu I (1990) Electrophysiological and mechanical effects of calcitonin gene-related peptide on guinea-pig atria. Br J Pharmacol 100:27–30

Ohsawa H, Kanatsuka A, Yamaguchi T, Makino H, Yoshida S (1989) Islet amyloid polypeptide inhibits glucose-stimulated insulin secretion from isolated rat pancreatic islets. Biochem Biophys Res Commun 160:961–967

Ohtani R, Kaneko T, Kline LW, Labedz T, Tang Y, Pang PKT (1989) Localization of calcitonin gene-related peptide in the small intestine of various vertebrate species. Cell Tissue Res 258:35–42

Olgiati VR, Guidobono F, Netti C, Pecile A (1983) Localization of calcitonin binding sites in rat central nervous system: evidence of its neuroactivity. Brain Res 265:209–215

Ono K, Delay M, Nakajima T, Irisawa H, Giles W (1989) Calcitonin gene-related peptide regulates calcium current in heart muscle. Nature 340:721–724

Palmer JBD, Cuss FMC, Mulderry PK, Ghatei MA, Springall DR, Cadieux A, Bloom SR, Polak JM, Barnes PJ (1987) Calcitonin gene-related peptide is localised to human airway nerves and potently constricts human airway smooth muscle. Br J Pharmacol 91:95–101

Pappas T, Debas HT, Walsh JH, Rivier J, Taché Y (1986) Calcitonin gene-related peptide-induced selective inhibition of gastric acid secretion in dogs. Am J Physiol 250:G127–G133

Pecile A, Ferri S, Braga PC, Olgiati VR (1975) Effects of intracerebroventricular calcitonin in the conscious rabbit. Experientia 31:332–333

Pecile A, Guidobono F, Netti C, Sibilia V, Biella G, Braga PC (1987) Calcitonin gene-related peptide: antinociceptive activity in rats, comparison with calcitonin. Regul Pept 18:189–199

Peleg S, Abruzzese RV, Cote GJ, Gagel RF (1990) Transcription of the human calcitonin gene is mediated by a C cell-specific enhancer containing E-box-like elements. Mol Endocrinol 4:1750–1757

Pennefather JN, Reynoldson NA, Handberg GM (1990) Inhibition of rat uterine contractions by rat and human CGRP. Peptides 11:903–906

Perez Cano R, Girgis SI, Galan Galan F, MacIntyre I (1982a) Identification of both human and salmon calcitonin-like molecules in birds suggesting the existence of two calcitonin genes. J Endocrinol 92:351–355

Perez Cano R, Girgis SI, MacIntyre I (1982b) Further evidence for calcitonin gene duplication: the identification of two different calcitonins in a fish, a reptile and two mammals. Acta Endocrinol (Copenh) 100:256–261

Peterfreund RA, Vale WW (1986) Local anesthetics inhibit veratridine-induced secretion of calcitonin gene-related peptide (CGRP) from cultured rat trigeminal ganglion cells. Brain Res 380:159–161

Petermann JB, Born W, Chang JY, Fischer JA (1987) Identification in the human central nervous system, pituitary, and thyroid of a novel calcitonin gene-related peptide, and partial amino acid sequence in the spinal cord. J Biol Chem 262:542–545

Pettersson M, Ahrén B (1988) Insulin and glucagon secretion in rats: effects of calcitonin gene-related peptide. Regul Pept 23:37–50

Pontiroli AE (1985) Intranasal calcitonin and plasma calcium concentrations. Br Med J 291: 54–55

Popper P, Micevych PE (1990) Steroid regulation of calcitonin gene-related peptide mRNA expression in motoneurons of the spinal nucleus of the bulbocavernosus. Mol Brain Res 8:159–166

Pöschl E, Lindley I, Hofer E, Seifert J-M, Brunowsky W, Besemer J (1987) The structure of procalcitonin of the salmon as deduced from its cDNA sequence. FEBS Lett 226:96–100

Primi MP, Bueno L (1986) Centrally mediated stimulation of jejunal water and electrolyte secretion by calcitonin in dogs. Am J Physiol 250:G172–G176

Rattan S, Gonnella P, Goyal RK (1988) Inhibitory effect of calcitonin gene-related peptide and calcitonin on opossum esophageal smooth muscle. Gastroenterology 94:284–293

Reginster JY, Albert A, Lecart MP, Labelin P, Denis D, Deroisy R, Fontaine MA, Franchimont P (1987) 1-year controlled randomised trial of prevention of early postmenopausal bone loss by intranasal calcitonin. Lancet 2:1481–1483

Reinecke M, Forssmann WG (1988) Neuropeptide (neuropeptide Y, neurotensin, vasoactive intestinal polypeptide, substance P, calcitonin gene-related peptide, somatostatin) immunohistochemistry and ultrastructure of renal nerves. Histochemistry 89:1–9

Réthelyi M, Metz CB, Lund PK (1989) Distribution of neurons expressing calcitonin gene-related peptide mRNAs in the brain stem, spinal cord and dorsal root ganglia of rat and guinea-pig. Neuroscience 29:225–239

Riley JH, Edbrooke MR, Craig RK (1986) Ectopic synthesis of high-M_r calcitonin by the BEN lung carcinoma cell line reflects aberrant proteolytic processing. FEBS Lett 198:71–79

Roos BA, Fischer JA, Pignat W, Alander CB, Raisz LG (1986) Evaluation of the in vivo and in vitro calcium-regulating actions of noncalcitonin peptides produced via calcitonin gene expression. Endocrinology 118:46–51

Rosenfeld MG, Mermod J-J, Amara SG, Swanson LW, Sawchenko PE, Rivier J, Vale WW, Evans RM (1983) Production of a novel neuropeptide encoded by the calcitonin gene via tissue-specific RNA processing. Nature 304:129–135

Russo AF, Nelson C, Roos BA, Rosenfeld MG (1988) Differential regulation of the coexpressed calcitonin/α-CGRP and β-CGRP neuroendocrine genes. J Biol Chem 263:5–8

Sabate MI, Stolarsky LS, Polak JM, Bloom SR, Varndell IM, Ghatei MA, Evans RM, Rosenfeld MG (1985) Regulation of neuroendocrine gene expression by alternative RNA processing. J Biol Chem 260:2589–2592

Sabbatini F, Fimmel CJ, Pace F, Tobler PH, Hinder RA, Blum AL, Fischer JA (1985) Distribution of intraventricular salmon calcitonin and suppression of gastric secretion. Digestion 32:273–281

Saito A, Masaki T, Uchiyama Y, Lee TJ-F, Goto K (1989) Calcitonin gene-related peptide and vasodilator nerves in large cerebral arteries of cats. J Pharmacol Exp Ther 248:455–462

Samuelson UE, Dalsgaard C-J, Lundberg JM, Hökfelt T (1985) Calcitonin gene-related peptide inhibits spontaneous contractions in human uterus and fallopian tube. Neurosci Lett 62:225–230

Sano Y, Hiroshima O, Yuzuriha T, Yamato C, Saito A, Kimura S, Hirabayashi T, Goto K (1989) Calcitonin gene-related peptide-binding sites of porcine cardiac muscles and coronary arteries: solubilization and characterization. J Neurochem 52:1919–1924

Saria A, Gamse R, Petermann J, Fischer JA, Theodorsson-Norheim E, Lundberg J-M (1986) Simultaneous release of several tachykinins and calcitonin gene-related peptide from rat spinal cord slices. Neurosci Lett 63:310–314

Sasayama Y, Matsuda K, Oguro C, Kambegawa A (1989) Immunohistochemical demonstration of calcitonin gene-related peptide in the ultimobranchial gland of some lower vertebrates and in the nervous tissues of some invertebrates. Zool Sci 6:423–426

Scherübl H, Schultz G Hescheler J (1990) A slowly inactivating calcium current works as a calcium sensor in calcitonin-secreting cells. FEBS Lett 273:51–54

Schiebinger RJ, Santora AC (1989) Stimulation by calcitonin gene-related peptide of atrial natriuretic peptide secretion in vitro and its mechanism of action. Endocrinology 124:2473–2479

Schifter S, Johannsen L, Aagaard MT, Goltermann N, Parkes HC, Craig RK (1989) Elevated serum levels of calcitonin gene-related peptide (CGRP) but no evidence for CGRP gene expression in non-small cell lung carcinomas. Clin Endocrinol (Oxf) 31:137–142

Scott Helton W, Mulholland MM, Bunnett NW, Debas HT (1989) Inhibition of gastric and pancreatic secretion in dogs by CGRP: role of somatostatin. Am J Physiol 256:G715–G720

Segond N, Legendre B, Tahri EH, Besnard P, Jullienne A, Moukhtar MS, Garel J-M (1985) Increased level of calcitonin mRNA after 1,25-dihydroxyvitamin D_3 injection in the rat. FEBS Lett 184:268–272

Segond N, Delehaye MC, Jullienne A, Taboulet J, Minvielle S, Milhaud G, Moukhtar MS (1989) Actinomycin D inhibits the rapid increase in translatable calcitonin mRNA provoked by acute calcium stimulation. Horm Metab Res 21:489–493

Seifert H, Chesnut J, de Souza E, Rivier J, Vale W (1985) Binding sites for calcitonin gene-related peptide in distinct areas of rat brain. Brain Res 346:195–198

Seitz PK, Cooper CW (1989) Cosecretion of calcitonin and calcitonin gene-related peptide from cultured rat medullary thyroid C cells. J Bone Miner Res 4:129–134

Sexton PM, McKenzie JS, Mason RT, Moseley JM, Martin TJ, Mendelsohn FAO (1986) Localization of binding sites for calcitonin gene-related peptide in rat brain by in vitro autoradiography. Neuroscience 19:1235–1245

Sexton PM, Adam WR, Moseley JM, Martin TJ, Mendelsohn FAO (1987) Localization and characterization of renal calcitonin receptors by in vitro autoradiography. Kidney Int 32:862–868

Sexton PM, McKenzie JS, Mendelsohn FAO (1988) Evidence for a new subclass of calcitonin/calcitonin gene-related peptide binding site in rat brain. Neurochem Int 12:323–335

Shah GV, Wang W, Grosvenor CE, Crowley WR (1990) Calcitonin inhibits basal and thyrotropin-releasing hormone-induced release of prolactin from anterior pituitary cells: evidence for a selective action exerted proximal to secretagogue-induced increases in cytosolic Ca^{2+}. Endocrinology 127:621–628

Shimizu N, Oomura Y (1986) Calcitonin-induced anorexia in rats: evidence for its inhibitory action on lateral hypothalamic chemosensitive neurons. Brain Res 367:128–140

Sigrist S, Franco-Cereceda A, Muff R, Henke H, Lundberg JM, Fischer JA (1986) Specific receptor and cardiovascular effects of calcitonin gene-related peptide. Endocrinology 119:381–389

Simmons RE, Hjelle JT, Mahoney C, Deftos LJ, Lisker W, Kato P, Rabkin R (1988) Renal metabolism of calcitonin. Am J Physiol 254:F593–F600

Singer FR, Mills BG (1984) Paget's disease of bone: etiologic and therapeutic aspects. Bone Miner Res 2:394–421

Singer FR, Habener JF, Greene E, Godin P, Potts JT Jr (1972a) Inactivation of calcitonin by specific organs. Nature [New Biol] 237:269–270

Singer FR, Aldred JP, Neer RM, Krane SM, Potts JT Jr, Bloch KJ (1972b) An evaluation of antibodies and clinical resistance to salmon calcitonin. J Clin Invest 51:2331–2338

Skofitsch G, Jacobowitz DM (1985) Autoradiographic distribution of ^{125}I calcitonin gene-related peptide binding sites in the rat central nervous system. Peptides 4:975–986

Stangl D, Born W, Fischer JA (1991) Characterization and photoaffinity labeling of a calcitonin gene-related peptide receptor solubilized from human cerebellum. Biochemistry 30:8605–8611

Steenbergh PH, Höppener JWM, Zandberg J, van de Ven WJM, Jansz HS, Lips CJM (1984) Calcitonin gene-related peptide coding sequence is conserved in the human genome and is expressed in medullary thyroid carcinoma. J Clin Endocrinol Metab 59:358–360

Steenbergh PH, Höppener JWM, Zandberg J, Cremers AFM, Jansz HS, Lips CJM (1985a) Structure of the human calcitonin gene and its transcripts in medullary thyroid carcinoma. In: Pecile A (ed) Calcitonin. Elsevier Amsterdam, pp 23–31

Steenbergh PH, Höppener JWM, Zandberg J, Lips CJM, Jansz HS (1985b) A second human calcitonin/CGRP gene. FEBS Lett 183:403–407

Steenbergh PH, Höppener JWM, Zandberg J, Visser A, Lips CJM, Jansz HS (1986) Structure and expression of the human calcitonin/CGRP genes. FEBS Lett 209:97–103

Stevenson JC, Adrian TE, Christofides ND, Bloom SR (1985) Effect of calcitonin on gastrointestinal regulatory peptides in man. Clin Endocrinol (Oxf) 22:655–660

Stief CG, Benard F, Bosch RJLH, Aboseif SR, Lue TF, Tanagho EA (1990) A possible role for calcitonin gene-related peptide in the regulation of the smooth muscle tone of the bladder and penis. J Urol 143:392–397

Stolarsky-Fredman L, Leff SE, Klein ES, Crenshaw EB III, Yeakley J, Rosenfeld MG (1990) A tissue-specific enhancer in the rat-calcitonin/CGRP gene is active in both neural and endocrine cell types. Mol Endocrinol 4:497–504

Struthers AD, Brown MJ, MacDonald DWR, Beacham JL, Stevenson JC, Morris HR, MacIntyre I (1986) Human calcitonin gene-related peptide: a potent endogenous vasodilator in man. Clin Sci 70:389–393

Su HC, Bishop AE, Power RF, Hamada Y, Polak JM (1987) Dual intrinsic and extrinsic origins of CGRP- and NPY-immunoreactive nerves of rat gut and pancreas. J Neurosci 7:2674–2687

Takamori M, Yoshikawa H (1989) Effect of calcitonin gene-related peptide on skeletal muscle via specific binding site and G protein. J Neurol Sci 90:99–109

Tannenbaum GS, Goltzman D (1985) Calcitonin gene-related peptide mimics calcitonin actions in brain on growth hormone release and feeding. Endocrinology 116:2685–2687

Tashjian AH Jr, Wright DR, Ivey JL, Pont A (1978) Calcitonin binding sites in bone: relationships to biological response and "escape". Recent Prog Horm Res 34:285–334

Tobler PH, Tschopp FA, Dambacher MA, Fischer JA (1984) Salmon and human calcitonin-like peptides in man. Clin Endocrinol (Oxf) 20:253–259

Tschirhart E, Bertrand C, Theodorsson E, Landry Y (1990) Evidence for the involvement of calcitonin gene-related peptide in the epithelium-dependent contraction of guinea-pig trachea in response to capsaicin. Naunyn Schmiedebergs Arch Pharmacol 342:177–181

Tschopp FA, Tobler PH, Born W, Dambacher MA, Pettengill OS, Sorenson G, Fischer JA (1982) Human calcitonin and carboxyl-terminal adjacent peptide

(PDN-21): identification of a common polyprotein in man. In: Cohn DV, Potts JT Jr, Fujita T (eds) Endocrine control of bone and calcium metabolism, Vol 8B. Elsevier, Amsterdam, pp 273–275

Tschopp FA, Tobler PH, Fischer JA (1984) Calcitonin gene-related peptide in the human thyroid, pituitary and brain. Mol Cell Endocrinol 36:53–57

Tschopp FA, Henke H, Petermann JB, Tobler PH, Janzer R, Hökfelt T, Lundberg JM, Cuello C, Fischer JA (1985) Calcitonin gene-related peptide and its binding sites in the human central nervous system and pituitary. Proc Natl Acad Sci USA 82:248–252

Twery MJ, Kirkpatrick B, Critcher EC, Lewis MH, Mailman RB, Cooper CW (1986) Motor effects of calcitonin administered intracerebroventricularly in the rat. Eur J Pharmacol 121:189–198

Uchida S, Yamamoto H, Iio S, Matsumoto N, Wang X-B, Yonehara N, Imai Y, Inoki R, Yoshida H (1990) Release of calcitonin gene-related peptide-like immunoreactive substance from neuromuscular junction by nerve excitation and its action on striated muscle. J Neurochem 54:1000–1003

Umeda Y, Arisawa M (1989) Characterization of the calcitonin gene-related peptide receptor in mouse T lymphocytes. Neuropeptide 14:237–242

Umeda Y, Okada T (1987) Inhibition of gastric acid secretion by human calcitonin gene-related peptide with picomolar potency in guinea-pig parietal cell preparations. Biochem Biophys Res Commun 146:430–436

Van Mansfeld ADM, Mosselman S, Höppener JWM, Zandberg J, van Teeffelen HAAM, Baas PD, Lips CJM, Jansz HS (1990) Islet amyloid polypeptide: structure and upstream sequences of the IAPP gene in rat and man. Biochim Biophys Acta 1087:235–240

Venesio T, Mulatero B, Fasolo A (1987) Coexistence of substance P and calcitonin gene-related peptide in the frog spinal cord. Neurosci Lett 80:246–250

Villar MJ, Roa M, Huchet M, Hökfelt T, Changeux J-P, Fahrenkrug J, Brown JC, Epstein M, Hersh L (1989) Immunoreactive calcitonin gene-related peptide, vasoactive intestinal polypeptide, and somatostatin in developing chicken spinal cord motoneurons. Distribution and role in regulation of cAMP in cultured muscle cells. Eur J Neurosci 1:269–287

Villarreal D, Freeman RH, Verburg KM, Brands MW (1988) Renal hemodynamic response to intrarenal infusion of calcitonin gene-related peptide in dogs. Peptides 9:1129–1135

Voelkel EF, Tashjian AH Jr, Davidoff FF, Cohen RB, Perlia CP, Wurtman RJ (1973) Concentrations of calcitonin and catecholamines in pheochromocytomas, a mucosal neuroma and medullary thyroid carcinoma. Endocrinol Metab 37: 297–307

Vora NM, Williams GA, Hargis GK, Bowser EN, Kawahara W, Jackson BL, Henderson WJ, Kukreja SC (1978) Comparative effect of calcium and of the adrenergic system on calcitonin secretion in man. J Clin Endocrinol Metab 46:567–571

Wada C, Hashimoto C, Kameya T, Yamaguchi K, Ono M (1988) Developmentally regulated expression of the calcitonin gene-related peptide (CGRP) in rat lung endocrine cells. Virchows Arch [B] 55:217–223

Westermark P, Wernstedt C, Wilander E, Sletten K (1986) A novel peptide in the calcitonin gene-related peptide family as an amyloid fibril protein in the endocrine pancreas. Biochem Biophys Res Commun 140:827–831

Wiesenfeld-Hallin Z, Hökfelt T, Lundberg JM, Forssmann WG, Reinecke M, Tschopp FA, Fischer JA (1984) Immunoreactive calcitonin gene-related peptide and substance P coexist in sensory neurons to the spinal cord and interact in spinal behavioral responses of the rat. Neurosci Lett 52:199–204

Wimalawansa SJ, Morris HR, MacIntyre I (1989) Both α- and β-calcitonin gene-related peptides are present in plasma, cerebrospinal fluid and spinal cord in man. J Mol Endocrinol 3:247–252

Wimalawansa SJ, Morris HR, Etienne A, Blench I, Panico M, MacIntyre I (1990) Isolation, purification and characterization of β-hCGRP from human spinal cord. Biochem Biophys Res Commun 167:993–1000

Wohlwend A, Malmström K, Henke H, Murer H, Vassalli J-D, Fischer JA (1985) Calcitonin and calcitonin gene-related peptide interact with the same receptor in cultured LLC-PK$_1$ kidney cells. Biochem Biophys Biophys Res Commun 131:537–542

Woloszczuk W, Reich-Kilcher B, Benke A, Dinstl K (1986) Effect of infusion of salmon calcitonin on the secretion of somatostatin and gastrin in man. Horm Metab Res 18:197–200

Yamamoto A, Kimura S, Hasui K, Fujisawa Y, Tamaki T, Fukui K, Iwao H, Abe Y (1988) Calcitonin gene-related peptide (CGRP) stimulates the release of atrial natriuretic peptide (ANP) from isolated rat atria. Biochem Biophys Res Commun 155:1452–1458

Yamatani T, Kadowaki S, Chiba T, Abe H, Chihara K, Fukase M, Fujita T (1986) Calcitonin gene-related peptide stimulates somatostatin release from isolated perfused rat stomach. Endocrinology 118:2144–2145

Yusufi ANK, Berndt TJ, Murayama N, Knox FG, Dousa TP (1987) Calcitonin inhibits Na$^+$ gradient-dependent phosphate uptake across renal brush-border membranes. Am J Physiol 252:F598–F604

Zabel M, Schäfer HJ (1988) Localization of calcitonin and calcitonin gene-related peptide mRNAs in rat parafollicular cells by hybridocytochemistry. J Histochem Cytochem 36:543–546

Zaidi M, Bevis PJR, Girgis SI, Lynch C, Stevenson JC, MacIntyre I (1985) Circulating CGRP comes from the perivascular nerves. Eur J Pharmacol 117:283–284

Zaidi M, Datta HK, Chambers TJ, MacIntyre I (1989) Production and characterisation of immunoreactive calcitonin gene-related peptide (CGRP) from a CGRP receptor-positive cloned osteosarcoma cell line (UMR 106.01). Biochem Biophys Res Commun 158:214–219

Zaidi M, Datta HK, Moonga BS, MacIntyre I (1990) Evidence that the action of calcitonin on rat osteoclasts is mediated by two G proteins acting via separate post-receptor pathways. J Endocrinol 126:473–481

Zhou Z-C, Villanueva ML, Noguchi M, Jones SW, Gardner JD, Jensen RT (1986) Mechanism of action of calcitonin gene-related peptide in stimulating pancreatic enzyme secretion. Am J Physiol 251:G391–G397

Zona C, Farini D, Palma E, Eusebi F (1991) Modulation of voltage-activated channels by calcitonin gene-related peptide in cultured rat neurones. J Physiol (Lond) 433:631–643

CHAPTER 17

Parathyroid Hormone-Related Protein: Molecular Biology, Chemistry, and Actions

T.J. MARTIN

A. Introduction

From observations made on patients with a high plasma calcium associated with cancer, it had long been suspected that the tumors were producing a factor with actions very similar to those of parathyroid hormone (PTH) (ALBRIGHT 1941; LAFFERTY 1966; MUNDY and MARTIN 1982). This issued was resolved in 1987 with the isolation and molecular cloning of a protein, PTH-related protein (PTHrP), which is most likely derived from the same ancestral gene as PTH (MOSELEY et al. 1987; SUVA et al. 1987). Its structural similarity to PTH around the amino-terminal region is enough to bestow on it the ability to reproduce virtually all of the physiological actions of PTH. Furthermore, it can explain the biochemical similarities between certain patients with hypercalcemia in cancer and those with primary hyperparathyroidism.

The humoral hypercalcemia of malignancy (HHM) is the term used to describe those hypercalcemic patients with cancer in whom the high plasma calcium levels cannot be explained by bone metastases or by elevated levels of PTH (MARTIN and ATKINS 1979; STEWART et al. 1980), but in whom there are several accompanying biochemical features identical with those in primary hyperparathyroidism, including especially low plasma phosphate levels and increased nephrogenous cyclic AMP. Certain biochemical similarities were recognized many years ago, and prompted the suggestion that such tumors were inappropriately producing PTH (ALBRIGHT 1941). This signaled the adoption of the "ectopic PTH" concept, which held sway until the late 1970s, when it was realized that the tumor product responsible for the excess bone resorption and other effects was not PTH itself, but most likely some other factor which was able to reproduce faithfully the actions of PTH. It was evident that such a factor could be isolated from an appropriate source by following purification with the use of a suitable bioassay for PTH-like activity. The early work on PTH extraction and purification had been carried out with relatively cumbersome and insensitive biological assays, but by the early 1980s it was possible to apply assays which were sensitive, reproducible, and robust, and capable of being executed in the very large numbers that were required for protein purification work. Thus several groups set out to purify the hypercalcemic factor from tumor material or culture media, monitoring purification with the use of sensitive assays for PTH-like activity, measuring cyclic AMP formation as a result of adenylate cyclase stimulation in osteoblasts or kidney cells, both of which are response systems for PTH in which specificity for the PTH receptor can be tested by peptide antagonists of PTH (Rodan et al. 1983; Stewart et al. 1983).

B. Molecular Biology

I. Isolation and Cloning

The earliest amino-terminal sequence of PTHrP revealed a very close structural relationship with PTH which seemed sufficient to account for the PTH-like actions of the protein, but it was clear that it was a distinct gene product, and most likely related to the PTH gene by a process of gene duplication (Moseley et al. 1987). Further amino acid sequencing established that this primary sequence similarity was confined to the amino-terminal region, with 8 of the first 13 amino acids of PTHrP identical with those of PTH, and that there was no further homology between the two proteins. This was fully confirmed in the predicted sequence by cDNA cloning (Suva et al. 1987; Mangin et al. 1988a), which revealed first a mature protein consisting of 141 amino acids, with a 36 amino acid leader sequence. In the initial cDNA cloning experiments from a cDNA library established from human lung cancer cells (Suva et al. 1987), it was noted that one of the clones contained a divergent 5' untranslated region. One possible explanation for this was that an alternative splicing mechanism might result in production of two mRNAs encoding the same protein. In other studies of cDNA for PTHrP it was clearly shown that 3' alternate mRNA splicing occurs (Thiede et al. 1988). Thus it was established at that stage that mature PTHrP could consist of the 141 amino acid protein, or as a result of alternate transcripts could consist either of a 139 amino acid protein, or a 173-residue PTHrP molecule (Thiede et al. 1988; Mangin et al. 1988b). This evidence for divergent mRNA both at the 3' and 5' ends of PTHrP of course stimulated great interest in the structure of the *PTHrP* gene.

II. Chromosomal Localization

The chromosomal localization of the human *PTHrP* gene on the short arm of chromosome 12 subbands 12p 11.1–12p 12.2 (Mangin et al. 1988a; Suva et al. 1989) provided further evidence consistent with an evolutionary relationship between PTHrP and PTH. The latter gene is localized on chromosome 11p 15 (Mannens et al. 1987). Chromosomes 11 and 12 are of similar size, centromere index, and banding pattern and are thought to have a common origin, perhaps in tetraploidy. There are several examples of related proteins, the genes for which are located one on chromosome 11 and

Table 1. Related genes located on chromosomes 11 and 12

Chromosome 11		Chromosome 12	
Location	Gene	Location	Gene
q13	Glutathione *S* transferase	q13-q14	Glutathione *S* transferase 3-like 1
p15.4	Parathyroid hormone	p11.2-p12.1	Parathyroid hormone-related protein
p14.1-p15	Lactate dehydrogenase A Lactate dehydrogenase C	p12.2-p12.1	Lactate dehydrogenase B
p15.5	Tyrosine hydroxylase	q22-q24.2	Phenyalanine hydroxylase
p15.5	Harvey *ras* sarcoma 1	p12.1	Kirsten *ras* sarcoma 2
q13	Murine mammary tumor virus integration site (v-*int*-2)	q12-q13	Murine mammary tumor virus integration site (v-*int*-1)
p15.5	Insulin-like growth factor II	q22-q24.2	Insulin-like growth factor 1
p15.1	Insulin		
p11-q12	Coagulation factor II (prothrombin)	p12	Coagulation factor VII (von Willebrand factor)
q12-q13.1	Complement component inhibitor 1	p13	Complement component 1 s

the other on chromosome 12. Some of these are listed in Table 1. Thus PTHrP as a protein is related to PTH, but is like PTH in its actions (to be discussed below) only in the region around the amino-terminus.

III. Genomic Structure

The genomic structure of the human *PTHrP* gene has been studied independently by three groups (MANGIN et al. 1989, 1990; SUVA et al. 1989; YASUDA et al. 1989a), and the following description is based on composite information from that work. In the coding region of the *PTHrP* gene there is no significant nucleotide sequence homology to the *PTH* gene within the intragenic region or in the flanking genomic sequences. The probable evolutionary relationship between *PTH* and *PTHrP* is further supported by the conservation of intron-exon boundaries in both genes and of course by their similar biological actions. The *PTHrP* gene is far more complex than the *PTH* gene, which has only three exons, whereas *PTHrP* has nine exons. The genes do share a common exonic region including the prepro sequence (Fig. 1, exon V for *PTHrP* and II for PTH). Of the nine exons of the *PTHrP* gene, exons V and VI (coding the prepro molecule and the majority of the coding region respectively) are invariant in mRNA transcripts. Exon VI comprises the majority of the coding region for the mature protein, up to residue 139, where a splice donor site is located. Read-through of exon VI

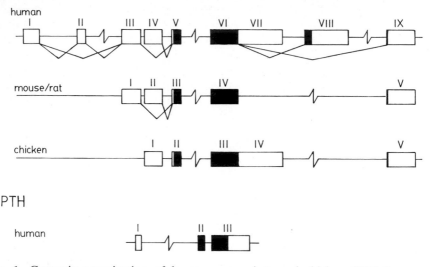

Fig. 1. Genomic organization of human, mouse/rat, and chicken *PTHrP* genes. *Closed and open boxes* indicate coding regions and untranslated sequences respectively. Potential alternate splicing events in *PTHrP* genes are indicated. See text for details

into exon VII results in the introduction of a termination signal producing a protein product of 139 amino acids in length, while participation of exons VIII and IX by alternate mRNA splicing results in protein products of 173 and 141 amino acids respectively. These alternate splice products leading to proteins with variable carboxy-termini had been predicted from the cDNA cloning data referred to earlier (Thiede et al. 1988; Mangin et al. 1988b). The genes for mouse (Mangin et al. 1991), rat (Yasuda et al. 1989b), and chicken (Thiede and Rutledge 1990) PTHrPs are all appreciably simpler than those of human, consisting of five exons in each case (Fig. 1).

In addition to the variable 3′ exonic regions, production of multiple mRNA species by the action of alternate 5′ promoters is evident, and explains the divergent clones noted during cDNA cloning (Suva et al. 1987). 5′ to exons I and IV are canonical TATA consensus sequences, while 5′ to exon III is a GC-rich region, containing a Sp1 and two AP-2 binding sites. Both of these elements are known to act as promoters in the absence of RNA II-dependent polymerase. It is possible that the different promoters are used in a tissue-specific manner, as is the case in the expression of for example the mouse α-amylase gene (Young et al. 1981), but no systematic studies have yet been published.

IV. Regulation of Gene

Primer extension studies support the idea that production of PTHrP mRNA species containing divergent 5′-untranslated regions occurs by initiation of transcription from three separate transcriptional start sites. Thus it is clear that there is potential for great heterogeneity in mRNAs for PTHrP, and this has indeed been the experience in studies of tumor and tissue mRNA for PTHrP (e.g., IKEDA et al. 1988a,b). It has also been suggested that 3'-untranslated sequences of some genes may play a role in development- or tissue-specific gene expression (e.g., YAFFE et al. 1985), and this could be true for PTHrP, especially because of its evident production by a number of fetal tissues. The presence of the motif ATTTA, which has been implicated in rapid turnover of many cytokines and some protooncogene mRNAs, in each of the 3' untranslated sequences (i.e., those specified by exons VII, VIII, and IX) is in agreement with the short half-life of PTHrP mRNA. There are a few reported examples of such complex genes that produce multiple mRNA species with different 5' and 3' ends. One of these is the mouse dihydrofolate reductase (*DHRF*) gene that produces multiple mRNA species by initiation from distinct nonconsensus promoters and alternate splicing (SETZER et al. 1982). The complex nature of the *PTHrP* gene will provide much interest in the details of its regulation. Such studies are in their early stage, but treatment with glucocorticoid hormone has resulted in decreased transcription of the *PTHrP* gene (IKEDA et al. 1989) and elevation of cyclic AMP in increased PTHrP mRNA production (ZAJAC et al. 1989).

V. Recombinant PTHrP

When the cDNA for PTHrP was cloned it was expressed transiently in mammalian cells, and biological activity was obtained (SUVA et al. 1987). Subsequently recombinant PTHrP was prepared by expression in bacteria (THORIKAY et al. 1989; HAMMONDS et al. 1989). PTHrP (1–141, 1–108) and (1–84) were expressed from recombinant DNA-derived clones, and expressed in E. coli as fusion proteins so that cyanogen bromide cleavage yielded the desired product, making use of the fact that the protein expressed by this cDNA contained no methionine residue (HAMMONDS et al. 1989). These recombinant preparations of PTHrP were characterized after purification and shown to be biologically active in several assay systems. In particular it was shown that the whole of the PTH-like activity was contained within the first 34 amino acids of PTHrP, and furthermore that antibodies against PTHrP (1–16) and PTHrP (1–34) were able to block fully the biological activity of full-length recombinant PTHrP (HAMMONDS et al. 1989).

C. Chemistry

I. Structure-Activity Relationships

Prediction of the structure of PTHrP revealed the existence of a previously unrecognized hormone, in which there was striking homology with PTH about the amino-terminal region. Since it seemed likely that this amino-terminal region was the functional PTH-like portion of the protein related in evolution to PTH, initial efforts were directed towards assessing biological activity of synthetic peptide analogs. Strategies were based on the fact that the biological activity of PTH was contained within the first 34 residues (TREGEAR et al. 1973). PTHrP (1–34) was found to stimulate cyclic AMP formation in osteogenic carcinoma cells with a potency four to six times greater than that of the human or bovine PTH (1–34) (KEMP et al. 1987). A similar greater potency had been found in the PTHrP which had been purified from lung cancer cell conditioned medium and used for sequence determination (MOSELEY et al. 1987). From this and other work (HORIUCHI et al. 1987; YATES et al. 1988; STEWART et al. 1988), it was clear that PTHrP (1–34) was at least as potent in PTH-responsive adenylate cyclase assays as PTH itself. Furthermore the structural requirements for PTH-like action within the amino-terminal portion of PTHrP resembled very closely those of PTH itself, in that PTHrP (1–29) had 10% of the activity of PTHrP (1–34), and peptides of shorter chain length were virtually inactive (KEMP et al. 1987). As predicted from the foregoing, studies of specific binding of PTHrP and PTH to bone and kidney cell targets indicated that the two peptides bind to the one receptor (JUEPPNER et al. 1988; SADI et al. 1989). Competition studies showed that PTH and PTHrP have approximately the same affinity, each ligand competes for the alternate ligand, and desensitization to one can be achieved by preincubation with the other. Furthermore cross-linking of either labeled PTH or PTHrP gave rise to receptor components of identical molecular weights (SHIGENO et al. 1988). The fact that some degree of competition for binding could be achieved with relatively high concentrations of PTHrP (15–34) (SADI et al. 1989), in which there is no sequence homology with PTH, implied that this portion of the molecule was involved in receptor interaction. This fits with previous conclusions regarding the receptor-binding component of PTH itself (NUSSBAUM et al. 1980).

II. Tertiary Structure

Analysis by nuclear magnetic resonance of the tertiary configuration of PTHrP (1–34) (BARDEN and KEMP 1989) revealed a surprisingly compact structure, containing multiple interactions between the N-terminal and C-terminal residues of the peptide. An α-helical structure existed between residues 4 and 14, which was followed by a series of bends comprising a hydrophobic cluster of residues, consisting of I-15, L-18, F-22, L-24, L-27, I-28, and I-31 (Fig. 2). Consistent with the observations in adenylate cyclase response, it is predicted from the structural analysis that removal of residues 30–34 would destabilize the end of the helix and reduce binding. Removal of residues 26–29 would be expected to destroy the second turn and virtually all binding, and this was the result of studies with the shorter synthetic peptides (KEMP et al. 1987). It is concluded from this NMR analysis that the amino-terminal region of the peptide (up to residue 14) is fairly mobile and

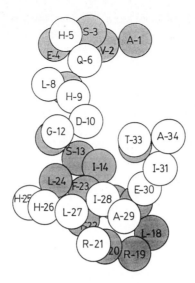

Fig. 2. Tertiary structure of human PTHrP (1–34), based on NMR analysis. See text for details

is thus able to reach the "agonist switch" following binding of the domain (14–29), perhaps with some swivel action around the I-15/S-14. This structural analysis is being extended to PTHrP (1–84), and preliminary data show that the configuration seen in PTHrP (1–34) is conserved in the longer molecule (BARDEN, personal communication).

III. Immunology

It is important to note that, although 8 of the first 13 residues of PTHrP are identical with those in PTH, antisera raised against PTHrP frequently show no measurable cross-reactivity with PTH (MARTIN et al. 1989; HAMMONDS et al. 1989; DANKS et al. 1989). Indeed, immunogenicity plots predicted that these two proteins would differ immunologically, despite this similarity in primary structure (WELLING et al. 1985; MOSELEY and SUVA 1990). Thus it is possible to obtain antisera against PTHrP which show no cross-reactivity against PTH under conditions of radioimmunoassay (BURTIS et al. 1990; GRILL et al. 1992), and even are found to be completely specific under the conditions of high antibody concentration used in immunoneutralization or immunohistology (DANKS et al. 1989, 1990). The same applies to antisera against PTH, which can be selected to show no cross-reactivity with PTHrP. However, in each case some antisera clearly do cross-react, and that is the most likely explanation for the fact that over many years in the 1960s and early 1970s certain PTH radioimmunoassays were able to detect immunoreactivity in plasma and tumor extracts of patients with HHM, and in media from cells cultured from such patients' tumors (Sherwood et al. 1967; Greenberg et al. 1973; Mayes et al. 1984; Palmieri et al. 1974; Ilardi and Faro 1975).

IV. Molecular Processing

Although there is no significant homology with PTH in any part of the PTHrP molecule other than the first 13 residues, the sequence of the prepro region of PTHrP is reminiscent of that of PTH. This sequence contains a hydrophobic core of amino acids surrounded by charged residues, characteristic of a secretory protein. Possible cleavage sites at G-8 or S-6 would leave a short pro sequence which could be cleaved during the secretory process. The sequence of mature PTHrP is clearly appreciably longer than that of mature PTH, and contains a sequence of many basic residues between amino acids 88 and 108. Among other potential cleavage sites in the molecule is the RRR at residues 19–21. The unusually strongly basic sequence between positions 88 and 108 might indicate that the peptide is cleaved at this region and released into the circulation shortly after secretion, leaving a primary circulating form of PTHrP no longer than about 86 amino acids. This is speculative since there is currently no information on the circulating form of PTHrP, but consistent with this suggestion is the presence of a potential amidation site at P-86. Certainly it seems likely that circulating PTHrP will be heterogeneous, chiefly because of the susceptibility to proteolytic digestion. It may also be that cleavage within tumors is tumor specific, and consistent with this possibility is the fact that certain tumors reproducibly released biologically active PTHrP of a particular molecular size. Thus the BEN lung cancer cell line released predominantly PTHrP corresponding in size approximately to PTHrP (1–108) (Hammonds et al. 1989), a renal cortical carcinoma cell line consistently released material into medium with an approximate M_R of 6000 (Strewler et al. 1983, 1987), and rat parathyroid cells in culture release material of size approximating that of PTHrP (1–84) (Zajac et al. 1989). Furthermore, Western blotting of PTHrP in extracts of human parathyroid adenomata indicated a molecular size approximately that of PTHrP (1–84) (Danks et al. 1990). If this does indeed prove to be the case, it is becoming increasingly important to define circulating forms of the molecule, and to bear this heterogeneity in mind especially when devising two-site assays for the hormone.

V. Structural Conservation

The structures of PTHrP of rat, mouse, and chicken have now been predicted on the basis of cDNA cloning (Yasuda et al. 1989b; Mangin et al. 1991; Thiede and Rutledge 1990). There is a remarkable degree of structural conservation within the first 111 residues among these species, suggesting that this portion of PTHrP molecule subserves an important function. Thus

hPTHrP	M Q R R L V Q Q W S V A V F L L S Y A V P S C G R S V E G L
rPTHrP	M L R R L V Q Q W S V L V F L L'S Y S V P S R G R S V E G L −6
cPTHrP	A K L F Q Q W S F A V F L L S Y S V P S Y G R S V E G I

hPTHrP	S R R L K R A V S E H Q L L H D K G K S I Q D L R R R F F L
rPTHrP	G R R L K R A V S E H Q L L H D K G K S I Q D L R R R F F L 24
cPTHrP	S R R L K R A V S E H Q L L H D K G K S I Q D L R R R I F L

hPTHrP	H H L I A E I H T A E I R A T S E V S P N S K P S P N T K N
rPTHrP	H H L I A E I H T A E I R A T S E V S P N S K P A P N T K N 54
cPTHrP	Q N L I E G V N T A E I R A T S E V S P N P K P A T N T K N

hPTHrP	H P V R F G S D D E G R Y L T Q E T N K V E T Y K E Q P L K
rPTHrP	H P V R F G S D D E G R Y L T Q E T N K V E T Y K E Q P L K 84
cPTHrP	Y P V R F G S E D E G R Y L T Q E T N K S Q T Y K E Q P L K

hPTHrP	T P G K K K K A K P G K R K E Q E K K K R R T R S A W L D S
rPTHrP	T P G K K K K A K P G K R R E Q E K K K R R T R S A W P G T 114
cPTHrP	V S G K K K K A K P G K R K E Q E K K K R R T R S A W L N S

hPTHrP	G V T G S G L E G D H L S D T S T T S L E L D S R R H *
rPTHrP	T G S G L L E D P Q P H T S P T S T S L E P S S R T H * 141
cPTHrP	G M Y G S N V T E S P V L D N S V T T H N H I L R *

Fig. 3. Amino acid sequences of human, rat, and chicken PTHrP molecules. Residues common to all three are *boxed*

for example, rat PTHrP (1–111) differs only in two residues from the sequence of human, and even chick PTHrP (1–111) differs only in 11 residues (Fig. 3). However, the remainder of the molecule in each case consists of a unique peptide sequence.

D. Actions

The discovery of PTHrP resulted from the search for a substance which appeared capable of having effects very similar to those of PTH. Therefore much of the early work on the actions of PTHrP has focussed upon studies in systems which are known to be PTH responsive. In this discussion the results from these studies will be summarized. Investigations with the amino-terminal region of PTHrP, usually with the synthetic peptide PTHrP (1–34), reveal actions that are indistinguishable from those of PTH (1–34). There are some differences in potencies in some assay systems, which may be explained by different susceptibility of the two to proteolytic cleavage. However, studies with longer forms of PTHrP, either partially purified or recombinant, suggest that there may be other actions within the PTHrP molecule not shared with PTH.

I. Second Messengers and Receptors

As is the case with PTH, PTHrP actives adenylate cyclase in kidney and osteoblasts (KEMP et al. 1987; HORIUCHI et al. 1987; YATES et al. 1988; NISSENSON et al. 1989), and the full expression of this biological activity is contained within the first 34 residues (HAMMONDS et al. 1989). It has been pointed out earlier that the structure-activity relationships within the amino-terminal region of PTHrP are very similar to those of PTH itself, and there is very strong evidence that the two proteins bind to the same receptor (JÜPPNER et al. 1988; SADI et al. 1989). Adenylate cyclase activation in membrane and in whole cell response systems is achieved as effectively by recombinant PTHrP (1–141), (1–108), and (1–84) as it is by the fully active synthetic peptides based on the amino-terminal sequence (HAMMONDS et al. 1989). In addition to affecting adenylate cyclase in PTH targets in an apparently identical manner to that of PTH itself, PTHrP has also been shown to affect cellular calcium uptake in osteogenic carcinoma cells (CIVITELLI et al. 1990). This is an action which has been clearly shown with PTH also, and represents an alternative initial pathway of action of both PTH and PTHrP. These data strongly indicate that the PTH-like effects of PTHrP are mediated through interactions with a receptor common to PTH. They do not exclude the possibility that either molecule might also contain separate biological activities which are mediated through separate receptors. Indeed it is highly likely that this is the case, at least for PTHrP, and this will be discussed later in this chapter.

Studies with PTH receptor antagonist peptides and direct binding experiments using photoaffinity labeling showed that PTHrP and PTH act through the one receptor (SHIGENO et al. 1988). The discovery of PTHrP might have raised further hopes for a particularly effective receptor antagonist, but the analogs of PTHrP with deletions of the amino-terminal residues, although they do have some antagonist activity, as do the corresponding PTH analogs, all have significant agonist activity, and studies to date have not yielded any particularly promising antagonists (McKEE et al. 1988; MOSELEY and SUVA 1990).

II. Postreceptor Events

In addition to their identical early signal responses, PTH and PTHrP exert similar actions on later events which have been studied in isolated cells. These include effects on renal ion transport, stimulation of plasminogen activator activity, inhibition of cell replication in osteogenic carcinoma cells, and relaxation of smooth muscle.

Both partially purified PTHrP (PIZURKI et al. 1988a) and synthetic PTHrP (1–34) (PIZURKI et al. 1988b) have been shown to inhibit Na-dependent Pi transport in kidney cells by a cAMP-dependent mechanism. This Pi transport system is similar to that operating in the brush-border membrane of the rat kidney proximal tubule. Furthermore, synthetic PTHrP (1–34) was found to be as effective as PTH (1–34) in inhibiting amiloride-sensitive sodium transport in cultured renal epithelia (CAVERZASIO et al. 1988), which is taken as an estimate of the Na^+/H^+ exchanger activity of the cells. The effect of longer, recombinant preparations of PTHrP was not tested in those experiments. As will be discussed later, PTHrP (1–141) treatment in prolonged infusions in rat kidney did lead to subtle differences in renal bicarbonate handling (ELLIS et al. 1990), which might contribute to the known differences in acid-basis status between patients with primary hyper-parathyroidism and those with the HHM syndrome.

It has been established that stimulation of plasminogen activator activity is a cyclic AMP-mediated response to PTH in osteoblasts (ALLAN et al. 1986), and this effect of PTHrP has been shown in osteogenic carcinoma cells with both PTHrP (1–34) and recombinant PTHrP (HAMMONDS et al. 1989). A further late effect of PTHrP which is identical to that of PTH is the stimulation of glucose-6-phosphate dehydrogenase activity in distal con-voluted tubules in a cytochemical bioassay (NAKAI et al. 1988). Just as PTH itself inhibits replication of either osteoblasts or osteogenic sarcoma cells (PARTRIDGE et al. 1985), so too does PTHrP (1–34) (RODAN et al. 1988) or PTHrP (1–141) (unpublished data). It has long been recognized that PTH acts directly on smooth muscle to cause its relaxation. This effect has been demonstrated with PTHrP (1–34) in relaxing rat gastric smooth muscle (MOK et al. 1989) and uterine smooth muscle (THIEDE et al. 1990). The evidence for production of PTHrP in uterus and in the chick oviduct during the egg-laying cycle has led to the suggestion that PTHrP may have a paracrine role in these situations, causing smooth muscle relaxation (THIEDE et al. 1991).

III. Actions on Bone

As soon as synthetic preparations of PTHrP were available, it was shown that the peptide was able to promote bone resorption (KEMP et al. 1987). This has been very clearly established by several groups and the only differences among the various results relate to the relative potencies of PTHrP (1–34) and PTH (1–34) in the bone resorption assays that have been used. Thus in some published work it is reported that PTHrP is significantly less effective than PTH in promoting bone resorption (KEMP et al. 1987; THORIKAY et al. 1989; RAISZ et al. 1990), whereas in some the two are equally potent (HORIUCHI et al. 1987; YATES et al. 1988; STEWART et al. 1989) and in others PTHrP is more potent (FUKAYAMA et al. 1988). PTHrP (1–141) clearly stimulates bone resorption in organ culture, and in isolated osteoclasts growing on cortical bone slices it has been found that, provided osteoclast cultures on bone slices are contaminated with significant numbers of osteoblasts or of added osteogenic sarcoma cells, PTHrP (1–34), (1–84), and (1–141) all promote bone resorption (EVELY et al. 1991).

Indeed, in that work, the structural requirements within the amino-terminal region of PTHrP for the stimulation of bone resorption were found to be identical with structural requirements for activation of adenylate cyclase. Thus PTHrP (1–29) or (1–25) was unable to stimulate bone resorption. This was consistent with the view that the bone-resorbing action of PTHrP is also contained within the amino-terminal 34 residues, and again illustrates the correlation between the stimulation of cyclic AMP effects in osteoblasts and the activation of osteoclastic resorption. In that work it was also shown using radiolabeled PTHrP (1–84) that PTHrP binds specifically to osteoblasts and not to osteoclasts, reflecting the indirect effects of these agents on osteoclastic resorption.

One of the interesting differences between the bone findings of patients with HHM and those with primary hyperparathyroidism is that in the latter case there is an osteoblastic response in bone, presumably because of the coupling of resorption to formation in hyperparathyroidism. In patients with HHM, however, the usual finding is that there is no such osteoblastic response, and the bone formation surfaces in patients with HHM are usually depressed (STEWART et al. 1982). These histological findings are reproduced in an experimental model of HHM in which hypercalcemic human cancers are grown in nude mice which become hypercalcemic, and the bones of which show greatly increased resorption and depressed osteoblastic activity (ABRAMSON et al. 1984). In this experimental model it has been shown that neutralizing antibodies against amino-terminal PTHrP are able to prevent and treat the hypercalcemia (KUKREJA et al. 1988). Furthermore, treatment with these antibodies can prevent the bone changes in these animals just as effectively as does surgical removal of the tumors (KUKREJA et al. 1990). This indicates an important role for PTHrP in the development both of the hypercalcemia and of the bone histological changes, but does not exclude the possible contribution of other factors. From what we know of the cellular actions of PTHrP at present, we cannot explain this apparent uncoupling between resorption and formation in HHM. The failure of osteoblastic response could have some other explanation, including possibly the action of other tumor products, e.g., cytokines such as TGFα or TNFα as suggested by MUNDY (1988), or could be related to other accompaniments of the syndrome, including perhaps the prolonged hypercalcemia which is often more severe in the patients with cancer than in those with primary hyperparathyroidism.

Both PTHrP (1–34) and recombinant PTHrP (1–141) can elevate the plasma calcium in animals. Perfusion of PTHrP (1–34) into thyroparathyroidectomized rats leads to elevation of plasma calcium and reduced calcium excretion (HORIUCHI et al. 1987; YATES et al. 1988). The dose-dependent hypercalcemic responses to PTHrP and PTH were equivalent in intact mice, but the hypercalcemia was more sustained than that in response to PTH (YATES et al. 1988). This could fit with the observations of HOCK et al. (1989), whose in vivo studies of the anabolic effects of PTHrP (1–34) and PTH (1–34) in rats suggested that PTHrP is significantly less effective than PTH in its ability to increase bone mass. Histomorphometry showed that the less potent effect of PTHrP on bone mass was not due to differences in bone turnover or a greater stimulation of osteoclastic resorption. PTH increased bone-forming surfaces by two- to three-fold, but PTHrP was significantly less effective. It did, however, evoke a qualitatively similar response in bone formation measures when either the dose was increased or the treatment time was extended. Clearly further in vivo studies of anabolic effects on bone are needed, and differences in pharmacokinetics between PTH and PTHrP will need to be taken into account in such in vivo studies.

There is ample clinical evidence that the renal contribution to hypercalcemia in the HHM syndrome is an important one, and it is now clear that PTHrP, like PTH, has important actions on the kidney. One which is of particular interest is that they both stimulate the activity of the 25-hydroxyvitamin D 1-hydroxylase (HORIUCHI et al. 1987).

IV. Actions on Kidney

In the isolated, perfused rat kidney, PTHrP (1–34) was shown to stimulate calcium reabsorption and the excretion of both phosphate and cyclic AMP (EBELING et al. 1988). These effects, identical to those of PTH, were also evident in vivo (YATES et al. 1988; ZHOU et al. 1989), and established clearly the PTH-like actions of PTHrP on the kidney. The renal responses were investigated further in subsequent work because of the fact recognized for some time that patients with HHM often have a mild hypokalemic alkalosis, whereas a mild hyperchloremic acidosis is more characteristic of primary hyperparathyroidism. It was found that, when infusions of the isolated perfused rat kidney with PTHrP (1–108) and PTHrP (1–141) were carried out for a short period, their effects on biocarbonate excretion were the same as those of PTHrP (1–34) and PTHrP (1–84) (ELLIS et al. 1990). However, when the infusions were prolonged beyond 1 h, there were significant differences in the responses to PTHrP (1–108) and PTHrP (1–141). Both of these peptides on prolonged infusion produced a sharp decline in bicarbonate concentration and excretion, without any significant difference in effects on GFR, fractional excretion of sodium, or urine volume. Although by no means conclusive, this type of experiment should be followed up to determine whether there is some influence of a carboxy-terminal portion of PTHrP which can result in effects on renal bicarbonate handling which differ from those which result from the direct actions of the amino-terminal portion and of PTH. There is no doubt that the renal effect of the hormone is important, and in vivo studies with infusions of PTHrP (1–34) and PTH (1–34) in rats in which resorption was inhibited with a bisphosphonate certainly established that both the bone and renal components of the hypercalcemia mechanism are important (RIZZOLI et al. 1989). This has therapeutic implications in the hypercalcemia of cancer, in that treatments need to consider the renal as well as the bone component of the hypercalcemic complication.

E. Physiological Functions

I. Parathyroid Hormone Related Protein as an Oncofetal Hormone

Most of the initial interest in PTHrP was in its role as a tumor product responsible largely or entirely for the high plasma calcium accompanying many cancers. Since its discovery, however, it seems likely that it is an oncofetal protein, which will turn out to have important physiological roles, perhaps as a paracrine regulator in some tissues and as a hormone in the fetus. While it is not appropriate for this review to consider in detail the evidence for these functions, certain aspects of them will be discussed in order to draw attention to the fact that there is increasing evidence that there may be some actions of PTHrP which are mediated by portions of the molecule other than the PTH-like sequence.

In the mammalian fetus the plasma concentration of calcium is significantly higher than that of the mother (CARE et al. 1988). It is maintained at this level by an active placental calcium pump which provides calcium from the mother to the fetus to make it available for the growing fetal skeleton. Removal of the parathyroid gland in the fetal lamb during the last month of pregnancy results in a decline in the plasma calcium over the subsequent 24–48 h to levels below those of the mother, and this is associated with loss of the placental calcium gradient. At term these lambs show evidence of gross impairment of mineralization of bone (CARE et al. 1986).

These experiments in the fetal lamb show that some factor secreted by the fetal parathyroid glands contributes to maintenance of the placental calcium gradient. In addition to these observations it was known that plasma levels of immunoreactive PTH are lower in the fetus than the mother, but, when PTH-like activity is measured by a sensitive cytochemical assay, activities are higher in the fetus than in the mother (ALLGROVE et al. 1985). Thus physiological hypercalcemia in the fetal lamb and the pathological hypercalcemia in the HHM syndrome are both associated with biologically active, yet immunologically undetectable, PTH-like activities. For that reason the hypothesis was tested that the fetal parathyroid factor apparently responsible for placental calcium transport was indeed PTHrP.

In experiments in which the placentae of previously thyroparathyroidectomized (and thyroxine-replaced) fetal lambs were perfused in situ, the transfer of calcium across the placenta was studied. Removal of the parathyroids was shown to be associated with impairment of the placental calcium transport mechanism which could not be restored by perfusion with PTH (1–84) or PTH (1–34), or with PTHrP (1–34). However, the gradient could be restored with either infusions of partially purified preparations of PTHrP from cancer cell culture media (RODDA et al. 1988) or in later experiments with recombinant PTHrP (1–84), PTHrP (1–108), and PTHrP (1–141) (ABBAS et al. 1989). The conclusion from this work is that PTHrP is a hormone in the fetus which can contribute to the transport of calcium across the placenta from mother to fetus. Furthermore the effect of PTHrP is one which is not associated with the PTH-like part of the molecule, but requires a portion of the PTHrP which is included at least within the 84-residue recombinant preparation. A different conclusion was reached by BARLET et al. (1990), who used an experimental model in which the pregnant ewe was labeled with calcium Ca^{45}, and fetuses treated with either PTH (1–34) or PTHrP (1–34). However, the kinetics of the model they used were validated only for undisturbed pregnancies, and not for studies in which fetal calcium metabolism is disturbed by treatment with the hormones, which would both restrict fetal renal calcium excretion and promote bone resorption.

In addition to the evidence that a portion of PTHrP contributes to placental calcium transport, results from PTHrP immunoassay of extracts of fetal lamb parathyroids (ABBAS et al. 1990) and immunohistology on the same tissue (MacISAAC et al. 1991) indicate that the fetal parathyroid produces PTHrP. There is also evidence that the placenta, particularly in early pregnancy, is capable of producing PTHrP (RODDA et al. 1988), and our current hypothesis is that PTHrP is a hormone of the fetal parathyroid gland which controls the placental calcium pump and makes calcium available for the fetal skeleton in that way. In addition to that we have shown that recombinant PTHrP (1–141) and PTHrP (1–34) decrease calcium excretion by the kidney of the fetal lamb (MacISAAC et al., in preparation). Thus the physiological role of PTHrP in the fetus is similar to that in the postnatal animal. The role of PTH is to be conservative of the extracellular fluid plasma calcium level, elevating calcium by the means available to it, which postnatally means stimulation of bone resorption, restriction of calcium excretion, and indirectly promotion of calcium absorption through activation of vitamin D. In the fetus the major means available for elevation of the fetus plasma calcium are the placental calcium pump and some contribution from renal conservation of calcium. Each of these seems to be stimulated by PTHrP, the placental effect requiring a portion of the molecule other than the PTH-like component, but the renal action being mediated through the PTH-like sequence. Thus we might consider the PTHrP molecule as a precursor of more than one biologically active peptide. As discussed previously in this chapter, the shared PTH/PTHrP receptor mediates the actions on bone and kidney of the PTH-like prototope of PTHrP. The portion of the PTHrP molecule which promotes placental calcium transfer may or may not require the amino-terminal region, and would be expected to have a distinct receptor to mediate its effects. Clearly it would not be appropriate to look for such a receptor with PTHrP (1–34) as the ligand.

II. Paracrine Agent in Smooth Muscle Relaxation

Not all of the nonbone, nonrenal actions of PTHrP are likely to be mediated by a unique portion of the molecule. For example, PTHrP has been shown to exert potent effects relaxing smooth muscle of rat fundus (MOK et al. 1989) or of vascular smooth muscle (WINQUIST et al. 1987). The actions of PTHrP and PTH are very similar in these respects, and therefore the local production of PTHrP around smooth muscle targets is likely to be the important determinant of its physiological role in this respect. Such a role has been proposed in the uterus (THIEDE et al. 1990), and also in the chicken oviduct, in which PTHrP production has been demonstrated and its action on relaxation of the oviduct smooth muscle (THIEDE et al. 1991).

III. Parathyroid Hormone Related Protein in Lactating Breast

The production of PTHrP by lactating mammary tissue has been demonstrated (THIEDE and RODAN 1988) and shown to be prolactin stimulated. The finding of very large amounts of immunoreactive PTHrP in milk of several species, including human milk (BUDAYR et al. 1989b), together with evidence correlating milk calcium with milk PTHrP levels (LAW et al. 1991), indicates that PTHrP production in the lactating breast may have an influence on calcium transport into milk, and is therefore analogous with its effect on the placental calcium-transporting mechanism (RODDA et al. 1988). There is no direct evidence at this stage showing any effect of PTHrP on milk calcium transport, but, if this does become apparent, it will obviously be extremely interesting to know whether this is a property of the PTH-like part of the PTHrP molecule or another portion, perhaps the same as that responsible for the placental effect.

IV. Location in Epithelia

Finally, the localization of PTHrP by immunohistology in the keratinocyte layer of normal skin (DANKS et al. 1989) has raised the possibility that it might play a role in keratinocyte differentiation. Furthermore, the finding of PTHrP in a number of different epithelia in the fetus (MOSELEY et al. 1991) has also raised the possibility of a differentiation effect. This would imply a paracrine role for PTHrP in skin and other epithelia, perhaps by regulating calcium transport. These remain at present as possibilities to be tested, and including the possibility that any paracrine effects are mediated not by the PTH-like part but by another portion of the molecule. Data indicating the presence or absence of PTH receptors in these epithelial tissues are not necessarily relevant to this question.

V. Endocrine and Paracrine Roles

The discovery of PTHrP and its obvious ability to mimic many (or all) of the actions of PTH reveals a previously unrecognized protein, related in evolution to PTH, which may have both endocrine and paracrine functions. Some of the latter possibilities have been mentioned, but in conclusion it is appropriate to reflect on the role of PTHrP as a hormone. There is no evidence yet that, in the postnatal animal (or man), PTHrP functions as a circulating hormone. The evidence that it may do so in the mammalian fetus is strong, but circumstantial, and needs to be proved by classic methods of endocrinology. There is no doubt that PTHrP functions as a hormone in those patients whose cancers produce and release it in excess, in whom circulating levels are clearly elevated (BUDAYR et al. 1989b; BURTIS et al. 1990; GRILL et al. 1992; HENDERSON et al. 1990), and have been shown to fall with removal of the tumor (BURTIS et al. 1990; GRILL et al. 1992). Assays for PTHrP with a sensitivity of 1–2 pmol/l either fail to detect PTHrP in normal human plasma (GRILL et al. 1992) or do so at levels which make interpretation of assay data difficult (BURTIS et al. 1990). It will need assays at least an order of magnitude more sensitive than those currently available to resolve this question. It is interesting to note also that, although production of PTHrP mRNA by parathyroid adenoma has been shown (IKEDA et al. 1988b) and PTHrP localized by immunohistology in parathyroid adenoma tissue (DANKS et al. 1990), elevated levels of plasma PTHrP have not been found in primary hyperparathyroidism with two well-validated assays (BURTIS et al. 1990; GRILL et al. 1992). Just as the PTHrP identified in the keratinocyte layer of normal skin may act in a paracrine manner, and reach the circulation only in very small amounts, very small amounts may be released from parathyroid adenomata. These observations raise interesting questions on the storage and processing of PTHrP.

References

Abbas SK, Pickard DW, Rodda CP, Heath JA, Hammonds RG, Wood WI, Caple IW, Martin TJ, Care AD (1989) Stimulation of ovine placental calcium transport by purified natural and recombinant parathyroid hormone-related protein (PTHrP) preparations. Q J Exp Physiol 74:549
Abbas SK, Pickard DW, Illingworth D, Storer J, Purdie DW, Moniz C, Dixit M, Caple IW, Ebeling PR, Rodda CP, Martin TJ, Care AD (1990) Measurement of parathyroid hormone-related protein in extracts of fetal parathyroid glands and placental membranes. J Endocrinol 124:139
Abramson EC, Kukla LJ, Shevrin DH, Lad TE, McGuire WP, Kukreja SC (1984) Model for malignancy-associated humoral hypercalcemia. Calcif Tissue Int 36:563
Albright F (1941) Case records of the Massachusetts General Hospital (case 27401). N Engl J Med 225:789
Allan EH, Hamilton JA, Medcalf RL, Kubota M, Martin TJ (1986) Cyclic AMP-dependent and -independent effects on tissue-type plasminogen activator activity in osteogenic sarcoma cells; evidence from phosphodiesterase inhibition and parathyroid hormone antagonist. Biochem Biophys Acta 888:199
Allgrove J, Admini S, Manning RM, O'Riordan JLH (1985) Cytochemical bioassay of parathyroid hormone in maternal and cord blood. Arch Dis Child 60:110
Barden JA, Kemp BE (1989) NMR study of a 34-residue N-terminal fragment of the parathyroid hormone related protein secreted during humoral hypercalcemia of malignancy. Eur J Biochem 184:379

Barlet JP, Davicco MJ, Coxam V (1990) Synthetic parathyroid hormone-related peptide (1–34) fragment stimulates calcium transfer in ewes. J Endocrinol 127:33

Budayr AA, Halloran BP, King JC, Diep D, Nissenson RA, Strewler GJ (1989a) High levels of a parathyroid hormone-like protein in milk. Proc Natl Acad Sci USA 86:7183

Budayr AA, Nissenson RA, Klein RF, Pun KK, Clark OH, Diep D, Arnaud CD, Strewler GJ (1989b) Increased serum levels of a parathyroid hormone-like protein in malignancy-associated hypercalcemia. Ann Intern Med 111: 807

Burtis WJ, Wu J, Bunch CM, Wysolmerski JJ, Insogna KL, Weir EC, Broadus AE, Stewart AF (1987) Identification of a novel 17 000-dalton parathyroid hormone-like adenylate cyclase-stimulating protein from a tumor associated with humoral hypercalcemia of malignancy. J Biol Chem 262:7151

Burtis WJ, Brady TG, Orloff JJ, Ersbak JB, Warrell RP, Olson BR, Wu TL, Mitnick ME, Broadus AE, Stewart AE (1990) Immunochemical characterization of circulating parathyroid hormone-related protein in patients with humoral hypercalcemia of cancer. N Engl J Med 322:1106

Care AD, Caple IW, Abbas SK, Pickard DW (1986) The effect of fetal thyropara-thyroidectomy on transport of calcium across the ovine placenta to the fetus. Placenta, 7:417

Care AD, Caple IW, Pickard DW (1988) The roles of the parathyroid and thyroid glands on calcium homeostasis in the ovine fetus. In: Jones CT, Nathaniels P (eds) The physiological development of the fetus and newborn. Academic, New York, p 135

Care AD, Abbas SK, Pickard DW, Barri M, Drinkhill M, Findlay JBC, White IR, Caple IW (1990) Stimulation of ovine placental transport of calcium and magnesium by mid-molecule fragments of human parathyroid hormone-related protein. Exp Physiol 75:605

Caverzasio J, Rizzoli R, Martin TJ, Bonjour P (1988) Tumoral synthetic parathyroid hormone-related peptide inhibits amiloride-sensitive sodium transport in cultured renal epithelia. Pflugers Arch 413:96

Civitelli A, Martin TJ, Hruska KA, Avioli LV (1990) Parathyroid hormone-related peptide (PTHrP) transiently increases intracellular calcium in osteoblastic-like cells. Endocrinology 125:1204

Danks JA, Ebeling PR, Hayman J, Chou ST, Moseley JM, Dunlop J, Kemp BE, Martin TJ (1989) Parathyroid hormone-related protein of cancer: immuno-histochemical localization in cancers and in normal skin. J Bone Miner Res 4: 273

Danks JA, Ebeling PR, Hayman JA, Diefenbach-Jagger H, Collier F, Grill V, Southby J, Moseley JM, Chou ST, Martin TJ (1990) Immunohistochemical localization of parathyroid hormone-related protein in parathyroid adenoma and hyperplasia. J Pathol 16:27

Ebeling PR, Adam WR, Moseley JM, Martin TJ (1988) Actions of parathyroid hormone-related protein on the isolated rat kidney. J Endocrinol 12:45

Ellis AG, Adam WR, Martin TJ (1990) Comparison of the effects of parathyroid hormone (PTH) and recombinant PTH-related protein on bicarbonate excretion by the isolated, perfused rat kidney. J Endocrinol 126:403

Evely RS, Bonomo A, Schneider H-G, Moseley JM, Gallagher J, Martin TJ (1991) The action of parathyroid hormone-related protein (PTHrP) on bone resorption by isolated osteoclasts. J Bone Miner Res 6:85

Fukayama S, Bosma TJ, Goaad DL, Voelkel EF, Tashjian AH Jr (1988) Human parathyroid hormone (PTH)-related protein and human PTH: comparative biological activities on human bone cells and bone resorption. Endocrinology 128:2841

Greenberg PB, Martin TJ, Sutcliffe HS (1973) Synthesis and release of parathyroid hormone by a renal carcinoma in cell culture. Clin Sci Mol Med 45:183

Grill V, Diefenbach-Jagger H, Ebeling PR, Glatz JA, Moseley JM, Hammonds GR, Wood WI, Martin TJ (1989) Characterization of parathyroid hormone-related protein with region specific antisera. J Bone Miner Res 3 Suppl 1:A779

Grill V, Ho P, Body JJ, Johanson, N, Lee S, Kukreja S, Moseley J, Martin TJ (1991) Parathyroid hormone-related protein: elevated levels both in humoral hypercalcemia of malignancy and in hypercalcemia complicating metastatic breast cancer. J Clin Endocrinol Metab 73:1309

Hammonds RG, McKay P, Winslow GA, Diefenbach-Jagger H, Grill V, Glatz JA, Rodda CP, Moseley JM, Wood WI, Martin TJ (1989) Purification and characterization of recombinant human parathyroid hormone-related protein. J Biol Chem 264:14806

Henderson JE, Shustik C, Kremer R, Rabbani SA, Hendy GN, Goltzman D (1990) Circulating concentrations of parathyroid hormone-like peptide in malignancy and hyperparathyroidism. J Bone Miner Res 5:105

Hock JM, Fonseca J, Gunness-Hey M, Kemp BE, Martin TJ (1989) Comparison of the anabolic effects of synthetic parathyroid hormone-related protein (PTHrP) 1–34 and PTH 1–34 on bone in rats. Endocrinology 125:2022

Horiuchi N, Caulfield MP, Fisher JE, Goldman ME, McKee RL, Reagan JE, Levy JJ, Nutt RF, Rodan SB, Scholfield TL, Clemens TL, Rosenblatt M (1987) Similarity of synthetic peptide from human tumor to parathyroid hormone in vivo and in vitro. Science 238:1566

Ikeda K, Mangin M, Dreyer BE, Webb AC, Posillico JT, Stewart AF, Bander NH, Weir EC, Insogna KL, Broadus AE (1988a) Identification of transcripts encoding a parathyroid hormone-like peptide in messenger RNAs from a variety of human and animal tumors associated with humoral hypercalcemia of malignancy. J Clin Invest 81:2010

Ikeda K, Weir E, Mangin M, Dannies PS, Kinder B, Deftos LJ, Brown E, Broadus AE (1988b) Expression of messenger ribonucleic acids encoding a parathyroid hormone-like peptide in normal human and animal tissues with abnormal expression in human parathyroid adenomas. Mol Endocrinol 2:1230

Ikeda K, Lu C, Weir EC, Mangin M, Broadus AE (1989) Transcriptional regulation of the parathyroid hormone-related peptide gene by glucocorticoids and vitamin D in a human C-cell line. J Biol Chem 264:15743

Ilardi CF, Faro JC (1975) Localization of parathyroid hormone-like substance in squamous cell carcinoma. Arch Pathol Lab Med 109:752

Isales C, Carcangiu ML, Stewart AF (1987) Hypercalcemia in breast cancer: reassessment of the mechanism. Am J Med 82:1143

Jueppner H, Abou-Samra AB, Uneno S, Gu WX, Potts JT, Segre GV (1988) The parathyroid hormone-like peptide associated with humoral hypercalcemia of malignancy and parathyroid hormone bind to the same receptor on the plasma membrane of ROS 17/2.8 cells. J Biol Chem 263:8557

Kemp BE, Moseley JM, Rodda CP, Ebeling PR, Wettenhall REH, Stapleton D, Diefenbach-Jagger H, Ure F, Michelangeli VP, Simmons H, Raisz LG, Martin TJ (1987) Parathyroid hormone-related protein of malignancy: active synthetic fragments. Science 238:1568

Kukreja SC, Schavin DH, Wimbuscus S, Ebeling PR, Danks JA, Rodda CP, Wood WI, Martin TJ (1988) Antibodies to parathyroid hormone-related protein lower serum calcium in athymic mouse models of malignancy associated hypercalcemia due to human tumors. J Clin Invest 82:1798

Kukreja SC, Rosol TJ, Wimbiscus SA, Shevrin DH, Grill V, Barengolts L, Martin TJ (1990) Tumor reaction and antibodies to parathyroid hormone-related protein cause similar changes on bone histomorphometry in hypercalcemia of cancer. Endocrinology 127:305

Lafferty FW (1966) Pseudohyperparathyroidism. Medicine (Baltimore) 45:247

Law FMK, Moate PJ, Leaver DD, Diefenbach-Jagger H, Grill V, Ho PWM, Martin TJ (1991) Parathyroid hormone-related protein in milk and its correlation with bovine milk calcium. J Endocrinol 128:21

MacIsaac RJ, Caple IW, Danks JA, Diefenbach-Jagger H, Grill V, Moseley JM, Southby J, Martin TJ (1991) Ontogeny of parathyroid hormone-related protein in the ovine parathyroid gland. Endocrinology 129:757

Mangin M, Webb AC, Dreyer BE, Posillico JT, Ikeda K, Weir EC, Stewart AF, Bander NH, Milstone L, Barton DE, Francke U, Broadus AE (1988a) Identification of a cDNA encoding a parathyroid hormone-like peptide from a human tumor associated with humoral hypercalcemia of malignancy. Proc Natl Acad Sci USA 85:597

Mangin M, Ikeda K, Dreyer BE, Milstone L, Broadus AE (1988b) Two distinct tumor-derived parathyroid hormone-like peptides result from alternative ribonucleic acid processing. Mol Endocrinol 2:1049

Mangin M, Ikeda K, Dreyer BE, Broadus AE (1989) Isolation and characterization of the human parathyroid hormone-like peptide gene. Proc Natl Acad Sci USA 86:2408

Mangin M, Ikeda K, Dreyer B, Broadus AE (1990) Identification of an upstream promoter of the human parthyroid hormone-related peptide gene. Mol Endocrinol 4:851

Mangin M, Ikeda K, Broadus AE (1991) Structure of the mouse parathyroid hormone-related peptide gene. Gene 95:195

Mannens M, Slater RM, Heyting C, Guerts van Kessel A, Goedde-Salz B, Frants RR, van-Ommen GJB, Pearson PL (1987) Regional localization of DNA probed on the short arm of chromosome 11 using anirdia-Wilms' tumor associated deletions. Hum Genet 75:180

Martin TJ, Atkins D (1979) Biochemical regulators of bone resorption and their significance in cancer. Essays Med Biochem 4:49

Martin TJ, Allan EH, Caple IW, Care AD, Danks JA, Diefenbach-Jagger H, Ebeling PR, Gillespie MT, Hammonds RG, Heath JA, Hudson PJ, Kemp BE, Kubota M, Kukreja SC, Moseley JM, Ng KW, Raisz LG, Rodda CP, Simmons HA, Suva LJ, Wettenhall REH, Wood WI (1989) Parathyroid hormone-related protein: isolation, molecular cloning and mechanism of action. Recent Prog Horm Res 45:467

Mayes LC, Kasselberg AG, Rolott JS, Lukens JN (1984) Hypercalcemia associated with immunoreactive parathyroid hormone in a malignant rhabdoid tumor of the kidney (rhabdoid Wilm's tumor). Cancer 54:882

McKee RL, Goldman ME, Caulfield MP, de Haven PA, Levy TJ, Nutt RF, Rosenblatt M (1988) The 7–34 fragment of human hypercalcemia factor is a partial agonist/antagonist for parathyroid stimulated cAMP production. Endocrinology 122:3008

Mok LLS, Ajiwe E, Martin TJ, Thompson JC, Cooper CW (1989) Parathyroid hormone-related protein relaxes smooth muscle and shows cross-desensitization with PTH. J Bone Miner Res 4:433

Moseley JM, Suva LJ (1990) Isolation, biochemistry and molecular biology of the PTH-related protein of malignant hypercalcemia. Bone Miner Res 7:175

Moseley JM, Kubota M, Diefenbach-Jagger H, Wettenhall REH, Kemp BE, Suva LJ, Rodda CP, Ebeling PR, Hudson PJ, Zajac JD, Martin TJ (1987) Parathyroid hormone-related protein purified from a human lung cancer cell line. Proc Natl Acad Sci USA 84:5048

Moseley JM, Hayman JA, Danks JA, Alcorn D, Grill V, Southby J, Horton MA (1991) Immunohistochemical detection of parathyroid hormone-related protein (PTHrP) in human fetal epithelia. J Clin Endocrinol Metab 73:478

Mundy GR (1988) Hypercalcemia of malignancy revisited. J Clin Invest 82:1

Mundy GR, Martin TJ (1982) The hypercalcemia of malignancy: pathogenesis and treatment. Metabolism 31:1247

Mundy GR, Ibbotson KJ, D'Souza SM, Simpson EL, Jacobs JW, Martin TJ (1984) The hypercalcemia of cancer. N Engl J Med 310:1718

Nakai M, Kukase M, Sakaguchi K et al. (1988) Human PTHrP fragment (1–34) had glucose-β-phosphate dehydrogenase activity on distal convoluted tubules in cytochemical bioassay. Biochem Biophys Res Commun 154:146

Nissenson RA, Diep D, Strewler GJ (1989) Synthetic peptides comprising the amino-terminal sequence of a parathyroid hormone-like protein from human malignancies. J Biol Chem 263:12866

Nussbaum SR, Rosenblatt M, Potts JT Jr (1980) Parathyroid hormone-renal receptor interactions. Demonstration of two receptor binding domains. J Biol Chem 255:10183

Palmieri GMA, Nordquist RE, Omenn GS (1974) Immunochemical localization of parathyroid hormone in cancer tissue from patients with ectopic hyperparathyroidism. J Clin Invest 53:1726

Partridge NC, Opie AL, Opie RT, Martin TJ (1985) Inhibitory effects of parathyroid hormone on growth of osteogenic sarcoma cells. Calc Tissue Int 37:519

Percival RC, Yates AJP, Gray RES, Galloway J, Rogers K, Neal FE, Kanis JA (1985) Mechanisms of malignant hypercalcemia in carcinoma of the breast. Br Med J 2:7766

Pizurki L, Rizzoli R, Caverzasio J, Bonjour JP (1988a) Factor derived from human lung carcinoma associated with hypercalcemia mimics the effects of parathyroid hormone on phosphate transport in cultured epithelia. J Bone Miner Res 3:233

Pizurki L, Rizzoli R, Moseley J, Martin TJ, Caversasio J, Bonjour JP (1988b) Effect of synthetic tumoral PTH-related peptide on cAMP production and Na-dependent Pi transport. Am J Physiol 255:F957

Raisz L, Simmons HA, Vargus SJ, Kemp BE, Martin TJ (1990) Comparison of the effects of amino-terminal synthetic parathyroid hormone related peptide (PTHrP) of malignancy and parathyroid hormone on resorption of cultured fetal rat long bones. Calcif Tissue Int 46:233

Rizzoli R, Caverzasio J, Chapuy MC, Martin TJ, Bonjour J-P (1989) Role of bone and kidney in parathyroid hormone-related peptide-induced hypercalcemia in rats. J Bone Miner Res 4:759

Rodan SB, Insogna KL, Vignery AM-C, Stewart AF, Broadus AE, D'Souza S, Bertolini DR, Mundy GR, Rodan GA (1983) Factors associated with humoral hypercalcemia of malignancy stimulate adenylate cyclase in osteoblastic cells. J Clin Invest 72:1511

Rodan SB, Noda M, Wesolowski G, Rosenblatt M, Rodan GA (1988) Comparison of postreceptor effects of 1–34 human hypercalcemic factor and 1–34 human parathyroid hormone in rat osteosarcoma cells. J Clin Invest 81:924

Rodda CP, Kubota M, Heath JA, Ebeling PR, Moseley JM, Care AD, Caple IW, Martin TJ (1988) Evidence for a novel parathyroid hormone-related protein in fetal lamb parathyroid glands and sheep placenta: comparisons with a similar protein implicated in humoral hypercalcemia of malignancy. J Endocrinol 117:261

Sadi A, Samra A, Uneno S, Jueppner H, Keutmann H, Potts JT Jr, Segre GV, Nussbaum SR (1989) Non-homologous sequences of parathyroid hormone related peptide bind to a common receptor in ROS 17/2.8 cells. Endocrinology 125:2215

Setzer DR, McGrogan M, Schimke RT (1982) Nucleotide sequences surrounding multiple polyadenylation sites in the mouse dihydrofolate reductase gene. J Biol Chem 257:5143

Sherwood LM, O'Riordan JLH, Aurbach GD (1967) Production of parathyroid hormone by non-parathyroid tumors. J Clin Endocrinol Metab 27:140

Shigeno C, Hiraki Y, Westerberg DP, Potts JT Jr, Segre GV (1988) Photoaffinity labeling of parathyroid hormone receptors in clonal rat osteosarcoma cells. J Biol Chem 263:3864

Stewart AF, Horst R, Deftos LJ, Cadman EC, Lang R, Broadus AE (1980) Biochemical evaluation of patients with cancer-associated hypercalcemia. Evidence for humoral and non-humoral groups. N Engl J Med 303:1377

Stewart AF, Vignery A, Silvergate A, Ravin ND, Li Volsi V, Broadus AE, Baron R (1982) Quantitative bone histomorhometry in humoral hypercalcemia of malignancy: uncoupling of bone cell activity. J Clin Endocrinol Metab 55:219

Stewart AF, Insogna KL, Goltzman D, Broadus AE (1983) Identification of adenylate cyclase-stimulating activity and cytochemical glucose-6-phosphate dehydrogenase stimulating activity in extracts of tumors from patients with humoral hypercalcemia of malignancy. Proc Natl Acad Sci USA 80:1454

Stewart AF, Wu T, Goumas D, Burtis WJ, Broadus AE (1987) N-terminal amino-acid sequence of two novel tumor-derived adenylate cyclase-stimulating proteins: identification of parathyroid hormone-like and unlike domains. Biochem Biophys Res Commun 146:672

Stewart AF, Mangin M, Wu T, Goumas D, Insogna KL, Burtis WJ, Broadus AE (1988) Synthetic human parathyroid hormone-like protein stimulates bone resorption and causes hypercalcemia in rats. J Clin Invest 81:596

Stewart AF, Elliot J, Burtis WJ, Wu F (1989) Synthetic parathyroid hormone-like protein (1–74): biochemical and physiological characterization. Endocrinology 24:642

Strewler GJ, Williams RD, Nissenson RA (1983) Human renal carcinoma cells produce hypercalcemia in the nude mouse and a novel protein recognised by parathyroid hormone receptors. J Clin Invest 71:769

Strewler GJ, Stern PH, Jacobs JW, Eveloff J, Klein RF, Leung SC, Rosenblatt M, Nissenson RA (1987) Parathyroid hormone-like protein from human renal carcinoma cells. Structural and functional homology with parathyroid hormone. J Clin Invest 80:1803

Suva LJ, Winslow GA, Wettenhall REH, Kemp BE, Hudson PJ, Diefenbach-Jagger H, Moseley JM, Rodda CP, Martin TJ, Wood WI (1987) A parathyroid hormone-related protein implicated in malignant hypercalcemia: cloning and expression. Science 237:893

Suva LJ, Mather KA, Gillespie MT, Webb GC, Ng KW, Winslow GA, Wood WI, Martin TJ, Hudson PJ (1989) Structure of the 5' flanking region of the gene encoding human parathyroid-hormone-related protein (PTHrP). Gene 77:95

Thiede MA, Rodan GA (1988) Expression of a calcium-mobilizing parathyroid hormone-like peptide in lactating mammary tissue. Science 242:278

Thiede MA, Rutledge SJ (1990) Nucleotide sequence of a parathyroid hormone-related protein expressed by the 10 day chicken embryo. Nucleic Acids Res 18:3062

Thiede MA, Strewler RA, Nissensen RA, Rosenblatt M, Rodan GA (1988) Human renal carcinoma expresses two messages encoding a parathyroid hormone like peptide: evidence for the alternate splicing of a single copy gene. Proc Natl Acad Sci USA 85:4605

Thiede MA, Daifotis AG, Weir EC, Brines ML, Burtis WJ, Ikeda K, Dreyer BE, Garfield RE, Broadus AE (1990) Intrauterine occupancy controls expression of the parathyroid hormone-related peptide gene in preterm rat myometrium. Proc Natl Acad Sci USA 87:6969

Thiede MA, Harm SC, McKee RL, Grasser W, Duong LT, Leach RM (1991) Expression of the parathyroid hormone-related protein gene in the avian oviduct: potential role as a local modulator of vascular smooth muscle tension and shell gland motility during the egg-laning cycle. Endocrinol 129

Thorikay M, Kramer S, Reynolds FH, Sorvillo JM, Doescher L, Wu T, Morris CA, Burtis WJ, Insogna KL, Valenzuela DM, Stewart AF (1989) Synthesis of a gene encoding parathyroid hormone-like protein (1–141). Purification and biological characterization of the expressed protein. Endocrinology 124:111

Tregear GW, van Reitschotten J, Greene E, Keutman HT, Niall HD, Reit B, Parsons JA, Potts JT Jr (1973) Bovine parathyroid hormone: minimum chain length of synthetic peptide required for biological activity. Endocrinology 93:1349

Welling GW, Wejser WJ, van der Zee R, Welling-Webster S (1985) Production of sequential antigenic regions in proteins. FEBS Lett 188:215

Winquist RJ, Baskin EP, Vlasuk GP (1987) Synthetic tumor-derived human hypercalcemic factor exhibits PTH-like vasorelaxation in renal arteries. Biochem Biophys Acta 149:227

Yaffe D, Nudel U, Mayer Y, Neuman S (1985) Highly conserved sequences in the 3' untranslated regions of mRNAs coding for homologous proteins in distantly related species. Nucleic Acids Res 13:372

Yasuda T, Banville D, Hendy GN, Goltzman D (1989a) Characterization of the human parathyroid hormone-like peptide gene. J Biol Chem 264:7720

Yasuda T, Banville D, Rabbani SA, Hendy G, Goltzman D (1989b) Rat parathyroid hormone-like peptide: comparison with the human homologue and expression in malignant and normal tissue. Mol Endocrinol 3:519

Yates AJP, Gutierrez GE, Smoleus P, Travis PS, Katz MS, Aufdemorte TB, Boyce BF, Hymer TK, Poser JW, Mundy GR (1988) Effects of a synthetic peptide of a parathyroid hormone-related protein on calcium homeostasis, renal tubular calcium reabsorption and bone metabolism in vivo and in vitro in rodents. J Clin Invest 81:932

Young RA, Hägenbuchle O, Schibler V (1981) A single mouse α-amylase gene specifies two different tissue-specific mRNAs. Cell 23:451

Zajac JD, Callaghan J, Eldridge C, Diefenbach-Jagger H, Suva LJ, Hudson P, Moseley JM, Michelangeli VP, Pasquini G (1989) Production of parathyroid hormone-related protein by a rat parathyroid cell line. Mol Cell Endocrinol Metab 67:107

Zhou H, Leaver DD, Moseley JM, Kemp BE, Ebeling PR, Martin TJ (1989) Actions of parathyroid hormone-related protein on the rat kidney in vivo. J Endocrinol 122:227

CHAPTER 18

Pathophysiology of Skeletal Complications of Cancer

G.R. MUNDY and T.J. MARTIN

A. Introduction

Tumors frequently affect the skeleton and alter the function of normal bone cells. In most patients, they increase the activity and probably the formation of bone-resorbing osteoclasts. The result is a destructive or osteolytic bone lesion. Occasionally they lead to an increase in activation of osteoblasts or bone-forming cells. In a relatively small number of patients, this increase in osteoblastic activity is profound and the result is an area of newly formed bone around the tumor cell deposit which can be detected radiologically and is referred to as an osteoblastic or sclerotic metastasis. In this chapter, we plan to review what is known of the mechanisms responsible for development of osteolytic and osteoblastic bone lesions.

B. Frequency of the Skeleton as a Site for Malignant Disease

The skeleton is probably the third most common site of distant spread of solid tumors, after the liver and the lung. There are no available satisfactory figures for the frequency of bone metastases. Bone metastases may be very subtle and are difficult to detect when they are small and particularly when they are present in the appendicular skeleton. All studies which have been performed can be criticized because none of the methods used in detection of bone metastases are entirely reliable, and of course the frequency always depends on the stage of the disease at the time of assessment. However, it can be estimated that there are approximately 500 000 deaths per year in the United States from malignant disease and probably one-half to two-thirds of these patients die with bone lesions. Possibly the only entirely reliable figures would be those obtained from careful and meticulous autopsy studies performed on patients who die from cancer. As an example of the variability of the reported frequency of bone metastases in specific tumors, estimates in the literature on the frequency of bone metastases in breast cancer vary from 47% to 85% (GALASKO 1986a,b). Although most tumors have the capacity to metastasize to bone, and the actual sites of bone metastases are similar for different tumors, nevertheless there are specific patterns of metastasis to the skeleton for different tumors. Moreover, there are some relatively less common tumors which seem to metastasize to bone more frequently than others, so that the capacity to metastasize avidly to bone seems not to be a simple random or stochastic process, but rather a complex sequence of essential steps determined by specific properties of the cancer cells and the target organ, in this case bone. These issues will be discussed in more detail in the following pages.

The clinical detection of bone metastases is difficult when they are subtle. X-rays will not detect lesions less than 1 cm in diameter, and require loss of 40% of mineral for detection. In older people, lytic lesions in the vertebrae may be difficult to distinguish from osteopenia. In cancer, a ragged outline of the lesion and destruction of the pedicles are clues which may help. X-rays are not very sensitive, since cortical bone is usually not involved in metastatic bone disease. X-rays show metastatic bone lesions to be lytic, blastic, or mixed. Lytic and mixed are far more common than predominantly blastic lesions. Larger (>1 cm) lesions usually have well-defined edges and are often solitary. More rapidly growing tumors often form multiple smaller lytic lesions with ill-defined edges (Lodwick 1964). Radionuclide scans are more sensitive than X-rays if lesions have a blastic component, but the limit of resolution is 2–3 mm, and false positives are more frequent. CAT scans or MRI provide little additional help except under special circumstances. The CAT scan may be useful in distinguishing metastatic bone disease from degenerative joint disease in the periphery. It gives an indication of the amount of bone lost and is particularly helpful in the vertebral column. It also gives useful information about tumor extension into adjacent structures such as the spinal canal or the pelvic cavity. MRI is not very helpful with mineralized tissues, although it may be helpful in clarifying adjacent structures such as the spinal canal. Markers such as

Table 1. Frequency of skeletal metastases at autopsy. (Modified from Galasko 1986b)

Tumor	Frequency of skeletal metastasis [%]
Breast	50–85
Prostate	60–85
Thyroid	28–60
Kidney	33–60
Lung	32–64
Esophagus	6
Gastrointestinal tract	3–10
Rectum	8–60
Bladder	42
Uterine cervix	50
Ovaries	9
Liver	16
Melanoma	7

fasting urine calcium, urine hydroxyproline, or deoxypyridinolone cross-links may give indications of increased bone resorption, but are non-specific. They are useful for monitoring potential treatments, but not for diagnosis. Table 1 shows the different types of bone metastases and their characteristics.

C. Cancers Which Involve the Skeleton

Table 2 shows the frequency of solid tumors which are associated with metastatic bone lesions. For reasons already indicated, these figures are greatly influenced by the time in the course of the disease the examination is made. The most common solid tumors of man, namely lung tumors and breast tumors, are also frequently associated with bone metastases. However, there are also some tumors which metastasize to bone out of proportion to their frequency in the general population. The most notable of these is thyroid cancer, which frequently attacks the skeleton. Thus, there must be specific properties of certain tumors which allow this predilection for skeletal metastases. The reported incidence of skeletal metastases for various tumors has been reviewed in detail by GALASKO (1986), and the reader is referred to this source for more complete information.

Table 2. Frequency of skeletal metastases, as detected by scintigraphy. (Modified from GALASKO 1986b)

Primary site	Percentage with metastases
Breast	84
Prostate	70
Thyroid	43
Kidney	60
Bronchus	64
Rectum	61
Uterine cervix	56

Table 3. Destruction of bone metastases detected by scintigraphy. (From TOYE et al. 1975)

Primary tumor	Distribution of skeletal metastases (%)				
	Skull	Spine	Rib cage	Pelvis	Appendicular skeleton
Breast	28	60	59	38	32
Lung	16	43	65	25	27
Prostate	14	60	50	57	38
Cervix	26	26	22	43	43
Bladder	13	47	53	47	7
Rectum	21	36	29	43	43

D. Favored Skeletal Sites of Malignancy

The most common sites of skeletal metastases are in the axial skeleton, and are characterized by rich blood supply and red bone marrow. Thus, most tumor cells metastasize to the pelvis, the ribs, and the vertebral column. Table 3 shows the distribution of skeletal metastases as detected by scintigraphy.

The ribs are a frequent site of tumor cell metastasis. Tumors also frequently metastasize to the proximal ends of long bones. Metastases to the skull occur, but are less common. Although metastases in the appendicular skeleton are less frequent, they do occur occasionally. In particular, melanoma and renal carcinoma may metastasize to distal extremities. The distribution of skeletal metastases from various primary cancers has been reviewed in detail by Galasko (1986a,b). The actual sites to which tumor cells metastasize is determined to some degree by blood flow from the primary site. For example, prostate cancer seems to metastasize particularly to the vertebral column, and in this situation Batson's vertebral venous plexus may be important. Batson's vertebral plexus is a low-pressure, high-volume system of vertebral veins which was demonstrated when dye was injected into the dorsal vein of the penis in cadavers and experimental animals (Batson 1940). It communicates fully with the intercostal veins. Although dye traverses this system as it runs up the spine, little gets into the caval system. It has been linked particularly to the distribution of tumor cell metastasis in patients with prostate cancer. This system has extensive intercommunications which may function independently of other major venous systems such as the pulmonary, caval, and portal systems (Batson 1940). Other evidence also suggests that this system in fact may be important for the spread of tumor cells to the skeleton and particularly to the axial skeleton (Coman and DeLong 1951; Van den Brenk et al. 1975; Galasko 1986). However, not all urologists have accepted the importance of this paravertebral plexus, and have questioned whether prostate cancer does spread preferentially to the pelvis, lumbar spine, and sacrum (Dodds et al. 1981).

E. Complications of the Metastatic Process

When tumors metastasize to bone, there are a number of important implications for patients. The most important is that, under these circumstances, tumors are rarely curable and only palliative therapy is possible. An exception may be renal cell carcinoma, where occasionally a solitary metastasis occurs which can be removed surgically with a reasonable prognosis. When tumor cells metastasize to bone, patients frequently develop bone pain at the site of metastasis. The mechanisms responsible for bone pain are not clear, since bone pain may fluctuate without apparent changes in the size or nature of the underlying lesion. Bone is always significantly weakened by the presence of metastasis, and pathologic fractures may result. This is particularly likely to occur in patients with predominantly lytic lesions. Pathologic fractures are most common in the vertebrae. Other common sites of pathologic fracture are the pelvis and femur. Nerve compression syndromes may occur in patients with severe destructive lesions. These are most common in diseases such as myeloma, where spinal cord compression can occur as a consequence of vertebral body collapse and deformity. In patients with blastic lesions, bony overgrowth may also lead to subsequent nerve compression syndromes. These are particularly associated with prostate cancer, which in metastasizing to the vertebrae can cause spinal cord compression, cauda equina syndromes, and paraparesis, or to the base of the skull can impinge on the cranial nerves.

Hypercalcemia frequently occurs in patients with osteolytic bone destruction due to metastatic bone disease. It is present in approximately 30% of patients with breast cancer some time during the course of the disease (Galasko and Burn 1971). A similar number of patients with myeloma also develop hypercalcemia (Mundy 1990). It is possible that in some of these patients the increase in bone resorption is due to the production of systemic factors by the tumor cells. However, in many of these patients hypercalcemia is rare unless the tumor is widely metastatic and it is likely in these circumstances that the local destruction of bone is the major pathogenetic mechanism. Although definitive evidence is not available, it is probable that the major mechanism by which bone is destroyed is by an increase in osteoclast activity. There are two arguments for this notion, although neither is conclusive. Firstly, when looked for, osteoclasts are always found adjacent to tumor cells at bone-resorbing margins, and scanning electron microscopy studies of endosteal bone surfaces in patients with osteolytic bone destruction show evidence of Howship's lacunae made by osteoclasts (Boyde et al. 1986). Although it has been shown that breast cancer cells have the capacity to release ^{45}Ca from devitalized bone and lead to degradation of bone matrix (Eilon and Mundy 1978), the role of tumor cells as mediators of bone resorption does not appear to be major and has not been verified by scanning electron microscopy views of the bone surface. The second argument is that drugs which inhibit osteoclast activity such as bisphosphonates and plicamycin are effective anti-hypercalcemic agents, and decrease parameters of increased bone resorption such as hydroxyproline excretion and fasting urine calcium in normocalcemic patients with osteolytic disease (Siris et al. 1980; Van Breukelen et al. 1979).

For a number of years, it has been conventional to classify patients with solid tumors and hypercalcemia into those with the humoral hypercalcemia of malignancy, where a systemic or circulating factor is responsible, and those with localized osteolysis, where either local factors produced by tumor cells which have metastasized to bone or the tumor cells themselves are responsible for localized bone destruction which leads to hypercalcemia.

This has been a practical classification, but one which is no longer particularly helpful. The relative contribution of local osteolytic bone destruction relative to systemic osteoclastic bone resorption has never been possible to discern. In some patients, it is clear that both local and systemic bone resorption contribute to the hypercalcemia. In some patients with localized osteolytic bone destruction and hypercalcemia, it is now apparent that systemic mediators are produced by the tumor cells and are likely to play a major role in the pathophysiology of hypercalcemia. These factors are likely to be even more important if they are produced in relatively larger concentrations at the bone site by metastatic tumor cells than if they are produced by distant tumor cells at the primary site in the same concentration. Obviously, under the latter circumstances the factors will be diluted by the time they reach bone-resorbing cells. Some groups have made a distinction between these two groups based on the measurement of nephrogenous cyclic AMP (STEWART et al. 1980). This may be misleading, since PTH-rP is not the only factor associated with the humoral hypercalcemia of malignancy, and, indeed, some patients with the humoral hypercalcemia of malignancy do not have increased nephrogenous cyclic AMP. Moreover, if PTH-rP is produced locally by metastatic tumor cells and plays an important role in the hypercalcemia, it may not be produced in sufficient amounts to cause an increase in nephrogenous cyclic AMP, which is due to the effects of circulating PTH-rP on the renal tubular cells.

It is also possible that increased renal tubular calcium reabsorption is important in the pathophysiology of hypercalcemia in patients with metastatic bone disease. PERCIVAL et al. (1985) and GALLACHER et al. (1990) showed that in patients with breast cancer there was frequently an increase in renal tubular calcium reabsorption which could not be ascribed to PTH-rP. The mechanisms by which hypercalcemia itself or other mediators associated with hypercalcemia could enhance renal tubular calcium reabsorption are unknown, but have not been thoroughly investigated as yet.

TUTTLE et al. (1991) found that when extracellular fluid volume and hydration status were carefully controlled and hypercalcemic patients were compared with controls with similar rates of glomerular filtration, enhanced renal tubular calcium reabsorption was almost universal in hypercalcemic cancer patients, and occurred even in patients with myeloma. GALLACHER et al. (1990) similarly found no correlation between renal tubular calcium reabsorption and urinary cyclic AMP excretion, a marker of PTH-rP activity. Thus, decreased calcium excretion in the urine is not necessarily a reflection of a circulating mediator. An alternative mechanism suggested by HARINCK et al. (1987) is that calcium excretion is altered by changes in renal tubular handling of sodium in hypercalcemia, although the data of TUTTLE et al. (1991) do not support this hypothesis.

More information on the relative frequency, possible mechanisms, and arguments on local versus systemic factors will be reviewed in the section under breast cancer later in this chapter.

F. Pathophysiology of the Metastatic Process

PAGET (1889) first suggested that there were specific patterns of metastasis of certain tumors to distant organs. He noted that some tumors metastasize preferentially to the lung and liver, whereas others spread to the brain or to bone. In particular, bone appears to be a preferred site of metastasis for breast and prostate cancers, neuroblastoma, and thyroid and kidney cancers. With considerable insight, PAGET concluded that "in cancer of the breast the bones suffer in a special way, which cannot be explained by any theory of embolism alone." It has been estimated that in 40% of tumors the distribution of metastases in distant organs can be predicted from the anatomic route of the blood flow from the primary site (originally referred to as the Ewing hypothesis for tumor cell dissemination), but that in 50%–60% of tumors the distribution of metastases cannot be forecast from anatomic considerations alone (LIOTTA and KOHN 1990). To explain the nonrandom nature of tumor metastasis, Paget developed the concept known as the "seed and soil" hypothesis (PAGET 1889), regarding the organ to which a tumor metastasized preferentially as a congenial soil. Certain tissues are unfavorable sites for tumor metastasis, for example cartilage. Although this may be partly because cartilage is avascular, several groups (BREM and FOLKMAN 1975; LANGER et al. 1980; EISENSTEIN et al. 1975) have shown that cartilage contains a factor or factors which inhibits proliferation of new vessels. Thus, as proposed by Paget, the environment of the target organ is an important determinant of metastasis. The tumor cells represented the seed for this soil, since they presumably have specific properties which favor metastasis to that site.

It is now apparent that tumor cell metastasis is a multistage process in which discrete steps are involved, each of which is due to specific determinants of both the tumor and the tissue (Fig. 1) (LIOTTA and KOHN 1990; ZETTER 1990). Each of these steps can potentially be interrupted. Only a relatively small proportion of tumor cells in the primary site may have the potential to metastasize to distant organs. The steps involved in systemic metastasis include local invasion, which involves angiogenesis, the capacity of the cells to traverse the capillary wall to reach the circulation (WEISS et al. 1989), and the capacity of the metastasizing cells to survive physical trauma in the circulation and the host-defense mechanisms that they will encounter including activated lymphocytes and macrophages, and natural killer cells (NK cells) (LIOTTA et al. 1974). The tumor cells stop in the capillary bed of the target organ, traverse the vascular wall of these capillaries, adhere to structures in the target organ, and then survive and proliferate at this distant site. Their survival and subsequent proliferation at this site may depend on local growth factors produced in that organ. Those factors which determine the success of a metastasis will be discussed in more detail below.

Thus, tumors do in fact preferentially metastasize to specific organ sites. A good example is the prostate, which almost invariably metastasizes to

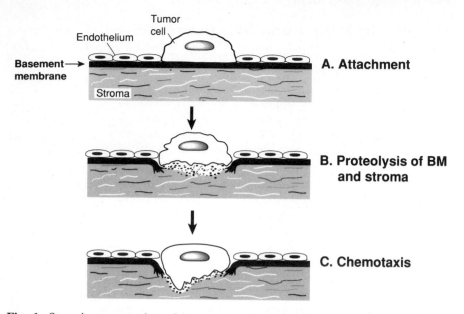

Fig. 1. Stepwise progression of breast cancer cell metastasis from primary site to bone. Two cellular mechanisms of bone destruction have been described. The molecular events at each step are described in detail in the text

bone. This presumably occurs because of mechanisms which make bone a congenial soil for prostate cancer cells. However, this is not to preclude that tumor cells also metastasize to distant organs preferentially due to mechanical reasons based in part on blood supply. In the case of prostate cancer, one of the most common sites of metastasis is to the vertebral column, possibly because Batson's plexus carries the tumor cells from the prostate to this site (see earlier). Once in the vertebral bodies, tumor cell growth may be influenced by factors produced at this site, which can enhance their growth. Evidence in support of this notion is that growth of prostatic cancer cells can be enhanced by factors produced by stromal cells (CHACKAL-ROY et al. 1989).

I. Properties of Tumor Cells Which Favor Metastasis

Primary tumors comprise heterogeneous populations of cells with differing metastatic capabilities (CARR and ORR 1983; HEPPNER 1984; POSTE 1986; FIDLER and POSTE 1985; FIDLER 1978). These differences occur because of rapid clonal diversification during tumor growth and progression (REEDY and FIALKOW 1980). The mechanisms responsible for the phenotypic instability of tumors are not completely understood, although they have been addressed many times (NOWEL 1976; MILLER 1983). Several of the possibilities include a host selection process, possibly due to immune defense mechanisms selecting for survival of certain tumor cells, or acquired genetic variability occurring, for example, following treatment with anticancer drugs. However, observations made on cells in culture may not always be relevant to in vivo situations. Cells which are cloned from a tumor may differ from the cells in the original population or cells in situ because the cultured cells are not in contact with the environment of the host, and are removed from possible interactions with other tumor cells (POSTE et al. 1981) or other properties of the target organ which may influence their capacity to survive and grow.

Some light has recently been shed on genetic factors which may influence a tumor cell's capacity to metastasize. The observation that mouse melanoma cells may contain a gene which suppresses the capacity of cells to metastasize to distant organs has generated considerable interest (KALEBIC et al. 1988; STEEG et al. 1988; BIGGS et al. 1990; LIOTTA and STEEG 1990; STEEG 1989; BEVILACQUA et al. 1989; ROSENGARD et al. 1989). This gene is referred to as NM23 (nonmetastatic, 23rd gene clone). Melanoma cells expressing this gene do not form metastases. This gene was detected during observations of genes preferentially expressed by highly metastatic mouse melanoma cells compared with normal mouse cells. Based on these observations, Steeg, Liotta and colleagues transfected mouse melanoma cells with this NM23 gene and found that the capacity of these transfected cells to metastasize was markedly reduced. Since at least one of the alleles of the *NM23* gene is deleted in some human malignancies (including breast, lung, colon, and kidney cancers), it is possible that this gene also suppresses metastasis in human tumors (BEVILACQUA et al. 1989).

The *NM23* gene shares considerable homology at the amino acid level with a gene called *awd* (LIOTTA and STEEG 1990; ROSENGARD et al. 1989). Defects in the *awd* gene in *Drosophilia* larvae can result in abnormal development. The *NM23* gene also shares considerable homology at the amino acid level with an NDP kinase which is responsible for converting nucleoside diphosphates to triphosphates. These kinases are energy sources for nucleic acids which maintain pools of nucleoside triphosphates. They are also necessary for microtubule polymerization and they supply GTP, which is important for the activation of coupling proteins during signal transduction. Should it be possible to show that human tumors also contain this or similar genes which suppress the capacity of these cells to metastasize, this may in part account for heterogeneity in tumor cell metastasis in humans. An interesting additional facet of this work is that there are now suggestions of differences in responses of the mouse melanoma cells which express the *NM23* gene, compared with those which do not. In particular, these cells respond to transforming growth factor β with an increase in proliferation. Transfection with the *NM23* gene makes these cells unresponsive to TGFβ. Since TGFβ is present in bone and is released when bone is resorbing or remodeling (HAUSCHKA et al. 1986; PFEILSCHIFTER and MUNDY 1987; CANALIS et al. 1989), it is possible that local concentrations of TGFβ may be important in causing proliferation of those cells which are in the vicinity of the bone surface (see later).

There are other genetic factors which may influence a tumor cell's capacity to metastasize. Expression of some oncogenes has been linked to metastatic potential. It is important to realize that oncogenes which affect the tumorigenic phenotype do not necessarily alter metastatic potential. For example, transfection of rat embryo fibroblasts with the *ras* oncogene increases both tumorigenicity and metastatic potential in these cells, whereas other oncogenes or combinations of oncogenes may suppress the metastatic phenotype, but be fully tumorigenic (Garbisa et al. 1987; Liotta and Kohn 1990). Some oncogenes have been linked to aggressive metastatic tumors in humans. The *HER-2/neu* oncogene is amplified in some patients with aggressive breast cancer (Slamon et al. 1987). Deletions of chromosomal material on chromosome 11p is found in some aggressive breast cancers (Ali et al. 1987) and deletions on chromosomes 17 and 18 are found in colon carcinomas arising from colonic polyps (Vogelstein et al. 1988; Baker et al. 1989).

There are other less clearly defined reasons why some primary tumors may have low metastatic potential (Sanchez et al. 1986). Activated host immune cells in the vicinity of the tumor can reduce the number of metastatic tumors in experimental models by mechanisms which at least in part include the local production of cytokines (Tsuchida et al. 1981; Hanna et al. 1972). Proteinase inhibitors may limit the number of metastases, suggesting that proteolytic degradative enzymes enhance the capacity of tumor cells to form growing colonies at distant sites (Stahl et al. 1985). There are clear links between the capacity of tumor cells to metastasize and the blood coagulation mechanism, including the capacity of embolic tumor cells to form thrombi (Warren and Vales 1972; Winterbauer et al. 1968; Hilgard and Gordon-Smith 1974). There have been suggestions that both platelet inhibitors and anticoagulants of the coumarin class influence metastatic potential, although the data remain conflicting and controversial.

II. Tumor Cell Invasion at the Primary Site

At the primary site, the first step in metastasis is tumor cell invasion of the stroma of the primary organ, and in particular the invasion of the local basement membrane of the organs of the primary site, and that which surrounds the vascular endothelium at this site. Tumor cells are invasive because they have the capacity to modify this extracellular matrix or basement membrane at the primary site. This requires the production of proteolytic enzymes either by tumor cells or by host cells. The concept of invasion espoused by Liotta (1986; Liotta et al. 1980) suggests that there are three steps involved in local tumor invasion (Fig. 1). These are tumor cell attachment to the basement membrane, tumor cell production of degradative enzymes to break down the basement membrane, and tumor cell migration so the tumor cell penetrates the basement membrane. The corresponding cellular events are tumor cell attachment to specialized cell adhesion molecules such as laminin and fibronectin, the secretion of hydrolytic enzymes by the tumor cells which can lyse the matrix and make basement membranes permeable so cells can pass, and the capacity of the tumor cells to migrate. In part, cell migration and motility is mediated by chemotactic signals. Each of these steps will now be described in more detail.

1. Adhesion

There is now considerable evidence to suggest that organ-specific adhesion molecules are important in tumor cell invasion. Tumor cells have been shown to attach preferentially to endothelial cells at the metastatic site (AUERBACH et al. 1987) by specific cell adhesion molecules such as fibronectin and laminin. The adhesion of tumor cells at these sites may enhance motility, may also enhance the production of proteolytic enzymes by the tumor cells, and may protect the tumor cells from the normal host-defense mechanisms which would otherwise endanger them. It is almost certainly significant that the expression of some of these adhesion molecules on endothelial cells can be enhanced by cytokines such as interleukin-1, tumor necrosis factor, and γ-interferon, as well as by the extracellular matrix of certain organs. This may be another important means of interaction between tumor cells and host cells.

One of the initial factors in tumor cell adhesion may be the presence of laminin receptors on tumor cells. These receptors bind laminin, a glycoprotein which is present only in basement membranes, and which in turn binds to type IV collagen in the basement membrane (ENGEL et al. 1981). Highly invasive and metastatic tumor cells may have a 50-fold increase in laminin receptors on the cell surface (WEWER et al. 1987). Competitive binding of the laminin receptor with laminin fragments can reduce the metastatic capacity of tumor cells (BARSKY et al. 1984; MCCARTHY et al. 1988).

2. Secretion of Enzymes

Recently, BASSET et al. (1990) have shown that invasive breast carcinomas express a gene which encodes a metalloproteinase. This gene is not encoded by noninvasive breast cancers or nonmalignant breast lesions. Surprisingly, the gene is not expressed by breast cancer cells themselves, but rather by fibroblasts and stromal cells adjacent to the breast cancer cells. The expression of this gene is enhanced by growth factors produced by breast cancer cells such as PDGF, TGFα, and basic FGF. These data highlight the important interactions which can occur between tumor cells and the neighboring stroma, and suggest that the mechanisms by which tumor cells affect distant organs may involve products of normal host cells stimulated by the presence of the tumor as well as the tumor cells themselves.

An enzyme which is clearly important in the invasive capacity of a tumor cell is type IV collagenase. This enzyme can degrade basement membranes, and its expression correlates well with invasive capacity of some tumors (Garbisa et al. 1987). ·

3. Cell Motility

The capacity of the tumor cell to metastasize depends at least in part on its motility. A number of chemotactic factors have now been identified for tumor cells. Some of these chemotactic factors are produced by tumor cells themselves (Liotta and Schiffmann 1988). It has also been shown that organs to which tumor cells metastasize may contain chemoattractants for tumor cells. For example, the products of resorbing bone harvested from bone organ cultures contain factors which may influence the motility of breast cancer cells (Orr et al. 1979, 1980). Other potential chemotactic factors have been found in extracts of tumors (Hujanen and Terranova 1985) as well as other cellular molecules or fragments of molecules such as collagen, fibronectin, laminin, and elastin (Hujanen and Terranova 1985; McCarthy et al. 1985; Juliano 1987; Mundy et al. 1981; Yusa et al. 1989; Blood et al. 1988; Magro et al. 1985).

Recently, Liotta et al. (1986) identified a new class of cytokines which are referred to as autocrine motility factors. These factors may act in an autocrine or paracrine fashion and increase random motility and subsequent migration of tumor cells, and possibly be responsible for enhancing their movement through defects in the basement membrane.

III. Tumor Cells in the Bloodstream

Once in the general circulation, tumor cells will travel to organs with the richest blood supply. However, within the general circulation they are at risk from physical trauma and the mechanisms by which host cells defend against invasion of foreign or abnormal cells or microorganisms. The majority of tumor cells do not reach the circulation. It should be appreciated that most tumor cells at the primary site do not have the capacity to metastasize, and that even of the tumor cells that do leave the primary site, less than 1% become viable metastases (Weiss 1985; Liotta et al. 1974). Tumor cells do not usually leave the primary site until the primary tumor has reached a volume of at least 10^9 cells (Weiss 1982). However, there are great variations. Some very large tumors do not form metastases, whereas small or even occult primary tmors may form metastases. The reasons the tumor cells are destroyed in the circulation include mechanical shear forces, host-defense mechanisms, and anoxia or removal from the favorable growth environment at the primary site. It is possible that the major host-defense mechanism mounted to the presence of the metastasizing tumor is mediated by natural killer or NK cells which are activated macrophages. These are the cells which are responsible for the destruction of most tumor cells which are inoculated intravenously (GORELIK et al. 1979).

IV. Tumor Cell Arrest at the Metastatic Site

Although tumor cells are most likely to lodge in organs with the richest blood supply (FIDLER 1970; WEISS and GLANES 1974), other factors are clearly important. Aggregates of tumors metastasize much more frequently than do single cells (FIDLER 1973; THOMPSON 1974). It is likely that aggregates by their physical nature are protected from mechanical forces or host-defense mechanisms which destroy the majority of metastasizing cells. However, another important factor in metastasis to specific organs is the capacity of tumor cells to adhere at certain organ sites. Thus, the lodging of a tumor cell in a distant organ is dependent on tumor cell adhesion at that site, production of proteolytic enzymes, and sequentially the digestion of extracellular matrix by these proteolytic enzymes. This is the same cascade of events which determined the capacity of the tumor cell to invade adjacent tissue and leave the primary site. This may cause the release of chemotactic factors and possibly growth factors which can regulate tumor cell migration and growth.

V. Growth Regulatory Factors at Metastatic Sites

The capacity of the tumor to grow at a metastatic site will depend at least in part on growth regulatory factors which are present at that site. This has been relatively unexplored in bone but may be very important. For example, it is now realized that bone is a storehouse for many growth factors which have important regulatory effects on tumor cells such as acidic fibroblast growth factor, transforming growth factor β, and platelet-derived growth factor (HAUSCHKA et al. 1986). Presumably, these factors could be released either during normal bone remodeling or possibly by the invasive effects of the metastatic tumor, and thereby favor the growth of the metastasis at that tumor site. Alternatively, in the case of some tumors, growth inhibitors for the tumor may be released. These could include transforming growth factor β, which may have growth inhibitory effects on some tumor cells as well as other factors such as tumor necrosis factor which are produced by activated macrophages. In these circumstances, responsive tumor cells may be prevented from forming a successful metastasis. Recently, it has been shown that bone marrow stroma contains a growth factor which enhances the growth of human prostatic cancer cells in vitro (CHACKAL-ROY et al. 1989). This phenomenon may account for the capacity of prostatic cancer cells to grow so readily in bone.

Thus, tumor cells in a foreign site are exposed to many influences which may inhibit their growth and protect the patient from the development of a metastasis. In the case of tumor cells which metastasize to the marrow cavity, the tumor cells may interact through various mechanisms with adjacent cells and influence the process of bone remodeling. The major interaction is probably via the production of factors which influence bone cell activity, and particularly the activity of osteoclasts which cause bone resorption. As a consequence of bone resorption, chemotactic factors, growth regulatory factors, and proteolytic enzymes are all produced, and, as indicated above, these may favor the formation of a viable metastasis in bone.

G. Potential Mechanisms for the Metastatic Process in Bone

There are special features of the bone metastasis which may be important for successful lodging of metastatic cancer cells at the bone site. To form a metastasis in bone, tumor cells reach the bone marrow. Since the bone marrow is a very vascular organ, it is not surprising that tumor cells should effectively reach this site. Most bone metastases occur in the axial skeleton and the proximal ends of long bones, both of which are highly vascularized. In the marrow cavity, tumor cells traverse wide-channeled marrow sinusoids. There are a number of influences which may be relevant in the subsequent formation of the metastasis adjacent to an endosteal bone surface.

I. Chemotactic Factors

Bone which is resorbing has been shown to produce chemotactic factors for cancer cells. Conditioned media harvested from resorbing organ cultures of bone contain activity which causes unidirectional migration of rat and human cancer cells (ORR et al. 1979, 1980). Fragments of type-I collagen cause unidirectional migration of breast cancer cells (MUNDY et al. 1981), and fragments of osteocalcin have also been shown to cause the chemotaxis of tumor cells and monocytes (MUNDY and POSER 1983).

II. Growth Regulatory Factors

Bone is a repository for growth regulatory factors (HAUSCHKA et al. 1986). Transforming growth factors βI and II, bone morphogenetic proteins, acidic and basic fibroblast growth factors, platelet-derived growth factor, and insulin-like growth factors I and II are all stored within the proteinaceous bone matrix. These factors are presumably released when bone is degraded or resorbed and are available locally to influence tumor cell growth. Most of these factors have been implicated as growth regulatory factors for tumor cells. TGFβ can have either stimulatory or inhibitory effects on tumor cells, but platelet-derived growth factor, insulin-like growth factor-1, and the fibroblast growth factors may all have effects on tumor cell growth and behavior.

III. Calcium

Calcium has also been linked to tumor cell proliferation. In fact, it is possible that the increased extracellular calcium concentrations presumably present at the metastatic site in bone may favor tumor cell proliferation (RIZZOLI and BONJOUR 1989). Data on this topic are rather limited and still speculative.

IV. Proteolytic Enzymes

Proteolytic enzymes are produced at sites of bone resorption. Organ cultures of resorbing bones produce proteolytic enzymes (VAES 1968; EILON and RAISZ 1978), and are presumably produced by osteoclasts. Moreover, activated host immune cells such as macrophages may produce proteolytic enzymes in response to tumor cells. As reviewed earlier, tumor cells may produce type IV collagenase and other degradative enzymes which assist in disruption of basement membrane collagen. Recently, it has been shown that breast cancer cells which have invasive capabilities induce the expression of a metalloproteinase in adjacent stromal cells (BASSET et al. 1990). As indicated above, the production of these degradative enzymes may be important for a number of features of the metastatic process including tumor cell migration, tumor cell adhesion, and protection of tumor cells from a hostile environment.

Finally, it is possible that bone itself provides a very favorable niche for a tumor cells. Thus, in this site it may be protected from some of the factors which would endanger it in a more accessible organ site. Again there is little information on this point.

Clearly it would help our understanding of the pathogenesis of bone metastases if suitable animal models were available for its study, such as have been used in investigating pulmonary metastases (FIDLER and POSTE 1985). Only in the last few years has any progress been made with bone models, however. SHEVRIN et al. (1988) induced bone metastases from prostatic cancer cells (PC3) injected intravenously into nude mice in which the inferior vena cava had been obstructed. Bone metastases occurred in 53% of the animals, whereas subcutaneous injection achieved metastases in lymph nodes and lungs but not the skeleton. Intracardiac injection of B16 melanoma cells into mice resulted in colonization of bone in regions containing hemopoietic bone marrow (ARGUELLO et al. 1988). The recent development of a nude rat model of skeletal metastases might provide the most significant recent advance (KJONNIKSEN et al. 1990). Reproducible skeletal metastases were obtained at high frequency in animals injected with LOX human melanoma cells into the left ventricle. The relative case of working with the immune-deficient rats should lead to experiments in which cells colonizing bone as metastases can be studied, looking for enrichment in those properties which may facilitate growth in bone.

H. Factors Which May Be Involved in Osteolysis

We will consider several of the factors which, alone or cooperatively, might contribute to the osteolysis which seems essential for tumor establishment in bone.

I. Parathyroid Hormone Related Protein

Although parathyroid hormone-related protein (PTHrP) is generally thought of as a systemic factor, it is also likely that it can act under some circumstances as a local mediator of osteoclastic bone destruction. Since most patients with breast cancer have extensive osteolytic bone destruction (Mundy and Martin 1982) and patients with breast cancer usually do not develop hypercalcemia unless they have extensive bone destruction and they are late in the course of the disease, it has always seemed likely that hypercalcemia in breast cancer is related to the degree of metastatic bone involvement. However, one of the groups who purified PTHrP did so from extracts of a patient with breast cancer (Stewart et al. 1987), and PTHrP has been detected in normal rat lactating breast tissue (Thiede and Rodan 1988) as well as in breast milk (Budayr et al. 1989), and some cells have been reported of hypercalcemia in association with breast enlargement, in which PTHrP has been implicated (Khosla et al. 1990; Braude et al. 1991). Recently, PTHrP has been identified in 60% of 102 samples of breast cancer tissue by immunohistochemistry (Southby et al. 1990), and plasma levels of PTHrP were elevated in 16 of 26 patients with hypercalcemia in breast cancer, associated with lytic skeletal metastases (Grill et al. 1991). In those series reported, 30%–45% of patients with breast cancer have increased urinary cyclic AMP excretion (Stewart et al. 1980; Isales et al. 1987; Gallacher et al. 1990; Corbett et al. 1983), possibly reflecting PTHrP effects.

If PTHrP production by breast cancer cells is significant in the bone metastasis process, it could contribute by providing the tumor cells in marrow with the ability to promote bone resorption, and hence aid tumor establishment. In a preliminary study of a small number of cancers, Powell et al. (1991) identified PTHrP by immunohistochemistry in 12 of 13 bone metastases, and 3 or 18 nonbone metastases from breast cancers. It is possible that one of the properties contributing to the ability of breast cancers to grow in bone is PTHrP production. Prospective studies will be needed to determine conclusively whether PTHrP is involved in bone metastasis formation, and whether it requires in addition any of the several other factors to be considered below.

II. Transforming Growth Factor α

Transforming growth factor α (TGFα) is a powerful stimulator of osteoclastic bone resorption (Ibbotson et al. 1985; 1986; Stern et al. 1985; Tashjian et al. 1985) which stimulates proliferation of osteoclast progenitors and increases osteoclast formation (TAKAHASHI et al. 1986). In vivo, we have found that it has synergistic effects with PTHrP on increasing the plasma calcium (YATES et al. 1991).

Transforming growth factor α transcripts have frequently been detected in breast cancer tissue and TGFα has been measured in the conditioned media harvested from breast cancer cell lines (PERROTEAU et al. 1986; DERYNCK et al. 1987). TGFα production by breast cancer cells may be regulated when the breast cancer cells contain estrogen receptors. The synthesis and secretion seems to be enhanced by treatment with estrogens (LIPPMAN et al. 1986; SALOMON et al. 1986), thus providing an autocrine mechanism by which estrogen can mediate proliferative effects on breast cancer cells, making use of their EGF receptors.

Although TGFα can cause hypercalcemia when administered systemically, it may also be a local mediator of bone destruction and hypercalcemia. Membrane-bound TGFα may be the means by which some cancer cells stimulate osteoclasts or other cells involved in the bone resorption process by cell-cell communication. It is now well known that TGFα can exert its biological effects as either a soluble or membrane-anchored factor (MASSAGUE 1990). Pro-TGFα is a membrane glycoprotein which comprises 160 amino acids with a hydrophobic transmembrane sequence (DERYNCK et al. 1984). The transmembrane and the cytoplasmic regions of pro-TGFα comprise 63 amino acids. TGFα is released from the cell through a proteolytic process which has not yet been well described, but in most cells seems to be inefficient. This may be an important site of regulation of TGFα activity. Some cells fail to release soluble TGFα, a process required for TGFα to function in an endocrine manner at distant sites. Pro-TGFα is glycosylated heterogeneously and this may account for differing capacities of some cell types to release biologically active TGFα. Membrane anchored pro-TGFα is biologically active, and may be responsible for the adhesion of cells expressing TGFα with other cells which possess EGF receptors, and may activate the target cell through cell-cell contact. MASSAGUE (1990) has referred to this mechanism of cell-cell communication as juxtacrine stimulation. Other cytokines with similar properties include TNFα and colony-stimulating factor-1. It is interesting to note that all of these factors have been linked to osteoclast formation and activation. The significance of these observations to either normal bone resorption or osteoclastic bone resorption mediated by metastatic tumor cells has not been studied as yet.

III. Transforming Growth Factor β

Transforming growth factor β (TGFβ) is another common autocrine or paracrine growth factor which is produced by breast cancer cells. Like transforming growth factor α, its production by breast cancer cells can be modulated by estrogens. In the case of transforming growth factor β, its production is inhibited by estrogen, but enhanced by tamoxifen (Derynck et al. 1987; Knabbe et al. 1987). However, its role as a bone active factor in metastatic breast cancer is unclear. It seems to have dual effects on osteoclasts. Under some circumstances it inhibits osteoclast formation and activity (Pfeilschifter et al. 1988; Chenu et al. 1988), but, under other conditions in vitro, it has been shown to increase osteoclast formation both in vitro and in vivo (Tashjian et al. 1985; Pfeilschifter et al. 1988; Marcelli et al. 1990). Its stimulatory effects on osteoclasts may be mediated by prostaglandins (Tashjian et al. 1985; Pfeilschifter et al. 1988).

Transforming growth factor β has profound effects on osteoblasts to cause new bone formation (Noda and Camilliere 1989; Marcelli et al. 1990), and it may become important as a stimulator of osteoblastic metastasis than a regulator of resorption. In this regard, $TGF\beta_2$ is expressed in large amounts by the prostate carcinoma cell line PC-3 (Marquardt et al. 1987).

Transforming growth factor β is usually produced in a latent form bound to a binding protein which masks its biological effects. This is also so in breast cancer, although there is some evidence that breast cancer cells release some $TGF\beta$ which is biologically active (Knabbe et al. 1987). The release of the active moiety from binding proteins is essential, but there are many mechanisms in the bone and tumor microenvironment which could achieve this process. For example, acid production under the ruffled border of the osteoclast (Pfeilschifter et al. 1990a), plasminogen activator production by bone cells or tumor cells (Allan et al. 1990; Pfeilschifter et al. 1990b), or the production of other proteolytic enzymes by invasive tumor cells could all be involved.

Transforming growth factor β may be important at the bone metastatic site not only for its effects on bone cells, but also for its effects on tumor cells. It is stored in bone and its local release as bone is resorbed (Pfeilschifter and Mundy 1987) could be responsible for regulating tumor cell proliferation, mobility, and even expression of specific proteins at that site.

IV. Prostaglandins of the E Series

It has been known for many years that prostaglandins of the E series can stimulate osteoclastic bone resorption (Klein and Raisz 1970). In the 1970s, several investigators examined the role of prostaglandins as potential mediators of bone destruction in patients with metastatic breast cancer. Powles et al. (1976) and Bennett et al. (1975) showed that cultured breast cancer cells and breast cancer extracts contained prostaglandins of the E series. Coculture of these cells stimulated osteoclastic bone resorption in organ cultures of neonatal mouse calvariae. Breast cancer cells produce prostaglandins in vitro and this was inhibited by treatment with aspirin or drugs which inhibit prostaglandin synthesis. Similarly, the bone resorption in the organ cultures caused by the breast cancer cells was inhibited. This led to a number of studies on the potential role of prostaglandin synthesis inhibitors in the treatment of bone metastases caused by breast cancer, which were uniformly disappointing (Powles et al. 1982). Furthermore, a study indicating a higher incidence of bone metastasis formation in patients with increased PGE production by primary breast cancers (Bennett et al. 1976) has not been extended or confirmed.

It seems unlikely that prostaglandins of the E series provide a major mechanism by which breast cancer cells destroy bone. However, this does not mean that they cannot be part of the mechanism. Cultures of human MCF-7 cells, which are frequently used as a model of estrogen-receptor positive breast cancer cells, were shown by Valentin et al. (1985) to release increased amounts of prostaglandins of the E series when treated with estrogens or tamoxifen, as well as bone-resorbing activity. Production of bone-resorbing activity and the prostaglandins was inhibited by treatment with indomethacin.

Prostaglandins of the E series have very complex effects on osteoclastic bone resorption. They stimulate bone resorption in organ cultures of fetal rat long bones and neonatal mouse calvariae (Klein and Raisz 1970; Tashjian et al. 1972). Prostaglandins may also be generated within bones themselves and this may be the mechanism whereby some other factors can stimulate bone resorption (Lerner 1987; Garrett and Mundy 1989; Boyce et al. 1989a,b). In marrow culture systems, they appear to have biphasic effects on the formation of cells with osteoclast characteristics (Chenu et al. 1990; Akatsu et al. 1989). They have transient effects on isolated osteoclasts to cause cell contraction and inhibit bone resorption (Chambers and Ali 1983).

V. Parathyroid Hormone

Although there were earlier reports suggesting a role for ectopic parathyroid hormone (PTH) in the hypercalcemia associated with breast cancer and other malignancies associated with extensive osteolysis, these results were never confirmed and it is likely to be due to the assays being used at that time to measure PTH (Benson et al. 1974). PTH can now be dismissed as anything but a rare cause of hypercalcemia associated with cancer, except in those infrequent cases where the two diseases may coexist. There have been several convincing recent reports of ectopic PTH production by nonparathyroid cancers (Yoshimoto et al. 1989; Nussbaum et al. 1990), but the vast majority of cancers do not express PTH (Simpson et al. 1983). There has been no reported role for ectopic PTH production in skeletal metastasis, but presumably those rare tumors which do produce ectopic PTH may cause localized bone destruction by a PTH-mediated mechanism if the tumor metastasizes to the bone marrow cavity.

VI. Vitamin D Sterols

Many years ago, it was suggested by Gordan et al. (1967) that vitamin D sterols present in breast cancer tissue may account for the bone-resorbing activity and hypercalcemia associated with breast cancer. However, later it was found that these sterols were ubiquitous and may be found in many tissues including breast tissue and others not associated with hypercalcemia (HADDAD et al. 1970). This issue has not been reopened, and it appears unlikely that these compounds are important. However, it should be noted that the argument used to dismiss these studies is not really valid. The occurrence of hypercalcemia may be related to tumor cell burden, special capacity of tumor cells to secrete the factor, or other mechanisms. For example, PTH-rP has been noted frequently in nonhypercalcemic tumors (DANKS et al. 1989).

VII. Platelet-Derived Growth Factor

Although it is possible that PDGF is produced by some breast cancer cells in vitro and in vivo, its role in the mediation of bone destruction associated with cancer remains completely uninvestigated.

VIII. Procathepsin D

Procathepsin D is a ubiquitous housekeeping lysosomal protease which is produced in large amounts by many breast cancer cells, but not by normal cells. This increased secretion by breast cancer cells is due to both over-expression of the gene and altered processing of the protein. The precursor, which is of 52 kDa, has been found in breast cancer cells in culture as well as in many cancer cell lines (WESTLEY and MAY 1987). In those with estrogen receptors, its production seems to be regulated by estrogens. VIGNON et al. (1986) have shown that it has mitogenic action for breast cancer cells, indicating an autocrine or paracrine growth regulatory mechanism, and clinical studies identify it as an independent predictor of metastasis at any site (SPYRATOS et al. 1989). Human MCF-7 and 2R75-1 cells produce aberrant forms of procathepsin D. These abnormalities may represent aberration in glycosylation of the precursor region as well as in amino acid substitutions. We have tested the aberrant form of procathepsin D purified by affinity purification from human MCF-7 cells and found that it has some interesting properties on bone cells in vitro. It increases bone resorption in fetal rat long bone cultures (Wo et al. 1990). It also affects isolated avian and rat osteoclasts and stimulates tartrate-resistant acid phosphatase activity as well as the capacity to form pits on calcified matrices such as sperm whale dentine (Wo et al. 1990). Its effects on avian osteoclasts appear to occur independent of the addition of osteoblasts or extraneous cells, as pro-cathepsin D may be a direct effector of osteoclastic activity. The conclusion from these studies is that the 52-kDa protein purified from MCF-7 cells stimulates osteoclasts to resorb bone. Normal cells do not secrete pro-cathepsin D. The importance of procathepsin D as a mediator of osteoclast activity in breast cancer and other cancers will need to be confirmed and determined relative to other mediators.

IX. Bone-Resorbing Cytokines

Bone-resorbing cytokines such as interleukin-1, tumor necrosis factor, and interleukin-6 could be involved in local bone destruction associated with bone metastases in two ways. They can either be produced directly by the tumor cells, or by normal host immune cells in response to the presence of the tumor. Interleukin-1α (IL-1α) has been detected in a number of solid tumors including squamous cell carcinomas of the head and neck (SATO et al. 1989; FRIED et al. 1989; NOWAK et al. 1990) but not so far from human breast cancer cells. Other bone-resorbing factors are frequently produced in conjunction with IL-1α. For example, in the tumor studied by SATO et al. (1989), PTHrP was produced together with IL-1α and together the two factors were shown to produce synergistic effects on hypercalcemia.

There have been a number of instances now where solid tumors have been shown to stimulate normal host immune cells to produce osteotropic cytokines such as tumor necrosis factor (SABATINI et al. 1990a,b; YONEDA et al. 1991). This has been demonstrated in the human melanoma, the A375 tumor, in the rat Leydig tumor, and in the MH-85 human squamous cell carcinoma of the maxilla. In each of these situations, the tumor cells produce soluble factors which can stimulate normal host immune cells, and particularly cells in the monocyte-macrophage family, to release tumor necrosis factor (TNF). In the case of the A375 tumor, the mediator is GM-CSF (SABATINI et al. 1990b). However, in the case of the MH-85 tumor, another factor is involved (YONEDA et al. 1991). TNF produced by normal immune cells appears to be the major mediator in the MH-85 tumor.

Nude mice carrying this tumor develop hypercalcemia and have a four-fold increase in circulating TNF levels. Hypercalcemia has been reversed by passive inoculation with neutralizing antibodies to tumor necrosis factor and it has also been reversed by splenectomy. The spleen is the site in the mouse where most of the normal host immune cells reside (YONEDA et al. 1991). The tumor cells themselves do not produce TNF (YONEDA et al. 1991). Since bone metastases usually are composed of tumor cells and host immune cells, these bone-resorbing cytokines produced in excess by the host immune cells in this manner are likely important in the pathophysiology of localized bone loss.

The production of cytokines by host cells may be a defense mechanism to protect the host from the tumor invader. However, these same cytokines could also be responsible for some of the paraneoplastic syndromes associated with tumors. For example, cachexia, leukocytosis, anemia, and hypertrigly-ceridemia can all be attributed to these factors. In addition, the hypercalcemia can be enhanced in those tumors which produce other mediators such as PTHrP and TGFα, as happens in the rat Leydig tumor, since these factors have synergistic effects on bone resorption (SABATINI et al. 1990; STASHENKO et al. 1987). In the case of the MH-85 tumor, where the tumor cells do not produce these factors, the production of cytokines by host cells is presumably the mechanism responsible for hypercalcemia (YONEDA et al. 1991).

I. Factors Involved in Osteoblastic Effects

Occasionally, tumors metastatic to bone are associated with a predominant increase in new bone formation. The most frequent examples of tumors which form osteoblastic metastases are prostate cancer, neuroblastoma, breast cancer, and some lymphomas such as Hodgkin's disease. Serum alkaline phosphatase, reflecting osteoblast activity, is usually increased in these patients. The increase in osteoblast activity is not due to the normal coupling phenomenon of bone remodeling, which is responsible for the increase in local bone formation to repair and replace the defects in bone made by resorptive episodes. In these patients, the newly formed bone may be laid down directly on trabecular bone surfaces without a preceding resorptive episode (Charhon et al. 1983). These are important metastases in prostate cancer because most patients with this malignancy will develop predominantly osteoblastic bone metastases if they live long enough.

The mechanism by which these metastases form is not entirely clear. From the histomorphometric studies of Charhon et al. (1983), it appears most likely they are due to soluble factors which are produced by the metastasizing cancer cells which stimulate directly the bone formative process on trabecular surfaces without the requirement for prior resorption. Most studies have concentrated on prostate cancer, since this is the malignancy most frequently associated with blastic metastases. There have now been a number of studies in which prostate cancer cells have been shown to produce proliferative factors for cells with the osteoblast phenotype in vitro. This was first shown by Jacobs and Lawson (1980), who reported that extracts of a well-differentiated prostatic carcinoma stimulated [³H]thymidine incorporation into fibroblasts. Similar effects were seen with extracts of benign prostatic hyperplasia. Preliminary characterization of this activity showed it to have an apparent molecular weight of >67 kDa.

More recently, others including Simpson et al. (1985) and Koutsilieries et al. (1987) also found osteoblast-stimulating activity produced by prostatic cancer tissue. Simpson et al. (1985) took extracts from the human prostate cancer cell line PC3, injected total RNA into *Xenopus* oocytes, and then examined the conditioned media for bone stimulatory activity. These extracts stimulated both mitogenesis and alkaline phosphatase activity in osteosarcoma cells with the osteoblast phenotype. In contrast, Koutsilieries et al. (1987) took extracts of prostate cancer tissue as well as extracts of normal prostatic tissue and found growth proliferative activity which has not yet been characterized. One of the problems in this area is that there are very few well-characterized human prostate cancer cell lines available for study. A number of factors have been suggested as potential mediators of osteoblastic metastasis associated with prostate cancer.

I. Transforming Growth Factor β_2

Recently, it has been shown that TGFβ_2 is abundant in PC3 prostatic cancer cells (MARQUARDT et al. 1987). Since both TGFβ_1 and TGFβ_2 have profound effects on bone cells including the stimulation of proliferation, chemotaxis, and differentiated function, TGFβ_2 must be a potential bone growth factor in patients with this type of malignancy.

II. Fibroblast Growth Factor

Prostatic cancer cells express large amounts of both acidic and basic fibroblast growth factors and these are potential mediators of osteoblast proliferation in patients with this disease (CANALIS et al. 1987, 1988).

III. Plasminogen Activator Sequence

Recently, there has been a report of purification of mitogenic activity for rat calvarial osteoblastic cells from the human prostatic cancer cell line PC3 (RABBANI et al. 1990a,b). This factor is similar or identical to the urokinase type of plasminogen activator. The first ten amino acids were sequenced and shown to be identical.

References

Akatsu T, Takahashi N, Debari K, Morita I, Murota S, Nagata N, Takatani O, Suda T (1989) Prostaglandins promote osteoclast like cell formation by a mechanism involving cyclic adenosine 3',5'-monophosphate in mouse bone marrow cell cultures. J Bone Miner Res 4:29–35

Ali IU, Lidereau R, Theillet C, Callahan R (1987) Reduction to homozygosity of genes on chromosome 11 in human breast neoplasia. Science 238:185–188

Allan EH, Gough NH, Gelehrter TD, Zeheb R, Martin TJ (1990) Transforming growth factor β and leukemia inhibitory factor increase mRNA and protein for plasminogen activator inhibitor-1 in osteoblasts. Excerpta Med Int Congr Ser 886:285–290

Arguello F, Baggs RB, Frantz CN (1988) A murine model of experimental metastasis to bone and bone marrow. Cancer Res 48:6876–6881

Auerbach R, Iu WC, Pardon E, Gumkowski F, Kaminska G, Kaminski M (1987) Specificity of adhesion between murine tumor cells and capillary endothelium: an in vitro correlate of preferential metastasis in vivo. Cancer Res 47:1492–1496

Baker SJ, Fearon ER, Nigro JM, Hamillon SR, Preisinger AC, Jessup JM, van Tuinen P, Ledbetter DH, Barker DF, Nakamura Y (1989) Chromosome 17 deletions and p53 gene mutations in colorectal carcinomas. Science 244:217–221

Barsky SH, Rao CN, Williams JE, Liotta LA (1984) Laminin molecular domains which alter metastasis in a murine model. J Clin Invest 74:843–848

Basset P, Bellocq JP, Wolf C, Stoll I, Hutin P, Limacher JM, Podhajcer OL, Chenard MP, Rio MC, Chambon P (1990) A novel metalloproteinase gene specifically expressed in stromal cells of breast carcinomas. Nature 348:699–704

Batson OV (1940) The function of the vertebral veins and their role in the spread of metastases. Ann Surg 112:138–149

Bennett A, McDonald AM, Simpson JS, Stanford IF (1975) Breast cancer, prostaglandins, and bone metastases. Lancet 1:1218–1220

Bennett A, Charber EM, McDonald AM, Simpson JS, Stamford IF, Zebro T (1976) Prostaglandins and breast cancer. Lancet 2:624

Benson RC, Riggs BL, Pickard BM, Arnaud CD (1974) Radioimmunoassay of parathyroid hormone in hypercalcemic patients with malignant disease. Am J Med 56:821–826

Bevilacqua G, Sobel ME, Liotta LA, Steeg PS (1989) Association of low nm23 RNA levels in human primary infiltrating ductal breast carcinomas with lymph node involvement and other histopathological indicators of high metastatic potential. Cancer Res 49:5185–5190

Biggs J, Hersperger E, Steeg PS, Liotta LA, Shearn A (1990) A *Drosophila* gene that is homologous to a mammalian gene associated with tumor metastasis codes for a nucleoside diphosphate kinase. Cell 63:933–940

Blood CH, Sasse J, Brodt P, Zetter BR (1988) Identification of a tumor cell receptor for VGVAPG, an elastin-derived chemotactic peptide. J Cell Biol 107:1987–1993

Boyce BF, Aufdemorte TB, Garrett IR, Yates AJP, Mundy GR (1989a) Effects of interleukin-1 on bone turnover in normal mice. Endocrinology 125:1142–1150

Boyce BF, Yates AJP, Mundy GR (1989b) Bolus injections of recombinant human interleukin-1 cause transient hypocalcemia in normal mice. Endocrinology 125:2780–2783

Boyde A, Maconnachie E, Reid SA, Delling G, Mundy GR (1986) Scanning electron microscopy in bone pathology: review of methods. Potential and applications. Scanning Electron Microsc 4:1537–1554

Braude S, Graham A, Mitchell D (1991) Lymphoedema/hypercalcaemia syndrome-mediated by parathyroid-hormone-related protein. Lancet 337:140–141

Brem SS, Folkman J (1975) Inhibition of tumor angiogenesis mediated by cartilage. J Exp Med 141:427–439

Budayr AA, Halloran BP, King JC, Diep D, Nissenson RA, Strewler GJ (1989) High levels of a parathyroid hormone-like protein in milk. Proc Natl Acad Sci 86:7183–7185

Canalis E, Lorenzo J, Burgess WH, Maciag T (1987) Effects of endothelial cell growth factor on bone remodeling in vitro. J Clin Invest 79:52–58

Canalis E, Centrella M, McCarthy T (1988) Effects of basic fibroblast growth factor on bone formation in vitro. J Clin Invest 81:1572–1577

Canalis E, McCarthy T, Centrella M (1989) Growth factors and the regulation of bone remodeling. J Clin Invest 81:277–281

Carr I, Orr FW (1983) Current reviews: invasion and metastasis. Can Med Assoc J 128:1164–1167

Chackal-Roy M, Niemeyer C, Moore M, Zetter BR (1989) Stimulation of human prostatic carcinoma cell growth by factors present in human bone marrow. J Clin Invest 84:43–50

Chambers TJ, Ali NN (1983) Inhibition of osteoclastic motility by prostaglandins I2, E1, E2 and 6-oxoE1. J Pathol 139:383–397

Charhon SA, Chapuy MC, Delvin EE, Valentin-Opran A, Edouard CM, Meunier PJ (1983) Histomorphometric analysis of sclerotic bone metastases from prostatic carcinoma with special reference to osteomalacia. Cancer 51:918–924

Chenu C, Pfeilschifter J, Mundy GR, Roodman GD (1988) Transforming growth factor beta inhibits formation of osteoclast-like cells in long-term human marrow cultures. Proc Natl Acad Sci USA 85:5683–5687

Chenu C, Valentin-Opran A, Chavassieux P, Saez S, Meunier PJ, Delmas PD (1990) Insulin like growth factor-1 hormonal regulation by growth hormone and by 1,25(OH)2D3 and activity on human osteoblast-like cells in short term cultures. Bone 11:81–86

Coman DR, DeLong RP (1951) The role of the vertebral venous system in the metastasis of cancer to the spinal column; experiments with tumour cell suspension in rats and rabbits. Cancer 4:610–618

Corbett JR, Nicod PH, Huxley RL, Lewis SE, Rude RE, Willerson JT (1983) Left ventricular functional alterations at rest and during submaximal exercise in patients with recent myocardial infarction. Am J Med 74:577–591

Danks JA, Ebeling PR, Hayman J, Chou ST, Moseley JM, Dunlop J, Kemp BE, Martin TJ (1989) Parathyroid hormone-related protein: immunohistochemical localization in cancers and in normal skin. J Bone Miner Res 4:273–278

Derynck R, Roberts AB, Winkler ME, Chen EY, Goeddel DV (1984) Human transforming growth factor-alpha: precursor structure and expression in E. coli. Cell 38:287–297

Derynck R, Goeddel DV, Ullrich A, Gutterman JU, Williams RP, Bringman TS, Berger WH (1987) Synthesis of messenger RNAs for transforming growth factors alpha and beta and the epidermal growth factor receptor by human tumors. Cancer Res 47:707–712

Dodds PR, Caride VJ, Lytton B (1981) The role of vertebral veins in the dissemination of prostatic carcinoma. J Urol 126:753–755

Eilon G, Mundy GR (1978) Direct resorption of bone by human breast cancer cells in vitro. Nature 276:726–728

Eilon G, Raisz LG (1978) Comparison of the effects of stimulators and inhibitors of resorption on the release of lysosomal enzymes and radioactive calcium from fetal bone in organ culture. Endocrinology 103:1969–1975

Eisenstein R, Kuettner KE, Neapolitan C, Soble LW, Sorgente N (1975) The resistance of certain tissues to invasion II cartilage extracts inhibit the growth of fibroblasts and endothelial cells in culture. Am J Pathol 81:337–347

Engel J, Odermatt E, Engel A, Madri JA, Furthmayr H, Rohde H, Timpl R (1981) Shapes, domain organization and flexibility of laminin and fibronectin: two multifunctional proteins of the extracellular matrix. Mol Biol 150:97–120

Fidler IJ (1970) Metastasis: quantitative analysis of distribution and fate of tumor emboli labeled with ^{125}I-5-IODO-7'-deoxyuridine. JNCI 45:773–782

Fidler IJ (1973) The relationship of embolic homogeneity, number, size and viability to the incidence of experimental metastasis. Eur J Cancer 9:223–227

Fidler IJ (1978) Tumor heterogeneity and the biology of cancer invasion and metastasis. Cancer Res 38:2651–2660

Fidler IJ, Poste G (1985) The cellular heterogeneity of malignant neoplasms: implications for adjuvant chemotherapy. Semin Oncol 12:207–221

Fried RM, Voelkel EF, Rice RH, Levine L, Gaffney EV, Tashjian AII (1989) Two squamous cell carcinomas not associated with humoral hypercalcemia produce a potent bone resorption-stimulating factor which is interleukin-1 alpha. Endocrinology 125:742–751

Galasko CSB (1986a) Skeletal metastases. Clin Orthop 210:18–30

Galasko CSB (1986b) Skeletal metastases. Butterworth, London

Galasko CSB, Burn JI (1971) Hypercalcemia in patients with advanced mammary cancer. Br Med J 3:573–577

Gallacher SJ, Fraser WD, Patel U, Logue FC, Soukop M, Boyle IT, Ralston SH (1990) Breast cancer-associated hypercalcaemia: a reassessment of renal calcium and phosphate handling. Ann Clin Biochem 27:551–556

Garbisa S, Pozzatti R, Muschel RJ, Safflotti V, Ballin M, Goldfarb RH, Khoury G, Liotta LA (1987) Secretion of type IV collagenolytic protease and metastatic phenotype: induction by transfection with c-Ha-ras but not c-Ha-ras plus AD2-Ela. Cancer Res 47:1523–1528

Garrett IR, Mundy GR (1989) Relationship between interleukin-1 and prostaglandins in resorbing neonatal calvariae. J Bone Miner Res 4:789–794

Gordan GS, Fitzpatrick ME, Lubich WP (1967) Identification of osteolytic sterols in human breast cancer. Trans Assoc Am Physicians 80:183–189

Gorelik E, Foggl M, Feldman M, Segal S (1979) Differences in resistance of metastatic tumor cells and cells from local tumor growth to cytotoxicity of natural killer cells. JNCI 63:1397–1404

Grill V, Ho P, Body JJ, Donohoo G, Ferber I, Johanson N, Orf JW, Lee SC, Kukreja SC, Moseley JM, Martin TJ (1991) Parathyroid hormone-related protein: elevated levels in hypercalcemia of malignancy and in hypercalcemia complicating metastatic breast cancer. J Clin Endocrinol Metab 73:1309–1315

Haddad JG, Cowranz SJ, Avioli LV (1970) Circulating phytosterols in normal females, lactating mothers, and breast cancer patients. J Clin Endocrinol Metab 30:174–180

Hanna MG, Zbar B, Rapp HJ (1972) BCG treatment reduced experimental metastases. JNCI 48:441–455

Harinck HI, Bijvoet OL, Plantingh AS, Body JJ, Elte JW, Sleeboom HP, Wildiers J, Neijt JP (1987) Role of bone and kidney in tumor-induced hypercalcemia and its treatment with bisphosphonate and sodium chloride. Am J Med 82:1133–1142

Hauschka PV, Mavrakos AE, Iafrati MD, Doleman SE, Klagsbrun M (1986) Growth factors in bone matrix. J Biol Chem 261:12665–12674

Heppner G (1984) Tumor heterogeneity. Cancer Res 214:2259–2265

Hilgard P, Gordon-Smith EL (1974) Microangiopathic hemolytic anemia and experimental tumor-cell emboli. Br J Haematol 26:651–659

Hujanen ES, Terranova VP (1985) Migration of tumor cells to organ-derived chemoattractants. Cancer Res 45:3517–3521

Ibbotson KJ, Twardzik DR, D'Souza SM, Hargreaves WR, Todaro GJ, Mundy GR (1985) Stimulation of bone resorption in vitro by synthetic transforming growth factor-alpha. Science 228:1007–1009

Ibbotson KJ, Harrod J, Gowen M, D'Souza S, Smith DD, Mundy GR (1986) Human recombinant transforming growth factor alpha stimulates bone resorption and inhibits formation in vitro. Proc Natl Acad Sci USA 83:2228–2232

Isales C, Carcangiu ML, Stewart AF (1987) Hypercalcemia in breast cancer: reassessment of the mechanism. Am J Med 82:1143–1147

Jacobs SC, Lawson R (1980) Mitogenic factors in human prostate extracts. Urology 16:488–491

Juliano RL (1987) Membrane receptors for extracellular matrix macromolecules: relationship to cell adhesion and tumor metastasis. Biochim Biophys Acta 907:261–278

Kalebic T, Williams JE, Talmadge JE, Kao-Shan CS, Kravitz B, Locklear K, Siegal GP, Liotta LA, Sobel ME, Steeg PS (1988) A novel method for selection of invasive tumor cells: derivation and characterization of highly metastatic K1735 melanoma cell lines based on in vitro and in vivo invasive capacity. Clin Exp Metastasis 6:301–318

Khosla S, van Heerden JA, Gharib H, Jackson IT, Danks J, Hayman JA, Martin TJ (1990) Parathyroid hormone-related protein and hypercalcemia secondary to massive mammary hyperplasia. N Engl J Med 322:1157

Kjonniksen I, Nesland JM, Pihl A, Fodstad O (1990) Nude rat model for studying metastasis of human tumor cells to bone and bone marrow. JNCI 82:408–412

Klein DC, Raisz LG (1970) Prostaglandins: stimulation of bone resorption in tissue culture. Endocrinology 86:1436–1440

Knabbe C, Lippman ME, Wakefield LM, Flanders KC, Kasid A, Derynck R, Dickson RB (1987) Evidence that transforming growth factor β is a hormonally regulated negative growth factor in human breast cancer cells. Cell 48:417–428

Koutsilieris M, Rabbani SA, Bennett HP, Goltzman D (1987) Characteristics of prostate-derived growth factors for cells of the osteoblast phenotype. J Clin Invest 80:941–946

Langer R, Conn H, Vacanti J, Haudenschild C, Folkman J (1980) Control of tumor growth in animals by infusion of angiogenesis inhibitor. Proc Natl Acad Sci USA 77:4331–4335

Lerner UH (1987) Modifications of the mouse calvarial technique improve the responsiveness to stimulators of bone resorption. J Bone Miner Res 2:375–383

Liotta LA (1986) Tumor invasion: role of the extracellular matrix. Cancer Res 46:1–7

Liotta LA, Kohn E (1990) Cancer invasion and metastases. JAMA 263:1123–1126

Liotta LA, Schiffmann E (1988) Tumour motility factors. Cancer Surv 7:631–652

Liotta LA, Steeg PS (1990) Clues to the function of Nm23 and Awd proteins in development, signal transduction, and tumor metastasis provided by studies of *Dictyostelium discoideum*. JNCI 82:1170–1172

Liotta LA, Kleinerman J, Saidel GM (1974) Quantitative relationships of intravascular tumor cells, tumor vessels, and pulmonary metastases following tumor implantation. Cancer Res 34:997–1004

Liotta LA, Tryggvason K, Garbisa S, Hart I, Foltz C, Shafie S (1980) Metastatic potential correlates with enzymatic degradation of basement membrane collagen. Nature 284:67–68

Liotta LA, Mandler R, Murano G, Katz DA, Gordon RK, Chiang PK, Schiffmann E (1986) Tumor cell autocrine motility factor. Proc Natl Acad Sci USA 83: 3302–3306

Lippman ME, Dickson RB, Bates S, Knabbe C, Huff K, Swain S, McManaway M, Bronzert D, Kasid A, Gelmann EP (1986) Autocrine and paracrine growth regulation of human breast cancer. Breast Cancer Res Treat 7:59–70

Lodwick GS (1964) Reactive response to local injury in bone. Radiol Clin North Am 2:209–219

Magro C, Orr FW, Manishen WJ, Sivananthan K, Mokashi SS (1985) Adhesion, chemotaxis, and aggregation of Walker carcinosarcoma cells in response to products of resorbing bone. JNCI 74:829–838

Marcelli C, Yates AJP, Mundy GR (1990) In vivo effects of human recombinant transforming growth factor beta on bone turnover in normal mice. J Bone Miner Res 5:1087–1096

Marquardt H, Lioubin MN, Ikeda T (1987) Complete amino acid sequence of human transforming growth factor type beta 2. J Biol Chem 262:12127–12130

Massague J (1990) Transforming growth factor alpha. A model for membrane-anchored growth factors. J Biol Chem 265:21393–21396

McCarthy JB, Basara ML, Palm SL, Sas DF, Furcht LT (1985) The role of cell adhesion proteins – laminin and fibronectin – in the movement of malignant and metastatic cells. Cancer Metastasis Rev 4:125–152

McCarthy JB, Skubitz APN, Palm SL, Furcht LT (1988) Metastasis inhibition of different tumor types by purified laminin fragments and a heparin-binding fragment of fibronectin. JNCI 80:108–116

Miller FR (1983) Tumor subpopulation interactions in metastasis. Invasion Metastasis 3:234–242

Mundy GR (1990) Calcium homeostasis: hypercalcemia and hypocalcemia. Dunitz, London

Mundy GR, Martin TJ (1982) The hypercalcemia of malignancy: pathogenesis and management. Metabolism 31:1247–1277

Mundy GR, Poser JW (1983) Chemotactic activity of the gamma-carboxyglutamic acid containing protein in bone. Calcif Tissue Int 35:164–168

Mundy GR, DeMartino S, Rowe DW (1981) Collagen and collagen-derived fragments are chemotactic for tumor cells. J Clin Invest 68:1102–1105

Noda M, Camilliere JJ (1989) In vivo stimulation of bone formation by transforming growth factor beta. Endocrinology 124:2991–2994

Nowak RA, Morrison NE, Goad DL, Gaffney EV, Tashjian AH (1990) Squamous cell carcinomas often produce more than a single bone resorption-stimulating factor: role of interleukin-1 alpha. Endocrinology 127:3061–3069

Nowel PS (1976) The clonal evolution of tumor cell subpopulations. Science 194: 23–38

Nussbaum SR, Gaz RD, Arnold A (1990) Hypercalcemia and ectopic secretion of parathyroid hormone by an ovarian carcinoma with rearrangement of the gene parathyroid hormone. N Engl J Med 323:1324–1328

Orr W, Varani J, Gondek MD, Ward PA, Mundy GR (1979) Chemotactic responses of tumor cells to products of resorbing bone. Science 203:176–179

Orr FW, Varani J, Gondek MD, Ward PA, Mundy GR (1980) Partial characterization of a bone derived chemotactic factor for tumor cells. Am J Pathol 99:43–52

Paget S (1889) The distribution of secondary growths in cancer of the breast. Lancet 1:571–573

Percival RC, Yates AJP, Gray RES, Galloway J, Rogers K, Neal FE, Kanis JA (1985) Mechanisms of malignant hypercalcemia in carcinoma of the breast. Br Med J 291:776–779

Perroteau I, Salomon D, DeBortoli M, Kidwell W, Hazarika P, Pardue R, Dedman J, Tam J (1986) Immunological detection and quantitation of alpha transforming growth factors in human breast carcinoma cells. Breast Cancer Res Treat 7:201–210

Pfeilschifter JP, Mundy GR (1987) Modulation of transforming growth factor beta activity in bone cultures by osteotropic hormones. Proc Natl Acad Sci USA 84:2024–2028

Pfeilschifter JP, Seyedin S, Mundy GR (1988) Transforming growth factor β inhibits bone resorption in fetal rat long bone cultures. J Clin Invest 82:680–685

Pfeilschifter J, Bonewald L, Mundy GR (1990a) Characterization of the latent transforming growth factor β complex in bone. J Bone Miner Res 5:49–58

Pfeilschifter J, Erdmann J, Schmidt W, Naumann A, Minne HW, Ziegler R (1990b) Differential regulation of plasminogen activator and plasminogen activator inhibitor by osteotropic factors in primary cultures of mature osteoblasts and osteoblast precursors. Endocrinology 126:703–711

Poste G (1986) Pathogenesis of metastatic disease: implications for current therapy and for the development of new therapeutic strategies. Cancer Treat Rep 70:183–199

Poste G, Doll J, Fidler IJ (1981) Interactions between clonal subpopulations affect the stability of the metastatic phenotype in polyclonal populations of the B16 melanoma cells. Proc Natl Acad Sci USA 78:6226–6230

Powell GJ, Southby J, Danks JA, Stillwell RG, Hayman JA, Henderson MA, Bennett RC, Martin TJ (1991) Localization of parathyroid hormone-related protein in breast cancer metastases: increased incidence in bone compared with other sites. Cancer Res 51:3059–3061

Powles TJ, Dowsett M, Easty GC, Easty DM, Neville AM (1976) Breast cancer osteolysis, bone metastases, and anti-osteolytic effect of aspirin. Lancet 1:608–610

Powles TJ, Muindi J, Coombes RC (1982) Mechanisms for development of bone metastases and effects of anti-inflammatory drugs. In: Powles TJ, Bockman RS, Honn KV, Ramwell P (eds) Prostaglandins and related lipids, vol 2. Liss, New York, pp 541–553

Rabbani SA, Desjardins J, Bell AW, Banville D, Henkin J, Goltzman D (1990a) An amino-terminal fragment of urokinase isolated from a prostate cancer cell line (PC-3) is mitogenic for osteoblast-like cells. Biochem Biophys Res Commun 173:1058–1064

Rabbani SA, Desjardins J, Bell AW, Banville D, Goltzman D (1990b) Identification of a new osteoblast mitogen from a human prostate cancer cell line, PC-3. J Bone Miner Res 5:549

Reedy AL, Fialkow PJ (1980) Multicellular origin of fibrosarcomas in mice induced by the chemical carcinogen 3-methylcholanthrene. J Exp Med 150:878–886

Rizzoli R, Bonjour JP (1989) High extracellular calcium increases the production of a parathyroid hormone-like activity by cultured Leydig tumor cells associated with humoral hypercalcemia. J Bone Miner Res 4:839–844

Rosengard AM, Krutzsch HC, Shearn A, Biggs JR, Barker E, Margulies IM, King CR, Liotta LA, Steeg PS (1989) Reduced Nm23/Awd protein in tumour metastasis and aberrant *Drosophila* development. Nature 342:177–180

Sabatini M, Yates AJ, Garrett R, Chavez J, Dunn J, Bonewald LF, Mundy GR (1990a) Increased production of tumor necrosis factor by normal immune cells in a model of the humoral hypercalcemia of malignancy. Lab Invest 63:676–681

Sabatini M, Chavez J, Mundy GR, Bonewald LF (1990b) Stimulation of tmor necrosis factor release from monolytic cells by the A375 human melanoma via granulocyte-macrophage colony-stimulating factor. Cancer Res 50:2673–2678

Salomon DS, Kidwell WR, Liu S (1986) Presence of alpha TGF mRNA in human breast cancer cell lines and in human breast carcinomas. Breast Cancer Res Treat 8:106A

Sanchez J, Baker V, Miller DM (1986) Review: basic mechanisms of metastasis. Am J Med Sci 292:376–385

Sato K, Fujii Y, Kasono K, Ozawa M, Imamura H, Kanaji Y, Kurosawa H, Tsushima T, Shizume K (1989) Parathyroid hormone-related protein and inter-leukin-1α synergistically stimulate bone resorption in vitro and increase the serum calcium concentration in mice in vivo. Endocrinology 124:2172–2178

Shevrin D, Kukreja SC, Ghosh L, Lad TE (1988) Development of skeletal metastasis by human prostate cancer in athymic nude mice. Clin Exp Metastasis 6:401–409

Simpson EL, Mundy GR, D'Souza SM, Ibbotson KJ, Bockman R, Jacobs JW (1983) Absence of parathyroid hormone messenger RNA in non-parathyroid tumors associated with hypercalcemia. N Engl J Med 309:325–330

Simpson EL, Harrod J, Eilon G, Jacobs JW, Mundy GR (1985) Identification of a mRNA fraction in human prostatic cancer cells coding for a novel osteoblast stimulating factor. Endocrinology 117:1615–1620

Siris ES, Sherman WH, Baquiran DC, Schlatterer JP, Osserman EF, Canfield RE (1980) Effects of dichloromethylene diphosphonate on skeletal mobilization of multiple myeloma. N Engl J Med 302:310–315

Slamon DJ, Clark GM, Wong SG, Levin WJ, Ullrich A, McGuire WL (1987) Human breast cancer: correlation of relapse and survival with amplification of the HER-2/neu oncogene. Science 235:177–182

Southby J, Kissin MW, Danks JA, Hayman JA, Moseley JM, Henderson MA, Bennett RC, Martin TJ (1990) Immunohistochemical localization of para-thyroid hormone-related protein in human breast cancer. Cancer Res 50:7710–7716

Spyratos F, Maudelonde T, Brouillet JP, Brunet M, Defrenne A, Andrieu C, Hacene K, Desplaces A, Rouesse J, Rochefort H (1989) Cathepsin D: an independent prognostic factor for metastasis of breast cancer. Lancet 2:1115–1118

Stahl KW, Mathe G, Kovacs G (1985) Decrease of metastogenic potential by pregraft treatment of Lewis lung carcinoma cells with proteinase and protein kinase affinity labels. Cancer Res 45:5335–5340

Stashenko P, Dewhirst FE, Rooney ML, Desjardins LA, Heeley JD (1987) Interleukin-1A is a potent inhibitor of bone formation in vitro. J Bone Miner Res 2:559–565

Steeg PS (1989) Search for metastasis suppressor genes. Invasion Metastasis 9:351–359

Steeg PS, Bevilacqua G, Kopper L, Thorgeirsson UP, Talmadge JE, Liotta LA, Sobel ME (1988) Evidence for a novel gene associated with low tumor metastatic potential. JNCI 80:200–204

Stern PH, Krieger NS, Nissenson RA, Williams RD, Winkler ME, Derynck R, Strewler GJ (1985) Human transforming growth factor alpha stimulates bone resorption in vitro. J Clin Invest 76:2016–2019

Stewart AF, Horst R, Deftos LJ, Cadman EC, Lang R, Broadus AE (1980) Bio-chemical evaluation of patients with cancer-associated hypercalcemia: evidence for humoral and nonhumoral groups. N Engl J Med 303:1377–1383

Stewart AF, Wu T, Goumas D, Burtis WJ, Broadus AE (1987) N-terminal amino acid sequence of two novel tumor-derived adenylate cyclase-stimulating proteins: identification of parathyroid hormone-like and parathyroid hormone-unlike domains. Biochem Biophys Res Commun 146:672–678

Takahashi N, Mundy GR, Roodman GD (1986) Recombinant human interferon gamma inhibits formation of human osteoclast like cells. J Immunol 137:3544–3549

Tashjian AH, Voelkel EF, Levine L, Goldhaber P (1972) Evidence that the bone resorption-stimulating factor produced by mouse fibrosarcoma cells is prostaglandin E2: a new model for the hypercalcemia of cancer. J Exp Med 136:1329–1343

Tashjian AH, Voelkel EF, Lazzaro M, Singer FR, Roberts AB, Derynck R, Winkler ME, Levine L (1985) Alpha and beta transforming growth factors stimulate prostaglandin production and bone resorption in cultured mouse calvaria. Proc Natl Acad Sci USA 82:4535–4538

Thiede MA, Rodan GA (1988) Expression of a calcium-mobilizing parathyroid hormone-like peptide in lactating mammary tissue. Science 242:278–280

Thompson SL (1974) The colony forming efficiency of single cells and cell aggregates from a spontaneous mouse mammary tumor using the lung colony assay. Br J Cancer 30:332–336

Tofe AJ, Francis MD, Harvey WJ (1975) Correlation of neoplasms with incidence and localization of skeletal metastases. An analysis of 1355 diphosphonate bone scans. J Nucl Med 16:986–989

Tsuchida T, Fujiwara H, Tsuji Y, Hamaoka T (1981) Inhibitory effect of *Propionibacterium acnes*-activated macrophages on tumor metastases induced by tumor-specific immunosuppression. Gan 72:205–212

Tuttle KR, Kunau RT, Loveridge N, Mundy GR (1991) Altered renal calcium handling in the hypercalcemia of malignancy. J Am Soc Nephrol 2:191–199

Vaes G (1968) On the mechanisms of bone resorption. The action of parathyroid hormone on the excretion and synthesis of lysosomal enzymes and on the extracellular release of acid by bone cells. J Cell Biol 39:676–697

Valentin A, Eilon G, Saez S, Mundy GR (1985) Estrogens and anti-estrogens stimulate release of bone resorbing activity by cultured human breast cancer cells. J Clin Invest 75:726–731

Van Breukelen FJM, Bijvoet OLM, van Oosterom AT (1979) Inhibition of osteolytic bone lesions by (3-amino-1-hydroxypropylidene)-1. 1. bisphosphonate (A.P.D.). Lancet 1:803–805

Van den Brenk HAS, Burch WM, Kelley H, Orton C (1975) Venous diversion trapping and growth of blood-borne cancer cells en route to the lungs. Br J Cancer 31:46–61

Vignon F, Capony F, Chambon M, Freiss G, Garcia M, Rochefort H (1986) Autocrine growth stimulation of the MCF-7 breast cancer cells by the estrogen-regulated 52K protein. Endocrinology 118:1537–1545

Vogelstein B, Fearon ER, Hamilton SR, Kern SE, Preisinger AC, Leppert M, Nakamura Y, White R, Smits AM, Bos JL (1988) Genetic alterations during colorectal tumor development. N Engl J Med 319:525–532

Warren BA, Vales O (1972) The adhesion of thromboplastic tumor emboli to vessel walls in vivo. Br J Exp Pathol 53:301–313

Weiss L (1985) Metastatic inefficiency in principles of metastasis. In: Weiss L, Gilbert H (eds) Liver metastasis. Academic Press, p 148

Weiss L, Glanes D (1974) Waited, the influence of host immunity on the arrest of circulating cancer cells and its modification by neuraminidase. Int J Cancer 13:850–862

Weiss L, Orr FW, Honn KV (1989) Interactions between cancer cells and the microvasculature: a rate-regulator for metastasis. Clin Exp Metastasis 7:127–167

Westley BR, May FEB (1987) Oestrogen regulates cathepsin D mRNA levels in oestrogen responsive human breast cancer cells. Nucleic Acids Res 15:3771–3786

Wewer UM, Taraboletti G, Sobel ME, Albrechtsen R, Liotta LA (1987) Laminin receptor: role in tumor cell migration. Cancer Res 47:5691–5698

Winterbauer RH, Elfenbein IB, Ball WC (1968) Incidence and clinical significance of tumor embolization to the lungs. Am J Med 45:271–290

Wo Z, Bonewald L, Oreffo ROC, Chirgwin JW, Capony F, Rochefort H, Mundy GR (1990) The potential role of procathepsin D secreted by breast cancer cells in bone resorption. In: Cohn DV, Glorieux FH, Martin TJ (eds) Calcium regulation and bone metabolism. Basic and clinical aspects, vol 10. Elsevier, Amsterdam, pp 304–310

Yates AJP, Oreffo ROC, Mayor K, Mundy GR (1991) Inhibition of bone resorption by inorganic phosphate is mediated both by reduced osteoclast formation and by impaired activity of mature osteoclasts. J Bone Miner Res 6:473–478

Yoneda T, Alsina MM, Chavez JB, Bonewald L, Nishimura R, Mundy GR (1991) Evidence that splenic cytokines play a pathogenetic role in the paraneoplastic syndromes of cachexia, hypercalcemia and leukocytosis in a human tumor in nude mice. J Clin Invest 87:977–985

Yoshimoto K, Yamasaki R, Sakai H, Tezuka U, Takahashi M, Iizuka M, Sekiya T, Saito S (1989) Ectopic production of parathyroid hormone by small cell lung cancer in a patient with hypercalcemia. J Clin Endocrinol Metab 68:976–981

Yusa T, Blood CH, Zetter BR (1989) Tumor cell interactions with elastin: implications for pulmonary metastasis. Am Rev Respir Dis 140:1458–1462

Zetter BR (1990) The cellular basis of site-specific tumor metastasis. N Engl J Med 322:605–612

CHAPTER 19

The Proteins of Bone

P.D. Delmas and L. Malaval

A. Introduction

Bone comprises a unique calcified extracellular matrix which is the most abundant source of connective tissue components. It is mainly composed of type I collagen (90% of the organic matrix), which differs from the type I collagen present in other connective tissues by several posttranslational modifications. The non-collagenous component (10% of the organic matrix) has been extensively characterized in the past 15 years, due to progress in protein biochemistry and molecular biology techniques, as reviewed by GEHRON-ROBEY (1989). In particular, the alternate use of dissociating (EDTA) and nondissociating buffers leads to the differentiation of a mineral phase (hydroxyapatite crystals) and an organic phase (collagenous matrix), between which the proteins are distributed. The population of proteins present in bone is composed of exogenous and endogenous proteins (listed in Table 1). Exogenous proteins are synthesized in other organs, circulate in blood and tissue fluids, and are trapped in bone matrix because of their affinity for hydroxyapatite. Endogenous proteins are synthesized by the bone-forming cells – the osteoblasts – and incorporated into the complex three-dimensional scaffolding of bone matrix. These bone matrix proteins have raised considerable interest as they are thought to play an important role in several aspects of bone physiology (Fig. 1). Some of them might play a role in the nucleation and growth of hydroxyapatite crystals associated with type I collagen, a mineralization process which does not occur physiologically in most other collagen-containing connective tissues such as skin, tendon, and sclera. As discussed below, bone matrix proteins might also be involved in the proliferation and maturation of bone cells at different stages of bone development. Some of these proteins appear to be chemotactic for a variety of cells, and other proteins induce cell attachment and spreading through specific amino acid motifs such as the Arg-Gly-Asp amino acid sequence. These properties suggest that bone matrix proteins interact with bone cell recruitment and activity, participating in the local control of bone remodeling.

With one exception, bone matrix proteins are not unique to bone. They can be synthesized and secreted by other tissues, although their concentration in bone is much higher than in any other tissue. The specificity of bone

Table 1. Proteins of bone: structural properties, quantitative contribution, distribution, and potential role. The list given—by no means exhaustive—is restricted to proteins whose presence in mineralized matrix has been established. The quantitative

Origin	Proteins	Structural properties
Bone	*Collagens* Type I	Gly-X-Y repeats Fibrillar
	Type V *N*-propeptide of type I	a_1 (V), a_2 (V), a_1 (XI) Phosphorylated
	GLA-containing proteins	γ-Carboxylation of some Glu residues
	Osteocalcin	3 Gla, hydrophilic
	Matrix Gla-protein	5 Gla, hydrophobic
	Proteoglycans	Glycosaminoglycan (GAG): chondroïtin-4-sulfate
	Biglycan	2 GAG chains
	Decorin	1 GAG chain In both, ten repeats of a "leucin-rich" motif in the protein sequence
	PG-CS III	Highly acidic, does not bind to nitrocellulose
	Sparc/osteonectin	High affinity for calcium and hydroxyapatite
	RGD-containing proteins	Present of the consensus sequence for binding to intergrin-type receptors
	Osteopontin	Mainly phosphorylated; Sulfated; highly sialylated
	Bone sialoprotein	Mainly sulfated; phosphorylated; highly sialylated
	BAG-75?	Not yet shown to contain an RGD sequence; highly sialylated
	Thrombospondin	Multidomain protein
	Proteases MMP-1	Present in a latent form
	Growth factors Bone morphogenetic proteins TGFβ	See Chaps. 5 and 20, this volume
	IGF	
Plasma	Albumin a_2-HS glycoprotein	
	IgG Transferrin a_1-Antitrypsin Apo A1 lipoprotein Hemoglobin	

contributions to the matrix are indicative; values may vary according to the species investigated (most studies concern bovine and human bone) and the age of the subjects (maximal values are observed in fetuses and young subjects)

Quantitative contribution	Distribution	Role, established or presumed
~90% of proteins	Creates an organized scaffold of fibers, secondarily mineralized	Tensile strength, elasticity
~3% of collagen ~5% of noncollagenous protein (fetus)	Two pools, one bound to the organic matrix, one bound to the mineral phase	Regulation of collagen synthesis; regulation of fibrillogenesis? inhibition of mineralization?
Up to 20% of noncollagenous proteins	Bound to the mineral phase	Regulation of resorption? Used as a marker of formation
	Bound to the organic matrix (collagen)	Inhibition of mineralization?
Up to 10% of noncollagenous proteins	Bound to the mineral, pericellular	Cell differentiation?
Major proteoglycan of bone matrix	Bound to collagen fibers	Regulation of fibrillogenesis? Inhibition of mineralization?
	Bound to the mineral phase	
Up to 20% of noncollagenous proteins (fetus)	Bound mainly to mineral	Involved in cell/substrate and cell/cell interactions, and in cell proliferation: tissue remodeling?
	Bound mainly to the mineral phase	Cell adhesion; regulation of crystal growth?
~12% of noncollagenous proteins	Present in mineral and organic phase	Cell adhesion; crystal nucleation
		Modulation of cell adhesion and proliferation
		Preparation of bone surface for osteoclast adhesion? Resorption?
		Proliferation and differentiation of bone cells; osteogenesis
200 µg/KG; major storing site in the body		Promotion of bone formation and osteogenesis
Major components of plasma origin	All exogenous proteins are bound to the mineral phase	Cell migration?

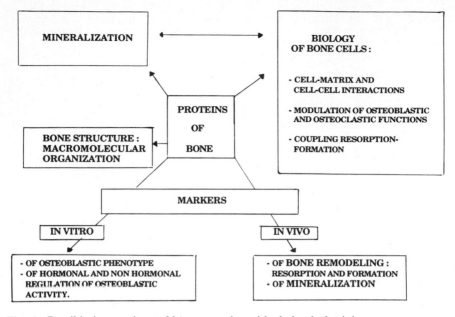

Fig. 1. Possible interactions of bone proteins with skeletal physiology

tissue is likely to rely on tissue-specific posttranslational modifications, and on interactions between these proteins, which are expressed at different stages of osteoblastic differentiation, and either type I collagen or hydroxy-apatite. In addition to their role in bone physiology, bone matrix proteins have been used as phenotypic markers of osteoblasts in culture and they are potential markers of bone turnover in the clinical investigation of metabolic bone diseases. Indeed, a fraction of newly synthesized proteins leak into the circulation, where they can be measured by radioimmunoassay. Serum levels of the major bone matrix proteins should reflect various aspects of osteoblastic functions, provided that the contribution from other tissues is negligible. Similarly, fragments of matrix proteins released into the circulation during bone resorption can be measured to assess osteoclastic activity, as is already done with collagen products.

B. Collagen

Collagen is the most abundant protein in the body and 90% of the protein content of bone is collagenous. Mineralized matrix contains mainly type I collagen, and small amounts of type V (VON DER MARK et al. 1976; REDDI et al. 1977; WIESTNER et al. 1981). Although type III collagen is synthesized by osteoblastic cells in culture (BELLOWS et al. 1986), it does not seem to be present in mineralized matrices. Fibril-associated collagens have been shown to be present in many connective tissues (SHAW and OLSEN 1991), but so far not in bone.

I. Structure and Synthesis of Bone Collagen

1. Structure of Collagens

Collagens are a large and expanding family of proteins (review in PROCKOP et al. 1979a,b; BORNSTEIN and SAGE 1980; HOLLISTER et al. 1983; FLEISCHMAJER et al. 1989), which are defined by the presence, in at least a part of their sequence, of repeats of the triplet Gly -X-Y, in which roughly one-third of the X repeats are proline and one-third of the Y repeats are hydroxyproline – the latter being specific to collagen molecules. This unique feature gives to the sequence a right-handed helical conformation. A collagen molecule is composed of three chains, whose helical portions are associated in a left-handed superhelix (Fig. 1). This "triple helix" structure is made possible by the regular repeat of Gly residues, and the presence of hydroxyproline residues is crucial to its stability. The number of triplets in the molecule, the sequence and position of the "noncollagenous" portions, and the sequence of the other residues present in X and Y vary from one type of collagen to another. In addition, different chains may exist for one type of collagen. This is the case for type I, in which molecules are made of two sets of chains, $\alpha_1(I)$ and $\alpha_2(I)$, in a 2:1 ratio ($[\alpha_1(I)]2\ \alpha_2(I)$). Molecules with an $[\alpha_1(I)]3$ composition have been described in mineralized tissues, such as growing dentin (SODEK and MANDELL 1982). Type I molecule is mainly triple helical, with short nonhelical portions at both ends. The "fibrillar" or "interstitial" collagens such as type I, type II (restricted to cartilage), and type III are organized in fibers. Apart from bone and dentine, type I fibers are present in tendon, skin, and many other connective tissues. In lamellar bone, type I collagen fibers are strictly parallel, and form successive sheets with alternate orientations. In woven bone (produced in primary ossification and in pathological situations such as Paget's disease of bone and renal osteodystrophy) the collagenous structure is less organized. In addition to type I collagen, bone contains minute amounts of type V collagen. Three α-chains have been described for type V collagen, and their ratio in the molecule seems to vary from one tissue to another. In bone, type V collagen seems to be heterogeneous, involving chains $\alpha_1(V)$, $\alpha_2(V)$, and $\alpha_1(XI)$, with a 1:1:1 ratio (NIYIBIZI and EYRE 1989). Type V collagen is present in most connective tissues in a pericellular location, but its distribution in bone is not known.

2. Type I Collagen Synthesis and Secretion

a) Synthesis

Type I collagen is by far the most extensively studied of bone proteins and its synthesis and assembly are regularly reviewed (PROCKOP et al. 1979a,b;

FLEISCHMAJER et al. 1989; CHEAH 1985). The genes for the $\alpha_1(I)$- and $\alpha_2(I)$-chains (located on chromosomes 7 and 17, respectively, in human) present the same number of exons (51), but have very different sizes (18 and 40 kbp, respectively) due to differences in the sizes of the introns. The helical domain is encoded by exons corresponding to exact multiples of the (Gly X-Y) triplet (45, 54, 99, and 108 bp, respectively). It is believed that the 54-bp exon would be the primordial gene, from which collagenous molecules would have evolved by duplication and recombination (CHEAN 1985). However, not all genes of nonfibrillar collagens contain this exon. $\alpha_1(I)$- and $\alpha_2(I)$-chains are synthesized in the rough endoplasmic reticulum as precursor molecules, containing a signal sequence and N- and C-propeptides. The amounts produced are in a $2:1$ ratio (α_1 versus α_2), as could be expected from the composition of the molecule. Several posttranslational modifications occur while the chains elongate in the cisternae: elimination of the signal sequence, hydroxylation of some proline and lysine residues, then glycosylation of some hydroxylysine residues by addition of galactose or galactose and glucose. After completion of the elongation, disulfide bonds are formed between the C-terminal propeptides of two α_1-chains and one α_2-chain, and the triple-helix forms, progressing to the N-terminal end, and preventing and further modification of the helical part. Hydroxylation of proline and formation of the interchain bonds are absolute requirements for the spontaneous folding of the triple helix. Glycosylation of asparagine residues of the C-terminal propeptide occurs in the Golgi apparatus. After secretion of the procollagen molecule, specific proteinases cleave the N- and C-terminal propeptides. The specific fate of these fragments in bone matrix is discussed below.

b) Fiber Organization and Cross-linking

As soon as the propetides are removed, the collagen molecules ($\sim$95 kDa) assemble spontaneously in fibers. Studies on the sequence of fibrillar collagen chains have shown that the residues in X- and Y-positions in the triplets present a pattern such that alternate hydrophilic and hydrophobic clusters are organized along the collagen molecule, allowing lateral self-assembly (PIEZ 1982). In fibers, molecules are associated head to tail, separated by a gap of $\sim$45 nm (Fig. 2). In addition, each molecule is staggered by about one-fourth of its length (234 amino acids, 67 nm) relative to its lateral neighbors. The alternation of zones with and without "holes" (gaps) along the fibers explains the 67-nm banding pattern observed after contrasting with heavy metals in electron microscopy. The holes in type I collagen fibers play a crucial part in the theory of bone matrix mineralization, being held as the site of formation of hydroxyapatite crystals (WEINER and TRAUB 1986). Apart from these fundamental mechanisms, the formation and composition of collagen fibers in the extracellular matrix is also dependent on interactions with other components of the matrix, such as the propeptides or proteoglycans.

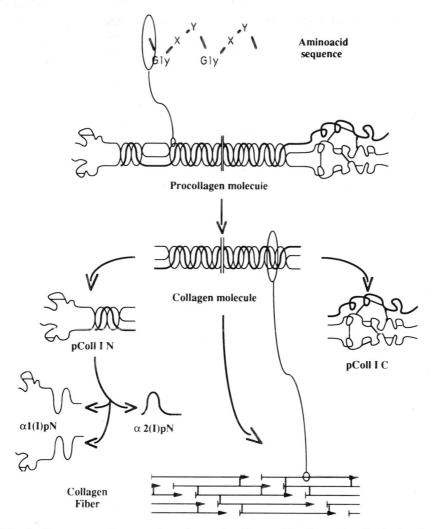

Fig. 2. Structure and processing of type I collagen. The figure details the levels of organization and the fate of fragments. See text for explanations. (▮), cross-links; (〜), α_1-chains; (〜), α_2-chains; (—), disulfide bridges

An important posttranslational modification that stabilizes the collagen molecules is the gradual formation of covalent cross-links. These cross-links form bridges between α-chains within the triple-helical molecule or between α-chains belonging to adjacent molecules (EYRE 1987). Lysyl oxidase induces the conversion of some lysyl and hydroxylysyl residues to the aldehydic derivatives allysine and hydroxyallysine. Three of these derivatives condense to form reducible, and subsequently nonreducible, cross-links between three α-chains. As discussed below, the urinary excretion of these cross-links has been recently proposed as a marker of bone collagen degradation.

c) Fate of the Propeptides

Maturation of type I collagen in bone seems to begin with the removal of the N-propeptide first, then the C-propeptide (DAVIDSON et al. 1977). C-Propeptides of α_1- and α_2-chains (termed α_1 and α_2(I)pC) are globular structures of about 250 amino acids ($\sim$30 kDa), stabilized by intrachain disulfide bridges. As previously mentioned, interchain bonds also link the three chains at this level. The N-propeptides of α_1-chains (α_1(I)pN, $\sim$25 kDa) present an N-terminal globular domain, containing intrachain disulfide bonds, a collagen domain involved in a triple-helix and a short nonhelical terminal part, near the cleavage site of the N-proteinase (Fig. 2). α_2-chains have a shorter N-propeptide, reduced to the matching collagenous domain and the noncollagenous tail. Several studies indicate that the cleavage of the propeptides may not be complete in type I collagen of bone (MORRIS et al. 1975), and that pN and pC collagens would be integrated in the fibers. Interestingly, the pN propeptide has been detected in smaller fibers, while to pC propeptide was present mainly in the larger fibers (FLEISCHMAJER et al. 1987). A component of mineralized matrix, originally named "24-kDa phosphoprotein" (TERMINE et al. 1981a), has been identified to the α_1(I) pN propeptide (FISHER et al. 1987a). A striking feature of this molecule is the phosphorylation of its unique serine residue, a posttranscriptional modification which has not been described in other tissues. Other results indicate that the N-propeptide population present in bone matrix is heterogeneous. Two pools have been identified, which differ in hydroxyapatite binding and in distribution between the mineral and collagenous components of the matrix. This suggests either the existence of truncated forms, or variations in glycosylation and/or phosphorylation (GOLDBERG et al. 1988a; SODEK et al. 1989).

Several hypotheses have been presented concerning the biological role that propeptides could play after cleavage. Strong evidence indicates that they could regulate type I collagen synthesis, in a negative feedback process. When added to cell cultures (WU et al. 1986) and to cell-free translation systems (KÜHN et al. 1982), the propeptides reduce the amount of mRNA and of collagen synthesized and/or secreted. Such a mechanism would directly affect bone formation. As suggested for other tissues, the propeptides could also play a role in fibril formation (FLEISCHMAJER et al. 1987). In the special case of bone matrix, an interesting suggestion is that the N-propeptide would occupy the "hole" regions of type I collagen fibers, preventing or enhancing the mineralization of the matrix (FLEISCHMAJER et al. 1987; FISHER et al. 1987a; GOLDBERG et al. 1988a).

d) Other Collagenous Components

Two minor collagenous peptides (named "small collagenous apatite binding proteins" = SCAB1 and 2, M_r 25 000 and 28 000, respectively) have been described in fetal porcine bone matrix (SODEK et al. 1989; KUWATA et al. 1987). About half of their sequence is not α-helical, and their immunologic and chromatographic properties seem to rule out a relationship with either α_1(I)pN or the type I collagen molecule itself (KUWATA et al. 1987). Further studies are necessary to assess whether these molecules belong to another type of collagen (propeptides of type V?) or to novel collagenous components of bone matrix.

II. Disorders of Collagen Synthesis: Osteogenesis Imperfecta

The complex process of synthesis and secretion of type I collagen offers many possibilities for genetic defects to affect tissue development, particularly in bone, in which this collagen is dominant. Osteogenesis imperfecta (OI) is a group of inherited diseases of bone characterized by bone fragility, but often associated with defects of dentin and nonmineralized tissues (fragility of joints or skin, deafness). OI is heterogeneous in gravity, clinical manifestation, heritability, genetic dominance, and molecular origins (reviews in HOLLISTER et al. 1983; CHEAH 1985; PROCKOP and KIVIRIKKO 1984). Four main categories have been defined by SILLENCE (1981) on clinical criteria, type I being the mildest and type II lethal before or at birth. Molecular studies of defects in type I collagen synthesis concentrate mainly on fibroblasts, which are easier to use as experimental material than bone cells. A large number of mutations in one or both structural genes of type I collagen have been described in patients with OI. The pattern includes substitution of amino acid (particularly glycine, which impairs helix formation), deletions of amino acids, including deletions of several exons within the helix-coding protions of the genes, splicing mutations, and other mutations that produce frameshifts. Increases in the degree of hydroxylation of proline and lysine residues are often observed. This reflects a reduced rate of formation of the triple helix, due to defects in the sequence, as hydroxylation is blocked only when the formation of the triple helix is completed. The outcome is the reduction of the amount of type I collagen produced and/or the production of an abnormal collagen (unstable helix, partly or exclusively α_1(I) trimer), which is stored in the cell or secreted at a reduced rate. A frequent observation is the increase in the tissues of the relative amount of type III collagen, which may also be present in bone matrix (POPE et al. 1980). This may be due either to the decrease in type I content or to compensation mechanisms. Few studies have focused on the effects of OI on other components of the mineralized matrix. The first studies on animal models (TERMINE et al. 1984; FISHER et al. 1986) and human subjects (FISHER et al. 1987b) suggested a large diversity of effects; a recent analysis of human subjects with all types of OI (VETTER et al. 1991) documents a consistent reduction of SPARC/osteonectin amounts in cortical bone and an increase in bone sialoprotein, osteocalcin, and α_2HS glycoprotein.

III. Markers of Collagen Metabolism

In search of specific circulating markers of bone metabolism, early attention was focussed on collagen, the most important organic component of bone matrix. Although type I collagen is not restricted to bone, the relative contribution of the skeleton and its continuous turnover indicate that circulating components assessing type I collagen synthesis or degradation would be fairly representative of bone formation or resorption. Among the markers developed, some are of routine use in some clinical laboratories (hydroxyproline), while others, though promising, are still in the course of development (pyridinoline).

1. Markers of Type I Collagen Synthesis: Propeptides

Specific assays for type I collagen N and C propetides have been developed since the mid-1970s (Rohde et al. 1976; Taubmann et al. 1976). An assay for the C propetide (pColl-I-C, three chains linked by disulfide bonds) was applied to subjects with Paget's disease of bone, showing an increase in the circulating concentrations (from 50–150 ng/ml in controls, up to 2 mg/ml) (Taubmann et al. 1976). The values correlated with the levels of serum alkaline phosphatase, and, after treatment with a bisphosphonate, decreased dramatically to normal values in most patients, reflecting the decrease in bone turnover. These observations were confirmed in recent work (Simon et al. 1984), in which a rapid decrease of circulating levels under treatment with calcitonin was also documented. Another study showed a decreased in circulating levels of pColl-I-C upon infusion of parathyroid hormone [1–34], reflecting an induced decrease of type I collagen synthesis (Simon et al. 1988). Serum levels of pColl-I-C correlate positively with serum alkaline phosphatase and bone formation rate (BFR) measured on transiliac biopsies, in patients with osteopenia (Parfitt et al. 1987). However, no strong correlation could be found with BFR in a subset of patients with postmenopausal osteoporosis.

A radioimmunoassay has been recently reported (Kraenzlin et al. 1989) that measures the levels of the N-propetide of the α_1-chain of type I collagen (α_1(I)pN), a single chain, which may aggregate in a trimer due to its collagenous part (Fisher et al. 1987a). Serum levels were increased in pagetic (~50 ng/ml) and osteoporotic (~16 ng/ml) patients as compared to controls (~10 ng/ml). A strong correlation with alkaline phosphatase was also observed, and treatment with a bisphosphonate induced a decrease in circulating levels parallel to the decrease of alkaline phosphatase activity.

The use of these assays presents three potential drawbacks: (a) part of the antigen detected could result from collagen degradation, and thus the values assayed would not specifically reflect bone formation, (b) the antigen detected could differ from the standard and tracer used in the assay due to different cleavage and/or posttranslational modification (Simon et al. 1984; cf. also N-propeptide in bone: Fisher et al. 1987a,c), and (c) the amounts assayed also reflect a contribution from nonmineralized tissues (GOLDBERG et al. 1988a).

2. Markers of Collagen Degradation

a) Urinary Hydroxyproline and Hydroxylysine Glycosides

Hydroxyproline represents about 13% of the amino acid content of the collagen molecule (PROCKOP and KIVIRIKKO 1968). Because free hydroxyproline released during degradation of collagen cannot be reutilized in collagen synthesis, most of the endogenous hydroxyproline present in biologic fluids is derived from the degradation of various forms of collagen (PROCKOP et al. 1979a,b). As half of human collagen resides in bone, where its turnover is probably faster than in soft tissues, excretion of hydroxyproline in urine is regarded as a marker of bone resorption. Actually, the C1q fraction of the complement contains significant amounts of hydroxyproline and could account for up to 40% of urinary hydroxyproline. The relationship of the urinary hydroxyproline to the metabolism of collagen is complex. Hydroxyproline is present in biologic fluids in different forms. About 90% of the hydroxyproline released by the breakdown of collagen in the tissues, and especially during bone resorption, is degraded to the free amino acid that circulates in plasma, is filtered, and is almost entirely reabsorbed by the kidney. It is eventually completely oxidized in the liver and is degraded to carbon dioxide and urea (KIVIRIKKO 1983; LOWRY et al. 1985). About 10% of the hydroxyproline released by the breakdown of collagen circulates in the peptide-bound form, and these peptides that contain hydroxyproline are filtered and excreted in urine with no further metabolism. Thus, the urinary total hydroxyproline represents only about 10% of total collagen catabolism. Hydroxyproline is present in urine in three forms: free hydroxyproline, small hydroxyproline-containing peptides that are dialyzable and represent over 90% of the total urinary excretion of this amino acid, and a small number of nondialyzable polypeptides containing hydroxyproline (PROCKOP and KIVIRIKKO 1968). Colorimetric assay of hydroxyproline is usually performed on a hydrolyzed urine sample and therefore reflects the total excretion of the amino acid. As a consequence of its tissue origin and metabolism pattern, urinary hydroxyproline may not be sensitive enough to assess subtle changes of bone resorption, such as in osteoporotic states. In patients with vertebral osteoporosis, urinary hydroxyproline is poorly correlated with bone resorption assessed by calcium kinetics or bone histomorphometry (DELMAS 1988) and there is an obvious need for a more sensitive marker of bone resorption. Hydroxylysine is another amino acid unique to collagen and proteins containing collagen-like sequences. Like hydroxyproline, hydroxylysine is not reutilized for collagen biosynthesis, and, although it is much less abundant than hydroxyproline, it is a potential marker of collagen degradation (CUNNINGHAM et al. 1967). Hydroxylysine is present in part as galactosylhydroxylysine and in part as glucosyl-galactosylhydroxylysine. The relative proportion and total content of both moieties vary in bone and soft tissues, which suggests that their urinary excretion might be a more sensitive marker of bone resorption than urinary hydroxyproline (Moro et al. 1988).

b) Urinary Excretion of Pyridinoline Cross-links

The HPLC assay of pyridinoline (Pyr) and deoxypyridinoline (D-Pyr), also called HP and LP, is presently the most promising marker of bone resorption. Pyr and D-Pyr are nonreducible cross-links which stabilize the collagen chains within the extra-cellular matrix (reviewed in Eyre 1987). Pyr is present in bone and cartilage matrix, and in minute amounts in some other connective tissues. Significant amounts of D-Pyr are only found in bone collagen, at a concentration of 0.07 mol/mol collagen. The relative proportion of Pyr and D-Pyr in bone matrix is variable according to the species. In human bone, the Pyr/D-Pyr ratio is 2 to 3. Pyr and D-Pyr are likely to be released from bone matrix during its degradation by the osteoclasts. As both cross-links result from a posttranslational modification of collagen, they cannot be reutilized during collagen synthesis. Available data suggest that Pyr and D-Pyr are not metabolized in vivo, and they are found in urine in free form (30%–40%) and in peptide-bound form (60%–70%). The total amount can be measured by fluorimetry after reverse-phase HPLC of cellulose-bound extract of hydrolyzed urine (Eyre 1987; Black et al. 1988). Urinary Pyr and D-Pyr are markedly higher in children than in adults, are increased by 50%–100% at the time of menopause, and go down to premenopausal levels after estrogen therapy (Uebelhart et al. 1991). In patients with vertebral osteoporosis, the urinary cross-link levels, especially of D-Pyr, are correlated with bone turnover measured by calcium kinetics and bone histomorphometry (Delmas et al. 1991). Pyr and D-Pyr appear to be more sensitive than hydroxyproline in Paget's disease of bone and are reduced markedly by bisphosphonate therapy (Uebelhart et al. 1990). Pyr and D-Pyr are also significantly increased in patients with primary hyperparathyroidism and malignant hypercalcemia. In summary, the measurement of urinary cross-links appears to have several potential advantages over hydroxyproline: they are relatively specific for bone turnover, they do not appear to be metabolized in vivo prior to their urinary excretion, and the absence of intestinal absorption of Pyr and D-Pyr contained in gelatine allows collection of urine with no food restriction. However, more information is needed about their clearance, especially when the glomerular filtration rate is decreased, a common finding in the elderly. The potential contribution of connective tissues other than bone in the urinary excretion also needs to be addressed. Finally, a more convenient assay is mandatory if this measurement is to be developed on a large scale.

C. Gamma-carboxyglutamic Acid Containing Proteins of Bone

I. Gamma-carboxyglutamic Acid (GLA)

The discovery of carboxyglutamic acid (GLA) is related to the study of the vitamin K-dependent clotting factors (factor II, VII, IX, X). In 1974, a new amino acid, GLA, was discovered in prothrombin. GLA was shown to derive from glutamic acid residues by a post-translational carboxylation that requires vitamin K and a specific carboxylase. GLA is responsible for the binding of calcium to prothrombin and of the other vitamin K-dependent factors and it promotes their binding to phospholipids (reviewed in GALLOP et al. 1980). Because of its unique calcium-binding features, GLA was searched for in mineralized tissues. A GLA-Containing protein (bone GLA-protein or osteocalcin) was discovered independently in chicken (HAUSCHKA et al. 1975) and calf bone (PRICE et al. 1976). More recently, another GLA-containing protein has been isolated from bone, matrix GLA-protein (PRICE et al. 1983). Actually, these two proteins account for most – but not all – of the GLA content of bone, and other vitamin K-dependent GLA-containing proteins are likely to be present in bone matrix.

II. Osteocalcin

1. Structure, Biosynthesis, and Tissular Distribution

Osteocalcin is a low molecular weight protein (6000 daltons), consisting of a single chain of 49–50 amino acids. It is an acidic protein showing on two-dimensional electrophoresis four isomeric forms of identical molecular weight with a pI ranging from 3.95 to 4.5 (DELMAS et al. 1984a). The entire covalent structure has been determined by amino acid sequencing in several species including human, swordfish, calf, chicken, rat, and monkey (reviewed in PRICE 1985; LIAN and GUNDBERG 1988; LIAN et al. 1989). Common features include three residues of GLA in positions 17, 21, and 24 with an associated disulfide bond and indicate that osteocalcin is highly conserved. The human osteocalcin gene has been localized on chromosome 1 and contains four exons. The gene predicts a protein of 125 amino acids (prepro-osteocalcin), including a 26 amino acid signal peptide and a 10-kDa proosteocalcin which is posttranslationally modified (vitamin K dependent carboxylation of some glutamic acid residues) and then processed into the mature 6-kDa form (CELESTE et al. 1986). The propeptide sequence, which is analogous to the propeptide of vitamin K dependent liver protein, is the recognition signal for g-carboxylation of glu residues (PAN and PRICE 1985). Administration of warfarin, which inhibits the vitamin K carboxylase enzyme complex, results in the intracellular accumulation of proosteocalcin, and in the secretion of a non-carboxylated osteocalcin which does not bind to hydroxyapatite. 1,25-Dihydroxyvitamin D, the most potent vitamin D metabolite, markedly stimulates osteocalcin synthesis (Price and Baukol 1980, 1981). The existence of a vitamin D responsive element in the osteocalcin gene promoter indicates that the 1,25-dihydroxyvitamin D-induced osteocalcin gene expression is transcriptionally regulated (Lian et al. 1989; Markose et al. 1990; Owen et al. 1990). The biosynthesis of osteocalcin by nontransformed osteoblast-like cells and by several osteo-sarcoma cell lines from various species and by tissue cultures has been demonstrated. The culture systems have been used to show the inhibition of osteocalcin secretion by parathyroid hormone and 17b-estradiol, and its stimulation by growth hormone, insulin-like growth factor I (IGF-I), and basic and acidic fibroblast growth factors (Lian et al. 1989; Canalis and Lian 1988; Chenu et al. 1990).

The tissue distribution of osteocalcin has been studied by immunocyto-chemistry and by Northern blot analysis of extracted RNA. All studies have failed to show the presence of osteocalcin in tissues other than bone and dentine. Osteocalcin is secreted by osteoblasts and odontoblasts, and is present in dentine and calcified bone matrix, but only occasionally in osteoid tissue. The temporal sequence of the occurrence of osteocalcin and mineral is controversial, as studies performed in developing embryonic bone of various species have produced conflicting results (Price et al. 1980a, 1981a; Hauschka et al. 1983; Hauschka and Reddi 1980). Osteocalcin deposition into bone and dentine increases with increasing mineral content (Lian et al. 1989), but the early stage of mineral deposition may precede osteocalcin expression (Price 1985).

2. Functional Role

Osteocalcin binds calcium and hydroxyapatite, with a relatively low affinity which depends primarily on the presence of GLA, and inhibits hydroxyapatite crystal growth in vitro (Poser et al. 1982; Romberg et al. 1986). The conformation of the molecule is highly dependent on the fixation of calcium on its GLA residues and its binding to calcium (Hauschka and Carr 1982; Delmas et al. 1984a). These properties, the fact that osteocalcin synthesis is highly dependent on $1,25(OH)_2D$, and its specificity for bone tissue suggested that osteocalcin might play a role in bone mineralization. Actually, such a role seems to be unlikely. Osteocalcin appears late in bone development, does not appear to precede the onset of mineralization (Price et al. 1981a), and is absent in the early stage of bone calcification. Histoimmunochemical detection of osteocalcin with light and electron microscopy has led to con-flicting results. Osteocalcin has been consistently found in osteoblasts of various origins and in the mineralized matrix, but is absent in early, non-mineralized osteoid matrix (Mark et al. 1987; Gorter De Vries et al. 1988) or is present in small amounts (Groot et al. 1986; Bronckers et al. 1987).

In addition, circulating osteocalcin is increased in patients with nutritional osteomalacia (DEMIAUX et al. 1992).

To better understand the potential role of osteocalcin, Price has developed an experimental model in which rats are maintained on high doses of warfarin and low doses of vitamin K1 for up to 8 months (PRICE and WILLIAMSON 1981; PRICE et al. 1982). Under these conditions, osteocalcin is secreted at a normal rate but is not incorporated into bone matrix because of its undercarboxylation. Despite osteocalcin bone levels which are only 2% of normal, long bones from rats maintained for 3 months in a vitamin K-deficient state are not different from controls in length, weight, and total mineral content, and the X-ray diffraction pattern of the mineral is not altered (PRICE and WILLIAMSON 1981). The response of metaphysal bone to a large dose of 1,25(OH)$_2$D, however, is modified by concurrent warfarin treatment through an unclear mechanism (PRICE 1985). Finally, rats maintained on warfarin during 8 months showed a dramatic closure of the epiphyseal growth plate, causing a cessation of longitudinal growth (PRICE et al. 1982; LEE et al. 1983). This excessive mineralization is likely to result

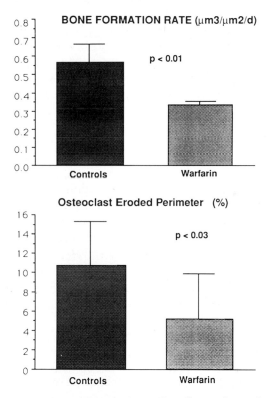

Fig. 3. Significant decrease of bone formation (bone formation rate) and bone resorption (*osteoclast-eroded perimeter*, osteoclast-covered eroded surfaces) in lambs on a high dose of warfarin for 3 months. (PASTOUREAU et al. 1989)

from the absence of osteocalcin and/or from the warfarin-induced decrease of matrix GLA-protein, another GLA-containing protein which is abundant in cartilage (see below). We have recently looked at the trabecular bone remodeling activity measured on iliac crest biopsy from lambs that were maintained on high doses of warfarin from birth to 3 months of age, and whose bone concentrations of osteocalcin were decreased by 90%. When compared to control animals, warfarin-treated lambs had a marked and significant decrease of trabecular bone mass. This was associated with a major impairment of trabecular bone turnover, a decrease of bone resorption, and a dramatic reduction of the bone formation rate, suggesting that osteocalcin, along with other GLA-containing proteins, is important in the maintenance of a normal bone turnover (Pastoureau et al. 1989) (Fig. 3).

A role of osteocalcin in the induction of bone resorption is suggested by in vitro experiments showing that osteocalcin along with osteocalcin fragments and L-GLA – which might be generated during the resorption process – are chemotactic for monocytes, a cell population that is believed to contain the precursor of osteoclasts (Malone et al. 1982a,b; Mundy and Poser 1983). Subsequent experiments have indeed shown that implants of bone particles from warfarin-treated rats are not degraded to the same extent as normal bone particles (Lian et al. 1984), and further experiments using this model have suggested that osteocalcin might function as a matrix signal in the recruitment and differentiation of bone-resorbing cells (Glowacki et al. 1991). This model, however, might not be optimal, because bone particles implanted subcutaneously are degraded by a mixed population of multinucleated cells containing more macrophages than osteoclasts (Marks and Chambers 1991).

3. Circulating Osteocalcin

The noninvasive assessment of bone formation and resorption can be achieved by measuring enzymatic activity predominantly associated with the bone-forming or -resorbing cells (such as serum alkaline phosphatase, reflecting bone formation) or by measuring bone matrix components released into the circulation during formation or resorption (such as urinary hydroxyproline, reflecting resorption). Conventional markers of bone turnover lack sensitivity and specificity in diseases characterized by subtle alterations of bone remodeling, such as osteoporosis. This has led to the search for more specific markers, especially among specific components of bone matrix.

Osteocalcin circulates in the blood, where it can be measured by radioimmunoassay (Price et al. 1980b), is cleared by kidney filtration, and has a short half-life in plasma (Price et al. 1981b; Delmas et al. 1983). Using the warfarin model in the rat, Price et al. (1981b) have clearly shown that circulating osteocalcin originates from new cellular synthesis and not from the release of extracellular matrix osteocalcin during resorption, a pattern subsequently confirmed by clinical investigation. Thus, a fraction of newly synthesized osteocalcin is not incorporated into extracellular matrix but leaks into the circulation, where it can be used as a marker of osteoblastic activity. Because antibodies directed against bovine osteocalcin cross-react with human osteocalcin, most systems have been developed with bovine osteocalcin as a tracer, standard, and immunogen. These assays recognize almost exclusively intact circulating osteocalcin in most metabolic bone diseases, with the exception of chronic renal failure, a condition in which significant amounts of osteocalcin fragments can be detected (Gundberg and Weinstein 1986). Several studies have shown that serum osteocalcin is significantly correlated with bone turnover, especially with the bone formation rate, assessed by bone histomorphometry and by calcium kinetics in a variety of metabolic bone diseases. Serum osteocalcin measurement is a sensitive marker of bone turnover when resorption and formation are coupled, and it is a specific marker of formation whenever both activities are uncoupled, such as in multiple myeloma, corticosteroid induced bone disease, and in some patients with vertebral osteoporosis (reviewed in Delmas 1990).

III. Matrix GLA-Protein

As previously mentioned, osteocalcin does not account for all the GLA content of bone. Another GLA-containing protein has been isolated from bone matrix, called matrix GLA-protein (MGP) (Price et al. 1983). MGP is a highly hydrophobic 79-residue protein (M_r — 15000) containing five residues of GLA and one disulfide bridge (Price and Williamson 1985). Although there is no immunological cross-reactivity between MGP and osteocalcin, osteocalcin and the carboxy-terminal end of MGP share sufficient homology to conclude that they result from gene duplication. The human gene of MGP has been identified. It contains four exons and three introns. Exon 1 codes for the signal peptide, exon 2 for an a-helical region of the molecule, exon 3 for the carboxylase recognition sequence, and exon 4 for the region which is carboxylated (Cancela and Price 1989). MGP appears much earlier than osteocalcin in developing bone (Otawara and Price 1986), suggesting that both proteins may be under different developmental regulation. The expression and secretion of osteocalcin and MGP by clonal rat osteosarcoma cell lines are mutually exclusive, suggesting that these proteins are markers for different osteoblastic phenotypes, although prolonged $1,25(OH)_2D_3$ treatment of the osteocalcin-secreting osteosarcoma cell line ROS 17/2 can induce MGP synthesis (Fraser et al. 1988; Fraser and Price 1990). MGP is not unique to bone: large amounts of mRNA, determined by Northern blot analysis, are found in cartilage, lung, heart, and kidney, although bone contains 40–50 times more protein than these other tissues (Fraser and Price, 1988). The precise physiological function of MGP is unknown. MGP can anchor in bone by association with the organic matrix as well as with hydroxyapatite. Because of its abundance in cartilage, MGP is thought to be responsible for the closure of the growth plate previously described in warfarin-treated rats, suggesting that MGP could prevent its mineralization under normal circumstances.

D. Proteoglycans

Proteoglycans (PGs, reviews in Ruoslahti 1988, 1989) are glycoproteins to which one or several glycosaminoglycans are attached. Glycosaminoglycans (GAGs) are polymers of disaccharide units, which exist in four main forms: hyaluronic acid, heparan sulfate and heparin, chondroitin sulfate/dermatan sulfate, and keratan sulfate. Hyaluronic acid is an unsulfated protein-free GAG, synthesized on the cell surface and present in all extracellular matrices. All other GAGs are sulfated and linked to protein cores; the GAG type carried by the same protein core may vary according to the cell type studied and/or the environmental conditions for a given cell type (see below). Several PGs of varying sizes have been described in bone (Fisher et al. 1983; Hunter et al. 1984; Franzen and Heinegard 1984a,b; Goldberg et al. 1988b). A large (M_r ~1 000 000) chondroitin sulfate PG called versican (Zimmermann and Ruoslahti 1989) is present in the mesenchyme surrounding calcified bone (Fisher et al. 1983), and in the supernatant of osteoblastic cells in culture (Beresford et al. 1987; Hunter et al. 1983). It is not, however, integrated in the mineralized compartment, and is thus not a component of bone matrix stricto sensu. Three small PGs have been described to date in the mineralized matrix of bone, of which the best known so far are biglycan and decorin.

I. Biglycan and Decorin

Biglycan (BGN) and decorin (DCN) are not unique to bone, but are also present in cartilage (Rosenberg et al. 1985), tendon (Vogel and Fisher 1986), skin (Choi et al. 1989), sclera (Cöster et al. 1981), and other tissues (Heinegard et al. 1985; Bianco et al. 1990). In bone, however, there two PGs have chondroitin-4-sulfate side chains, while in all other tissues and in bone cell cultures (Beresford et al. 1987; Fedarko et al. 1990) they carry dermatan sulfate side chains.

1. Structure

In SDS-PAGE, BGN and DCN present an M_r of 270 000 and 135 000, respectively, with protein cores of M_r ~38 000 and GAG chains of M_r ~40 000. BGN carries two GAG chains and DCN only one, which explains the different M_rs of the intact molecules (Fisher et al. 1983). Although the different immunoreactivities (Vogel and Fisher 1986; Fisher et al. 1987c) and N-terminal sequences (Fisher et al. 1989) of the protein cores showed that they were distinct proteins, cDNA cloning of BGN (Fisher et al. 1989; Neame et al. 1989) and DCN (Krusius and Ruoslahti 1986; Day et al.

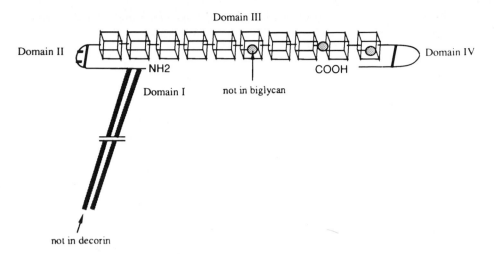

Fig. 4. Structure of biglycan and decorin (inspired by NEAME et al. 1989). The molecule drawn is a composite: differences between the two PGs are indicated. No attempt has been made to devise a three-dimensional structure. The position of the disulfide bonds is proposed. (▮), GAG chains; (—), cysteine residues and disulfide bridges; *boxes*, leucine-rich sequences; (●), glycosylation sites

1987) revealed strong structural homologies (Fig. 4). Fifty-five percent of the sequences are identical, and replacement by equivalent amino acids accounts for most of the differences. This strongly suggests that these two PGs evolved by duplication of the same gene. In human, the genes of BGN and DCN are located on chromosomes X and 12, respectively (YOUNG et al. 1989). BGN and DCN molecules are synthesized in a pro-form. The secreted proteins (332 amino acids for BGN, 331 for DCN) can be divided into four domains. Domain I, N-terminal (~23 amino acids), carries the GAG chains, bound to serine residues in Ser-Gly sequences (one chain in position 4 of DCN, two chains in positions 5 and 11 in BGN). As already mentioned, and apart from the GAG-binding sites, domain I presents the highest sequence differences between the two proteins. Domain II (~28 amino acids) contains four cysteines, and at least one, perhaps two, disulfide bonds (NEAME et al. 1989). Domain III spans most of the length of the proteins (~232 amino acids). This most remarkable section consists of 10 repeats of very similar leucine-rich motifs of 14 amino acids, separated by less-conserved sequences (~10 amino acids each). This domain also contains binding sites for N-linked oligosaccharides (two for BGN and three for DCN). Domain III and part of domain II (including two or four cysteines) present structural similarities with a serum protein ("leucine-rich a_2-glycoprotein"), two platelet membrane glycoproteins (Gp Iba and b) and chaoptin, a protein from Drosophila involved in morphogenesis regulation. Similarities restricted to the leucine-rich domain III can be observed with another Drosophila protein, produced by a homeodomain gene (*Toll*) and with two cytoplasmic proteins, liver RNAse, and yeast adenylate cyclase. In all cases, the "leucine-rich repeat" domain seems to be involved in binding to other proteins. Domain IV of BGN and DCN (~49 amino acids) is another region of the sequence in which BGN and DCN present an important sequence divergence. This domain also includes two cysteines, probably forming a disulfide bond (Neame et al. 1989). On the whole, the amino acid sequence differences between DCN and BGN result in a higher percentage of hydrophobic amino acids in the latter (Neame et al. 1989).

2. Distribution

Immunocytochemistry and in situ hybridization for BGN and DCN in human fetal bone show a strong expression of both PGs in osteoblasts, and in bone matrix (Bianco et al. 1990). In bovine fetal bone, the PGs account for up to 10% of the noncollagenous proteins (Fisher et al. 1983). The amount decreases in aging bone, as for other proteins of the matrix. In vitro studies of matrix production by porcine calvariae suggest that DCN is associated with the collagenous matrix, before mineralization (Nagata et al. 1991b). Histochemical and immunocytochemical studies on bone (Scott 1988) and nonmineralized tissues (Scott et al. 1981; Pringle and Dodd 1990) have shown the association of DCN with type I collagen fibers. DCN was pre-ferentially localized in the "hole" zone of the fibers in nonmineralized tissues, but not in mineralized bone. A close association of DCN with fibrillar matrix is in accordance with the results of pulse-chase studies on human bone cells in culture (Beresford et al. 1987). Likewise, the expression of DCN outside bone in human fetus (Bianco et al. 1990) was shown to concern mainly the matrix of most collagen(type I and II)-rich connective tissues. The distribution of BGN is clearly different. In pulse-chase studies on in vitro bone cell cultures, BGN appears as a cell-associated component, with a high rate of turnover (Beresford et al. 1987). In fetal bone, BGN, and not DCN, is present in periosteocytic lacunae (Bianco et al. 1990). From a developmental point of view, BGN seems to be associated with osteoblast differentiation, whereas DCN is more uniformly expressed. In fetal nonmineralized tissues, BGN presents a different distribution than DCN, being more associated with several cell types: chondrocytes, myofibers, endothelial cells, renal epithelium, and keratinocytes (Bianco et al. 1990). Distribution is sometimes mutually exclusive, as in bone articular ends of human fetus, where BGN is present in the articular cartilage and DCN is expressed in the resting cartilage underneath (Bianco et al. 1990).

3. Properties and Potential Role

Decorin binds to collagen fibers (Scott 1988; Scott et al. 1981; Pringle and Dodd 1990) through its protein core (Vogel et al. 1984) and inhibits their formation in vitro (Vogel et al. 1984). These properties, in accordance with its distribution, suggest a role for this protein in fibril formation, stability, and/or growth. In bone tissue, the specific absence of DCN from the "hole" region of type I collagen fibers, where it is present in nonmineralized tissues (SCOTT 1988), is striking. Mineralization is thought to be initiated in the gap region (WEINER and TRAUB 1986). It has been suggested that DCN may act as an inhibitor of crystal seeding, which would have to be removed from the hole region before mineralization begins (NAGATA et al. 1991b).

The association of BGN with several specialized cell types, along with its kinetic of secretion and incorporation in pulse-chase studies (BERESFORD et al. 1987), hints at a role in pericellular environment, perhaps more specifically in differentiating events (BIANCO et al. 1990). For both PGs, interaction with other components of the matrix is likely (DCN binds to fibronectin, through its protein core; SCHMIDT et al. 1987). Another field of action for PGs in the intercellular matrix is the binding of growth factors and cytokines, an important aspect of the local regulation of these agonists (RUOSLAHTI and YAMAGUSHI 1991). The protein core of DCN binds TGFβ, and, in culture, DCN inhibits the effects of TGFβ on Chinese hamster ovary cells (YAMAGUSHI et al. 1990). As TGFβ, a key factor in bone turnover regulation, stimulates BGN and DCN synthesis (BASSOLS and MASSAGUE 1988), this effect may represent a negative feedback mechanism (RUOSLAHTI and YAMAGUSHI 1991).

II. CS-PGIII

A third small chondroitin sulfate PG, named CS-PGIII, has been described from porcine bone (GOLDBERG et al. 1988b). This component of M_r ~110 000 (protein core M_r ~38 000) may have been overlooked in previous studies since it does not stain with coomassie blue and does not bind to nitrocellulose blotting membranes. CS-PGIII is not recognized by antibodies directed to DCN (GOLDBERG et al. 1988b), but its protein core is not characterized. Kinetic studies of radiolabeled proteins in porcine calvariae indicated a binding to the mineral phase rather than the organic matrix (NAGATA et al. 1991b).

III. Other Proteoglycans

The plasticity of the correspondence between core protein and GAG chain is exemplified by bone sialoprotein, which is usually not a PG, but was found to carry a keratan sulfate chain in rabbit bone (KINNE and FISHER 1987). The opposite case could be represented by fibromodulin, a 59-kDa protein of cartilage and other connective tissues, which has been reported to be present in bone (HEINEGARD et al. 1986; HEINEGARD and OLDBERG 1989). Fibromodulin is not a proteoglycan, but its structure is highly homologous to BGN and DCN (OLDBERG et al. 1989). Like DCN, fibromodulin binds to collagen fibrils and inhibits their formation in vitro, as its name suggests (HEDBOM and HEINEGARD 1989). The presence of this protein in bone matrix has not been thoroughly documented (HEINEGARD and OLDBERG 1989), and the amounts are probably low (HEINEGARD et al. 1986).

Studies on osteoblastic cell culture suggest the presence of a cell-associated a heparan sulfate PG (BERESFORD et al. 1987; HUNTER et al. 1983; FEDARKO et al. 1990), which has not yet been characterized. Cell-bound heparan sulfate PGs such as syndecan (SAUNDERS et al. 1989), involved in cell/substrate interactions and growth factor binding (RUOSLAHTI and YAMAGUSHI 1991), are present in many cell types. One receptor for TGFβ, betaglycan, is also a heparan sulfate PG (ANDRES et al. 1989).

E. SPARC/Osteonectin

Osteonectin (review in TRACY et al. 1988) is a 29-kDa glyco- and phospho-protein, originally described from bovine fetal bone, where it constitutes 15%–20% of the noncollagenous proteins (TERMINE et al. 1981a). Although osteonectin was originally believed to be specific to bone tissue, immunocytochemical studies (TUNG et al. 1985) and northern blot (YOUNG et al. 1986), radioimmunoassay (MALAVAL et al. 1987), and in vitro synthesis (WASI et al. 1984) have shown its presence and synthesis in many non-mineralized tissues and in platelets (STENNER et al. 1986). Osteonectin was also found to be identical to an M_r 43000 "culture shock" protein secreted by bovine endothelial cells (SAGE et al. 1984), a protein isolated from a tumor-secreted murine basement membrane ("BM 40"; DZIADEK et al. 1986), and another murine protein originally described from mouse parietal endoderm (termed SPARC, secreted protein, acidic and rich in cysteine; MASON et al. 1986). Considering the wide distribution of this protein in cell and tissue types, the name osteonectin is somewhat misleading. The compound name "SPARC/osteonectin" is a compromise between history, biological data, and practical usage.

I. Structure

The cDNA and/or genes of murine (McVEY et al. 1988), bovine (FINDLAY et al. 1988), human (SWAROOP et al. 1988; VILLAREAL et al. 1989), and *Xenopus* (DAMJANOVSKI et al. 1992) SPARC/osteonectin have been cloned. In all species studied, the haploid genome contains a single copy of the gene; in humans it is localized on chromosome 5 (SWAROOP et al. 1988). SPARC/ osteonectin is a highly conserved protein, with more than 90% identity in the exon sequence within all the species studied so far (VILLAREAL et al. 1989). This protein is encoded by nine exons (McVEY et al. 1988), of similar sizes (~130 bp), coding for four distinct domains, as confirmed by physico-chemical studies (ENGEL et al. 1987) (Fig. 5). SPARC/osteonectin is synthesized as a pre-protein (KUWATA et al. 1985), including a leader sequence of 17 amino acids encoded in exon 2. The amino-terminal domain

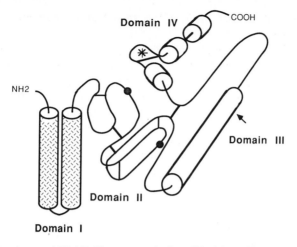

Fig. 5. Structure of SPARC/osteonectin (modified from ENGEL et al. 1987; BOLANDER et al. 1988). No attempt has been made to devise a three-dimensional structure. The position of disulfide bonds is proposed, by analogy with ovomucoid. *Cylinders*, α-helix regions; ( ), glutamic acid rich region; (—), disulfide bridges; (●), glycosylation site;( ), trypsin cleavage site;(✳), "E-F hand" calcium-binding site. Two glycosylation sites have been described in bovine and human, only one in mouse

of the secreted protein (domain I, ~50 amino acids) is encoded in exons 3 and 4. This glutamic acid rich segment binds calcium (>8 calcium ions; ENGEL et al. 1987) and undergoes a conformational transition to a helix upon calcium binding (ENGEL et al. 1987). Exon 3 is the more variable region of the SPARC/osteonectin gene, concentrating most interspecific differences (BOLANDER et al. 1988). Domain II (~100 amino acids), encoded by exons 5 and 6, contains 11 cysteines and is probably highly disulfide bonded. Part of the sequence of this domain presents homologies with ovomucoid, a serine-proteinase inhibitor (ENGEL et al. 1987; BOLANDER et al. 1988). Exons 7 and 8 code for domain III (~100 amino acids), an α-helix containing one site susceptible to cleavage by trypsin-like proteases (ENGEL et al. 1987), as confirmed by fragmentation studies (MANN et al. 1987; DOMENICUCCI et al. 1988). Studies on bovine and human cDNA and gene have identified in this domain a sequence homologous to an EF-hand type calcium-binding site (ENGEL et al. 1987; VILLAREAL et al. 1989). However, such homology has not been found in mouse (McVEY et al. 1988). Domain IV (~50 amino acids), encoded by exon 9, contains an EF-hand calcium-binding site, stabilized by a disulfide bond, and present in all species studied. High-affinity binding of calcium to this site has been confirmed by physico-chemical techniques ($K_d = 3 \times 10^{-7}M$; ENGEL et al. 1987; ROMBERG et al. 1985) and direct binding of ^{45}Ca on blotted fragments (SAGE et al. 1989a; DOMENICUCCI et al. 1988).

Although SPARC/osteonectin is the product of a single gene, several data suggest the existence of structural variants of the protein. Platelet SPARC/osteonectin is unique in presenting a slightly higher apparent molecular weight in SDS-PAGE (Kelm and Mann 1990; Malaval et al. 1991) and a different glycosylation (Kelm and Mann 1991) than SPARC/osteonectin from bone. Furthermore, a monoclonal antibody directed to bone SPARC/osteonectin presents 100-fold reduced affinity for platelet SPARC/osteonectin (Malaval et al. 1991). Treatment with N-glycosidases does not affect the binding of this antibody, suggesting that the epitope is not dependent on N-glycosylation (Maillard et al. 1992). Screening of nonmineralized tissues confirmed that these properties are specific to platelet SPARC/osteonectin (Maillard et al. 1992). Two types of SPARC/osteonectin, on the basis of antibody recognition, have also been identified in human bone cells after treatment with antisense mRNA (Gehron-Robey et al. 1989a). Phosphorylation was described as a conspicuous feature of SPARC/osteonectin purified from bovine bone, which contained about 0.5%–0.6% phosphorus (Romberg et al. 1985). This was also documented in endothelial mouse SPARC/osteonectin (Hughes et al. 1987). However, work on porcine (Domenicucci et al. 1988) and rat (Nagata et al. 1991a) calvariae cells, as well as bovine endothelial cells (Sage et al. 1984, 1989a), failed to detect phosphorylation of SPARC/osteonectin. A high homology (65%) has recently been shown between the sequence of domains III–IV of SPARC/osteonectin and the C-terminal part of SC-1, an extracellular protein of rat brain (Johnston et al. 1990), suggesting the existence of a family of "SPARC/osteonectin-like" proteins.

II. Binding to Hydroxyapatite and to Other Proteins

The affinity of SPARC/osteonectin for hydroxyapatite was an early discovery (Termine et al. 1981a). SPARC/osteonectin from bone binds to hydroxyapatite with a K_d of $8 \times 10^{-8}M$ (Romberg et al. 1985) and, among a wide spectrum of calcium-binding proteins tested (including osteocalcin), it appeared as the most potent inhibitor of hydroxyapatite crystal growth (Romberg et al. 1986). This property is attributed to the highly acidic domain I of the protein. Early reports also documented the binding of bone SPARC/osteonectin to gelatin and purified intact collagen (Termine et al. 1981a,b). Binding to both collagen and hydroxyapatite was combined in in vitro experiments showing that SPARC/osteonectin could promote the mineralization of collagen (Termine et al. 1981b). The calcium phosphate deposited was found to be a form of hydroxyapatite. However, the ability of SPARC/osteonectin to bind collagen was not confirmed with material purified from porcine bone (Domenicucci et al. 1988) or from endothelial cells (Sage et al. 1984), and the question is controversial. A report suggests that cleavage by a specific protease may enhance the binding of SPARC/osteonectin to type I collagen (Tyree1989). Calcium-dependent binding to collagens type

III, V, II, IV, and I – in decreasing order of affinity – was shown in solid phase assay, for SPARC/osteonectin purified from endothelial cells (SAGE et al. 1989a). A conspicuous feature reported for the "43 K protein" – the form of SPARC/osteonectin found in bovine endothelial cells – was a high-affinity binding to albumin (SAGE et al. 1984). This has been confirmed with SPARC/osteonectin isolated from porcine bone (DOMENICUCCI et al. 1988). The binding was calcium dependent. Preparations of SPARC/osteonectin from bovine bone and human platelets were shown to bind equally to thrombospondin, in both solid and liquid phase assay (CLEZARDIN et al. 1988). In contrast, platelet SPARC/osteonectin did not bind to type I, III, and V collagens in a solid phase assay, unlike bone SPARC/osteonectin (KELM and MANN 1991).

III. Tissular Distribution

Immunocytochemistry (TUNG et al. 1985; WASI et al. 1984; WEVER et al. 1988; SAGE et al. 1989), northern blot (YOUNG et al. 1986), radio-immunoassay (MALAVAL et al. 1987), and in situ hybridization (HOLLAND et al. 1987; NOMURA et al. 1988; METSARANTA et al. 1989) have established the expression of SPARC/osteonectin in both mineralized and nonmineralized tissues. In bovine fetus, the highest concentration is found in bone, where SPARC/osteonectin is roughly 100 times more abundant than in non-mineralized tissues ($\sim$150 μg/mg proteins; MALAVAL et al. 1987), the amount decreasing with age. However, rat bone contains much lower amounts (ZUNG et al. 1985), which could be due to sequence differences in domain I, resulting in a lower affinity of rat SPARC/osteonectin for hydroxyapatite (DOMENICUCCI et al. 1988). Electron microscopic studies have shown that SPARC/osteonectin is not integrate to the matrix prior to mineralization (ROMANOWSKI et al. 1990), suggesting that it is trapped by the mineral phase (hydroxyapatite) rather than by the organic phase (collagen and other matrix proteins). Another hypothesis is that the relatively high percentage of woven bone present throughout life in rats would store lower amounts of SPARC/osteonectin than lamellar bone (GEHRON-ROBEY 1989), as was observed in developing bovine fetal bone (CONN and TERMINE 1985). Immunocyto-chemical and in situ hybridization studies on human (METSARANTA et al. 1989; BIANCO et al. 1988) and murine (SAGE et al. 1989a; NOMURA et al. 1988) fetuses showed a high level of expression of SPARC/osteonectin in bone cells (osteoblasts, osteocytes, odontoblasts, cells of the periosteum), in bone matrix (osteoid, mineralizing parts of bone and dentin), and in hypertrophic chondrocytes. In addition, SPARC/osteonectin was highly expressed in areas of somatogenesis and in many nonmineralized tissues (SAGE et al. 1989a). In adult mouse, many nonmineralized tissues expressing significant SPARC/osteonectin (gut, skin, glands) presented a high rate of turnover (SAGE et al. 1989a). A pattern emerges, showing SPARC/osteonectin associated with actively remodeling tissues, or injured tissues undergoing repair (cf. its secretion by platelets, active in hemostasis; STENNER et al. 1986). This would fit with a constitutive expression in bone, a tissue undergoing a continuous remodeling.

IV. Biological Properties and Potential Role

Soon after its discovery, the "mineralizing properties" of SPARC/osteonectin in in vitro studies led to the suggestion that this protein would be the specific factor responsible for the mineralization of type I collagen in bone matrix (TERMINE et al. 1981b). A converse hypothesis was that SPARC/osteonectin would act as an inhibitor of mineralization (ENGEL et al. 1987). However, the discovery of very low levels of SPARC/osteonectin in rat bone (ZUNG et al. 1985) and the expression of this protein in nonmineralized tissues made any tissue-specific function unlikely. The possibility of serine protease inhibitor activity, suggested by sequence analogies (see Sect. I), has been ruled out by experiments (VILLAREAL et al. 1989; SAGE et al. 1989a).

The only positive biological effects of SPARC/osteonectin have been obtained in nonmineralized systems. SAGE et al. (1989b) have shown that SPARC/osteonectin induced a rounded morphology, without detachment, in endothelial cells, fibroblasts, and smooth muscle cells. In addition, cells newly plated in the presence of SPARC/osteonectin did not spread on the substrate. The effect seemed to be cell specific, as several cell lines tested were not affected. The same group has shown that the effect was mimicked by synthetic peptides corresponding to the N-terminal part (beginning or domain I) and the EF-hand calcium-binding segment (in domain IV) of SPARC/osteonectin (LANE and SAGE 1990); the latter domain also seemed to be involved in the interaction with collagens. In a recent paper (FUNK et al. 1991), these authors have shown an inhibition by SPARC/osteonectin of the progression from G1 to S phase of the cell cycle in bovine endothelial cells, which would be mediated by domain II. This effect, combined with detachment, would allow either migration or further differentiation of the cells. Considering these results, and the high expression of SPARC/ osteonectin in remodeling tissues, these authors suggest that SPARC/ osteonectin may facilitate cell movements, by interacting with macromolecules at the cell surface, in a calcium-dependent manner (SAGE et al. 1989; SAGE and BORNSTEIN 1992). Another set of data was obtained in studying the role of SPARC/osteonectin in platelets. SPARC/osteonectin is synthesized by megakaryocytes (TRACY et al. 1988). stored in platelets (CLEZARDIN et al. 1991), and secreted upon stimulation (STENNER et al. 1986). SPARC/ osteonectin binds to the surface of platelets (KELM and MANN 1990; CLEZARDIN et al. 1991), the number of binding sites being roughly 1500–2000/ platelet. Interestingly, the binding of thrombospondin to the platelet surface is specifically reduced by an anti-SPARC/osteonectin antiserum, suggesting a cooperation between these two proteins on this site (CLEZARDIN et al. 1991). An anti-SPARC/osteonectin antiserum also inhibits collagen-induced platelet aggregation, in a dose-dependent manner (CLEZARDIN et al. 1991). Data obtained on cell culture and on platelets hint at the involvement of SPARC/osteonectin in cell/substrate and cell/cell interactions, perhaps by cooperating with other macromolecules. A similar role could be played in bone, in which cell movements play an important part in the coupling between formation and resorption.

V. Circulating SPARC/Osteonectin

The levels of SPARC/osteonectin detected in serum range from 200 to 1.5 μg/ml, according to the authors (STENNER et al. 1986; MALAVAL et al. 1987, 1990). This is mainly platelet SPARC/osteonectin (STENNER et al. 1986). Work with thrombocytopenic patients, presenting a wide range of platelet counts, has shown a linear correlation of serum SPARC/osteonectin with the number of platelets in blood (MALAVAL et al. 1990). The zero intercept of the curve (giving the theoretical basal level of SPARC/osteonectin when no platelet is activated) was ~20 ng/ml, one-half of the values obtained in plasma. This suggests that even a careful preparation may not prevent all platelet activation in plasma. Assays were also made with a monoclonal antibody presenting 100 fold reduced affinity for platelet SPARC/osteonectin SPARC/osteonectin as compared to bone SPARC/osteonectin (MALAVAL et al. 1991). The results indicate that most of the basal circulating level of SPARC/osteonectin may still be of platelet origin, and that the actual contribution of other tissues (including bone) to the circulating pool may be very low (MALAVAL and DELMAS, unpublished results). Thus, despite the high level of constitutive expression of SPARC/osteonectin in bone, its use as a specific marker of bone metabolism in vivo seems to be ruled out.

F. Bone RGD-Containing Proteins

Cell-cell and cell-matrix recognition occurs by means of the expression of specific adhesion molecules. Many adhesive proteins present in the extra-cellular metrices and circulating in the blood contain and arginine-glycine-aspartic acid (RGD) sequence, a tripeptide which is essential for the cell-binding properties of these proteins. Cell surface receptors that recognize the RGD sequence have been isolated and characterized. They form a family of structurally related receptors, integrins, that are transmembrane heterodimeric proteins with two membrane-spanning subunits. some of these receptors bind to the RGD sequence of a single adhesion protein, whereas others recognize several of them. Over ten RGD-containing proteins, including fibronecting, vitronectin, collagen, fibrinogen, thrombospondin, and Von Willebrand factor, and at least as many integrin receptors binding these proteins have been identified. Adhesion proteins and their integrin receptors play an important role in many physiological processes such as

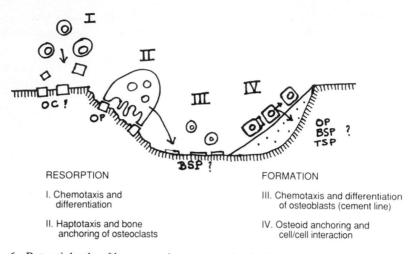

RESORPTION

I. Chemotaxis and
   differentiation

II. Haptotaxis and bone
    anchoring of osteoclasts

FORMATION

III. Chemotaxis and differentiation
     of osteoblasts (cement line)

IV. Osteoid anchoring and
    cell/cell interaction

Fig. 6. Potential role of bone attachment proteins in the process of bone remodeling. *OC*, osteocalcin; *OP*, osteopontin; *BSP*, bone sialoprotein; *TSP*, thrombospondin

embryological development, hemostasis, thrombosis, immune and non-immune defense mechanisms, and oncogene transformation (reviewed in RUOSLAHTI and PIERSCHBACHER 1987). The characterization of two RGD-containing proteins isolated from bone, osteopontin, and BSP (bone sialoprotein II), and the discovery that bone matrix contains thrombospondin and perhaps fibronectin, has shed new light on the potential role of nocollagenous proteins in the physiology of bone. By analogy with other organs, these RGD-containing proteins might be involved in cell precursor displacement in osteoblast and osteoclast anchorage onto bone matrix, and possibly in cell differentiation (Fig. 6).

I. Bone Sialoproteins

The presence of a high concentration of sialic acid in bone protein extract obtained after demineralization was reported many years ago. HERRING (1972) described a sialic acid rich protein of approximately 25 000 daltons from bovine bone, which was subsequently shown to be a proteolytic fragment of a larger bone sialoprotein (FISHER et al. 1983). During the last decade, two major noncollagenous proteins enriched in sialic acid have been isolated from bone, osteopontin (also called bone sialoprotein I or 44-kDa phosphoprotein) (FRANZEN and HEINEGARD 1985) and BSP (bone sialoprotein II). Both contain an RGD sequence that accounts for their cell attachment features. Recently, another sialic acid containing protein has been identified in rat bone, BAG-75 (bone acidic glycoprotein). Partial characterization of BAG-75 revealed an N-terminal sequence which is distinct from both osteopontin and BSP (GORSKI and SHIMIZU 1988). BAG-75 has been shown to be restricted in its synthesis and distribution to calcified tissues (GORSKI et al. 1990). Proteolytic cleavage of BAG-75 produces a fragment of 50 kDa which is present in extracts of calcific tissues and in serum (GORSKI et al. 1990). The function of BAG-75 is not known yet, but initial experiments indicate that BAG-75 exhibits osteosarcoma cell adhesive activity (GORSKI et al. 1989), although it has not been shown to have an RGD sequence.

1. Osteopontin

a) Structure and Distribution

Osteopontin, also called 44-kDa bone phosphoprotein, bone sialoprotein I, and 2 ar is an acidic phosphorylated glycoprotein with an isoelectric point of 5.0 described initially by FRANZEN and HEINEGARD (1985; reviewed by BUTLER 1988). The protein has a molecular weight of 41500, contains 301 amino acids, and is rich in aspartic acid, serine, and glutamic acid. In bone, it contains 12 phosphoserine and one phosphothreonine, 5–6 O-linked oligosaccharide, and one N-linked oligosaccharide. Several forms, differing in posttranslational modifications, have been described (KUBOTA et al. 1989). The amino acid sequence for osteopontin predicted from a cDNA sequence was determined in murine, rat, chicken, porcine, and human species (OLDBERG et al. 1986; CRAIG et al. 1989; MOORE et al. 1991; WRANA et al. 1989; KIEFER et al. 1989). In humans, the osteopontin gene is located on chromosome 4 (YOUNG et al. 1989).

Osteopontin has been detected immunohistochemically in new-born rats in the bone estracellular matrix, in osteoid tissue, and in bone forming cells: preosteoblasts, osteoblasts, and osteocytes (MARK et al. 1987b). The appearance of osteopontin in preosteoblasts several hours before the formation of osteoid and bone indicates that osteopontin is expressed early during osteogenesis (MARK et al. 1988) but probably later than alkaline phosphatase (WEINREB et al. 1990). Immunolocalization and in situ hybridization experiments as well as Northern blots have shown that the protein is also synthesized by several cell types other than bone cells such as odontoblasts, hypertrophic chondrocytes, some neural and neurosensory cells of the inner ear and brain as well as kidney, deciduum, and placental cells (NOMURA et al. 1988). Studies on in vitro models of osteogenesis (NAGATA et al. 1991b) and immunoelectron microscopy (MCKEE et al. 1990) indicate that OP is a component of the mineral phase of bone matrix, bound to interfiber mineral deposits. Immunolocalization in fetal porcine bone shows a preferential localization along the surface of the trabeculae (CHEN et al. 1991b).

b) Secretion and Properties

The regulation of the secretion of osteopontin has been studied using the rat osteosarcoma cell line ROS 17/2.8. The levels of osteopontin and osteopontin mRNA production are increased in response to $1,25(OH)_2$ D_3, whereas dexamethasone decreases the level of osteopontin mRNA in the same cells (PRINCE et al. 1987; YOON et al. 1987). NODA et al. (1988) reported that TGFβ1 and TGFβ2 stimulate the production of osteopontin in these cells by a mechanism which involves transcriptional control. Il-1 has been shown to increase the expression of osteopontin mRNA by osteoblasts (JIN et al. 1990). In contrast, human parathyroid hormone (1–34) suppresses the de novo secretion of osteopontin by osteoblasts, at least in part through a transcriptional control. Similar studies on rat calvaria cell cultures and on a clonal rat calvarial cell line showed a stimulation of osteopontin expression and secretion by growth factors (PDGF, EFG, TGFβ) and $1,25(OH)_2$ D_3, and inhibition by PTH (KASUGAI et al. 1991a).

OLDBERG et al. (1986) and SOMERMAN et al. (1988) have shown that osteopontin has the ability to promote attachement and spreading of human osteosarcoma cells ROS 17/2.8 and of human gingival fibroblasts to plastic in a dose-dependent manner. This attachment is inhibited by RGD-containing peptides, indicating that osteopontin binds to a cell surface integrin recognizing the Arg-Gly-Asp (RGD) sequence of the protein. The attachment properties of osteopontin are different from those of fibronectin, as osteopontin does not promote cell attachment onto type I collagen. In summary, osteopontin is an adhesion molecule that might play a role in the regulation of osteoblast attachment and spreading at the site of osteogenesis. The affinity of this protein for HAP – due to its high content in aspartic acid and its high level of phosphorylation – along with its binding to the mineral phase suggest a role in the mineralization of bone matrix, perhaps the regulation of crystal growth (NAGATA et al. 1991b).

2. Bone Sialoprotein II

a) Structure and Distribution

Bone sialoprotein has not been extensively studies. In calf cortical bone, BSP is more abundant than osteopontin and constitutes about 12% of the noncollagenous proteins extracted with guanidine HCl/EDTA. It has a molecular weight of 33 000 and undergoes extensive posttranslational modifications in the forms of glycosylation, sulfation, and phosphorylation (FISHER et al. 1983, 1990; OLDBERG et al. 1988; ECARROT-CHARRIER et al. 1989; ZHANG et al. 1990). The protein contains clusters of up to ten consecutive glutamic acid residues. These negatively charged domains, together with the sialic acid residues and phosphate groups, are likely to be responsible for the high affinity of BSP for hydroxyapatite. Human BSP differs from human osteopontin by its amino acid sequence and does not cross-react on western blot analysis with an anti-osteopontin antiserum (FISHER et al. 1987c) although a partial cross-reactivity has been reported (FRANZEN and HEINEGARD 1985). In rabbit, BSP is known to be a keratan sulfate proteoglycan, while, in human, bovine, and rat, BSP does not appear to contain keratan sulfate chains. The nucleotide sequence of the cDNA corresponding to rat BSP has been determined and predicts a 320-residue protein including a 16-residue propeptide and a mature protein with a molecular weight of 33 6000. As well as for osteopontin, the human gene is located on chromosome 4.

Contrasting with the wide distribution of osteopontin, BSP is almost bone specific. BSP is present in bone matrix and in dentin. BSP and its messenger RNA have been localized in fetal epiphyseal cartilage cells, particularly in hypertrophic chondrocytes of growth plates, in human decidua and trophoblasts but not in other connective and nonconnective tissues such as aorta, kidney, liver, muscle, skin, and tendon (OLDBERG et al. 1988; BIANCO et al. 1992). In bone, BSP is present in mature osteoblasts, in osteocytes, but not in immature osteoblasts, suggesting that it is expressed at late stages of differentiation. The expression of BSP in bone is essentially restricted to cells directly involved in the formation of mineralizing connective tissue matrices, indicating that BSP could have a specific role in mineralization (CHEN et al. 1991a). In situ hybridization and immunostaining have also revealed a high level of expression in osteoclast, suggesting a possible role of BSP as a mediator of osteoclast adhesion to bone (BIANCO et al. 1991). In addition, BSP has been recently found to be a constituent of cementum, which is responsible for the attachment of periodontal ligament fibers to the root surface (SOMERMAN et al. 1990). In vitro studies (NAGATA et al. 1991a) suggest that BSP would be mainly bound to HAP in bone matrix, but that a part of it would be present in the collagen matrix. Finally, BSP has been shown by Western blooting to be present in platelets, and released into the medium after thrombin stimulation of platelets (CHENU and DELMAS 1990). Study of platelets from a patient with a gray platelet syndrome suggests that BSP is not synthesized endogenously by megakaryocytes but rather originates from plasma by endocytosis (CHENU and DELMAS 1992).

b) Biosynthesis and Properties

Bone sialoprotein mRNA levels are increased after dexamethasone treatment of rat osteosarcoma cells ROS 17/2.8, through an increase in the transcription rate, and decreased by $1,25(OH)_2 D_3$ (OLDBERG et al. 1989b), while these two hormones have opposite effects on the regulation of osteopontin synthesis. In an in vitro model of osteogenesis from rat bone marrow cultures, BSP expression and secretion are induced by dexamethasone, in association with bone nodule formation (KASUGAI et al. 1991b).

Bone sialoprotein has cell attachment properties that differ from osteopontin. The cell attachment sequence is GRGDN, as compared to GRGDS for osteopontin. In fibroblastic cells, BSP is less effective and for a shorter period than osteopontin, but is equally active in bone cell attachment (Fig. 7). The membrane receptor of BSP has been identified in ROS 17/2.8 cells and is an RGD-directed receptor which appears to be identical to the

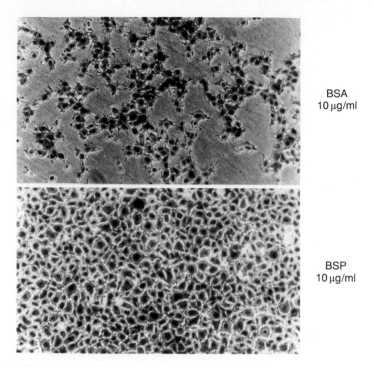

Fig. 7. Adhesion of MG-63 osteosarcoma cells to solid-phase absorbed bone sialoprotein (*BSP*) as compared to bovine serum albumin (*BSA*)

vitronectin receptor based on size, binding specificity, and immunological reactivity (Oldberg et al. 1988). Osteoclasts also express a vitronectin receptor which is responsible for their attachment to the RGD-containing proteins of bone matrix (Alvarez et al. 1990). Taken together, these data suggest that BSP is involved in the anchoring processes of bone cells (osteoblasts and osteoclasts), and might play a major role in the local mechanism of bone remodeling. As for OP, the acidic character of the molecule induces a high affinity for HAP. Based on the binding of BSP to collagen and HAP, it has been suggested (Nagata et al. 1991a) that it could act as a nucleator-inducing crystal formation at the surface of collagen fibers (Glimcher 1989). The restricted tissular distribution of BSP makes it a better candidate for such a role than SPARC/osteonectin.

II. Thrombospondin

Thrombospondin (TSP, review in Lawler 1986; Frazier 1987) is a 450-kDa glycoprotein, which is a major component of platelet α-granules, and is released by platelets upon thrombin stimulation. TSP is also synthesized by many other cell types, including fibroblasts, endothelial cells, smooth muscle cells, monocytes, macrophages, osteoblasts, and osteosarcoma cells (LAWLER 1986; FRAZIER 1987; GEHRON-ROBEY et al. 1989b; CLEZARDIN et al. 1989). TSP is present in mineralized bone matrix, and is incorporated into the extracellular matrix synthesized by human osteoblasts in culture in increasing amounts upon treatment with TGFβ (GEHRON-ROBEY et al. 1989b).

Thrombospondin is a trimer of identical chains (M_r ~150–160 kDa each). Each chain can be divided into three domains: an N-terminal globular part (~30 kDa), a thin connecting stalk (~85 kDa), and a second, C-terminal, globular domain (~70 kDa). Each domain binds specifically different components of the extracellular matrix. The N-terminal globular part binds to heparin and sulfated glycolipids. The stalk region contains, in its N-terminal side, a disulfide-rich segment, where the three chains are connected. This zone binds to collagen (mainly type V, less strongly types I and III; GALVIN et al. 1987). The following zone contains three incomplete repeats of a 57-amino acid sequence presenting homologies with two malarial proteins, the complement protein, properdin, and factors C6–C9 of the complement (LAWLER and HYNES 1986; KOBAYASHI et al. 1986). This properdin-like repeat contains a cell attachment site (PRATER et al. 1991). This zone is followed by three incomplete repeats of a 50–60 amino acid sequence homologous to the epidermal growth factor precursor (LAWLER and HYNES 1986). This region binds fibronectin, laminin, fibrinogen, plasminogen, plasminogen activator, and histidine-rich glycoprotein. A third type of repeat sequence – eightfold 38 residues – is present within the C-terminal globular domain. This sequence presents analogies with the EF-hand calcium-binding sites of parvalbumin and calmodulin. The Arg-Gly-Asp integrin-binding sequence is inserted within the last repeat. The conformation of this domain is calcium dependent, and it is possible that the Arg-Gly-Asp cell-binding sequence is accessible only in a low-calcium environment, when the C-terminal globular part is "unfolded." The last C-terminal segment contains a platelet-binding site. There is evidence of the existence of isoforms of TSP (CLEZARDIN et al. 1986), due to alternate splicing of the mRNA, in which exons may be included in or excluded from the expressed sequence (PAUL et al. 1992).

Thrombospondin is thought to be involved in platelet aggregation, through its N- and C-terminal sequences. Evidence is also increasing that it plays a part in cell adhesion processes, in a rather complex way. TSP would bind to the cell surface by at least three different mechanisms (ASCH et al. 1991): interaction with heparan sulfate PGs (inhibited by heparin), binding to integrin type receptors and/or binding to GPIV, a nonintegrin membrane protein. In vitro studies on endothelial cells document a reduction of the number of focal contacts (i.e., partial detachment) induced by TSP (MURPHY-ULRICH and HÖÖK 1989). Immunological study of developing mouse embryo has shown the association of TSP with basement membranes and cell surfaces, with a precise spatial and temporal pattern of distribution (O'SHEA and DIXIT 1988). TSP is also an autocrine growth factor: secreted

TSP binds to the cell surface and induces proliferation (MAJACK et al. 1988). This protein appears associated with cell proliferation and migration in morphogenetic processes. In bone tissue, TSP would thus be a potential modulator of cell adhesion and proliferation. Perhaps the most interesting aspect of the presence of TSP in bone is its binding to SPARC/osteonectin, which is also secreted by platelets (see Sect. D). The condistribution of these two proteins, which are both implicated in platelet and cell adhesion (SAGE et al. 1989b; CLEZARDIN et al. 1991), hints at a cooperative role, but further investigations are necessary to decide this point.

III. Fibronectin

Fibronectin (FN; review in HYNES 1985) is a ~500-kDa multidomain protein, present in many extracellular matrices, and active in cell/matrix interactions, cell proliferation, and cell displacements. This most studied of multidomain proteins is composed of two similar chains (~250 kDa each), which can be divided into several domains, made of three types of sequence repeats, in a manner similar to TSP. FN binds to fibrin (domains I and VIII), collagen and gelatin (domain II) and heparin (domains I and VII). A modification of a type 3 repeat in domain VI introduces an Arg-Gly-Asp sequence, which binds to cell receptors of the integrin type. Owing to its multiple binding properties, FN can behave as a bridge between cell surfaces and extracellular matrices of fibrin and collagen. Although FN is encoded by a single gene (in chromosome 7), alternate splicing of the mRNA allows the production of a family of proteins, differing in sequence and properties from one tissue to another and according to the development stage.

Fibronectin is produced by bone cells in culture, and its production is stimulated by TGFβ (WRANA et al. 1988). Its production has also been shown in fetal rat parietal bones, where it is downregulated by glucocorticoids, as is the case for collagen (GRONOWICZ et al. 1991). Studies with an in vitro model of osteogenesis have shown that FN secretion by osteoblasts decreases when the secretion of the more specialized proteins of bone tissue (such as osteopontin and alkaline phosphatase) increase (STEIN et al. 1990). Also, in ectopic osteogenesis studies, in which subcutaneous bone development is induced by the implantation of demineralized bone matrix, FN is present throughout the endochondral bone development, but not integrated to the bone matrix (WEISS and REDDI 1980). Likewise, immunofluorescence studies of FN distribution in bone and dentin (CONNOR et al. 1984) have shown the presence of FN in the vicinity of osteocytes and odontoblasts, and sometimes between the lamellae of bome, but not in the mineralized matrix. In bone, FN could be, along with type III collagen and the proteoglycan, versican, a component of the loose mesenchyme in contact with the mineralized tissue, or, alternatively, of the primary matrix deposited before the onset of bone development. Its association with the cell periphery in bone is logical in view of the cell-binding properties of this widespread protein.

G. Other Proteins in Bone

Bone matrix contains a large variety of growth factors that are synthesized by osteoblasts and/or trapped in bone from the circulation. These include insulin-like growth factors I and II, platelet-derived growth factor, fibroblast growth factors, $\beta 2$ microglobulin, and transforming growth factors (TGF)$\beta 1$ and 2. Bone is the largest reservoir of TGFβ in the body and TGFβ is likely to play a crucial role in the local control of both formation and resorption, acting either directly or through interaction with other components of the bone-marrow microenvironment (reviewed by MUNDY and CANALIS, this volume). Bone matrix also contains proteins that are able to induce mesenchymal cells to differentiate into bone and cartilage, including the bone morphogenetic protein family and osteoinductive factor, reviewed by WOZNEY and ROSEN in this volume. Among the other components of bone matrix, two groups of proteins deserve attention: proteases/protease inhibitors, which might play a role in the regulation of bone resorption, and the adsorbed plasma proteins, which represent a substantial fraction of the noncollagenous proteins present in bone (about 30%).

I. Proteases and Protease Inhibitors

An overview of the proteases produced by osteoblasts is not beyond the scope of this chapter, as they contribute to the turnover of all other components described previously, and at least one of them (procollagenase, MMP1) is integrated into the mineralized matrix. Osteoblasts have been shown to synthesize and secrete proteases belonging to two main groups: matrix metalloproteinases and plasmin-like serine proteases – and the corresponding inhibitors. None of these enzymes is specific to bone tissue, and they are produced in all connective matrices.

Matrix metalloproteinases (termed MMPs; review in EMONARD and GRIMAUD 1990; MATRISIAN 1990) are a family of Zn^{2+}-dependent enzymes, active at a neutral pH, which degrade proteins of the extracellular matrices. MMPs are secreted as proenzymes that can be activated by various agents, such as organomercuric compounds, or by proteolysis; active MMPs are inhibited by chelators. They present a highly homologous structure, including an N-terminal "pro" domain, which is cleaved when the enzyme is converted to an active form, and a catalytic Zn^{2+}-binding region. In vitro studies on rabbvit (SELLERS et al. 1978; MURPHY et al. 1981, 1985; GALLOWAY et al. 1983), mouse (VAES 1972; VAES et al. 1978), and rat (OTSUKA et al. 1984) bone cells have shown the synthesis of three MMPs: interstitial collagenase (MMP1), type IV collagenase (gelatinase, MMP2), and stromelysin (proteoglycanase, MMP3). MMP1 (52 kDa, review in HARRIS et al. 1984) cleaves intact fibrillar collagens between residues 775 and 776 (glycin and isoleucin) of α_1(I) chain (and at similar locations of α_1(II) and α_1(III) chains), i.e., at about one-fourth of the length of the molecule. This makes possible the unfolding of the triple helix (denaturation), which can then be cleaved by gelatinases, such as MMP2. As stated previously, MMP1 can be extracted from mineralized bone matrix (EECKHOUT et al. 1986). MMP2 (72 kDa in bone) degrades gelatins, and is not active on intact type I–III collagens, but displays significant activity on types IV, V, and VII, and on fibronectin. The MMP2 secreted by a rat osteoblastic cell line has been shown to degrade cross-linked collagen fragments (OVERALL and SODEK 1987). Stromelysin (MMP3, 53 kDa) has neither type I collagenase nor gelatinase activity. It cleaves the large aggregating proteoglycan of cartilage, laminin, fibronectin, and the extension peptides of procollagen (GALLOWAY et al. 1983), although it is different from the specific procollagen peptidases involved in procollagen maturation (see Sect. G.I.2.b). MMP3 also degrades type III and IV collagens (GALLOWAY et al. 1983). Bone cells also produce the tissue inhibitor of metalloproteinases (CAWSTON et al. 1981). This M_r 25 000–30 000 protein forms a stoichiometric (1:1) complex with the MMPs, which inactivates them irreversibly.

Rat (HAMILTON et al. 1985; PFEILSCHIFTER et al. 1990) and human (EVANS et al. 1990) bone cells have been shown to secrete a plasmin-like serine protease, named tissue type plasminogen activator (tPA). The serine proteases are so termed because of the presence of a serine residue within their active site. They are also synthesized in a proactive form, which has to be cleaved for activation. They are inactivated by lysine analogues such as ε-aminocaproic acid, or by paramethylsulfonyl fluoridate. The main target of tPA (M_r 68 000) is plasminogen, which it cleaves to form active plasmin. Plasmin is another serine protease which is mainly known for its ability to lyse fibrin clots, but also cleaves a wide spectrum of proteins (see below). The possible production of urokinase-type plasminogen activator (=uPA), along with tPA, by rat osteoblasts has recently been reported (LASCHINGER et al. 1991). Apart from their role in the blood clot, plasminogen activators bind to the cell surface, where they play an important part in cell/matrix interactions and cell movements. In contrast to uPA, no cell receptor for tPA has been characterized so far. Osteoblastic cells also produce an inhibitor of plasminogen activator, PAI-1 (OVERALL et al. 1989; PFEILSCHIFTER et al. 1990), which, like TIMP, inactivates its target enzyme by irreversible binding.

A functional connection can be made between these two groups of proteases, as the activation of procollagenase seems to be made in vivo by plasmin, generated by tPA from circulating plasminogen (HE et al. 1989). Secondarily, cleavage of preactivated plasmin by stromelysin would "superactivate" this enzyme (MATRISIAN 1990).

Studies on bone explants (EECKHOUT et al. 1986) and bone cells in culture (HAMILTON et al. 1985; OVERALL et al. 1989; PFEILSCHIFTER et al. 1990; PARTRIDGE et al. 1987) reveal a pattern of hormonal regulation in which resorbing hormones (1,25(OH)$_2$ D$_3$, parathyroid hormone, prostaglandin E2) stimulate procollagenase (PARTRIDGE et al. 1987) and tPA

(Cawtson 1981) secretion, while PAI secretion is inhibited and TIMP secretion presents a delayed stimulation (Partridge et al. 1987). In contrast, TGFβ, an anabolic factor, inhibits the secretion of procollagenase and tPA, while stimulating PAI, TIMP, and gelatinase synthesis (Overall et al. 1989; Pfeilschifter et al. 1990). This would fit with a role for proteases produced by osteoblasts in the preliminary steps to resorption (extensive discussion in Vaes 1988). In this model, withdrawing osteoblasts and/or lining cells would have to remove an osteoid layer covering uniformly mineralized bone before osteoclasts could begin resorption (Chambers et al. 1985; Chambers and Fuller 1985). This would explain the stimulation of proteases by resorbing agents; the delayed stimulation of TIMP could reflect a negative feedback regulation. The stimulation of formation induced by TGFβ would logically inhibit the secretion of proteases. The special case of gelatinase (stimulated by TGFβ) can be explained through another possible role for these protease, i.e., the "cleaning" of resorption lacunae, by removal of denatured collagen fragments, before a new deposition of osteoid (Overall et al. 1989). However, apart from primary bone and woven bone produced in fracture repair and some pathological conditions, the existence of an osteoid layer on mineralized matrix is discussed (Vaes 1988). Collagenase trapped in the matrix may also be activated by lysosomal enzymes secreted by osteoclasts, and play a direct part in the resorption process. It has also been recently proposed that plasmin would be an activator of latent TGFβ (Lyons et al. 1990). Specific proteases, targeted to precise components of bone matrix, have also been described, such as an MMP specifically cleaving SPARC/osteonectin (Tyree 1989) and an "osteopontinase" (Sato et al. 1989).

II. Plasma Proteins

Through its hydroxyapatite component, bone represents a major interface tissue for circulating molecules. By two-dimensional electrophoresis of a cortical bovine bone extract, we have identified 160 different spots representing at least 40 different protein families (Delmas et al. 1984b). Comparison with mapping of serum proteins indicated that only 14 of them were not serum proteins. These adsorbed serum proteins include albumin and α_2HS-glycoprotein, which are by far the two most abundant, IgG, transferrin, α_1-acid glycoprotein, α_1-antitrypsin, apo A-1 lipoprotein, and hemoglobin. It is not known if these proteins have a function in bone. α_2HS-glycoprotein is a disulfide-linked dimer with an M_r of 49 000. It is coded by a single gene located on chromosome 3. α_2HS-glycoprotein is synthesized in the liver, but it is accumulated in bone. Circulating levels in adults range from 400 to 800 μg/ml, suggesting a preferential accumulation of the protein in bone (Dickson et al. 1975; Ashton et al. 1976; Triffit et al. 1976). α_2HS-glycoprotein has a relatively high affinity for calcium, and is chemotactic for monocytes (Malone et al. 1982a). Because of its abundance, α_2HS-glycoprotein has been postulated to play a role in bone metabolism, but this needs to be documented.

H. Conclusion

In the past 15 years, the major constituents of bone matrix have been identified, cloned, and sequenced. With the exception of osteocalcin and to a lesser extent bone sialoprotein, noncollagenous proteins of bone are not unique to this tissue, but they are likely to interact specifically within each other and with type I collagen to form the scaffolding of bone matrix, a unique structure that promotes hydroxyapatite mineralization. The biosynthesis and secretion of bone proteins have been recently characterized, and are regulated by systemic hormones and growth factors. As discussed above, bone proteins are expressed at different stages of the multiple steps leading from the osteoblast precursor to the mature osteoblast, and perhaps the osteocyte. Studies on in vitro models of osteogenesis suggest a sequence in which early expression of type I collagen, secondarily downregulated, would be followed, during matrix maturation, by alkaline phosphatase and MGP; osteocalcin and osteopontin expression would parallel matrix mineralization (Stein et al. 1990). However, recent results indicate the existence of large differences in specific protein content (Nimomyia et al. 1990) and secretion (Heersche and Reimers 1991) between cortical and trabecular bone, suggesting differences related to the bone structure. The study of these patterns of secretion and incorporation, in addition to further characterization of the ability of bone proteins to influence cell-cell and cell-matrix interaction, is likely to provide crucial information for the understanding of their precise role in bone growth and remodeling.

Acknowledgements. We are grateful to Drs. Chantal Chenu, Philippe Clezardin, and Jaro Sodek for helpful discussions and comments on the manuscript, to Dr. Chantal Chenu for kindly providing Fig. 6, and to Véronique Fortaire for skillful secretarial assistance.

References

Alvarez JI, Teitelbaum SL, Chappel JC, Cheresh DA, Sander D, Farach Carson MC, Robey PG, Ross FP (1990) Osteoclast attachment to bone and its subsequent resorption depend upon the vitronectin receptor. J Bone Miner Res 5:S154

Andres JL, Stanley K, Cheifetz S, Massagué J (1989) Membrane-anchored and soluble forms of betaglycan, a polymorphic proteoglycan that binds transferring growth factor b. J Cell Biol 109:3137–3145

Asch AS, Tepler, Silbiger S, Nachman RL (1991) Cellular attachment of thrombospondin. Cooperative interactions between receptor system. J Biol Chem 266: 1740–1745

Ashton BA, Hohling HJ, Triffitt JT (1976) Plasma proteins present in cortical bone: enrichment of the α2HS glycoprotein. Calcif Tissue Res 22:27–33

Bassols A, Massagué J (1988) Transforming growth factor β regulates the expression and structure of extracellular matrix chondroitin/dermatan sulfate proteoglycans. J Biol Chem 263(6):3039–3045

Bellows CG, Aubin JE, Heersche JNM, Antosz ME (1986) Mineralized bone nodules formed in vitro from enzymatically released rat calvaria cell populations. Calcif Tissue Int 38:143–154

Beresford H, Fedarko NS, Fisher LW, Midura RJ, Yanaghishita M, Termine JD, Gehron-Robey P (1987) Analysis of the proteoglycans synthesized by human bone cells in vitro. J Biol Chem 262(35):17164–17172

Bianco P. Silvestrini G, Termine JD, Bonucci E (1988) Immunohistochemical localization of osteonectin in developing human bone using monoclonal antibodies. Calcif Tissue Int 43:155–161

Bianco P, Fisher LW, Young MF, Termine JD, Gehron-Robey P (1990) Expression and localization of the two small proteoglycans biglycan and decorin in developing human skeletal and non-skeletal tissues. J Histochem Cytochem 38(11):1549–1563

Bianco P, Fisher LW, Young MF, Termine JD, Gehron Robey P (1991) Expression of bone sialoprotein (BSP) in developing human tissues. Calcif Tissue Int 49:421–426

Black D, Duncan A, Robins SP (1988) Quantitative analysis of the pyridinium crosslinks of collagen in urine using ion-paired reversed-phase high-performance liquid chromatography. Anal Biochem 169:197–203

Bolander ME, Young MF, Fisher LW, Yamada Y, Termine JD (1988) Osteonectin cDNA sequence reveals potential binding regions for calcium and hydroxyapatite and shows homologies with both a basement membrane protein (SPARC) and a serine proteinase inhibitor (ovomucoid). Proc Natl Acad Sci USA 85:2919–2923

Bornstein P, Sage H (1980) Structurally distinct collagen types. Annu Rev Biochem 49:957–1003

Bronckers ALJJ, Gay S, Finkelman RD, Butler WT (1987) Developmental appearance of gla proteins (osteocalcin) and alkaline phosphatase in tooth germs and bones of the rat. Bone Miner 2:361–373

Brown J, Delmas PD, Malaval L, Edouard C, Meunier PJ (1984) Serum bone Glaprotein: a specific marker for bone formation in post-menopausal osteoporosis. Lancet 1:1091–1093

Butler WT, Prince CW, Mark MP, Somerman MJ (1988) Osteopontin: a bone derived cell attachment factor. In: Sikes CS, Wheeler AP (eds) Chemical aspects of regulation of mineralization. University of South Alabama Publication Services, Mobile, pp 29–31

Canalis E, Lian JB (1988) Effects of bone associated growth factors on DNA, collagen and osteocalcin synthesis in cultured fetal rat calvariae. Bone 9:243–246

Cancela L, Price PA (1989) Structural organization of the human matrix Gla protein gene. J Bone Miner Res 4 Suppl:S241

Cawston TE, Galloway WA, Mercer E, Murphy G, Reynolds JJ (1981) Purification of rabbit bone inhibitor of collagenase. Biochem J 195:159–165

Celeste AJ, Rosen V, Buecker JL, Kriz R, Wang EA, Wozney JM (1986) Isolation of the human gene for bone gla protein utilizing mouse and rat cDNA clones. EMBO J 5:1885–1890

Chambers TJ, Fuller K (1985) Bone cells predispose bone surfaces to resorption by exposure of mineral to osteoclastic contact. J Cell Sci 76:155–165

Chambers TJ, Darby JA, Fuller K (1985) Mammalian collagenase predisposes bone surfaces to osteoclastic resorption. Cell Tissue Res 241:671–675

Cheah KSE (1985) Collagen genes and inherited connective tissue disease. Biochem J 229:287–303

Chen J, Shapiro HS, Wrana JL, Reimers S, Heersche JNM, Sodek J (1991a) Localization of bone sialoprotein (BSP) expression to sites of mineralized tissue formation in fetal rat tissues by in situ hybridization. Matrix 11:133–143

Chen J, Zhang Q, McCullock CAG, Sodek J (1991b) Immunohistochemical localization of bone sialoprotein in foetal porcine bone tissues: comparisons with
secreted phosphoprotein 1 (SPP-1, osteopontin) and SPARC (osteonectin).
Histochem J 23:281–289
Chenu C, Delmas PD (1990) Radioimmunoassay for bone sialoprotein. II. Assessment of circulating levels. In: Cohn DV, Glorieux FH, Martin TJ (eds) Calcium
regulation and bone metabolism. Elsevier, Amsterdam, pp 247–253
Chenu C, Delmas PD (1992) Platelets contribute to circulating levels of bone
sialoprotein (BSP) in human. J Bone Miner Res 7:47–54
Chenu C, Valentin Opran A, Chavassieux P, Saez S, Meunier PJ, Delmas PD (1990)
Insulin like growth factor I hormonaly regulation by growth hormone and by
1,25(OH)$_2$ D$_3$ and activity in human osteoblast-like cells in short term cultures.
Bone 11:81–86
Choi HU, Johnson TL, Pal S, Tang LH, Rosenberg LC, Neame PJ (1989) Characterization of the dermatan sulfate proteoglycans, DS-PG I and DS-PG II from
bovine articular cartilage and skin isolated by octyl sepharose chromatography. J
Biol Chem 264:2876–2884
Clezardin P, Hunter N, Lawler J, Pratt D, McGregor JL, Pepper DS, Dawes J
(1986) Structural and immunological comparison of human thrombospondin
isolated from platelets and from culture supernatants of endothelial cells and
fibroblasts: evidence for a thrombospondin polymorphism. Eur J Biochem
159:569–579
Clezardin P, Malaval L, Ehrensperger AS, Delmas PD, Dechavanne M, McGregor
JL (1988) Complex formation of human thrombospondin with osteonectin. Eur
J Biochem 175:275–284
Clezardin P, Jouishomme H, Chavassieux P, Marie PJ (1989) Thrombospondin is
synthesized and secreted by human osteoblasts and osteosarcoma cells. A model
to study the different effects of thrombospondin in cell adhesion. Eur J Biochem
181:721–726
Clezardin P, Malaval L, Morel MC, Guichard J, Lecompte T, Trzeciak MC,
Dechavanne M, Breton-Gorjus J, Delmas PD, Kaplan C (1991) Osteonectin is
an α-granule component involved with thrombospondin in platelet aggregation.
J Bone Miner Res 6:1059–1070
Conn KM, Termine JD (1985) Matrix protein profiles in calf bone development.
Bone 6:33–36
Connor NS, Aubin JE, Melcher AH (1984) The distribution of fibronectin in rat
tooth and periodontal tissues: an immunofluorescence study using a monclonal
antibody. J Histochem Cytochem 32:565–572
Cöster L, Frannson LA, Shehan J, Nieduszynski IA, Phelps CF (1981) Self associa-
tion of dermatan sulfate proteoglycans from bovine sclera. Biochem J 197:
483–490
Craig AM, Smith JH, Denhardt DT (1989) Osteopontin, a transformation-associated
cell adhesion phosphoprotein, is induced by 12-O-Tetradecanoylphorbol
13-acetate in mouse epidermis. J Biol Chem 264:9682–9689
Cunningham LW, Ford JD, Segrest JP (1967) The isolation of identical hydroxylysyl
glucosides from hydrolysates of soluble collagen and from human urine. J Biol
Chem 242:2570–2571
Damjanovski S, Liu F, Ringuette M (1992) Molecular analysis of Xenopus laevis
SPARC (secreted protein, acidic, rich in cysteine) – a highly conserved acidic
calcium-binding extracellular-matrix protein. Biochem J 281:513–517
Davidson JM, McEneany LSG, Bornstein P (1977) Intermediates in the conversion
of procollagen to collagen – Evidence for limited proteolysis of the COOH-
terminal peptide extensions. Eur J Biochem 81:349–355
Day AA, McQuillan CI, Termine JD, Young MF (1987) Molecular cloning and
sequence analysis of the cDNA for small proteoglycan II of bovine bone.
Biochem J 248:801–805

Delmas PD (1988) Biochemical markers of bone turnover in osteoporosis. In: Riggs BL, Melton LJ (eds) Osteoporosis: etiology, diagnosis and management. Raven, New York, p 297

Delmas PD (1990) Biochemical markers of bone turnover for the clinical assessment of metabolic bone disease. Endocrinol Metab Clin North Am 19:1:1–18

Delmas PD, Wilson DM, Mann KG, Riggs BL (1983) Effect of renal function of plasma levels of bone GLA-protein. J Clin Endocrinol Metab 57:1028–1030

Delmas PD, Stenner D, Romberg R, Riggs B, Mann K (1984a) Immunochemical studies of conformational alterations in bone γ carboxyglutamic acid containing protein. Biochemistry 23:4720–4725

Delmas PD, Tracy R, Riggs B, Mann K (1984b) Identification of the non collagenous proteins of bovine bone by two-dimensional gel electrophoresis. Calcif Tissue Int 36:308–316

Delmas PD, Schlemmer A, Gineyts E, Riis B, Christiansen C (1991) Urinary excretion of pyridinoline crosslinks correlates with bone turnover measured on iliac crest biopsy in patients with vertebral therapy. J Bone Miner Res 6:639–644

Demiaux B, Arlot MA, Chapuy MC, Meunier PJ, Delmas PD (1992) Serum osteocalcin is increased in patients with osteomalacia. J Clin Endocrinol Metab 74(5):1146–1151

Dickson JR, Poole AR, Veis A (1975) Localization of plasma α2HS glycoprotein in mineralizing human bone. Nature 265:430–432

Domenicucci C, Goldberg H, Hofmann T, Isenman D, Wasi S, Sodek J (1988) Characterization of porcine osteonectin extracted from foetal calvariae. Biochem J 253:139–151

Dziadek M, Paulsson M, Aumailley M, Timpl R (1986) Purification and tissue distribution of a small protein (BM-40) extracted from a basement membrane tumor. Eur J Biochem 161:455–464

Ecarrot-Charrier B, Bouchard F, Delloyes C (1989) Bone sialoprotein II synthesized by cultured osteoblasts contains tyrosine sulfate. J Biol Chem 264:20049–20053

Eeckhout Y, Delaissé JM, Vaes G (1986) Direct extraction and assay of bone tissue collagenase and its relation to parathyroid-hormone-induced bone resorption. Biochem J 239:793–796

Emonard H, Grimaud JA (1990) Matrix metalloproteinases. A review. Cell Mol Biol 36:131–153

Engel J, Taylor W, Paulsson M, Sage H, Hogan B (1987) Calcium binding domains and calcium-induced conformational transition of SPARC/BM40/osteonectin, an extracellular glycoprotein expressed in mineralized and nonmineralized tissues. Biochemistry 26:6958–6965

Evans DB, Bunning RAD, Russel RGG (1990) The effects of recombinant human interleukin-1β on cellular proliferation and the production of prostaglandin E2, plasminogen activator, osteocalcin and alkaline phosphatase by osteoblast-like cells derived from human bone. Biochim Biophys Res Commun 166:208–216

Eyre D (1987) Collagen crosslinking amino-acids. Methods Enzymol 144:115–139

Fedarko NS, Termine JD, Young MF, Gehron-Robey P (1990) Temporal regulation of hyaluronan and proteoglycan metabolism by human bone cells in vitro. J Biol Chem 265:12200–12209

Findlay DM, Fisher LW, McQuillan CI, Termine JD, Young MF (1988) Isolation of the osteonectin gene: evidence that a variable region of the osteonectin molecule is encoded within one exon. Biochemistry 27:1483–1489

Fisher LW, Termine JD, Dejter S, Whitson W, Yanagishita M, Kimura JH, Hascall V, Kleinman HK, Hassel JR, Nilsson B (1983) Proteoglycans in developing bone. J Biol Chem 358:6588–6594

Fisher LW, Denholm LJ, Conn KM, Termine JD (1986) Mineralized tissue protein profiles in an Australian form of osteogenesis imperfecta. Calcif Tissue Int 38:16–20

Fisher LW, Gehron-Robey P, Tuross P, Otsuka AS, Tepen DA, Esch FS, Shimasaki S, Termine JD (1987a) The M_r 24 000 phosphoprotein from developing bone is the NH$_2$-terminal propeptide of the α1 chain of type I collagen. J Biol Chem 262:13457–13463

Fisher LW, Drum MA, Gehron-Robey R, Conn KM, Termine JD (1987b) Osteonectin content in human osteogenesis imperfecta bone shows a range similar to that of two bovine models of OI. Calcif Tissue Int 40:260–264

Fisher LW, Hawkins GR, Tuross N, Termine JD (1987c) Purification and partial characterization of small proteoglycans I and II, bone sialoproteins I and II, and osteonectin from the mineral compartment of developing human bone. J Biol Chem 262:9702–9708

Fisher LW, Termine JD, Young MF (1989) Deduced protein sequence of bone small proteoglycan I (biglycan) shows reduced homology with proteoglycan II (decorin) and several nonconnective tissue proteins in a variety of species. J Biol Chem 264(8):4571–4576

Fisher LW, McBride OW, Termine JD, Young MF (1990) Human bone sialoprotein: deduced protein sequence and chromosomal localization. J Biol Chem 265: 2347–2351

Fleischmajer R, Perlish JS, Olsen BR (1987) Amino and carboxy propetides in bone collagen fibrils during embryogenesis. Cell Tissue Res 247:105–109

Fleischmajer R, Olsen BR, Kuhn K (eds) (1989) Structure, molecular biology and pathology of collagen. New York Academy of Science, New York

Franzén A, Heinegård D (1984a) Characterization of proteoglycans from the calcified matrix of bovine bone. Biochem J 224:59–66

Franzén A, Heinegård D (1984b) Extraction and purification of proteoglycans from mature bovine bone. Biochem J 224:47–58

Franzén A, Heinegård D (1985) Isolation and characterization of two sialoproteins present only in bone calcified matrix. Biochem J 232:715–724

Fraser JD, Price PA (1988) Lung, heart and kidney express high levels of mRNA for the vitamin K-dependent matrix Gla protein: implications for the possible functions of matrix Gla protein and for the tissue distribution of the gamma carboxylase. J Biol Chem 263:11033

Fraser JD, Price PA (1990) Induction of matrix Gla protein synthesis during prolonged 1,25-dihydroxyvitamin D3 treatment of osteosarcoma cells. Calcif Tissue Int 46:270–279

Fraser JD, Otawara Y, Price PA (1988) 1,25-Dihydroxyvitamin D stimulates the synthesis of matrix gamma-carboxyglutamic acid protein by osteosarcoma cells: mutually exclusive expression of vitamin K dependent bone proteins by clonal osteoblastic cell lines. J Biol Chem 263:911

Frazier WA (1987) Thrombospondin: a modular adhesive glycoprotein of platelets and nucleated cells. J Cell Biochem 105:625–632

Funk SE, Sage EH (1991) The Ca^{2+}-binding glycoprotein SPARC modulates cell cycle progression in bovine aortic endothelial cells. Proc Natl Acad Sci USA 88:2648–2652

Gallop PM, Lian JB, Hauschka PV (1980) Carboxylated calcium binding proteins and vitamin K. N Engl J Med 302:1460–1466

Galloway WA, Murphy G, Sandy JD, Gavrilovic J, Cawtson TE, Reynolds JJ (1983) Purification and characterization of a rabbit bone metalloproteinase that degrades proteoglycan and other connective-tissue components. Biochem J 209: 741–752

Galvin NJ, Vance PM, Dixit VM, Fink B, Frazier A (1987) Interaction of human thrombospondin with types I–V collagen. Direct binding and electron microscopy. J Cell Biol 104:1413–1422

Gehron-Robey P (1989) The biochemistry of bone. Endocrinol Metab Clin North Am 18:859–902

Gehron-Robey P, Heferan TE, Zon G, Termine JD (1989a) Manipulations of protein synthesis with anti-sense DNA reveals two forms of osteonectin. J Bone Miner Res 4:S322

Gehron-Robey P, Young MF, Fisher LW, McClain TD (1989b) Thrombospondin is an osteoblast-derived component of mineralized extracellular matrix. J Cell Biol 108:719–727

Glimcher MJ (1989) Mechanisms of calcification in bone: role of collagen fibrils and collagen-phosphorprotein complexes in vitro and in vivo. Anat Rec 224:139–153

Glowacki J, Rey C, Glimcher MJ, Cox KA, Lian J (1991) A role for osteocalcin in osteoclast differentiation. J Cell Biochom 45:292–302

Goldberg HA, Maeno M, Domenicucci C, Zhang Q, Sodek J (1988a) Identification of small collagenous proteins with properties of procollagen α1pN-propeptide in fetal porcine calvaria bone. Coll Relat Res 8:187–197

Goldberg HA, Domenicucci C, Pringle G, Sodek J (1988b) Mineral-binding proteoglycans of fetal porcine calvarial bone. J Biol Chem 263:12092–1201

Gorski JP, Shimizu K (1988) Isolation of new phophorylated glycoprotein from mineralized phase of bone that exhibits limited homology to adhesive protein osteopontin. J Biol Chem 263:15938–15945

Gorski JP, Frost C, Griffin D, Dudley G (1989) J Cell Biol 109:16a

Gorski JP, Griffin D, Dudley G, Standford C, Thomas R, Huang C, Lai E, Karr B, Solursh M (1990) Bone acidic glycoprotein 75 is a major synthetic product of osteoblastic cells and localized as 75- and/or 50 kDa forms in mineralized phases of bone and growth plate in serum. J Biol Chem 265:14956–14963

Gorter de Vries I, Coomans D, Wisse E (1988) Ultrastructural localization of osteocalcin in rat tooth germs by immunogold staining. Histochemistry 89:509–514

Gronowicz GA, Derome ME, McCarthy MBV (1991) Glucocorticoids inhibit fibronectin synthesis and messenger ribonucleic acid levels in cultured fetal rat parietal bones. Endocrinology 185:1107–1114

Groot CG, Danes JK, Block J, Hoogendijk A, Hauschka PV (1986) Light and electron microscopic demonstration of osteocalcin antigenicity in embryonic and adult rat bone. Bone 7:379–385

Gundberg C, Weinstein RS (1986) Multiple immunoreactive forms in uremic serum. J Clin Invest 77:1762–1767

Hamilton JA, Lingelbach S, Partridge NC, Martin TJ (1985) Regulation of plasminogen activator production by bone-resorbing hormones in normal and malignant osteoblasts. Endocrinology 116:2186–2191

Harris ED, Welgus HG, Krane SM (1984) Regulation of mammalian collagenases. Coll Relat Res 4:493–512

Hauschka PV, Carr SA, Biemann K (1982) Primary structure of monkey osteocalcin. Biochemistry 21:638

Hauschka PV, Reddi AH (1980) Correlation of the appearance of γ-carboxyglutamic acid with the onset of mineralization in developing endochondral bone. Biochem Biophys Res Commun 92:1037

Hauschka PV, Lian JB, Gallop PM (1975) Direct indentification of the calcium binding amino acid γ-carboxyglutamate, in mineralized tissue. Proc Natl Acad Sci USA 72:3925–3929

Hauschka PV, Frenkel J, DeMuth R, Gundberg CM (1983) Presence of osteocalcin and related higher molecular weight γ-carboxyglutamic acid-containing proteins in developing bone. J Biol Chem 258:176–182

He C, Wilhelm SM, Pentland AP, Marmer BL, Grant GA, Eisen AZ, Goldberg GI (1989) Tissue cooperation in a proteolytic cascade activating human interstitial collagenase. Proc Natl Acad Sci USA 86:2632–2636

Hedbom E, Heinegård D (1989) Interaction of a 59-kDa connective tissue matrix protein with collagen I and II. J Biol Chem 264:6898–6905

Heersche JNM, Reimers S (1991) Osteoblasts are heterogeneous with regard to the expression of mRNA for several bone matrix proteins. J Bone Miner Res 6:485

Heinegård D, Oldberg Å (1989) Structure and biology of cartilage and bone matrix noncollagenous molecules. FASEB J 3:2042–2051

Heinegård D, Bjorne-Person A, Cöster L, Franzén A, Gardell S, Malmström A, Paulsson M, Sandfalk R, Vogel K (1985) The core proteins of the large and small interstitial proteoglycans from various connective tissues form distinct subgroups. Biochem J 230:181–194

Heinegård D, Larsson T, Franzén A, Paulsson M, Hedbom E (1986) Two novel matrix proteins isolated from articular cartilage show wide distributions among connective tissues. J Biol Chem 261:13866–13872

Herring GM (1972) In: Bourne GH (ed) The biochemistry and physiology of bone, vol 1. Academic New York, p 127

Holland PWH, Harper SJ, McVey JH, Hogan BLM (1987) In vivo expression of mRNA for the Ca^{2+}-binding protein SPARC (osteonectin) revealed by in situ hybridization. J Cell Biol 105:473–482

Hollister DW, Byers PH, Holbrook KA (1983) Genetic disorders of collagen metabolism. Adv Hum Genet 13:1–87

Hughes RC, Taylor A, Sage H, Hogan BLM (1987) Distinct patterns of glycosylation of colligin, a collagen binding glycoprotein, and SPARC (osteonectin), a secreted Ca^{2+}-binding glycoprotein. Eur J Biochem 163:57–65

Hunter GK, Heersche JNM, Aubin JE (1983) Isolation of three species of proteoglycans synthesized by cloned bone cells. Biochemistry 22:831–837

Hunter GK, Heersche JNM, Aubin JE (1984) Proteoglycan synthesis and depostition in fetal rat bone. Biochemistry 23:1572–1576

Hynes RO (1985) Molecular biology of fibronectin. Annu Rev Cell Biol 1:67–90

Jin CH, Miyaura C, Ishimi Y, Hua Hong M, Sato T, Abe E, Suda T (1990) Interleukin l regulates the expression of osteopontin mRNA by osteoblasts. Mol Cell Endocrinol 74:221–228

Johnston IG, Paladino T, Gurd JW, Brown IR (1990) Molecular cloning of SC1: a putative brain extracellular matrix glycoprotein showing partial similarity to osteonectin/BM40/SPARC. Neuron 2:165–176

Kasugai S, Zhang Q, Overall CM, Wrana JL, Butler WT, Sodek J (1991a) Differential regulation of the 55 and 44 kDa forms of secreted phosphoprotein 1 (SPP-1, osteopontin) in normal and transformed rat bone cells by osteotropic hormones, growth factors and a tumor promoter. Bone Miner 13:235–250

Kasugai S, Todescan R, Nagata T, Yao KL, Butler W, Sodek J (1991b) Expression of bone matrix proteins associated with mineralized tissue formation by adult rat bone marrow cells in vitro: inductive effects of dexamethasone on the osteobastic phenotype. J Cell Physiol 147:111–120

Kelm RJ, Mann KG (1990) Human platelet osteonectin: release, surface expression and partial characterization. Blood 75:1105–1113

Kelm RJ, Mann KG (1991) The collagen binding specificity of bone and platelet osteonectin is related to differences in glycosylation. J Biol Chem 266:9632–9639

Kiefer MC, Bauer DM, Barr PJ (1989) The cDNA and derived amino acid sequence for human osteopontin. Nucleic Acids Res 17(8):3306

Kinne RW, Fisher LW (1987) Keratan sulfate proteoglycan in rabbit compact bone is sialoprotein II. J Biol Chem 262:10206–10211

Kivirikko KI (1983) Excretion of urinary hydroxyproline peptide in the assessment of bone collagen deposition and resorption. In: Frame B, Potts JT Jr (eds) Clinical disorders of bone and mineral metabolism. Excerpta Medica, Amsterdam, pp 105–107

Kobayashi S, Eden-McCutchan F, Framson P, Bornstein P (1986) Partial amino acid sequence of human thrombospondin as determined by analysis of cDNA clones: homology with malarial sporozoite proteins. Biochemistry 25:8418–8425

Kraenzlin ME, Mohan S, Singer F, Baylink DJ (1989) Development of a radio-immunoassay for the N-terminal type I procollagen: potential use to assess bone formation. Eur J Clin Invest 19(2):A86

Krusius T, Ruoslahti E (1986) Primary structure of an extracellular matrix proteoglycan core protein deduced from cDNA. Proc Natl Acad Sci USA 83: 7683–7687

Kubota T, Zhang Q, Wrana JL, Ber R, Aubin JE, Butler WT, Sodek J (1989) Multiple forms of SppI (secreted phosphoprotein, osteopontin) synthesized by normal and transformed rat bone cell populations: regulation by TGF-β. Biochem Biophys Res Commun 162:1453–1459

Kühn K, Wiestner M, Krieg T, Müller PK (1982) Structure and function of the amino terminal propeptide of type I and III collagen. Connect Tissue Res 10:43–50

Kuwata F, Yao KL, Sodek J, Ives S, Pulleyback D (1985) Identification of pre-osteonectin produced by cell-free translation of fetal porcine calvarial mRNA. J Biol Chem 260:6993–6998

Kuwata F, Maeno M, Kam-Ling Y, Domenicucci C, Goldberg H, Wasi S, Aubin JE, Sodek J (1987) Characterization of a monoclonal antibody recognizing small collagenous proteins in fetal calf bone. Coll Relat Res 7:39–55

Lane TF, Sage H (1990) Functional mapping of SPARC: peptides from two distinct Ca^{2+}-binding sites modulate cell shape. J Cell Biol 111:3065–3076

Laschinger CA, Bellows C, Wasi S (1991) Modulation of plasminogen activators and plasminogen inhibitors by TGF-β, IL-1α and EGF in fetal rat calvaria cells at different times in culture. Bone Miner 13:23–34

Lawler J (1986) The structural and functional properties of thrombospondin. Blood 67:1197–1209

Lawler J, Hynes RO (1986) The structure of human thrombospondin, an adhesive glycoprotein with multiple calcium binding sites and homologies with several different proteins. J Cell Biol 103:1635–1648

Lee WSS, Haba T, Price PA (1983) Time course of growth plate mineralization in chronically warfarin treated rats. Calcif Tissue Int 35:658

Lian JB, Gundberg CM (1988) Osteocalcin. Biochemical considerations and clinical applications. Clin Orthop 226:267–291

Lian JB, Tassinari M, Glowacki J (1984) Resorption of implanted bone prepared from normal and warfarin treated rats. J Clin Invest 73:1223–1226

Lian JB, Coutts M, Canalis E (1988) Studies of hormonal regulation of osteocalcin synthesis in cultured fetal rat calvariae. J Biol Chem 260:8706–8710

Lian JB, Stein GS, Gerstenfeld L, Glowacki J (1989) Gene expression and functional studies of the vitamin K-dependent protein of bone, osteocalcin. In: Lindh E, Torell JJ (eds) Clinical impact of bone and connective tissue markers. Pharmacia Diagnostas Symposie, Academic Press, pp 121–132

Lowry M, Hall DE, Brosnan JJ (1985) Hydroxyproline metabolism by the rat kidney: distribution of renal enzymes of hydroxyproline catabolism and renal conversion of hydroxyproline to glycine and serine. Metabolism 34:955

Lyons RM, Gentry LE, Purchio AF, Moses HL (1990) Mechanism of activation of latent recombinant transforming growth factor β1 by plasmin. J Cell Biol 110: 1361–1367

Maillard C, Malaval L, Delmas PD (1992) Immunological screening of osteonectin in nonmineralized tissues. Bone 13:257–264

Majack RA, Goodman LV, Dixit VM (1988) Cell surface thrombospondin is functionally essential for vascular smooth muscle cell proliferation. J Cell Biol 106:415–422

Malaval L, Fournier B, Delmas PD (1987) Radioimmunoassay for osteonectin. Concentrations in bone, non mineralized tissues and blood. J Bone Miner Res 2:457–465

Malaval L, Ffrench M, Delmas PD (1990) Circulating levels of osteonectin in normal subjects and patients with thrombocytopenia. Bone Miner 9:129–135

Malaval L, Darbouret B, Preaudat C, Jolu JP, Delmas PD (1991) Intertissular variations in osteonectin: a monoclonal antibody directed to bone osteonectin shows reduced affinity for platelet osteonectin. J Bone Miner Res 6:315–323

Malone JD, Teitelbaum GL, Griffin GL, Senior RM, Kahn AJ (1982a) Recruitment of osteoclast precursors by purified bone matrix constituents. J Cell Biol 92: 227–238

Malone JD, Teitelbaum SL, Hauschka PV, Kahn AJ (1982b) Presumed osteoclast precursors (monocytes) recognize two or more regions of osteocalcin. Calcif Tissue Int 84:511

Mann K, Deutzmann R, Paulsson M, Timpl R (1987) Solubilization of protein BM40 from a basement membrane tumor with chelating agents and evidence for its identity with osteonectin and SPARC. FEBS Lett 218:167–172

Mark MP, Butler WT, Finkelman RD, Ruch JV (1987a) Bone gamma-carboxyglutamic acid-containing protein (osteocalcin) expression by osteoblasts during mandibular bone development in fetal rats: absence of correlation with the mineralization process. Med Sci Res 15:1299–1300

Mark MP, Prince CW, Oosawa T, Gay S, Bronckers ALJJ, Butler WT (1987b) Immunohistochemical demonstration of a 44-KD phosphoprotein in developing rat bones. 35:707–715

Mark MP, Butler WT, Prince CW, Finkelman RD, Ruch JV (1988) Developmental expression of 44-kDa bone phosphoprotein (osteopontin) and bone γ-carboxyglutamic acid (Gla)-containing protein (osteocalcin) in calcifying tissues of rat. Differentiation 37:123–136

Markose ER, Stein JL, Stein GS, Lian JB (1990) Vitamin D-mediated modifications in protein-DNA interactions at two promoter elements of the osteocalcin gene. Proc Natl Acad Sci USA 87:1701–1705

Marks SC, Chambers TJ (1991) The giant cells recruited by subcutaneous implants of mineralized bone particles and slices in rabbits are not osteoclasts. J Bone Miner Res 6(4):395–400

Mason IJ, Taylor A, Williams JG, Sage H, Hogan BLM (1986) Evidence from molecular cloning that SPARC, a major product of mouse embryo parietal endoderm, is related to a endothelial cell "culture shock" glycoprotein of M_r 43 000. EMBO J 5:1465–1472

Matrisian LM (1990) Metalloproteinases and their inhibitors in matrix remodelling. Trends Genet 6:121–125

McKee MD, Nanci A, Landis WJ, Gotoh Y, Gerstenfeld LC, Glimscher MJ (1990) Developmental appearance and ultrastructural immunolocalization of a major 66 kDa phosphoprotein in embryonic and post-natal chicken bone. Anat Rec 28:77–92

McVey JH, Nomura S, Kelly P, Mason IJ, Hogan BLM (1988) Characterization of the mouse SPARC/osteonectin gene. Intron/exon organization and an unusual promoter region. J Biol Chem 263(23):11111–11116

Metsarànta M, Young MF, Sandberg M, Termine JD, Vuorio E (1989) Localization of osteonectin expression in human fetal skeletal tissues by in situ hybridization. Calcif Tissue Int 45:146–152

Moore MA, Gotoh Y, Rafidi K, Gerstenfeld LC (1991) Characterization of a cDNA for chicken osteopontin: expression during bone development, osteoblast differentiation and tissue distribution. Biochemistry 30:2501–2508

Moro L, Mucelli RSP, Gazzarrini C et al. (1988) Urinary β-1-galactosyl-O-hydroxylysine (GH) as a marker of collagen turnover of bone. Calcif Tissue Int 42:87–90

Morris NP, Fessler LI, Weinstock A, Fessler JH (1975) Procollagen assembly and secretion in embryonic chick bone. J Biol Chem 250:5719–5726

Mundy GR, Poser JW (1983) Chemotactic activity of γ-carboxyglutamic and containing protein in bone. Calcif Tissue Int 35:164–168

Murphy G, Cawtson TE, Galloway WA, Barnes MJ, Bunning RAD, Mercer E, Reynolds JJ, Burgeson RE (1981) Metalloproteinases from rabbit bone culture medium degrade type IV and V collagens, laminin and fibronectin. Biochem J 199:807–811

Murphy G, McAlpine CG, Poll CT, Reynolds JJ (1985) Purification and characterization of a bone metalloproteinase that degrades gelatin and types IV and V collagen. Biochim Biophys Acta 831:49–58

Murphy-Ulrich JE, Höök M (1989) Thrombospondin modulates focal adhesions in endothelal cells. J Cell Biol 109:1309–1319

Nagata T, Bellows CG, Kasugai S, Butler WT, Sodek J (1991a) Biosynthesis of bone proteins [SPP-1 (secreted phosphoprotein-1, osteopontin), BSP (bone sialoprotein) and SPARC (osteonectin)] in association with mineralized-tissue formation by fetal-rat calvarial cell culture. Biochem J 274:513–520

Nagata T, Goldberg HA, Zhang Q, Domenicucci C, Sodek J (1991b) Biosynthesis of bone proteins by fetal porcine calvariae in vitro. Rapid association of sulfated sialoproteins (secreted phosphoprotein-1 and bone siaoprotein) and chondroitin sulfate proteoglycan (CS-PGIII) with bone mineral. Matrix 11:86–100

Neame PJ, Choi HU, Rosenberg LC (1989) The primary structure of the core protein of the small, leucin-rich proteoglycan (PG I) from bovine articular cartilage. J Biol Chem 264:8653–8661

Nimomiya JJ, Tracy RP, Calore JD, Gendreau MA, Kelm RJ, Mann KG (1990) Heterogeneity of human bone. J Bone Miner Res 5:933–939

Niyibizi C, Eyre DR (1989) Bone type V collagen: chain composition and location of a trypsin cleavage site. Connect Tissue Res 20:247–250

Noda M, Yoon K, Prince CW, Butler WT, Rodan GA (1988) Transcriptional regulation of osteopontin production in rat osteosarcoma cells by type B transforming growth factor. J Biol Chem 263(27):13916–13921

Nomura S, Wills A, Edwards DR, Heath JK, Hogan BLM (1988) Developmental expression of 2ar (osteopontin) and SPARC (osteonectin) RNA as revealed by in situ hybridization. J Cell Biol 106:441–450

Oldberg A, Franzén A, Heinegård D (1986) Cloning and sequence analysis of rat bone sialoprotein (osteopontin) cDNA reveals an ARG-GLY-ASP cell-binding sequence. Proc Natl Acad Sci USA 83.8819–8823

Oldberg A, Franzén A, Heinegård D (1988) The primary structure of a cell-binding bone sialoprotein. J Biol Chem 263(36):19430–19432

Oldberg A, Jirskog-Hed B, Axelsson S, Heinegard D (1989a) Regulation of bone sialoprotein mRNA by steroid hormones. J Cell Biol 109:3183–3186

Oldberg Å, Antonsson P, Lindblom K, Heinegård D (1989b) A collagen-binding 59kd protein (fibromodulin) is structurally related to the small interstitial proteoglycans PG-S1 and PG-S2 (decorin). EMBO J 8:2601–2604

O'Shea KS, Dixit VM (1988) Unique distribution of the extracellular matrix component thrombospondin in the developing mouse embryo. J Cell Biol 107:2737–2748

Otawara Y, Price PA (1986) Developmental appearance of matrix Gla protein during calcification in the rat. J Biol Chem 261:10828

Otsuka K, Sodek J, Limeback HF (1984) Collagenase synthesis by osteoblast-like cells. Calcif Tissue Int 36:722–724

Overall CM, Sodek J (1987) Initial characterization of a neutral metalloproteinase, active on native 3/4-collagen fragments, synthesized by ROS 17/2.8 osteoblastic cells, periodontal fibroblasts, and identified in gingival crevicular fluid. J Dent Res 66:1271–1282

Overall CM, Wrana JL, Sodek J (1989) Transforming growth factor-β regulation of collagenase, 72 kDa-progelatinase, TIMP and PAI-1 expression in rat bone cell populations and human fibroblasts. Connect Tissue Res 20:289–294

Owen TA, Bortell R, Yocum SA, Smock SL, Zhang M, Abate C, Shalhoub V, Aronin V, Wright KL, van Wijnen AJ, Stein JL, Curran T, Lian JB, Stein GS (1990) Coordinate occupancy of AP-1 sites in the vitamin D responsive and CCAAT box elements by Fos-Jun in the osteocalcin gene: a model for phenotype suppression of transcription. Proc Natl Acad Sci USA 87:9990–9994

Pan LC, Price PA (1985) The propeptide of rat bone gamma-carboxyglutamic acid protein shares homology with other vitamin K-dependent protein precursors. Proc Natl Acad Sci USA 82:6109

Parfitt AM, Simon LS, Villanueva AR, Krane SM (1987) Procollagen type I carboxyterminal extension peptide in serum as a marker of collagen biosynthesis in bone. Correlation with iliac bone formation rates and comparison with total alkaline phosphatase. J Bone Miner Res 2:427–435

Partridge NC, Jeffrey JJ, Ehlich LS, Teitelbaum SL, Fliszar C, Welgus HG, Kahn AJ (1987) Hormonal regulation of the production of collagenase and a collagenase inhibitor activity by rat osteogenic sarcoma. Endocrinology 120: 1956–1962

Pastoureau P, Arlot ME, Caulin F, Barlet JP, Meunier PJ, Delmas PD (1989) Effects of oophorectomy on biochemical and histological indices of bone turnover in ewes (Abstr). J Bone Miner Res 4 Suppl 1:164

Paul LL, Boeing JM, Finn MB, Frazier WA (1992) Identification of a human TSP isoform generated by alternative splicing. J Cell Biol (in press)

Pfeilschifter J, Erdmann J, Schmidt W, Naumann A, Minne HW, Ziegler R (1990) Differential regulation of plasminogen activator and plasminogen activator inhibitor by osteotropic factors in primary cultures of mature osteoblasts and osteoblast precursors. Endocrinology 126:703–711

Piez KA (1982) Structure and assembly of the native collagen fibril. Connect Tissue Res 10:25–36

Pope FM, Nicholls AC, Eggleton C, Narcissi P, Hey E, Parkin JM (1980) Osteogenesis imperfecta (lethal) bones contain types III and V collagens. J Clin Pathol 33:534–538

Poser JW, Sunberg RT, Francis SL, Benedict JJ (1982) The bone Gla protein as an inhibitor of seeded crystal growth. Calcif Tissue Int 34:S26

Prater CA, Plotkin J, Jaye D, Frazier WA (1991) The properdin-like type I repeats of human thrombospondin contain a cell attachment site. J Cell Biol 112: 1031–1040

Price PA (1985) Vitamin K-dependent formation of bone gla protein (osteocalcin) and its function. Vitam Horm 42:65–108

Price PA, Baukol SA (1980) 1,25-Dihydroxyvitamin D3 increases synthesis of the vitamin K-dependent bone protein by osteosarcoma cells. J Biol Chem 255: 11660–11663

Price PA, Baukol SA (1981) 1,25-Dihydroxyvitamin D3 increases serum levels of the vitamin K-dependent bone protein. Biochem Biophys Res Commun 99:928–935

Price PA, Williamson MK (1981) Effects of warfarin on bone. Studies on the vitamin K-dependent protein of rat bone. J Biol Chem 256:12760–12766

Price PA, Williamson MK (1985) Primary structure of bovine matrix Gla protein, a new vitamin K-dependent bone protein. J Biol Chem 260:14971

Price PA, Otsuka AS, Poser JW, Kristaponis J, Raman N (1976) Characterization of a γ-carboxyglutamic acid-containing protein from bone. Proc Natl Acad Sci USA 73:1447–1451

Price PA, Lothringer JW, Nishimoto SK (1980a) Absence of the vitamin K-dependent bone protein in fetal rat mineral. Evidence for another γ-carboxyglutamic acid-containing component in bone. J Biol Chem 255: 2938–2942

Price PA, Parthemore JG, Deftos LJ (1980b) New biochemical marker for bone metabolism. J Clin Invest 66:878–883

Price PA, Lothringer JW, Baukol SA, Reddi AH (1981a) Developmental appearance of the vitamin K-dependent protein of bone during calcification. J Biol Chem 256:3781–3784

Price PA, Williamson MK, Lothringer JW (1981b) Origin of vitamin K-dependent bone protein found in plasma and its clearance by kidney and bone. J Biol Chem 256:12760–12766

Price PA, Williamson MK, Haba T, Dell RB, Jee WSS (1982) Excessive mineralization with growth plate closure in rats on chronic warfarin treatment. Proc Natl Acad Sci USA 79:7734–7738

Price PA, Urist MR, Otawara Y (1983) Matrix Gla protein, a new gamma-carboxyglutamic acid-containing protein which is associated with the organic matrix of bone. Biochem Biophys Res Commun 117:765

Prince CW, Oosawa T, Butler WT, Tomana M, Bhown A, Bhown M, Schrohenloher RE (1987) Isolation, characterization and biosynthesis of a phosphorylated glycoprotein from rat bone. J Biol Chem 262(6):2900–2907

Pringle GA, Dodd CM (1990) Immunoelectron microscopic localization of the core protein of decorin near the d and e bands of tendon collagen fibrils by use of monoclonal antibodies. J Histochem Cytochem 38:1405–1411

Prockop DJ, Kivirikko KI (1984) Heritable diseases in collagen. N Engl J Med 311(6):376–386

Prockop DJ, Kivirikko KI, Tudermann L, Guzman NA (1979a) The biosynthesis of collagen and its disorders. N Engl J Med 301(1):13–23

Prockop DJ, Kivirikko KI, Tudermann L, Guzman NA (1979b) The biosynthesis of collagen and its disorders. N Engl J Med 301(2):77–85

Prockop OJ, Kivirikko KI (1968) Hydroxyproline and the metabolism of collagen. In: Gould BS (ed) Treatise on collagen, vol 2. Academic, New York, pp 215–246

Reddi H, Gay R, Gay S, Miller EJ (1977) Transitions in collagen types during matrix-induced cartilage, bone, and bone marrow formation. Proc Natl Acad Sci USA 74:5589–5592

Rohde H, Becker U, Nowack H, Timpl R (1976) Antigenic structure of the amino-terminal region in type I procollagen. Characterization of sequential and conformational determinants. Immunochemistry 13:967–974

Romanowski R, Jundt G, Termine JD, von der Mark K, Schultz A (1990) Immunoelectron microscopy of osteonectin and type I collagen in osteoblasts and bone matrix. Calcif Tissue Int 46:353–360

Romberg D, Werness PG, Lollar P, Riggs L, Mann KG (1985) Isolation and characterization of native adult osteonectin. J Biol Chem 260:2728–2736

Romberg RW, Werness PG, Riggs BL, Mann KG (1986) Inhibition of hydroxyapatite crystal growth by bone-specific and other calcium binding proteins. Biochemistry 25:1176–1180

Rosenberg LG, Choi HU, Tank LH, Johnson TL, Pal S, Webber C, Reiner A, Poole AR (1985) Isolation of dermatan sulfate proteoglycans from mature bovine articular cartilages. J Biol Chem 260:6304–6313

Ruoslahti E (1988) Structure and biology of proteoglycans. Annu Rev Cell Biol 4:229–255

Ruoslahti E (1989) Proteoglycans in cell regulation. J Cell Biol 264:13369–13372

Ruoslahti E, Pierschbacher MD (1987) New perspectives in cell adhesion: RGD and integrins. Science 238:491–497

Ruoslahti E, Yamagushi Y (1991) Proteoglycans as modulators of growth factor activites. Cell 84:867–869

Sage E, Bornstein P (1992) Extracellular proteins that modulate cell-matrix interactions: SPARC, tenascin and thrombospondin. J Biol Chem 266:14831–14834

Sage H, Johnson C, Bornstein P (1984) Characterization of a novel serum albumin-binding glycoprotein secreted by endothelial cells in culture. J Biol Chem 259:3993–4007

Sage H, Vernon RB, Decker J, Funk S, Iruela-Arispe ML (1989a) Distribution of the calcium binding protein SPARC in tissues of embryonic and adult mice. J Histochem Cytochem 37(6):819–829

Sage H, Vernon RB, Funk SE, Everitt EA, Angello J (1989b) SPARC, a secreted protein associated with cellular proliferation, inhibits cell spreading and exhibits Ca^{2+}-dependent binding to the extracellular matrix. J Cell Biol 109:341–356

Saksela O, Rifkin DB (1988) Cell-associated plasminogen activator: regulation and physiological functions. Annu Rev Cell Biol 4:93–126

Sato S, Kubota T, Sodek J (1989) Purification and properties of a phosphoprotein proteinase (osteopontinase) activity from bovine periodontal ligament and rat calvarial bone and its relationship to alkaline phosphatase. J Bone Miner Res 4:S247

Saunders S, Jalnaken M, O'Farrel S, Bernfield M (1989) Molecular cloning of syndecan, an integral membrane proteoglycan. J Cell Biol 108:1547–1556

Schmidt G, Robenek H, Harrach B, Glössl J, Nolte V, Hörmann H, Richter H, Kresse H (1987) Interaction of small dermatan sulfate proteoglycan from fibroblasts with fibronectin. J Cell Biol 104:1683–1691

Scott JE (1988) Proteoglycan-fibrillar collagen interactions. Biochem J 252:313–323

Scott JE, Orford CR, Hughes EW (1981) Proteoglycan-collagen arrangements in developing rat tail tendon. An electron microscopic and biochemical investigation. Biochem J 195:573–581

Sellers A, Reynolds JJ, Meikle MC (1978) Neutral metallo-proteinases of rabbit bone. Separation in latent forms of distinct enzymes that when activated degrade collagen, gelatin and proteoglycans. Biochem J 171:493–496

Shaw LM, Olsen BR (1991) FACIT collagens: diverse molecular bridges in extracellular matrices. Trends Biochem Sci 16:191–194

Sillence D (1981) Osteogenesis imperfecta: an expanding panorama of variants. Clin Orthop 159:11–25

Simon LS, Krane SM, Wortmann PD, Krane IM, Kovitz KL (1984) Serum levels of type I and III procollagen fragments in Paget's disease of bone. J Clin Endocrinol Metab 58(1):110–120

Simon LS, Slovik DM, Neer RM, Krane SM (1988) Changes in serum levels of type I and III procollagen extension peptides during infusion of human parathyroid hormone fragment (1–34). J Bone Miner Res 3:241–246

Sodek J, Mandell SM (1982) Collagen metabolism in rat incisor predentine in vivo: synthesis and maturation of type I, al(I) trimer, and type V collagens. Biochemistry 21:2011–2015

Sodek J, Goldberg H, Domenicucci C, Zhang Q, Kwon B, Maeno M, Kuwata F (1989) Characterization of multiple forms of small collagenous apatite-binding proteins in bone. Connect Tissue Res 20:233–240

Somerman MJ, Fisher LW, Foster RA, Sauk JJ (1988) Human bone sialoprotein I and II enhance fibroblast attachment in vitro. Calcif Tissue Int 43:50–53

Somerman MJ, Sauk JJ, Foster RA, Norris K, Dickerson K, Argraves WS (1991) Cell attachment activity of cementum: bone sialoprotein II identified in cementum. J Periodont Res 26:10–16

Stein GS, Lian JB, Owen TA (1990) Relationship of cell growth to the regulation of tissue-specific gene expression during osteoblast differentiation. FASEB J 4:3111–3123

Stenner DD, Tracy RP, Riggs BL, Mann KG (1986) Human platelets contain and secrete osteonectin, a major protein of mineralized bone. Proc Natl Acad Sci USA 83:6892–6896

Swaroop A, Hogan BLM, Francke U (1988) Molecular analysis if the cDNA for human SPARC/osteonectin/BM40: sequence, expression and localization of the gene to chromosome 5 q31–q33. Genomics 2:37–47

Taubmann MB, Kammerman S, Goldberg B (1976) Radioimmunoassay of procollagen in serum of patients with Paget's disease of bone. Proc Soc Exp Biol Med 152:284–287

Termine JD, Belcourt AB, Conn KM, Kleinman HK (1981a) Mineral and collagen-binding proteins of fetal calf bone. J Biol Chem 256:10403–10408

Termine JD, Kleinmann HK, Whitson SW, Conn KM, McGarvey ML, Martin GR (1981b) Osteonectin, a bone specific protein linking mineral to collagen. Cell 26:99–105

Termine JD, Gehron-Robey P, Shimokawa H, Drum MA, Conn KM, Hawkin GR, Cruz JB, Thompson KG (1984) Osteonectin, bone proteoglycan and phosphoryn defect in a form of bovine osteogenesis imperfecta. Proc Natl Acad Sci USA 81:2213–2217

Tracy R, Shull S, Riggs L, Mann KG (1988) The osteonectin family of proteins. Int J Biochem 20:653–660

Triffitt JT, Gebauer U, Ashton BA, Owen ME (1976) Origin of plasma α2HS glycoprotein and its accumulation in bone. Nature 262:226–227

Tung PS, Domenicucci C, Wasi S, Sodek J (1985) Specific immunohistochemical localization of osteonectin and collagen types I and III in fetal and adult porcine dental tissues. J Histochem Cytochem 33:531–540

Tyree B (1989) The partial degradation of osteonectin by a bone-derived metalloproteinase enhances binding to type I collagen. J Bone Miner Res 4:877–883

Uebelhart D, Gineyts E, Chapuy MC, Delmas PD (1990) Urinary excretion of pyridinium crosslinks: a new marker of bone resorption in metabolic bone disease. Bone Miner 8:87–96

Uebelhart D, Schlemmer A, Johansen JS, Gineyts E, Christiansen C, Delmas PD (1991) Effect of menopause and hormone replacement therapy on the urinary excretion of pyridinium cross-links. J Clin Endocrinol Metab 72:367–373

Vaes G (1972) The release of collagenase as an inactive proenzyme by bone explants in culture. Biochem J 126:275–289

Vaes G (1988) Cellular biology and biochemical mechanism of bone resorption. A review of recent developments on the formation, activation, and mode of action of osteoclasts. Clin Orthop 231:239–271

Vaes G, Eeckhout Y, Lenaers-Clayes C, Francois-Gillet C, Druetz JY (1978) The simultaneous release by bone explants in culture and the parallel activation of procollagenase and of a latent neutral proteinase that degrades cartilage proteoglycans and denatured collagen. Biochem J 172:261–274

Vetter U, Fisher LW, Mintz RP, Kopp JB, Turos N, Termine JD, Gehron Robey P (1991) Osteogenesis imperfecta: changes in noncollagenous proteins in bone. J Bone Miner Res 6:501–505

Villareal XC, Mann KG, Long GL (1989) Structure of human osteonectin based upon analysis of cDNA and genomic sequences. Biochemistry 28:6483–6491

Vogel KG, Fisher LW (1986) Comparisons of antibody reactivity and enzyme sensitivity between small proteoglycans from bovine tendon, bone, and cartilage. J Biol Chem 261:11334–11340

Vogel KG, Paulsson M, Heinegård D (1984) Specific inhibition of type I and type II collagen fibrillogenesis by the small proteoglycan of tendon. Biochem J 223: 587–597

Von der Mark K, Von der Mark H, Gay S (1976) Study of differential collagen synthesis during development of the chick embryo by immunofluorescence. II. Localization of type I and type II collagen during long bone development. Dev Biol 53:153–170

Wasi S, Otsuka K, Yao KL, Tung PS, Aubin JA, Sodek J, Termine JD (1984) An osteonectin like protein in porcine periodontal ligament and its synthesis by periodontal ligament fibroblasts. Can J Biochem Cell Biol 62:470–478

Weiner S, Traub W (1986) Organization of the hydroxyapatite crystals within collagen fibrils. FEBS Lett 206(2):262–266

Weinreb M, Shinar D, Rodan GA (1990) Different pattern of alkaline phosphatase, osteopontin, and osteocalcin expression in developing rat bone visualized by in situ hybridization. J Bone Miner Res 5:831–842

Weiss RE, Reddi AH (1980) Synthesis and localization of fibronectin during collagenous matrix-mesenchymal cell interaction and differentiation of the cartilage and bone in vivo. Proc Natl Acad Sci USA 77:2074–2078

Wiestner M, Fischer S, Dessau W, Müller PK (1981) Collagen tupes synthesized by isolated calvarium cells. Exp Cell Res 133:115–125

Wrana JL, Maeno M, Hawrylshyn B, Yao KL, Domenicucci C (1988) Differential effects of transforming growth factor-β on the synthesis of extracellular matrix proteins by normal fetal calvarial bone cell populations. J Cell Biol 106:915–924

Wrana JL, Zhang Q, Sodek J (1989) Full length cDNA sequence of porcine secreted phosphoprotein-I (SPP-I, osteopontin). Nucl Acids Res 17:10119

Wu CH, Donovan CB, Wu GY (1986) Evidence for pretranslational regulation of collagen synthesis by procollagen propeptides. J Biol Chem 261:10482–10484

Yamagushi Y, Mann DM, Ruoslahti E (1990) Negative regulation of transforming growth factor-β by the proteoglycan decorin. Nature 346:281–284

Yoon K, Buenaga R, Rodan GA (1987) Tissue specificity and developmental expression of rat osteopontin. Biochem Biophys Res Com 148;3:1129–1136

Young MF, Bolander ME, Day AA, Ramis CL, Gehron-Robey P, Yamada Y, Termine JD (1986) Osteonectin mRNA: distribution in normal and transformed cells. Nucl Acids Res 14:4483–4497

Young MF, Fisher LW, McBride OW, Termine JD (1989) Chromosomal localization of bone matrix PGI (biglycan), PGII (decorin), osteopontin and bone sialoprotein in the human genome. J Bone Miner Res 4:S380

Zhang Q, Domenicucci C, Goldberg HA, Wranas JL, Sodek J (1990) Characterization of fetal porcine bone sialoproteins, secreted phosphoprotein I (SPPI, osteopontin), bone sialoprotein, and a 23-kDa glycoprotein. J Biol Chem 265:7583–7589

Zimmermann DS, Ruoslahti E (1989) Multiple domains of the large fibroblast proteoglycan, versican. EMBO J 8:2975–2981

Zung P, Domenicucci C, Wasi S, Kuwata F, Sodek J (1985) Osteonectin is a minor component of mineralized connective tissues in rat. Biochem Cell Biol 64:356–362

CHAPTER 20

Bone Morphogenetic Proteins

J.M. Wozney and V. Rosen

A. Introduction

Production of new bone during embryogenesis occurs through a complex series of cellular interactions that integrate the information needed for correct pattern formation with the signals required for differentiation of cells into cartilage and bone. Most of the bones of the body are first laid down as cartilaginous models which are ultimately replaced by bone. This process, known as endochondral bone formation, begins when mesenchymal cells gather together at precise locations, condense into tightly packed groups, and begin to secrete an extracellular matrix rich in collagen type II and highly sulfated proteoglycans. The chondroblasts become surrounded by the extracellular matrix they produce, this matrix becomes calcified, and blood vessels invade the area and bring in cells capable of removing the cartilage matrix. At this time osteoprogenitor cells differentiate into active osteoblasts and bone formation begins. In contrast, bones of the craniofacial skeleton form directly by the conversion of mesenchymal progenitors into osteoblasts, foregoing the intermediate cartilage stage, in a process called intramembranous bone formation. The end result of either developmental path is a bone surrounded by a periosteal layer rich in progenitor cells and containing a mature marrow cavity and vascular supply.

In adults, remodeling of the existing skeleton is a continuous event that results in no net bone formation. This highly regulated process is sensitive to hormonal fluctuations and aging. Imbalances between bone resorption and bone formation can result in osteopenias and osteoscleroses that are the hallmark of many metabolic bone diseases. In addition, intense periods of new bone formation in adults occur during fracture healing when bone is made to replace that lost by injury. Interestingly, the repair process used in the adult has many similarities to bone formation during early development. Osteoprogenitor cells located in the periosteum actively undergo cell division, creating an expanded population of osteoblasts in the fracture area. These cells then differentiate into mature, secretory osteoblasts and produce large quantities of bone matrix, filling the gap in the periosteal surface created at the time of injury. A second component of the fracture-healing process is the differentiation of mesenchymal cells that migrate from the marrow stroma and surrounding connective tissues into chondroblasts that produce a cartilaginous extracellular matrix that fills the fracture gap. These two processes stabilize the area, and then the cartilage is subsequently replaced by bone in an endochondral bone formation cascade.

The act of fracture results in destruction of bone matrix and the liberation of many of the growth factors known to be stored in this matrix. An additional source of growth factors is the soft tissue repair that usually accompanies fracture healing. It is likely that some or all of the growth signals present in the fracture site are involved in wound repair. Recent studies have shown that TGFβ and FGF are increased in fracture callus and that injection of exogenous growth factors such as TGFβ into closed fractures results in increases in the cartilage and bone cell populations of the callus (Joyce et al. 1990; Jingushi and Bolander 1991; Jingushi et al. 1991). A unique, osteoinductive activity called bone morphogenetic protein (BMP) is also stored within bone; BMP-containing extracts from bone can initiate de novo bone formation in vivo. Since BMPs are known to be present in bone matrix, it is also possible that fracture results in the release of BMPs into the wound site, where they could provide the osteoinductive signals needed for new bone formation.

In addition to fracture healing, new bone formation in adults occurs at soft tissue injury sites (heterotopic ossification) such as those created during implantation of prostheses. In rodents, implantation of certain tumor cells, epithelial cells, or extracts of demineralized bone at subcutaneous or intra-muscular sites results in ectopic bone formation (Huggins 1931; Urist 1965; Wlodarski 1969; Wlodarski et al. 1971; Takaoka et al. 1981; Hall and van Exan 1982). The observed progression to bone in these instances follows the sequence described for endochondral bone formation during embryogenesis or fracture healing, suggesting that similar signals may be responsible for initiating these events. The focus of this chapter will be the identification of the inductive signals responsible for cartilage and bone formation in each of these instances.

B. Biochemistry and Molecular Biology of the BMPs

I. In Vivo Assay System

This osteoinductive activity present in bone could not be accounted for by any known single growth factor or combinations of growth factors, suggesting the existence of a novel bone-inductive protein. Because of the complexity of the activity of this protein, i.e., the formation of bone, the assay system of choice for use in the purification of BMP activity from bone has been the in vivo induction of ectopic bone. The use of in vitro assay systems has proven not to be predictive of bone formation in vivo, most probably because multiple growth factors such as FGF, TGF-β, the IGFs, and so on have effects on the proliferation and expression of markers of the differentiated state of bone cells in vitro (HAUSCHKA et al. 1988). In the in vivo assay systems, rodents have been typically used as the host animals due to the speed of response and ease of use. Rodent assays for BMP typically utilize either subcutaneous implantation (SAMPATH and REDDI 1981) or intramuscular injection of the material to be tested (URIST et al. 1979). Either method results in reproducible bone formation within 14 days of BMP delivery.

The complex cascade triggered by BMP in the rat ectopic assay consists of multiple cellular events (REDDI 1981) that are diagrammed in Fig. 1. By histological analysis, mesenchymal fibroblastic cells first infiltrate the area between days 1 and 3 following implantation. These cells begin to differentiate into chondroblasts and chondrocytes (cartilage-forming cells) between days 4 and 7. The cartilage formed gradually matures, with the chondrocytes becoming hypertrophic and calcified. Bone cells first appear within the implant site between days 10 and 12, and begin laying down bone matrix (osteoid). The bone mineralizes, and osteoclasts (bone-resorbing cells) appear in the implant along with hematopoietic marrow by day 12. Concurrent with the new bone formation, the cartilage template is gradually resorbed. The bone then remodels such that at late times only an ossicle of bone containing bone marrow remains. As in mature normal bone, the ectopically induced bone maintains the continuous remodeling sequence which includes both the formation and resorption of the bone tissue.

These events observed histologically have also been characterized biochemically (REDDI 1981; YU et al. 1991). The kinetics of the induction of cartilage have been quantified through measurement of the levels of the

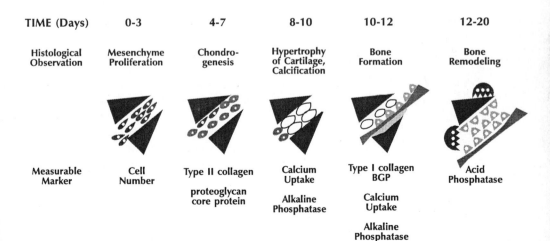

Fig. 1. Time course of events in the rat ectopic assay. Implantation of bone-derived extracts induce the formation of cartilage and bone in a time-dependent manner as shown pictorially. These histological observations can be confirmed by the examination of levels of various markers as detailed below

cartilage-specific markers type II collagen and the large aggregating cartilage proteoglycan. Bone formation has been assessed by measuring levels of the enzyme alkaline phosphatase and by direct measurement of calcium content. Iron incorporation into heme has also been used as a measure of the presence of hematopoietic marrow. Thus, bone-inductive extracts are able to initiate a series of events which are histologically and biochemically similar to those observed in both embryonic endochondral bone formation and adult fracture healing. While BMP can be implanted alone, the addition of a carrier matrix appears to enhance the bone-inductive response (Wang et al. 1988). In fact, because of the enhanced sensitivity and reproducibility, a reconstitution assay has been widely used to characterize the activities of BMP (Sampath and Reddi 1981; Sampath and Reddi 1984). This system utilizes rat bone matrix as a carrier. The matrix consists of demineralized rat bone particles of a defined size which have been extensively extracted with guanidine to remove all of the endogenous bone-inductive activity. BMPs absorbed to the matrix are implanted subcutaneously in a rat, where they are held for various times, up to 21 days or more. The samples are then removed and examined for the presence of newly formed bone. In this system, it is important to use allogeneic matrix carrier, most likely because immunogenic responses interfere with the bone-inductive activity (Sampath and Reddi 1983). Other investigators have used variations on the matrix carrier used in these implants. Collagen and proteoglycan have been added to the rat matrix carrier system (Muthukumaran et al. 1988) with some apparent enhancement of the bone-inductive activity. Others have used purified bovine dermal collagen combined with hydroxyapatite/tricalcium phosphate composite as a carrier system (Bentz et al. 1989), thereby eliminating the concern that the rat bone matrix may contain additional growth factors or other proteins that are required for the bone-inductive effect.

Quantitation with a complex assay system such as this is inherently difficult, especially since the amount of BMP implanted affects the kinetics of bone formation (Wang et al. 1988; Muthukumaran et al. 1988). Surrogate end points such as the amount of alkaline phosphatase activity or the calcium content of the implant have been used to signify bone induction. However, alkaline phosphatase can be synthesized by both chondrocytes and osteoblasts, as well as by a variety of other cell types. In addition, the calcium content of the implant increases during the calcification of the cartilage, continues to increase during the bone mineralization phase, but declines as the bone is remodeled and filled with bone marrow. Since the desired end point of the assay is the formation of new cartilage and bone, histological examination of sections from the implants has also been used in a semiquantitative manner for assessing bone-inductive activity. For example, scoring systems based on the percentage area of cartilage and bone observed in histological sections of the implant have been used as a measure of bone-inductive activity (Wang et al. 1990).

II. Discovery of Multiple Related Proteins

1. Purification from Bone

Within the last few years, there have been several reports of the purification of BMP activity from bovine bone using the in vivo assay system described above. Each of these purifications has begun with extracts of demineralized bone known to contain BMP activity (URIST et al. 1973). Many of these fractionations have employed heparin-affinity resins, as the bone-inductive activity binds to heparin in a manner analogous to other known growth factors such as acidic FGF, basic FGF, and PDGF (HAUSCHKA et al. 1986; KLAGSBRUN 1989). In addition, preparative SDS-PAGE has been used based on the finding that BMP activity electrophoreses with an approximate molecular weight of 30 000 (WANG et al. 1988). Purifications of greater than 300 000-fold with respect to the initial bone extract have been necessary to obtain protein of sufficient purity for protein sequence determination. In the most purified preparations, several related proteins have been identified, all of which are dimeric molecules with subunits of approximately 16 000–18 000 daltons. The quantity of these proteins present in bone is believed to be small; though yields have been difficult to calculate, there appears to be approximately $1 \mu g$ bone-inductive protein present in 1 kg bone (WANG et al. 1988; LUYTEN et al. 1989; SAMPATH et al. 1990). In comparison, TGFβ is present at approximately $460 \mu g/kg$, IGF-I at $85 \mu g/kg$, and IGF-II at $1260 \mu g/kg$ bone (FINKELMAN et al. 1990). We now know that multiple BMP proteins with similar molecular weights are present in even the most highly purified preparations and that these molecules are difficult to separate due to their biochemical similarities. Using fragmentary sequence information from these preparations, molecular clones for each of these proteins have been derived (see below). Synthesis of the corresponding recombinant proteins and examination of their in vivo activities have allowed the determination of their bone-inductive potential.

2. Bone Morphogenetic Protein Family

The first reported purification of bovine bone-derived bone-inductive protein (WANG et al. 1988) has led to the cloning of six related human proteins termed BMP-2 through BMP-7 (WOZNEY et al. 1988; WOZNEY 1989; CELESTE et al. 1990). Other investigations have subsequently identified bone-derived BMP activity as consisting of BMP-3, also known as osteogenin (LUYTEN et al. 1989), or as a combination of BMP-2 with BMP-7, also known as OP-1 (SAMPATH et al. 1990). BMP-7 and OP-1 are identical molecules identified in separate molecular cloning endeavors (CELESTE et al. 1990; ÖZKAYNAK et al. 1990). The molecule derived from bovine bone and identified by sequence analysis as osteogenin is the bovine homolog of human BMP-3. For the purposes of this review, the recombinant molecule will be termed BMP-3, while the bovine bone-derived entity will be referred to as osteogenin.

While these molecules should be comparable, it is possible that bone-derived materials may yet contain additional growth factors (e.g., other BMPs). The amino acid sequence of human BMP-6 indicates that it is the human homolog of the murine protein Vgr-1, isolated by cross-hybridization from an embryonic mouse cDNA library (Lyons et al. 1989a).

Analysis of the amino acid sequences derived from their respective cDNA clones indicates that BMP-2 through BMP-7 are all related molecules that share some common characteristics with the TGFβ superfamily (Fig. 2). Each BMP protein is synthesized in a precursor form, with a hydrophobic secretory leader sequence and a substantial propeptide region. Similar to the TGFβs, each mature protein is expected to consist of a dimer of the carboxy-terminal portion of the precursor molecules. The processing of these molecules to their mature forms probably involves cleavage at dibasic or other consensus basic residue sequences (see below) to create homodimeric BMP molecules. While it is possible that heterodimers of these proteins exist, as with other members of the TGFβ superfamily, it has been reported that the predominant forms of at least BMP-2 and BMP-7 (Sampath et al. 1990) as well as osteogenin (Luyten et al. 1989) found in bone are in fact homodimers. All of the mature regions of the molecules contain one or more N-linked glycosylation sites, at least one of which appears to be used, based on the sensitivity of bone-derived materials to deglycosylating enzymes. The primary sequence indicates that all of the BMPs contain seven cysteine residues conserved within all members of the superfamily; the TGFβs themselves contain nine cysteine residues within the mature region. TGFβ also contains three cysteine residues in the propeptide, which have been implicated in the formation of the latency-associated peptide or LAP (Brunner et al. 1989). The majority of TGFβ appears to be synthesized associated with LAP in a latent or inactive form (see Roberts and Sporn 1990). In contrast, three of the BMP proteins (BMP-2, BMP-4, BMP-7) do not contain cysteine residues within the propeptide regions. Since these BMP propeptides are unable to form dimers, these BMPs are unlikely to be secreted in latent forms.

Based on their primary amino acid sequences in the mature regions, the BMPs may be divided into subgroups (see Fig. 3). BMP-2 and BMP-4 are very closely related molecules, sharing 92% amino acid identity in their cysteine-rich carboxy-terminal regions. The 13- to 15-amino acid amino-terminal regions of mature BMP-2 and BMP-4 are more divergent, being less than 50% identical. One N-linked glycosylation site is present at corresponding positions in both molecules; BMP-4 contains an additional glycosylation site. BMP-5, BMP-6, and BMP-7 comprise another subgroup, sharing an average of 89% identity in the seven-cysteine region. The amino-terminal portions of these mature molecules are longer than those of BMP-2 and BMP-4 (36 or 37 amino acid residues), but again they still share less homology (59% identity or less) than in the seven cysteine region. BMP-5, BMP-6, and BMP-7 each contain three N-linked glycosylation sites present

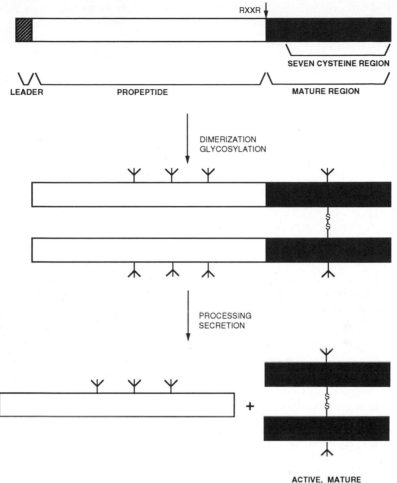

Fig. 2. Processing and secretion of BMP-2. The dimerization, glycosylation, and secretion of BMP-2 are presented as a model of the production of the BMP proteins. The leader sequence directs secretion of the protein from the cell. Cleavage at an arg-X-X-arg sequence results in removal of the propeptide sequence, leaving the mature dimeric BMP-2 protein. The mature molecule contains the seven-cysteine region, defined as the portion of the molecule from the first of seven cysteine residues conserved within the TGFβ family to the carboxy-terminus of the protein

at similar positions, two of which are in the amino-terminal domain. These two subgroups of the BMPs (BMP-2/4 and BMP-5/6/7) are related to each other by an average of 60% identity, and are therefore more closely related to each other than they are to BMP-3 (49% and 43%, respectively).

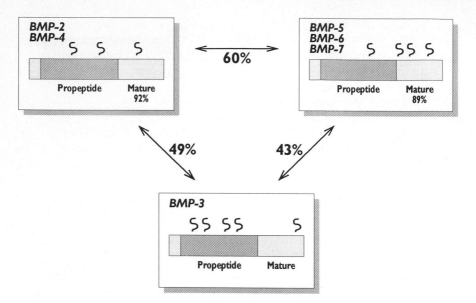

Fig. 3. The BMP family. The six BMPs of the TGFβ superfamily can be divided into subgroups based on their primary amino acid sequences. *Numbers given* are average percentages of amino acid identities in the seven-cysteine regions. Glycosylation sites conserved between all members of a subgroup are indicated

	TGF-β1,2,3	Vg1	dpp	BMP-5,6,7	BMP-3
BMP-2,4	35-39	56-58	74-76	58-61	48-49
BMP-3	34	49	43	42-44	
BMP-5,6,7	36-41	57-59	57-59		
dpp	37	48			
Vg1	36-39				

Fig. 4. Relationships of the BMPs to TGFβ family members. The primary sequences of the BMPs are compared to other TGFβ superfamily members. *Numbers* are the ranges of percentages of amino acid identities in the seven-cysteine region

A large number of proteins within the TGFβ superfamily have now been identified in a variety of species. Figure 4 displays the relationships of the BMPs to selected members of the superfamily. BMP-2 and BMP-4 display striking similarity to a protein identified in Drosophila, decapentaplegic or dpp (Padgett et al. 1987). In addition to the high amino acid similarity in the carboxy-terminal region (75%), similarities can be observed to extend through the propeptide region. In addition, the gene structures of BMP-2, BMP-4, and dpp are similar in that each contains a single intron within the coding region, placed at analogous positions in all three genes. Therefore, it is probable that these genes are derived from a common ancestral gene. From extensive genetic analysis, it is known that dpp is necessary for several events during Drosophila development, including at early times in dorsal-ventral specification and later in the development of the imaginal disks. Though these BMPs are known to induce bone formation in the adult, their relationship to dpp implicates them as potential regulatory molecules during embryogenesis (see also Sect. C.III). The BMPs are next most closely related to the Xenopus protein Vg1 (WEEKS and MELTON 1987). Though the function of this protein remains unknown, the presence of its mRNA specifically localized to the vegetal hemisphere of the Xenopus oocyte suggests a role in delivering positional information during development. It is perhaps interesting to note that the BMPs are only distantly related to the TGFβs themselves. In spite of the known abundance of TGFβ in bone and its multiple effects on bone cells in vitro and in vivo, it is clear that the BMPs have very distinct and sometimes opposite effects from those of TGFβ (see Sect. C.II).

There is considerable conservation of the amino acid sequences of at least some of the BMPs among different species. The amino acid sequence of the entire mature region of BMP-2 is identical in the mouse and human, while murine and human BMP-4 are identical in the seven-cysteine region (WOZNEY et al. 1988; DICKINSON et al. 1990). Two homologs of BMP-4 have been isolated from Xenopus (KÖSTER et al. 1991). One of these is identical to human BMP-4 in the seven-cysteine region, while the other contains a single amino acid difference. Overall, including the propeptide region, the Xenopus BMP-4 proteins are 80% homologous to human BMP-4. The human and mouse BMP-6 amino acid sequences are 92% identical overall, with only two amino acid differences in the seven-cysteine region (LYONS et al. 1989a; CELESTE et al. 1990).

3. Recombinant Expression

Some of the BMPs have been produced in a recombinant form, and much of the information regarding the biochemistry and activities of these molecules has come from the recombinant molecules, since significant amounts of the natural BMPs have been difficult to obtain. Most of the reported production of active BMPs has been done in mammalian cells. For example, BMP-2 has been overexpressed in Chinese hamster ovary (CHO) cells and stable cell lines have been derived which secrete the mature dimeric rhBMP-2 into the conditioned medium (WANG et al. 1990). Dimerization and processing to the mature molecule appears to occur intracellularly or upon secretion (see Fig. 2). The major processing of the propeptide occurs after an arg-glu-lys-arg site, yielding the mature molecule as a dimer of two 114 amino acid subunits. Small amounts of partially processed forms are also found, i.e., the primary translation product minus its secretory leader dimerized with either itself or with the mature monomer peptide. As expected, since there are no cysteine residues, the propeptide is secreted in a monomeric form which does not associate with the mature dimer.

Recently, rhBMP-4 has been expressed in a transient expression system utilizing human embryonic kidney 293 cells (Hammonds et al. 1991). Enhanced expression of BMP-4 was achieved using a construction of the mature region of the BMP-4 cDNA combined onto the BMP-2 propeptide region. The BMP-4 propeptide is processed in an analogous position to the closely related molecule BMP-2; the resulting mature molecule is a dimer of two 116 amino acid subunits. In addition, stable CHO cell lines expressing active BMP-4 have been established (LaPan et al. 1991). BMP-5 has also been expressed in CHO cells, yielding a mature homodimeric peptide of 138 amino acids (D'Alessandro et al. 1991). rhBMP-2, rhBMP-4, and rhBMP-5 are all glycosylated in these mammalian expression systems, though it has been reported that activity of bone-derived BMPs is unaffected by deglycosylation (Sampath et al. 1990). In all these systems, processing of the precursors to the mature molecules occurs predominantly after an arg-X-X-arg sequence. The reported processing sites of all other TGFβ family members also conform to this consensus sequence. BMP-7 has also been reported to be expressed as a 36-kDa dimer in a mammalian cell system (Sampath et al. 1991).

4. Expression of BMPs in Other Tissues

While the BMPs have been identified by their presence in bone-inductive extracts derived from bone, and some of the recombinant molecules have the capacity to induce cartilage and bone formation in the adult animal, the activities of the BMP proteins are probably not restricted to the domain of bone formation. In embryogenesis, the expression of the mRNAs for BMP-2, BMP-4, and BMP-6/vgr-1 have been localized in many developing tissues (see Sect. C.III). Many of the BMP mRNAs have also been found in adult tissues and cell lines derived from adult tissues. As shown in Table 1, though BMP-2, BMP-4, BMP-6, and BMP-7 are more abundantly expressed in bone, they are also found in many other tissues, some with substantial levels of the mRNAs (Wozney et al. 1990). BMP-3 mRNA is unusual in its distribution with high levels of expression in brain and lung. Multiple BMP mRNAs have been detected in osteosarcoma cell lines. For example, all of the known BMPs except BMP-3 are expressed by U-2 OS human osteosarcoma cells (Wozney et al. 1988; Celeste et al. 1990; Özkaynak et al. 1990; Harris et al. 1991a; Bonewald et al. 1991). In addition, BMP-4 and BMP-3 mRNAs have been detected in prostate carcinoma cell lines (Harris et al. 1991b). Taken together, these results suggest that this set of related molecules is involved in processes distinct from the induction and maintenance of bone. While little is known about the role(s) that the BMPs may play in these other tissues, by analogy with their purported role in bone,

Table 1. Bone morphogenetic protein mRNAs detected in tissues and cell lines

BMP	Tissue	Cell line
BMP-2	Bone, spleen, liver, brain, lung, kidney, heart	U-2 OS (osteosarcoma) MG-63 (osteosarocoma)
BMP-3	Lung, brain	PC-3 (prostate), H128 (small cell lung carcinoma)
BMP-4	Bone, lung, kidney, brain, spleen, liver, heart	U-2 OS (osteosarcoma), MG-63 (osteosarcoma), PC-3 (prostate), DU-145 (prostate)
BMP-5		U-2 OS (osteosarcoma)
BMP-6	Calvaria, lung, brain, placenta, kidney, uterus, muscle, skin	U-2 OS (osteosarcoma), F9 (+RA+cAMP)
BMP-7	Calvaria, placenta, brain	U-2 OS (osteosarcoma)

the BMPs may interact with extracellular matrix components and remain localized in the tissue matrices of many organs. It may also explain the observation that devitalized cells or extracts from other tissue types, e.g., WISH cells, HeLa cells, transitional epithelium of the bladder, and prostate cells, contain bone-inductive activity (ANDERSON 1990).

5. Chromosomal Localization of the BMP Genes

Some of the BMP genes have been assigned to their respective chromosomes in both the mouse and the human. In all cases examined to date they are not physically linked to each other (DICKINSON et al. 1990; TABAS et al. 1991; COHEN et al. 1991). In addition, they have been proposed to be candidates for several morphogenetic loci in mouse or for defective genes in human disorders. BMP-2 is located on chromosome 2 in the mouse, where it is a candidate for tight skin (tsk), which leads to a disorder of loose connective tissue, bone, cartilage, and tendons. As predicted by synteny, BMP-2 localizes to chromosome 20 in the human. The BMP-3 gene is located on chromosome 5 in the mouse and chromosome 4 in human. Dentinogenesis imperfecta type II has been linked to chromosome 4. The BMP-4 gene is located on chromosome 14 in the mouse, and could be a candidate for the pug-nose (pn) locus, associated with defects in the growth and development of the skull bones. A BMP-4-related sequence present on the X chromosome may represent yet another related gene or a pseudogene. The human BMP-4 gene is on chromosome 14. Holt-Oram syndrome, associated with defects in skeletal and cardiac development, has been linked to chromosome 14. BMP-6 (*Vgr*-1) is located on mouse chromosome 13 and could be a candidate for the congenital hydrocephalus (ch) locus.

C. Activities of Individual BMP Molecules

I. In Vivo Activities

The use of recombinant DNA technology to express individual BMP proteins has allowed for the investigation of the osteogenic potential of these molecules in a number of in vivo systems. At present, rhBMP-2, rhBMP-4, rhBMP-5, and rhBMP-7 have been shown to initiate new ectopic cartilage and bone formation in rats. The data obtained suggest that each of the BMPs tested to date is by itself sufficient to induce de novo bone formation. Once implanted subcutaneously with an appropriate carrier, the BMPs initiate a series of events beginning with the differentiation of mesenchymal cells into chondroblasts. The cartilaginous matrix produced by these cells then calcifies and is removed and replaced by bone. The osteoblasts and osteoclasts required to maintain remodeling of the mature bone are present within 10–14 days of BMP implantation. In general, the sequence of events obtained with implantation of each recombinant protein is strikingly similar to the development cascade observed with bovine bone-derived BMP. With all of the BMPs tested to date, early chondrogenesis is the hallmark of osteogenesis at later time points.

As shown in Table 2, the amount of new bone formed and the rate of completion of the bone development progression are dependent upon the amount of BMP-2 implanted (Wang et al. 1990). The ability of increasing doses of rhBMP-2 protein to alter the rate of new cartilage and bone formation suggests that BMPs act not only as initiators of bone formation but are also regulatory signals for other steps in the osteoinduction sequence.

Table 2. Time course of cartilage (C) and bone (B) formation by various amounts of rhBMP-2 in rat ectopic assay system

Dose of rhBMP-2	Day 5	Day 7	Day 10	Day 14
1.2	C ±	C + 2	C + 3	C ±
	B = 0	B = 0	B + 1	B + 3
12	C + 3	C + 3	C + 2	C = 0
	B = 0	B + 2	B + 3	B + 4
24	C + 3	C + 4	C + 1	C = 0
	B ±	B + 3	B + 4	B + 4
115	C + 4	C + 4	ND	C = 0
	B + 2	B + 5	ND	B + 5

Since results of in vivo activities for other BMPs have used different quantitation methods, their relative activities are difficult to determine.

While synergy between individual BMP proteins is unproven at present, the recombinant proteins have been reported to be, at least in the ectopic bone formation assay, less potent bone inductive agents than the mixture of native BMPs making up highly purified bovine bone-derived BMP (WANG et al. 1990). Since each BMP protein can initiate the bone formation cascade, it is possible that individual BMP proteins are regulators of specific steps in the cartilage and bone development process and may regulate the transition from cartilage to bone or other developmental decisions which would, in turn, lead to increased potency as measured by the ectopic bone formation assay.

The use of rhBMPs has greatly increased our understanding of the role of matrix or carrier in ectopic bone formation. While it is probably true that bone matrix provides a substratum for BMP responsive cells to adhere to and move against (SAMPATH and REDDI 1984), this component is not a requirement for bone formation, as implantation of rhBMP-2 without a matrix results in bone formation (WOZNEY et al. 1990). It appears likely that matrix serves as a slow release system for BMPs, allowing the inductive signals to remain available to responsive cells for greater time intervals. This idea is supported by the increased sensitivity of the ectopic assay in the presence of bone matrix. Detailed release studies for characterization of the interactions of specific BMPs with bone matrix will help clarify this matter. Matrix may also increase the potency of BMPs by providing an environment that maximizes presentation of the inductive signal to the responsive cell. Osteogenin has been reported to bind avidly to type IV collagen and to a lesser extent to both type I and type IX collagens (PARALKAR et al. 1990). These data, along with the well-established ability of many BMP proteins to bind to heparin, suggest that bone matrix is an important component of the BMP response and interactions of BMPs with extracellular matrix may modulate their local actions in vivo. Since TGFβ is known to be a major component of bone matrix, some interaction between the BMPs and TGFβ may occur. In fact, CARRINGTON et al. (1988) have reported that TGFβ is synthesized and stored in large quantities in the extracellular matrix during the progression from cartilage to bone in the rat ectopic assay system. More investigation is required to determine the roles of matrix in BMP-mediated bone formation.

II. In Vitro Activities

An increasing body of data indicates that treatment of mesenchymal cells with BMPs in vitro results in the expression of osteoblast and chondroblast phenotypes. Using the C20 and C26 cell lines isolated from newborn mouse calvaria, YAMAGUCHI et al. (1991) have shown that BMP-2 stimulates alkaline phosphatase activity, PTH-specific cAMP responsiveness, and BGP synthesis, all characteristics of the osteoblast phenotype. Treatment of C26 cells for 6 days resulted in a 16-fold increase in alkaline phosphatase activity and a 156-fold increase in PTH-stimulated cAMP. Osteocalcin mRNA was also induced after 6 days of incubation of C26 cells in rhBMP-2. In contrast, BMP-2 treatment of C26 cells reduces the expression of desmin, a marker associated with the muscle phenotype. In C20 cells, a model for the differentiated osteoblast, similar treatments did not significantly increase the already high basal alkaline phosphatase activity, but rhBMP-2 activated the PTH-stimulated cAMP production by these cells in a dose-dependent manner. By comparison, TGFβ treatment inhibited alkaline phosphatase activity in both C20 and C26 cells and did not induce PTH-stimulated cAMP or osteocalcin synthesis in C26 cells. These data indicate that rhBMP-2 is able to induce differentiation of osteoblast precursor cells into more mature osteoblast-like cells in vitro.

In a preliminary study with MC3T3 E1 cells, BMP-2 treatment stimulated alkaline phosphatase activity and this stimulation was potentiated by cotreatment with β-estradiol, dexamethasone, and $1,25(OH)_2$ vitamin D_3 (TAKUWA et al. 1991). Collagen type I synthesis was also somewhat increased in MC3T3 E1 cells in response to BMP-2. Taken together with the effects on C26 cells, for all calvarial-derived cells to date, BMP-2 treatment results in increases in osteoblast-like characteristics in osteoprogenitor cells. The effects of rhBMP-4 on MC3T3 E1 cells appear to be similar to results obtained with rhBMP-2. An inhibition of [^{3}H]thymidine incorporation occurs after 24 h, while increases in alkaline phosphatase production by MC3T3 E1 cells require approximately 72 h of BMP-4 treatment (HAMMONDS et al. 1991). Treatment of these same cells, as well as primary calvarial cells, with osteogenin also results in increased expression of the osteoblast phenotype similar to that observed with BMP-2 or BMP-4 (VUKICEVIK et al. 1989, 1990a; PARALKAR et al. 1991). Since these osteogenin preparations may also have contained significant amounts of native BMP-2 and BMP-4, it is difficult to evaluate which, if any, of the reported effects were specific to osteogenin. These results are in contrast to the effects of TGFβ on these cells. Again, TGFβ treatment results in inhibition of alkaline phosphatase activity of MC3T3 E1 cells (NODA and RODAN 1986; KATAGIRI et al. 1990a).

Another target for BMPs is the osteoprogenitor population located in bone marrow stroma. Many investigators have shown that, under the proper culture conditions, a small subset of cells within the stromal population will differentiate into osteoblasts (HOWLETT et al. 1986). THIES et al. (1992) have reported that BMP-2 treatment of W-20 cells, a multipotent cell line derived from adult mouse stroma, results in increased expression of alkaline phosphatase, enhanced production of cAMP in response to PTH, and induction of osteocalcin expression, suggesting that BMPs are able to promote differentiation of stromal cells into osteoblast-like cells. Osteogenin has also been reported to increase alkaline phosphatase production by primary bone marrow stromal cells in vitro (PARALKAR et al. 1991).

In vitro, BMPs are able to induce expression of the chondroblast phenotype in cells isolated from embryonic limb bud. Treatment of several 13 dpc mouse limb bud cell lines with BMP-2 results in the expression of alkaline phosphatase activity, PTH-stimulated cAMP, and incorporation of sulfate into proteoglycan, though the responses of the different lines are somewhat heterogeneous (ROSEN et al. 1991). When primary cells isolated from stage 24–25 chick embryo limb are cultured in BMP-4, chondrogenic and non-chondrogenic precursors differentiate into cartilage cells as measured by increases in type II collagen and cartilage-specific proteoglycan synthesis. Osteogenin treatment also increases the expression of cartilage-specific markers in chick limb bud cells in vitro (CARRINGTON et al. 1991). Preliminary evidence with 10T1/2 cells, derived from early mouse mesoderm, shows that BMP-2 treatment increases both alkaline phosphatase activity and PTH-stimulated cAMP levels, suggesting that BMP-2 modulates the differentiation of these cells into cells of the osteoblastic phenotype (KATAGIRI et al. 1990b).

In summary, treatment of osteoblast-like and chondroblast-like cells, and also their progenitors with BMPs, results in the differentiation of these cells along the cartilage and bone cell pathways.

III. Bone Morphogenetic Proteins in Embryogenesis

Since the earliest site of osteogenesis is the embryonic skeleton, there is much interest in the role of BMPs in primary skeletal formation. Detailed in situ hybridization analysis has shown that BMPs are present during fetal and embryonic development in a spatial and temporal pattern consistent with their involvement in early skeletal formation (ROSEN et al. 1989; LYONS et al. 1989b; LYONS et al. 1990; JONES et al. 1991). A high level of BMP-2 transcript is found in developing limb buds (ventral ectoderm and apical ectodermal ridge), tooth buds, and craniofacial mesenchyme, as well as nonskeletal tissues such as heart myocardium, whisker follicles, and skin. BMP-4 transcripts are also found in elevated levels in developing limbs and facial processes. BMP-2 and BMP-4 are present in embryos prior to overt chondrogenesis and osteogenesis. Once these processes have begun, the BMP-2 and BMP-4 mRNAs are associated with sites thought to contain progenitor cells for bone and cartilage. In contrast, BMP-6 mRNA has been localized to hypertrophic cartilage but not to earlier stages of bone formation. TGFβ mRNA is expressed at very high levels in differentiated osteoblasts and chondroblasts, and activin mRNA has also been localized to sites of bone formation (ROBERTS and SPORN 1990; ROBERTS et al. 1991). These data support the hypothesis that specific BMP molecules, as well as other TGFβ superfamily members, are involved in individual steps in the bone developmental cascade. Genetic analysis employing knockout and transgenic technology will allow correlation of these localization patterns with specific functions for the individual BMP genes.

Indirect evidence for the involvement of BMPs in early skeletal formation has been provided by autoradiographic localization of radiolabeled osteogenin to multiple sites undergoing bone formation in the developing mouse embryo (Vukicevik et al. 1990b). The ability of osteogenin to bind with high affinity to many components of the extracellular matrix may also account for the increase in localization over the developing skeleton (Paralkar et al. 1990).

D. Clinical Utility of BMPs

I. Clinical Indications

While bone has a significant capacity for regeneration and healing, these processes are limited by the size of the defect and the age of the patient, as well as by other pathological conditions. Currently, bone loss due to acute trauma and surgical intervention is routinely treated by grafting bone from various sources. Autologous graft, while the most successful, is limited by the amount of bone that can be removed from a secondary site. Allogeneic bone transplantation carries considerable risk of infection by viruses such as HIV or hepatitis. It is also limited by the fact that the bone is not living and therefore, rather than being osteoinductive, it is merely osteoconductive and capable of lending physical support.

The bone-inductive capacity of the BMPs is expected to allow them to be used clinically to replace the bone lost due to trauma and surgical procedures. The use of the BMPs is not expected to be limited by site, that is, it may be used in craniofacial areas, dental indications, and orthopedics. Indications include catastrophic bone loss or complex fracture sites, removal of osteosarcomas, and removal of other tumors which invade bone and require bone resection. BMPs additionally may be used in other procedures that currently use bone grafting, such as spinal fusions and repair of nonunion fractures, where the normal repair processes of bone have failed. The ability of synthetic implants to integrate into the surrounding bone may also be increased by the use of a bone-inductive protein. The BMPs may be used both in primary fixation of implants to gain stability and during procedures for replacement of failed prostheses, where remaining bone is frequently insufficient to adequately stabilize the new device.

Bone morphogenetic proteins are also likely to significantly impact the practices of dentistry and oral surgery. For example, the BMPs may be able to replace the bone lost due to periodontal disease. They may also find application in the filling of extraction sockets with bone, and in enhancing the rate of implant fixation. BMPs additionally may be useful in alveolar ridge augmentation, where synthetic bone replacements such as hydroxyapatite are now commonly used. Each of these indications may require unique physical properties of the matrix to which the protein is attached; for example, certain procedures may require shaping of the bone replacement while others demand instant physical stability.

II. Animal Studies

At present, various bone-derived bone-inductive extracts have been used in various preclinical models of bone repair and in clinical settings. In addition, there are some recent reports of the use of recombinant single BMP factors for the replacement of large bone defects in several animal models.

1. Bone-Derived Extracts

The efficacy of bone extracts in bone induction and growth has been investigated in a number of different animals. It must be realized that the hormonal environment and the architecture of bone is unique to each animal species. For instance, while rodent systems are convenient and easy to manipulate, their metabolism rate and constant bone growth vary significantly from humans. Canine and ovine models are thought to more closely represent the human situation in terms of bone architecture, size, and growth regulation.

The bone extracts used in these animal studies have either been combined with a carrier matrix for implantation or merely utilized protein impurities in the material as the carrier. In one study, partially purified xenogeneic (bovine) bone extracts alone have been shown to heal critical-sized defects in the long bones (ulna) of dogs (NILSSON et al. 1986; JOHNSON et al. 1989). In these studies, 100 mg bone extract was implanted in 2.5- to 3.5-cm defect sites. While bone induction was seen in all studies, bony union was achieved with variable success. This may be associated with the size of the defect or the dose of bone-inducing protein in the crude extract. Other studies have used bone extracts implanted into surgically introduced holes in the skulls (trephine defects) of dogs and sheep (URIST et al. 1987; LINDHOLM et al. 1988). Bone extract in quantities of 10–100 mg implanted alone or with tricalcium phosphate carrier materials were shown to heal 1.4- to 2.0-cm defects. In a canine spinal fusion model, addition of 25 mg bovine bone extract in a polylactic acid polymer was shown to augment bone formation by bone graft (LOVELL et al. 1989). A study of bone growth in drill holes in femoral condyles showed that 5 mg allogeneic (rabbit) bone extract combined with hydroxyapatite and/or fibrin carriers augmented bone formation in 3.5-mm femoral defects (SATO et al. 1991).

Primate studies have been limited to trephine defects in rhesus monkeys and baboons (FERGUSON et al. 1987; HOLLINGER et al. 1989). Implantation of 100 mg bovine bone extracts have healed 1.4- to 2.0-cm calvarial defects in both species. All of these studies demonstrate that bone extracts containing BMP activity will successfully induce bone formation and heal critical-sized bone defects. In addition, they demonstrate that the BMP effect does not appear to be species specific. However, observed suboptimal results may be due to use of xenogeneic bone extracts which may contain materials that are immunogenic and decrease the BMP effect.

2. Recombinant Human BMPs

Recent studies have shown that the bone-inductive molecule recombinant human BMP-2 is able to heal critical-sized defects in the rat femur, sheep femur, and dog mandible. In each study, rhBMP-2 was combined with an allogeneic, bone-derived inert carrier from which endogenous bone-inductive activity had been removed. In the rat femur model, a 0.5-cm defect implanted with 11 μg rhBMP-2 + 10 mg carrier resulted in union at 9 weeks in eight out of ten animals examined (YASKO et al. 1991). The induction of bone and the resulting union was assessed radiographically, biomechanically, and histologically. By each assessment criterion, bone formation was induced by BMP-2, and the bone formed successfully integrated into the surrounding bone yielding a successful union.

Much larger defects have been healed in sheep, where 1.5 mg rhBMP-2 was implanted with 3 g carrier into a 2.5-cm femoral defect (GERHART et al. 1991). The defect was then stabilized with a lateral metal fixation plate. Radiographs indicated the beginnings of visible bone formation at week 4, and enhanced bone formation continuing to the end of the study at 3 months. Biomechanical testing at the end of the study indicated that the test femurs had bending strengths comparable to contralateral untreated controls, and to identical defects treated with autologous bone graft. Similarly, 3.0-cm defects in the mandibles of dogs have been healed within 3 months by the implantation of 250 μg rhBMP-2 with 500 mg matrix (TORIUMI et al. 1991).

These studies indicate that this single BMP protein, rhBMP-2, which induces ectopic formation in rats, is capable of inducing functional bone which can integrate into the surrounding bone in a variety of animal models. This protein induces the cascade of cellular events which results in bone formation; once bone has been formed, it is subject to the normal physiological processes that cause it to remodel due to its physical environment and the mechanical stresses placed on it (Wolff's law). While in these studies animals were implanted with allogeneic bone matrix as the carrier, the development of synthetic or more defined carrier systems is awaited. In addition, similar studies with other single recombinant BMP molecules will determine whether they, like BMP-2, can be used in bone replacement indications.

III. Human Studies with Bone Extracts

There have been multiple reports of the use of human demineralized bone matrix (GLOWACKI et al. 1981) and bone extracts in the healing of bony defects in humans. Human bone extracts were combined with autologous cancellous bone grafts to successfully treat six patients with 3- to 17-cm tibial defects (JOHNSON et al. 1988a). Twelve patients with femoral nonunions were also treated with 50–100 mg partially purified human bone extract following internal fixation (JOHNSON et al. 1988b). In these studies, the bone extract was delivered in gelatin capsules or polylactic acid/polyglycolic acid strips, and in some cases the treatment was combined with autologous or allogeneic bone grafts. Eleven of the 12 nonunions were reported to be healed using these regimens. An additional four patients with nonunions of the tibia have recently been reported to have been treated with human bone extracts (JOHNSON et al. 1990). Again, union was achieved following delivery of human bone extract either in polylactic acid/polyglycolic acid strips or gelatin capsules. While these studies provide evidence that BMP activity will be useful in the treatment of human bone disorders, none is sufficiently controlled to allow for critical evaluation of the results. Controlled clinical trials using recombinant BMPs are eagerly awaited.

E. Summary

Significant progress has been made in understanding the nature of the bone-inductive signals stored in bone matrix. Isolation of the BMP genes and production of recombinant human BMP proteins has demonstrated that rhBMP-2, rhBMP-4, rhBMP-5, and rhBMP-7, when administered individually, initiate the complex developmental progression necessary for bone formation. Moreover, rhBMP-2-induced bone formation in critical-size defects in rats, dogs, and sheep suggests that the BMP proteins will show clinical utility in humans and in the near future may be part of the thera-peutic modality used in the treatment of skeletal defects. While knowledge of the mechanisms by which BMPs exert their effects is very preliminary, in vitro data support in vivo observations that BMP proteins act as differen-tiation factors, inducing differentiation of mesenchymal progenitor cells into osteoblasts and chondroblasts while inhibiting their conversion into muscle cells. The localization of BMPs at multiple sites undergoing morphogenesis during embryonic development suggests that BMPs may be the regulatory signals involved in initial skeletal formation as well as adult skeletal repair, but they may also play initial roles in the development of other tissues. The availability of recombinant probes and proteins has just allowed us to begin to unravel the biology of this important and exciting gene family.

References

Anderson HC (1990) The role of cells versus matrix in bone induction. Connec Tissue Res 24:3–12

Bentz H, Nathan RM, Rosen DM, Armstrong RM, Thompson AY, Segarini PR, Mathews MC, Dasch JR, Piez KA, Seyedin SM (1989) Purification and charac-terization of a unique osteoinductive factor from bovine bone. J Biol Chem 264:20805–20810

Bonewald LF, Mundy GR, Kester MB, Harris MA, Harris SE (1991) Transforming growth factor beta (TGFβ) and bone morphogenetic protein (BMP) 4 expression in human MG-63 bone cells is enhanced by TGF-β. J Bone Miner Res 6:S258

Brunner AM, Marquardt H, Malacko AR, Lioubin MN, Purchio AF (1989) Site-directed mutagenesis of cysteine residues in the pro region of the transforming growth factor β1 precursor. J Biol Chem 264:13660–13664

Carrington JL, Roberts AB, Flanders KC, Roche NS, Reddi AH (1988) Accumulation, localization, and compartmentation of transforming growth factor β during endochondral bone development. J Cell Biol 107:1969–1975

Carrington JL, Chen P, Yanagishita M, Reddi AH (1991) Osteogenin (bone morphogenetic protein-3) stimulates cartilage formation by chick limb bud cells in vitro. Dev Biol 146:406–415

Celeste AJ, Iannazzi JA, Taylor RC, Hewick RM, Rosen V, Wang EA, Wozney JM (1990) Identification of transforming growth factor β family members present in bone-inductive protein purified from bovine bone. Proc Natl Acad Sci USA 87:9843–9847

Cohen RB, Tabas JA, Seaunez HH, Wozney JM, Emanuel B, Zasloff M, Kaplan FS (1991) Chromosomal localization of the human gene for bone morphogenetic protein-4 (BMP-4). J Bone Miner Res 6:S156

D'Alessandro JS, Cox KA, Israel DI, LaPan P, Moutsatsos IK, Nove J, Rosen V, Ryan MC, Wozney JM, Wang EA (1991) Purification, characterization and activities of recombinant bone morphogenetic protein-5. J Bone Miner Res 6:S153

Dickinson ME, Kobrin MS, Silan CM, Kingsley DM, Justice MJ, Miller DA, Ceci JD, Lock LF, Lee A, Buchberg AM, Siracusa LD, Lyons KM, Derynck R, Hogan BLM, Copeland NG, Jenkins NA (1990) Chromosomal localization of seven members of the murine TGF-β superfamily suggest close linkage to several morphogenetic mutant loci. Genomics 6:505–520

Ferguson D, Davis WL, Urist MR, Hurt WC, Allen EP (1987) Bovine bone morphogenetic protein (bBMP) fraction-induced repair of craniotomy defects in the rhesus monkey. Clin Orthop 219:251–290

Finkelman RD, Mohan S, Jennings JC, Taylor AK, Jepsen S, Baylink SJ (1990) Quantitation of growth factors IGF-I, SGF/IGF-II, and TGF-β in human dentin. J Bone Miner Res 5:717–723

Gerhart TN, Kirker-Head CA, Kriz MJ, Hipp JA, Rosen V, Schelling S, Wozney JM, Wang EA (1991) Healing of large mid-femoral segmental defects in sheep using recombinant human bone morphogenetic protein (BMP-2). Trans Orthop Res Soc 16:172

Glowacki J, Kaban LB, Murray JE, Folkman J, Mulliken JB (1981) Application of the biological principle of induced osteogenesis for craniofacial defects. Lancet 8227:959–963

Hall BK, van Exan RJ (1982) Induction of bone by epithelial cell products. J Embryol Exp Morphol 69:37–46

Hammonds RG Jr, Schwall R, Dudley A, Berkemeier L, Lai C, Lee J, Cunningham N, Reddi AH, Wood WI, Mason AJ (1991) Bone-inducing activity of mature BMP-2b produced from a hybrid BMP-2a/2b precursor. Mol Endocrinol 5:149–155

Harris SE, Bonewald LF, Harris MA, Sabatini M, Mundy GR (1991a) Retinoic acid (RA) regulates expression of early growth response genes, BMP 4, and BMP 2 mRNA in human osteoblastic cells. J Bone Miner Res 6:S199

Harris SE, Harris MA, Mahy P, Sabatini M, Dunn J, Boyce B, Mundy GR (1991b) Expression of BMP-4 and BMP-3-like mRNA by human prostate carcinoma cells. J Bone Miner Res 6:S193

Hauschka PV, Mavrakos AE, Iafrati MD, Doleman SE, Klagsbrun M (1986) Growth factors in bone matrix: isolation of multiple types by affinity chromatography on heparin sepharose. J Biol Chem 261:12665–12674

Hauschka PV, Chen TL, Mavrakos AE (1988) Polypeptide growth factors in bone matrix. In: Evered D, Harnett S (eds) Cell and molecular biology of vertebrate hard tissues. Wiley, Chichester, pp 207–225

Hollinger J, Mark DE, Bach DE, Reddi AH, Seyfer AE (1989) Calvarial bone regeneration using osteogenin. J Oral Maxillofac Surg 47:1182–1186

Howlett CR, Cave J, Williamson M, Farmer J, Ali SY, Bab I, Owen ME (1986) Mineralization in in vitro cultures of rabbit marrow stromal cells. Clin Orthop 213:251–263

Huggins CB (1931) The formation of bone under the influence of epithelium of the urinary tract. Arch Surg 22:377–408

Jingushi S, Bolander ME (1991) Modulation of rat femoral fracture healing by in vivo injections of basic fibroblast growth factor and transforming growth factor-β1. Trans Orthop Res Soc 16:118

Jingushi S, Hjelmeland L, Joyce ME, Jaye M, Sugioka Y, Bolander ME (1991) A role of acidic fibroblast growth factor in rat fracture healing – induction of chondrogenesis. Trans Orthop Res Soc 16:382

Johnson EE, Urist MR, Finerman GAM (1988a) Bone morphogenetic protein augmentation grafting of resistant femoral nonunions: a preliminary report. Clin Orthop 230:257–265

Johnson EE, Urist MR, Finerman GAM (1988b) Repair of segmental defects of the tibia with cancellous bone grafts augmented with human bone morphogenetic protein. Clin Orthop 236:249–257

Johnson EE, Urist MR, Schmalzried TP, Chotivichit A, Huang HK, Finerman GAM (1989) Autogeneic cancellous bone grafts in extensive segmental ulnar defects in dogs. Clin Orthop Relat Res 243:254–265

Johnson EE, Urist MR, Finerman GAM (1990) Distal metaphyseal tibial nonunion: deformity and bone loss treated by open reduction, internal fixation, and human bone morphogenetic protein (hBMP). Clin Orthop 250:234–240

Jones CM, Lyons KM, Hogan BLM (1991) Involvement of bone morphogenetic protein-4 (BMP-4) and Vgr-1 in morphogenesis and neurogenesis in the mouse. Development 111:531–542

Joyce ME, Roberts AB, Sporn MB, Bolander ME (1990) Transforming growth factor-β and the initiation of chondrogenesis and osteogenesis in the rat femur. J Cell Biol 110:2195–2207

Katagiri T, Lee T, Takeshima H, Suda T, Tanaka H, Omura S (1990a) Transforming growth factor-β modulates proliferation and differentiation of mouse clonal osteoblastic MC3T3-E1 cells depending on their maturation stages. Bone Miner 11:285–293

Katagiri T, Yamaguchi A, Ikeda T, Yoshiki S, Wozney JM, Rosen V, Wang EA, Tanaka H, Omura S, Suda T (1990b) The non-osteogenic mouse pluripotent cell line, C3H10T1/2, is induced to differentiate into osteoblastic cells by recombinant human bone morphogenetic protein-2. Biochem Biophys Res Commun 172:295–299

Klagsbrun M (1989) The fibroblast growth factor family: structural and biological properties. Prog Growth Factor Res 1:207–235

Köster M, Plessow S, Clement JH, Lorenz A, Tiedemann H, Knochel W (1991) Bone morphogenetic protein 4 (BMP-4), a member of the TGF-β family, in early embryos of Xenopus laevis: analysis of mesoderm inducing activity. Mech Dev 33:191–200

LaPan P, Bauduy M, Cox KA, D'Alessandro JS, Israel DI, Nove J, Rosen V, Wozney JM, Moutsatsos IK, Wang EA (1991) Purification, characterization and activities of recombinant human bone morphogenetic protein 4. J Bone Miner Res 6:S153

Lindholm TC, Lindholm TS, Alitalo I, Urist MR (1988) Bovine bone morphogenetic protein (bBMP) induced repair of skull trephine defects in sheep. Clin Orthop 227:265–268

Lovell TP, Dawson EG, Nilsson OS, Urist MR (1989) Augmentation of spinal fusion with bone morphogenetic protein in dogs. Clin Orthop 243:266–275

Luyten FP, Cunningham NS, Ma S, Muthukumaran N, Hammonds RG, Nevins WB, Wood WI, Reddi AH (1989) Purification and partial amino acid sequence of osteogenin, a protein initiating bone differentiation. J Biol Chem 264:13377–13380

Lyons K, Graycar JL, Lee A, Hashmi S, Lindquist PB, Chen EY, Hogan BLM, Derynck R (1989a) Vgr-1, a mammalian gene related to Xenopus Vg-1, is a member of the transforming growth factor β gene superfamily. Proc Natl Acad Sci USA 86:4554–4558

Lyons KM, Pelton RW, Hogan BLM (1989b) Patterns of expression of murine Vgr-1 and BMP-2a RNA suggest that transforming growth factor-β-like genes coordinately regulate aspects of embryonic development. Genes Dev 3:1657–1668

Lyons KM, Pelton RW, Hogan BLM (1990) Organogenesis and pattern formation in the mouse: RNA distribution patterns suggest a role for bone morphogenetic protein-2A (BMP-2A). Development 109:833–844

Muthukumaran N, Ma S, Reddi AH (1988) Dose-dependence of and threshold for optimal bone induction by collagenous bone matrix and osteogenin-enriched fraction. Collagen Rel Res 8:433–441

Nilsson OS, Urist MR, Dawson EG, Schmalzried TP, Finerman GAM (1986) Bone repair induced by bone morphogenetic protein in ulnar defects in dogs. J Bone Joint Surg 68B:635–642

Noda M, Rodan GA (1986) Type-β transforming growth factor inhibits proliferation and expression of alkaline phosphatase in murine osteoblast-like cells. Biochem Biophys Res Commun 140:56–65

Özkaynak E, Rueger DC, Drier EA, Corbett C, Ridge RJ, Sampath TK, Oppermann H (1990) OP-1 cDNA encodes an osteogenic protein in the TGF-β family. EMBO J 9:2085–2093

Padgett RW, St. Johnston RD, Gelbart WM (1987) A transcript from a Drosophila pattern gene predicts a protein homologous to the transforming growth factor-β family. Nature 325:81–84

Paralkar VM, Nandedkar AKN, Pointer RH, Kleinman HK, Reddi AH (1990) Interaction of osteogenin, a heparin binding bone morphogenetic protein, with type IV collagen. J Biol Chem 265:17281–17284

Paralkar VM, Hammonds RG, Reddi AH (1991) Identification and characterization of cellular binding proteins (receptors) for recombinant human bone morphogenetic protein 2B, an initiator of bone differentiation cascade. Proc Natl Acad Sci USA 88:3397–3401

Reddi AH (1981) Cell biology and biochemistry of endochondral bone development. Collagen Rel Res 1:209–226

Roberts AB, Sporn MB (1990) The transforming growth factor-βs. In: Sporn MB, Roberts AB (ed) Peptide growth factors and their receptors, vol 1. Springer, Berlin Heidelberg New York, pp 419–472

Roberts VJ, Sawchenko RE, Vale W (1991) Expression of inhibin/activin subunit messenger ribonucleic acids during rat embryogenesis. Endocrinology 128:3122–3129

Rosen V, Wozney JM, Wang EA, Cordes P, Celeste A, McQuaid D, Kurtzberg L (1989) Purification and molecular cloning of a novel group of BMPs and localization of BMP mRNA in developing bone. Connec Tissue Res 20:313–319

Rosen V, Bauduy M, McQuaid D, Donaldson D, Thies S, Wozney J (1991) Expression of osteoblast-like phenotype in mouse embryo limb bud cell lines cultured in BMP-2 and retinoic acid. Proc Endocrine Soc 73:57

Sampath TK, Reddi AH (1981) Dissociative extraction and reconstitution of extracellular matrix components involved in local bone differentiation. Proc Natl Acad Sci USA 78:7599–7603

Sampath TK, Reddi AH (1983) Homology of bone-inductive proteins from human, monkey, bovine, and rat extracellular matrix. Proc Natl Acad Sci USA 80:6591–6595

Sampath TK, Reddi AH (1984) Importance of geometry of the extracellular matrix in endochondral bone differentiation. J Cell Biol 98:2192–2197

Sampath TK, Coughlin JE, Whetsone RM, Banach D, Corbett C, Ridge RJ, Özkaynak E, Oppermann H, Rueger DC (1990) Bovine osteogenic protein is composed of dimers of OP-1 and BMP-2A, two members of the transforming growth factor-β superfamily. J Biol Chem 265:13198–13205

Sampath TK, Özkaynak E, Jones WK, Sasak H, Tucker R, Tucker M, Kusmik W, Lightholder J, Pang R, Corbett C, Oppermann H, Rueger DC (1991) Recombinant human osteogenic protein (hOP-1) induces new bone formation with a specific activity comparable to that of natural bovine osteogenic protein. J Bone Miner Res 6:S155

Sato T, Kawamura M, Sato K, Iwata H, Miura T (1991) Bone morphogenesis of rabbit bone morphogenetic protein-bound hydroxyapatite-fibrin composite. Clin Orthop 263:254–262

Tabas JA, Zasloff M, Wasmuth JJ, Emanuel BS, Altherr MR, McPherson J, Wozney JM, Kaplan FS (1991) Bone morphogenetic protein: chromosomal localization of human genes for BMP-1, BMP-2A, and BMP-3. Genomics 9:283–289

Takaoka K, Yoshikawa H, Shimizu N, Ono K, Amitani K, Nakata Y, Sakamoto Y (1981) Purification of a bone-inducing substance (osteogenic factor) from a murine osteosarcoma. Biomed Res 2:466–471

Takuwa Y, Ohse C, Wang EA, Wozney JM, Yamashita K (1991) Bone morphogenetic protein-2 stimulates alkaline phosphatase activity and collagen synthesis in cultured osteoblastic cells, MC3T3-E1. Biochem Biophys Res Commun 174:96–101

Thies RS, Bauduy M, Ashton BA, Kurtzberg L, Wozney JM, Rosen V (1991) Recombinant human bone morphogenetic protein-2 induces osteoblastic differentiation in W-20-17 stromal cells. Endocrinology 130:1318–1324

Toriumi DM, Kotler HS, Luxenberg DP, Holtrop ME, Wang EA (1992) Mandibular reconstruction with a bone-inducing factor. Functional, histologic and biomechanical evaluation. Arch Otolaryngol Head Neck Surg 117:1101–1112

Urist MR (1965) Bone: formation by autoinduction. Science 150:893–899

Urist MR, Iwata H, Ceccotti PL, Dorfman RL, Boyd SD, McDowell RM, Chien C (1973) Bone morphogenesis in implants of insoluble bone gelatin. Proc Natl Acad Sci USA 70:3511–3515

Urist MR, Mikulski A, Lietze A (1979) Solubilized and insolubilized bone morphogenetic protein. Proc Natl Acad Sci USA 76:1828–1832

Urist MR, Nilsson O, Rasmussen J, Hirota W, Lovell T, Schmalzreid T, Finerman GAM (1987) Bone regeneration under the influence of a bone morphogenetic protein (BMP) beta tricalcium phosphate (TCP) composite in skull trephine defects in dogs. Clin Orthop 214:295–304

Vukicevic S, Luyten FP, Reddi AH (1989) Stimulation of the expression of osteogenic and chondrogenic phenotypes in vitro by osteogenin. Proc Natl Acad Sci USA 86:8793–8797

Vukicevic S, Luyten FP, Reddi AH (1990a) Osteogenin inhibits proliferation and stimulates differentiation in mouse osteoblast-like cells (MC3T3-E1). Biochem Biophys Res Commun 166:750–756

Vukicevic S, Paralkar VM, Cunningham NS, Gutkind JS, Reddi AH (1990b) Autoradiographic localization of osteogenin binding sites in cartilage and bone during rat embryonic development. Dev Biol 140:209–214

Wang EA, Rosen V, Cordes P, Hewick RM, Kriz MJ, Luxenberg DP, Sibley BS, Wozney JM (1988) Purification and characterization of other distinct bone-inducing factors. Proc Natl Acad Sci USA 85:9484–9488

Wang EA, Rosen V, D'Alessandro JS, Bauduy M, Cordes P, Harada T, Israel D, Hewick RM, Kerns K, LaPan P, Luxenberg DP, McQuaid D, Moutsatsos I, Nove J, Wozney JM (1990) Recombinant human bone morphogenetic protein induces bone formation. Proc Natl Acad Sci USA 87:2220–2224

Weeks DL, Melton DA (1987) A maternal mRNA localized to the vegetal hemisphere in *Xenopus* eggs codes for a growth factor related to TGF-β. Cell 51:861–867

Wlodarski K (1969) The inductive properties of epithelial established cell lines. Exp Cell Res 57:446–448

Wlodarski K, Poltorak A, Koziorowska J (1971) Species specificity of osteogenesis induced by WISH cell line and bone induction by vaccinia virus transformed human fibroblasts. Calcif Tissue Res 7:345–352

Wozney JM (1989) Bone morphogenetic proteins. Prog Growth Factor Res 1:267–280

Wozney JM, Rosen V, Celeste AJ, Mitsock LM, Whitters MJ, Kriz RW, Hewick RM, Wang EA (1988) Novel regulators of bone formation: molecular clones and activities. Science 242:1528–1534

Wozney JM, Rosen V, Byrne M, Celeste AJ, Moutsatsos I, Wang EA (1990) Growth factors influencing bone development. J Cell Sci [Suppl] 13:149–156

Yamaguchi A, Katagiri T, Ikeda T, Wozney JM, Rosen V, Wang EA, Kahn AJ, Suda T, Yoshiki S (1991) Recombinant human bone morphogenetic protein-2 stimulates osteoblastic maturation and inhibits myogenic differentiation in vitro. J Cell Biol 113:681–687

Yasko AW, Lane JM, Fellinger EJ, Rosen V, Wang EA, Wozney JM, Gross JM, Glasser DB (1991) Recombinant BMP-2a bone induction in a rat orthotopic model. Trans Orthop Res Soc 16:410

Yu YM, Becvar R, Yamada Y, Reddi AH (1991) Changes in the gene expression of collagens, fibronectin, integrin and proteoglycans during matrix-induced bone morphogenesis. Biochem Biophys Res Commun 177:427–432

Subject Index

Springer-Verlag
and the Environment

We at Springer-Verlag firmly believe that an international science publisher has a special obligation to the environment, and our corporate policies consistently reflect this conviction.

We also expect our business partners – paper mills, printers, packaging manufacturers, etc. – to commit themselves to using environmentally friendly materials and production processes.

The paper in this book is made from low- or no-chlorine pulp and is acid free, in conformance with international standards for paper permanency.

Printing: Mercedesdruck, Berlin
Binding: Buchbinderei Lüderitz & Bauer, Berlin

SCIENCE LIBRARY
UNIVERSITY OF THE PACIFIC
STOCKTON, CA 95211